NEUROIMAGING
PART I

HANDBOOK OF CLINICAL NEUROLOGY

Series Editors

MICHAEL J. AMINOFF, FRANÇOIS BOLLER, AND DICK F. SWAAB

VOLUME 135

ELSEVIER

AMSTERDAM BOSTON HEIDELBERG LONDON NEW YORK OXFORD
PARIS SAN DIEGO SAN FRANCISCO SINGAPORE SYDNEY TOKYO

NEUROIMAGING
PART I

Series Editors

MICHAEL J. AMINOFF, FRANÇOIS BOLLER, AND DICK F. SWAAB

Volume Editors

JOSEPH C. MASDEU AND R. GILBERTO GONZÁLEZ

VOLUME 135

3rd Series

ELSEVIER

AMSTERDAM BOSTON HEIDELBERG LONDON NEW YORK OXFORD
PARIS SAN DIEGO SAN FRANCISCO SINGAPORE SYDNEY TOKYO

ELSEVIER
Radarweg 29, PO Box 211, 1000 AE Amsterdam, Netherlands
The Boulevard, Langford Lane, Kidlington, Oxford OX5 1GB, UK
50 Hampshire Street, 5th Floor, Cambridge, MA 02139, USA

British Library Cataloguing-in-Publication Data
A catalogue record for this book is available from the British Library

Library of Congress Cataloging-in-Publication Data
A catalog record for this book is available from the Library of Congress

ISBN: 978-0-444-53485-9

For information on all Elsevier publications
visit our website at https://www.elsevier.com/

Publisher: Shirley Decker-lucke
Acquisition Editor: Mara Conner
Editorial Project Manager: Kristi Anderson
Production Project Manager: Sujatha Thirugnana Sambandam
Designer: Alan Studholme

Typeset by SPi Global, India

Handbook of Clinical Neurology 3rd Series

Available titles

Vol. 79, The human hypothalamus: basic and clinical aspects, Part I, D.F. Swaab, ed. ISBN 9780444513571
Vol. 80, The human hypothalamus: basic and clinical aspects, Part II, D.F. Swaab, ed. ISBN 9780444514905
Vol. 81, Pain, F. Cervero and T.S. Jensen, eds. ISBN 9780444519016
Vol. 82, Motor neurone disorders and related diseases, A.A. Eisen and P.J. Shaw, eds. ISBN 9780444518941
Vol. 83, Parkinson's disease and related disorders, Part I, W.C. Koller and E. Melamed, eds. ISBN 9780444519009
Vol. 84, Parkinson's disease and related disorders, Part II, W.C. Koller and E. Melamed, eds. ISBN 9780444528933
Vol. 85, HIV/AIDS and the nervous system, P. Portegies and J. Berger, eds. ISBN 9780444520104
Vol. 86, Myopathies, F.L. Mastaglia and D. Hilton Jones, eds. ISBN 9780444518996
Vol. 87, Malformations of the nervous system, H.B. Sarnat and P. Curatolo, eds. ISBN 9780444518965
Vol. 88, Neuropsychology and behavioural neurology, G. Goldenberg and B.C. Miller, eds. ISBN 9780444518972
Vol. 89, Dementias, C. Duyckaerts and I. Litvan, eds. ISBN 9780444518989
Vol. 90, Disorders of consciousness, G.B. Young and E.F.M. Wijdicks, eds. ISBN 9780444518958
Vol. 91, Neuromuscular junction disorders, A.G. Engel, ed. ISBN 9780444520081
Vol. 92, Stroke – Part I: Basic and epidemiological aspects, M. Fisher, ed. ISBN 9780444520036
Vol. 93, Stroke – Part II: Clinical manifestations and pathogenesis, M. Fisher, ed. ISBN 9780444520043
Vol. 94, Stroke – Part III: Investigations and management, M. Fisher, ed. ISBN 9780444520050
Vol. 95, History of neurology, S. Finger, F. Boller and K.L. Tyler, eds. ISBN 9780444520081
Vol. 96, Bacterial infections of the central nervous system, K.L. Roos and A.R. Tunkel, eds. ISBN 9780444520159
Vol. 97, Headache, G. Nappi and M.A. Moskowitz, eds. ISBN 9780444521392
Vol. 98, Sleep disorders Part I, P. Montagna and S. Chokroverty, eds. ISBN 9780444520067
Vol. 99, Sleep disorders Part II, P. Montagna and S. Chokroverty, eds. ISBN 9780444520074
Vol. 100, Hyperkinetic movement disorders, W.J. Weiner and E. Tolosa, eds. ISBN 9780444520142
Vol. 101, Muscular dystrophies, A. Amato and R.C. Griggs, eds. ISBN 9780080450315
Vol. 102, Neuro-ophthalmology, C. Kennard and R.J. Leigh, eds. ISBN 9780444529039
Vol. 103, Ataxic disorders, S.H. Subramony and A. Durr, eds. ISBN 9780444518927
Vol. 104, Neuro-oncology Part I, W. Grisold and R. Sofietti, eds. ISBN 9780444521385
Vol. 105, Neuro-oncology Part II, W. Grisold and R. Sofietti, eds. ISBN 9780444535023
Vol. 106, Neurobiology of psychiatric disorders, T. Schlaepfer and C.B. Nemeroff, eds. ISBN 9780444520029
Vol. 107, Epilepsy Part I, H. Stefan and W.H. Theodore, eds. ISBN 9780444528988
Vol. 108, Epilepsy Part II, H. Stefan and W.H. Theodore, eds. ISBN 9780444528995
Vol. 109, Spinal cord injury, J. Verhaagen and J.W. McDonald III, eds. ISBN 9780444521378
Vol. 110, Neurological rehabilitation, M. Barnes and D.C. Good, eds. ISBN 9780444529015
Vol. 111, Pediatric neurology Part I, O. Dulac, M. Lassonde and H.B. Sarnat, eds. ISBN 9780444528919
Vol. 112, Pediatric neurology Part II, O. Dulac, M. Lassonde and H.B. Sarnat, eds. ISBN 9780444529107
Vol. 113, Pediatric neurology Part III, O. Dulac, M. Lassonde and H.B. Sarnat, eds. ISBN 9780444595652
Vol. 114, Neuroparasitology and tropical neurology, H.H. Garcia, H.B. Tanowitz and O.H. Del Brutto, eds. ISBN 9780444534903
Vol. 115, Peripheral nerve disorders, G. Said and C. Krarup, eds. ISBN 9780444529022
Vol. 116, Brain stimulation, A.M. Lozano and M. Hallett, eds. ISBN 9780444534972
Vol. 117, Autonomic nervous system, R.M. Buijs and D.F. Swaab, eds. ISBN 9780444534910
Vol. 118, Ethical and legal issues in neurology, J.L. Bernat and H.R. Beresford, eds. ISBN 9780444535016
Vol. 119, Neurologic aspects of systemic disease Part I, J. Biller and J.M. Ferro, eds. ISBN 9780702040863
Vol. 120, Neurologic aspects of systemic disease Part II, J. Biller and J.M. Ferro, eds. ISBN 9780702040870
Vol. 121, Neurologic aspects of systemic disease Part III, J. Biller and J.M. Ferro, eds. ISBN 9780702040887
Vol. 122, Multiple sclerosis and related disorders, D.S. Goodin, ed. ISBN 9780444520012
Vol. 123, Neurovirology, A.C. Tselis and J. Booss, eds. ISBN 9780444534880

Vol. 124, Clinical neuroendocrinology, E. Fliers, M. Korbonits and J.A. Romijn, eds. ISBN 9780444596024
Vol. 125, Alcohol and the nervous system, E.V. Sullivan and A. Pfefferbaum, eds. ISBN 9780444626196
Vol. 126, Diabetes and the nervous system, D.W. Zochodne and R.A. Malik, eds. ISBN 9780444534804
Vol. 127, Traumatic brain injury Part I, J.H. Grafman and A.M. Salazar, eds. ISBN 9780444528926
Vol. 128, Traumatic brain injury Part II, J.H. Grafman and A.M. Salazar, eds. ISBN 9780444635211
Vol. 129, The human auditory system: Fundamental organization and clinical disorders, G.G. Celesia and G. Hickok, eds. ISBN 9780444626301
Vol. 130, Neurology of sexual and bladder disorders, D.B. Vodušek and F. Boller, eds. ISBN 9780444632470
Vol. 131, Occupational neurology, M. Lotti and M.L. Bleecker, eds. ISBN 9780444626271
Vol. 132, Neurocutaneous syndromes, M.P. Islam and E.S. Roach, eds. ISBN 9780444627025
Vol. 133, Autoimmune neurology, S.J. Pittock and A. Vincent, eds. ISBN 9780444634320
Vol. 134, Gliomas, M.S. Berger and M. Weller, eds. ISBN 9780128029978

Foreword

We are proud to present the first volumes dedicated to neuroimaging in the *Handbook of Clinical Neurology* series. Neurologists, not just those in training, may wonder at the kind of medical world that existed before modern imaging. Indeed, the neuroscience community has since its beginning attempted to understand the human mind and brain through imaging. As far back as 1880, the Italian physiologist Angelo Mosso introduced the "human circulation balance," which could noninvasively measure the redistribution of blood during emotional and intellectual activity. More recently, semi-invasive techniques such as pneumoencephalography (introduced by Dandy in 1918) and arteriography (pioneered by Moniz in 1927) allowed partial visualization of the brain and its surrounding structures. New methods enabling easier, safer, noninvasive, painless, and repeatable imaging have only been developed in the past 50 years or so, starting with computed tomography, some of whose developers won the 1979 Nobel Prize for medicine or physiology. The many subsequent developments in neuroimaging are masterfully presented in these two volumes.

The volumes deal with a variety of neuroimaging-related topics. They include thorough descriptions of the involved methods and their application to specific diseases of the brain, spinal cord, and peripheral nervous system. Emphasis is given to the most common disorders, such as tumors, strokes, multiple sclerosis, movement disorders, infections, dementia, and trauma, but less common conditions such as neurocutaneous syndromes are also discussed. The important questions of when and where to image, as well as the differential diagnosis of imaging findings, are discussed in the light of specific syndromes. A separate section covers pediatric neuroimaging. The volumes conclude with sections dedicated to interventional neuroimaging as well as to postmortem imaging and neuropathologic correlations.

We have been fortunate to have as volume editors two distinguished scholars, Dr. Joseph C. Masdeu, of the Department of Neurology, Methodist Hospital, Houston, Texas, and Dr. R. Gilberto González, from the Department of Radiology, Massachusetts General Hospital in Boston. Both have been at the forefront of neuroimaging research for many years. They have assembled a truly international group of authors with acknowledged expertise to contribute to the texts and have produced two authoritative, comprehensive, and up-to-date volumes. Their availability electronically on Elsevier's Science Direct site as well as in print format should ensure their ready accessibility and facilitate searches for specific information.

We are grateful to the volume editors and to all the contributors for their efforts in creating such an invaluable resource. As series editors we read and commented on each of the chapters with great interest. We are therefore confident that both clinicians and researchers in many different medical disciplines will find much in these volumes to appeal to them.

And last, but not least, it is always a pleasure to acknowledge and thank Elsevier, our publisher – and, in particular, Michael Parkinson in Scotland, and Mara Conner and Kristi Anderson in San Diego – for their unfailing and expert assistance in the development and production of these volumes.

Michael J. Aminoff
François Boller
Dick F. Swaab

Preface

Neuroimaging has become one of the most useful set of tools for understanding and diagnosing diseases of the nervous system. Fittingly, the present two volumes of the *Handbook of Clinical Neurology* review the extensive advances in the field. In the first volume, discussions of the various techniques used in neuroimaging are followed by reviews of the imaging findings caused by brain diseases. We have chosen not to include a chapter on brain anatomy because it would be quite long and extant atlases are excellent. The second volume begins with a description of the functional anatomy of the spine and of the imaging findings in diseases of the spine and spinal cord. Imaging of peripheral nerve and muscle follows. Then, there is a section on when and how to image the various clinical syndromes produced by diseases of the nervous system. Adequacy in the use of expensive neuroimaging tools has always been a priority, but it is becoming more acute as the application of neuroimaging expands more rapidly than the available resources. The next section is unusual in a book of this type: a description of the various imaging findings that should lead to consideration of the diseases causing them. Such information is particularly important when using techniques like computed tomography and magnetic resonance imaging, which offer a panoply of findings and are extensively used in clinical practice. Next is a section on pediatric neuroimaging, led by a chapter on imaging findings during normal development. After three chapters on the therapeutic use of endovascular imaging, the second volume concludes with a chapter on postmortem imaging as a tool to better define normal brain structure on imaging and its alteration by some disorders.

We hope that this book will be useful to all those who work with clinical imaging of the nervous system, such as neurologists, neuroradiologists, neurosurgeons, and nuclear medicine physicians. Some sections, for instance, the sections on the spine, peripheral nerve, and muscle, may be helpful to orthopedic surgeons and rehabilitation specialists. Neuropsychologists may find helpful the chapters on neurodegenerative disorders leading to cognitive impairment.

Neuroimaging is used not only clinically, but also by those interested in clarifying the still largely undiscovered landscape and functional intricacy of the brain. While the clinical literature of neuroimaging is extensive, even more extensive and more widely cited is the literature of neuroimaging applied to the study of the healthy human nervous system. Although human disease has traditionally led to a better understanding of normal structure and function, researchers looking primarily for information on the normal nervous system should look elsewhere.

We are most thankful to the authors, who have distilled their expertise in superbly written and illustrated chapters. Mr. Michael Parkinson, from Elsevier, has skillfully coordinated the gathering of information for these two volumes. We are also thankful to the three series editors and, particularly, to Dr. François Boller, for their excellent suggestions.

Joseph C. Masdeu
R. Gilberto González

Contributors

A. Alavi
Division of Nuclear Medicine, Hospital of the University of Pennsylvania, Philadelphia, PA, USA

C. Auger
MR Unit, Department of Radiology, Hospital Universitari Vall d'Hebron, Autonomous University of Barcelona, Barcelona, Spain

T. Batchelor
Departments of Neurology and Radiation Oncology, Division of Hematology/Oncology, Massachusetts General Hospital, Boston, MA, USA

W.G. Bradley
Department of Radiology, University of California San Diego Health System, San Diego, CA, USA

D.J. Brooks
Department of Medicine, Imperial College London, London, UK

B.R. Buchbinder
Department of Radiology, Division of Neuroradiology, Massachusetts General Hospital, Harvard Medical School, Boston, MA, USA

E.C.S. Camargo
Department of Neurology, Massachusetts General Hospital, Boston, MA, USA

J.J. Carroll
Department of Radiology, Massachusetts General Hospital, Boston, MA, USA

B. Cohen
Departments of Dermatology and Pediatrics, Johns Hopkins University School of Medicine, Baltimore, MD, USA

W.A. Copen
Division of Neuroradiology, Department of Radiology, Massachusetts General Hospital and Harvard Medical School, Boston, MA, USA

M.B. Cunnane
Department of Radiology, Harvard Medical School and Massachusetts Eye and Ear Infirmary; and Division of Neuroradiology, Massachusetts General Hospital, Boston, MA, USA

H.D. Curtin
Department of Radiology, Harvard Medical School and Massachusetts Eye and Ear Infirmary, Boston, MA, USA

F. Eichler
Departments of Neurology and Radiology, Massachusetts General Hospital, Harvard Medical School, Boston, MA, USA

M.D. Farwell
Department of Radiology, Perelman School of Medicine of the University of Pennsylvania, Philadelphia, PA, USA

M. Filippi
Neuroimaging Research Unit, Institute of Experimental Neurology, Division of Neuroscience, San Raffaele Scientific Institute, Vita-Salute San Raffaele University, Milan, Italy

B. Fischl
Athinoula A. Martinos Center for Biomedical Imaging, Massachusetts General Hospital, Charlestown, MA, USA

K. Goffin
Division of Nuclear Medicine, University Hospital Leuven and KU Leuven, Leuven, Belgium

R.G. González
Department of Radiology, Massachusetts General Hospital, Boston, MA, USA

R. Gupta
Division of Neuroradiology and Cardiac Radiology, Massachusetts General Hospital and Harvard Medical School, Boston, MA, USA

C. Habas
Neuroimaging Service, Centre National d'Ophtalmologie des Quinze-Vingts, Paris, France

V. Haughton
Section of Neuroradiology, Department of Radiology, University of Wisconsin, Madison, WI, USA

J.A. Hirsch
Neurointerventional Service, Massachusetts General Hospital, Boston, MA, USA

M. Ichise
Molecular Neuroimaging Program, Molecular Imaging Center, National Institute of Radiological Sciences, Anagawa, Inage, Chiba, Japan

S. Kamalian
Division of Neuroradiology, Department of Radiology, Massachusetts General Hospital and Harvard Medical School, Boston, MA, USA

H.R. Kelly
Department of Radiology, Harvard Medical School and Massachusetts Eye and Ear Infirmary; and Division of Neuroradiology, Massachusetts General Hospital, Boston, MA, USA

A.J.M. Kiruluta
Department of Radiology, Massachusetts General Hospital, Boston and Department of Biophysics, Harvard University, Cambridge, MA, USA

N. Klar
Division of Neuroradiology, Russell H. Morgan Department of Radiology, Johns Hopkins University School of Medicine, Baltimore, MD, USA

K. Lameka
Department of Radiology, Tufts University, Boston and Department of Radiology, Baystate Medical Center, Springfield, MA, USA

M. Larvie
Divisions of Neuroradiology and Nuclear Medicine and Molecular Imaging, Massachusetts General Hospital, Boston, MA, USA

T.M. Leslie-Mazwi
Neurointerventional Service, Massachusetts General Hospital, Boston, MA, USA

M.H. Lev
Division of Emergency Radiology and Division of Neuroradiology, Department of Radiology, Massachusetts General Hospital and Harvard Medical School, Boston, MA, USA

D.D.M. Lin
Division of Neuroradiology, Russell H. Morgan Department of Radiology, Johns Hopkins University School of Medicine, Baltimore, MD, USA

M. Manto
Department of Neurology, Université Libre de Bruxelles Erasme, Brussels, Belgium

K.-A. Mardal
Department of Mathematics, University of Oslo, Oslo, Norway

J.C. Masdeu
Department of Neurology, Houston Methodist Hospital, Houston, TX, USA

M. Moghbel
Department of Radiology, Hospital of the University of Pennsylvania, Philadelphia, PA, USA

N. Nagornaya
Department of Radiology, University of Miami Miller School of Medicine, Miami, FL, USA

A. Newberg
Myrna Brind Center of Integrative Medicine, Thomas Jefferson University and Hospital, Philadelphia, PA, USA

B. Pascual
Department of Neurology, Houston Methodist Hospital, Houston, TX, USA

N. Pavese
Division of Brain Sciences, Imperial College London, UK and Aarhus University, Denmark

R. Pizzolato
Department of Neuroradiology, Massachusetts General Hospital, Harvard Medical School, Boston, MA, USA

S.R. Pomerantz
Department of Neuroradiology, Massachusetts General Hospital, Boston, MA, USA

M.J.D. Post
Department of Radiology, University of Miami Miller School of Medicine, Miami, FL, USA

P. Preziosa
Neuroimaging Research Unit, Institute of Experimental Neurology, Division of Neuroscience, San Raffaele Scientific Institute, Vita-Salute San Raffaele University, Milan, Italy

T. Ptak
Division of Neuroradiology and Division of Emergency Radiology, Massachusetts General Hospital, Boston, MA, USA

J.D. Rabinov
Neurointerventional Service, Massachusetts General Hospital, Boston, MA, USA

O. Rapalino
Division of Neuroradiology, Department of Radiology, Massachusetts General Hospital and Harvard Medical School, Boston, MA, USA

E.-M. Ratai
Division of Neuroradiology, Department of Radiology, Massachusetts General Hospital and Harvard Medical School, and Athinoula A. Martinos Center for Biomedical Imaging, Boston, MA, USA

S. Rincon
Division of Neuroradiology, Massachusetts General Hospital, Boston, MA, USA

M.A. Rocca
Neuroimaging Research Unit, Institute of Experimental Neurology, Division of Neuroscience, San Raffaele Scientific Institute, Vita-Salute San Raffaele University, Milan, Italy

J.M. Romero
Department of Neuroradiology, Massachusetts General Hospital, Harvard Medical School, Boston, MA, USA

J. Rosand
Neuroscience Intensive Care Unit, Department of Neurology, Massachusetts General Hospital, Boston, MA, USA

Á. Rovira
MR Unit, Department of Radiology, Hospital Universitari Vall d'Hebron, Autonomous University of Barcelona, Barcelona, Spain

A. Rovira
Corporació Sanitària Parc Taulí, CD-UDIAT, Sabadell, Spain

G. Saigal
Department of Radiology, University of Miami Miller School of Medicine, Miami, FL, USA

P.W. Schaefer
Department of Radiology, Massachusetts General Hospital, Boston, MA, USA

L.H. Schwamm
Department of Neurology, Massachusetts General Hospital and Harvard Medical School, Boston, MA, USA

A.B. Singhal
Department of Neurology, Massachusetts General Hospital, Boston, MA, USA

J.G. Smirniotopoulos
Department of Radiology and Radiological Sciences, Uniformed Services University of the Health Sciences, Bethesda, MD, USA

Y.F. Tai
Division of Brain Sciences, Imperial College London, UK

K. Van Laere
Division of Nuclear Medicine, University Hospital Leuven and KU Leuven, Leuven, Belgium

Contents of Part I

SECTION 2 Brain diseases

Contents of Part II

Section 1

Neuroimaging methods

Handbook of Clinical Neurology, Vol. 135 (3rd series)
Neuroimaging, Part I
J.C. Masdeu and R.G. González, Editors

Chapter 1

Computed tomography imaging and angiography – principles

SHERVIN KAMALIAN[1]*, MICHAEL H. LEV[2], AND RAJIV GUPTA[1]

[1]*Division of Neuroradiology, Department of Radiology, Massachusetts General Hospital and Harvard Medical School, Boston, MA, USA*

[2]*Division of Emergency Radiology and Division of Neuroradiology, Department of Radiology, Massachusetts General Hospital and Harvard Medical School, Boston, MA, USA*

Abstract

The evaluation of patients with diverse neurologic disorders was forever changed in the summer of 1973, when the first commercial computed tomography (CT) scanners were introduced. Until then, the detection and characterization of intracranial or spinal lesions could only be inferred by limited spatial resolution radioisotope scans, or by the patterns of tissue and vascular displacement on invasive pneumoencaphalography and direct carotid puncture catheter arteriography. Even the earliest-generation CT scanners – which required tens of minutes for the acquisition and reconstruction of low-resolution images (128 × 128 matrix) – could, based on density, noninvasively distinguish infarct, hemorrhage, and other mass lesions with unprecedented accuracy. Iodinated, intravenous contrast added further sensitivity and specificity in regions of blood–brain barrier breakdown. The advent of rapid multidetector row CT scanning in the early 1990s created renewed enthusiasm for CT, with CT angiography largely replacing direct catheter angiography. More recently, iterative reconstruction postprocessing techniques have made possible high spatial resolution, reduced noise, very low radiation dose CT scanning. The speed, spatial resolution, contrast resolution, and low radiation dose capability of present-day scanners have also facilitated dual-energy imaging which, like magnetic resonance imaging, for the first time, has allowed tissue-specific CT imaging characterization of intracranial pathology.

COMPUTED TOMOGRAPHY IMAGING AND ANGIOGRAPHY: PRINCIPLES

Introduction

The evaluation of patients with diverse neurologic disorders was forever changed in the summer of 1973, when the first commercial computed tomography (CT) scanners were introduced. Until then, the detection and characterization of intracranial or spinal lesions could only be inferred by limited spatial resolution radioisotope scans, or by the patterns of tissue and vascular displacement on invasive pneumoencaphalography and direct carotid puncture catheter arteriography (Taveras et al., 1969). Even the earliest-generation CT scanners – which required tens of minutes for the acquisition and reconstruction of low-resolution images (13 mm slice thickness, 80 × 80 matrix) – could, based on density, noninvasively distinguish infarct, hemorrhage, and other mass lesions with unprecedented accuracy (New et al., 1974). The addition of iodinated, intravenous contrast material added further sensitivity and specificity, highlighting pathologic regions with blood–brain barrier breakdown (Wing et al., 1976).

Although, for a short time in the early 1990s, it seemed that magnetic resonance imaging (MRI) might cause CT neuroimaging to become obsolete, the advent of rapid, multidetector row CT scanning created renewed enthusiasm (Sorensen et al., 1996; Jones et al., 2001). Indeed, since then, CT angiography (CTA) has largely replaced direct catheter arteriography for routine diagnosis and

*Correspondence to: Shervin Kamalian, M.D. M.Sc, Division of Neuroradiology, Department of Radiology, Massachusetts General Hospital and Harvard Medical School, 55 Fruit Street, Boston MA 02114, USA. E-mail: mkamalian@mgh.harvard.edu

screening (Napel et al., 1992; Schwartz et al., 1992). Thinner slices (0.6 mm, 512–1024 × 512–1024 matrix) and increased scanning speed have facilitated more widespread adoption of coronal and sagittal image reformatting – improving detection of subtle contusion and subarachnoid hemorrhage (SAH) in the anterior frontal and temporal lobes and cortical sulci (Baker, 1981; Wei et al., 2010). Moreover, CT perfusion (CTP) imaging has increasingly been utilized at many centers for qualitative assessment to improve differential diagnosis, determine stroke subtype, guide hypertensive management, and sort treatment options for vasospasm following aneurysmal SAH (Koenig et al., 1998; Eastwood et al., 2002).

Advances in CT neuroimaging have paralleled advances in computer processing speed and in efficiency of image reconstruction algorithms. Most recently, iterative reconstruction techniques – the first genuinely novel CT image-processing development since Hounsfield's filtered backprojection methodology (for which he was awarded the Nobel Prize in 1979) – have made possible high spatial resolution, reduced noise, very low radiation dose CT scanning (Rapalino et al., 2012). The improved scanning speed, *z*-direction coverage, spatial resolution, contrast resolution, and low radiation dose capability of present-day CT scanners have also facilitated dual-energy imaging, which – for the first time, like MRI – has allowed tissue-specific characterization of intracranial pathology, including dedicated CT imaging that can reliably distinguish calcium, iodine, fat, water, and hemorrhage (Gupta et al., 2010). Virtual monochromatic dual-energy CT images also have the potential to help reduce the posterior fossa beam hardening artifact caused by dense bone at the skull base (Pomerantz et al., 2013).

PRINCIPLES

Noncontrast computed tomography (NCCT)

The physical basis of CT scanning is that the attenuation of an X-ray beam through living tissue is proportional to the electron density of that tissue, generally corresponding to the physical density of the tissue, and that a gray-scale image – reflecting the relative densities of different voxels of such tissue – can be reconstructed from the attenuation values obtained when rotating an X-ray source around a patient, using a mathematical technique known as filtered backprojection (FBP). The gray-scale values are assigned an arbitrary linear value, the Hounsfield unit (HU), named after Sir Godfrey Hounsfield, the physicist who was awarded the 1979 Nobel Prize in Medicine (as well as earning a knighthood) for his invention of CT scanning in the late 1960s–early 1970s, while he was an employee of the British music company EMI (the first record label for the Beatles).

The Hounsfield scale is defined as the attenuation value of the X-ray beam in a given voxel, minus the attenuation of water, divided by the attenuation of water, multiplied by 1000. Hence, water is arbitrarily assigned an HU value of zero, with materials more dense than water having positive values and materials less dense than water having negative values. Although roughly linearly proportional to physical density (based on so-called Compton scatter), the Hounsfield scale is relative, rather than absolute, in that different-energy X-ray beams will result in different attenuation values and hence different HU values. Moreover, because some elements – such as iodine – preferentially absorb photons of certain specific energies based on the photoelectric effect (so-called *k*-edge or characteristic radiation), they will appear to have disproportionately large attenuation values relative to their actual physical density. Indeed, this is why iodine-based intravascular contrast agents are ideally suited to CT imaging.

For example, at routine CT X-ray beam energies of 120–140 kV, the HU value of air is approximately –1000 and the HU value of dense cortical bone is approximately +1000. Fat, which floats on water (i.e., is less dense) is typically in the –30 to –70 HU range. White matter is about 25 HU, gray matter about 35 HU, and soft tissue about 20–30 HU. The standard deviation of HU values is usually in the ±10–20% range. The HU value of *in vivo* blood is (not surprisingly) proportional to the hematocrit level, and typically about 30. Extravascular, intracranial blood, however, clots rapidly, and as plasma is extruded and resorbed from the clot, the concentration of the hemoglobin protein can double and triple, so that intracranial hemorrhage typically measures 60–90 HU (but rarely >100) (Fig. 1.1). An important caveat with regard to evaluating trauma patients is that not all potential foreign bodies are high-density, high-HU structures. The CT number of a dry, wooden foreign body, for example, is typically in the –100 to –170 HU range, due to dry wood's air-filled porous microstructure (Yamashita et al., 2007) (Fig. 1.2).

In CT image display, higher HU values appear brighter and lower HU values appear darker. Because the human eye can only distinguish approximately 128 shades of gray, the dynamic range of the CT image display must be adjusted so as to be appropriate to the tissue being evaluated. The mid-value of this gray scale is termed the center level, and the full dynamic range is known as the window width. For example, with standard head CT image display parameters of center level 30 HU and window width 100 HU, each pixel greater than 80 HU (=30+50) would be equally bright, whereas each pixel less than –20 HU (=30 – 50) would be equally dark. With

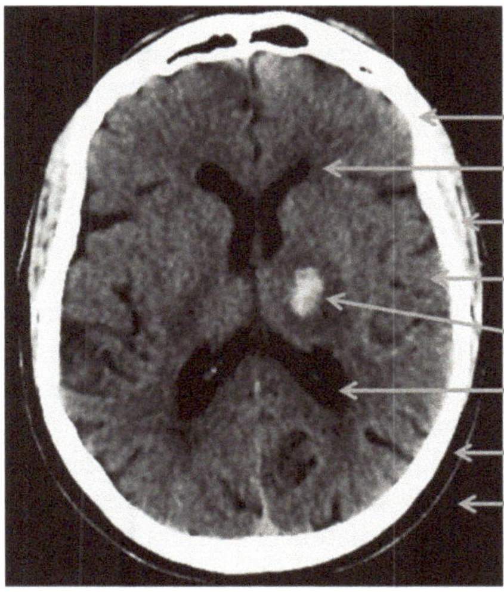

CT Number Ranges in Hounsfield Units (HU)	
Bone	+1000
White matter	+20 to 30
Muscle	+20 to 40
Gray matter	+30 to 40
Hemorrhage	+65 to +95
CSF (water)	0
Fat	-30 to -70
Air	-1000

Fig. 1.1. Axial computed tomography (CT) image with sample typical CT numbers in HU. CSF, cerebrospinal fluid.

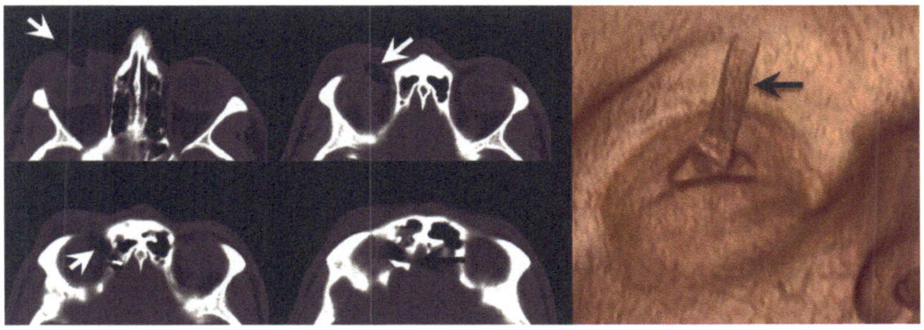

Fig. 1.2. Hypodense foreign body – a wooden pencil – penetrating the superior medial orbit, with perforation into the anterior cranial fossa. Note that the wood has a similar computed tomography appearance to air.

such settings, a subtle crescentic subdural hematoma (~90 HU) would appear equally as bright as the adjacent skull (~1000 HU), and hence be undetectable. Conversely, fat (~–30 HU) and air (~–1000 HU) would appear equally dark, and hence, air within intraorbital fat resulting from a paranasal sinus fracture would also be undetectable (Fig. 1.3). By expanding the window width display and centering the gray scale at a higher HU level, the difference in density between the same subdural hematoma and adjacent bone can be made visually apparent. Similarly, it has been suggested that subtle vasogenic edema in acute stroke can be more sensitively detected by soft copy image review using narrowed window width display settings that exaggerate the HU differences between gray and white matter (Lev et al., 1999).

Given its speed, convenience, low cost relative to MRI, and widespread availability, head CT has become a first-line method for assessment of focal neurologic symptoms, and has largely become an extension of the routine physical exam. CT, unlike MRI, is ideal for evaluating fractures and calcifications. A major strength of CT is the rapid and accurate diagnosis of intracranial hemorrhage, which appears hyperdense (i.e., bright) relative to normal brain tissue. Indeed, current guidelines for thrombolytic therapy within 4.5 hours of acute stroke

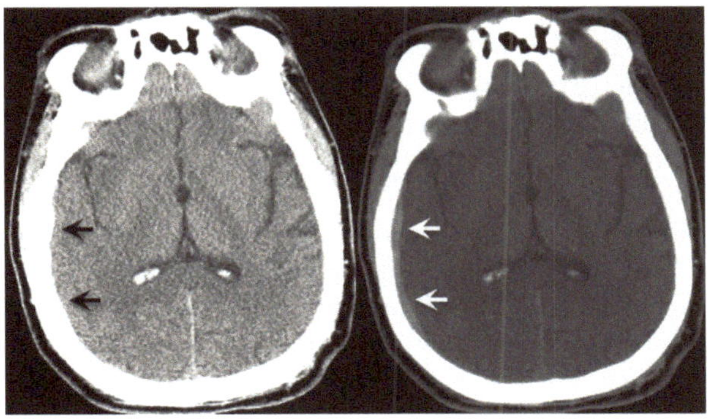

Fig. 1.3. Computed tomography image at left has center-level display setting of 30 HU and window width of 100 HU. The image at right has center-level 80 HU and window width 200 HU. With the display settings on the right, the subtle crescentic subdural hematoma adjacent to bone becomes visually apparent.

Table 1.1

Pearls and pitfalls of unenhanced head computed tomography

Pearls	Pitfalls
Widely available Accurate method for: • Intracranial hemorrhage • Fracture • Temporal bone evaluation • Spinal stenosis • Sinusitis • Calcification in central nervous system lesions • Pre- and postoperation evaluation Soft-tissue evaluation when magnetic resonance imaging is contraindicated or not available	Radiation exposure Limited sensitivity for soft-tissue resolution (early ischemic changes, multiple sclerosis lesions, early neoplastic changes) Anatomy and pathology may be obscured due to partial volume averaging, patient motion, beam hardening, and metallic streak artifacts

onset require an unenhanced head CT to rule out hemorrhage as the only absolute contraindication to intravenous tissue plasminogen activator (IV-tPA) administration. With current-generation head CT scanners, whole-brain images can be obtained in seconds, so that image review can take place in real time at the scanner console, expediting clinical management. Some strengths and weaknesses of CT are outlined in Table 1.1.

Weaknesses of CT include radiation exposure, reconstruction artifacts, limited sensitivity for detecting subtle differences in soft-tissue density (e.g., the early edema associated with hyperacute stroke), and poor interobserver reliability. Indeed, objective measures of CT image quality typically distinguish between high- versus low-contrast resolution capability (Table 1.2). Lesion conspicuity is a function of size and density relative to that of surrounding normal tissues, as well as the degree of image noise (so-called quantum mottle). High-contrast (spatial) resolution refers to the ability to resolve small objects but of widely different densities that are very close together as distinct structures, such as the bony trabeculae of the mastoid air cells, nondisplaced skull fractures, or punctate intracranial hemorrhage. High-contrast resolution structures can typically be more sensitively detected with thinner slices (less volume averaging) and sharper image reconstruction algorithms (e.g., bone kernel) (Fig. 1.4). Low-contrast resolution refers to the ability to resolve adjacent objects of similar densities that differ only minimally in HU, such as demyelinative white-matter plaques, or early stroke edema. Low-contrast resolution conspicuity is proportional to image noise; therefore, techniques that reduce noise can improve sensitivity for lesion detection. Such techniques include using soft-tissue kernel image reconstruction algorithms, thick-slice axial images (2.5–5 mm) for greater signal relative to noise, optimized center level and window width display settings, and the use of newer iterative reconstruction algorithms (Fig. 1.5) (discussed in further detail below).

Additional user-defined specific scan parameters, such as X-ray beam energy in milliamperes (mA) and kilovoltage (kV), as well as table speed and helical pitch, can also be optimized for maximal image quality at minimal radiation dose. Detailed discussion of these important parameters, however, is beyond the scope of this chapter.

Computed tomography angiography (CTA)

Neurovascular imaging is critical for locating arterial occlusions, determining degree of stenosis, and identifying dissections, aneurysms, venous sinus thrombosis, and other vascular lesions such as arteriovenous malformations (AVMs). CTA, with CT venography (CTV), is the most accurate widely available minimally invasive imaging method to evaluate the vessels of the head and neck, and, with greater than 95% sensitivity and specificity for diagnosing proximal artery occlusion, has largely replaced direct catheter arteriography as the diagnostic method of choice for emergency vascular assessment of stroke and other cerebrovascular disorders. CTA requires intravenous administration of iodinated contrast solution via a power injector. The CT scanner is programmed to detect the arrival of the radiopaque contrast within the aortic arch, and then triggers scanning for optimal vascular opacification. CTA can be tailored to optimally delineate either the arterial or venous phase of contrast enhancement, or both. With modern multidetector row scanners, images of the head and neck arteries can be obtained in under 15 seconds, minimizing motion artifact.

Disadvantages of CTA include radiation exposure and utilization of iodinated contrast, which may result in allergic reactions or renal injury (the latter especially in patients with diabetes or preexisting kidney impairment) (Table 1.3). Advantages of CTA include high-resolution images from the aortic arch to the vertex. Indeed, CTA is often used as the confirmatory test or tie breaker when there is discordance between carotid duplex ultrasound imaging and magnetic resonance angiography for evaluating the degree of carotid stenosis. Unlike ultrasound and magnetic resonance angiography, CTA images are not flow-weighted, and hence,

Table 1.2

Computed tomography (CT) neuroimaging image quality assessment: low- versus high-contrast resolution lesions

Image quality metric	Definition	Alternative nomenclature	Neuroanatomic example	Neuropathologic example	Relevant imaging parameters
Low-contrast resolution	Ability to distinguish lesions with only small differences in density	- Low-contrast detectability - Sensitivity of the system - Soft-tissue resolution	Gray–white-matter differentiation (GWMD)	- Loss of GWMD due to cytotoxic versus vasogenic edema in acute ischemic stroke - Early neoplastic lesions	- Lesion size - Image noise related to: 1. Reconstruction algorithm (iterative reconstruction vs filtered backprojection) 2. Reconstruction kernels (i.e., soft vs sharp) 3. Slice thickness - Gray-scale display
High-contrast resolution	Ability to distinguish very small lesions as distinct, rather than confluent	- Spatial resolution - Detail resolution	Fine osseous trabeculae, aqueduct of Sylvius	- Fractures - Punctate hemorrhage	- Pixel/voxel size related to: 1. Matrix size (typically 512 × 512 for CT) 2. Field-of-view (FOV: typically 20–25 cm for head CT) 3. Reconstruction kernels (sharp vs soft) 4. Slice thickness (volume averaging) - Gray-scale display

CTA assessment of luminal diameter is not routinely influenced by turbulent or slow flow. Similarly, CTA with delayed imaging is the most accurate vascular imaging test – short of performing a catheter arteriogram – for distinguishing true total occlusion from slow flow with a hairline residual lumen in cervical carotid disease (Lev et al., 2003). Delayed carotid artery imaging (typically by about 20–40 seconds after peak arterial phase) is required to assure that contrast has sufficient time to fully opacify the vessel lumen, in the setting of a very tight proximal stenosis.

One challenge for CTA imaging of carotid atherosclerotic disease is heavy circumferential calcification, which can obscure the adjacent vessel lumen due to beam-hardening effects and cause overestimation of the degree of vessel stenosis. Another challenge is that most current CT scanners do not have sufficient temporal resolution to capture dynamic blood flow through such lesions as AVMs, which have rapid artery-to-vein shunting. The newest generation of mega multidetector row CT scanners, however, has sufficient speed, *z*-axis coverage, and spatial resolution to allow – at acceptably low total radiation doses – dynamic 4D volume acquisition with temporal resolution approaching 0.2 second per CT gantry rotation. The resulting datasets can not only be used to accurately assess rapid filling of AVMs and delayed collateral flow patterns in patients with major intracranial stenoses and occlusions, but can also be postprocessed to create CT perfusion images (see Chapter 6).

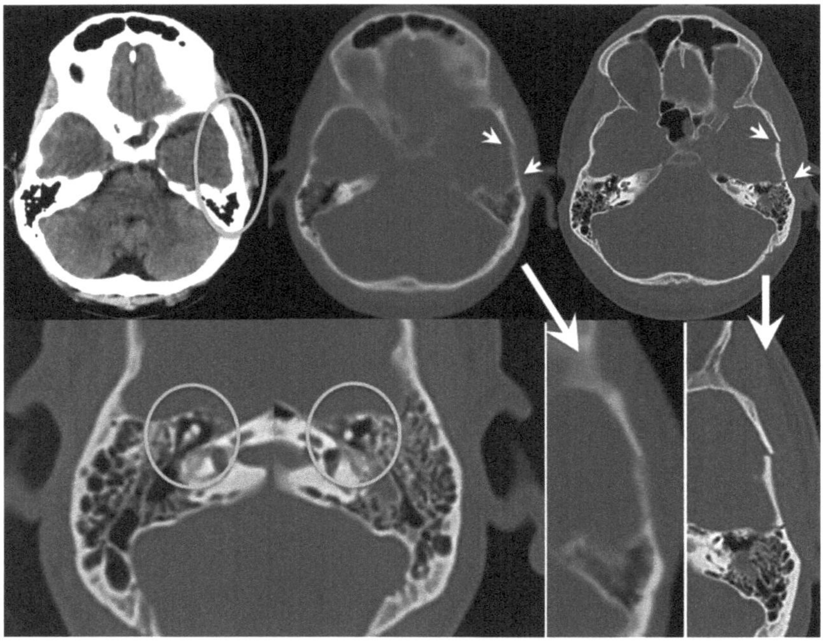

Fig. 1.4. Importance of sharp reconstruction kernel, thin slice images, with bone window-level display settings, for the detection of minimally displaced posttraumatic skull fractures. Upper left panel is a 5-mm thick axial computed tomography image reconstructed with soft kernel at standard brain display settings. Upper central panel is the same image with bone display settings of center level 600 HU and window width 3250 HU. The fracture is best visualized on the right upper and lower panels using thin-slice, sharp kernel, and bone display settings.

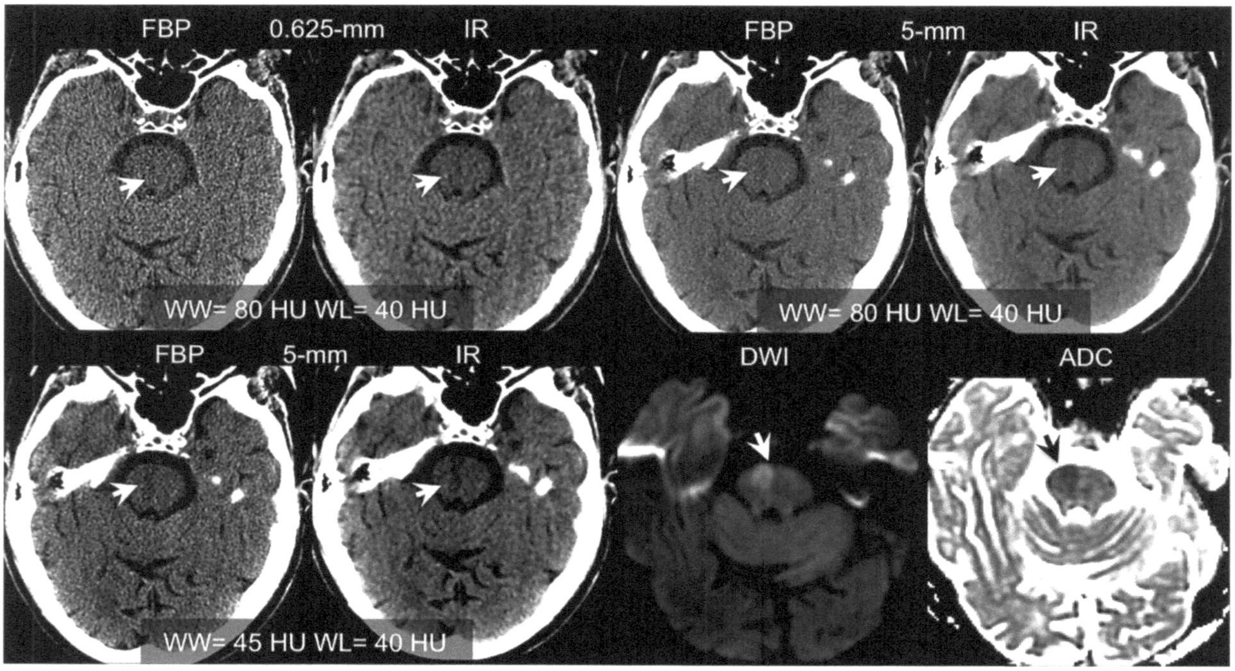

Fig. 1.5. Improved low-contrast resolution lesion detectability with iterative reconstruction (IR) algorithm compared to filtered backprojection (FBP); acute right pontine infarct proven on reference standard diffusion-weighted magnetic resonance imaging (DWI: lower right panel) is best visualized on the thick slice, IR, narrow window width (WW) computed tomography images (lower left panel). ADC, apparent diffusion coefficient. (Courtesy of Stuart R. Pomerantz, MD, Massachusetts General Hospital.)

Table 1.3

Advantages versus disadvantages of computed tomography (CT) angiography

Advantages	Disadvantages
Widely available	Additional radiation exposure
Excellent noninvasive method to evaluate vascular anatomy and pathologies: • Arterial occlusion and stenosis • Aneurysm • Arterial-venous malformations • Venous occlusive disease • Vasospasm • Blood–brain barrier disruption (neoplasm, infection)	Requires iodinated contrast administration (limitation in patients with allergy or renal impairment)
More sensitive than noncontrast CT to evaluate parenchymal ischemic changes	No flow information; provides a static snapshot of vascular anatomy (not reliable to assess brain tissue viability)
Fast and critical reconstructions can be performed at the scanner console without need for complex postprocessing	Vessel patency may be obscured due to heavy calcification, beam hardening, and metallic streak artifacts

Given these potentially very large axial imaging datasets, image postprocessing is required to efficiently visualize vessel abnormalities and facilitate diagnoses (Fig. 1.6). In particular, maximum-intensity projection (MIP) images of the intracranial circulation provide an easy way to detect proximal arterial occlusions in stroke patients, for example, that may be amenable to catheter-based treatments. These MIP images depict the highest density along a particular imaging ray. For evaluation of the intracranial arteries, MIP images reformatted to 20–30 mm thickness with 3–5 mm overlap can be created in axial, coronal, and sagittal planes quickly at the scanner console by the CT technologist. More complex postprocessing techniques include curved reformats, multiplanar volume reformats, and volume-rendered images. Curved reformats depict the entire course of a particular vessel in a single two-dimensional image, and provide a good evaluation of arterial steno-occlusive disease in the neck, such as at the carotid bifurcation. The 3D volume-rendered and other surface techniques are less helpful for ischemic stroke evaluation, but are routinely used in aneurysm detection and treatment planning (Fig. 1.7).

In addition to information regarding vessel patency, CTA source images (CTA-SI) can provide a sensitive evaluation of ischemic changes within the brain parenchyma. Parenchymal hypoattenuation on CTA-SI represents decreased contrast opacification within the capillary bed, and is more readily detectable than an unenhanced CT hypodensity (Camargo et al., 2007). One caveat is that the type and degree of the perfusion weighting of these CTA source images are highly variable, depending on circulation time and a number of other factors related to collateral flow, so that they cannot be used to reliably distinguish tissue likely to infarct (core) from highly ischemic but still salvageable tissue (penumbra) (Schramm et al., 2002; Coutts et al., 2004).

Indeed, there have been numerous studies regarding the utility of CTA for grading the robustness of pial collateral flow in patients with acute embolic stroke. These grading schemes have not been generally useful for making management decisions in individual patients, as their accuracy for predicting tissue and clinical outcome – in the absence of early, robust recanalization – is typically poor. An exception to this, however, is the malignant CTA collateral profile, which – again, in the absence of early, robust reperfusion – correlates strongly with the concurrent MR diffusion-weighted imaging findings of irreversible infarction (Souza et al., 2012). This malignant CTA collateral pattern is defined as the complete absence of vascular enhancement within a large cortical area (typically >33–50% of a middle cerebral artery division). As noted above, time-resolved CTA with 4D volume dynamic CTA scanning should prove useful for more accurate characterization of such delayed collateral flow patterns. Specifically, if intracranial collateral flow is imaged too early in arterial phase, arrival time delays caused by slow flow (in the setting of proximal extracranial or circle-of-Willis major artery occlusions/stenoses) can result in a false-positive malignant collateral pattern (Fig. 1.8).

CT/CTA selected technical-clinical pearls and pitfalls

Detailed discussion regarding the imaging evaluation of specific neurologic disorders is provided in subsequent chapters. In what follows, selected technical pearls and pitfalls for common clinical situations will be highlighted.

All head CT interpretation should follow a consistent search pattern, to insure that incidental findings are not overlooked. The symmetry of the ventricles, sulci, and cisterns should be assessed; midline shift, sulcal effacement, herniation, mass lesions, and bleeds in the epidural, subdural, subarachnoid, and parenchymal compartments of the supratentorial and infratentorial spaces should be excluded. Extracranially, the globes, orbits, paranasal

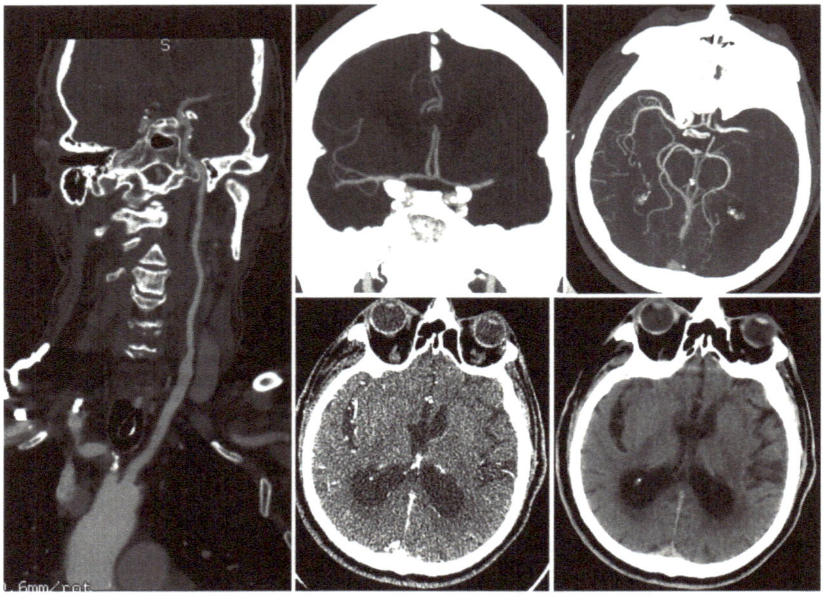

Fig. 1.6. Computed tomography (CT) angiogram provides high-resolution images of vascular anatomy from aortic arch to the cranial vertex. Left: curved reformat image of left common carotid artery to (occluded) proximal middle cerebral artery; upper middle: coronal thick slab collapsed maximum-intensity projection (MIP) reconstruction showing left middle cerebral artery occlusion, performed at the scanner console by the CT technologist; upper right: axial thick slab collapsed MIP reconstruction, also performed at the scanner console; lower middle: CT angiogram source image showing relative decreased contrast in the left versus right hemisphere; and lower right: unenhanced head CT without bleed or large parenchymal hypodensity suggestive of established infarction.

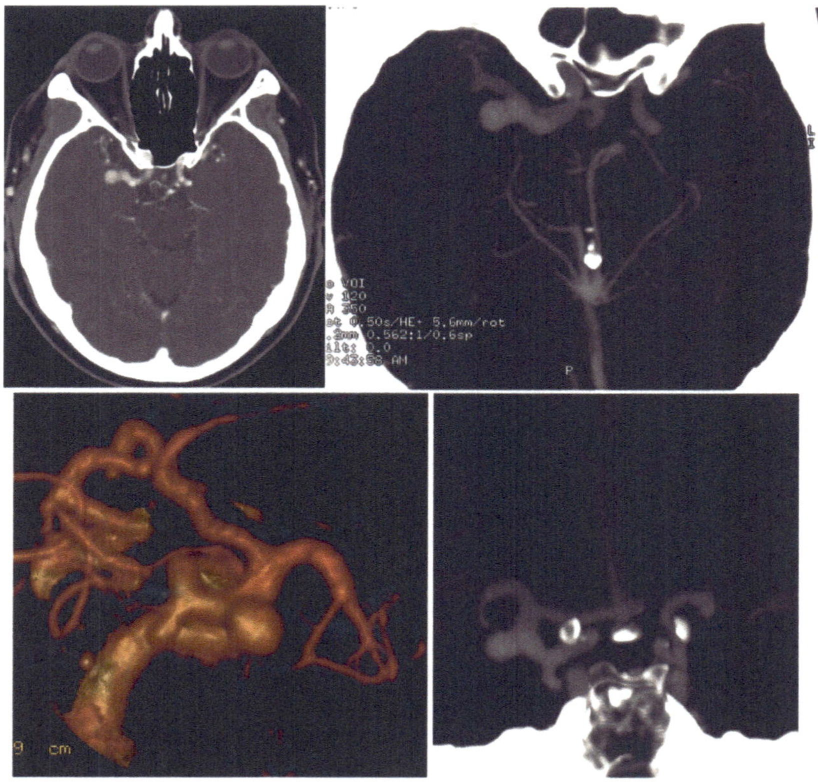

Fig. 1.7. Computed tomography (CT) angiogram of unruptured aneurysm. Top left: axial CT angiogram source image showing right proximal middle cerebral artery aneurysm pointing laterally; top right: axial thick slab collapsed maximum-intensity projection (MIP) reconstruction also showing aneurysm, performed at the scanner console by the CT technologist; bottom left: volume-rendered view of aneurysm used for surgical planning; and bottom right: coronal thick slab collapsed MIP reconstruction showing aneurysm, also performed at the scanner console by the CT technologist.

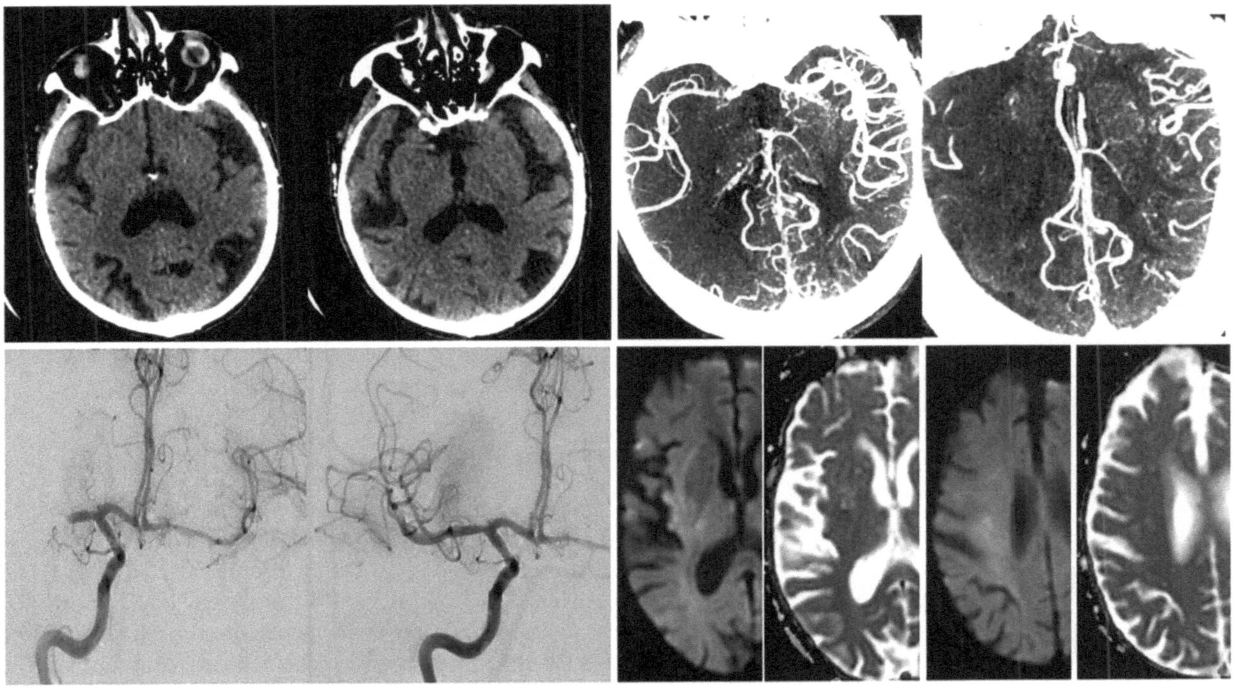

Fig. 1.8. A 45-year-old woman presenting to emergency department approximately 30 minutes after stroke onset. Top left: no evidence of infarct on unenhanced computed tomography (CT); however, origin of right middle cerebral artery (MCA) shows hyperdense vessel sign; top right: CT angiogram source images show filling defect at right MCA origin and a malignant collateral pattern in the right hemisphere; bottom left: catheter cerebral arteriogram shows right MCA occlusion prior to clot retrieval, with fully recanalized vessel within 1.5 hours of stroke onset; bottom right: follow-up diffusion-weighted MRI shows only minimal right-hemisphere infarct 2 days following treatment.

sinuses, fossa of Rosenmuller, masticator space (a.k.a. infratemporal fossa), Waldeyer's tonsillar ring, and visualized portions of the nasopharyngeal and parapharyngeal spaces should be reviewed. Air in a place it does not belong adjacent to a paranasal sinus – either intracranially or extracranially – is generally a clue to a fracture (Fig. 1.2, lower left panel, black arrow).

With regard to the sensitive detection of intracranial hemorrhage, review of coronal and sagittal images – reformatted from thin-slice helically acquired axial CT source images – is essential (Wei et al., 2010). Volume averaging of subtle SAH, for example, may only be apparent in the imaging plane that is perpendicular to the long axis of the involved sulcus (Fig. 1.9). In direct trauma, the anteriormost portions of the frontal and temporal lobes (the most freely mobile parts of the brain) are a common location for contusion. With thick-slice axial images, however, these regions are often obscured by streak artifact from the adjacent surrounding bony skull base. Coronal images, again, typically provide more sensitive detection of subtle hemorrhage in these locations (Fig. 1.9, arrows).

For CTA image review of the intracranial circulation, as noted previously, MIP reformatted axial, coronal, and sagittal images (30 mm slice thickness at 5 mm overlapping intervals) can be rapidly created at the scanner console – typically in under a minute – by the CT technologist. These MIP reformatted images allow for quick, efficient screening for occlusions, stenoses, and aneurysms of the major intracranial arteries. The para- and supraclinoid carotid arteries should also be checked for aneurysms on the axial CTA source images because overlapping bony and vascular structures in these regions could obscure detection of lesions on the MIP reformats. Because the extracranial carotid and vertebral arteries are perpendicular to the axial imaging plane, they can be rapidly screened for stenoses, dissections, or occlusions by scrolling through the axial CTA source images. Finally, with regard to not overlooking incidental findings, the lungs, thyroid gland, lymph nodes in the neck, larynx, pharynx, bones, and skull base should always additionally be reviewed. Care must be taken, however, to only evaluate the patency of the venous structures if an appropriate delay has been built into the CTA protocol – otherwise, incomplete venous opacification secondary to early arterial phase imaging might be mistaken for a venous sinus thrombosis.

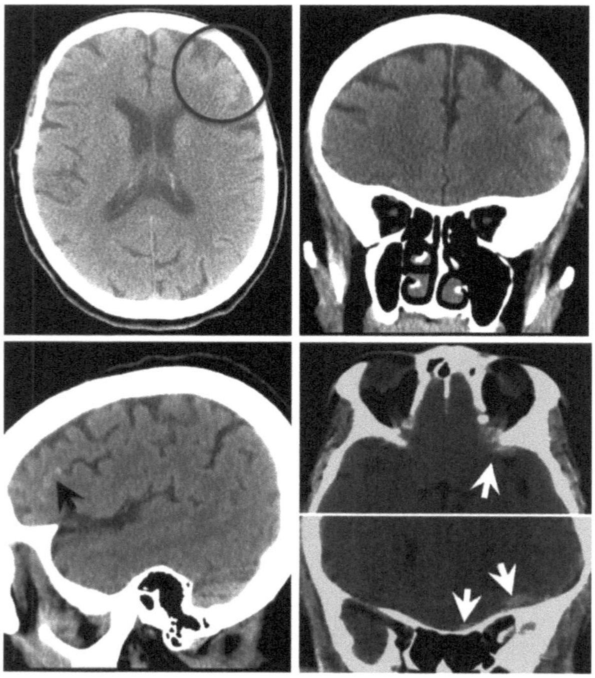

Fig. 1.9. Coronal and sagittal reformatted images can mitigate volume averaging and streak artifacts from adjacent bony structures, improving the conspicuity of subtle hemorrhage compared to that of thick-slice axial images alone.

When interpreting CTA images, care must also be taken to not confuse certain imaging artifacts commonly seen in association with direct catheter arteriography with CTA artifacts. For example, the differential diagnosis of circumferential irregularity of the carotid artery wall in the setting of blunt carotid trauma includes carotid intimal injury, fibromuscular dysplasia, atheromatous disease, or potentially a poor-contrast bolus (Fig. 1.10). Standing waves that are caused by vibrations from high-pressure power injection of contrast during selective catheter arteriography are not included in this differential diagnosis.

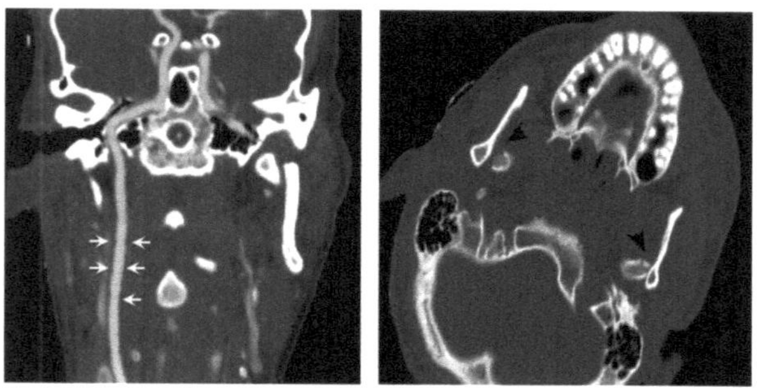

Fig. 1.10. Subtle internal carotid intimal irregularity (arrows) caused by blunt trauma, with bilateral displaced mandibular condyle fractures (arrowheads).

Similarly, an intraluminal filling defect in the proximal and mid basilar artery on CTA is likely to represent a free-floating thrombus, or potentially beam-hardening artifact, but should never be mistaken for mixing artifact, which again is a phenomenon exclusively associated with direct catheter arteriography (Fig. 1.11). Mixing artifact occurs during selective injection of contrast into one vertebral artery, when unopacified blood from the contralateral vertebral artery mixes with the contrast column in the basilar lumen. With CTA, for which contrast is administered intravenously, mixing occurs in the heart and lungs, with uniformly opacified blood exiting the aorta.

Stroke – technical pearls and pitfalls

Imaging indications are driven by the available management options. Hence, it was not until Food and Drug Administration approval of thrombolytic treatment for stroke using IV-tPA in 1996 that the use of CT for stroke assessment became the standard of care (NINDS, 1995). Intracranial hemorrhage is an absolute contraindication to IV-tPA administration (von Kummer et al., 1997). A large (>30%) middle cerebral artery territory low-density lesion suggesting established infarct is a relative contraindication, owing to increased hemorrhagic risk (von Kummer et al., 2001). Given the low sensitivity and specificity of the early CT signs of stroke, compared to that of MR diffusion-weighted imaging, obtaining a correlative clinical history of abrupt onset of focal neurologic symptoms – prior to CT image interpretation – is essential (Mullins et al., 2002).

An early CT sign of embolic stroke that might help guide patient selection for intra-arterial clot retrieval therapy is the hyperdense vessel sign (Fig. 1.12). More distal clots in third-order branches may be identified as dot signs. A recent retrospective study showed that patients with CT hyperdense clot lengths > 8 mm, as measured on thin-section CT, have a near-zero probability of responding to IV-tPA alone; hence, such patients might benefit from intra-arterial clot retrieval (Somford et al., 2002; Riedel et al., 2011; Kamalian et al., 2013).

A classic early ischemic CT sign is focal cortical swelling. Other early CT imaging signs of stroke include obscuration of the lentiform nucleus and insular ribbon (Fig. 1.13) sign, both attributable to loss of gray/white-matter differentiation with hypodensity related to vasogenic edema (Tomura et al., 1988; Truwit et al., 1990). The detection of these early stroke signs varies between observers, but they are typically seen in less than two-thirds of patients imaged at 3 hours post stroke onset. Parenchymal hypoattenuation is related to increased water content from vasogenic edema and appears to

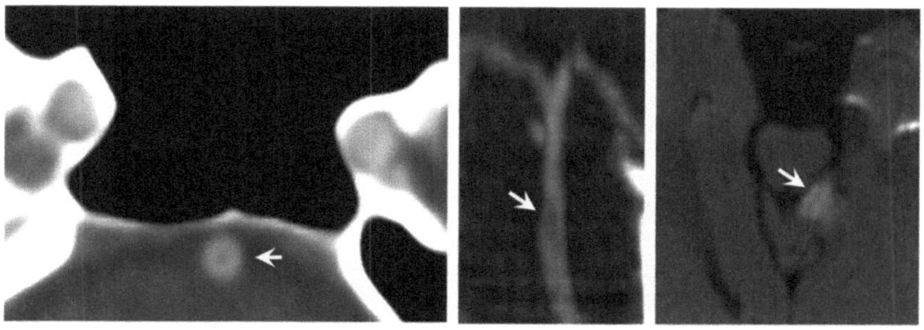

Fig. 1.11. Filling defect within basilar artery due to intraluminal free-floating thrombus, with associated left superior cerebellar infarct seen on diffusion-weighted magnetic resonance imaging. The filling defect should not be attributed to mixing artifact in the absence of direct catheter arteriography.

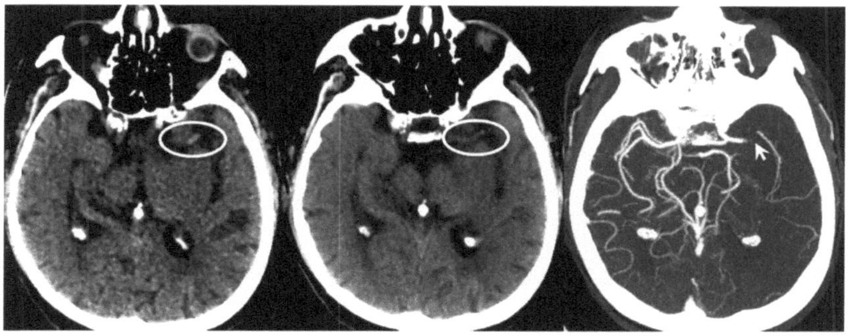

Fig. 1.12. Hyperdense left middle cerebral artery clot is visible on the axial thin, 1.25-mm computed tomography (CT) slice, but only as a dot sign on the thick, 5-mm CT slice due to partial volume averaging; confirmed on the axial CT angiography maximum-intensity projection image.

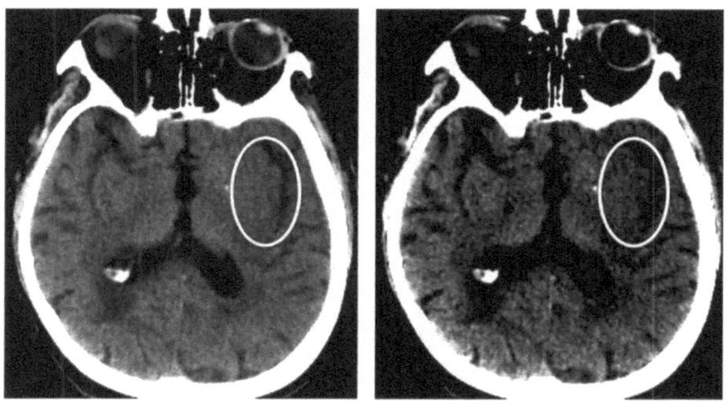

Fig. 1.13. Hypoattenuation of the left insular ribbon, an early ischemic computed tomography sign of stroke, better visualized with narrow window width display settings (35 HU, right), than at standard window width display settings (70 HU, left).

be a sign of irreversible tissue injury, while recent studies suggest that focal swelling alone may be reversible. A 10% increase in tissue water corresponds to a 20–30 HU decrease in tissue density.

Nontraumatic intracranial hemorrhage – technical pearls and pitfalls

This group includes intraparenchymal hemorrhage (IPH) and SAH. Acute SAH is detected on CT as hyperdensity (blood clot density) in the cerebrospinal fluid spaces surrounding the brain. Although the primary cause of SAH is ruptured aneurysm, it can also be due to intracranial dissection, trauma, vasculitis, dural AVM, or cervical fistulas. CTA is highly accurate to detect aneurysms, with accuracies approaching that of digital subtraction catheter arteriography (the detection rate for aneurysms $\geq$3 mm is close to 100%). Of note, aneurysm rupture need not necessarily present as SAH; for example, if the dome of a top-of-internal carotid artery aneurysm is pointing superiorly into the brain parenchyma, aneurysm rupture can dissect into the adjacent brain tissue causing the appearance of an IPH, which can mimic a hypertensive hemorrhage (Fig. 1.14).

The vast majority of IPHs are primary; these are often related to hypertension and/or anticoagulation. Hypertensive bleeds typically affect the basal ganglia, pons, and deep cerebellar nuclei. Imaging is critical for identifying potential causes of secondary IPH, which include AVM, aneurysm, venous sinus thrombosis, tumor, and vasculitis. On CTA, clues to the diagnosis of AVM include numerous enlarged vessels corresponding to feeding arteries, the vascular nidus or draining veins, as well as associated phleboliths.

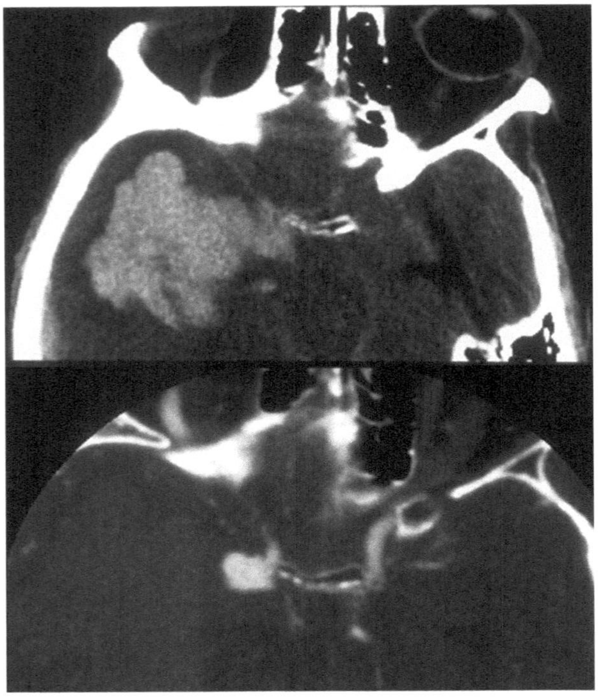

Fig. 1.14. Intraparenchymal hemorrhage due to ruptured aneurysm; not all aneurysms result in subarachnoid hemorrhage. Top: unenhanced computed tomography (CT) scan showing right parenchymal hemorrhage; bottom: CT angiogram showing top-of-internal carotid artery aneurysm.

Dural sinus or cortical vein thrombosis is a less common cause of IPH, but should always be considered as a diagnosis of exclusion, especially in young/middle-aged females who are postpartum or on oral contraceptives. If rounded and heterogeneous, hemorrhagic lesions from cortical vein thrombosis can sometimes mimic tumor (Thaler and Frosch, 2002) (Fig. 1.15). If an adequate venous-phase intracranial CTA has been obtained – even if the CT exam was not ordered or protocoled as a dedicated CTV – both the arteries and veins should always be screened for filling defects or occlusion. Important mimics of dural venous sinus thrombosis include arachnoid granulations, which are often seen on CTA as lobulated filling defects in the lateral aspects of the transverse sinuses, as well as hypoplasia of a transverse sinus. Suspected thrombosis should be confirmed on unenhanced CT as hyperdense clot within the vein or sinus (Fig. 1.15). Dedicated CT or MR venography may be performed. Gradient echo imaging is often helpful for cortical vein thrombosis, which appears as a tortuous, dysplastic area of signal loss (blooming artifact). Diffusion-weighted imaging may reveal restricted diffusion from intravascular clot.

In our emergency department practice, CTA is typically obtained for every intracranial hemorrhage that

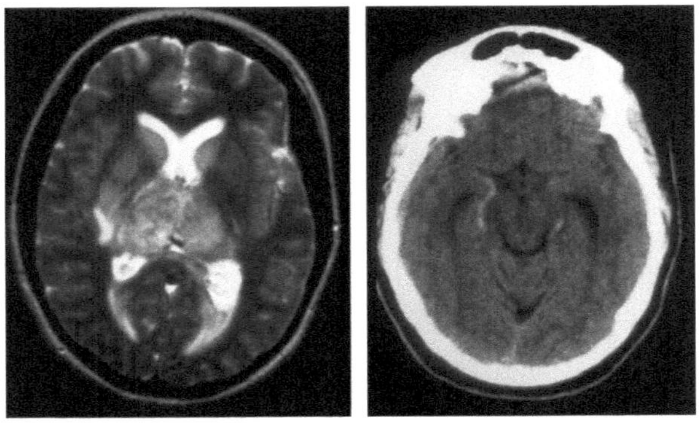

Fig. 1.15. Complex, heterogeneous, hemorrhagic bithalamic mass on T2-weighted magnetic resonance imaging (MRI) in a young postpartum female, initially thought to represent a glioblastoma multiforme tumor (left). Unenhanced head computed tomography (CT) revealed hyperdense right greater than left internal cerebral veins, later confirmed on CT and MR venography to be deep-vein thrombosis.

is not clearly attributable to mechanical trauma. The goal is to exclude an unusual presentation of an aneurysm, another vascular lesion such as an AVM, or a spot sign that would help identify patients at high risk of hematoma expansion (Delgado Almandoz et al., 2009a; Romero et al., 2009). Large hematoma volume at presentation (>60 mL) and intraventricular blood are predictors of poor outcome. Spot sign reflects active contrast extravasation of contrast into the hematoma; obtaining a delayed venous-phase CTA can increase sensitivity for spot sign detection (Delgado Almandoz et al., 2009b; Brouwers et al., 2014). Spot sign characteristics with high positive predictive value for hematoma expansion include $\geq$3 spots, maximum diameter of the largest spot $\geq$5 mm, and maximum attenuation of the largest spot $\geq$180 HU.

NEW DEVELOPMENTS AND FUTURE DIRECTIONS

Although there have been many recent advancements in the CT imaging chain – from improved X-ray beam generation to more efficient detectors and more advanced image reconstruction and postprocessing techniques – we will highlight two important new developments in the following paragraphs: dual-energy CT (Gupta et al., 2010; Rapalino et al., 2011; Pomerantz et al., 2013) and iterative reconstruction (Ramachandran and Lakshminarayanan, 1971; Rapalino et al., 2012; Corcuera-Solano et al., 2014).

Dual-energy CT (DECT)

Conventional CT assigns a CT number (also known as a linear attenuation coefficient or Hounsfield unit), to each imaged voxel. The CT number depends on the energy of the X-ray beam used for imaging: the higher the energy, lower the linear attenuation coefficient. In addition, how the CT number changes as a function of energy is unique to each material. This fact can be used for characterizing the material in each voxel. Many newer scanners allow dual-energy imaging for tissue characterization. Two images are acquired at low and high energies (typically, 80 and 140 kV). These are then postprocessed to answer specific clinical questions about the underlying anatomy and/or physiology. DECT can be implemented using any one of the following four paradigms.

1. Dual-spin scanners sequentially acquire two independent image sets of the same anatomy at two different energy settings.
2. Fast kVp switching scanners employ a special X-ray tube that is capable of rapidly switching between high and low voltage settings on a projection-by-projection basis, as the scanner rotates around the patient.
3. Dual-source scanners, as the name implies, have two independent imaging chains mounted on a single CT gantry. One imaging chain is operated in the low-energy mode and the other imaging chain is operated in the high-energy mode.
4. Dual-layer detector-based scanners use the inherent polychromatic nature of the X-ray beam to acquire a low- and high-energy spectral band from a single exposure by using a specialized detector that can provide two spectral bands from the same X-ray illumination.

The postprocessing steps, irrespective of how the low- and high-energy images are acquired, are the same and are schematically shown in Figure 1.16. As mentioned before, for each voxel, the total attenuation decreases with increasing X-ray photon energy, and the decrease is characteristic of the material composition of each voxel. Material density images, for any two preselected materials, are created based on the theory of basis material decomposition. The attenuation coefficients of any material can be calculated as a weighted sum of the attenuation coefficients of two materials

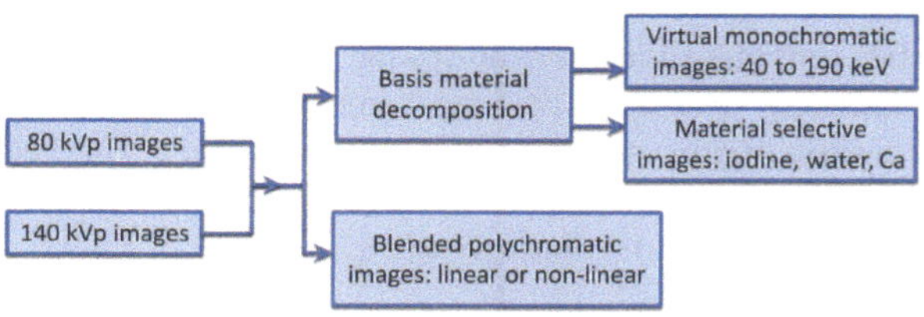

Fig. 1.16. Steps in dual-energy computed tomography (DECT) postprocessing.

as long as the *k*-edge of the material is not within the evaluated energy range. This works best if the two materials have sufficiently different atomic numbers.

The preselected material pairs could be, for example, water versus contrast material or calcium versus hemorrhage. In this decomposition, each image represents materials that have spectral signature close to that of the selected material.

Material decomposition can be used to advantage in multiple clinical situations. For example, in a noncontrast head CT scan after trauma, a parenchymal hyperdensity may represent acute hemorrhage or chronic calcification. Because the spectral signatures of hemorrhage and calcification are quite distinct, one can use a DECT to make this differentiation.

As shown in Figure 1.16, one can also split the attenuation of each voxel into its two main components, the photoelectric effect and the Compton scattering. Since the energy dependence of each of these components is known, one can generate a simulated or virtual monochromatic image of the anatomy at any desired energy level.

The following applications of DECT have been described in the literature (Gupta et al., 2010; Rapalino et al., 2011; Pomerantz et al., 2013):

- automatic bone removal
- virtual monochromatic images for optimal contrast viewing and posterior fossa artifact reduction
- differentiation of hemorrhage from iodinated-contrast extravasation
- calcified plaque and bone subtraction for CTA in order to discern the contrast-opacified vessels from adjacent bone, particularly in the skull base and vertebrae
- evaluation of extracranial–intracranial bypass surgery
- metal artifact reduction.

Some clinical examples of these indications follow in the paragraphs below.

Figure 1.17 shows the attenuation of iodine and water as a function of X-ray energy. As can be seen, the attenuation of iodine declines markedly as the X-ray photon energy increases; the attenuation of water, on the other hand, remains relatively constant. This fact can be used to increase the conspicuity of contrast-enhanced vessels against the background of the brain parenchyma or drastically cut down the amount of contrast that is administered, with obvious benefits in terms of renal health.

While the contrast of iodine increases as the X-ray photon energy is lowered, the opposite is true of metal artifacts. Any piece of metallic hardware either completely blocks the X-ray beam, or substantially hardens the beam. After CT reconstruction, this

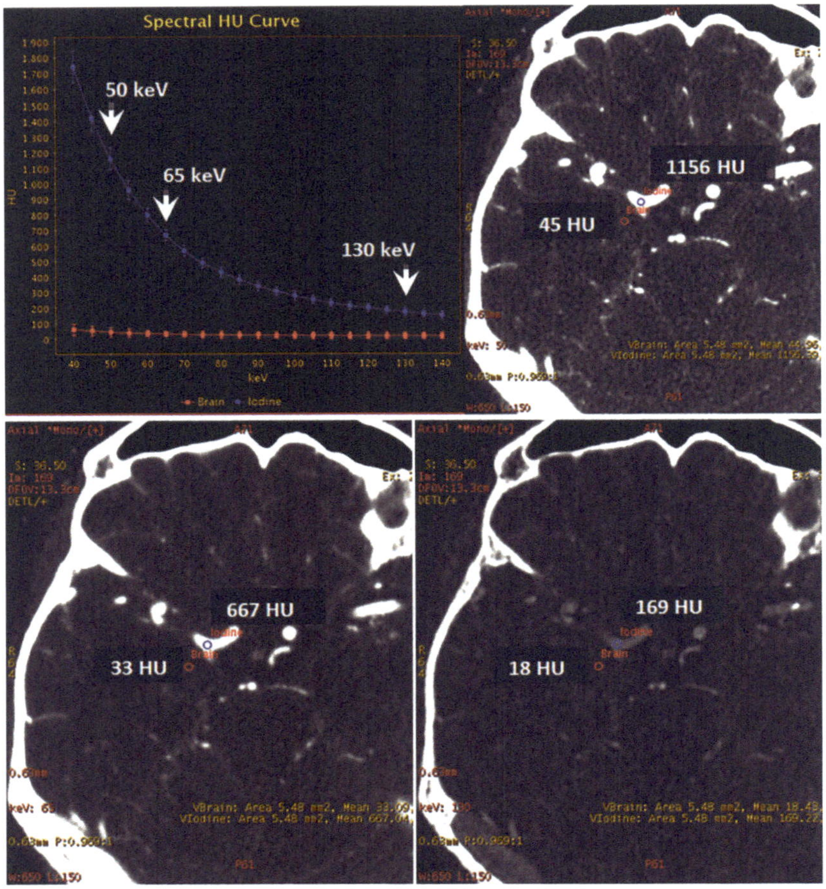

Fig. 1.17. Dual-energy virtual monochromatic images of a contrast-enhanced brain at three different energy levels: 50 keV (top right), 65 keV (bottom left), and 130 keV (bottom right). With dual-energy computed tomography, virtual monochromatic reconstruction at lower keV levels improves intravascular enhancement and contrast-to-noise ratio as the X-ray photon energy moves closer to the *k*-edge of iodine (33.2 keV). As can be seen, the attenuation with the vessel jumps from 169 HU to 1156 HU when we move from 130 keV to 50 keV. With this change, the brain parenchyma only goes from 18 HU to 45 HU. This fact can be used to drastically cut down the amount of contrast that is administered, with obvious benefits in terms of renal health.

phenomenon manifests itself as linear streaks in the images, as shown in the case of a surgical fixation frame in Figure 1.18. As this figure illustrates, one can substantially reduce these artifacts by increasing the simulated monochromatic energy level. Another example of this use of DECT is shown in a trauma CTA, performed for assessing potential involvement of the carotid artery by a foreign body with substantial metal in it (Fig. 1.19). The single-energy images in this case were unrevealing because of excessive spray artifact from the metal. High-keV virtual monochromatic images, however, clearly demonstrated that the cavernous carotid was not involved.

The same trick, in fact, can be used with any substance with high density that causes beam hardening. For example, the visualization of the posterior fossa contents, especially the brainstem, is severely degraded by beam-hardening artifact arising from the petrous ridges laterally and the clivus anteriorly. As shown in Figure 1.20, one can considerably reduce this artifact using the virtual monochromatic images.

Iterative reconstruction algorithms

An X-ray image provides a superposition of all the structures in the path of the X-ray beam. In CT, close to 1000 such projection images are acquired and converted into tomographic slice data using a specialized reconstruction algorithm. Johann Radon, an Austrian mathematician, provided the mathematic basis for this conversion process almost a century ago. Radon proved that a 2-D function (e.g., an image of a tomographic slice through the body) is mathematically equivalent to its projections. It was not until the early 1970s that Sir Godfrey Hounsfield recognized that X-rays provided an experimental method for obtaining a set of projection images

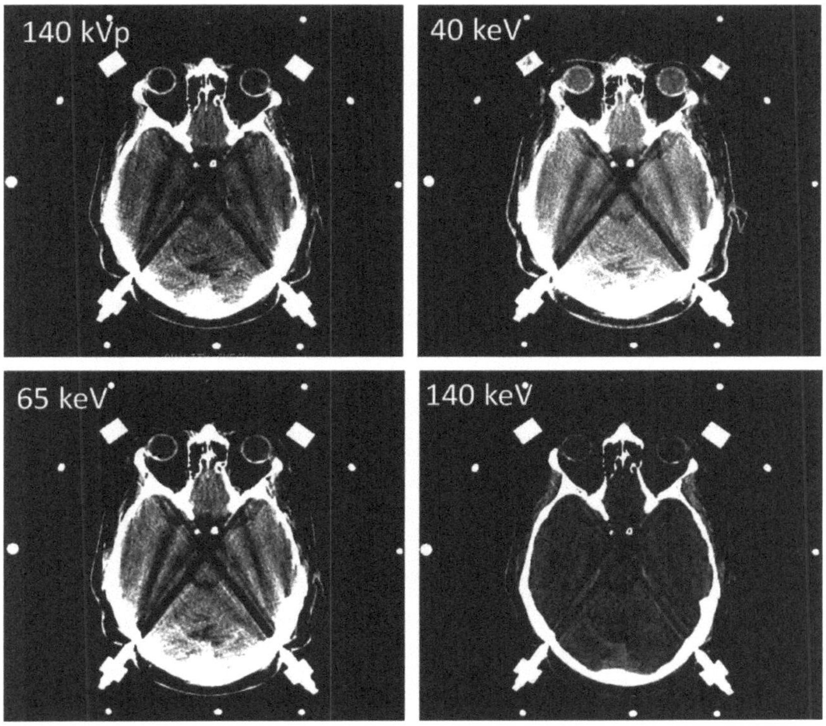

Fig. 1.18. Dual-energy computed tomography of stereotactic frame imaging for pre-op measurements; reduction of beam hardening due to metallic frame.

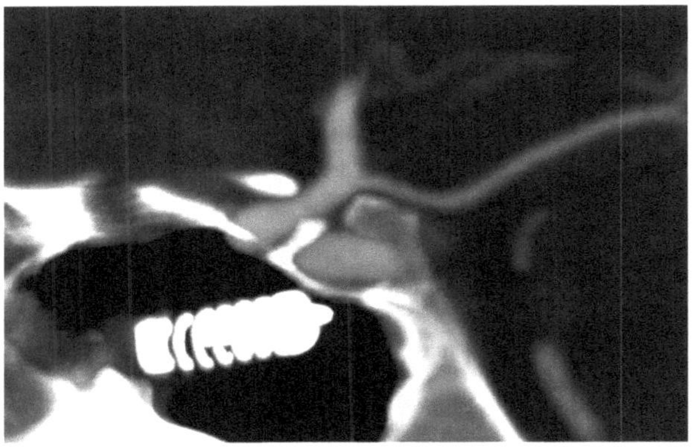

Fig. 1.19. An example of virtual monochromatic imaging at 180 keV for metal artifact reduction in a patient with a foreign body (a ballpoint pen) in the sphenoid sinus. Despite the presence of metal, one can clearly discern that the carotid artery is not involved by the trauma.

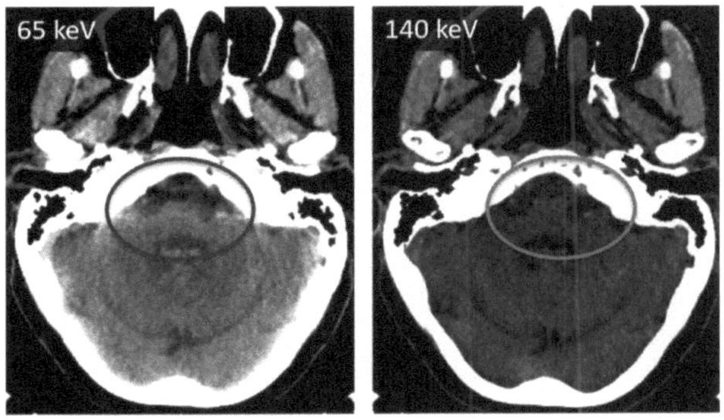

Fig. 1.20. An example of virtual monochromatic imaging for posterior fossa beam-hardening artifact reduction.

of any object, that are, in a fundamental mathematic sense, equivalent to the tomographic images of that object.

The most common method for converting a set of projection images into the corresponding set of tomographic slices is via an algorithm called filtered backprojection or FBP (Ramachandran and Lakshminarayanan, 1971). In this algorithm, the set of projections are convolved with a function called a kernel, and then projected into the tomographic plane. FBP provides an analytic method for image reconstruction; no attempt is made to minimize the overall error between the reconstructed tomographic image and its corresponding set of projection images. Such analytic reconstruction algorithms provide a single-pass solution to the reconstruction task: each projection is convolved with the kernel and then backprojected with no attempt at error minimization. As a result, FBP is very fast and nearly universally available on all CT scanners. However, this algorithm is prone to noise and artifacts, especially in the presence of beam hardening and metallic objects in the field of view. FBP

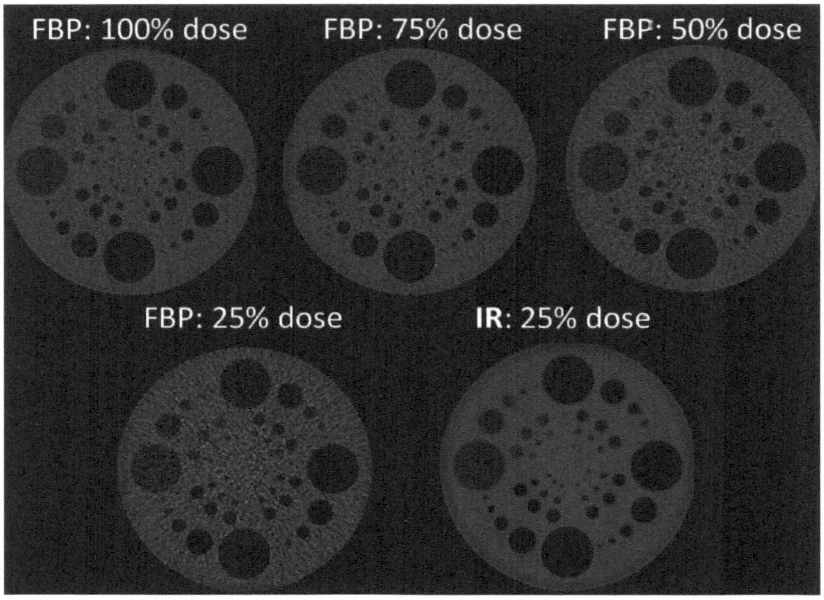

Fig. 1.21. Effect of dose reduction on filtered backprojection (FBP) reconstruction algorithm and iterative reconstruction (IR) algorithm. (Courtesy of Synho Do, PhD, Massachusetts General Hospital.)

also requires a large number of projections, increasing the radiation dose to the patient.

Recently, a new class of algorithms called iterative reconstruction algorithms has been increasingly used to improve image quality and to minimize radiation dose. These algorithms, unlike their analytic counterparts, explicitly minimize projection error between a reconstructed slice and its corresponding projection set. The nomenclature iterative reconstruction derives from the fact that this error minimization proceeds iteratively, with incremental improvements in the reconstructed slice, until the overall error is minimized. Typically, anywhere from 1 to 30 iterations may be needed to accomplish this. Iterative reconstruction algorithms reduce image noise, increase image resolution, and decrease radiation dose.

The major drawback of iterative reconstruction algorithms is their slow computational speed: it may take several hours to arrive at the global minimum on a single processor machine. However, given the computational power available on most multicore processors and graphical processing units, this drawback is fast becoming a nonissue. Many of the computational steps required by these algorithms, for example, ray tracing, are available in the high-end processors designed for video game industry. With the advent of such processing power, the computational time can be reduced to less than 1 minute, making iterative reconstruction feasible in current clinical practice. Most vendors of CT equipment have introduced specialized iterative reconstruction algorithms to reduce radiation dose associated with scanning. These algorithms go by specialized names, such as: Adaptive Statistical Iterative Reconstruction or ASIR and Veo (both by GE Healthcare); IRIS, Sinogram Affirmed Iterative Reconstruction (SAFIRE), and Admire (all by Siemens Medical Solutions); iDose and IMR (Philips); and AIDER-3D (Toshiba). A detailed discussion of these algorithms is beyond the scope of this chapter.

One can understand the effect of iterative reconstruction algorithm on the noise profile with the help of a CT resolution phantom, shown in Figure 1.21. In this figure, the dose was monotonically reduced from full-dose (100%) to 75%, 50%, and 25% and the images were reconstructed using FPB. As can be seen, the noise, as manifested by the quantum mottle in the image, increases as the dose is reduced. As a result, the smallest low-density inserts in the phantom become invisible at lower doses. The projection set for the case with the lowest dose (25% of the full dose) was reconstructed with a custom iterative reconstruction algorithm. As can be seen, the quality of this iterative reconstruction image is considerably superior to that of the corresponding FBP image. In fact, a case could be made that it is better than the FBP reconstruction with 100% of the dose. In general, iterative reconstruction algorithms can reduce dose while preserving or improving image quality.

The same phenomenon can also be demonstrated clinically, as shown in Figures 1.22 and 1.23. These figures illustrate the affect of two popular iterative reconstruction algorithms on image quality with varying levels of iterative reconstruction applied. In Figure 1.22, ASIR

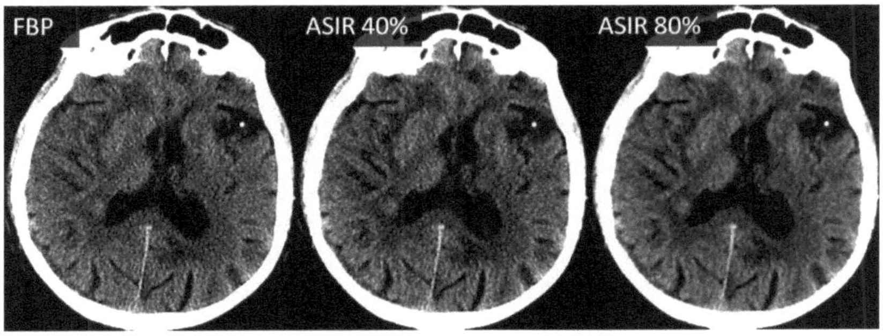

Fig. 1.22. Filtered backprojection (FBP)), ASIR 40%, ASIR 80%, less image noise and improved gray–white-matter differentiation.

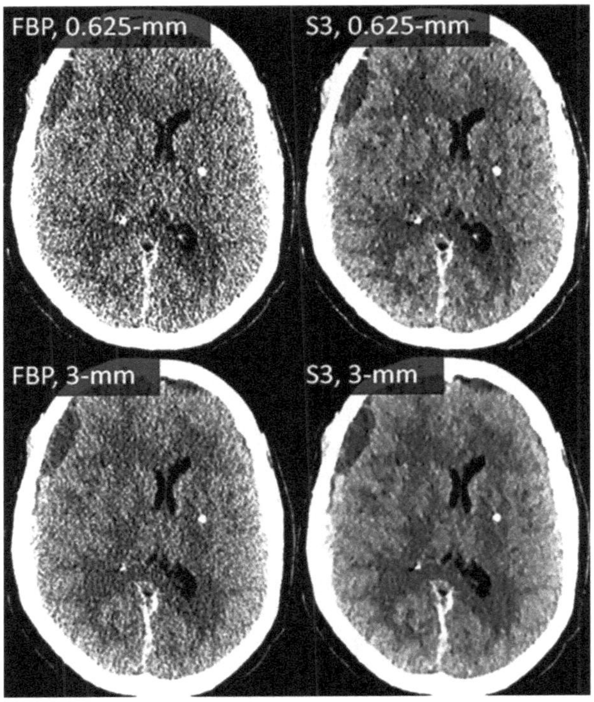

Fig. 1.23. Filtered backprojection (FBP), Sinogram-Affirmed Iterative Reconstruction (SAFIRE) level 3 with less image noise and improved gray–white-matter differentiation.

(GE Healthcare) was used at 40% and 80% levels. As can be seen, there is corresponding decrease in the quantum mottle in the last image that uses the highest percentage of ASIR. Similar effect is seen with SAFIRE (Siemens Medical Solutions). Figure 1.23 shows the level S3 of SAFIRE applied to two different slice thicknesses. In each case, the application of SAFIRE improved the gray–white differentiation and reduced the image noise.

References

Baker Jr HL (1981). The clinical usefulness of routine coronal and sagittal reconstructions in cranial computed tomography. Radiology 140: 1–9.

Brouwers HB, Chang Y, Falcone GJ et al. (2014). Predicting hematoma expansion after primary intracerebral hemorrhage. JAMA Neurol 71: 158–164.

Camargo EC, Furie KL, Singhal AB et al. (2007). Acute brain infarct: detection and delineation with CT angiographic source images versus nonenhanced CT scans. Radiology 244: 541–548.

Corcuera-Solano I, Doshi AH, Noor A et al. (2014). Repeated head CT in the neurosurgical intensive care unit: feasibility of sinogram-affirmed iterative reconstruction-based ultra-low-dose CT for surveillance. AJNR Am J Neuroradiol 35: 1281–1287.

Coutts SB, Lev MH, Eliasziw M et al. (2004). ASPECTS on CTA source images versus unenhanced CT: added value in predicting final infarct extent and clinical outcome. Stroke 35: 2472–2476.

Delgado Almandoz JE, Schaefer PW, Forero NP et al. (2009a). Diagnostic accuracy and yield of multidetector CT angiography in the evaluation of spontaneous intraparenchymal cerebral hemorrhage. AJNR Am J Neuroradiol 30: 1213–1221.

Delgado Almandoz JE, Yoo AJ, Stone MJ et al. (2009b). Systematic characterization of the computed tomography angiography spot sign in primary intracerebral hemorrhage identifies patients at highest risk for hematoma expansion: the spot sign score. Stroke 40: 2994–3000.

Eastwood JD, Lev MH, Azhari T et al. (2002). CT perfusion scanning with deconvolution analysis: pilot study in patients with acute middle cerebral artery stroke. Radiology 222: 227–236.

Gupta R, Phan CM, Leidecker C et al. (2010). Evaluation of dual-energy CT for differentiating intracerebral hemorrhage from iodinated contrast material staining. Radiology 257: 205–211.

Jones TR, Kaplan RT, Lane B et al. (2001). Single- versus multi-detector row CT of the brain: quality assessment. Radiology 219: 750–755.

Kamalian S, Morais LT, Pomerantz SR et al. (2013). Clot length distribution and predictors in anterior circulation stroke: implications for intra-arterial therapy. Stroke 44: 3553–3556.

Koenig M, Klotz E, Luka B et al. (1998). Perfusion CT of the brain: diagnostic approach for early detection of ischemic stroke. Radiology 209: 85–93.

Lev MH, Farkas J, Gemmete JJ et al. (1999). Acute stroke: improved nonenhanced CT detection – benefits of soft-copy interpretation by using variable window width and center level settings. Radiology 213: 150–155.

Lev MH, Romero JM, Goodman DN et al. (2003). Total occlusion versus hairline residual lumen of the internal carotid arteries: accuracy of single section helical CT angiography. AJNR Am J Neuroradiol 24: 1123–1129.

Mullins ME, Lev MH, Schellingerhout D et al. (2002). Influence of availability of clinical history on detection of early stroke using unenhanced CT and diffusion-weighted MR imaging. AJR Am J Roentgenol 179: 223–228.

Napel S, Marks MP, Rubin GD et al. (1992). CT angiography with spiral CT and maximum intensity projection. Radiology 185: 607–610.

New PF, Scott WR, Schnur JA et al. (1974). Computerized axial tomography with the EMI scanner. Radiology 110: 109–123.

NINDS (1995). Tissue plasminogen activator for acute ischemic stroke. The National Institute of Neurological Disorders and Stroke rt-PA Stroke Study Group. N Engl J Med 333: 1581–1587.

Pomerantz SR, Kamalian S, Zhang D et al. (2013). Virtual monochromatic reconstruction of dual-energy unenhanced head CT at 65-75 keV maximizes image quality compared with conventional polychromatic CT. Radiology 266: 318–325.

Ramachandran GN, Lakshminarayanan AV (1971). Three-dimensional reconstruction from radiographs and electron micrographs: application of convolutions instead of Fourier transforms. Proc Natl Acad Sci U S A 68: 2236–2240.

Rapalino O, Kamalian S, Gupta R et al. (2011). Neurological applications. In: T Johnson, C Fink, SO Schönberg et al. (Eds.), Dual Energy CT in Clinical Practice. Springer, Berlin, pp. 127–142.

Rapalino O, Kamalian S, Kamalian S et al. (2012). Cranial CT with adaptive statistical iterative reconstruction: improved image quality with concomitant radiation dose reduction. AJNR Am J Neuroradiol 33: 609–615.

Riedel CH, Zimmermann P, Jensen-Kondering U et al. (2011). The importance of size: successful recanalization by intravenous thrombolysis in acute anterior stroke depends on thrombus length. Stroke 42: 1775–1777.

Romero JM, Artunduaga M, Forero NP et al. (2009). Accuracy of CT angiography for the diagnosis of vascular abnormalities causing intraparenchymal hemorrhage in young patients. Emerg Radiol 16: 195–201.

Schramm P, Schellinger PD, Fiebach JB et al. (2002). Comparison of CT and CT angiography source images with diffusion-weighted imaging in patients with acute stroke within 6 hours after onset. Stroke 33: 2426–2432.

Schwartz RB, Jones KM, Chernoff DM et al. (1992). Common carotid artery bifurcation: evaluation with spiral CT. Work in progress. Radiology 185: 513–519.

Somford DM, Nederkoorn PJ, Rutgers DR et al. (2002). Proximal and distal hyperattenuating middle cerebral artery signs at CT: different prognostic implications. Radiology 223: 667–671.

Sorensen AG, Buonanno FS, Gonzalez RG et al. (1996). Hyperacute stroke: evaluation with combined multisection diffusion-weighted and hemodynamically weighted echo-planar MR imaging. Radiology 199: 391–401.

Souza LC, Yoo AJ, Chaudhry ZA et al. (2012). Malignant CTA collateral profile is highly specific for large admission DWI infarct core and poor outcome in acute stroke. AJNR Am J Neuroradiol 33: 1331–1336.

Taveras JM, Gilson JM, Davis DO et al. (1969). Angiography in cerebral infarction. Radiology 93: 549–558.

Thaler DE, Frosch MP (2002). Case records of the Massachusetts General Hospital. Weekly clinicopathological exercises. Case 16-2002. A 41-year-old woman with global headache and an intracranial mass. N Engl J Med 346: 1651–1658.

Tomura N, Uemura K, Inugami A et al. (1988). Early CT finding in cerebral infarction: obscuration of the lentiform nucleus. Radiology 168: 463–467.

Truwit CL, Barkovich AJ, Gean-Marton A et al. (1990). Loss of the insular ribbon: another early CT sign of acute middle cerebral artery infarction. Radiology 176: 801–806.

von Kummer R, Allen KL, Holle R et al. (1997). Acute stroke: usefulness of early CT findings before thrombolytic therapy. Radiology 205: 327–333.

von Kummer R, Bourquain H, Bastianello S et al. (2001). Early prediction of irreversible brain damage after ischemic stroke at CT. Radiology 219: 95–100.

Wei SC, Ulmer S, Lev MH et al. (2010). Value of coronal reformations in the CT evaluation of acute head trauma. AJNR Am J Neuroradiol 31: 334–339.

Wing SD, Norman D, Pollock JA et al. (1976). Contrast enhancement of cerebral infarcts in computed tomography. Radiology 121: 89–92.

Yamashita K, Noguchi T, Mihara F et al. (2007). An intraorbital wooden foreign body: description of a case and a variety of CT appearances. Emerg Radiol 14: 41–43.

Handbook of Clinical Neurology, Vol. 135 (3rd series)
Neuroimaging, Part I
J.C. Masdeu and R.G. González, Editors

Chapter 2

MR imaging: deconstructing timing diagrams and demystifying *k*-space

ANDREW J.M. KIRULUTA[1,2]* AND R. GILBERTO GONZÁLEZ[1]

[1]*Department of Radiology, Massachusetts General Hospital, Boston, MA, USA*

[2]*Department of Biophysics, Harvard University, Cambridge, MA, USA*

Abstract

Magnetic resonance imaging (MRI) works on the principle that hydrogen molecules, which are abundant in organic tissue, have a magnetic moment arising from the spin of the protons in the nucleus. All atoms consist of a nucleus made of protons and neutrons. When a sample is put in a large magnet field, the hydrogen atoms become magnetized resulting in a bulk magnetization of the sample. Each of these hydrogen atoms acts like a bar magnet, spinning at a frequency about the applied main magnetic field. The frequency of spin is proportional to the applied main field and hence to encode position, we apply an additive field that increases linearly with position in a given direction. Hence, the spins in that direction will precess at a linearly increasing frequency and can be resolved by matching each resolvable frequency bin to a given position. This allows one direction to be resolved. By repeating the same procedure for the other dimension, a 2D image can be resolved by averaging over the third dimension.

INTRODUCTION

Magnetic resonance imaging (MRI) works on the principle that hydrogen molecules, which are abundant in organic tissue, have a magnetic moment arising from the spin of the protons in the nucleus (see, for example, Wehrli et al., 1988). All atoms consist of a nucleus made of positively charged protons and of neutrons. The positively charged nucleus is balanced by a cloud of electrons of opposite charge that render the atom neutral. Protons, neutrons, and electrons have intrinsic angular momentum, meaning that they inherently spin about their axis. For example, the single proton that makes up a hydrogen atom spins about its axis as shown in Figure 2.1B.

Rotating or moving charges (protons or electrons) give rise to an electric current. Associated with currents is a magnetic field so that each nuclear spin is like a magnetic dipole or bar magnet and will align with an applied field in a manner that is analogous to a compass needle. In the absence of an external magnetic field, each of these dipoles is randomly oriented such that the net magnetization of the sample is zero, as shown in Figure 2.1C. When a sample is placed in a magnetic field, a slightly higher number of these dipoles align in the direction of the field while the remainder align in a direction opposite to the main applied field. The net result is that the sample is slightly magnetized in the direction of the applied field, much like a paper clip becomes magnetized when it is attached to a magnet for a sufficient period of time. This net bulk magnetization of the sample is represented by a vector **M**, as shown in Figure 2.1D. Note that it takes some time for the net magnetization of the sample to reach its final or steady-state value. This rate of magnetization is the so-called T1 relaxation of a given sample or the time it takes the sample to reach 63% of its final magnetization steady state, as shown in Figure 2.1E (Bottomley et al., 1987).

In addition to the alignment with the applied field, each one of these spin dipoles precesses or oscillates about the main applied field B_0 at a frequency

*Correspondence to: Andrew J.M. Kiruluta, Massachusetts General Hospital, 55 Fruit St, Ellison 229D, Boston MA 02114, USA. Tel: +1-617-724-6536, E-mail: kiruluta@physics.harvard.edu

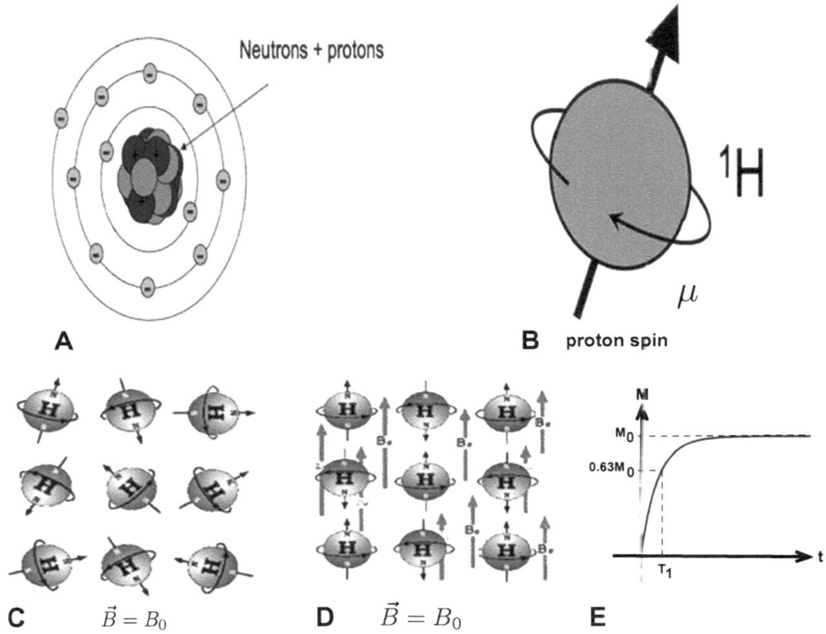

Fig. 2.1. (**A**) Simplified model of atomic structure showing a nucleus consisting of protons and neutrons surrounded by electrons in a shell structure. (**B**) Neutrons, protons, and electrons spin about their axis, and, for charged particles like protons and electrons, this results in a magnetic moment vector analogous to a campus needle. Spins, analogous to bar magnets, are normally oriented randomly in thermal equilibrium, as in (**C**). (**D**) Much like a compass aligns itself with the earth's magnetic field, in the presence of an applied polarizing magnetic field B_0, some spins align with the magnetic field while some align themselves against the magnetic field, thus canceling each other out. (**E**) The excess number of spins in the direction of the main field results in the net bulk magnetization of the sample, represented here as vector M. The growth in magnetization of the sample is asymptotic till it reaches its steady-state value, determined by the relaxation rate T_1 of the material.

proportional to the strength of this main field, the so-called larmor frequency. The higher the strength of the main field, the higher the frequency of precession of the spins. This relationship is given by the simple equation:

$$\omega = \gamma B_0 \tag{1}$$

where γ is a constant which depends on the size of nuclei. For hydrogen nuclei with a single proton, this constant is equal to a precession rate of 42 MHz per tesla, where tesla is a unit of measure of field strength, so that for the most common clinical scanner at 1.5 T, the spins oscillate at 64 million cycles per second. Now, the radio broadcast band, which includes AM, FM, and TV transmissions, spans the frequency range 3 Hz to 300 GHz so that MRI spin precession frequencies are well within the radio broadcast band, and hence the need for a radiofrequency (RF)-shielded room to isolate the scanner from broadcast contamination.

So what happens if we try to image an object based on what we have done so far? To recap, we have put a sample in a magnetic field where it has become magnetized. In addition, all these spins precess around the main applied field. We have essentially three fundamental problems that need to be resolved. First, the spins are all precessing at about the same larmor frequency, so that all points in a 3D volume contribute to the same signal at a single frequency and hence no spatial localization is possible from this frequency information. The second problem is that, even though all the spins are precessing at about the same frequency, they started precessing at slightly different times and are thus not in phase with each other. The third problem is related to limitation of detecting magnetic fields directly. However, changing magnetic fields (due to larmor precession in this case) will lead to the induction of a current in an appropriately placed receiver coil. Let us begin by addressing the spin localization problem.

SPIN LOCALIZATION

The solution to this problem is intrinsic to the larmor relationship, which states that spins precess at a frequency proportional to the field strength (eq. 1). The solution then is to add a small field, pointing in the same direction as the main field B_0, but which linearly increases the total field as a function of position to one side of the center of the magnet bore and linearly decreases the field as a function of position on the opposite side of the magnet center. The result is that spins experience a linearly increasing or decreasing field with distance and hence precess faster with distance on one side and slower on the other side from the center of the magnet bore. This encoding scheme allows us to identify different positions by the rate at which the spins in those respective positions precess.

The idea is illustrated in Figure 2.2, where spins at four different locations along the x-axis are precessing at four distinct frequencies and hence can be resolved with this gradient encoding scheme. Because each resolvable location in a given direction is precessing at a specific frequency, this spin localization scheme is referred to as frequency encoding when data are collected during this interval. This encoding scheme allows us to encode spins in a single direction only so that imaging in the presence of this gradient reduces a 3D object to a line. When data are collected when the gradient is turned off, the spins resort to precess at the same frequency but at different phases. This is then phase-encoded data (more on this later). We shall discuss later how to unfold this line into two dimensions based on several extensions of this basic gradient encoding idea.

SPIN SYNCHRONIZATION

The second problem is one of spin synchronization. To understand this idea, we need to understand the concept of phase. Consider the single-frequency signal shown as four separate traces in Figure 2.3, all with the same amplitude and frequency. The time origin is defined by the vertical line in the figure at $t = 0$. We see that, even though the frequency of oscillation is identical for all four traces, their starting point is different relative to reference waveform 1. The waveforms are thus delayed relative to the reference waveform and this delay is a measureable quantity, referred to as phase delay. As long as the phase is preserved in the measurement of the signal relative to a given reference, and we have the means to recover this phase, then all four traces can be distinguished from each other based on this relative phase delay. This is thus the basis of phase encoding.

The concept of phase is extremely important in MR. As we have seen, MR consists of an ensemble of spin frequencies that have been spatially encoded. The strength of the detected signal will depend on whether these different frequencies add up in phase (constructive interference: Fig. 2.4A), resulting in a larger signal, or out of phase (destructive interference: Fig. 2.4B), resulting in a smaller signal. The concept is similar to an analogy between a laser and a light bulb, as shown in Figure 2.4C. A light bulb illuminates with a wide range of frequencies that are for the most part out of phase with each other and hence the intensity of the illumination is not as pronounced. By contrast, a laser has only a very limited range of frequencies which are produced at a very precise phase, such that all components add coherently, resulting in a very intense output beam. For MRI to work, given that the bulk magnetization of

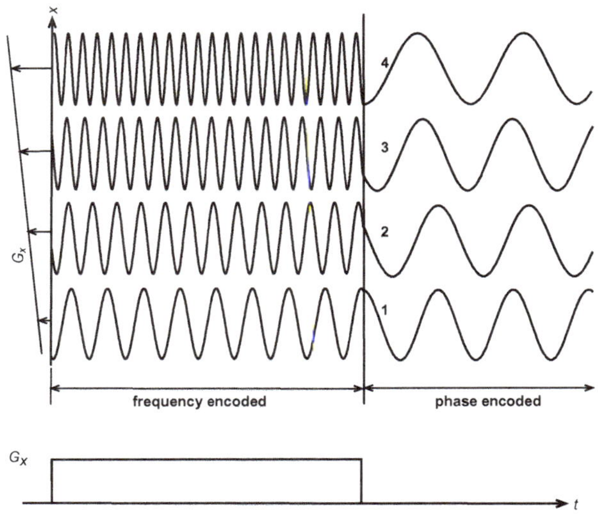

Fig. 2.2. Frequency encoding of spins by the superposition of a linear gradient on to the main field, B_0. The figure shows four spin positions precessing at linearly increasing frequencies along x. The data are said to be frequency-encoded. When the gradient pulse is switched off, the spins resume to precessing at the same rate, determined by the main polarization field B_0 but with different phases. The spins when detected in this range are said to be phase-encoded.

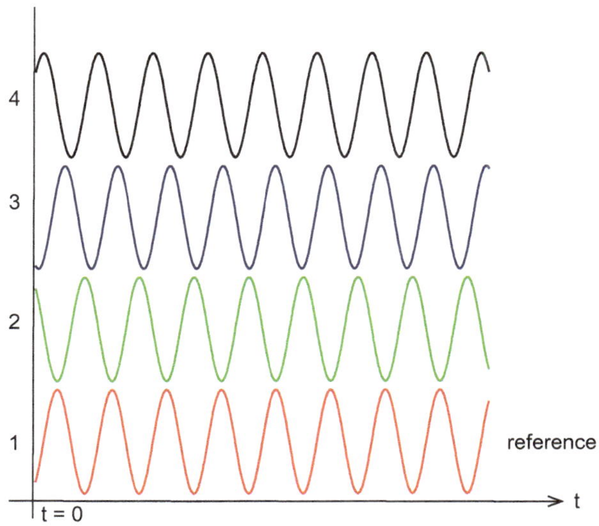

Fig. 2.3. Single-frequency waveforms referenced to a common point showing that, from this vantage point, the four traces can be discriminated from each other based on their delay relative to reference waveform 1. The waveforms are thus phase-encoded.

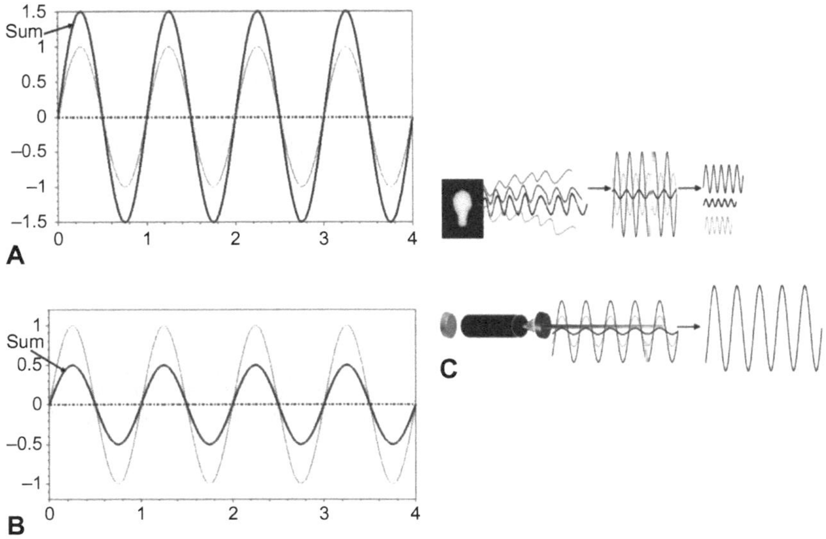

Fig. 2.4. The concept of adding frequencies in phase, referred to as constructive interference (**A**), results in a larger output signal, while that of adding out-of-phase signals results in destructive interference and a reduced output (**B**). (**C**) In analogous fashion, the random generation of out-of-phase frequencies from a light bulb and hence the illumination is not as intense as that of a laser from which a narrow range of frequencies is generated with a precise phase relationship. The result is a very coherent and intense laser beam.

the sample represented by the vector **M** is very small, even with a strong polarizing B_0 field, we need it to operate like a laser.

Hence, a mechanism has to be devised to bring all the precessing spins in synchronism or in phase. This is achieved by using an RF excitation pulse. To see how the RF excitation achieves this, consider Figure 2.5A, where the spins (represented by the off-axis vectors) are shown to precess about the main field in a random fashion, resulting in a component of magnetization along the *z*-axis, but none in the transverse *xy*-plane. Using an RF excitation pulse applied in the transverse plane and at the same frequency as the precessing spins, they can thus be brought in phase, as shown in Figure 2.5B). A direct consequence of this rephrasing is the emergence of a component of magnetization in the transverse plane (the vector sum of all spins) which will continue to precess about the main field B_0, while inducing a detectable current in a coil placed in the transverse plane, as shown in Figure 2.5C. The RF excitation thus serves two roles: to rephase the spin precessions and in so doing create a transverse component of the magnetization which is responsible for the MR signal.

An analogy of spin synchronization can be drawn from an orchestra, where a multitude of instruments and voices generating an ensemble of frequencies that comprise a symphony have to be synchronized to make beautiful music. That is the role of the conductor in ensuring that the timing of musical events is properly synchronized. The conductor synchronizes the start/end of music pieces to produce a symphony; otherwise the composition would fall apart as the composition loses coherence (dephases). The same holds true for precessing spins that we have encoded with a linear variation of frequencies in order to resolve positions.

Now let us put it all together. First, we need to reduce the 3D imaging problem to 2D by selecting only a slice to image. We do this by applying a gradient so that spins precess at linearly increasing frequencies along the direction of the applied gradient. We then apply an RF pulse to synchronize spins only in a restricted frequency range so that spins precessing at frequencies outside this range are not affected by the RF pulse. To accomplish this we need the RF pulse to carry the range of frequencies corresponding to the slice width we are interested in. This range of frequencies is referred to as the bandwidth of the RF pulse. Figure 2.6 shows the basic components of this process. A linear gradient is applied (Fig. 2.6A), for example along the *z*-direction, resulting in frequency encoding along that dimension. An RF pulse with a frequency bandwidth (Fig. 2.6C) corresponding to the desired slice thickness is applied at the same time. To get the RF pulse to yield a rectangular slice profile, corresponding to the bandwidth of interest, the RF pulse should be shaped as in Figure 2.6D, referred to as a sinc pulse. This is a requirement of Fourier transform theory, which we will revisit in a subsequent section.

We can thus represent the excitation phase of the sequence as shown in the timing diagram in Figure 2.6E, which shows a sinc RF pulse coincident with an applied

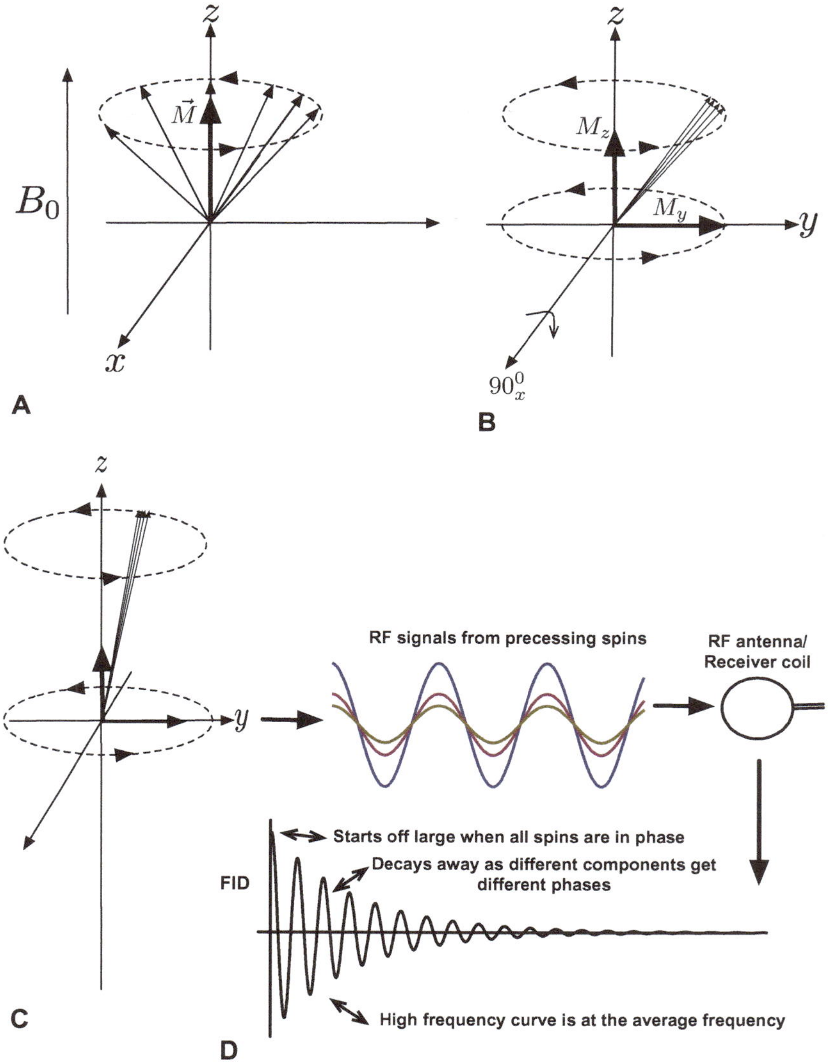

Fig. 2.5. Spin precession about the main field B_0, showing the lack of phase coherence between the various spins (**A**) and the effect of the radiofrequency (RF) pulse in refocusing the spins and creating a transverse component of magnetization (**B**). It is this precessing transverse component (**C**) that induces a current in a coil (**D**). The various frequency components in the transverse magnetization are initially in phase, resulting in a large signal which decays as the various frequency components eventually lose phase coherence over time (**D**). The rate at which this phase coherence is lost is the relaxation time constant, T_2. The detected signal is called a free induction decay (FID). GBM, glioblastoma; Cho, choline; NAA, *N*-acetyl aspartate.

gradient in the slice selection direction. The extra negative gradient lobe is a subtlety to compensate for the residual phase arising from the slice selection gradient. We will build the entire timing diagram for generating an image via this step-by-step approach while introducing the basics of *k*-space.

Now that we have all the spins that make up a slice in the transverse plane where we can detect the MR signal, we need to resolve the remaining two dimensions with some type of encoding scheme. We know that the spins are detectable through their precession about the applied field B_0. Precession signals can be characterized by their amplitude, frequency, and phase. The amplitude of the signal is determined by the concentration of the spins, ρ, and by the relaxation time constants, T1 and T2. Hence, we cannot use the amplitude of these oscillations to resolve x from y since it carries our contrast information. We are thus left with only two degrees of freedom to exploit: that of frequency and phase of the precessing spins. Hence, we will resolve one dimension with frequency while the other is encoded with phase.

The idea behind phase encoding is similar to frequency encoding in that a linear gradient is applied which makes spin precession frequencies change linearly along

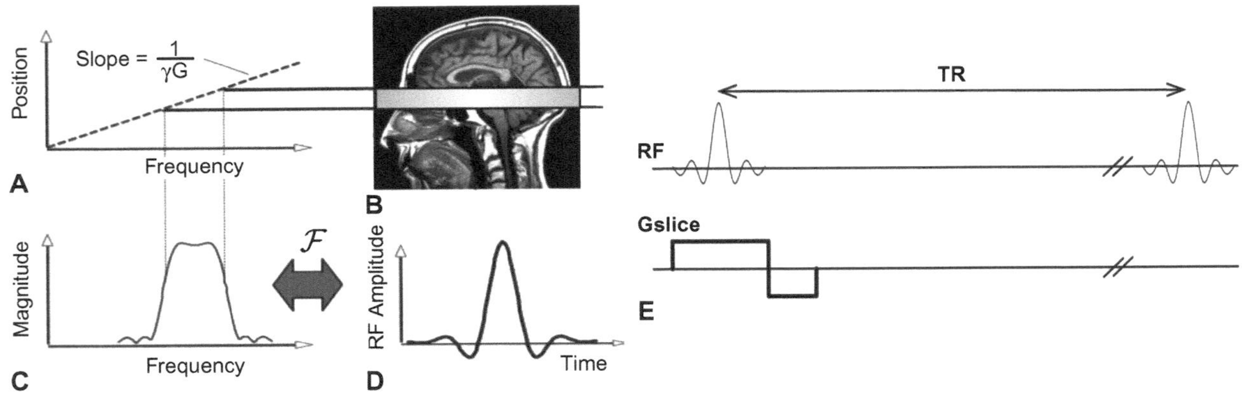

Fig. 2.6. A gradient is applied along one direction, as shown, which makes the spins along that direction precess with frequencies that linearly increase with position. A radiofrequency (RF) excitation pulse applied at the same time will rephase only those spins which are within its bandwidth, as shown in (**A–C**). The corresponding spins will then have a component in the transverse plane so that only signals in that slice are detectable. Note that the size of the slice is determined by the frequency content of the RF pulse as well as by the gradient strength, which determines the frequency-encoding resolution of the spins, given by the slope in (**A**). Applying an RF excitation pulse coincident with the slice selection gradient thus reduces the imaging problem from 3D to 2D. The timing diagram extract for slice selection is shown in (**E**). We will repeat this structure to adequately sample the 2D plane and the repetition time is denoted by TR (time to repeat).

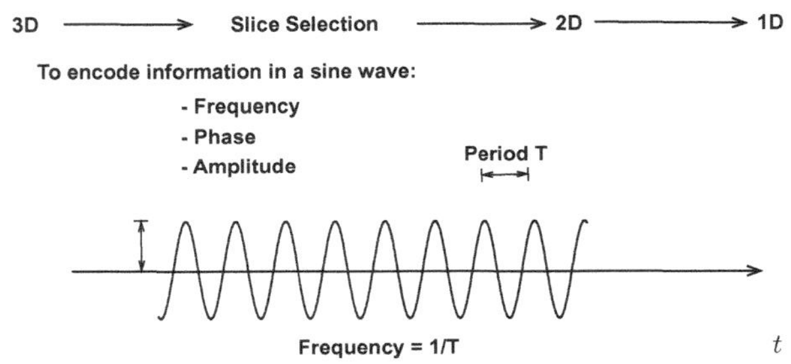

Fig. 2.7. Spin populations in magnetic resonance are detectable through their oscillations, which can be characterized by their frequency, phase, and amplitude.

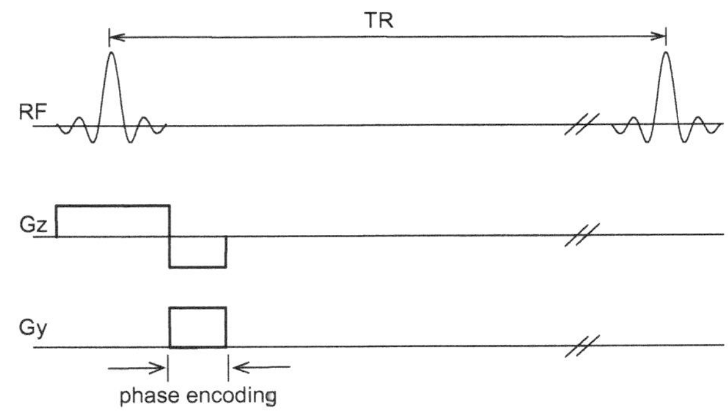

Fig. 2.8. Addition of a phase-encoding gradient to the timing diagram. After slice selection, one dimension is phase-encoded as shown, leaving the other dimension to be encoded separately. TR, time to repeat; RF, radiofrequency.

the direction of the applied gradient. During the interval when the gradient is on, the spins are frequency-encoded, as shown in Figure 2.7. When the gradient is turned off, the spins return to precessing at the same frequency. Notice, however, that the waveform starts at different temporal location or phase at each resolvable position. Hence, the spins are said to be phase-encoded in the direction of the previously applied gradient. The partially built sequence with the addition of a phase-encoding step is shown in Figure 2.8.

We still need one dimension to fully encode the 2D image. As shown in Figure 2.7, we used slice selection to choose a plane and then encoded one dimension as phase. We will thus encode the other dimension with the only remaining degree of freedom of spin oscillation: that of frequency. What distinguishes frequency from phase encoding is that data should be collected while the gradient is still on so that spins are recorded with their individual frequencies.

The full timing diagram for collecting a slice is shown in Figure 2.9. For each phase-encoding step, a line in *k*-space is collected corresponding to each resolvable frequency along the *x*-direction. The experiment is then repeated (at time-to-repeat (TR) intervals) for another increment in phase-encoding gradient. *k*-space is thus a way of arranging the collected frequencies and their respective phases in a 2D plot. This sequence is called a gradient echo because the signal reaches its maximum value when the frequency-encoding gradient passes through the origin of *k*-space at point 3 and hence the applied gradient along that direction is identical to zero.

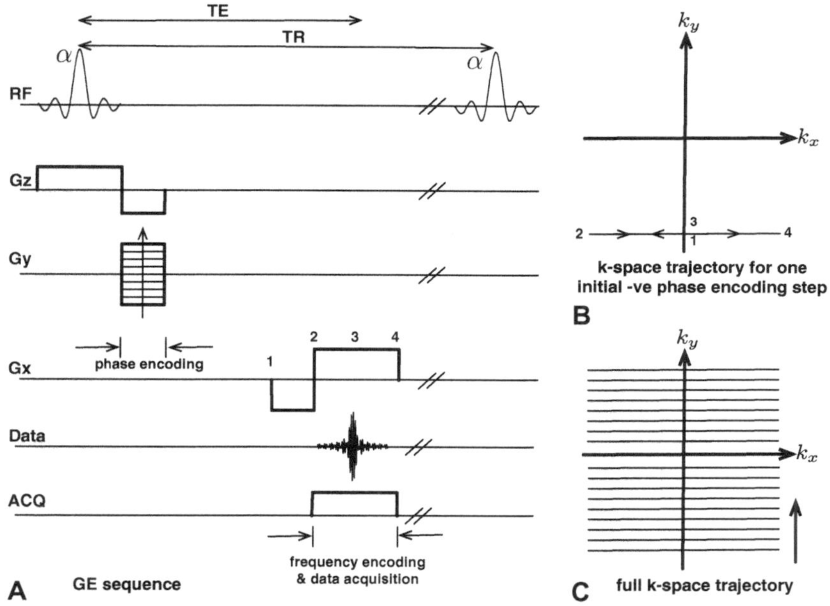

Fig. 2.9. Timing diagram for a single acquisition of a line in k-space along the frequency-encoding direction k_x for a gradient echo (GE) sequence. The analog-to-digital converter (ACQ) line represents timing of when the data are actually acquired, which corresponds to when the frequency-encoding gradient (G_x in this case) is turned on. Initially, for each phase-encoding step, we have an increasingly negative-going gradient along k_x from point 1 to point 2, then we have a positive-going gradient from 2 through the center of k-space at 3 and finally to point 4. Data are acquired during the interval 2–4, so that the line from 1 to 2 is collected only once. The experiment then repeats by increasing the phase-encoding area k_y, so that k-space is filled in the direction from the bottom to the top. The reasons for how much k-space is needed to be filled will be discussed in a later section. TE, time to echo; TR, time to repeat; RF, radiofrequency.

The location of this maximum signal point in k-space is the time to echo (TE), as defined in the timing diagram.

In this formulation, k-space is a way of organizing, in two dimensions, the distribution of spin-encoding frequencies and phases as we collect them. First, the phase for each of the precessing spins is set by the phase-encoding gradient, which yields a point along the k_y-axis. When the frequency-encoding gradient is applied along k_x, spins along the x-direction have a linear change in frequency and are collected simultaneously with this gradient encoding. The resulting signal is displaced in phase along the k_y-axis and consists of individual frequencies along the k_x-axis. The intensity of each oscillation, which is a measure of contrast, is contained in the amplitude of each point in the 2D space. Without loss of generality, k_x and k_y are interchangeable in terms of which one is phase and which one is frequency.

An equivalent coverage of k-space can also be accomplished using a spin-echo sequence, shown in Figure 2.10. In this case the trajectory from point 1 to 2 in k-space is mirrored by the application of the 180° pulse to the opposite quadrant at point 3, where it is then frequency-encoded from points 3 to 4.

The meaning of each point in (k_x, k_y) space is further illustrated in Figure 2.11. Each point in k-space corresponds to a specific frequency with an associated phase (Twieg, 1983). Once the entire k-space is filled, the image is generated by Fourier transforming the entire space. Along a fixed ky-axis, we see that each resolvable point has a different spatial frequency k_x, represented by the horizontal points. Similarly, for a fixed k_x, we have signals with a fixed frequency for each point but a linearly increasing phase between them as we track along k_y (represented by the vertical x points).

CONCEPT OF AN ECHO AND k-SPACE

The signals in the transverse plane consist of a collection of frequencies arising from both the spatial encoding with gradients as well as field inhomogeneities due to imperfections in the system. After a period of time longer than T2, these different frequencies, which are precessing at different rates, lose phase coherence with each other so that the transverse component of the magnetization is substantially reduced. If we wait long enough, the signal will entirely decay to zero. However, there are ways to recover signal decay caused by the spreading out of the signals due to imperfections in the system. In one case, we can use a gradient echo to recover the signal. As discussed earlier, applying a gradient changes the spin

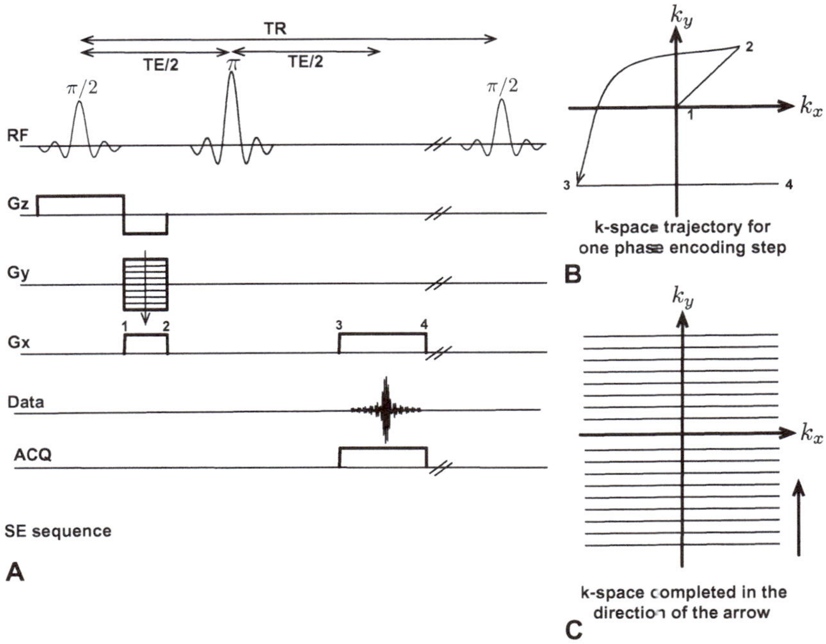

Fig. 2.10. Corresponding timing diagram for a spin-echo (SE) sequence. For example, for an initial positive *y*-gradient lobe and a positive gradient along k_x from point 1 to point 2, we have a tilted line in *k*-space from the origin at point 1 to point 2. The effect of the 180° pulse is to invert the phase in *k*-space by 180° to a new location at point 3. We then apply a frequency-encoded gradient from point 3 to 4 while reading out the data at the same time, so that *k*-space is recorded as a line from 3 to 4, as shown. TE, time to echo; TR, time to repeat; RF, radiofrequency; ACQ, analog-to-digital converter.

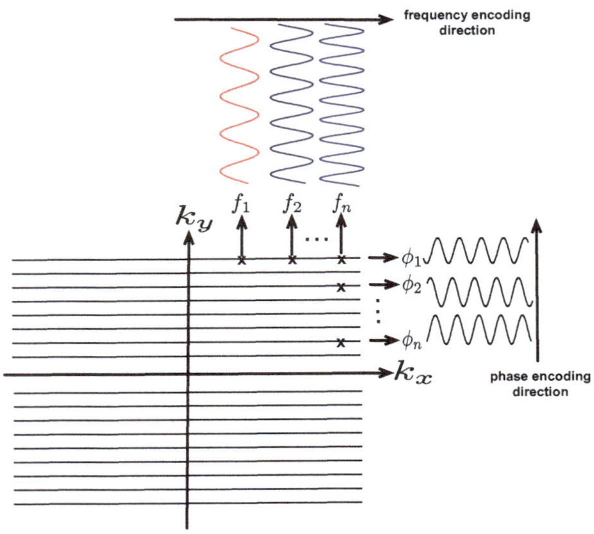

Fig. 2.11. Along the k_y axis, phase increases linearly, as shown by the vertical crosses and the corresponding signals which are at the same frequency on the k_x axis. *k*-space is filled by fixing the phase with a phase-encoding gradient along k_y and then collecting spin frequencies along the frequency-encoding gradient direction k_x.

precession linearly in the direction of the gradient field. This corresponds to a translation along the applied gradient direction in *k*-space. Now, signal strength is highest at the center of *k*-space, where all spins are precessing in phase, so that any deviation from the center of *k*-space due to the applied gradients results in a reduction in signal intensity. The gradient echo results whenever we reverse the gradient direction so that we transverse back to the center of *k*-space, resulting in an echo, as shown in Figure 2.12A.

Alternatively, we can return to the center of *k*-space by inverting the phase of the spins to the opposite side of *k*-space, as shown in Figure 2.12B, where we invert the spin *k*-space location from point 1 to point 2. If we now allow the spins to continue to precess as before, then they will be at the origin of *k*-space in the same time that it took them to reach point 1 and thus we get an echo (Wehrli, 1990). This inversion is independent of the field inhomogeneities that are causing the traversal of *k*-space and as long as the conditions for this traversal (due to field inhomogeneities, chemical shift, gradients, and other system imperfections) remain the same over time, then an echo will form when the spins transverse the same *k*-space distance in equal time after the inversion

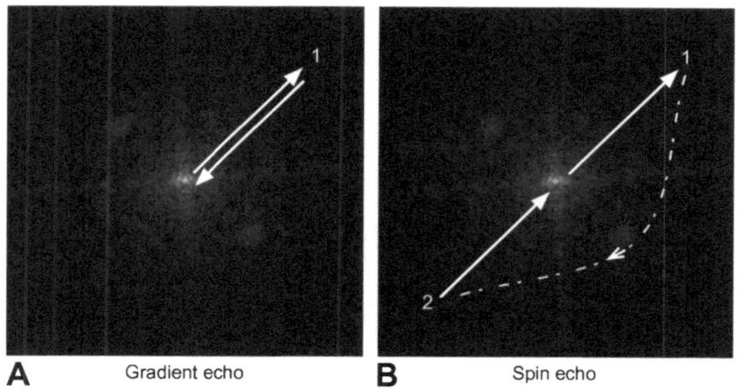

Fig. 2.12. Dynamics of echo formation in k-space. The signal intensity is highest at the center of k-space and falls off as we increase the frequency or phase of the spins. (**A**) For the gradient echo, the deviation from the center of k-space to point 1 is reversed by applying an opposite gradient which brings us back to the center and hence forms a gradient echo. (**B**) For a spin echo, a 180° pulse inverts the accumulated phase to its conjugate point 2, so that with the same rate of phase accrual due to field inhomogeneities as for moving from the center to point 1, the net magnetization returns to the center of k-space in the same time, resulting in a spin echo.

pulse. This is the basis of a spin-echo sequence, which achieves the inversion from point 1 to point 2 in k-space with a 180° RF pulse.

There is one very substantial difference between a gradient echo and a spin echo. Gradient echoes only reverse spin phases resulting from the applied gradients, while the spin echo inverts all spin phase differences regardless of the field inhomogeneity source. Spin echoes thus yield larger echo amplitudes than gradient echoes. Hence, in the presence of other field inhomogeneities, gradient echoes do not return to the precise origin of k-space. As well, in gradient-based echo imaging sequences, echoes are formed when either $k_x = 0$ or $k_y = 0$ or both.

A commonly used analogy is that of a foot race. Suppose all runners line up in a starting line, and at the sound of the starter's gun they begin to run clockwise around a track. Because they all run at somewhat different speeds, the pack of runners spreads out until eventually (after many laps) they are distributed nearly evenly, and seemingly randomly, around the track. At this time another gun is fired, commanding all runners to turn around and run counterclockwise. Now, the fast runners who were ahead of the others are suddenly behind, and the slow runners who were behind the others are miraculously ahead. As time goes on, the fast runners catch up to the slow ones, and eventually they all meet in one tight pack as they run past the starting line. This unexpected regrouping of the runners is the echo. The analogy is not perfect, because the spins always precess in the same direction. Nevertheless, the 180° pulse has the effect of placing the fast spinners behind the slow spinners, which is the essence of both the spin-echo effect and the runner analogy.

For the gradient echo, the respective speeds of the runners are assumed to be only due to the applied gradients. If at some point in time we switch the speed of the runners (the fastest runner becomes the slowest runner, and so on), then we would expect them to catch up with each other in the same amount of time that it took for them to separate out. This works as long as they are no other sources of speed uncertainty (field inhomogeneities, chemical shift, etc.) and hence the gradient echo is only capable of refocusing spins by removing phase differences arising out of the applied gradients.

A CLOSER LOOK AT IMAGE SPACE AND k-SPACE

For a more comprehensive and intuitive understanding of how MR images are formed, we need to further explore the relationship between an MR image and its "k-space" representation. As shown in Figure 2.13, we see that the image has coordinates x and y while k-space data has coordinates k_x and k_y. The units of x and y are in units of distance (centimeters (cm)) while the units of k_x and k_y are in units of 1/distance (1/cm), representing number of oscillation cycles per distance or a spatial frequency. The gray scale of the k-space data reflects the value of the data at positions k_x and k_y which is our contrast, primarily determined by the proton density, T1 and T2 (Bottomley et al., 1987).

In order to represent a two-dimensional function, such as a head image, one needs to use sine functions in two directions. Thus, k-space reflects that any continuous object can be decomposed or reconstructed from its frequency content. This is demonstrated in Figure 2.13, where we show the k-space representation of the head image. Again, the relation between the k-space data and the image data is through Fourier transformation. The brightness of a single point in the k-space domain reports the amplitude of the sine function, while the location of the point tells us its frequency and orientation. If we consider varying points we can see that sine patterns of varying frequency and orientation are represented by specifically oriented stripes. Hence, the Fourier transform of each individual point in k-space results in a stripe pattern with the orientation of the pattern determined by the location of the point in k-space. The intersection of the dotted lines represent the points of $k_x = k_y = 0$. For points on the k_x-axis the stripes are vertical. For points on the ky-axis the strips are horizontal. For points with arbitrary k_x and

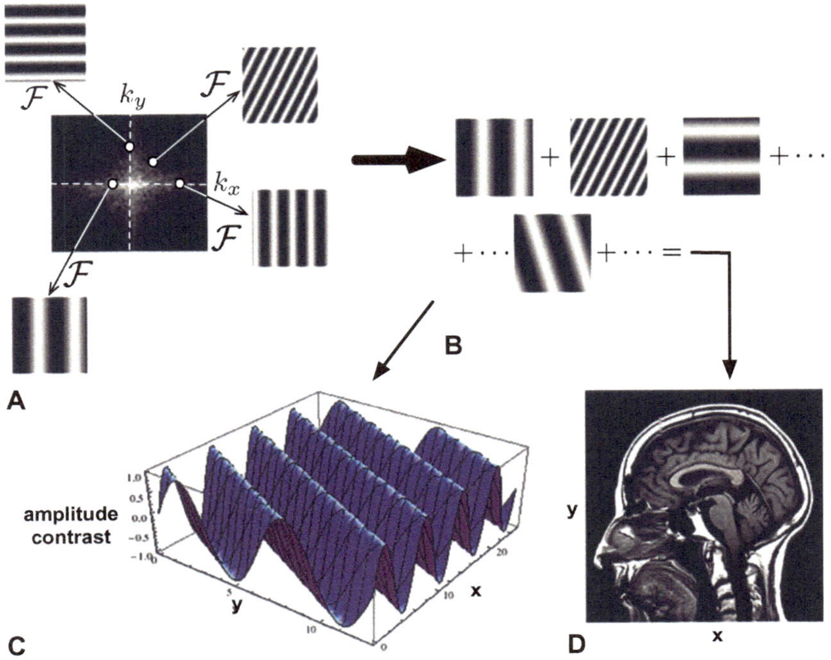

Fig. 2.13. (**A**) Various points in k-space (center) and their corresponding Fourier transform that results in a "stripe" pattern for each point in k-space. Each point in k-space corresponds to a spatial frequency value given by the corresponding frequency and phase coordinates (k_x, k_y), while the intensity of the point corresponds to the amplitude of the oscillation or "stripe" pattern. A sum of all these "stripe" patterns, shown in (**B**), results in the reconstruction of an image (**C**). (**D**) 3D depiction of a sample "stripe" function showing a harmonic oscillation along the x-axis at linearly increasing phase along the y-axis. Each object is thus composed of a large sum of its constituent frequencies.

k_y coordinates the stripes are oblique. The angle of the stripe pattern is such that the stripe density in x and y corresponds to the spatial frequency of the k_x and k_y component of the point in k-space. Fourier transformation is thus the generation of stripe patterns for each point in k-space. By combining all the points in k-space with their corresponding stripe amplitudes and frequencies, we generate the head image shown. Detailed discussion on the concept of stripe patterns can be found in a treatment by Plewes and Kucharczyk (2006) in an annual lecture at the International Society of Magnetic Resonance in Medicine, physics for clinician section.

In summary, we see that the k-space representation is simply a shorthand graphical notation which tells us the family of "stripe" functions, such that, when added together, they provide the desired image. The relationship between the k-space representation of the image and the image itself is through a two-dimensional Fourier transform. If we need to create an image with $256 \times 256 = 2^{16}$ pixels in the image domain, the number of points in the k-space domain needed to characterize this image must also be 2^{16} points.

IMAGE DETECTION AND RESOLUTION CONSIDERATIONS

As in any digital imaging method, the challenge for MRI is to define the intensity of the MRI signal for an array of pixels corresponding to differing points throughout the anatomy. However, unlike all other imaging methods in current use in medical imaging, the signal-detecting device (receiver coils) cannot be collimated to restrict the signal to a specific location, as is done in X-ray imaging, ultrasound, or radionuclide imaging. Rather, the MRI task is unique, as the detected signals originate from the entire object rather than a single point within it. As we discussed earlier, this corresponds to an ensemble of frequencies encoding each resolvable position in the object. The coil detects this sum of frequencies as a signal, which is sampled, and the resulting points used to fill k-space until a sufficient number of the stripe patterns of the object is acquired (Fig. 2.13). To reconstruct the image, we need to decompose the signals into their individual frequencies and phases to map to the corresponding image space. In fact, this is exactly what the ear does in practice (Fig. 2.14A).

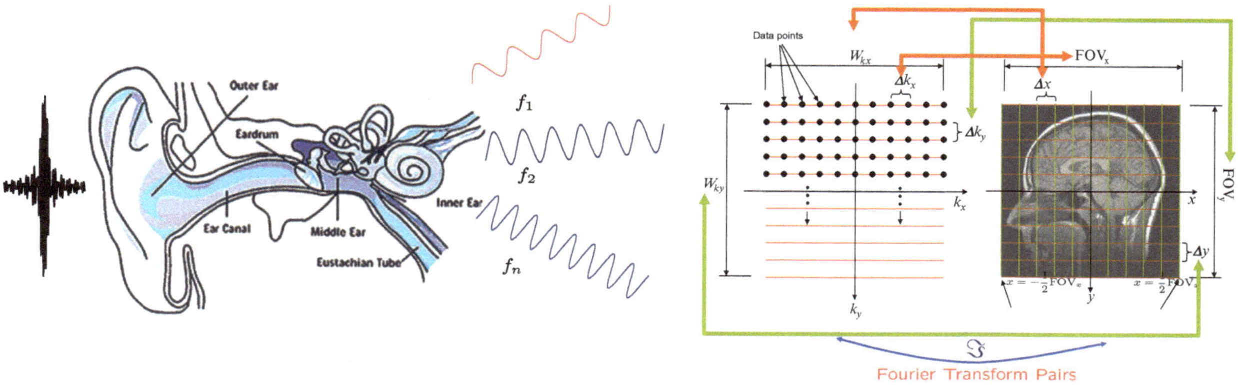

A **Ear Transformer** **B** **Fourier Image Transformer**

Fig. 2.14. (**A**) The ear: anatomy of a Fourier transformer decomposing a multifrequency, multiphase signal into individual frequencies, intensity, and timbre. (**B**) *k*-space and image space are Fourier transform pairs are well as reciprocal spaces. Resolution in one space corresponds to extent in the other, and vice versa. We see that the inverse of *k*-space resolution is given by $1/\Delta k = FOV$ and that the spatial extent of *k*-space $W_{kx,ky} = 1/\Delta x, \Delta y$ which is the inverse of the image space resolution and vice versa. FOV, field of view.

In the inner ear, the cochlea enables us to hear subtle differences in the sounds coming to our ears. The cochlea consists of a spiral of tissue filled with liquid and thousands of tiny hairs, which gradually get smaller from the outside of the spiral to the inside. Each hair is connected to a nerve that feeds into the auditory nerve bundle to the brain. The longer hairs resonate with lower-frequency sounds, and the shorter hairs with higher frequencies. Thus, the cochlea serves to Fourier transform the air pressure signal experienced by the eardrum into frequency information that can be interpreted by the brain as tonality and texture.

After repeated applications of all the G_y and G_x field gradients, resulting in a sufficient sample of stripe patterns to fill *k*-space, Fourier transformation, analogous to the harmonic decomposition by the ear, is used to generate the image, as shown in Figure 2.14B.

The question then arises as to how far in *k*-space we should sample and how closely should the samples be placed. Alternatively, how many different "stripe" patterns are required to accurately reconstruct the image? Once the field of view (FOV) necessary to cover the required anatomy is selected, we then need to determine the number of frequencies and phases required to achieve a given resolution. As shown in Figure 2.14B, this corresponds to going out further in *k*-space so that the resolution in a given direction is determined by the highest frequency, or phase, encoded. This is intuitively satisfying since the more frequencies or phases we set aside for spatial encoding in a given direction, the more resolution we should expect. Hence, resolution in image space is determined by the maximum frequency/phase encoded in *k*-space. Once the extent of *k*-space encoding is established, what then determines the spacing of frequency and phase samples in *k*-space? It turns out that the FOV itself is determined by the spacing between samples in *k*-space. Figure 2.14 shows that *k*-space and image space are reciprocals of each other. Resolution in *k*-space corresponds to FOV in image space, while FOV in *k*-space (W_{kx}, W_{ky}) corresponds to resolution in image space (Δx, Δy) and vice versa.

If the sampling criterion is not met (i.e., if Δk_x or Δk_y, the change in *k*-space sampling along *x* or *y* respectively, is too large, $> 1/FOV_{x,y}$), then the FOV will not be enough to contain the image and we will get aliasing, as shown in Figure 2.15. On the other hand, if we reduce the maximum frequency sampled in *k*-space (W_{kx}, W_{ky}), we see that the resolution in the resulting image decreases starting with edges in the image, which contain the high-frequency components, resulting in a blurred image. The center of *k*-space contains contrast information while the outer frequencies determine the resolution of the resulting image. As shown in Figure 2.16, when the higher frequencies are filtered out of *k*-space, we have a contrast-rich image but blurred due to the loss of resolution. Similarly, when the center of *k*-space is filtered out, we end up with a high-resolution image with well-defined boundaries but with no contrast.

PARALLEL IMAGING

As we discussed, aliasing results whenever *k*-space is undersampled. However, undersampling may be advantageous because it reduces imaging time. One approach that has gained a lot of applicability in clinical practice is to sample fewer lines in *k*-space and unalias the resulting

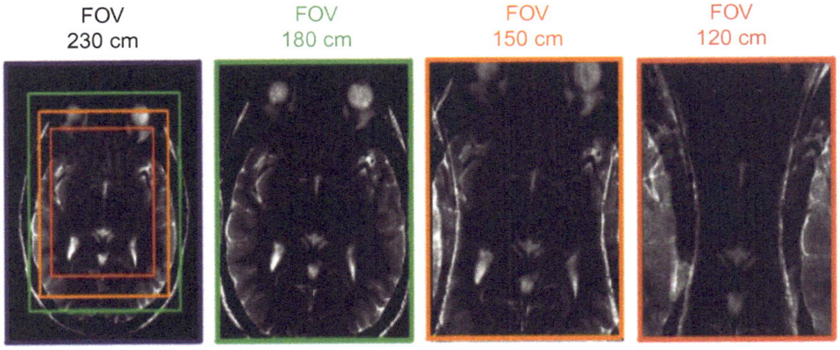

Fig. 2.15. Aliasing due to selection of an insufficient field of view (FOV) to support the physical dimension of the object being imaged. The object then wraps into the small FOV, as shown.

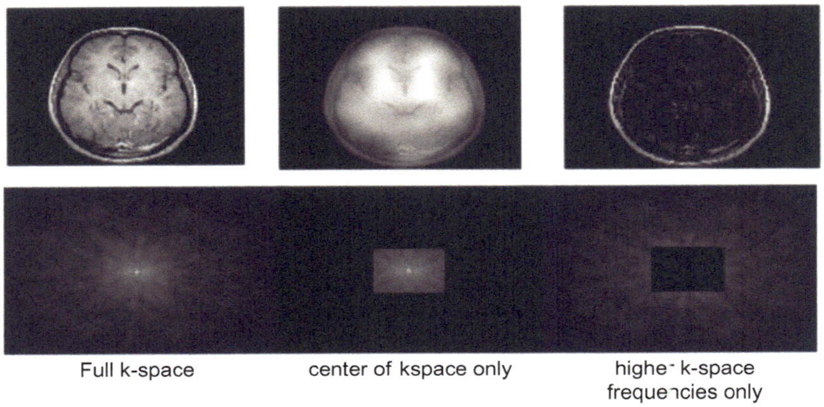

Fig. 2.16. The center of *k*-space is composed of low spatial frequencies which define an intensity-heavy image while the outer edges of *k*-space consisting of high spatial frequencies result in a detail heavy image. The center of *k*-space thus defines image contrast, while the higher spatial frequencies at the edge of *k*-space give us more resolution in the image.

image using postprocessing techniques. Consider a simple case where we skip every other line in *k*-space, as depicted in Figure 2.17, so that each coil data when reconstructed results in two images that are aliased as shown. Since we skipped every other line, the resulting image will have two separate pixels in the image overlap. If we correct for this aliasing in the frequency domain, the approach is referred to as GRAPPA (Sodickson and Manning, 1997; Griswold et al., 2002) while if we do it after Fourier transformation in the object domain, it is referred to as SENSE (Pruessmann et al., 1999).

The basic idea exploits differences in the sensitivity of individual coils, as depicted in Figure 2.17. Consider pixels A and B in a phantom as shown. Each of the four coils in the receiver array has slightly different spatially varying sensitivity S, which scales the intensity of the respective pixel as shown. The resulting four images are thus uniquely different in the spatially varying sensitivities on a pixel-by-pixel basis. Thus, to unalias an image involves solving a system of equations for the unknown A and B, in this case given the sensitivity profiles of the coils S_1 to S_4, which are known and usually determined *a priori* during an initial calibration scan. The steps to unaliasing an object are shown in Figure 2.18. The number of coil elements determines the minimum number of phase encodes to collect. For example, for a four-element coil, the number of phase encodes can be reduced by up to a factor of 4, also called the acceleration factor. The signal-to-noise ratio also decreases with increasing acceleration factors.

A WORD ABOUT CONTRAST

The most basic contrast determinants in MR are water concentration (proton density) in the tissue, time for tissue to magnetize/demagnetize (T1), and the time it takes the spins to lose the ability to precess in phase as an ensemble (T2). There are many other contrast mechanisms achievable in MRI, such as magnetization transfer, flow, susceptibility, diffusion, and blood oxygen level-dependent (BOLD), some of which are covered in subsequent chapters in this handbook, but for this introductory section we will just concentrate on these

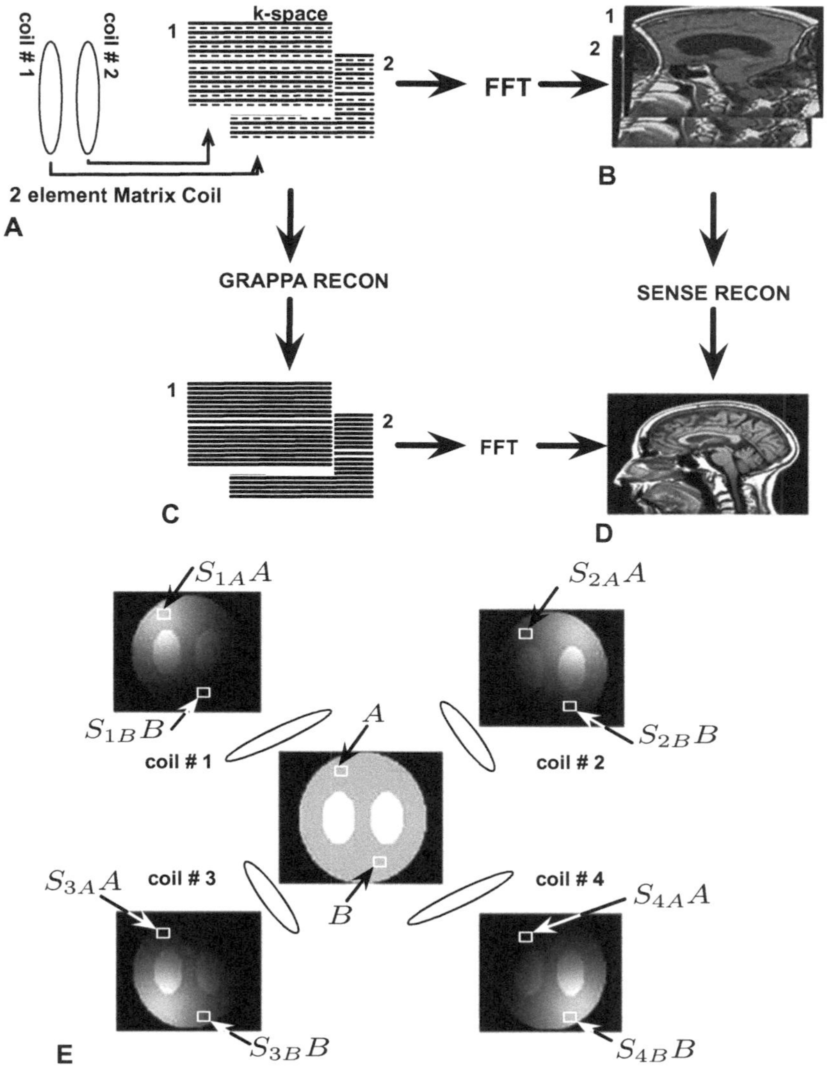

Fig. 2.17. Techniques for unaliasing magnetic resonance images when using multichannel coils. When the aliased image is corrected in the *k*-space domain, the approach is referred to as GRAPPA, while if it is carried out in the object domain, it is referred to as SENSE reconstruction. FFT, fast Fourier transformation.

three fundamental mechanisms, as they are by far the most relevant and widely applied for clinical work.

Of the three basic contrast mechanisms – proton, T1, and T2 – we should get an image that is primarily dominated by one of these contrasts at the expense of the other two. For example, to get a proton-weighted image, we need to minimize differences due to T1 and T2 of different tissue types such as between white/gray matter and cerebrospinal fluid (CSF) in the brain. Both white and gray matter have shorter T2 values than CSF as well as shorter T1 values relative to CSF. We can reduce the differences in T1 between white/gray matter and CSF by increasing TR so that both tissue types have had enough time to recover before the next excitation. Similarly, to reduce T2 weighting between these tissue types, we require a short TE time before the spins have dephased for either of these tissue types. The resulting image is said to be proton-weighted (Fig. 2.19), since contrast is dominated by water concentration in tissue. Similarly, to get a T1-weighted image, we require a short TE to minimize T2 effects and a modest TR where white/gray matter are distinguishable, as shown in Figure 2.20 for TR1. Note that if we wait too long till TR2, then CSF has recovered considerably, resulting in poor T1 weighting, as shown in Figure 2.20D. A T2-weighted image is obtained by using a long TR and a modest TE that maximizes the required contrast, as shown in Figure 2.21C for TE1.

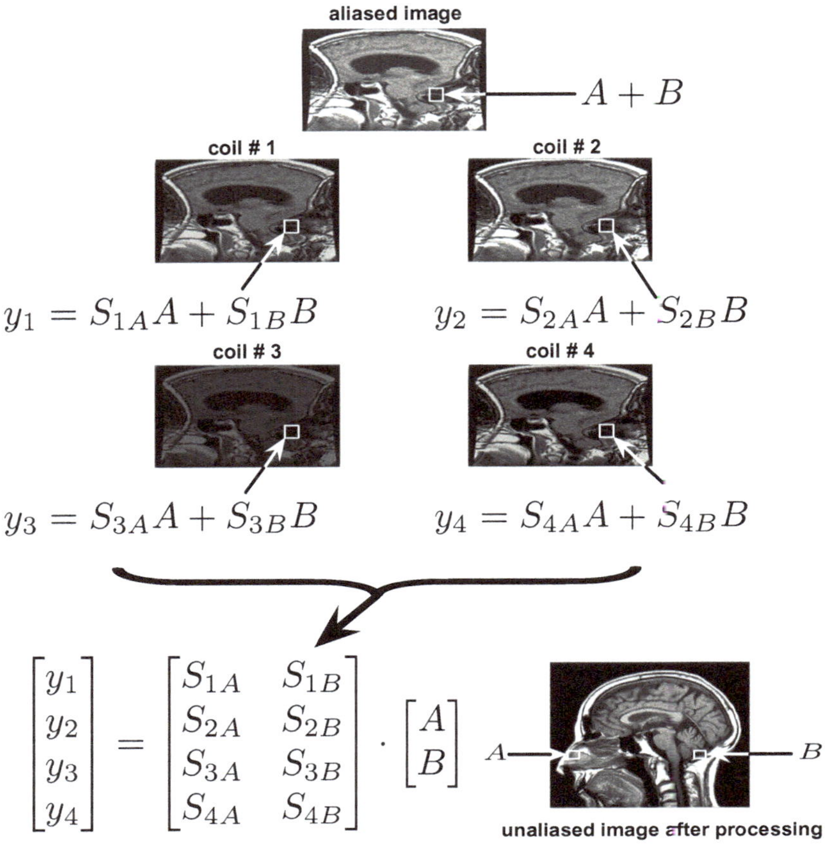

Fig. 2.18. Steps for unaliasing a magnetic resonance imaging image when using multiple channel coils. For example, in this case using four channels, when every other line in *k*-space is not collected (an acceleration factor of 2), will result in an aliased image where two individual pixels, *A* and *B*, overlap. By using a calibration test to determine the coil sensitivities, the problem is then reduced to solving four equations with two unknowns, *A* and *B*. This overdetermined system is then solved to yield the unaliased image, shown with the two pixels *A* and *B* unwrapped from each other.

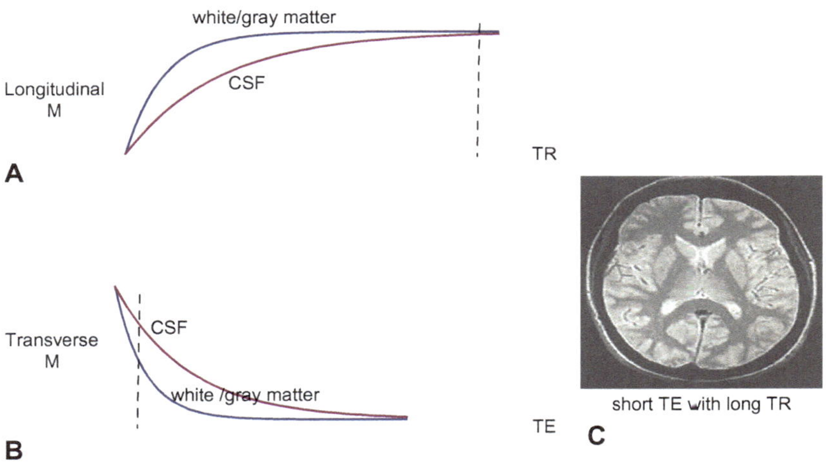

Fig. 2.19. Proton density contrast timing consideration showing little variation in normal soft tissue at short time to echo (TE) and long time to repeat (TR). CSF, cerebrospinal fluid.

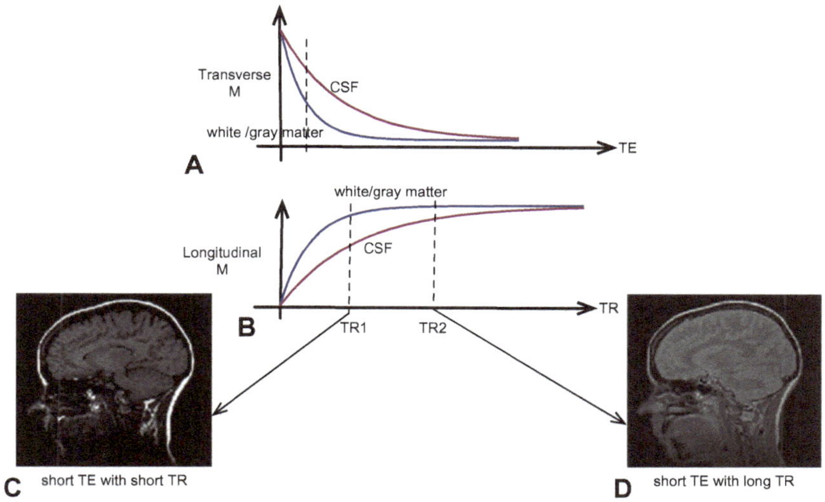

Fig. 2.20. T1-weighted image obtained at short time to echo (TE) and two different time to repeat (TR), showing cerebrospinal fluid (CSF) recovery in (**D**) for longer TR values.

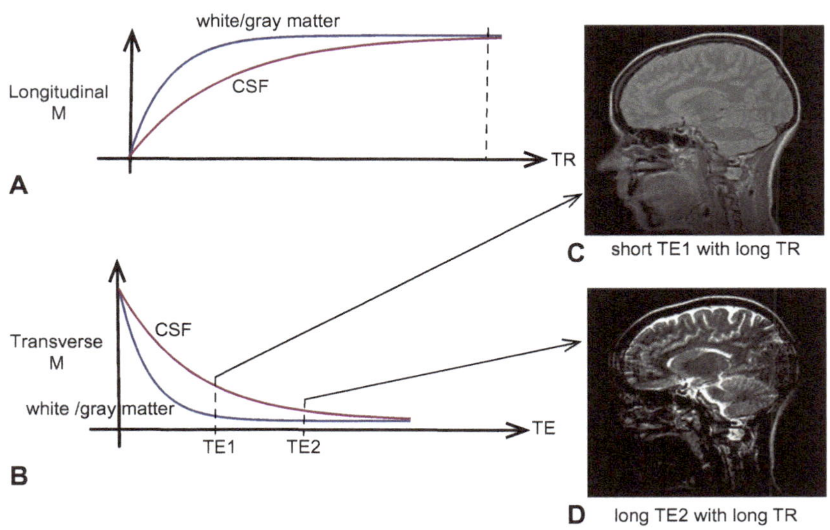

Fig. 2.21. To obtain a T2-weighted image requires a long time to repeat (TR). Images (**C**) and (**D**) are obtained at two different time to echo (TE) values. At long TEs, this T2-weighted image is dominated by cerebrospinal fluid (CSF), while most of the signal from white/gray matter has decayed away. Similarly, at short TE (**C**), white/gray-matter T2 contrast becomes noticeable, since it has a very short T2 relative to CSF.

k-SPACE MAPPING STRATEGIES

The spin-echo and gradient-echo sequences are the two fundamental building blocks of all sequences in MR. One modification of either of these building blocks is on the acquisition side of the sequence, where gradient encoding is optimized to cover *k*-space more efficiently, such as in the trajectories shown in Figure 2.22 and their corresponding sequences.

There are many ways of sampling *k*-space, too many to discuss here, but all are driven by two requirements: to reduce imaging time and/or to recover data by means of the well-established digital signal-processing technique of fast Fourier transformation (Hahn, 1950; Wehrli, 1991). We saw in the previous section that we need to cover *k*-space adequately to satisfy our resolution requirements and FOV limits. How we cover *k*-space then becomes a matter of how quickly we can satisfy these limits. Figure 2.22 shows some sample *k*-space trajectories that aim to cover the whole *k*-space quickly and thus reduce total imaging time.

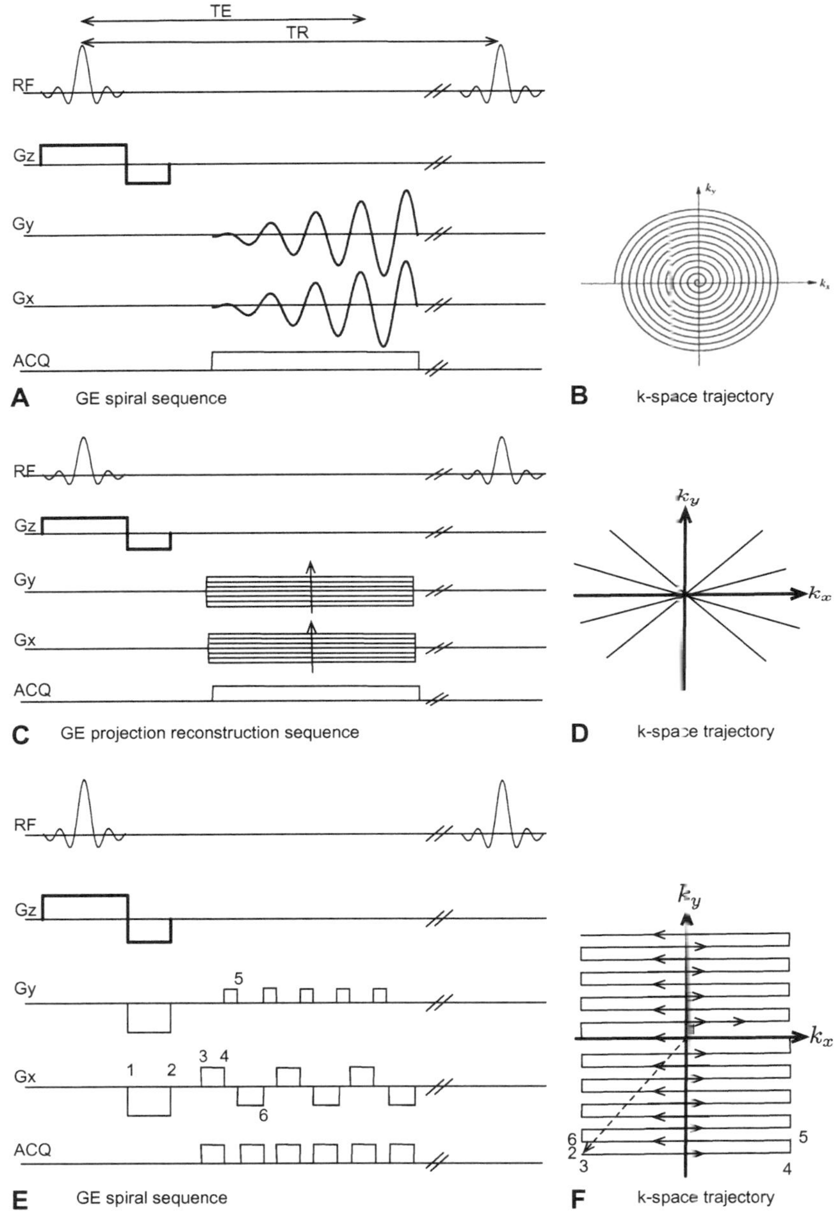

Fig. 2.22. Various techniques of fast sampling of *k*-space. (**A**) Spiral trajectory, where oscillating gradients on both G_x and G_y cover *k*-space in a circular pattern. (**B**) By progressively increasing the gradient amplitudes, we obtain a spiral trajectory in k-space. (**C**) Projection reconstruction, where the simultaneous application of linear gradients on G_y and G_x covers a projection in *k*-space, as in (**D**). By increasing the amplitude of both encoding gradients per time to repeat (TR), we obtain (**D**). In (**E**), we have a gradient echo (GE)-based echo planar sequence, in which *k*-space is acquired in a single time to repeat (TR), as shown in (**F**). TE, time to echo; RF, radiofrequency; ACQ, analog-to-digital converter.

CONCLUSIONS

In this chapter, we have attempted to introduce MR concepts using a unique perspective of deconstructing from timing diagrams and their consequent impact on *k*-space coverage. In doing so, we have explored further the concept of stripe patterns (Plewes and Kucharczyk, 2006–2012).

References

Bottomley PA, Hardy CJ, Argersinger RE et al. (1987). A review of H-1 nuclear magnetic resonance relaxation in pathology: are T1 and T2 diagnostic? Med Phys 14: 1–37.

Griswold MA, Jakob PM, Heidemann RM et al. (2002). Generalized autocalibrating partially parallel acquisitions (GRAPPA). MRM 47: 1202–1210.

Hahn EL (1950). Spin Echoes. Phys Rev 80: 580–594.

Plewes DB, Kucharczyk W (2006–2012). The physics of MRI-Basic Spin Gymnastics. Annual ISMRM lecture, Physics for Clinicians. Proceedings of the ISMRM.

Pruessmann KP, Weiger M, Scheidegger MB et al. (1999). SENSE: sensitivity encoding for fast MRI. MRM 42: 952–962.

Sodickson DK, Manning WJ (1997). Simultaneous acquisition of spatial harmonics (SMASH): fast imaging with radiofrequency coil arrays. MRM 38: 591–603.

Twieg DB (1983). The k-trajectory formulation of the NMR imaging process with application in analysis and synthesis of imaging methods. Med Phys 10: 610–621.

Wehrli FW (1990). Fast-scan magnetic resonance: principles and applications. Magn Reson 6: 165–236.

Wehrli FW (1991). Fast-Scan Magnetic Resonance: Principles and Applications. Raven Press, New York.

Wehrli FW, Shaw D, Kneeland JB (1988). Biomedical Magnetic Resonance Imaging: Principles, Methodology, and Applications. VCH Publishers, New York.

Handbook of Clinical Neurology, Vol. 135 (3rd series)
Neuroimaging, Part I
J.C. Masdeu and R.G. González, Editors

Chapter 3

Volumetric and fiber-tracing MRI methods for gray and white matter

MYKOL LARVIE[1]* AND BRUCE FISCHL[2]
[1]*Divisions of Neuroradiology and Nuclear Medicine and Molecular Imaging, Massachusetts General Hospital, Boston, MA, USA*
[2]*Athinoula A. Martinos Center for Biomedical Imaging, Massachusetts General Hospital, Charlestown, MA, USA*

Abstract

Magnetic resonance imaging (MRI) is capable of generating high-resolution brain images with fine anatomic detail and unique tissue contrasts that reveal structures that are not visible to the eye. Sharply defined gray- and white-matter interfaces allow for quantitative anatomic analysis that can be accurately performed with largely automated segmentation methods. In an analogous fashion, diffusion MRI in the brain provides structural information based on contrasts derived from the diffusivity of water in brain tissue, which can highlight the orientation of neuronal axons. Also using largely automated methods, diffusion MRI can be used to generate models of white-matter tracts throughout the brain, a method known as tractography, as well as characterize the microstructural integrity of neuronal axons. Tractographic analysis has helped to define connectivity in the brain that powerfully informs understanding of brain function, and, together with other diffusion metrics, is useful in evaluation of the normal and diseased brain. The quantitative methods of brain segmentation, tractography, and diffusion MRI extend MRI into a realm beyond visual inspection and provide otherwise unachievable sensitivity and specificity in the analysis of brain structure and function.

INTRODUCTION

The diagnosis of disease involving the central nervous system has traditionally relied heavily upon detailed investigation of a patient's history, meticulous physical examination, and often extensive laboratory testing, frequently requiring invasive sampling of blood and cerebrospinal fluid (CSF). These methods were developed and refined when neuroimaging was relatively unrevealing and often required invasive methods to generate contrast, such as catheter angiography and pneumoencephalography. Major intracranial pathology, such as large tumors and intracranial hemorrhage, were frequently manifest as subtle findings on these early methods, and interpretation of images from these examinations required attention to the smallest detail. A similar attention to minute detail was required for interpretation of early cross-sectional imaging, such as computed tomography (CT) and magnetic resonance imaging (MRI), since these methods produced images that were much lower resolution and had far less contrast compared to the photographic methods previously employed.

With current equipment and methods in widespread use, neuroimaging now routinely produces images with resolution of better than 1 mm, which is the same order of magnitude as the unaided human eye. A routine brain MRI examination includes images with contrasts derived from T1, T2, T2*, and diffusion signals, and often a wide variety of others. These images are intrinsically digital and are typically reviewed for interpretation using interactive video displays in which the images are dynamically manipulated. Despite these advances, interpretation of neuroimaging continues to be performed principally through visual inspection of

*Correspondence to: Mykol Larvie, MD, PhD, Massachusetts General Hospital, Divisions of Neuroradiology and Nuclear Medicine and Molecular Imaging, 55 Fruit Street, Boston MA 02114, USA. Tel: +1-617-726-8320, E-mail: mlarvie@gmail.com

these digital images, which are increasingly detailed and voluminous in number.

Compelled principally by research applications, methods for quantitative analysis of neuroimaging, primarily MRI, have been developed that are capable of discerning features that may be otherwise imperceptible using visual inspection only. Using these methods, brain structure and morphometry can be analyzed, compared to normative standards, and sensitively assayed for subtle changes over time. Results derived from these methods have yielded important insights into brain development (Yu et al., 2007), function (Kanai and Rees, 2011), and disease processes (Fischl et al., 2002; Rosas et al., 2002; Kuperberg et al., 2003), and increasingly are being exploited for application in the diagnosis of individual patients. With increasing experience and refinement of these methods, it is likely that a new diagnostic paradigm will emerge in which diagnostic imaging supported by quantitative analysis is an essential adjunct to traditional methods of visual inspection. In this paradigm, it is likely that neuroimaging will become more reliable and may come to play an increasingly larger role in the clinical evaluation of patients.

The following discussion of quantitative methods is divided into two sections. The first covers morphometric and volumetric analyses based on structural MRI, while the second reviews white-matter analyses based on diffusing imaging, including fiber tracing (tractography) and diffusivity measurements. These are fundamentally analogous methods in that they both represent quantitative, computational analyses of brain structure derived from different high-resolution MR contrast mechanisms. The success of these methods raises the prospect of the development of new imaging techniques based on different contrast mechanisms, from MRI or other modalities, that rely upon digital data and signal-processing methods to reveal fundamentally new information regarding brain function.

BRAIN MACROSTRUCTURE AND MICROSTRUCTURE

The human brain is comprised of a relatively small number of basic tissue types, principally gray matter and white matter, connective tissues such as dura mater, pia mater, and blood vessels, and CSF that circulates both inside the brain, within the ventricles, and outside the brain, within the sulci and cisterns. The distinct chemical properties of these tissues allow them to be reliably visualized with MRI, although precisely distinguishing their boundaries is a considerable challenge. Brain segmentation is a process that uses high-resolution, high-contrast images to classify brain parenchymal macrostructure, including identification of pia, gray matter, white matter, and CSF (Kikinis et al., 1996; Wells et al., 1996; Kapur et al., 1998; Fischl et al., 1999, 2002; Van Leemput et al., 1999, 2003, 2009; Ashburner and Friston, 2000; Amato et al., 2003; Anbeek et al., 2005; Van Leemput, 2006; Han and Fischl, 2007; Patenaude, 2007; Akselrod-Ballin et al., 2009; Sabuncu et al., 2010). Further, the macrostructure can be analyzed topologically to classify regions according to sulcal, gyral, and lobar anatomy.

In this context, brain microstructure refers to the organization of white-matter tracts within the brain, including the tracing of fiber tracts and analysis of axonal size and packing density. The data that informs this analysis are derived from diffusion imaging methods that are tailored to provide the highest possible spatial resolution and the most accurate measurement of diffusion properties.

The macrostructure and microstructure of the brain are highly related, although congenital and acquired abnormalities may affect them differently. Consequently, methods to analyze these features independently provide unique information that separately informs understanding of brain health, function, and disease.

QUANTITATIVE VOLUMETRIC BRAIN ANALYSIS: SEGMENTATION

Structural segmentation methods

Brain segmentation is a process of classifying regions made up of individual voxels in a brain image according to the type of tissue or structure that it represents. The two principal brain tissues of interest are gray and white matter, and these must be distinguished from CSF and the meninges covering the brain, particularly the dura and the pia. Since the MRI image consists of discrete voxels of limited resolution, a given voxel can, and often does, represent a combination of different tissue types, which is known as partial voluming or the partial volume effect (Fig. 3.1). Accurate segmentation requires that the

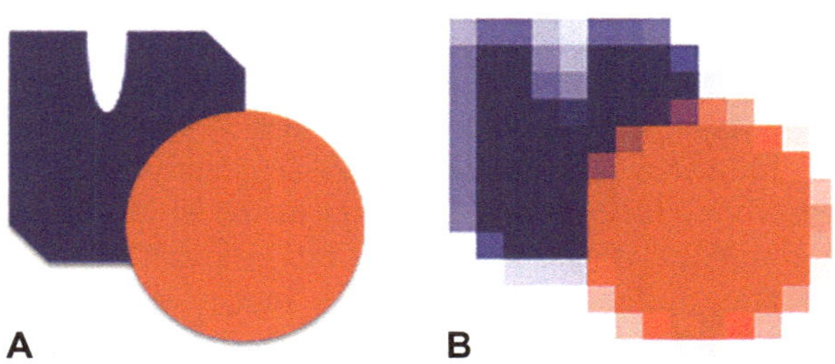

Fig. 3.1. Demonstration of partial volume effect. (**A**) Ideal image, with areas of fine detail and interface between objects. (**B**) Acquired image, with blurring of fine details and obscuration of the boundary between objects.

tissue boundaries be accurately designated and that the tissue types be properly classified.

The classification of a given voxel is informed by both the signal intensity and its position within the brain. For a T1-weighted image, CSF has the lowest signal intensity, white matter has the highest intensity, and gray matter has an intermediate intensity. Depending on the details of the MR sequence, the dura may have a variable intensity, which is important for distinguishing its boundary with the adjacent cortex. There are many different approaches to classifying the voxel contents. With the simplest approach, a voxel is designated as entirely a single tissue type. This leads to obvious errors, as the arbitrarily linear boundaries of the image voxels do not respect tissue borders. With more refined methods, partial volume modeling may be used, allowing each voxel to contain a mixture of different tissue types. In this approach, each voxel is assigned a fraction according to the composition of the tissues it contains, or equivalently, each voxel is assigned a probability of being a given tissue type.

The features of the voxels surrounding a given voxel can be used to improve the accuracy of classification. In a simple case, spatial neighborhood information can be used to aid in determining the classification of adjacent voxels. For example, a voxel that is near other white-matter voxels is likely to be white matter also. Statistical models have been used for this approach, such as the Markov random-field model employed in FSL (Kapur, 1999; Zhang et al., 2001) and in FreeSurfer (Fischl et al., 2002), resulting in significantly improved segmentation.

In addition to assessing the neighborhood surrounding a voxel, its position within the brain can be used to aid in classification. To identify the region of brain containing a given voxel, the subject brain must be aligned with an atlas (or template) of known brain structures, a process known as registration. In its simplest form, the registration may be done using only linear transformations. Because of the wide variation in size and configuration of normal brains, this type of transformation may result in significant discrepancies between the subject brain and the atlas brain. Nonlinear transformations, in which the brain is deformed to better fit the atlas, can greatly improve registration, although the size and shape variation can introduce systematic error.

Following registration of a subject brain to a standard atlas, the classification of voxels can be aided by knowledge of brain anatomy, based on correlation with the known anatomy of the atlas. Using these methods, the probability of a voxel containing a specific tissue type can be derived with good confidence from comparison with the atlas. This atlas-based classification can also significantly improve segmentation results (Cabezas et al., 2011). There are several atlases that are freely available and in widespread use, such as the Talairach atlas (Fischl et al., 2004b; Desikan et al., 2006), the MNI atlases (http://www.bic.mni.mcgill.ca/ServicesAtlases/HomePage), and the International Consortium for Brain Mapping atlas (Mazziotta et al., 2001). Additionally, an atlas may be made based on a set of subjects in a given study or based on a single subject with multiple scans, in which case there is reduced error in transforming the imaging to the atlas space (Reuter and Fischl, 2011).

The pial surface cannot be distinguished from the cortical surface using conventional imaging, and so the pia is taken as the external boundary of the cortex. Image contrast is generally sufficient to accurately distinguish between CSF and brain, so the boundaries between brain tissues, both white and gray matter, and CSF are typically reliably established (Fig. 3.2). There are notable exceptions, however. For example, areas of the cortex that are folded in close proximity, such as adjacent gyri, may be separated by a layer of CSF that is thinner than

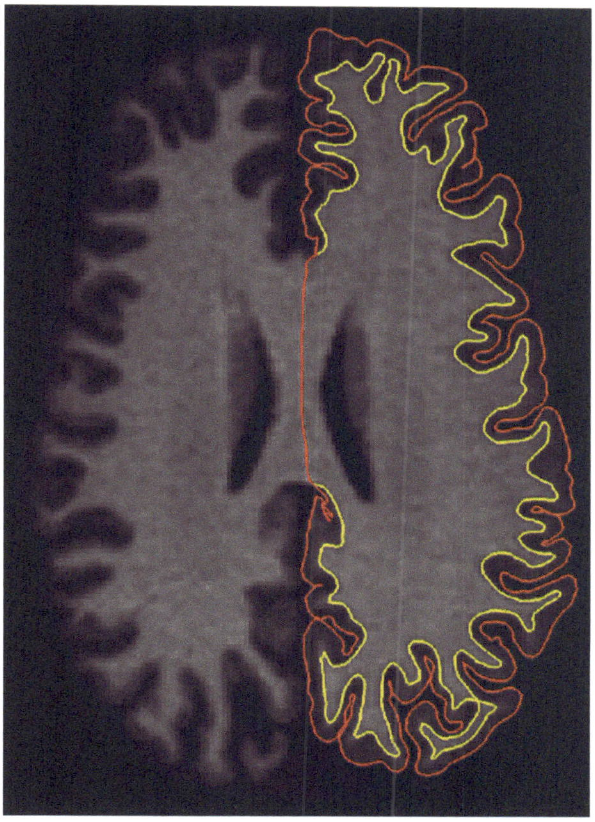

Fig. 3.2. T1-weighted brain magnetic resonance imaging image following segmentation using FreeSurfer. Segmentation is demonstrated in the left cerebral hemisphere, with the white-matter surface depicted by the yellow outline and the pial surface depicted by the red outline.

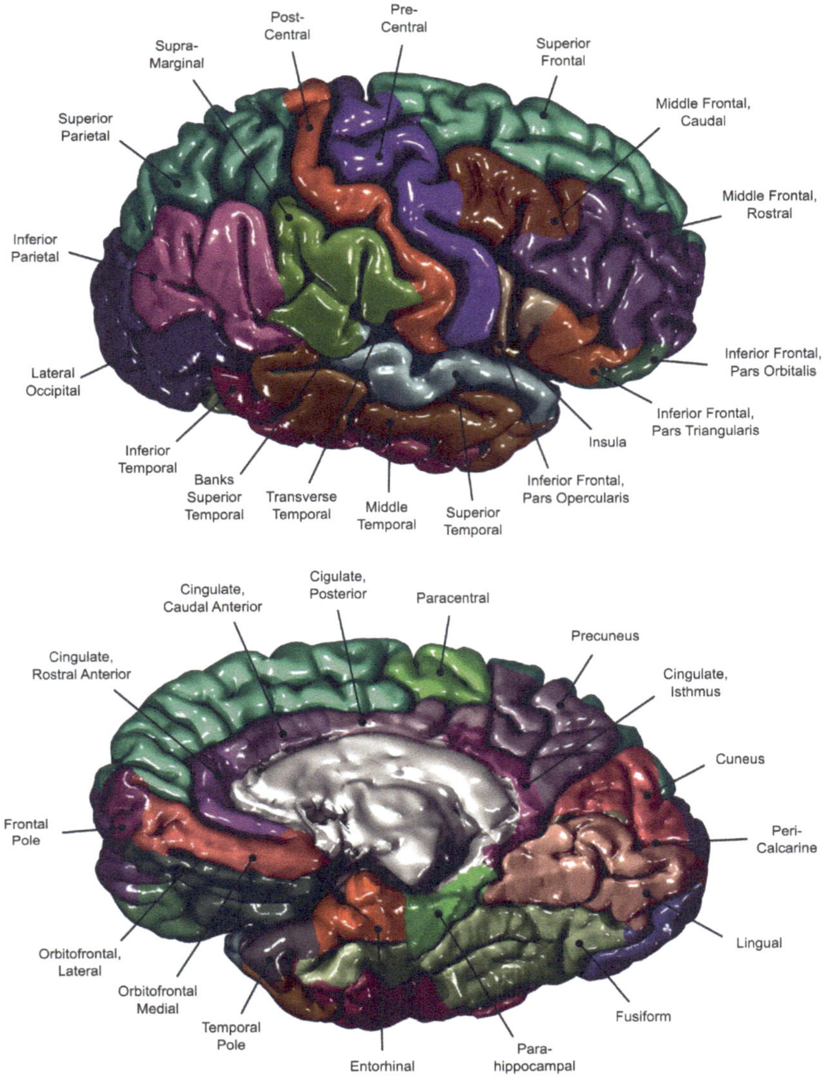

Fig. 3.3. Demonstration of labeled segmentation using tools developed in Fischl (2004a) using the atlas from (Desikan et al., 2006). Thirty-four cortical regions are identified, although some are not visible, as they are buried within sulci. Reproduced from Winkler et al. (2010).

the width of a voxel. In this case, a single image voxel will contain both CSF and cortex. The application of the methods described above, including the use of spatial neighborhood information and atlas-based segmentation methods, is valuable in minimizing errors of this sort.

The process of assigning an anatomic definition to a specific brain region is called labeling. Although labeling may be performed independently of segmentation, atlas-based segmentation methods permit automated labeling that can be highly accurate (Fischl et al., 2002; Cabezas et al., 2011). Labeling is extremely useful for the subsequent definition of regions of interest (ROIs) and anatomically informed analysis of brain structures (Fischl et al., 2004b; Desikan et al., 2006). Figure 3.3 demonstrates the results of automated segmentation and labeling.

Imaging requirements

Accurate and robust segmentation requires imaging with well-defined tissue contrasts that optimally distinguish CSF, gray matter, and white matter. Additionally, the best possible spatial resolution and the lowest possible spatial distortion are critical. Different MR sequences have been employed for segmentation, including T1-weighted, T2-weighted, T2*-weighted, and multispectral methods (Fischl et al., 2004a), with different advantages and disadvantages for each. Recently there has been increasing convergence on volumetric imaging using a T1-weighted contrast (Jack et al., 2008), including multispectral sequences such as MEMPRAGE (van der Kouwe et al., 2008).

Imaging should be performed with isotropic resolution on the order of 1 mm^3, with poorer resolution resulting in less accurate segmentation. Higher-field scanners provide better-quality images, with 3 T imaging superior to 1.5 T, although with increased image distortion. High-resolution head coils, typically achieved with an increased number of active elements, have been a major innovation in improving image quality (Wiggins et al., 2006; Lattanzi et al., 2010).

Sources of error

Studies of cortical thickness have reported differences in the range of 2% and even less (for example, Rosas et al., 2002; Kuperberg et al., 2003; Han et al., 2006; Fjell et al., 2009b). In order to measure brain structures with such precision, it is necessary to control for sources of error, which may occur at every step, including image acquisition and processing, segmentation, and comparative analysis.

For image acquisition, error may be related to the scanner-related factors, MR sequence factors, and image reconstruction factors. Important scanner factors include the specific manufacturer and model, field strength and stability, and coil design (Han et al., 2006; Jovicich et al., 2009). With the increasing application of segmentation methods, major manufacturers are addressing these issues and most have developed standard and reproducible systems for the acquisition of high-resolution structural images suitable for segmentation.

Accurate segmentation relies upon classification of voxels in part by their signal intensity. There are systematic differences in signal intensity throughout an image, due in largest part to inhomogeneity of the radiofrequency fields. This inhomogeneity can be characterized as a bias field, and its effects are more pronounced at higher field strengths. Bias field correction results in significantly improved segmentation and is routinely performed in major segmentation systems such as FreeSurfer and FSL (Sled et al., 1998; Dale et al., 1999).

Error arising from the segmentation methods and data processing may be both systematic, related to the methods employed, and spurious, such as those arising from subject motion and anatomic anomalies. The systematic error may be discerned through analysis and testing of the methods employed. Spurious error is challenging, and is best investigated by manual inspection of results from each stage, although this may be infeasible for large-scale studies.

Analysis of brain segmentation results

Segmentation results can be broadly considered in two categories, quantitative volumetric data and regional anatomic labeling. The quantitative data are derived from the definitions of the gray- and white-matter boundaries and their CSF interface. From this, volumes of cortical gray matter, deep gray matter, and white matter can be derived. Additionally, cortical thickness, or a related metric, cortical density, can be calculated. The anatomic labeling information can be used to define ROIs for comparative purposes and for analysis of other image-based data, such as positron emission tomography or functional MRI data projected on to an ROI or cortical surface.

Beyond analysis of a single brain, segmentation enables comparison between groups or between an individual and a group average. As there is remarkable individual variation in size and shape even among brains that fall within the limits of normal, precise comparison requires complex transformation and analysis. The same concept of atlas-based comparison described above for segmentation methods can be used for analysis. That is, a subject brain may be transformed to a common atlas space for comparison with other brains, which may be the same individual at different points in time, different individuals, or a group average.

For quantitative volumetric analysis it is necessary to establish an appropriate basis for comparison. This may be achieved by transformation of the brains to be compared into a common atlas space, in which case a scale factor is applied such that the data are normalized to a common total brain volume. This approach is limited in subjects with atrophy, which is a common feature of older individuals. Since atrophy often occurs in region-specific patterns, such as the temporoparietal dominant atrophy of Alzheimer's disease (AD), normalizing based on brain volume would lead to a systematic error related to underrepresentation of the atrophic regions (Sanfilipo et al., 2004). An alternative approach to normalization is to use the estimated total intracranial volume as a normative factor (Whitwell et al., 2001). The use of estimated total intracranial volume has the advantage that it is not biased by acquired brain defects and provides correction for differences in the sizes of brains across the lifespan (Buckner et al., 2004).

Volumetric analysis

The simplest approach to volumetric analysis is based on voxel-based morphometry (VBM) (Ashburner and Friston, 2000). In this approach, each voxel of the image data is assigned a unique tissue type and the volume of a given tissue is determined through counting the number of voxels in the ROI. As discussed in the methods section above, this leads to partial volume errors, since voxels frequently contain more than one tissue type. Refinements of VBM techniques employed in most segmentation systems employ partial volume corrections and smoothing techniques so that the resulting tissue boundaries are smoothed across the voxel elements. One caveat with VBM is that, in contrast to volume, the neurobiologic interpretation of differences in density is difficult as they can arise from multiple sources (segmentation errors, registration errors, or true differences in amount of gray matter).

Starting from the same segmentation results, different approaches may be used for quantitative analyses. Gray-matter density (or, equivalently, gray-matter concentration or gray-matter probability) is a metric defined to take into account the uncertainty regarding the tissue type in a given region that arises from partial volume effects and bias induced by transformation and registration of the image data to an atlas (Good et al., 2001). Alternatively, surface-based analyses may be performed to calculate cortical surface area, cortical thickness (Fischl and Dale, 2000), and cortical volume, each of which has relative strengths and weaknesses, so that it may be useful to evaluate these parameters separately (Dickerson et al., 2009b; Winkler et al., 2010). Similarly, cortical volume may be calculated by integrating the cortical thickness in an ROI (Fig. 3.4). In contrast to these volumetric approaches, tensor-based morphometry methods can be used to calculate differences in shape between image sets based on deformation fields (Ashburner and Friston, 2004; Hua et al., 2013).

Surface analysis

Brain cortex is regionally organized into specific domains that serve a wide range of neurologic function, including sensory and motor, vision, hearing, taste,

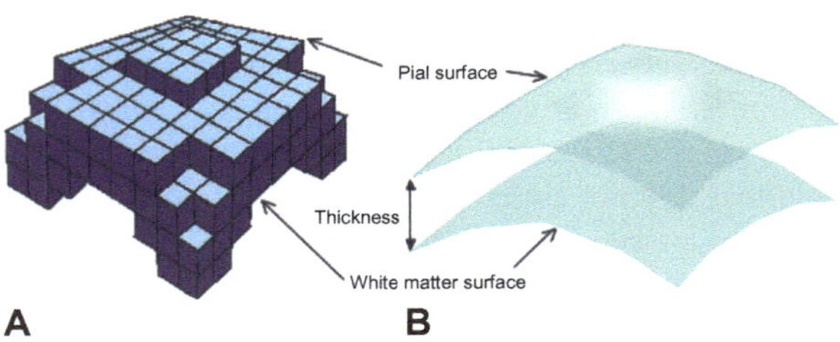

Fig. 3.4. Representations of white- and gray-matter boundaries for volumetric analysis. (**A**) Volume-based, voxel-wise representation. Volumes are calculated by summing the voxels, taking into account partial volume effects. Surface areas cannot be explicitly derived. (**B**) Surface-based representation. Gray-matter volume is calculated based on thickness, measured as the distance between the gray- and white-matter surfaces. Reproduced from Winkler et al. (2010).

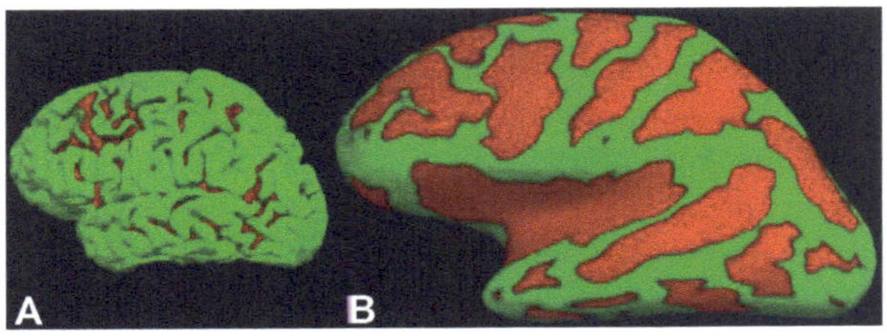

Fig. 3.5. Cortical inflation, performed by FreeSurfer. (**A**) Normal patterns of sulcation and gyration obscure a large fraction of the cortex from view. (**B**) The inflated brain reveals the entire cortical surface, which better demonstrates the spatial arrangement of cortical regions. Green represents gyri and red represents sulci.

memory, and attention. Many of these cortical domains are arranged in a topographic mapping of the sensory modality, such as somatotopic maps (somatic motor and sensation), retinotopic maps (vision), and tonotopic maps (hearing). The complex geometry and variability of the cortical surfaces make analysis of the cortex exceedingly complicated. To simplify this analysis, the cortex may be represented by a surface transformed by a combination of flattening and warping (DeYoe et al., 1996; Engel, 1997; Van Essen and Drury, 1997; Fischl et al., 1999). The transformed cortical surface can more simply depict the otherwise complex spatial arrangements of functional areas, allowing patterns of function and connectivity to be more readily discerned (Fig. 3.5).

Segmentation methods: practical approaches

Segmentation workflow

Brain segmentation can be broken down into a multi-step process, with the steps including: (1) image optimization, such as motion and bias field correction; (2) removal of nonbrain tissues (also termed skull stripping or brain extraction); (3) classification of brain tissue into gray matter, white matter, and CSF; (4) transformation into a common (atlas) space for atlas-based refinement of classification; (5) anatomic labeling; and (6) analysis of resulting data. These processes can be performed independently, although segmentation systems typically perform these in an integrated approach, which can produce more accurate results (Ashburner and Friston, 2005).

Brain segmentation systems

There are several packages available to perform brain segmentation analyses with a range of features aimed at specific user groups. At one end of the spectrum are packages and services targeted to clinical practitioners that are fully automated and produce tabular and graphic output quantitatively and qualitatively assessing areas of atrophy. Some of these systems have achieved regulatory approval for clinical use and are available for purchase or subscription. At the other end of the spectrum are software packages that require greater user input and which are capable of customized, sophisticated analyses using state-of-the-art methods. Many of these systems are made available for free to the public for nonclinical use. The most widely used of these segmentation systems are listed in Table 3.1.

Applications of brain segmentation analysis

There are numerous applications of volumetric and surface-based analysis, including in the areas of cognitive impairment, tumor analysis, traumatic brain injury, stroke, and brain connectivity analysis. MR scanner development, particularly refinements in the design of radiofrequency coils and MR pulse sequences, are providing imaging with higher spatial resolution and improved tissue contrast. Simultaneously, improvements in computational methods and implementation are providing highly accurate and reproducible results more quickly. Consequently, segmentation analysis is becoming a more routine method with more widespread application in research and clinical practice.

Evaluation of normal aging

The brain changes throughout the lifespan, with rapid development beginning *in utero* and continuing in infancy and through early adulthood, followed by slower changes in adulthood and then predominantly involutional changes in older ages. Because human life is long, and humans are enormously varied with respect to their acquired diseases and life histories, it is extremely difficult to characterize the changes of normal human aging. Normal aging is determined in part by diet, exercise

Table 3.1

Brain segmentation systems

System	Availability	Description	Reference
NeuroQuant (CorTechs Labs, La Jolla, USA)	Commercial (FDA-approved)	Fully automated, atlas-based, numeric and graphical output	Brewer (2009) Desikan et al. (2013) www.cortechslabs.com
SyMRI Neuro (SyntheticMR, Linköping, Sweden)	Commercial (CE-marked)	Fully automated, calculates user defined region of interest volumes for structural and lesion analysis	Ambarki et al. (2012) www.syntheticmr.com
Neuroreader (Brainreader ApS, Horsens, Denmark)	Commercial (CE-marked)	Fully automated	brainreader.net
BrainSuite	Free software for noncommercial use	Segmentation, labeling, and analysis packages	Shattuck and Leahy (2002) brainsuite.org
BrainVISA	Free software	Suite contains packages for brain image manipulation, including segmentation	brainvisa.info
FreeSurfer	Open source, free for noncommercial use	Suite contains packages for cortical and subcortical segmentation and analysis	Dale et al. (1999) Fischl et al. (1999) surfer.nmr.mgh.harvard.edu
FSL	Free for noncommercial research use	Library contains tools for segmentation and analysis	Smith et al. (2004) Jenkinson et al. (2012) fsl.fmrib.ox.ac.uk/fsl/fslwiki/
INSECT	Freely available	Undocumented	www.bic.mni.mcgill.ca/ServicesSoftwareAdvancedImageProcessingTools/HomePage
SepINRIA	Free for noncommercial research use	Segmentation package with ability to detect T1, T2, Parkinson's disease, and FLAIR lesions and evaluate atrophy	www-sop.inria.fr/asclepios/software/SepINRIA/

FDA, Food and Drug Administration; FLAIR, fluid-attenuated inversion recovery.

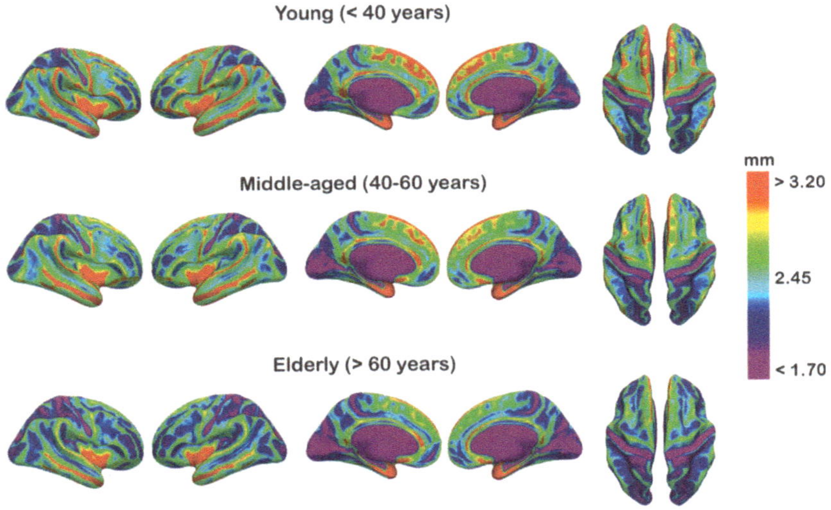

Fig. 3.6. Mean cortical thickness is mapped on to an inflated template brain based on an average of multiple subjects in three age cohorts. A pattern of decreasing cortical thickness is discernible, corresponding to increasing age. Reproduced from Fjell et al. (2009b).

habits, gender, and the presence of diseases such as diabetes, hypertension, and hypercholesterolemia, among many other variables. Certain genetic features are known to have strong correlations with brain health, with ApoE among the best characterized of these (Farrer, 1997; Caselli et al., 2004; Schilling et al., 2013).

Volumetric analyses based on brain segmentation have demonstrated a pattern of cortical thinning in adults that is most pronounced in the frontal, parietal, and temporal cortices (Sowell et al., 2003; Salat et al., 2004; Fjell et al., 2009b; McKay et al., 2014). This atrophy begins as early as the fifth decade of life, and progressive cortical thinning may be observed at intervals as short as 1 year (Fjell et al., 2009a), as depicted in Figure 3.6.

Neurodegenerative disease

Alzheimer's disease

AD is the most common neurodegenerative disease, and its investigation has been a principal motivation in the development of brain imaging and analysis tools. The earliest volumetric analyses in AD were based on CT imaging and compared changes between normal control subjects and patients with advanced AD (Sandor et al., 1988). This work identified changes diffusely within the brain, although more pronounced in the temporal lobes. Further refinement of volumetric analysis using MRI revealed patterns of atrophy, also in the temporal lobe, that were statistically significant features of early AD (Killiany et al., 1993). With improvements in MRI and processing methods, patterns of gray- and white-matter change have been revealed that are strongly associated with AD, such as atrophy involving the hippocampus, superior temporal gyrus, and inferior parietal lobe (Fig. 3.7). Unfortunately, these findings are difficult to apply sensitively and specifically to the diagnosis of individuals (Bozzali et al., 2006), and so computational methods

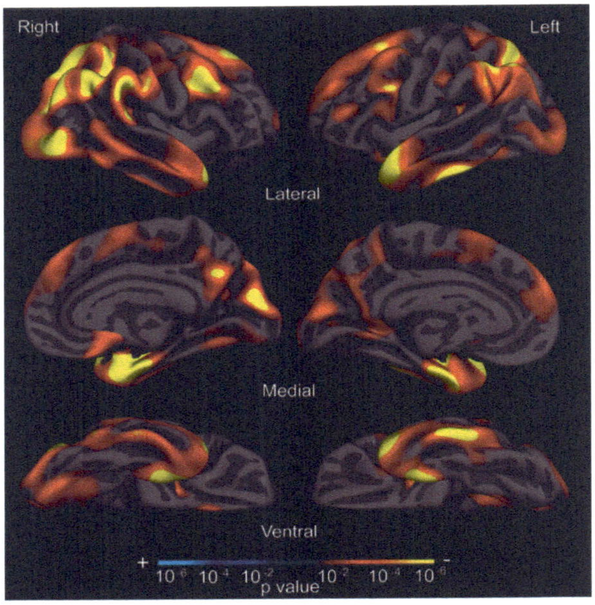

Fig. 3.7. Cortical thinning in a group of subjects with Alzheimer's disease compared to a group of control subjects of similar age. The color indicates the *p*-value derived from a general linear model, assessing the influence of Alzheimer's disease on cortical thickness, and is projected on a semi-inflated average brain. Light gray represents gyri and dark gray represents sulci. Reproduced rom Dickerson et al. (2009a).

have been developed based on multivariate comparison of an individual patient with an ensemble developed from a large number of subjects with AD (Vemuri et al., 2008; Desikan et al., 2010; Cuingnet et al., 2011). Generally, these methods are most accurate in distinguishing normal from AD, and less reliable in distinguishing normal from mild cognitive impairment.

The success of classifying individual patients according to the presence or absence of AD has spurred efforts to identify those who are at risk of AD but do not yet have evidence of cognitive decline. It is possible that anti-AD therapy may be most meaningfully directed at this group of preclinical AD patients, who have molecular pathology within the brain that may eventually result in AD, but who do not yet have a significant burden of neurodegeneration. Additionally, identification of subjects who are at risk for AD would enable clinical trials to be conducted with smaller numbers of research subjects, both lowering the cost and decreasing the time required to achieve a significant result (Holland et al., 2012).

Frontotemporal dementia

There has been a relative efflorescence of research and new insights into frontotemporal dementia (FTD) that has been substantially driven by neuroimaging. FTD has been a challenging clinical diagnosis in part because of the enormously variable clinical manifestations of the disease. Quantitative brain analyses have revealed corresponding patterns of brain abnormality, involving both gray and white matter, correlating with specific clinical subtypes (Seeley et al., 2009; Zhang et al., 2013). Perhaps even more intriguingly, the rate of atrophy has been measured with sufficient accuracy to distinguish the relatively more rapid progression of FTD pathology compared to AD (Krueger et al., 2010). These and other such results make the case that quantitative image analysis deserves a prominent role in the diagnosis and evaluation of FTD.

Epilepsy

One of the earliest applications of brain segmentation was the analysis of electroencephalographic and magnetoencephalography (MEG) data (Dale and Sereno, 1993). Further refinements of this technique provide a much more accurate representation of cortical electric activity and corresponding improved spatial resolution of measured electric activity, and are now routinely used for MEG analysis (Tanaka et al., 2013). In addition to such cortical surface-based analyses, volumetric analysis has been applied to the evaluation of epilepsy, and particularly the identification of hippocampal sclerosis (McDonald et al., 2008).

QUANTITATIVE ANALYSIS OF WHITE-MATTER INTEGRITY: DIFFUSION AND TRACTOGRAPHIC ANALYSIS

Introduction

Diffusion MRI (dMRI) is a method of directly measuring the ability of protons, principally those of water, to diffuse within tissues (Le Bihan et al., 1986). The movement of water within a biologic organism is constrained, or restricted, by the shape features of the organ system (for example, the gray- and white-matter contours of the brain), the organization of the extracellular spaces, and the subcellular structures of the intracellular spaces. The relative contribution to the diffusion signal is determined in large part by the space in which a water molecule is located and the physiologic properties of that space. Within the brain, the principal location of water demonstrating normal, physiologically restricted diffusion is within the intracellular space.

The dMRI signal is measured voxel-wise throughout the brain. Analogous to the interpretation of structural MRI data, maps derived from dMRI can be used to characterize tissue locally. For example, restricted diffusion within a vascular territory may represent ischemic infarction, restricted diffusion within a mass lesion may indicate a highly cellular tumor such as lymphoma, and increased diffusion within a mass lesion may reflect a low-grade primary brain neoplasm such as ganglioglioma. In addition to analysis of local structures, dMRI data can be used to discern large-scale features of brain structure. Chief among these features are the white-matter tracts, which can be tractographically modeled based on dMRI images.

Diffusion properties differ in intraneuronal water depending on whether it is located in the cell bodies or the axons. The axonal processes of neurons constitute a large portion of white-matter volume, and the water contained within them makes the largest contribution to restricted diffusion within normal white matter (Fig. 3.8A). The unrestricted length along the axis of an axon is much greater than the length of its radius. Consequently, there is relatively greater diffusivity of water along the long axis (axial diffusivity) than along the radius (radial diffusivity). dMRI can be used to measure axial diffusivity and radial diffusivity, and these can be informative regarding axonal structure and integrity.

Local diffusion analysis

An enormous amount of data can be derived using routine diffusion-weighted imaging, including the most commonly employed echoplanar imaging sequences. Several parameters may be calculated for each voxel

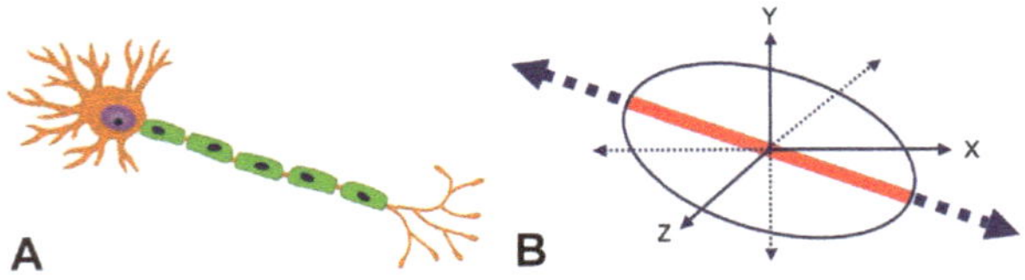

Fig. 3.8. (**A**) Schematic representation of a neuron. A single myelinated axon connects the cell body at one end with the axon terminus and associated synaptic connections at the other. Although this figure depicts a linear axon, axons may include both linear and highly curved segments. (**B**) An ellipsoid corresponding to the diffusion tensor corresponding to a diffusion magnetic resonance imaging voxel. The red line indicates the principal eigenvector (λ_1), while the largest vectors in the plane orthogonal to the principal eigenvector represent λ_2 and λ_3.

and displayed as maps, as summarized in Table 3.2. Diffusion within the voxel may be approximated by an ellipsoid (Fig. 3.8B), with the long axis of the ellipsoid indicating the direction of greatest diffusivity and the aspect ratio (that is, the ratio of the longest and shortest axes) of the ellipsoid representing the degree of diffusion anisotropy. The diffusion tensor is the principal theoretic construct underlying the simplest diffusion analysis, and indicates the principal direction and magnitude of diffusion in a voxel. The diffusion tensor trace is the sum of diffusivity along all three principal Cartesian axes. Mean diffusivity is the average of diffusivity along the three axes and is equal to trace divided by 3. Axial diffusivity represents diffusion along the axis

Table 3.2

Parameters derived from diffusion magnetic resonance imaging

Parameter	Description	Physical connotation	Application
Diffusion tensor	Geometric construct describing the magnitude and directionality of diffusion in a given voxel	The diffusion tensor can be represented as the sum of components (eigenvalues, λ) along the 3 Cartesian axes, λ_1, λ_2, and λ_3	Tractographic methods determine the course of white-matter tracts based upon analysis of diffusion tensors measured throughout the brain
Trace and mean diffusivity	Trace is the sum of diffusivity along the three Cartesian axes: Trace $= \lambda_1 + \lambda_2 + \lambda_3$. Mean diffusivity = trace ÷ 3, and is the average diffusivity along an axis	Maps of the trace or mean diffusivity depict the magnitude of restricted diffusion in the brain. Directionality is not indicated by this scalar value	Provides high sensitivity for the evaluation of stroke, and for tumor analysis, among many other applications. Typically represented as diffusion-weighted imaging or trace maps
Apparent diffusion coefficient (ADC)	A scalar value approximating the diffusion coefficient, D, in Einstein's diffusion equation	ADC is a quantitative estimate of the diffusivity of a water molecule within a biologic tissue	ADC is useful for depicting the degree of restricted diffusion in stroke, tumors, and other brain lesions
Axial (longitudinal) diffusivity	Diffusivity along the principal axis of diffusion, taken to be λ_1	Within white-matter tracts, axial diffusivity represents diffusion in the direction of the long axis of the axon	Axial diffusivity correlates with axonal integrity, and is increased in the setting of axonal injury
Radial diffusivity	Measurement of diffusivity orthogonal to the principal axis of diffusion. Radial diffusivity $= (\lambda_2 + \lambda_3)/2$	Radial diffusivity in axons is decreased by myelination, hence low radial diffusivity is expected in myelinated axons	Radial diffusivity correlates with the degree of axonal myelination, and is increased in axons with myelin damage
Fractional anisotropy (FA)	Scalar value representing the degree to which diffusion is restricted to specific axes. 0 = isotropic diffusion; 1 = diffusion restricted to a single axis	White-matter tracts can be characterized by a normal range of FA. Injury to tracts typically results in decreased FA. FA correlates with axonal diameter, myelination, and fiber density	FA can be analyzed visually, such as with FA maps derived from diffusion-weighted imaging, or quantitatively using tractographic methods

of greatest diffusivity (corresponding to the orientation of the long axis of the axon), whereas radial diffusivity represents diffusion orthogonal to the direction of axial diffusivity. Fractional anisotropy (FA) is a measure of the degree to which diffusion is not completely isotropic, and is expressed as a scalar value ranging from 0 (corresponding to no anisotropy) to 1 (perfectly anisotropic, indicating diffusion along a line). The more common dMRI maps are depicted in Figure 3.9.

The tensor is a convenient mathematic representation of regions in which there is a single dominant fiber orientation, but does not have the flexibility to model more complex fiber architectures in which different orientations cross. This has given rise to models and image acquisition techniques that allow the representation of multiple orientations within a voxel (Frank, 2001; Tuch, 2004; Jensen et al., 2005; Wedeen et al., 2005) at the cost of increased imaging time and more sophisticated modeling.

Regional diffusion analysis: tractography

Brain function is determined in large part by the organization and interactivity of billions of neurons, and this connectivity has been the subject of intense study for hundreds of years, dating to anatomists of the 18th century. In addition to gross anatomy investigations, studies using tracers to follow the migration and connectivity of neurons and axons through the brain have further informed understanding of connectivity, although these require invasive methods and usually sacrifice of the study animals. With the development of MRI diffusion tensor imaging (DTI) in 1994 (Basser et al., 1994), it has become possible to noninvasively chart the course of white-matter tracts in a living brain. Moreover, tractographic connectivity can be simultaneously correlated with cortical connectivity, as assessed by functional MRI, allowing real-time evaluation of brain structure and function in living subjects.

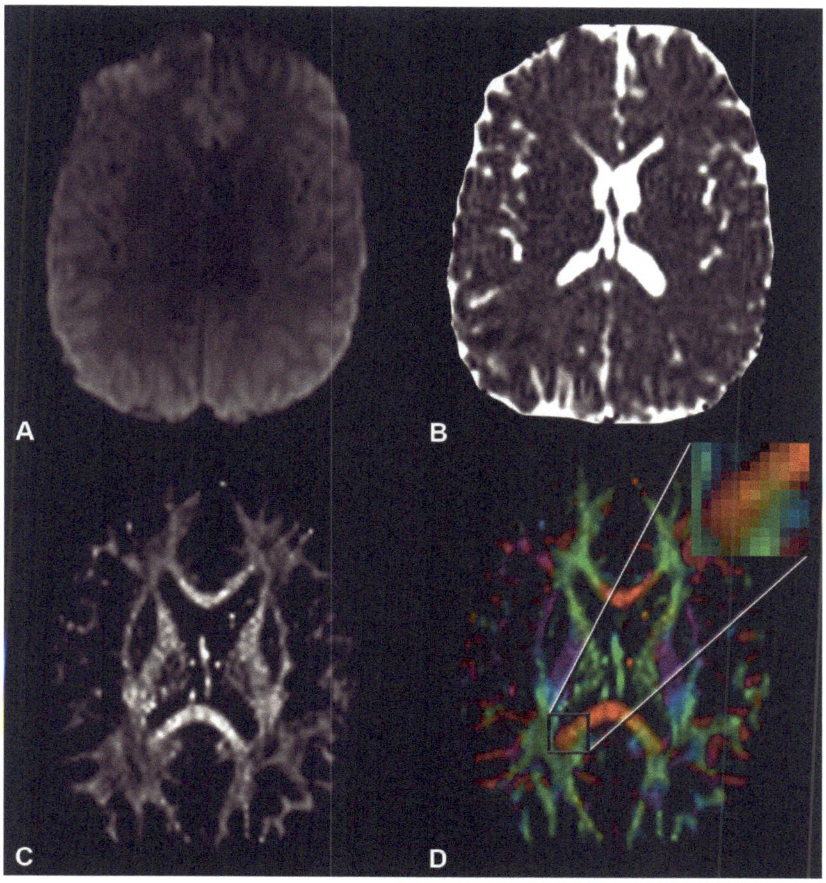

Fig. 3.9. Commonly used maps derived from diffusion magnetic resonance imaging. (**A**) Trace. (**B**) Apparent diffusion coefficient. (**C**) Fractional anisotropy (FA). (**D**) Color fractional anisotropy. A magnified view of the color FA map (inset) demonstrates the image voxelation. The color scheme reflects the dominant direction of the principal eigenvector in each voxel: red corresponds to right/left, green corresponds to anterior/posterior, and blue corresponds to superior/inferior.

Tractography, or fiber tracing, is a mathematic modeling technique based on the measurement of diffusion properties throughout the brain, such as the diffusion tensor. Essentially, tractography is the process of stitching together voxel-wise orientation information to recover the tracts that gave rise to them. Measures derived from the tensor may be depicted in a color FA map in which the color (red, green, or blue) indicates the orientation of the principal eigenvector of the diffusion tensor and brightness indicates the FA (Fig. 3.9D).

These tensor arrays can be used for modeling of white-matter tracts. Fibers can be modeled along the average trajectory of diffusion tensors within a local region, based on the similarity of eigenvectors in adjacent voxels (Fig. 3.10). Model tracts, representing the inferred path of bundles of axonal fibers, are defined based on alignment of tensors in neighboring voxels. Specified regions of interest may define fiber start and end points, with the fibers traced through these regions based on tensor fields. Additional criteria may be imposed on fiber tracing, such as minimum fiber length, minimum FA threshold, and maximum curvature thresholds.

Individual axons are on the order of 1–3 μm in diameter, and so necessarily the resolution of dMRI, which at best is on the order of 1 mm, will be much less than the anatomic dimensions of the objects of interest. Consequently, all voxels will contain numerous axons, some of which are traveling together as a fiber bundle, and some of which may be associated with other bundles coursing in different directions. Partial volume averaging results from a single voxel containing tracts with different trajectories, resulting in a diffusion measurement weighted by the proportion of each tract in the given voxel. Large bundles of nonparallel fibers occur frequently throughout the brain, such as in the corpus callosum and optic chiasm, resulting in large-scale partial volume averaging. Additionally, it is now clear that crossing fibers are a ubiquitous feature of white matter throughout much of the brain (Wedeen et al., 2005), also contributing to partial volume averaging on a smaller scale (Fig. 3.11).

Different approaches to fiber tracing have been developed to overcome the challenges imposed by the complexity of neuroanatomy and the imprecision of dMRI methods. The first tractography methods to be widely utilized were based on a streamline approach, in which a path is traced tangential to the DTI vectors in a three-dimensional field (Conturo et al., 1999; Mori et al., 1999). Streamline fiber tracing may be performed with different methods, varying principally in the function used to calculate the fiber path through the vector field. Initially, deterministic line propagation methods were employed (e.g., Conturo et al., 1999), which result in a simplification of the vector field by depicting the dominant fiber trajectory. Subsequent refinement of streamline methods led to the development of probabilistic line propagation (e.g., Hagmann et al., 2003), in which a greater number of smaller fibers could be traced, although with less certainty about their precise course. Other techniques seek to incorporate the uncertainty that is implicit in trying to track a noisy, limited-resolution representation of the underlying fibers to generate probability maps of the connectivity arising from a given point (Behrens et al., 2003).

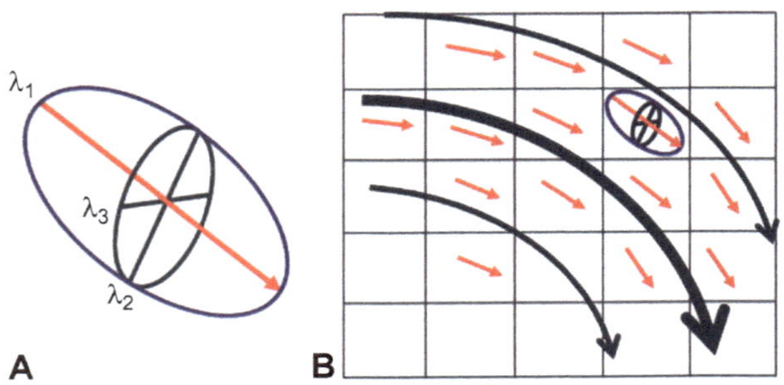

Fig. 3.10. Fiber tracking from diffusion tensor data. (**A**) An ellipsoid represents the diffusion tensor within a voxel (see Fig. 3.8 for comparison with an axon). The eigenvectors, λ_1, λ_2, and λ_3, define orthogonal components of the diffusion tensor. (**B**) Fibers may be traced through a tensor field using the average direction in each voxel. Termination of fiber tracking may be determined by a minimum fractional anisotropy threshold, minimum fiber length and curvature thresholds, among other criteria. A single representative ellipsoid is represented within the tensor field for illustration.

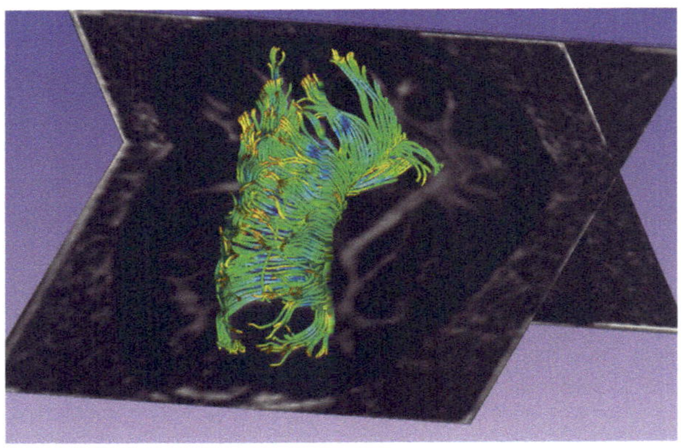

Fig. 3.11. Tractographic model of white-matter fibers of the corpus callosum. The orthogonal reference planes depict the fractional anisotropy values that were used to generate the diffusion tensors from which the tracts are derived. Image created with Slicer (Malcolm et al., 2010).

Diffusion MRI methods

Both 1.5 and 3.0 T commercial MRI scanners are capable of excellent-quality dMRI for many purposes, particularly for analysis of trace and apparent diffusion coefficient maps. It is worth noting that the diffusion signal is not proportional to the B_0 field strength, but rather to the applied gradient field, although there are other factors, particularly lower thermal noise, that contribute to improved image quality at higher B_0. Typical parameters for routine diffusion include a matrix size of 128×128, 5-mm slice thickness, and 5–10 diffusion direction-encoding gradient orientations, resulting in scan times less than 3 minutes. For tractography applications on commercial scanners, higher-resolution sequences can be performed using a matrix up to 256×256, slice thickness approximately 2 mm, and 15–30 diffusion direction-encoding gradients, with scan times of 7–10 minutes.

For specialized applications, such as the Human Connectome Project, scanners have been modified for improved diffusion image quality (Setsompop et al., 2013). Custom gradient coils produce much larger gradients that can be changed quickly and repeatedly, resulting in increased diffusion signal. Head coils with higher numbers of active elements improve signal-to-noise ratios and accelerate scan times. Pulse sequences capable of simultaneous multi-slice acquisition accelerate scan times. With these modifications, dMRI scans may be achieved in 5 minutes with resolution and signal-to-noise ratios far exceeding that which can be achieved in conventional scanners for the high-angular resolution imaging needed to properly characterize complex fiber architecture.

An alternative to DTI, which is limited to a single tensor per voxel, is diffusion spectrum imaging (DSI) (Wedeen et al., 2005). Analogous to the spatial representation of *k*-space, these techniques sample the images in a *q*-space, which represents the space of spin displacements caused by diffusion-encoding gradients in echo-planar MRI. DSI therefore requires sampling three dimensions in *k*-space as well as three dimensions in *q*-space, which leads to long scan times. To help overcome this limitation, alternative MR techniques such as high angular resolution diffusion imaging (HARDI) (Frank, 2002) and q-ball (Tuch et al., 2002) can be used in place of DSI. These techniques rely on sampling along one or more spherical shells, as opposed to sampling throughout Cartesian space, markedly decreasing scan times. These MR methods, used together with the scanner modifications described above, yield higher angular resolution data that have resulted in striking advances in the understanding of both white-matter anatomy and brain connectivity (Wedeen et al., 2012).

Application of diffusion MRI in the evaluation of white-matter integrity

Local dMRI measures of white-matter integrity and injury

dMRI is among the most sensitive methods for evaluation of brain parenchyma, often showing large changes well before abnormality is apparent in T1- or T2-weighted images. The use of dMRI in this capacity is most commonly applied in the assessment of infarction, relying principally upon trace and apparent diffusion coefficient maps, and has also become essential to the assessment of brain lesions such tumors, infection, and seizure, among others. Beyond these indications, dMRI has broad application in the evaluation of more subtly altered brain parenchyma, particularly white-matter tracts. A decrement in restricted diffusion (that is, increased diffusion) compared to normal white matter, revealed by increased mean diffusivity and corresponding decreased FA, can be a sensitive indicator of axonal abnormality. Changes in both axial and radial diffusivity may contribute to changes in mean diffusivity, and the relative contributions of these components may reflect specific axonal abnormality.

Patterns of axonal injury have been experimentally assessed using a murine model of optic nerve injury (Song et al., 2003). In this model, retinal ischemia leads to axonal injury in the optic nerve that at earlier time points manifests as axonal disruption with preservation of the myelin sheath. This results in decreased axial diffusivity with no alteration in radial diffusivity. At later time points, as the myelin is disrupted, radial diffusivity increases with little corresponding change in axial diffusivity. These results provide the basis for the hypothesis that alterations in axial and radial diffusivity reflect changes in axon and myelin integrity, respectively.

It is essential to recognize that this hypothesis is certainly an oversimplification, and its broad application in the human brain has not yet been definitively demonstrated. There are important limitations of this model, as axial and radial diffusivity are highly correlated metrics. For example, there is a range of normal axon diameter in the brain that corresponds in part to axon function, with larger-diameter axons specialized for higher speed, as found in visual and motor pathways. As radial diffusivity is strongly correlated with axonal diameter, these parameters should be assessed coordinately. Similarly, demyelinating processes may contribute both to decreased myelination, leading to increased radial diffusivity, as well as axonal disruption, leading to decreased axial diffusivity. In this manner, axial diffusivity and radial diffusivity are not independent variables, but are often highly correlated in both normal and abnormal brain tissue.

dMRI metrics have also been found to be correlated with volumetric measurements, based on brain segmentation: decreasing white-matter volume correlates with declining white-matter integrity, indicated by decreased FA. However, FA has been found to be a more sensitive measure of loss of white-matter integrity than white-matter volume (Fjell et al., 2008).

Local measures of dMRI in demyelinating disease

The conventional understanding of demyelinating disease, most extensively investigated in multiple sclerosis (MS), is that abnormal brain parenchyma is reflected by increased T2 hyperintensity. However, particularly through the application of dMRI methods, it has been demonstrated that the T2 lesion burden markedly underestimates the extent of brain abnormality (Roosendal et al., 2009). The most sensitive local measure of white-matter abnormality is FA, although this is a nonspecific finding, as FA is decreased in white-matter lesions arising from a broad array of etiologies, including demyelinating processes. FA has been shown to be decreased diffusely throughout white matter in patients with MS, as well as more focally decreased within T2 hyperintense lesions (Werring et al., 1999).

Conceptually, decreased FA may result from reduced axial diffusivity, increased radial diffusivity, or a combination of these. In keeping with the hypothesis of demyelinating disease predominantly affecting radial diffusivity, the FA abnormality in MS patients has been seen to relate principally to increased radial diffusivity, with either unchanged or increased axial diffusivity (Roosendal et al., 2009).

Local measures of dMRI changes in normal aging

The brain undergoes extensive myelination in the course of brain maturation, including development of myelin sheaths in associative areas continuing into middle age. Subsequently, and perhaps beginning as early as the fourth decade of life, a pattern of myelin breakdown and axonal loss begins to occur (Walhovd et al., 2005), some of which may be regarded as within the spectrum of normal aging. Additionally, other features of cerebral health were found to correlate with FA. Specifically, cortical gray-matter thickness, which slowly decreases with age, is positively correlated with FA, and the total burden of white-matter T2 hyperintense lesions, which increases in age in some subjects, is negatively correlated with FA (Kochunov et al., 2007).

Local measures of dMRI in neurodegenerative disease

The most common cerebral neurodegenerative processes, particularly AD, are considered as principally affecting cortical neurons, which, in the case of AD, are subject to the highest burdens of abnormal amyloid plaque and related neuropathology. Despite the asymmetric burden of molecular pathology in the cortex, abnormality involving cerebral white matter has also been demonstrated. In a study correlating dMRI metrics with disease state and cognitive ability, white-matter abnormality was identified involving brain regions known to be involved with Alzheimer pathology (Bosch et al., 2012), as shown in Figure 3.12. In this study, the pattern of white-matter degeneration was highly correlated with thinning of adjacent cortices, suggesting that the white matter may be secondary to cortical gray-matter neurodegeneration. FA was found the most sensitive measure of white-matter abnormality, and decreased FA was also found to correlate with decreased memory performance.

A similar study correlated white-matter degeneration with hippocampal structural connectivity (Rowley et al., 2013). In this work, a similar pattern of white-matter abnormality, characterized by increased mean diffusivity and decreased FA, was seen in AD patients, predominantly involving posterior parietal and temporal lobes, including the posterior cingulate gyri. Additionally, metrics of hippocampal structural connectivity were assessed, demonstrating decreased connectivity of the hippocampi to temporal and parietal cortices, consistent with and presumably related to the pattern of white-matter abnormality.

Beyond the few examples cited here, local metrics of dMRI have been evaluated in many other conditions, including traumatic brain injury, hypertension, seizure, human immunodeficiency virus (HIV) infection, neoplasm, and migraine, among many others. The findings of these studies have been largely concordant, with markers of diminished white-matter integrity associated with increased burden of neuropathology.

Regional measures of white-matter integrity: tractography

Fiber-tracing methods can be used to model white-matter tracts throughout the cerebrum, cerebellum, brainstem, and spinal cord. These results have identified short- and long-range connections within the brain, helping to define connectivity within and between functional cortical domains that powerfully inform understanding of brain function. Tractography is helpful for understanding patterns of normal brain function and has also provided new insights into normal brain aging and neuropathology, such as neurodegenerative disease,

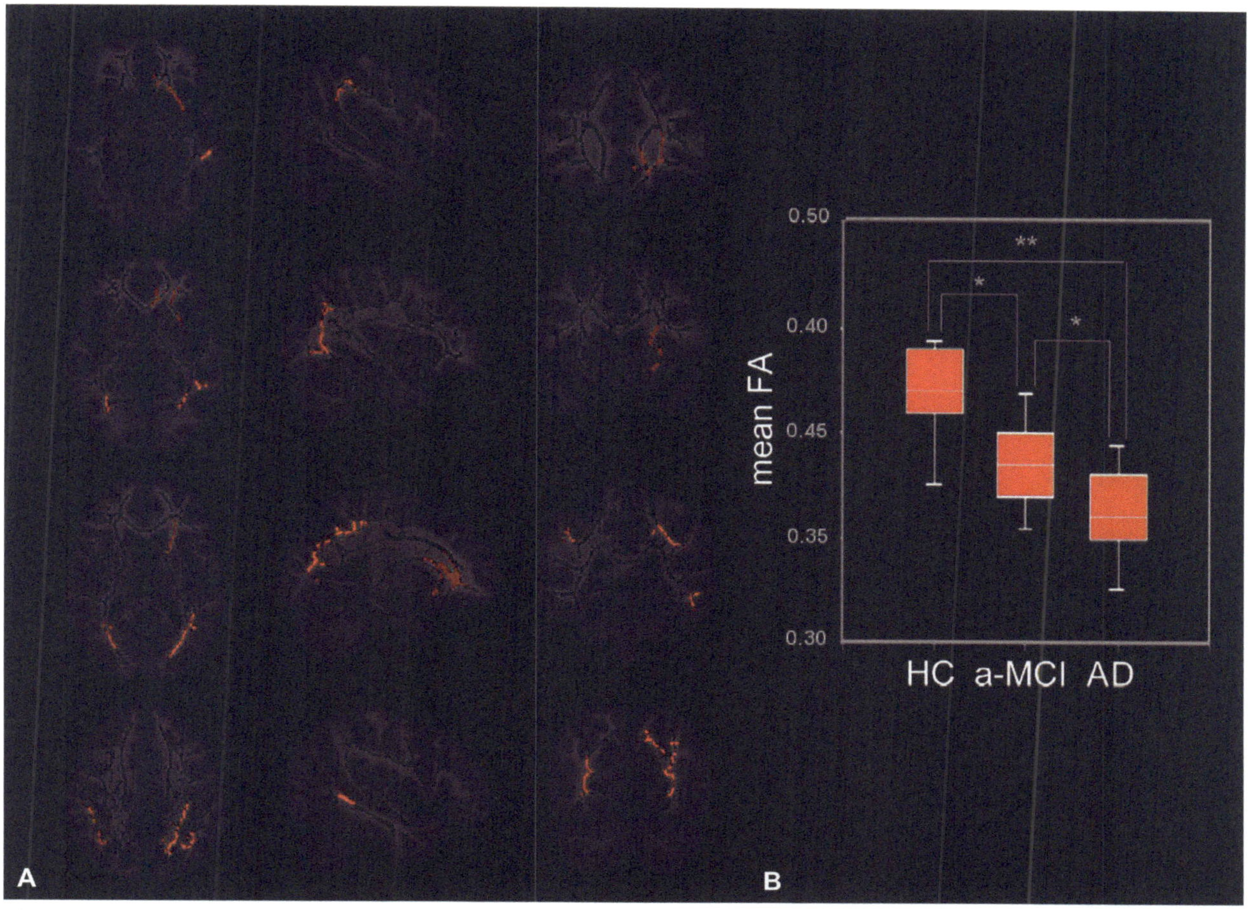

Fig. 3.12. Decreased fractional anisotropy (FA) in Alzheimer's disease (AD). (**A**) Anatomic projection of white-matter regions in which FA is decreased in AD subjects compared to healthy controls. (**B**) Plots of mean FA in healthy controls (HC), subjects with amnestic mild cognitive impairment (a-MCI), and subjects with AD. Modified from Bosch et al. (2012).

demyelinating diseases, brain tumors, and vascular disease, among others.

Tractography in normal brain can reliably and robustly detect major white-matter tracts. These may be classified as association pathways (superior longitudinal fasciculus, inferior longitudinal fasciculus, superior fronto-occipital fasciculus, inferior fronto-occipital fasciculus, uncinate fasciculus. and cingulum), commissural pathways (corpus callosum, anterior commissure, posterior commissure, hippocampal commissure of the fornix, habenular commissure, and tectal commissure) and projection pathways (corticospinal tracts, corticobulbar tracts, internal capsule, acoustic radiations, and optic radiations). The major cerebral and cerebellar white-matter pathways are depicted in Figure 3.13.

As fiber tracing is carried out using the same MRI data as used for local analysis, the results of regional tractographic analysis are generally concordant with voxel-wise analyses. Quantitative metrics have been developed for the evaluation of tractography results, including measures of connectivity (Poupon et al., 2001) and fiber density (Roberts et al., 2005), and these tend to correlate with local dMRI measures such as FA.

Tractography: axonal patterning

High spatial and angular resolution, high signal-to-noise ratio data obtained with a scanner optimized for dMRI, help to overcome partial volume averaging resulting from crossing fibers within a single voxel. Tractography performed with this data has revealed details of white-matter anatomy that had not previously been apparent from conventional anatomic studies (Wedeen et al., 2008, 2012). These DSI results have demonstrated a pattern of predominantly orthogonal fiber crossing that is manifest at multiple scales, ranging from cerebral hemisphere to lobe to dMRI voxel.

The pattern of crossing fibers is hypothesized to form a curvilinear three-dimensional grid that corresponds to the three principal chemotactic axes of embryogenesis

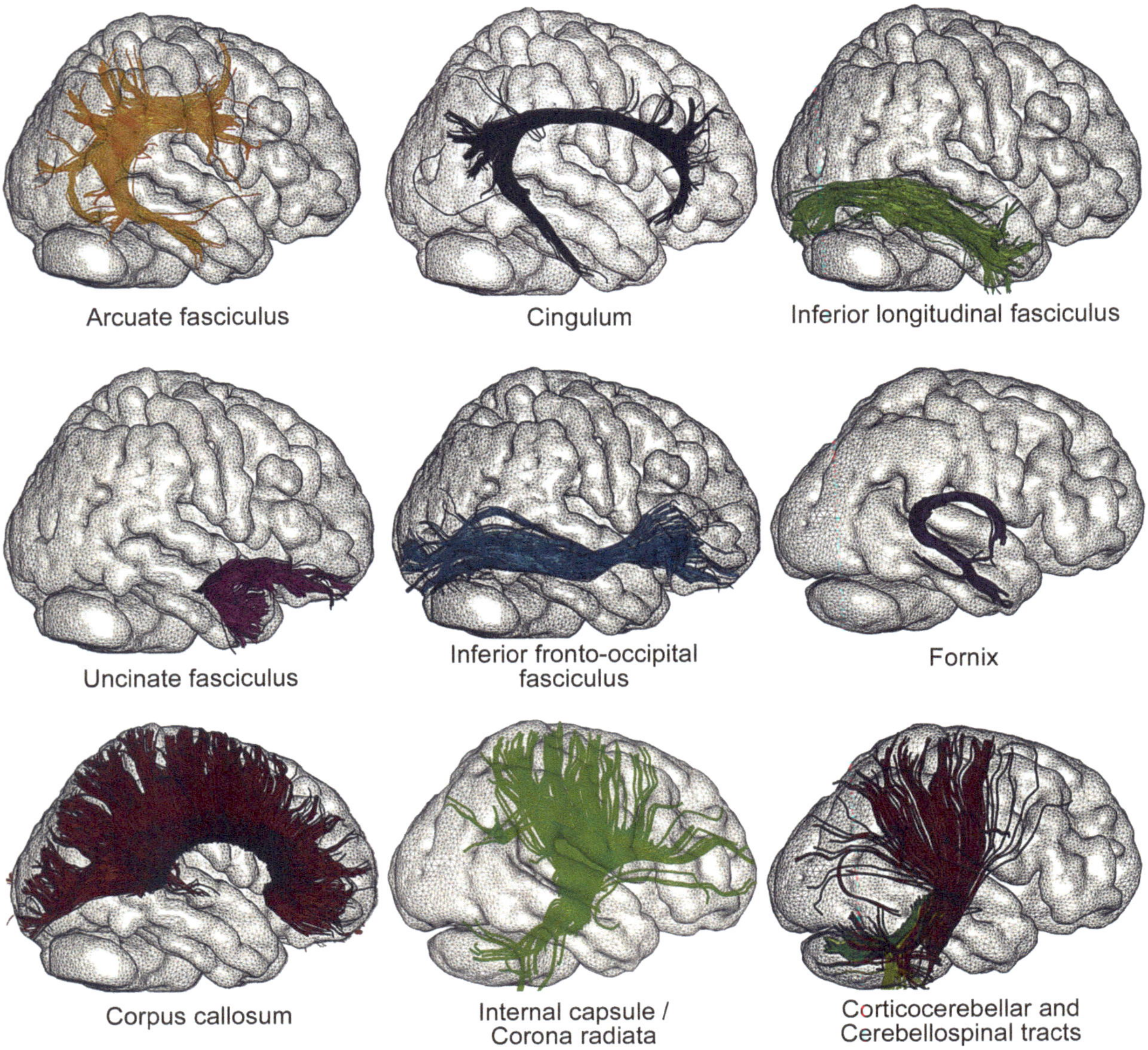

Fig. 3.13. Major cerebral and cerebellar white-matter tracts modeled from diffusion tensor imaging data. Modified from Catani and Thiebaut de Schotten (2008).

and brain organogenesis. This organization forms a pattern of "default connectivity" that may provide a structural basis upon which variations arising from evolution, development, and functional plasticity may result in functional adaptation (Wedeen et al., 2012). This model of brain architecture now informs understanding of brain function and has many applications in investigations of brain development and brain injury.

Tractography: brain connectivity

Brain function is increasingly understood to be a result of extensively interconnected neurons arranged both laterally and hierarchically within cerebral cortex and deep brain nuclei. This structure permits essentially continuous input, integration, and output of numerous multimodal sensory and physiologic streams simultaneously. The ability to obtain an anatomic map of brain connectivity has greatly informed understanding of brain function, and, it is hoped, may enable the better diagnosis and treatment of abnormal brain function. Together with segmentation and labeling, DTI methods are now essential tools for discerning brain connectivity, as depicted in Figure 3.14.

Tractography: applications

For evaluation of white-matter microstructural integrity, voxel-wise metrics such as FA, mean diffusivity, axial

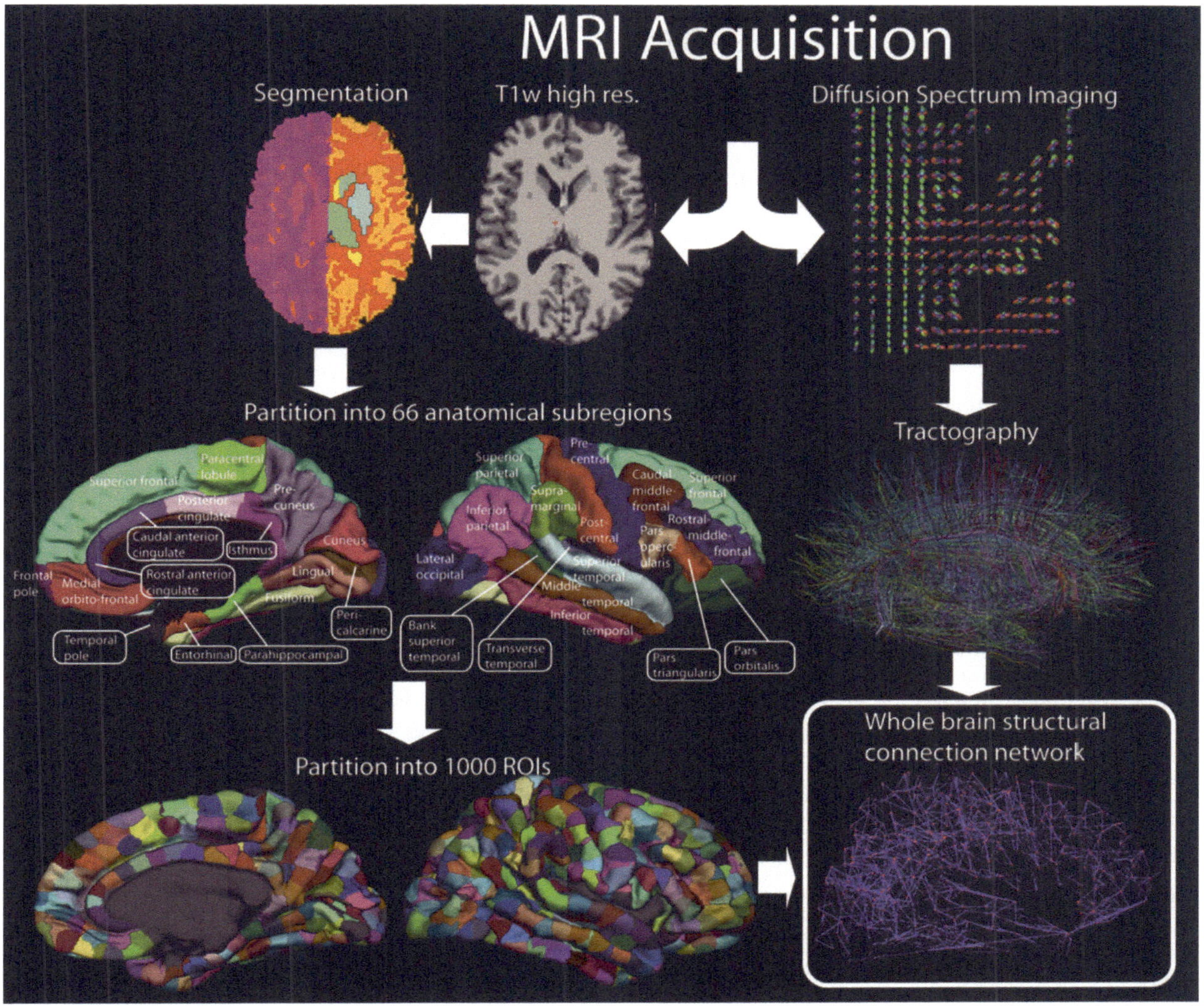

Fig. 3.14. Whole-brain structural connectivity derived from segmentation of high-resolution T1-weighted imaging and tractographic analysis of diffusion spectrum imaging. Regions of interest (ROIs) on the cortical surface are correlated with underlying white-matter tracts, resulting in a connection weight between each pair of cortical ROIs. The whole-brain structural connection network relating cortical ROIs and their underlying connectivity is depicted in the lower right image. MRI, magnetic resonance imaging. Reproduced from Hagmann et al. (2010).

diffusivity, and radial diffusivity are preferred for quantitative analysis. As described above, these metrics can be used to compare specific brain regions, with anatomy precisely defined by brain segmentation methods. Longitudinal analyses can be performed using highly automated workflows that result in highly reproducible measurements. These methods are now the foundation of white-matter microstructural studies. Assessment of tractographic results is more challenging, in part due to the difficulty of precisely defining white-matter tracts. Currently the definition of tracts typically requires the manual definition of ROIs, although automated methods have been developed (Gong et al., 2005). Once defined, tracts can be reasonably replicated in repeated interval scans of the same subject, although definition of the same tracts in different subjects is more challenging (Aarnink et al., 2014). Consequently, fiber tracing is currently most useful in the definition of brain connectivity, while voxel-wise metrics are more useful for quantitative analysis of white-matter microstructural integrity and longitudinal studies.

One of the most common clinical applications of tractography is planning surgical resection of brain lesions, such as tumors or cortical malformations. Brain lesions may disrupt or displace white-matter tracts. To the extent that the tracts are disrupted, most commonly by infiltration of tumor, edema, and/or gliosis, modeling of the affected tracts is impaired. Recognition of the disrupted tracts and the altered anatomy can be used to identify functional brain tissue that should be preserved as well as tumor-involved tissue that may be safely resected.

Diffusion MRI and tractography methods: practical approaches

Diffusion MRI and tractography workflows

As with brain segmentation, dMRI analysis can also be broken down into a multi-step process. These steps include:

1. application of corrections to the raw data, principally for head motion and eddy currents. This may be achieved by registering to other structural sequences and by applying corrections derived from field maps or gradient residuals;
2. removal of extracranial structures using a brain extraction process;
3. using the corrected brain data, a diffusion model is applied to each voxel. Currently, the most commonly employed are based on diffusion tensor models, although DSI models may be used with more advanced data acquisition methods. Both voxel-wise metrics and vector fields can be derived from the diffusion data;
4. using the vector field derived from the diffusion model, fiber-tracing algorithms are applied to model fiber pathways.

Various methods, including deterministic and probabilistic streamline methods, may be applied and compared to identify a method best suited for the intended application.

Tractographic results can be compared using measures based on voxels or ROIs, or tract-based statistical measures. Other dMRI metrics such as mean diffusivity, axial diffusivity, and radial diffusivity can be calculated and analyzed on a voxel-wise basis.

Diffusion MRI and tractography systems

As with brain segmentation systems, several different systems are available for dMRI analyses, also spanning a range of applications, from research to clinical practice. The research-oriented systems tend to be more flexible and allow for greater user-defined input, while the clinical systems are generally more automated. Several of the systems, both for research and clinical use, are integrated with other systems for brain analysis, including structural segmentation and analysis of function MRI data. The dMRI systems in most common use are listed in Table 3.3.

Table 3.3

Diffusion and tractography analysis systems

System	Availability	Description	Reference
FSL FDT (bedpostx)	Free for noncommercial research use	Bayesian estimation of diffusion parameters; model allows crossing fibers	Behrens et al. (2003) FMRIB Technical Report TR03TB1
iPlan FiberTracking (Brainlab, Munich, Germany)	Commercial (CE-marked and approved by the Food and Drug Administration)	Integrated fiber tracking and segmentation system for surgical planning	www.brainlab.com
MedINRIA	Open source, free for noncommercial use	Deterministic fiber-tracing algorithm	med.inria.fr
MITK Diffusion	Open source, free for research use	Diffusion tensor and Q-Ball reconstruction	www.mitk.org/MITK
NordicBrainEx (Nordic NeuroLab, Bergen Norway)	Commercial (CE-marked and approved by the Food and Drug Administration)	Integrated fiber tracking and fMRI analysis system	www.nordicneurolab.com
TRACULA	Open source, free for noncommercial use	TRActs Constrained by UnderLying Anatomy; global probabilistic streamline algorithm	Yendiki et al. (2011) surfer.nmr.mgh.harvard.edu/fswiki/Tracula
UKFTractography (Slicer Package)	Open source, free for noncommercial use	Applies an unscented Kalman filter using one, two, or three tensor methods	Malcolm et al. (2010) www.slicer.org

fMRI, functional magnetic resonance imaging.

Future developments

dMRI methods have developed very rapidly, and it remains necessary to correlate dMRI measures with anatomy and pathophysiology, to understand the range of normal and abnormal findings. This applies both to regional fiber-tracing results as well as to local voxel-wise measurements. Such correlation may be achieved through comparison with other experimental analyses as well as postmortem examinations (Dell'Acqua and Catani, 2012). Understanding of the physiologic correlates of dMRI measures can be expected to provide improved diagnostic utility in a range of specific pathology.

The Human Connectome Project is dedicated to the investigation of brain connectivity, and has as one of its priorities the development of improved methods. To this end, MR scanners have been optimized for diffusion imaging, and imaging methods, particularly DSI, have been developed for use with these scanners (Fjell et al., 2009a; Setsompop et al., 2013). High-resolution dMRI data from specialized as well as conventional scanners is aiding the development of computational methods, particularly with respect to the development of methods for automated analysis.

SUMMARY

Current-generation MR scanners in widespread, routine use are capable of producing images with spatial resolution approaching that of the unaided human eye. Additionally, due to the physical mechanisms underlying MRI, tissue contrasts can be achieved that are beyond those that can be achieved with human vision. Quantitative computational methods are available to make more complete use of the extraordinary data available from MRI.

Segmentation techniques are the basis of quantitative volumetric analysis of the brain, which can be used to identify subtle differences in cortical thickness and deep gray- and white-matter volumes. This analysis is useful for the analysis of patterns of atrophy, such as in neurodegenerative disease, traumatic brain injury, inflammatory disease, and metabolic disease. Additionally, segmentation has been useful for the identification and characterization of brain lesions such as cortical malformations and tumors. Longitudinal imaging data can be processed to assess for subtle patterns of change, and this has powerfully informed understanding of normal and abnormal brain aging.

Fiber-tracing methods, based on high-resolution dMRI, provide fundamentally different information regarding the structure of white matter that is correlated with, although substantially independent of, white-matter volume (Ly et al., 2014). Diffusion methods yield data on the integrity of the microstructure of the brain, specifically axons and their larger tract assemblies that reflect the connectivity of the cortical and deep gray-matter neurons. The connectivity patterns can help to inform our understanding of intrinsic connectivity networks in the brain that are also informed from data acquired using functional MRI studies. Understanding of white-matter tract integrity may be helpful in identifying patterns of disease such as neurodegenerative, inflammatory, traumatic, and neoplastic. Further, the ability to model tracts in a brain with a lesion, such as tumor or developmental abnormality, can inform surgical planning so as to achieve the most complete possible resection while sparing vital structures.

Advances in quantitative computational methods, including segmentation and tractography, have been achieved in conjunction with advances in MR techniques, leading to improvement both in imaging methods and computational approaches. This cycle of cooperative and collaborative development has substantially extended the capability of noninvasive imaging beyond the range of unaided human vision. This area of analysis has been termed computational functional anatomy, and is at least implicitly an element of most neuroimaging research at present (Miller and Qiu, 2009). Beyond research applications, these methods are certain to play an increasing role in clinical neuromedicine.

References

Aarnink SH, Vos SB, Leemans A et al. (2014). Automated longitudinal intra-subject analysis (ALISA) for diffusion MRI tractography. Neuroimage 86: 404–416.

Akselrod-Ballin A, Galun M, Gomori JM et al. (2009). Automatic segmentation and classification of multiple sclerosis in multichannel MRI. IEEE Trans Biomed Eng 56: 2461–2469.

Amato U, Larobina M, Antoniadis A et al. (2003). Segmentation of magnetic resonance brain images through discriminant analysis. J Neurosci 131: 165–174.

Ambarki K, Lindqvist T, Wåhlin A et al. (2012). Evaluation of automatic measurement of the intracranial volume based on quantitative MR imaging. AJNR Am J Neuroradiol 33: 1951–1956.

Anbeek P, Vincken KL, Van Bochove GS (2005). Probabilistic segmentation of brain tissue in MR imaging. Neuroimage 27: 795–804.

Ashburner J, Friston KJ (2000). Voxel-based morphometry – the methods. Neuroimage 11: 805–821.

Ashburner J, Friston KJ (2004). Morphometry. In: RSJ Frackowiak, KJ Friston, C Frith et al. (Eds.), Human Brain Function, Academic Press, San Diego, CA.

Ashburner J, Friston KJ (2005). Unified segmentation. Neuroimage 26: 839–851.

Basser PJ, Mattiello J, LeBihan D (1994). Estimation of the effective self-diffusion tensor from the NMR spin echo. J Magn Reson B 103: 247–254.

Behrens TEJ, Woolrich MW, Jenkinson M et al. (2003). Characterization and propagation of uncertainty in diffusion-weighted MR imaging. Magn Reson Med 50: 1077–1088.

Bosch B, Arenaza-Urquijo EM, Rami L et al. (2012). Multiple DTI index analysis in normal aging, amnestic MCI and AD. Relationship with neuropsychological performance. Neurobiol Aging 33: 61–74.

Bozzali M, Filippi M, Magnani G et al. (2006). The contribution of voxel-based morphometry in staging patients with mild cognitive impairment. Neurology 67: 453–460.

Brewer JB (2009). Fully-automated volumetric MRI with normative ranges: translation to clinical practice. Behav Neurol 21: 21–28.

Buckner RL, Head D, Parker J et al. (2004). A unified approach for morphometric and functional data analysis in young, old, and demented adults using automated atlas-based head size normalization: reliability and validation against manual measurement of total intracranial volume. Neuroimage 23: 724–738.

Cabezas M, Oliver A, Lladó X et al. (2011). A review of atlas-based segmentation for magnetic resonance brain images. Comput Methods Programs Biomed 104: e158–e177.

Caselli RJ, Reiman EM, Osborne D et al. (2004). Longitudinal changes in cognition and behavior in asymptomatic carriers of the APOE e4 allele. Neurology 62: 1990–1995.

Catani M, Thiebaut de Schotten M (2008). A diffusion tensor imaging tractography atlas for virtual in vivo dissections. Cortex 44: 1105–1132.

Conturo TE, Lori NF, Cull TS et al. (1999). Tracking neuronal fiber pathways in the living human brain. Proc Natl Acad Sci U S A 96: 10422–10427.

Cuingnet R, Gerardin E, Tessieras et al. (2011). Automatic classification of patients with Alzheimer's disease from structural MRI: a comparison of ten methods using the ADNI database. Neuroimage 56: 766–781.

Dale AM, Sereno MI (1993). Improved localization of cortical activity by combining EEG and MEG with MRI cortical surface reconstruction: a linear approach. J Cogn Neurosci 5: 162–176.

Dale AM, Fischl B, Sereno MI (1999). Cortical surface-based analysis. I. Segmentation and surface reconstruction. Neuroimage 9: 179–194.

Dell'Acqua F, Catani M (2012). Structural human brain networks: hot topics in diffusion tractography. Curr Opin Neurol 25: 375–383.

Desikan RS, Ségonne F, Fischl B et al. (2006). An automated labeling system for subdividing the human cerebral cortex on MRI scans into gyral based regions of interest. Neuroimage 31: 968–980.

Desikan RS, Cabral HJ, Settecase F et al. (2010). Automated MRI measures predict progression to Alzheimer's disease. Neurobiol Aging 31: 1364–1374.

Desikan RS, Rafii MS, Brewer JB et al. (2013). An expanded role for neuroimaging in the evaluation of memory impairment. AJNR Am J Neuroradiol 34: 2075–2082.

DeYoe EA, Carman GJ, Bandettini P et al. (1996). Mapping striate and extrastriate visual areas in human cerebral cortex. Proc Natl Acad Sci U S A 93: 2382–2386.

Dickerson BC, Bakkour A, Salat DH et al. (2009a). The cortical signature of Alzheimer's disease: regionally specific cortical thinning relates to symptom severity in very mild to mild AD dementia and is detectable in asymptomatic amyloid-positive individuals. Cereb Cortex 19: 497–510.

Dickerson BC, Feczko E, Augustinack JC et al. (2009b). Differential effects of aging and Alzheimer's disease on medial temporal lobe cortical thickness and surface area. Neurobiol Aging 30: 432–440.

Engel S (1997). Retinotopic organization in human visual cortex and the spatial precision of functional MRI. Cereb Cortex 7: 181–192.

Farrer LA (1997). Effects of age, sex, and ethnicity on the association between apolipoprotein E genotype and Alzheimer disease. JAMA 278: 1349–1356.

Fischl B, Dale AM (2000). Measuring the thickness of the human cerebral cortex from magnetic resonance images. Proc Natl Acad Sci U S A 97: 11050–11055.

Fischl B, Sereno MI, Dale AM (1999). Cortical surface-based analysis. II: Inflation, flattening, and a surface-based coordinate system. Neuroimage 9: 195–207.

Fischl B, Salat DH, Busa E et al. (2002). Whole brain segmentation: automated labeling of neuroanatomical structures in the human brain. Neuron 33: 341–355.

Fischl B, Salat DH, van der Kouwe AJW et al. (2004a). Sequence-independent segmentation of magnetic resonance images. Neuroimage 23 (Suppl 1): S69–S84.

Fischl B, van der Kouwe A, Destrieux C et al. (2004b). Automatically parcellating the human cerebral cortex. Cereb Cortex 14: 11–22.

Fjell AM, Westlye LT, Greve DN et al. (2008). The relationship between diffusion tensor imaging and volumetry as measures of white matter properties. Neuroimage 42: 1654–1668.

Fjell AM, Walhovd KB, Fennema-Notestine C et al. (2009a). One-year brain atrophy evident in healthy aging. J Neurosci 29: 15223–15231.

Fjell AM, Westlye LT, Amlien I et al. (2009b). High consistency of regional cortical thinning in aging across multiple samples. Cereb Cortex 19: 2001–2012.

Frank LR (2001). Anisotropy in high angular resolution diffusion-weighted MRI. Magn Reson Med 45: 935–939.

Frank LR (2002). Characterization of anisotropy in high angular resolution diffusion-weighted MRI. Magn Reson Med 47: 1083–1099.

Gong G, Jiang T, Zhu C et al. (2005). Asymmetry analysis of cingulum based on scale-invariant parameterization by diffusion tensor imaging. Hum Brain Mapp 24: 92–98.

Good CD, Johnsrude I, Ashburner J et al. (2001). Cerebral asymmetry and the effects of sex and handedness on brain structure: A voxel-based morphometric analysis of 465 normal adult human brains. Neuroimage 14: 685–700.

Hagmann P, Thiran JP, Jonasson L et al. (2003). DTI mapping of human brain connectivity: statistical fibre tracking and virtual dissection. Neuroimage 19: 545–554.

Hagmann P, Cammoun L, Gigandet X et al. (2010). MR connectomics: Principles and challenges. J Neurosci Methods 194: 34–45.

Han X, Fischl B (2007). Atlas renormalization for improved brain MR image segmentation across scanner platforms. IEEE Trans Med Imaging 26: 479–486.

Han X, Jovicich J, Salat D et al. (2006). Reliability of MRI-derived measurements of human cerebral cortical thickness: the effects of field strength, scanner upgrade and manufacturer. Neuroimage 32: 180–194.

Holland D, McEvoy LK, Desikan RS et al. (2012). Enrichment and stratification for predementia Alzheimer disease clinical trials. PLoS One 7: e47739.

Hua X, Hibar DP, Ching CRK et al. (2013). Unbiased tensor-based morphometry: improved robustness and sample size estimates for Alzheimer's disease clinical trials. Neuroimage 66C: 648–661.

Jack CR, Bernstein MA, Fox NC et al. (2008). The Alzheimer's Disease Neuroimaging Initiative (ADNI): MRI methods. J Magn Reson Imaging 27: 685–691.

Jenkinson M, Beckmann CF, Behrens TEJ et al. (2012). FSL. Neuroimage 62: 782–790.

Jensen JH, Helpern JA, Ramani A et al. (2005). Diffusional kurtosis imaging: the quantification of non-gaussian water diffusion by means of magnetic resonance imaging. Magn Reson Med 53: 1432–1440.

Jovicich J, Czanner S, Han X et al. (2009). MRI-derived measurements of human subcortical, ventricular and intracranial brain volumes: Reliability effects of scan sessions, acquisition sequences, data analyses, scanner upgrade, scanner vendors and field strengths. Neuroimage 46: 177–192.

Kanai R, Rees G (2011). The structural basis of inter-individual differences in human behaviour and cognition. Nat Rev Neurosci 12: 231–241.

Kapur T (1999). Model based three dimensional medical image segmentation. Massachusetts Institute of Technology, Cambridge, MA.

Kapur T, Eric W, Grimson L et al. (1998). Enhanced spatial priors for segmentation of magnetic resonance imagery. In: Medical Image Computing, Lecture Notes in Computer Science, Springer-Verlag, Berlin/Heidelberg, pp. 457–468.

Kikinis R, Shenton ME, Iosifescu DV et al. (1996). A digital brain atlas for surgical planning, model-driven segmentation, and teaching. IEEE Trans Visual Comput Graphics 2: 232–241.

Killiany RJ, Moss MB, Albert MS et al. (1993). Temporal lobe regions on magnetic resonance imaging identify patients with early Alzheimer's disease. Arch Neurol 50: 949–954.

Kochunov P, Thompson PM, Lancaster JL et al. (2007). Relationship between white matter fractional anisotropy and other indices of cerebral health in normal aging: tract-based spatial statistics study of aging. Neuroimage 35: 478–487.

Krueger CE, Dean DL, Rosen HJ et al. (2010). Longitudinal rates of lobar atrophy in frontotemporal dementia, semantic dementia, and Alzheimer's disease. Alzheimer Dis Assoc Disord 24: 43–48.

Kuperberg GR, Broome MR, McGuire PK et al. (2003). Regionally localized thinning of the cerebral cortex in schizophrenia. Arch Gen Psychiatry 60: 878–888.

Lattanzi R, Grant AK, Polimeni JR et al. (2010). Performance evaluation of a 32-element head array with respect to the ultimate intrinsic SNR. NMR Biomed 23: 142–151.

Le Bihan D, Breton E, Lallemand D et al. (1986). MR imaging of intravoxel incoherent motions: application to diffusion and perfusion in neurologic disorders. Radiology 161: 401–407.

Ly M, Canu E, Xu G (2014). Midlife measurements of white matter microstructure predict subsequent regional white matter atrophy in healthy adults. Hum Brain Mapp 35: 2044–2054.

Malcolm JG, Shenton ME, Rathi Y (2010). Filtered multitensor tractography. IEEE Trans Med Imaging 29: 1664–1675.

Mazziotta J, Toga A, Evans A et al. (2001). A probabilistic atlas and reference system for the human brain: International Consortium for Brain Mapping (ICBM). Philos Trans R Soc B Biol Sci 356: 1293–1322.

McDonald CR, Hagler Jr DJ, Ahmadi ME et al. (2008). Subcortical and cerebellar atrophy in mesial temporal lobe epilepsy revealed by automatic segmentation. Epilepsy Res 79: 130–138.

McKay DR, Knowles EEM, Winkler AAM et al. (2014). Influence of age, sex and genetic factors on the human brain. Brain Imaging Behav 8: 143–152.

Miller MI, Qiu A (2009). The emerging discipline of computational functional anatomy. Neuroimage 45: S16–S39.

Mori S, Crain BJ, Chacko VP et al. (1999). Three-dimensional tracking of axonal projections in the brain by magnetic resonance imaging. Ann Neurol 45: 265–269.

Patenaude B (2007). Bayesian Statistical Models of Shape and Appearance for Subcortical Brain Segmentation. University of Oxford, Oxford.

Poupon C, Mangin J, Clark CA et al. (2001). Towards inference of human brain connectivity from MR diffusion tensor data. Med Image Anal 5: 1–15.

Reuter M, Fischl B (2011). Avoiding asymmetry-induced bias in longitudinal image processing. Neuroimage 57: 19–21.

Roberts TPL, Liu F, Kassner A et al. (2005). Fiber density index correlates with reduced fractional anisotropy in white matter of patients with glioblastoma. AJNR Am J Neuroradiol 26: 2183–2186.

Roosendal S, Geurts J, Vrenken H et al. (2009). Regional DTI differences in multiple sclerosis patients. Neuroimage 44: 1397–1403.

Rosas HD, Liu AK, Hersch S et al. (2002). Regional and progressive thinning of the cortical ribbon in Huntington's disease. Neurology 58: 695–701.

Rowley J, Fonov V, Wu O et al. (2013). White matter abnormalities and structural hippocampal disconnections in amnestic mild cognitive impairment and Alzheimer's disease. PLoS One 8: e74776.

Sabuncu MR, Yeo BTT, Van Leemput K et al. (2010). A generative model for image segmentation based on label fusion. IEEE Trans Med Imaging 29: 1714–1729.

Salat DH, Buckner RL, Snyder AZ et al. (2004). Thinning of the cerebral cortex in aging. Cereb Cortex 14: 721–730.

Sandor T, Albert M, Stafford J et al. (1988). Use of computerized CT analysis to discriminate between Alzheimer patients and normal control subjects. AJNR Am J Neuroradiol 9: 1181–1187.

Sanfilipo MP, Benedict RHB, Zivadinov R et al. (2004). Correction for intracranial volume in analysis of whole brain atrophy in multiple sclerosis: the proportion vs. residual method. Neuroimage 22: 1732–1743.

Schilling S, DeStefano AL, Sachdev PS et al. (2013). APOE genotype and MRI markers of cerebrovascular disease: systematic review and meta-analysis. Neurology 81: 292–300.

Seeley WW, Crawford RK, Zhou J et al. (2009). Neurodegenerative diseases target large-scale human brain networks. Neuron 62: 42–52.

Setsompop K, Kimmlingen R, Eberlein E et al. (2013). Pushing the limits of in vivo diffusion MRI for the Human Connectome Project. Neuroimage 80: 220–233.

Shattuck DW, Leahy RM (2002). BrainSuite: an automated cortical surface identification tool. Med Image Anal 6: 129–142.

Sled JG, Zijdenbos AP, Evans AC (1998). A nonparametric method for automatic correction of intensity nonuniformity in MRI data. IEEE Trans Med Imaging 17: 87–97.

Smith SM, Jenkinson M, Woolrich MW et al. (2004). Advances in functional and structural MR image analysis and implementation as FSL. Neuroimage 23 (Suppl 1): S208–S219.

Song S-K, Sun S-W, Ju W-K et al. (2003). Diffusion tensor imaging detects and differentiates axon and myelin degeneration in mouse optic nerve after retinal ischemia. Neuroimage 20: 1714–1722.

Sowell ER, Peterson BS, Thompson PM et al. (2003). Mapping cortical change across the human life span. Nat Neurosci 6: 309–315.

Tanaka N, Liu H, Reinsberger C et al. (2013). Language lateralization represented by spatiotemporal mapping of magnetoencephalography. AJNR Am J Neuroradiol 34: 558–563.

Tuch DS (2004). Q-ball imaging. Magn Reson Med 52: 1358–1372.

Tuch DS, Reese TG, Wiegell MR et al. (2002). High angular resolution diffusion imaging reveals intravoxel white matter fiber heterogeneity. Magn Reson Med 48: 577–582.

van der Kouwe AJW, Benner T, Salat DH et al. (2008). Brain morphometry with multiecho MPRAGE. Neuroimage 40: 559–569.

Van Essen DC, Drury HA (1997). Structural and functional analyses of human cerebral cortex using a surface-based atlas. J Neurosci 17: 7079–7102.

Van Leemput K (2006). Probabilistic brain atlas encoding using Bayesian inference. Med Image Comput Comput Assist Interv 9: 704–711.

Van Leemput K, Maes F, Vandermeulen D et al. (1999). Automated model-based tissue classification of MR images of the brain. IEEE Trans Med Imaging 18: 897–908.

Van Leemput K, Maes F, Vandermeulen D et al. (2003). A unifying framework for partial volume segmentation of brain MR images. IEEE Trans Med Imaging 22: 105–119.

Van Leemput K, Bakkour A, Benner T et al. (2009). Automated segmentation of hippocampal subfields from ultra-high resolution in vivo MRI. Hippocampus 19: 549–557.

Vemuri P, Gunter JL, Senjem ML et al. (2008). Alzheimer's disease diagnosis in individual subjects using structural MR images: validation studies. Neuroimage 39: 1186–1197.

Walhovd KB, Fjell AM, Reinvang I et al. (2005). Effects of age on volumes of cortex, white matter and subcortical structures. Neurobiol Aging 26: 1261–1270. discussion 1275–1278.

Wedeen VJ, Hagmann P, Tseng W-YI et al. (2005). Mapping complex tissue architecture with diffusion spectrum magnetic resonance imaging. Magn Reson Med 54: 1377–1386.

Wedeen VJ, Wang RP, Schmahmann JD et al. (2008). Diffusion spectrum magnetic resonance imaging (DSI) tractography of crossing fibers. Neuroimage 41: 1267–1277.

Wedeen VJ, Rosene DL, Wang R et al. (2012). The geometric structure of the brain fiber pathways. Science 335: 1628–1634.

Wells WM, Grimson WL, Kikinis R et al. (1996). Adaptive segmentation of MRI data. IEEE Trans Med Imaging 15: 429–442.

Werring DJ, Clark CA, Barker GJ et al. (1999). Diffusion tensor imaging of lesions and normal-appearing white matter in multiple sclerosis. Neurology 52: 1626–1632.

Whitwell JL, Crum WR, Watt HC et al. (2001). Normalization of cerebral volumes by use of intracranial volume: implications for longitudinal quantitative MR imaging. AJNR Am J Neuroradiol 22: 1483–1489.

Wiggins GC, Triantafyllou C, Potthast A et al. (2006). 32-channel 3 Tesla receive-only phased-array head coil with soccer-ball element geometry. Magn Reson Med 56: 216–223.

Winkler AM, Kochunov P, Blangero J et al. (2010). Cortical thickness or grey matter volume? The importance of selecting the phenotype for imaging genetic studies. Neuroimage 53: 1135–1146.

Yendiki A, Panneck P, Srinivasan P et al. (2011). Automated probabilistic reconstruction of white-matter pathways in health and disease using an atlas of the underlying anatomy. Front Neuroinform 5: 23.

Yu P, Grant PE, Qi Y et al. (2007). Cortical surface shape analysis based on spherical wavelets. IEEE Trans Med Imaging 26: 582–597.

Zhang Y, Brady M, Smith S (2001). Segmentation of brain MR images through a hidden Markov random field model and the expectation-maximization algorithm. IEEE Trans Med Imaging 20: 45–57.

Zhang Y, Tartaglia MC, Schuff N et al. (2013). MRI signatures of brain macrostructural atrophy and microstructural degradation in frontotemporal lobar degeneration subtypes. J Alzheimers Dis 33: 431–444.

Handbook of Clinical Neurology, Vol. 135 (3rd series)
Neuroimaging, Part I
J.C. Masdeu and R.G. González, Editors

Chapter 4

Functional magnetic resonance imaging

BRADLEY R. BUCHBINDER*

Department of Radiology, Division of Neuroradiology, Massachusetts General Hospital, Harvard Medical School, Boston, MA, USA

Abstract

Functional magnetic resonance imaging (fMRI) maps the spatiotemporal distribution of neural activity in the brain under varying cognitive conditions. Since its inception in 1991, blood oxygen level-dependent (BOLD) fMRI has rapidly become a vital methodology in basic and applied neuroscience research. In the clinical realm, it has become an established tool for presurgical functional brain mapping. This chapter has three principal aims. First, we review key physiologic, biophysical, and methodologic principles that underlie BOLD fMRI, regardless of its particular area of application. These principles inform a nuanced interpretation of the BOLD fMRI signal, along with its neurophysiologic significance and pitfalls. Second, we illustrate the clinical application of task-based fMRI to presurgical motor, language, and memory mapping in patients with lesions near eloquent brain areas. Integration of BOLD fMRI and diffusion tensor white-matter tractography provides a road map for presurgical planning and intraoperative navigation that helps to maximize the extent of lesion resection while minimizing the risk of postoperative neurologic deficits. Finally, we highlight several basic principles of resting-state fMRI and its emerging translational clinical applications. Resting-state fMRI represents an important paradigm shift, focusing attention on functional connectivity within intrinsic cognitive networks.

INTRODUCTION

Functional neuroimaging techniques map the spatiotemporal distribution of neural activity under varying cognitive conditions. Among functional magnetic resonance methodologies, blood oxygen level-dependent (BOLD) functional magnetic resonance imaging (fMRI) is dominant. Since its discovery in 1992 (Kwong et al., 1992; Ogawa et al., 1992), BOLD fMRI has grown explosively, with myriad applications in the basic and clinical neurosciences (Rosen and Savoy, 2012). This chapter briefly reviews physiologic, biophysical, and methodologic principles that underlie these applications, and briefly illustrates its most prevalent clinical role, presurgical brain mapping.

PHYSIOLOGIC PRINCIPLES UNDERLYING BOLD fMRI

Metabolic and hemodynamic signals are surrogates for neural activity

Functional neuroimaging techniques, such as BOLD fMRI, [^{18}F]fluorodeoxyglucose positron emission tomography (FDG-PET), and [^{15}O]H_2O-PET reflect neural activity indirectly, through associated colocalizing metabolic and hemodynamic parameters, including the cerebral metabolic rate of oxygen consumption ($CMRO_2$), cerebral metabolic rate of glucose consumption (CMRGlc), cerebral blood flow (CBF), and cerebral blood volume (CBV). BOLD fMRI, in particular, reflects interplay

*Correspondence to: Bradley R. Buchbinder, MD, Director, Clinical Functional Magnetic Resonance Imaging, Division of Neuroradiology, Massachusetts General Hospital; Assistant Professor of Radiology, Harvard Medical School, Gray 2, 55 Fruit Street, Boston MA 02114, USA. Tel: +1-617-726-8320, Fax: +1-617-724-3338, E-mail: BBUCHBINDER@mgh.harvard.edu

between neural activity, $CMRO_2$, CBF, and CBV. The neurophysiologic and biophysical origins of the coupling between neural activity, metabolism, and blood flow critically inform the genesis, significance, and interpretation of the BOLD fMRI signal.

Neurometabolic and neurovascular coupling

Synaptic activity dominantly drives signaling-related energy metabolism

Functional neuroimaging has often been assumed to reflect the regional intensity of action potentials (APs) (Raichle and Mintun, 2006). However, APs only represent the output of the postsynaptic neuron, while excitatory and inhibitory postsynaptic potentials (EPSPs, IPSPs) represent its input. The relative contributions of the input synaptic activity and output spike activity to functional neuroimaging signals are important to their meaningful interpretation.

The relative energies consumed by postsynaptic potentials and APs inform their contributions to functional neuroimaging signals. Most signaling-related energy (91%) is expended by Na^+/K^+ ATPase to restore transmembrane ion gradients, which are dissipated by excitatory, primarily glutamatergic, synaptic signaling and to maintain the resting potential (Attwell and Laughlin, 2001; Howarth et al., 2012). Processes related to neurotransmitter release, recycling, and vesicular repackaging account for the remaining 9%. Inhibitory synaptic activity, most commonly mediated by γ-aminobutyric acid (GABA), consumes negligible energy itself. Of the signaling-related energy expenditures, EPSPs account for 50%, APs for 21%, the resting potential for 20%, presynaptic glutamate release for 5%, and glutamate recycling for 4%. Thus, compared with output spike activity (21%), excitatory input synaptic activity accounts for the majority (59%) of cortical signaling-related energy expenditure.

Classic model: neural activity is linearly coupled to CMRGlc, $CMRO_2$, and CBF

Adenosine triphosphate (ATP) demand is proportional to combined synaptic activity and spike activity, dominated by synaptic activity. ATP is generated from glucose through glycolysis, the tricarboxylic acid (TCA) cycle, and the electron transport chain. Glycolysis converts 1 molecule of glucose to 2 pyruvate, yielding 2 ATP. Under most aerobic conditions, pyruvate enters the TCA cycle and is oxidized through the electron transport chain, yielding approximately 30 additional ATP (Hertz et al., 2007; Berg et al., 2012). Under anaerobic conditions, lactate dehydrogenase (LDH) converts pyruvate to lactate. Thus, complete oxidation of glucose, in the net reaction $C_6H_{12}O_6 + 6O_2 \rightarrow 6CO_2 + 6H_2O$, yields approximately 32 ATP while glycolysis alone yields only 2 ATP. Since glucose oxidation is so much more efficient than glycolysis alone, it is expected to supply the vast majority of ATP required to fuel the Na^+/K^+ pump. Therefore, it is reasonable to hypothesize that neural activity is linearly coupled to both $CMRO_2$ and CMRGlc in the fixed stoichiometric ratio of 6:1, characterized by a constant oxygen-glucose index (OGI) of 6, where $OGI = CMRO_2/CMRGlc$. Moreover, the classic model predicts that CBF is also linearly coupled to $CMRO_2$ and CMRGlc, since it supplies both of these substrates to the brain. Linear coupling between CBF and $CMRO_2$ is also characterized by a ratio: the oxygen extraction fraction (OEF). OEF is the fraction of oxygen extracted from the capillaries per unit time per unit volume (or mass). It is equal to the ratio of the rate of oxygen consumption to the rate of oxygen delivery. The rate of oxygen delivery is $CBF \cdot [O_2]_{art}$, where $[O_2]_{art}$ is the arterial oxygen concentration. So,

$$OEF = \frac{CMRO_2}{CBF \cdot [O_2]_{art}}.$$

Since $[O_2]_{art}$ can be considered constant, linear coupling between CBF and $CMRO_2$ is characterized by a constant OEF (typically about 40%). In summary, the classic model predicts that neural activity, dominantly excitatory synaptic activity, is linearly coupled to $CMRO_2$, CMRGlc, and CBF, characterized by a constant OGI = 6, and a constant OEF.

Experiment: at rest neural activity is linearly coupled to $CMRO_2$, CMRGlc, and CBF

Indeed, in the awake, resting state, $CMRO_2$, CMRGlc, and CBF vary regionally, but they are locally coupled, and paired measurements in different brain regions are linearly correlated (Raichle et al., 1976; Baron et al., 1984). Also, as predicted, OEF and OGI are nearly uniform across the brain, and OGI is near 6. Average reported values are in the range of 5.3 (Raichle and Mintun, 2006). The fact that OGI is not exactly 6 indicates that a small fraction of glucose is not oxidized at rest, and is diverted to biosynthetic or other less energy-productive pathways that will be considered below.

A feedback model has long been hypothesized to coordinate CBF with neural activity and its metabolic demand (Roy and Sherrington, 1890; Attwell et al., 2010): neural activity consumes oxygen and glucose in proportion to its energy demand. In turn, CBF increases to supply the metabolic substrates glucose and oxygen, and to remove metabolic byproducts, such as CO_2 and lactate. In this model, substrate depletion and metabolite excess increase CBF, maintaining a balance between metabolic supply and demand (Fig. 4.1A).

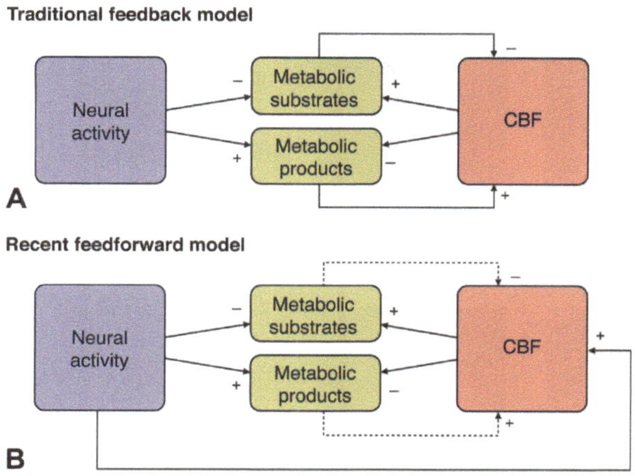

Fig. 4.1. A feedforward model has replaced the traditional feedback model for regulation of blood flow and metabolism during neural activation. (**A**) Traditional feedback model: neural activity consumes energy to restore ion gradients and neurotransmitters. Depletion of metabolic substrates (O_2, glucose, adenosine triphosphate) and accumulation of metabolic products (CO_2, lactate, H^+) drives increased cerebral blood flow (CBF). Increased flow supplies metabolic substrates and removes metabolic waste, maintaining a metabolic steady state through a negative-feedback loop. (**B**) Feedforward model supported by recent evidence: neural activity directly drives CBF in parallel with metabolism (solid lines). Metabolic substrates (O_2, adenosine) and products (CO_2, lactate, H^+) modulate CBF but are not the primary drivers of functional hyperemia (interrupted lines).

Experiment: with activation, neural activity is nonlinearly coupled to CMRGlc and CBF, but nearly linearly coupled to $CMRO_2$

Given the documented linear coupling between blood flow and metabolism at rest, it was long suspected that linear coupling would also characterize focal neural activation. However, seminal PET experiments measuring local changes in $CMRO_2$, CMRGlc, and CBF during vibrotactile stimulation (Fox and Raichle, 1986) and visual stimulation (Fox et al., 1988) challenged this assumption. If linear coupling between $CMRO_2$, CMRGlc, and CBF were to hold during activation, as it does at rest, their relative (percent) changes would be equivalent: a 5% rise in $CMRO_2$ would be coupled to a 5% rise in both CMRGlc and CBF. However, vibrotactile stimulation augmented CBF by 29% but $CMRO_2$ only by 5%; similarly, visual stimulation augmented CBF and CMRGlc by approximately 50%, but $CMRO_2$ also only by 5% (Fig. 4.2). Therefore, focal activation induces nonlinear coupling between $CMRO_2$ and CMRGlc, characterized by a disproportionate rise in CMRGlc relative to the rise in $CMRO_2$, and a decrease in OGI. Likewise, focal activation induces nonlinear coupling between $CMRO_2$ and CBF, characterized by a disproportionate rise in CBF relative to the rise in $CMRO_2$, and a decrease in OEF. Fox, Raichle, and colleagues called this shift from linear to nonlinear coupling physiologic "uncoupling" between blood flow, glucose consumption, and the demand for oxidative energy production (Fox and Raichle, 1986; Fox et al., 1988).

The key question is: what do these changes in metabolism and blood flow say about the change in underlying neural activity? ATP demand is the link between $CMRO_2$, CMRGlc, and neural activity. The decline in OGI indicates that much more glucose is consumed than can be accounted for by oxidative metabolism. Among the other possible metabolic fates for glucose, Fox, Raichle, and colleagues reasoned that most would go to glycolysis and lactate production, while some might go to glycogen synthesis; they did not consider other biosynthetic pathways (Fox et al., 1988). In this setting, glycolysis is often called aerobic glycolysis, since the shift away from oxidative phosphorylation is driven by factors other than oxygen debt (Raichle and Mintun, 2006). While their experiments did not determine the exact metabolic pathways behind the decline in OGI, a simplified model indicates its essential significance. Assume that: (1) the baseline OGI is 6; (2) activation causes CMRGlc and $CMRO_2$ to increase by 50% and 5% respectively; (3) all nonoxidative glucose consumption in the activated state goes entirely to glycolysis and lactate production; and (4) the lactate is not further metabolized. With these assumptions, activation reduces the OGI from 6 to 4.2, and 90% of the increase in glucose consumption is glycolytic. Despite this large rise in glucose consumption, ATP production increases by only 8%, since the ATP yield from glycolysis is so low. It is tempting to conclude that glycolysis supplies most of the relatively small amount of activation-induced energy demand, in contrast to oxidative phosphorylation, which supplies most of the energy required by the resting state. However, oxidative phosphorylation still accounts for 64% of the increased rate of ATP production in this example, since it generates ATP 16 times more efficiently than glycolysis. Since the 50% change in CMRGlc is markedly greater than the 8% change in ATP production, CMRGlc has strongly nonlinear coupling to neural activity. In contrast, since the 5% change in $CMRO_2$ is close to the 8% change in ATP, $CMRO_2$ has closer to linear coupling in this example. Subsequent studies have repeatedly confirmed a disproportionate rise in CMRGlc relative to $CMRO_2$, but with a smaller difference between them, implying that most of the increased ATP production during neural activation is due to oxidative phosphorylation (Attwell et al., 2010; Lin et al., 2010). This simplified model captures an essential prediction regarding the difference between $CMRO_2$, on the one hand, and CMRGlc and CBF, on the other, as neurometabolic and neurovascular signals: neural activation should be nonlinearly coupled to CMRGlc

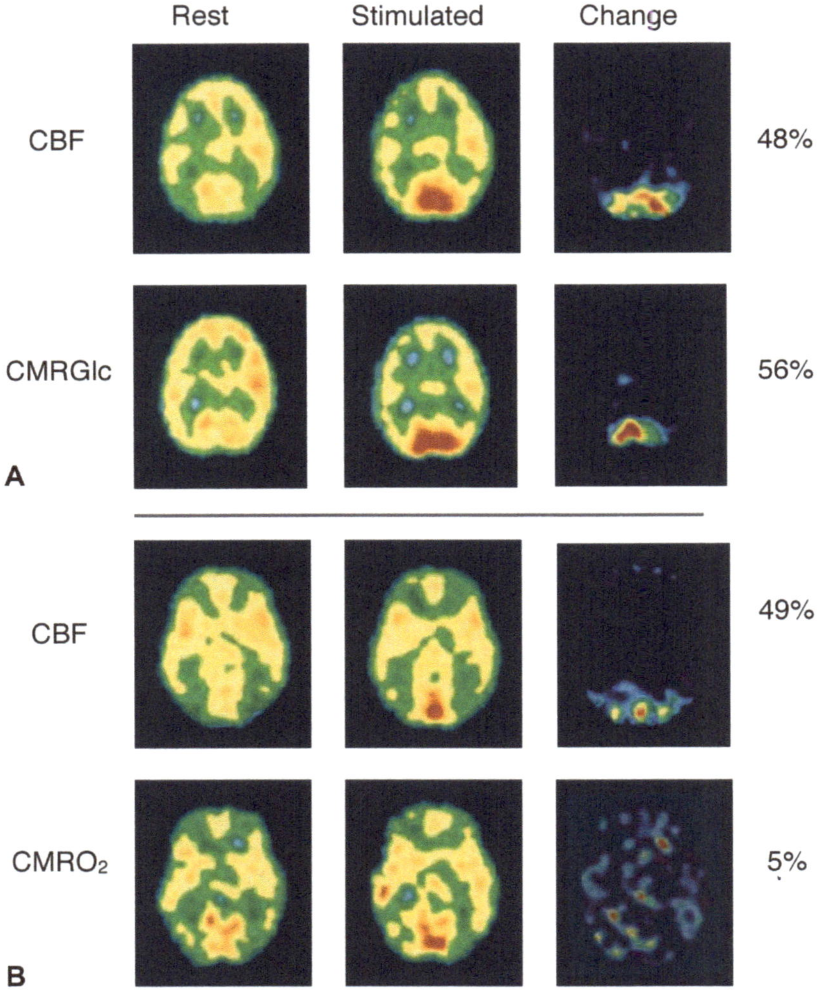

Fig. 4.2. Cerebral metabolic rate of glucose consumption (CMRGlc) and cerebral blood flow (CBF) couple nonlinearly with cerebral metabolic rate of oxygen consumption ($CMRO_2$) during visual stimulation in human subjects. (**A**) Simultaneous measurements of CBF and CMRGlc using positron emission tomography (PET): CBF and CMRGlc both increased by approximately 50% in visual cortex. (**B**) Simultaneous measurements of CBF and $CMRO_2$: CBF increased by approximately 50% but $CMRO_2$ increased only by 5% in visual cortex. (Modified from Fox et al., 1988, with permission from American Association for the Advancement of Science.)

and CBF, but it should be at least approximately linearly coupled to $CMRO_2$.

Indeed, recent *in vivo* experimental evidence strongly supports linear coupling between neural activity and $CMRO_2$ (Sheth et al., 2004; Offenhauser et al., 2005; Mathiesen et al., 2011) (Fig. 4.3A). While these experiments could not distinguish the individual contributions of EPSPs and APs to $CMRO_2$, *in vivo* ^{13}C nuclear magnetic resonance (NMR) measurements have consistently demonstrated a linear correlation between the cerebral metabolic rate of oxidative glucose consumption (CMRglc-ox) and the rate of glutamate recycling (Sibson et al., 2001; Hyder et al., 2006) (Fig. 4.3B). Since CMRglc-ox is directly proportional to $CMRO_2$ and the rate of glutamate recycling is directly proportional to synaptic glutamate release, these results further suggest that $CMRO_2$ is linearly coupled to glutamatergic synaptic activity, as predicted by the energy budget analysis. Similarly, recent *in vivo* experiments have also confirmed generally nonlinear coupling between synaptic activity and CBF (Hoffmeyer et al., 2007; Enager et al., 2009) (Fig. 4.3C). In summary, $CMRO_2$ is approximately proportional to synaptic activity, while CBF and CMRGlc are related to synaptic activity in a more complex way.

The results of Fox, Raichle, and colleagues have two additional broad implications. First, since blood flow and glucose consumption increased much more than the demand for ATP, neurometabolic and neurovascular coupling must be regulated by factors other than

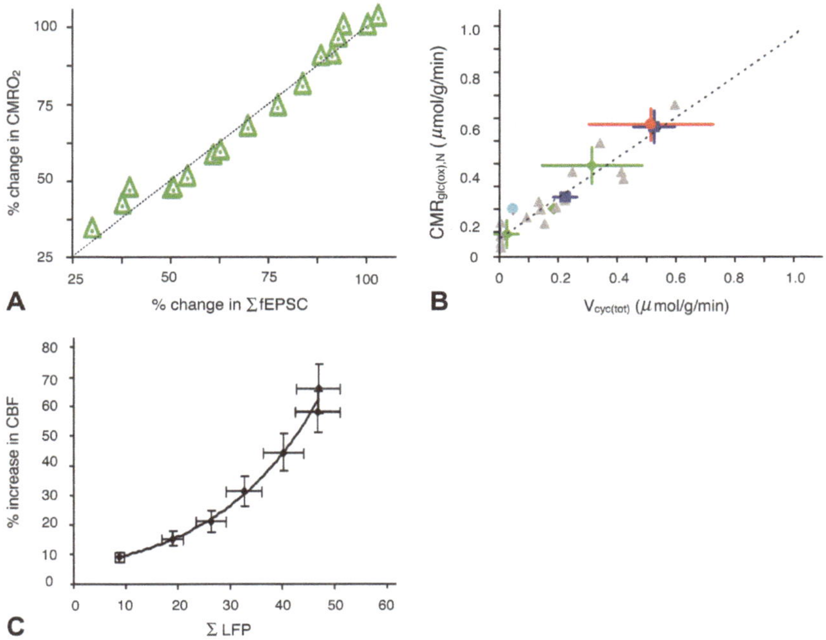

Fig. 4.3. Synaptic activity is linearly coupled to cerebral metabolic rate of oxygen consumption ($CMRO_2$), but nonlinearly coupled to cerebral blood flow (CBF). (**A**) Percent change in $CMRO_2$ vs percent change in mouse Purkinje cell (PC) synaptic activity in response to electric stimulation of the climbing fiber pathway. Synaptic activity was estimated by the field (i.e., extracellular) excitatory postsynaptic current (fEPSC). The total synaptic activity during the stimulation period was estimated by the summed fESPCs (ΣfESPC), equal to the fESPC amplitude per stimulus × stimulation frequency × duration of stimulation train, which is proportional to the total transmembrane Na^+ flux into PCs during the stimulation period. Local fEPSPCs were recorded by a microelectrode. Local $CMRO_2$ was computed from local tissue po_2 and local CBF, measured by oxygen microelectrode and laser Doppler flowmetry, respectively. The slope of the graph is approximately 1, indicating that $CMRO_2$ is directly proportional to synaptic activity. (Modified from Mathiesen et al., 2011, with permission from the Society for Neuroscience.) (**B**) Rate of neuronal oxidative glucose consumption ($CMR_{glc(ox),\ N}$) vs rate of total glutamate-glutamine neurotransmitter recycling ($V_{cyc(tot)}$) in rat brain, measured by ^{13}C magnetic resonance spectroscopy. The graph combines the results of five studies, detailed in Hyder et al. (2006), from which it is reproduced, with permission. Astrocytes take up glutamate from the perisynaptic zone and recycle it to neurons through glutamine. Above a basal metabolic rate, represented by the *y*-axis intercept, the rate of glutamate-glutamine recycling is proportional to the rate of synaptic glutamate release, and hence, synaptic activity. (**C**) Percent increase in CBF vs synaptic activity in rat primary somatosensory cortex due to electric stimulation of the homologous contralateral sensory cortex, mediated by a transcallosal corticocortical pathway. Synaptic activity is estimated by local field (i.e. extracellular) potentials (LFPs). The total synaptic activity during the stimulation period is estimated by the summed LFPs (ΣLFP), equal to the LFP amplitude × stimulation frequency × duration of stimulation train. LFPs were measured by a microelectrode while local CBF was measured by laser Doppler flowmetry. The nonlinear relationship between CBF and synaptic activity was best fit by an exponential. (Reproduced from Hoffmeyer et al., 2007, with permission.)

energy demand, arguing against the traditionally postulated negative-feedback, substrate-sensing mechanism. Multiple additional lines of evidence substantiate the argument against the traditional feedback model, by demonstrating experimentally induced dissociations between glucose availability, oxygen availability, and blood flow (Powers et al., 1996; Cholet et al., 1997; Wolf et al., 1997; Mintun et al., 2001; Lindauer et al., 2010). Together, these physiologic and experimental dissociations support a feedforward model, in which neural activity drives metabolism and blood flow in parallel (Fig. 4.1B) (Attwell et al., 2010).

Second, these observations form the physiologic basis for BOLD fMRI. The BOLD signal arises from linear coupling of neural activity to $CMRO_2$ combined with nonlinear coupling to CBF. Since focal neural activity augments CBF in excess of $CMRO_2$, the rate of oxygen delivery to activated cortex exceeds its rate of consumption, resulting in locally increased capillary-venous oxygen saturation, and, therefore, an increased ratio of oxygenated to deoxygenated hemoglobin. Diamagnetic oxyhemoglobin (oxy-Hb) negligibly affects the magnetic resonance (MR) signal, while paramagnetic deoxyhemoglobin (dHb) strongly attenuates it. Thus, the activity-induced increase in oxy-Hb / dHb ratio augments the MR signal, constituting the BOLD response.

Cortical architecture supports neurometabolic and neurovascular coupling

Cortical architecture is exquisitely adapted to coordinate local neural activity, metabolism, and blood flow. While highly heterogeneous, neuronal and synaptic density, mitochondrial density, and capillary density are locally correlated (Dunning and Wolff, 1937; Klein et al., 1986; Iadecola and Nedergaard, 2007). Examples include correlations within cortical layers, within functional cortical modules, and at cytoarchitectonic boundaries (Duvernoy et al., 1981; Humphrey and Hendrickson, 1983; Klein et al., 1986; Zheng et al., 1991; Woolsey et al., 1996; Iadecola and Nedergaard, 2007). Moreover, it has been recently recognized that astrocytes play a critical role in neurometabolic and neurovascular coupling: they cooperatively interact with neurons and blood vessels in the neurogliovascular unit (Iadecola and Nedergaard, 2007). Protoplasmic gray-matter astrocytes have fine perisynaptic processes that closely appose synapses, and they have larger vascular processes (endfeet) that closely appose vessels. The perisynaptic and endfoot processes envelop nearly all synapses and vessels. The astrocytes parcellate the neuropil into highly organized, largely nonoverlapping, roughly polyhedral spatial domains (Bushong et al., 2002; Nedergaard et al., 2003). Each astrocyte, along with its associated synapses and vessels, forms a neurogliovascular unit (Fig. 4.4). Each astrocytic domain encompasses on the order of 4 neuronal soma, 300–600 dendrites, and 140 000 synapses (Bushong et al., 2002; Halassa et al., 2007). In addition, gap junctions interconnect the astrocytic domains, forming an astroglial network or syncytium (Escartin and Rouach, 2013). The gap junctions exchange small molecules, including ions, second messengers, neurotransmitters, and energy metabolites. The astrocytic domain represents a bridge between synapses and vessels, which is well tailored to coordinate local synaptic, metabolic, and hemodynamic function (Iadecola and Nedergaard, 2007). In this fashion, the neurogliovascular unit plays an important role in the genesis of neurometabolic and neurovascular signals, including BOLD fMRI.

Mechanisms for neurometabolic coupling

Cooperative interactions between neurons and astrocytes couple neural activity to metabolism within the neurogliovascular unit (Barros and Deitmer, 2010; Bélanger et al., 2011; Bouzier-Sore and Pellerin, 2013). These interactions undergird the shifts in oxidative and glycolytic energy metabolism that characterize neural activation, and in turn, the decline in OGI. The conventional metabolic model predicts that neurons and astrocytes take up glucose in proportion to their individual energy demands (Barros and Deitmer, 2010). Since restoration of ion gradients after their dissipation by postsynaptic currents accounts for the great majority of ATP consumption, neuronal energy demand dwarfs that of astrocytes (80–95%) (Nehlig et al., 2004). Hence, the conventional model predicts that neuronal glucose uptake should far exceed that of astrocytes, especially with increasing neural activity (Attwell and Laughlin, 2001; Howarth et al., 2012). However, even in the resting awake (rat) brain, astrocytic and neuronal glucose uptake are approximately equal (Nehlig et al., 2004; Chuquet et al., 2010). Therefore, astrocytic glucose uptake appears excessive while neuronal uptake appears insufficient, relative to their individual energy demands. An alternative model could resolve this paradox: The apparently excessive glucose uptake in astrocytes could be explained by a preferentially activated glycolytic pathway and inhibited oxidative pathway. Since the glycolytic ATP yield is 16 times lower than the oxidative yield, the astrocyte would consume much more glucose to meet its ATP demand. Due to inhibition of the oxidative pathway, pyruvate would be diverted from the TCA cycle, and instead be converted to lactate by LDH. Conversely, the apparently deficient glucose uptake in neurons could be explained by a preferentially inhibited glycolytic pathway and activated oxidative pathway, combined with an astrocyte-neuron lactate shuttle (ANLSH) (Pellerin and Magistretti, 1994; Bélanger et al., 2011) (Fig. 4.5). This model hypothesizes that astrocytes export lactate to neurons, where it augments glucose as a substrate for oxidation. In the neuron, lactate is converted to pyruvate by LDH, and thereby enters the activated TCA cycle. Thus, the net effect of the ANLSH is preferential compartmentation of glycolysis in astrocytes and oxidation in neurons, with lactate serving as a metabolic intermediate. This model could explain disproportionate astrocytic glucose uptake relative to neuronal glucose uptake, while yielding large quantities of ATP in neurons and small quantities in astrocytes, appropriate to their energy needs.

Synaptic activation further modulates the complementary metabolic cooperation between neurons and astrocytes. Briefly, synaptic K^+ and glutamate release stimulate astrocytic glycolysis (Bittner et al., 2011; Ruminot et al., 2011) while glutamate simultaneously stimulates glucose uptake (Loaiza et al., 2003). The resulting bolus of astrocytic lactate is shuttled to neurons in the neurogliovascular unit, where it is oxidized to meet neuronal ATP demand. Thus, in this model, synaptic activity drives metabolism in a feedforward fashion through the ANLS.

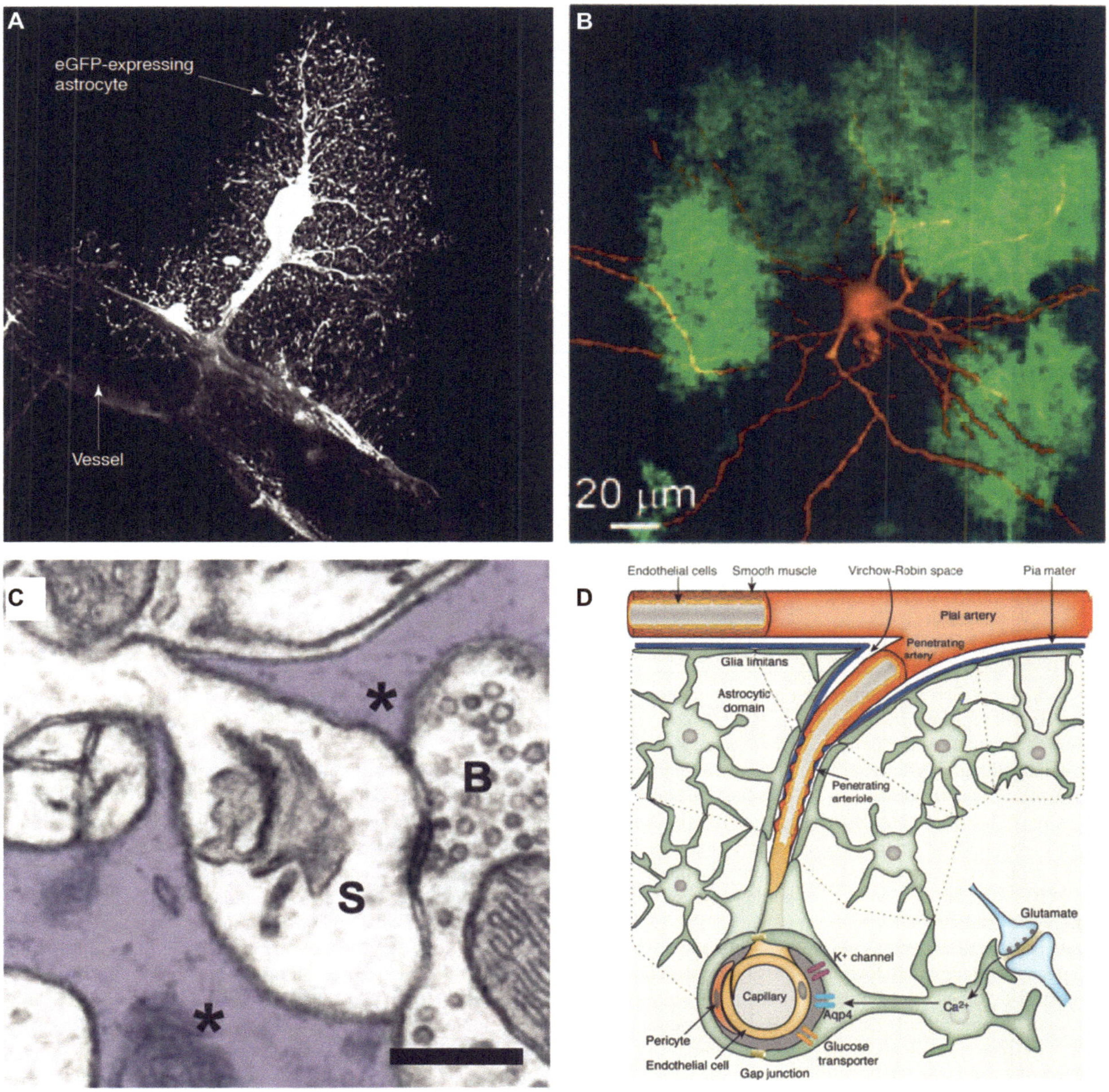

Fig. 4.4. The neurogliovascular unit. (**A**). Two-photon confocal imaging of a single astrocyte expressing enhanced green-fluorescent protein (eGFP) within a cortical slice. Dense perisynaptic processes suffuse a three-dimensional polyhedral shape. An endfoot process invests a small vessel. (Reproduced from Nedergaard et al., 2003.) (**B**) Two-photon confocal imaging of a cortical slice. Nonoverlapping astrocytic domains (green dye) ensheath different dendrites from a single neuron (red dye). (Reproduced from Halassa et al., 2007, with permission from the Society for Neuroscience.) (**C**) Electron micrograph. Perisynaptic astrocytic processes (blue, asterisk) enwrap a synapse, formed by an axonal terminal bouton (B) and a dendritic spine (S). (Reproduced from Genoud et al., 2006.) (**D**) Schematic diagram illustrating the overall architecture of the neurogliovascular unit. Perisynaptic astrocytic processes invest synapses, while endfoot processes invest penetrating arterioles and capillaries. Nonoverlapping polygonal astrocytic microdomains integrate local neuronal activity, mediating functional neurometabolic and neurovascular coupling. Aqp4, aquaporin 4. (Reproduced from Iadecola and Nedergaard, 2007, with permission.)

Recent evidence elucidates mechanisms that may promote aerobic glycolysis in astrocytes and lactate oxidation in neurons via the ANLS. Central to the model are cell type-specific expression patterns of key genes that regulate bioenergetic pathways, endowing astrocytes and neurons with complementary metabolic profiles (Bélanger et al., 2011). However, important issues remain open, including the physiologic benefits of this

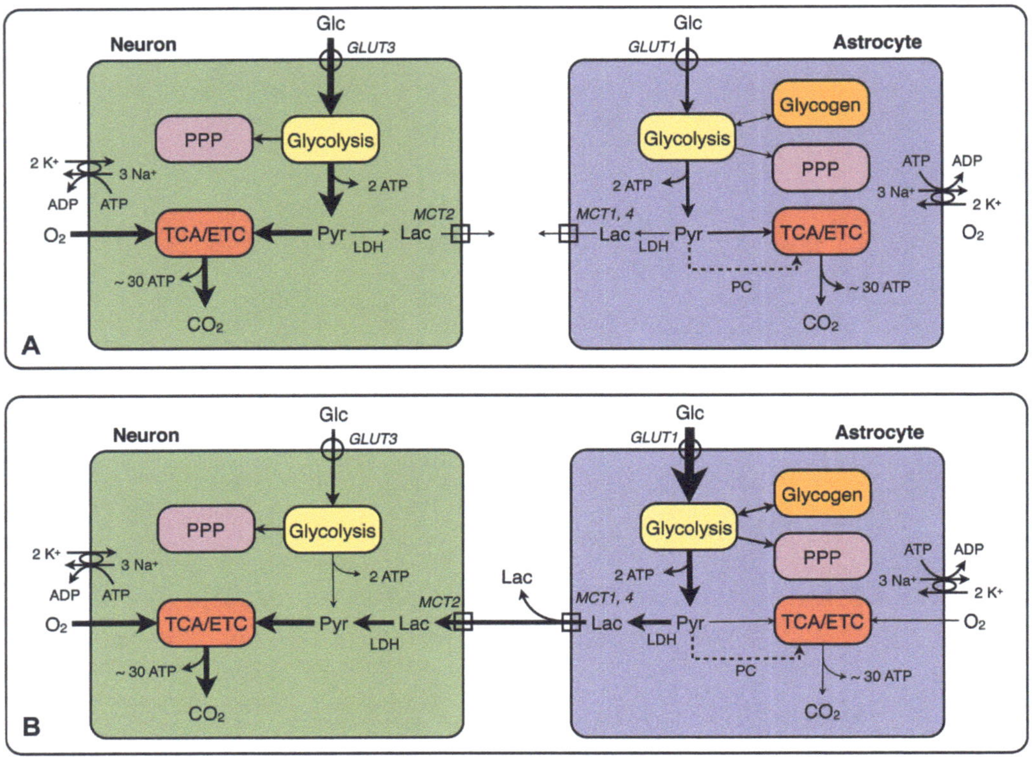

Fig. 4.5. Simplified mechanisms for neurometabolic coupling. (**A**) Conventional model: glucose (Glc) enters neurons and astrocytes via cell type-specific transporters (GLUTs) in proportion to adenosine triphosphate (ATP) demand. Therefore glucose consumption is much greater in neurons than astrocytes. In both cell types, most glucose is consumed by oxidative phosphorylation through the tricarboxylic acid (TCA) cycle and electron transport chain (ETC), with minimal conversion of pyruvate (Pyr) to lactate (Lac), efficiently generating ATP to fuel the Na^+/K^+ pump. Some glucose equivalents are diverted to the pentose phosphate pathway (PPP), where NADPH is generated for biosynthesis and detoxification of reactive oxygen species. Astrocytes, but not neurons, divert some glucose to glycogen formation and to anaplerosis via pyruvate carboxylase (PC). Despite its pedagogic simplicity, evidence argues against the conventional model, as discussed in the text. (Thicker (thinner) arrows indicate larger (smaller) flux.) (**B**) Astrocyte-neuron lactate shuttle (ANLS) model: while controversial, this model has accumulated considerable support from recent studies. Astrocytes upregulate aerobic glycolysis and downregulate oxidative phosphorylation. Abundant astrocytic lactate is shuttled to neurons via cell type-specific monocarboxylate transporters (MCTs). Conversely, neurons upregulate oxidative phosphorylation and downregulate glycolysis, consuming lactate over glucose. As a result of this metabolic compartmentation, most oxidative metabolism still occurs in neurons but most glucose is consumed by astrocytes. Despite the high rate of astrocytic aerobic glycolysis, most ATP is still produced by oxidative metabolism, both at rest and during neural activation. Diversion of glucose equivalents to the glycogen shunt, PPP, and lactate efflux (to the circulation and astrocytic syncytium), lowers the oxygen-glucose index (OGI) below its theoretical maximum of 6. The effect of synaptic glutamate on these pathways is discussed in the text, but is not illustrated here.

more complex arrangement and the origins of the activation-induced decline in OGI. Decline in the OGI indicates that some glucose is consumed but not oxidized within the activated region. Two likely contributors are efflux of lactate and activation of the glycogen pathway (Hertz et al., 2007). Instead of shuttling to neurons, some lactate is lost to the venous circulation and some spreads away from the active zone through gap junctions in the astrocytic syncytium, though its ultimate metabolic fate remains uncertain (Hertz et al., 2007; Barros, 2013; Escartin and Rouach, 2013). The net effect is that egress of nonoxidized lactate from the active zone lowers the OGI. Shunting of glucose through glycogen reduces the net glycolytic ATP yield by half, requiring twice the glucose uptake to maintain the same glycolytic ATP flux. This also increases lactate production, some of which may shuttle to neurons, but the remainder of which is lost to the circulation or astrocytic syncytium. Glucose consumption in biosynthetic pathways that have reduced or no oxidation potential also lowers the OGI, including the pentose phosphate and anaplerotic pathways.

Finally, the mechanisms coupling neural activity with cellular metabolism are complex. While much *in vitro*, *ex vivo*, and *in vivo* data has accumulated to support the ANLSH, it has engendered spirited debate and alternative models (Chih and Roberts, 2003; Dienel and Cruz, 2004; Simpson et al., 2007; Mangia et al.,

2009; Figley, 2011). Further investigation is necessary to resolve open questions.

Mechanisms for neurovascular coupling

Contradicting the classic metabolic feedback control hypothesis, a feedforward control mechanism mediates localized activity-induced increases in CBF, often called functional hyperemia: synaptic glutamate drives functional hyperemia via signaling pathways through neurons and astrocytes within the neurogliovascular unit (Attwell et al., 2010). This arrangement represents a paradigm shift in the physiology of functional neuroimaging. It undergirds the generally nonlinear coupling between CBF and neural activity, which forms the fundamental basis for the BOLD signal.

The astrocytic pathway couples synaptic activity to arteriolar dilation through a mechanism that involves glutamate, Ca^{2+}, K^+, and arachidonic acid derivatives. During synaptic activity, glutamate diffuses from the synaptic cleft to bordering astrocytes, and activates metabotropic glutamate receptors (mGluR), opening Ca^{2+} channels, increasing intracellular Ca^{2+} concentration ($[Ca^{2+}]i$), and triggering a cascade of events leading to the release of vasodilators from the astrocytic endfeet: K^+ and two classes of arachidonic acid derivates: prostaglandins (especially PGE_2) and epoxyeicosatrienoic acids (EETs) (Zonta et al., 2003; Filosa et al., 2006; Takano et al., 2006; Wang et al., 2006; Attwell et al., 2010) (Fig. 4.6).

The neuronal pathway couples synaptic activity to arteriolar dilation through a mechanism that involves Ca^{2+}, nitric oxide (NO), and prostaglandins. Synaptic glutamate activates postsynaptic ionotropic *N*-methyl-D-aspartate (NMDA) receptors, triggering an influx of Ca^{2+}, increasing $[Ca^{2+}]_i$, and triggering the release of vasodilators into the perivascular space: NO and prostaglandins (especially PGE_2) (Attwell et al., 2010). In cerebellar cortex, NO appears to be the main mediator of functional hyperemia (Akgören et al., 1996; Yang et al., 2003), while in cerebral cortex, it appears to play a more modulatory role (Lindauer et al., 1999) (Fig. 4.6).

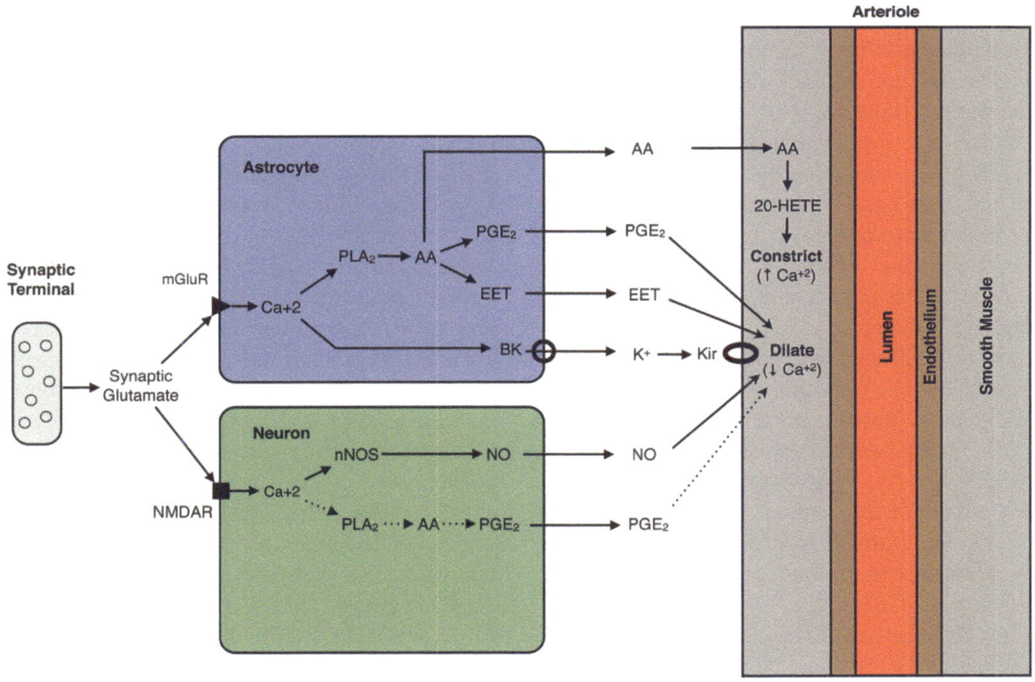

Fig. 4.6. Mechanisms for neurovascular coupling. Synaptic glutamate couples neural activity to cerebral blood flow, mediated by astrocytes and neurons within the neurogliovascular unit. In the astrocyte, glutamate activates metabotropic glutamate receptors (mGluR), raising $[Ca^{2+}]_i$, and triggering a cascade of events that ultimately releases vasoactive molecules from the astrocyte endfoot. Ca^{2+} activates phospholipase A_2 (PLA_2), which cleaves arachidonic acid (AA) from membrane-bound phospholipids. Prostaglandins, particularly PGE_2, are produced from AA via the cyclooxygenase (COX) pathway, while epoxyeicosatrienoic acids (EETs) are produced via the cytochrome P450 pathway. PGE_2 and EETs relax vascular smooth muscle, resulting in vasodilation. Ca^{2+}-activated potassium channels (BK) release K^+, which acts on smooth-muscle cell inward-rectifying K^+ channels (Kir), also leading to vasodilation. Under some conditions, AA is converted to 20-hydroxyeicosatetraenoic acid (20-HETE) in vascular smooth-muscle cells, resulting in vasoconstriction. Synaptic glutamate also activates neuronal *N*-methyl-D-aspartate receptors (NMDAR), increasing $[Ca^{2+}]_i$, triggering production and release of the vasodilator nitric oxide (NO), via neuronal nitric oxide synthase (nNOS). Ca^{2+} may also trigger production of PGE_2 in neurons. (Modified after Attwell et al., 2010, with permission.)

Additional factors modulate neurovascular coupling and/or the baseline CBF, including but not limited to the following:

1. The relative contributions between the astrocytic and neuronal signaling pathways modulate the vascular response to synaptic input; they vary between brain regions and even between different cell populations within the same region (Enager et al., 2009).
2. Metabolites, including oxygen, CO_2/H^+, adenosine, and lactate, may modulate neurovascular coupling, even if they are not the primary mediators (Iadecola and Nedergaard, 2007). Thus, lactate, in particular, may play complementary roles as metabolite in neurometabolic coupling and as a signaling molecule in neurovascular coupling.
3. Local inhibitory interneurons may be vasodilating or vasoconstricting (Cauli et al., 2004; Rancillac et al., 2006) and contribute to integration of local vascular responses (Drake and Iadecola, 2007).
4. Local arteriolar vasodilation is accompanied by graded dilation of larger upstream arterioles, which may serve to match proximal supply to distal demand, and mitigate vascular steal by activated cortex (Iadecola et al., 1997; Buxton, 2009).
5. Central pathways arising from the brainstem (raphe nuclei, locus coeruleus, ventral tegmental area) or basal forebrain (nucleus basalis) terminate near cortical microvessels and exert direct neuronal control on arteriolar dilation at distant sites (Drake and Iadecola, 2007).

In summary, synaptic activity drives functional hyperemia by feedforward signaling pathways through the neurogliovascular unit. Synaptic glutamate activates Ca^{2+} waves in postsynaptic neurons and perisynaptic astrocytes, promoting release of vasodilators, including K^+, PGE_2, EETs, and NO. Astrocytes integrate synaptic activity within their microdomains and orchestrate the local hemodynamic response. Additional local, regional, and central processes modulate the coupling between synaptic activity and CBF.

These complex feedforward mechanisms underlie the variable, and generally nonlinear coupling between synaptic activity and CBF (Lauritzen, 2001; Devor et al., 2003; Sheth et al., 2004). Nevertheless, they do not specifically explain the disproportionate activation-induced rise in CBF relative to $CMRO_2$ that is the *sine qua non* of BOLD fMRI. Although the underlying mechanism has been elusive, recent evidence suggests that the consequent rise in microvascular oxygenation is necessary to maintain adequate oxygen levels at tissue locations furthest from the feeding vessels (in between them), where baseline po_2 is low due to fall-off of diffusive oxygen delivery (Devor et al., 2011; Kasischke et al., 2011). These locations are most vulnerable to hypoxia during periods of sustained and/or intense neural activity. Increasing vascular po_2 drives oxygen diffusion to these sites of low tissue po_2. Thus, it is suggested that the disproportionate rise in CBF relative to $CMRO_2$ has been calibrated by evolution to ensure that these most vulnerable neurons maintain just enough oxygen supply to avoid activity-related hypoxia (Devor et al., 2011). In turn, it may resolve the paradox, first noted by Fox and Raichle (1986), that neural activity causes oxygen supply to rise in excess of its apparent demand.

What neural information is encoded in the BOLD signal?

The mechanisms for neurometabolic and neurovascular coupling suggest that metabolic and vascular functional imaging signals are causally correlated with integrated synaptic input activity, rather than spike output activity. Indeed, in autoradiography studies, 2-deoxyglucose localizes to the terminal synaptic zones of the activated pathways, rather than the cell bodies or axons of the spiking afferent neurons (Sokoloff, 1999; Raichle and Mintun, 2006). Similarly, in simultaneous fMRI and electrophysiology experiments, the BOLD signal correlates more closely with synaptic input activity than spike output activity (Logothetis et al., 2001; Goense and Logothetis, 2008). Moreover, for a given magnitude of synaptic activation within a small cortical area, the induced changes in CBF and $CMRO_2$ vary with the afferent pathways terminating in that area and the subpopulations of neurons on which they terminate. For example, even within a small localized region of somatosensory cortex, a given level of synaptic activity produces different changes in CBF and $CMRO_2$ depending on whether the afferent input projects from the thalamus (thalamocortical pathway) or from the contralateral homologous somatosensory cortex (corticocortical pathway) (Enager et al., 2009). These differences in neurometabolic and neurovascular response arise at least partly because the two pathways terminate on different subpopulations of pyramidal cells and inhibitory interneurons within the same small cortical region, and these cells also release different vasodilators. As a result, the neural information encoded by the BOLD signal is causally correlated with synaptic input activity, but in a nuanced fashion that depends on the sources of afferent input, the neuronal subpopulations that they target, and the vasodilators that they release. Moreover, the nonlinear coupling between synaptic activity and CBF complicates quantitative interpretation of the BOLD signal – without knowing the precise nature of the nonlinear relationship, the change in

BOLD signal could underestimate or overestimate the change in underlying synaptic activity.

Even though neurometabolic and neurovascular signals causally correlate with synaptic input activity, correlations with the spike output activity do occur and are not surprising. The effects of afferent synaptic activity and efferent spike activity on the functional neuroimaging signal can only be easily distinguished when the afferent neurons are widely separated from their targets (Schwartz et al., 1979). However, the great majority of excitatory and inhibitory axon terminals in a small cortical region arise from nearby cells; surprisingly, relatively few arise from more distant sites (Raichle and Mintun, 2006). For example, only 5% of axon terminals in primary visual cortex (V1) arise from the lateral geniculate nucleus in the cat (Peters and Payne, 1993). Therefore, the BOLD signal may correlate with the spike activity of the efferent neuronal population, even though it is causally driven by the spike activity of the afferent neurons, since the afferent neurons and their targets reside within the same voxel. Indeed, in the experiments of Logothetis et al., the BOLD signal correlated best with synaptic activity, but still correlated moderately with spike activity (Logothetis et al., 2001; Goense and Logothetis, 2008). Similarly, some experiments have reported strong linear correlations between the BOLD response and spike activity (Mukamel et al., 2005). Nevertheless, these correlations do not represent a direct cause-and-effect relationship and are not universal; they are context-sensitive and depend on interactions between excitatory and inhibitory cortical pathways (Lauritzen, 2001; Lauritzen et al., 2012). The complex relationships between synaptic activity, spike activity, and functional neuroimaging signals inform a nuanced interpretation of the neural information encoded by BOLD fMRI.

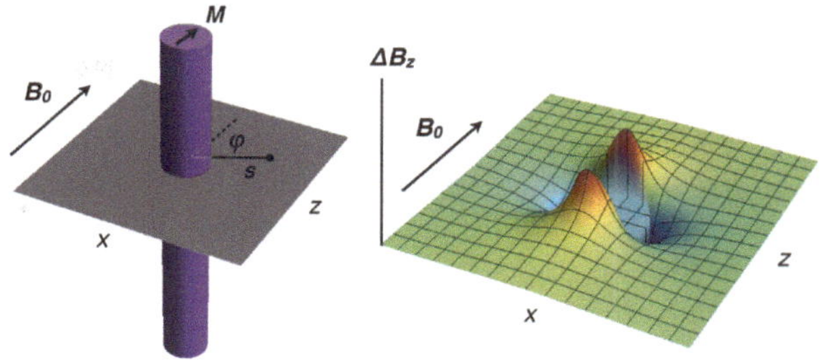

Fig. 4.7. Intravascular paramagnetic deoxyhemoglobin perturbs the otherwise uniform applied magnetic field B_0. Left: A vessel is modeled by an infinite cylinder with uniform internal magnetic susceptibility χ_i surrounded by a medium with uniform external susceptibility χ_e. Internal compartmentalization of hemoglobin within red blood cells is not included in the model. The paramagnetic cylinder perturbs the magnetic field in a way that depends on its orientation with respect to B_0. In this example, the cylinder is perpendicular to the field. B_0 induces a magnetization **M** within the cylinder due to alignment of atomic and molecular magnetic dipole moments with B_0. In turn, the magnetization produces a field $\mathbf{\Delta B}$ that perturbs the previously uniform B_0. Only the component along the axis of B_0 (ΔB_z) is significant for MR. The magnitude of ΔB_z is proportional to the difference between internal and external susceptibilities ($\Delta\chi = \chi_i - \chi_e$), B_0, and a geometric factor determined by the shape of the perturber. Right: Graph of ΔB_z in a plane perpendicular to the vessel. In this example, $\Delta B_{z,\,\mathrm{out}} = (1/2)\Delta\chi B_0 (R/s)^2 \cos 2\varphi$ and $\Delta B_{z,\,\mathrm{in}} = -(1/6)\Delta\chi B_0$, where $\Delta B_{z,\,\mathrm{out}}$ and $\Delta B_{z,\,\mathrm{in}}$ are the field shifts outside and inside the cylinder, respectively, relative to the background field that would otherwise exist in the surrounding medium absent the cylinder. s is the perpendicular distance from the center of the cylinder and φ is the angle subtended from the B_0 axis. Note that the field is uniform inside the cylinder but varies with angle relative to B_0 outside the cylinder. (These expressions include so-called Lorentz sphere corrections, which account for the effect that the granular origin of magnetic fields in matter from discrete point dipoles has on the nuclear resonance frequency.)

BIOPHYSICS OF THE BOLD SIGNAL

Many investigators have contributed to the biophysics of the BOLD effect, beginning with seminal contributions by Thulborn et al. (1982), Ogawa et al. (1990, 1992), and Kwong et al. (1992). Among discussions of BOLD physics in the literature, those by Buxton are especially lucid, and guide this précis (Buxton et al., 2004; Buxton, 2009, 2010).

Magnetic susceptibility

The BOLD signal physically derives from magnetic field perturbations within and around small blood vessels, caused by dHb. Because it contains unpaired electrons, which have a strong magnetic dipole moment, dHb is paramagnetic; it strongly perturbs the surrounding magnetic field. In contrast, because oxyhemoglobin does not contain unpaired electrons, it is diamagnetic, comparable to plasma and surrounding tissues; it does not perturb the surrounding field. When immersed in an otherwise uniform magnetic field, the vessel perturbs the field by an amount that is proportional to three factors: (1) the difference between the internal and external magnetic susceptibilities $\Delta\chi = \chi_i - \chi_e$; (2) the applied field strength B_0 (by convention, taken to be aligned along the z-axis), and (3) a factor describing the spatial variation of the field that depends only on the geometric shape and orientation of the vessel: $\Delta B_z(\mathbf{r}) = \Delta\chi B_0 g(\mathbf{r})$, where ΔB_z is the z-component of the magnetic field, and the vector $\mathbf{r}$ denotes the position in space where the field is being evaluated (Ogawa et al., 1993; Yablonskiy and Haacke, 1994) (Fig. 4.7). (Note that since B_0 is in the z

direction, only the z component of the field perturbations, ΔB_z contributes significantly to the NMR physics.) For our purposes, the key point is that $\Delta B_z \propto \Delta\chi B_0$. Since dHb is paramagnetic while oxyhemoglobin is not, $\Delta\chi$ is proportional to the intravascular dHb concentration, $\Delta\chi \propto [dHb]$. Thus, the magnitude of the local field perturbations fluctuates with intravascular oxygen saturation, and in proportion to the strength of the external field:

$$\Delta B_z \propto [dHb] \cdot B_0.$$

T_2^* relaxation

In turn, these oxygen-sensitive perivascular magnetic field perturbations alter the T_2^* relaxation time of the tissue. Thus, the BOLD effect is measured by a T_2^*-weighted MRI pulse sequence. The T_2^* relaxation effect results directly from the fundamental NMR relationship between resonance frequency and magnetic field strength: $\omega = \gamma B$, where ω is the (angular) frequency (radians/second) of a proton and B is the field experienced precisely at the location of that proton (the Larmor equation). Thus, the perivascular magnetic field perturbations create a spread of resonance frequencies around the Larmor frequency $\omega_0 = \gamma B_0$. As a result, after radiofrequency excitation, the spins within an imaging voxel precess about B_0 at varying frequencies, causing them to lose phase coherence, resulting in a faster rate of signal decay. The decay envelope is approximately exponential, characterized by the relaxation time T_2^*, or equivalently, its reciprocal, the relaxation rate R_2^*: $S(t) = S_0 e^{-t/T_2^*} = S_0 e^{-R_2^* t}$, where S_0 is the initial signal amplitude at $t = 0$. Since the perivascular field perturbations are proportional to [dHb], a high (low) level of [dHb] leads to faster (slower) signal decay (Fig. 4.8 A–C). In turn, [dHb] is affected by three factors: the rate at which oxygen is delivered to the microvasclature (CBF), the rate at which oxygen is extracted from the vessels ($CMRO_2$), and the relative fractional vascular volume (CBV). Since CBF delivers oxygen to the vessels, increased CBF tends to decrease [dHb]. Since oxygen metabolism removes oxygen from the vessels, increased $CMRO_2$ tends to increase [dHb]. Finally, since CBV includes a sizeable fraction of relatively deoxygenated venous blood, increased CBV also tends to increase [dHb]. The net effect depends on the physiologic interplay between these three parameters. Since CBF rises disproportionately to $CMRO_2$ during brain activation, and since the CBV effect is relatively small, the CBF effect dominates, resulting in a net decrease in [dHb], and a slower rate of T_2^* relaxation (Fig. 4.9). Therefore, when the T_2^*-weighted signal is measured at a fixed echo time (TE), the T_2^*-weighted signal is higher in the activated condition than in the control condition (Fig. 4.8C). The activation-induced rise in T_2^*-weighted signal intensity is the last link in the chain from neural activity, through neurometabolic and neurovascular coupling, to BOLD fMRI response.

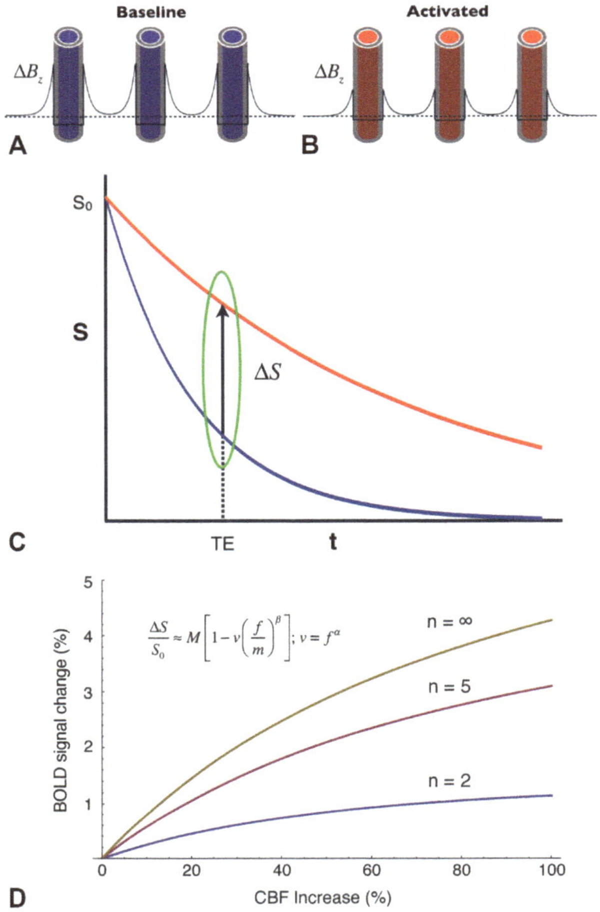

Fig. 4.8. Effect of local magnetic field perturbations on T_2^* relaxation rate. (**A**) Cartoon illustrating vessels with relatively high deoxyhemoglobin concentration [dHb] at baseline (**B**). Cartoon illustrating vessels with relatively lower [dHb] during neural activation. Lower [dHb] concentration results in smaller local field perturbations, due to the lower intravascular magnetic susceptibility. (**C**) T_2^* relaxation rate is proportional to the intravascular vs extravascular susceptibility difference, $\Delta\chi$, because larger field perturbations accelerate spin dephasing. Neural activation decreases [dHb], reducing the T_2^* relaxation rate, resulting in a higher signal at any given measurement time echo time (TE: arrow within green ellipse) (The magnitude of the signal change is exaggerated for purposes of illustration.) (**D**) Graph of fractional blood oxygen level-dependent (BOLD) signal increase vs fractional cerebral blood flow (CBF) increase predicted by the Davis model, computed with $M = 8\%$, $\beta = 1.5$, and $\alpha = 0.4$. The strength of the BOLD effect increases with n, the ratio of fractional CBF change to fractional cerebral metabolic rate of oxygen consumption change, especially at lower values of n, but with diminishing effect as n gets larger. At typical values of $n \sim 2$–3, the predicted BOLD signal change is only 0.8%–1.5%. (Adapted after Buxton, 2009.)

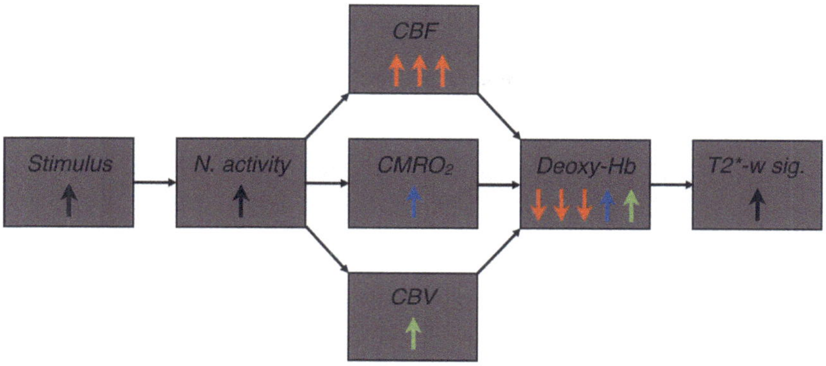

Fig. 4.9. Schematic summary of contributions made by cerebral blood flow (CBF), cerebral metabolic rate of oxygen consumption ($CMRO_2$), and CBV to voxel deoxyhemoglobin content and the T2*-weighted blood oxygen level-dependent (BOLD) signal. Increased CBF delivers oxygen to the tissue and decreases deoxyhemoglobin [dHB]. Increased $CMRO_2$ extracts O_2 from the vessels and increases [dHB]. Increased cerebral blood volume (CBV) augments the density of capillaries and venules more than arterioles, and increases [dHb]. On balance, the CBF increase is disproportionate to the $CMRO_2$ and CBV increases, resulting in a net decrease in [dHb], and increased T2*-weighted BOLD signal.

A basic model for the BOLD signal

A basic model illuminates the interplay between CBF, $CMRO_2$, CBV, and the BOLD signal (Davis et al., 1998; Buxton et al., 2004; Buxton, 2009). The relative signal change between the baseline and activation conditions is

$$\frac{\Delta S}{S_0}=\frac{S_a-S_0}{S_0}=\frac{S_a}{S_0}-1=\frac{e^{-R^*_{2\,(a)}\cdot TE}}{e^{-R^*_{2\,(0)}\cdot TE}}-1=e^{-\Delta R^*_2\cdot TE}-1 \approx -\Delta R^*_2\cdot TE$$

where S_0 and S_a are the signals in the baseline and activated conditions, respectively, $R^*_{2,\,(0)}$ and $R^*_{2,\,(a)}$ are the baseline and activated relaxation rates, respectively, $\Delta R^*_2=R^*_{2\,(a)}-R^*_{2\,(0)}$, and the (linear) approximation applies because ΔR^*_2 is small. Thus, the fractional change in T^*_2-weighted signal is proportional to the absolute change in T^*_2 relaxation rate. Here it is helpful to note that R^*_2 is the total transverse relaxation rate; it has two components: (1) intrinsic T_2 relaxation due to thermodynamic spin–spin interactions, R_2, and (2) relaxation due to the spatial magnetic field perturbations, R_2', where $R^*_2=R_2+R_2'$. Since R_2 is fixed, the change in R^*_2 with neural activation depends only on the change in the perivascular field perturbations: $\Delta R^*_2=\Delta R_2'$. Thus, the intrinsic T_2 relaxation rate factors out of the analysis, and we can focus on the activation-induced changes in R_2'. How does R_2' depend on the local magnetic field perturbations? Analytical models (Yablonskiy and Haacke, 1994), Monte Carlo simulations (Ogawa et al., 1993; Boxerman et al., 1995b), and experiments (Ogawa et al., 1993; Boxerman et al., 1995b) show that, as a first approximation, R_2' is proportional to the magnitude of the field perturbations, ΔB_z, and the vascular volume fraction CBV, denoted by V, for brevity: $R_2'\propto \Delta B_z\cdot V$; ΔB_z determines the contribution of each individual vessel, while V factors in the number of vessels in the voxel. Since $\Delta B_z\propto [dHb]B_0$, the relaxation rate is directly proportional to dHb concentration, vascular volume fraction, and magnetic field strength:

$$R_2'\propto [dHb]B_0V.$$

While this relationship is a reasonable first estimate, it ignores two important physical processes. First, it only applies to the so-called static dephasing regime, in which spins are relatively immobile during the dephasing process. However, if spin diffusion is fast enough, each spin samples a wide range of fields around the vessel, modifying its phase history. On the average, the spins experience similar net phase shifts, effectively narrowing phase dispersion and decreasing the net rate of T^*_2 relaxation. In this motional narrowing regime, the relaxation rate is approximately quadratic in ΔB_z (Ogawa et al., 1993). The diffusion effect is significant around small vessels – capillaries and small venules – while it is minimal around larger veins (Ogawa et al., 1993; Boxerman et al., 1995b). Therefore, the average effect of ΔB_z on R^*_2 is a balance between the linear effect of the larger veins and the quadratic effect of the smaller capillaries and venules. Second, the first approximation also excludes the effects of intravascular spins, on the principle that they account for only a few percent of the total MR signal. However, Monte Carlo modeling and experiments have shown that this small volume fraction actually accounts for over 50% of the BOLD signal, because the intravascular field perturbations around the red cells are much stronger than the extravascular field gradients around the vessels (Boxerman et al., 1995a).

The effects of both diffusion and intravascular spins can be incorporated into the model by a power law relationship:

$$R_2' \propto ([dHb]B_0)^\beta V,$$

where $\beta \approx 1.5$ is a good approximation for 1.5 – 3 T (Davis et al., 1998; Buxton et al., 2004; Buxton, 2009).

The link between BOLD physics and physiology is in the dependence of [dHb] on CBF and $CMRO_2$, which is most directly expressed through the OEF: [dHb] is equal to the total hemoglobin concentration ([Hb]) times the fraction of Hb that is deoxygenated. Assuming that arterial oxygen saturation is 100%, the fractional deoxygenation is equal to the OEF. Thus, $\Delta\chi \propto [dHb] = [Hb] \cdot E$, where E denotes OEF for brevity. Combining this with the prior result,

$$R_2' \propto ([Hb] \cdot E \cdot B_0)^\beta \cdot V.$$

Therefore, after minor algebraic rearrangement, the change in R_2^* between baseline and activated states is

$$\Delta R_2^* = \Delta R_2' = R'_{2,\,(a)} - R'_{2,\,(0)}$$
$$\propto (B_0[Hb]E_0)^\beta V_0 \left[\left(\frac{E_a}{E_0}\right)^\beta \left(\frac{V_a}{V_0}\right) - 1\right].$$

Since the OEF (E) is related to CBF by $E = CMRO_2/(CBF \cdot [O_2]_{art})$,

$$\frac{E_a}{E_0} = \left(\frac{CMRO_{2,\,(a)}}{CMRO_{2,\,(0)}}\right) \Big/ \left(\frac{CBF_a}{CBF_0}\right) = \frac{m}{f},$$

where m and f are $CMRO_2$ and CBF normalized to their baseline values. Similarly, denoting the normalized blood volume by $v = V_a/V_0$, and substituting into the expression for fractional BOLD signal change, we have (Fig. 4.8D)

$$\frac{\Delta S}{S_0} = M\left[1 - v\left(\frac{m}{f}\right)^\beta\right], \text{ where } M = k \cdot TE \cdot V_0 \cdot (B_0[Hb]E_0)^\beta.$$

This expression, first derived by Davis et al. (1998), relates the fractional change in T_2^*-weighted BOLD signal to the activation-induced changes in blood flow, blood volume, and oxygen metabolism. All of the parameters are conveniently dimensionless, as they are normalized to their baseline values. The ratio m/f can be related to the ratio of fractional change in CBF to fractional change in $CMRO_2$ that was discussed earlier, often designated by n.

$$n = \frac{f-1}{m-1}$$

While n was approximately 10 in Fox et al. (1988), subsequent studies have shown typical values closer to 2–3. The dimensionless constant M has important interpretations for the BOLD experiment (Buxton, 2009). First, it sets a ceiling on the BOLD effect that represents the limiting case in which CBF increases so much relative to $CMRO_2$ and CBV that it virtually washes out all of the baseline dHb ($\Delta S/S_0 \rightarrow M$ as $f, n \rightarrow \infty$). Second, M is set by three factors related to the underlying anatomy, physiology, and physics: (1) the vessel geometry (through k); (2) the total baseline dHb content (through [Hb], E_0, and V_0.); and (3) the NMR measurement (through TE and B_0). Generally, experimental values for M are in the range of 0.08, at 1.5 T, implying a theoretic maximal BOLD effect of 8%. Importantly, regional variations in M, n, and possibly β would lead to regional variations in the BOLD response, which could reflect differences in neurometabolic and neurovascular coupling, rather than differences in neural activity.

Additionally, the Davis model goes one step further by incorporating an empiric power law relationship between CBF and CBV: $v = f^\alpha$, where $\alpha \approx 0.4$ (Grubb et al., 1974; Davis et al., 1998). With this substitution, the relative BOLD signal change can be reduced to dependences on the relative changes in blood flow and metabolism:

$$\frac{\Delta S}{S_0} = M\left[1 - f^{\alpha-\beta} m^\beta\right].$$

For any given value of n, the fractional change in BOLD signal increases monotonically with the fractional change in CBF. For any given fractional change in CBF, the fractional change in BOLD signal increases with n but with diminishing returns due to the ceiling effect (Fig. 4.8D). While M represents the asymptotic maximal BOLD response, the actual BOLD response for typical values of n is much smaller. For example, with a typical empirical value of $M = 8\%$ at 1.5 T, a typical value of n in the range of 2–3, and an activation-induced increase in CBF of 50%, the model predicts a BOLD signal change of only 0.8%–1.5% (Fig. 4.8D). Thus, BOLD signals are relatively small and noisy.

Time course of the BOLD response

Thus far, the discussion has focused on relative changes between the baseline and activated states, without considering the temporal evolution of those changes. A detailed discussion of the physiology, models, and controversies behind the BOLD signal time course is beyond the scope of this discussion. Several basic points are highlighted (Buxton, 2009). The BOLD response to a brief neural impulse is delayed and dispersed on a time scale of seconds compared with the neural time scale of milliseconds. Some studies have shown an initial

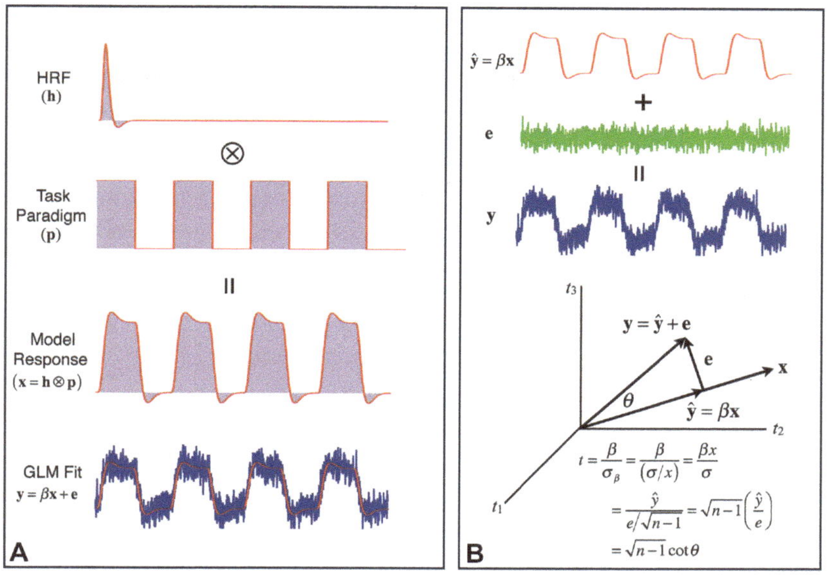

Fig. 4.10. Application of the general linear model (GLM) to the statistical analysis of functional magnetic resonance imaging (fMRI) data. (**A**) A model for the blood oxygen level-dependent (BOLD) response (**x**) is computed by convolution of the hemodynamic response function (**h**) with the task paradigm function (**p**). The hemodynamic response function (HRF) used here includes the peak response and poststimulus undershoot, but excludes the initial dip, which is not consistently observed (and is small). In this simple example using simulated data, the only regressor in the GLM is **x**, and the model equation is $\mathbf{y} = \beta\mathbf{x} + \mathbf{e}$, where **y** is the vector of voxel signal measurements at the sampled time points and **e** is the residual error between the model estimate and the actual data. The GLM computes the value of β that yields the best approximation of the data vector **y** by the model in the sense of minimizing the magnitude of the error **e** (the least-squares error). (**B**) The GLM decomposes the signal **y** into two components: the model estimate $\hat{\mathbf{y}} = \beta\mathbf{x}$ and the residual error **e**. A geometric interpretation illuminates the mathematic relationships (Buxton, 2009). The vectors occupy an n-dimensional space – one dimension for each point in the time series, of which only three dimensions can be schematically illustrated, labeled t_1, t_2, t_3. The model response **x** spans only one dimension. The closest approximation of **y** in the space spanned by **x** is the vector $\hat{\mathbf{y}}$, its perpendicular projection. β is therefore determined, such that $\hat{\mathbf{y}} = \beta\mathbf{x}$. The error vector **e** is perpendicular to the model vector $\hat{\mathbf{y}}$. The closer **y** is to the line spanned by **x**, the better the approximation, reflected by a smaller error **e** and narrower angle θ. The t-test can be interpreted in the context of this geometry. t is the ratio of the effect of interest, β, to its estimated standard deviation σ_β. The standard deviation of β, σ_β, is equal to the standard deviation of the BOLD signal noise, σ, scaled down by the overall magnitude of the model vector **x**: $\sigma_\beta = \sigma/x$. The noise standard deviation is estimated from the magnitude of **e**, scaled down by the square root of the number of degrees of freedom: $\sigma = e/\sqrt{n-1}$. Rearranging the relationships shows that t is proportional to the ratio of two legs of the right triangle: the magnitude of the model estimate $\hat{\mathbf{y}}$ to the magnitude of the error **e**: $t = \sqrt{n-1}(\hat{y}/e)$, and it is also related to the angle θ through $t = \sqrt{n-1}\cot\theta$. (The correlation coefficient r is even more directly related to the geometry: $r = \hat{y}/y = \cos\theta$.) (Geometric diagram modified after Buxton, 2009, Figure 15.4.)

dip, lasting 1–2 seconds, reflecting an initial increase in [dHb] (Menon et al., 1995). It is likely due to a burst of oxidative metabolism that precedes the rise in CBF and associated influx of oxygen (Malonek and Grinvald, 1996; Devor et al., 2003; Buxton, 2010). As CBF rises disproportionately to $CMRO_2$ and CBV, [dHb] declines, and the BOLD signal rises to a peak at about 5–6 seconds. Subsequently, the CBF and $CMRO_2$ responses dissipate and the BOLD signal declines toward baseline at about 10 seconds. Later, the signal typically falls below baseline, forming an undershoot, which peaks at about 15 seconds. Both hemodynamic and metabolic effects have been hypothesized for the undershoot, yet its precise origin remains elusive (Buxton, 2010). The entire BOLD response may last as long as about 20 seconds. This BOLD impulse response is often modeled by the sum of two gamma-variate functions (Boynton et al., 1996; Friston et al., 1998) (Fig. 4.10). A model for the hemodynamic response to an arbitrary stimulus paradigm is usually computed from the gamma-variate model for the impulse response, assuming that the system is approximately linear. With this assumption, the estimated BOLD response is the convolution of the impulse response with the stimulus time course (Friston et al., 1994) (Fig. 4.10A).

BOLD FMRI METHODOLOGY

The fMRI experiment includes three components: (1) design of the cognitive or behavioral task paradigm; (2) MR data acquisition; and (3) data analysis. Introductory overviews include Goebel (2007), Buxton (2009), Huettel et al. (2009), and Poldrack et al. (2011), while Friston et al. (2007) is an advanced source.

Experimental design

Task-based fMRI detects neural activity based on comparison between one or more activation conditions relative to one or more control conditions, using a blocked design or event-related design. Blocked designs are simpler, and are often appropriate for clinical applications. Event-related designs are more flexible, and have advantages for many cognitive fMRI applications. In blocked designs, one or more control conditions alternate with one or more activation conditions, in blocks that are typically 15–30 seconds in duration. In the simplest blocked design, one control condition alternates with one activation condition. During each block, the subject either performs a continuous task (such as hand movement) or responds to serial stimuli in relatively rapid succession (such as responding to a word or picture presented every 5 seconds). Activated cortex is identified by block-to-block periodic BOLD signal changes that are correlated with the task paradigm. Advantages of blocked designs include their simplicity and power for detection of an activation response. In particular, blocked paradigms summate the hemodynamic response over multiple neural events within each block, yielding relatively high BOLD contrast-to-noise ratio. Excessively low block frequencies are vulnerable to low-frequency noise (such as scanner drift) while excessively high block frequencies are vulnerable to attenuation of the BOLD response amplitude. A choice between 15 and 30 seconds often represents a reasonable compromise.

In event-related designs, stimuli are presented in brief individual trials similar to the strategy of event-related potentials. Trials of various activation and control stimuli are presented in randomized order. The responses to trials belonging to each condition are selectively averaged and statistically compared. Responses can also be sorted according to the nature of the response: for example, correct responses can be separated from incorrect responses. The slow time course of the hemodynamic response complicates the implementation and analysis of event-related paradigms. Ideally, the trials would be sufficiently separated in time (long intertrial interval [ITI]) that their BOLD time courses would remain independent (slow event-related design). However, the rate of data collection is inefficient with this strategy. Alternatively, the trials can be closely spaced in time (short ITI) to increase efficiency, but then the individual BOLD time courses overlap each other, making it more difficult to distinguish them. Nevertheless, methods exist to tease out the individual responses in rapid event-related designs, including randomization of the ITI (jitter) and deconvolution analysis. Advantages of event-related designs include greater control over cognitive stimuli, avoidance of cognitive adaptation that may occur during extended blocks, more flexible analysis strategies, and greater power to measure the hemodynamic response.

Data acquisition

BOLD fMRI studies require rapid acquisition of multiple brain slices through the whole brain at high temporal resolution. Echo-planar imaging is by far the most widely used imaging technique to achieve these goals. Since the nuclear magnetization and BOLD contrast increase with magnetic field strength, high magnetic field is advantageous. The current standard field strength is 3 T, while it can be performed at 1.5 T and specialized centers are also using higher fields (e.g., 7 T). In addition, multichannel head coils (e.g., 32 channels) and parallel imaging are valuable to increase acquisition speed and signal-to-noise ratio. These techniques can acquire whole-brain volumes every 2–3 seconds with a typical voxel size of 3 mm^3. High-resolution volumetric structural images are typically acquired with 1 mm^3 isotropic voxels, on which fMRI and diffusion tensor imaging (DTI) tractography data can be overlaid. In research settings, volumetric T_1-weighted sequences are typical for this purpose; in clinical settings, volumetric T_1-weighted, T_2-weighted, and/or T_2-weighted fluid-attenuated inversion recovery (FLAIR) sequences are frequently acquired, as well as a contrast-enhanced T_1-weighted sequence to define cortical venous anatomy and lesion enhancement.

Data analysis

The data analysis pipeline involves three steps: (1) preprocessing; (2) statistical analysis; and (3) visualization.

Preprocessing

Preprocessing typically includes these components:

- An automated algorithm detects and corrects head motion to minimize motion-related artifacts.
- An automated procedure is often applied to improve signal dropout and geometric distortions due to magnetic susceptibility effects, especially near air–bone–tissue interfaces at the skull base.

- An automated algorithm is used to account for the fact that the individual slices in each imaging volume are not acquired at the same time. In one approach to this problem, called slice timing correction, the slices are interpolated to estimate the voxel values that would be present if all slices were all acquired at the same point in time. In a second approach, the slice-dependent time shifts relative to the task paradigm are accounted for in the statistical analysis. The latter approach avoids potential adverse effects associated with slice interpolation.
- Low-pass spatial filtering is usually applied to remove high spatial frequency noise. A typical example is image convolution using a Gaussian smoothing kernel in the range of 4–8 mm.
- High-pass temporal filtering is usually applied to remove low temporal frequency drifts. Alternatively, low-frequency components can also be removed during the statistical analysis.

STATISTICAL ANALYSIS

Statistical analysis of fMRI data is a rich and complex field, beyond the scope of review here. However, several basic points are highlighted. Statistical analysis is used to assess the likelihood of activation for each voxel. The result of the analysis is a statistical parametric map, in which each voxel is assigned a statistic indicating the probability that the voxel time series would be observed under the null hypothesis that the voxel is not activated. While many statistical approaches have been used, by far the most prevalent is the general linear model (GLM). In the GLM, a model for the voxel time course is constructed from a linear combination of regressors (also called explanatory variables, predictors, covariates, or model functions). The GLM involves two steps: estimation of model parameters and hypothesis testing on the estimated parameters. The simplest example employs a single regressor, consisting of the predicted (idealized) hemodynamic response to the task paradigm. As mentioned earlier, it is computed by the convolution of the paradigm design function (e.g., a square wave in a blocked paradigm) with the idealized hemodynamic impulse response (e.g., a gamma-variate function) (Fig. 4.10). If $\mathbf{y}$ represents the vector of values measured at each sampled time point for one voxel, and $\mathbf{x}$ represents the vector of values predicted at each time point by the hemodynamic response model, then the voxel data can be modeled by the linear equation

$$\mathbf{y} = \beta\mathbf{x} + \mathbf{e},$$

where β is the coefficient that minimizes the residual least-squares error vector $\mathbf{e}$, and it is computed by linear regression. (For convenience, we assume that both $\mathbf{x}$ and $\mathbf{y}$ have been adjusted to have 0 means.) In a more complex example, regressors representing the predicted responses to other potential paradigm stimuli could be incorporated, along with nuisance regressors that account for other sources of variance in the signal, including a zero-frequency offset, low-frequency drifts, and head motion parameters, among others. Labeling the model regressor vectors by $\mathbf{x}_1, \ldots, \mathbf{x}_m$ and the corresponding coefficients by $\beta_1, \ldots, \beta_m$, the GLM is described by the linear combination

$$\mathbf{y} = \beta_1\mathbf{x}_1 + \beta_2\mathbf{x}_2 + \ldots + \beta_m\mathbf{x}_m + \mathbf{e},$$

which can be more compactly expressed by the matrix equation

$$\mathbf{y} = \mathbf{Xb} + \mathbf{e},$$

where $\mathbf{x}_i$ forms the ith column of the matrix $\mathbf{X}$, called the design matrix, and the β_i form the vector $\mathbf{b}$ of coefficients that minimizes the magnitude of the error vector $\mathbf{e}$ (the least-squares error) (Fig. 4.11). If n images are acquired, then the column vectors $\mathbf{y}$, $\mathbf{e}$, and $\mathbf{x}_i$ are all of dimension n, the column vector $\mathbf{b}$ is of dimension m, and the matrix $\mathbf{X}$ is of dimensions $n \times m$. It is not difficult to show that the solution for $\mathbf{b}$ is:

$$\mathbf{b} = \left(\mathbf{X}^T\mathbf{X}\right)^{-1}\mathbf{X}^T\mathbf{y}$$

where $\mathbf{A}^{\mathrm{T}}$ and $\mathbf{A}^{-1}$ denote transposition and inversion of matrix $\mathbf{A}$, respectively. A unique solution exists (i.e., the matrix $\mathbf{X}^T\mathbf{X}$ is invertible) as long as the columns of the design matrix $\mathbf{X}$ (the regressors) are linearly independent. These coefficients guarantee that the vector $\hat{\mathbf{y}} = \mathbf{Xb}$ is the best linear unbiased estimator of the data vector $\mathbf{y}$ in the sense of minimizing the least-squares error $\mathbf{e} = \mathbf{y} - \hat{\mathbf{y}}$.

Hypothesis testing is performed on contrasts between model parameters (the β_i) of interest. A contrast is defined by a column vector $\mathbf{c}$, of weights for each of the regressors. The contrast is defined by $c = c_1\beta_1 + \ldots + c\beta_m = \mathbf{c}^T\mathbf{b}$. The null hypothesis can generally be expressed by $H_0 : c = 0$. The contrast represents a hypothesized activation event, and acceptance of the null hypothesis indicates absence of evidence that the evident occurred. For example, consider a model that includes three regressors: regressor $\mathbf{x}_1$ is the predicted hemodynamic response to a series of light flashes, regressor $\mathbf{x}_2$ is the predicted hemodynamic response to a series of auditory clicks, and regressor $\mathbf{x}_3$ is a nuisance regressor for linear drift. The light flashes and auditory clicks are commingled in the task paradigm. If $\mathbf{c}^T = [1, 0, 0]$, then $\mathbf{c}^T\mathbf{b} = \beta_1$, and the null hypothesis is $H_0 : \beta_1 = 0$. The null hypothesis is rejected if β_1 differs from 0 sufficiently that it is unlikely to occur by chance

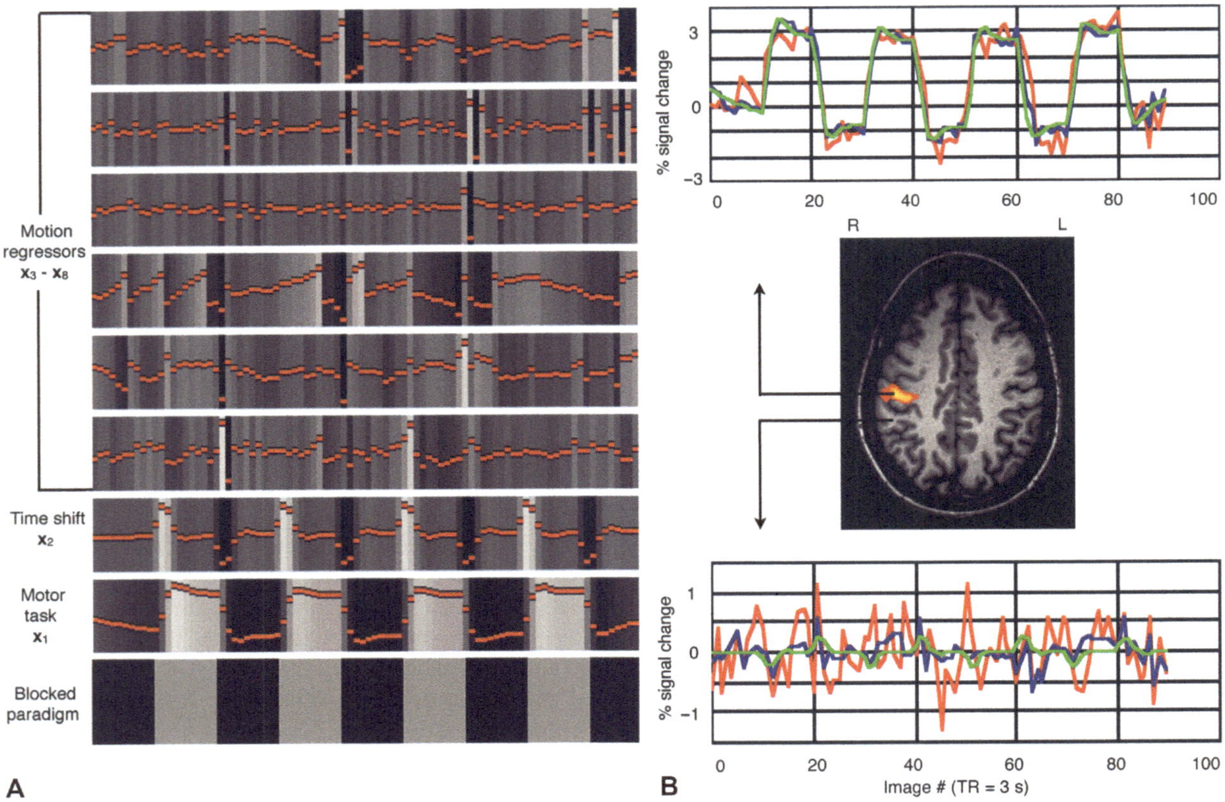

Fig. 4.11. Application of the general linear model (GLM) to sample data. (**A**) In this example, eight regressors are used in the GLM model: $\mathbf{x}_1$ is the predicted response to left-hand finger tapping in a blocked paradigm. $\mathbf{x}_2$ is the derivative of $\mathbf{x}_1$, which allows adjustment for slight time shifts in the paradigm. The remaining six regressors are head motion parameters (three translation, three rotation) that were measured by the automated motion correction algorithm. Their inclusion as nuisance regressors sometimes helps to reduce residual motion-related variance in the signal. These vectors constitute the columns of the design matrix, shown here as rows for graphic convenience. (**B**) Statistical parametric map through the center of the left-hand activation, computed from the β_1 contrast (the contrast vector in this case is simply $\mathbf{c} = [1, 0, 0, 0, 0, 0, 0, 0]$, reflecting finger tapping vs rest). The activation is centered on the right central sulcus. The signal time course and GLM model are illustrated for two illustrative voxels. A voxel near the activation peak shows strong blood oxygen level-dependent (BOLD) signal that is highly correlated to the task paradigm (upper graph). The BOLD signal (red) is well approximated by the smooth hemodynamic response model ($\mathbf{x}_1$, green). Inclusion of all eight regressors accounts for even more of the variance (blue). In contrast, a nonactivated voxel shows no significant correlation with the task paradigm, and does not statistically differ from noise. Data were analyzed using fMRI Expert Analysis Tool (FEAT) and related tools in FMRIB's Software Library (www.fmrib.ox.ac.uk/fsl) (Smith et al., 2004).

alone, indicating that the voxel was activated by the light stimuli. A statistical map of this contrast would show voxels that are activated by the light stimuli. Similarly, if $\mathbf{c}^T = [0, 1, 0]$, then $\mathbf{c}^T\mathbf{b} = \beta_2$ and the null hypothesis is $H_0 : \beta_2 = 0$. A statistical map of this contrast would show voxels that are activated by the auditory stimuli. Finally, if we would like to test the hypothesis that the voxel response to the light stimuli differed significantly from the auditory stimuli, then we could test the contrast $\mathbf{c}^T = [1, -1, 0]$, so that $\mathbf{c}^T\mathbf{b} = \beta_1 - \beta_2$, and the null hypothesis is $H_0 : \beta_1 - \beta_2 = 0$, or equivalently, $H_0 : \beta_1 = \beta_2$. One-tailed tests could be employed to reject the null hypothesis in favor of the alternatives $H_1 : \beta_1 > \beta_2$ or $H_1 : \beta_1 < \beta_2$. For example, a statistical map corresponding to $H_1 : \beta_1 > \beta_2$ would show voxels that were activated more by the light stimuli than the auditory stimuli. In each of these examples, the third component of the contrast vector is held at 0, since we are not interested in doing inference on the nuisance regressor. Nevertheless, the nuisance regressors are important, since they account for predicted sources of nonstimulus-related variance, thus decreasing the residual error and increasing statistical power.

While a variety of statistical tests can be employed, the t-test is an illustrative example. An appropriate statistic for hypothesis testing on the contrast is the ratio of the effect of interest ($\mathbf{c}^T\mathbf{b}$) to its standard deviation:

$$z = \frac{\mathbf{c}^T\mathbf{b}}{\sqrt{\mathrm{var}(\mathbf{c}^T\mathbf{b})}}$$

Assuming that the noise contributing to the signal at different time points is independent and identically normally distributed with 0 mean and variance σ^2, it can be shown that under the null hypothesis, the contrast $\mathbf{c}^T\mathbf{b}$ is also normally distributed with 0 mean and variance $\sigma^2\mathbf{c}^T\left(\mathbf{X}^T\mathbf{X}\right)^{-1}\mathbf{c}$. Therefore,

$$z = \frac{\mathbf{c}^T\mathbf{b}}{\sigma\sqrt{\mathbf{c}^T\left(\mathbf{X}^T\mathbf{X}\right)^{-1}\mathbf{c}}},$$

where z is distributed as a standard normal distribution. However, since the actual noise variance σ^2 is unknown, it is estimated from the measured residual error by $\hat{\sigma}^2 = \mathbf{e}^T\mathbf{e}/v$, where $v = n - m$ is the number of degrees of freedom. Substituting this estimate, the statistic

$$t = \frac{\mathbf{c}^T\mathbf{b}}{\hat{\sigma}\sqrt{\mathbf{c}^T\left(\mathbf{X}^T\mathbf{X}\right)^{-1}\mathbf{c}}},$$

is distributed as a t-distribution with $v = n - m$ degrees of freedom. For any given contrast of interest, computing the t-statistic for every voxel in the fMRI run yields a statistical parametric map. Voxels are then considered "activated" if their t-statistic achieves a sufficient threshold to ensure that the probability of falsely rejecting the null hypothesis is less than a desired level of significance: explicitly, if the level of significance is α (e.g., 0.05 or 0.01), then the threshold T is chosen such that the probability that $t \geq T$ under the null hypothesis (i.e., due to noise alone) is less than α (Fig. 4.10).

Several statistical issues challenge fMRI. First, the assumption that the error residuals e_i and e_j are independent for different scan times i and j is violated by correlations in the noise at nearby points in time. These temporal autocorrelations reduce the effective number of degrees of freedom; ignoring them does not bias the estimates of the β coefficients, but it does overestimate the t-statistic, and it therefore overestimates the number of apparently activated voxels at any given statistical threshold. There are several approaches to this problem. One popular choice is to estimate the autocorrelation structure from the error residuals, and then to remove the estimated autocorrelations by prewhitening, after which the GLM is recomputed, yielding a more accurate t-statistic. Second, the large number of voxels in the whole brain markedly increases the number of false positives in the brain for any given voxel-level statistical threshold.

There are two general strategies to this multiple comparison problem. The first is to control the probability of having at least one false-positive voxel in the brain (the familywise error rate (FWER), type I errors). The simplest approach to controlling the FWER is the Bonferroni correction, which scales the threshold by a factor equal to the number of voxels in the brain. However, this criterion is overly conservative, leading to low power for detection of activation due to many false-negative voxels (type II errors). A more powerful approach to controlling the FWER recognizes that the voxels are not independent and that activations tend to occur in clusters, employing various approaches to cluster analysis (Forman et al., 1995), including Gaussian random field theory (Worsley et al., 1992; Worsley, 2007). An important new approach to the multiple comparison problem is to control the rate of false-positive results among all positive results (the false discovery rate) (Benjamini and Hochberg, 1995). This surprisingly simple method is powerful, advantageous in fMRI, and gaining popularity. Finally, statistical analysis combining multiple datasets within and across individuals is essential for research studies. GLM methods for such higher-level analyses are also well developed, incorporating both fixed effects and random effects models (Beckmann et al., 2003).

Visualization

An automated algorithm is used to coregister BOLD fMRI data with associated DTI white-matter tractography data and high-resolution volumetric structural images. The fused datasets can be reviewed in multiplanar slices and in 3D volume renderings. In a major advance for neurosurgery, the structural, fMRI, and DTI datasets can be imported into systems for neurosurgical planning and intraoperative navigation, to assist in the resection of lesions near eloquent cortex and major white-matter tracts, as discussed next.

ILLUSTRATIVE CLINICAL APPLICATION: PRESURGICAL PLANNING

Rationale for presurgical fMRI

As a research tool, fMRI has touched nearly all facets of cognitive neuroscience (Rosen and Savoy, 2012). In the realm of clinically oriented research, many translational applications are being explored, involving a broad gamut of neuropsychiatric disorders (Matthews et al., 2006). To date, its dominant clinical application is presurgical functional mapping in patients with tumors, vascular malformations, epilepsy, and occasional other lesions. It is the only billable indication for fMRI in the USA (Bobholz et al., 2007). The overarching neurosurgical goal is to maximize resection of a pathologic lesion while minimizing risk to essential brain structures, including critical functional cortical areas and white-matter tracts. Presurgical fMRI is mainly used to map sensorimotor and language areas, while memory and visual studies are less frequent. DTI tractography is used to map related major projection and long association pathways. Together, these tools create a presurgical road map, which defines the three-dimensional relationships between lesion and nearby structural, functional, and tract anatomy. Preoperatively, the road map facilitates evaluation of surgical safety, choice of treatment strategy, planning of surgical approach, and anticipation of dangerous surgical margins. Intraoperatively, it guides navigation, accelerates electric cortical and white-matter mapping (when necessary), and overall, aims to help minimize the risk of a neurologic deficit.

Sensorimotor mapping

Motor and somatosensory mapping is widely used to map cortical foot, hand, face, and tongue representations for lesions near the central sulcus (Fig. 4.12). Typical task paradigms include repetitive toe flexion–extension, finger–thumb opposition, lip pursing, and forward–backward tongue movements in a closed mouth. The task paradigm usually employs a simple block design and the control condition is usually rest or visual fixation. Primary sensorimotor cortex and the associated corticospinal tract are the usual targets of

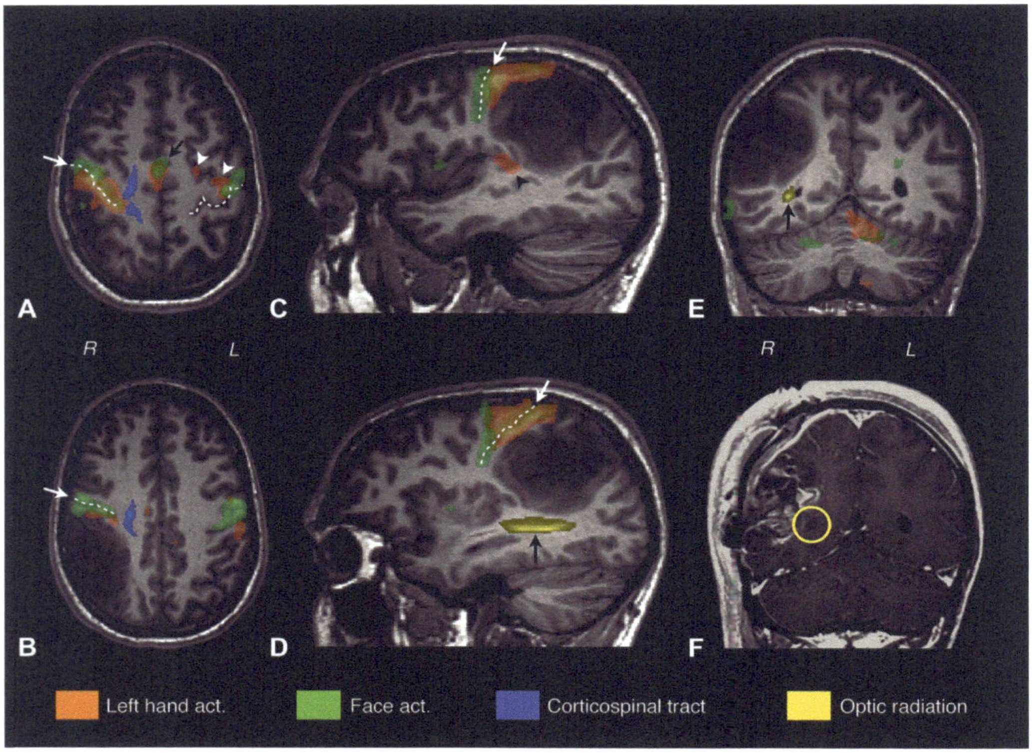

Fig. 4.12. Integration of sensorimotor functional magnetic resonance imaging with diffusion tensor imaging tractography in the evaluation of a 21-year-old male presenting with several days of confusion, and two generalized seizures. Preoperative axial (**A, B**), sagittal (**C, D**), and coronal (**E**) T_1-weighted images without contrast, overlaid with areas of left-hand (orange) and face (green) sensorimotor activation, the right corticospinal tract (blue), and the right optic radiation (yellow). Postoperative coronal (**F**) contrast-enhanced T_1-weighted image. Axial slice (**A**) is superior to (**B**). Sagittal slice (**C**) is lateral to (**D**). Coronal slices (**E**) and (**F**) are at comparable locations. A large T_1-hypointense right parietal tumor (oligoastrocytoma, World Health Organization grade II/IV) abuts and anteriorly displaces the left-hand and face primary sensorimotor areas (white arrows, **A, B, C, D**). The activations are centered along the central sulcus (CS) (interrupted lines). The left-hand primary sensorimotor activation localizes to the "omega" configuration of the right CS (**A**); the right omega is stretched and distorted by tumor mass effect, while the left omega demonstrates a typical appearance (interrupted lines). The face primary sensorimotor activation is represented bilaterally (**A, B**). On the right, the face primary sensorimotor activation localizes just inferior to, and slightly overlaps with, the hand activation, demonstrating expected somatotopy. Both tasks also activate the supplementary motor area in the medial aspects of the superior frontal gyri (black arrow, **A**). The left-hand task also activates smaller ipsilateral primary motor and premotor activations (white arrowheads, **A**) and contralateral secondary somatosensory activation (black arrowhead, **C**). The right corticospinal tract courses from the Rolandic region (**A**) through the centrum semiovale (**B**), where it lies in close proximity to the anteromedial tumor margin. The tumor is large enough that its inferior margin abuts the optic radiation (black arrows, **D, E**). Tumor resection disrupted the optic radiation (yellow circle, **F**), resulting in a postoperative left visual field cut.

greatest surgical interest, since their disruption can lead to permanent hemiparesis or hemiplegia. The supplementary motor area is also of surgical interest, since its disruption can lead to temporary motor and speech deficits (Krainik et al., 2001, 2003). Multiple studies have shown that motor mapping by BOLD fMRI strongly correlates with other noninvasive methods (Krings et al., 1997, 2001; Bittar et al., 1999; Reinges et al., 2004), and most importantly, with intraoperative direct electrocortical stimulation (ECS) (Yetkin et al., 1997; Pujol et al., 1998; Roux et al., 1999; Lehéricy et al., 2000; Krings et al., 2002b). Several factors make precise quantitative comparisons between fMRI and ECS localization challenging, including: (1) fMRI activations are often deep to the surface while cortical stimulation is always on the surface; (2) the extents of fMRI and ECS activation vary with statistical and electric thresholds, respectively; (3) intraoperative brain shift introduces quantitative error; (4) methodologies used for measurement (e.g., a neuronavigation system) and ECS (e.g., grids and strips) introduce their own variances. With attention to these limitations, one quantitative assessment of fMRI accuracy relative to ECS in 21 patients (Krings et al., 2002b) found that fMRI and ECS localizations were within 1 cm on the same gyrus in 15 patients, within 1–2 cm on the same gyrus in 5 patients, and further than 2 cm or on a different gyrus in 1 patient. By comparison, FDG-PET and ECS localizations were within 1 cm on the same gyrus in 18 patients, within 1–2 cm on the same gyrus in 1, and further than 2 cm or on a different gyrus in 1. The slightly better correlation with PET was attributed to the effect of draining veins in fMRI: BOLD signal in veins draining an activated area is slightly displaced relative to the locus of parenchymal activation. This effect was confirmed in a subsequent study comparing preoperative sensorimotor localization by fMRI and [^{15}O] H_2O-PET, which showed that the fMRI activation locus was shifted superolaterally relative to the PET activation locus by a mean of 8.1 ± 4.6 mm (Reinges et al., 2004). On balance, sensorimotor fMRI is considered quite accurate, but the confounding effects of draining veins and other potential MRI artifacts must be borne in mind. Finally, DTI tractography is proving to be accurate and valuable for mapping the corticospinal tract in relation to cortical sensorimotor activation, lesion margins, and potential surgical approach, especially when integrated into an intraoperative neuronavigation system (Coenen et al., 2003; Berman et al., 2007; Wu et al., 2007; Bello et al., 2008; Pillai, 2010) (Fig. 4.12).

Language mapping

Language mapping is used to lateralize (Fig. 4.13) and localize (Fig. 4.14) language areas. Language processing is complex, involving both linguistic and other associated cognitive processes. Intrinsically linguistic processes include those involved with phonetic, phonologic, orthographic, lexical, semantic, and syntactic operations (Binder, 2011a). Participating processes include those involved with lower-level visual or auditory input, attention, memory, executive function, and motor output (Binder, 2011a). Studies employing lesion-deficit correlations (Dronkers et al., 2004), intraoperative direct ECS (Ojemann, 1991), and functional neuroimaging (Binder et al., 1997) have shown that the classic language model (Geschwind, 1971) is oversimplified. Language processing encompasses a widely distributed perisylvian network, involving regions within the frontal, parietal, and temporal lobes, exceeding classic Broca's and Wernicke's areas (Vigneau et al., 2006; Bookheimer, 2007; Binder et al., 2009). Because of its complexity, models of language processing are still evolving (Hickok and Poeppel, 2007). These considerations make the performance and interpretation of language fMRI studies more difficult than motor studies.

A standard collection of paradigms for presurgical language mapping has not been universally adopted (Stippich et al., 2007; Binder, 2011a). Covert word generation and semantic decision tasks are particularly common. Covert (nonvoiced) responses avoid motion and susceptibility-related artifacts associated with overt speaking. Clinical language studies are usually performed using block design paradigms. The choice of control condition is important (Binder, 2011a). Simple rest or visual fixation does not control for participating nonlinguistic processes during the active condition, and does not control for default mode processing during the control condition. Therefore, a control condition that better isolates intrinsic language areas generally yields more robust, lateralized, and reliable language activation. Using two or more language paradigms also improves reliability (Pouratian et al., 2002; Bookheimer, 2007).

Despite the complexity and attendant challenges of language fMRI, multiple studies indicate a high level of concordance with the Wada test for hemispheric language dominance (Binder et al., 1996; FitzGerald et al., 1997; Benson et al., 1999; Woermann et al., 2003; Binder, 2011a; Janecek et al., 2013). It is increasingly accepted as a noninvasive alternative to Wada testing (Binder, 2011b). However, the relatively small sample sizes in published studies, particularly with respect to the low prevalence of atypical language lateralization, advises careful interpretation of the results in each case.

Encouraging correlations have also been reported between language fMRI and ECS (FitzGerald et al., 1997; Hirsch et al., 2000; Pouratian et al., 2002, 2003; Rutten et al., 2002; Roux et al., 2003). However, these

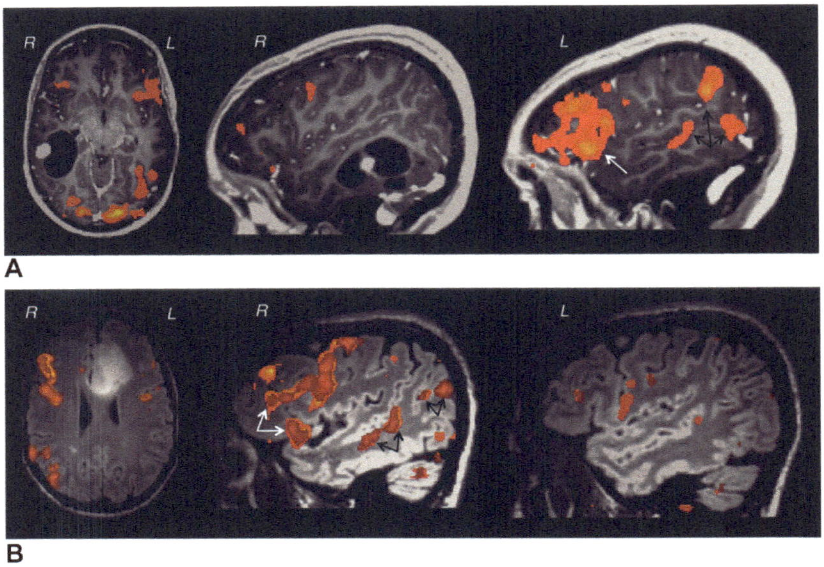

Fig. 4.13. Value of functional magnetic resonance imaging language lateralization in two left-handed patients. (**A**) A 15-year-old left-handed female presenting with a generalized seizure. Axial and sagittal contrast-enhanced T_1-weighted images overlaid with sites of mean language activation from two verb generation runs and one abstract vs concrete semantic decision run (vs visual fixation). Axial and right sagittal images show a right temporal-lobe cystic mass with an enhancing mural nodule (ganglioglioma). The axial, right sagittal, and left sagittal images demonstrate clear left-hemisphere language lateralization. The left sagittal image shows a typical distribution of activations associated with these tasks, including: (1) putative Broca's region and adjacent prefrontal and premotor areas (white arrow); (2) putative Wernicke's region involving posterior temporal lobe and inferior parietal lobe (supramarginal gyrus) (black arrows). Language function was completely intact after patient underwent resection under general anesthesia without a Wada test. (**B**) A 34-year-old left-handed male presenting with seizures. Axial and sagittal T_2-weighted fluid-attenuated inversion recovery (FLAIR) images overlaid with sites of mean language activation from two verb generation runs (dark orange) and two abstract vs concrete semantic decision runs (light orange). Axial image shows an expansile T_2-FLAIR-hyperintense left frontal lobe infiltrating glioma invading the corpus callosum. The axial, right sagittal, and left sagittal images demonstrate clear right-hemisphere language lateralization. The right sagittal image shows a typical distribution of activations, including: (1) putative Broca's region and its environs (white arrows); and (2) putative Wernicke's region, involving posterior temporal lobe and inferior parietal lobe (angular gyrus) (black arrows). Language function was completely intact after patient underwent debulking under general anesthesia without a Wada test.

studies are even more challenging. For example: (1) fMRI activates language function while cortical stimulation disrupts it; (2) in particular, electric disruption of language function is believed to predict essential language cortex, while fMRI activates both essential and participating areas; (3) activation patterns differ across task paradigms; (4) two-thirds of the cortex is enfolded within the sulci and is not accessible to ECS; and (5) language paradigms used in the operating room often differ from those used in fMRI. As a result, the reported correlations are more heterogeneous. False-negative and false-positive results occur. Moreover, quantitative assessments of sensitivity and specificity vary with fMRI technique, language task, matching criteria, and tissue pathology. In one study of 10 patients with arteriovenous malformations combining the results of five language paradigms, expressive language tasks had a sensitivity and specificity of up to 100% and 67%, respectively, in comparison with frontal-lobe ECS, while receptive language tasks had a sensitivity and specificity of up to 96% and 70%, respectively, in comparison with temporoparietal ECS (Pouratian et al., 2002). Conversely, a study of 14 patients with brain tumors combining the results of verb generation and naming paradigms found a sensitivity of 59% and specificity of 97%. On balance, language fMRI does not generally replace ECS (Roux et al., 2003). However, when used prudently, it often provides a guide to putative language areas, aiding presurgical evaluation and intraoperative mapping.

In addition to presurgical mapping, language fMRI has been used to predict postsurgical language outcome after left anterior temporal lobectomy in epilepsy patients. In a study using a semantic decision vs tone decision task, a laterality index based on fMRI activation in a temporal-lobe region of interest was strongly correlated with outcome (Sabsevitz et al., 2003). Stronger lateralization to the left (surgical) hemisphere predicted greater declines in scores on the Boston

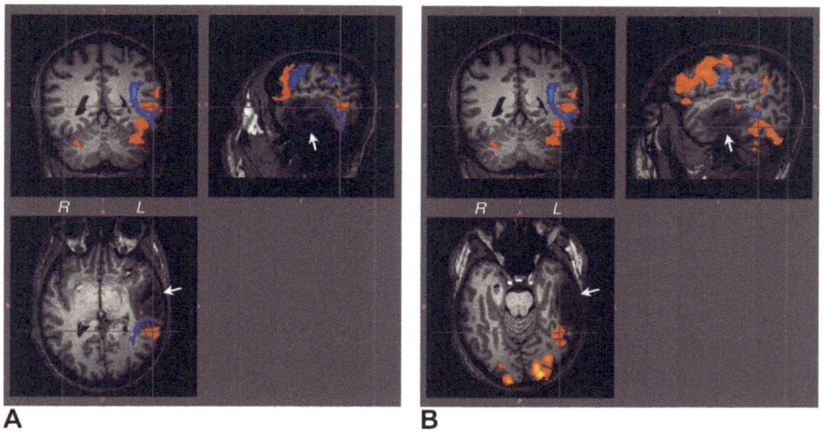

Fig. 4.14. Value of functional magnetic resonance imaging language localization and diffusion tensor imaging tract localization. A 30-year-old right-handed male presenting with new-onset seizure that started with "difficulty getting words out." Axial, sagittal, and coronal T_1-weighted images without contrast, overlaid with mean language activation (red) and the arcuate fasciculus (blue). Lines show mutual cross-registration between planes. A heterogeneous T_1-hypointense expansile mass infiltrates the left middle and inferior temporal gyri (arrows). (**A**) Cursor is centered on putative Wernicke's area, which abuts the posterior tumor margin. Arcuate fibers also abut the posterior tumor margin, and course in close proximity to putative Wernicke's area. (**B**) Cursor is centered on the putative visual word form area (VWFA), a functional module within the ventral visual stream that is selectively responsive to visual word forms; it participates in the transformation which endows low-level visual percepts with linguistic meaning, and is important in reading. It is lateralized to the dominant (left) hemisphere and located along the posterior aspect of the fusiform and inferior temporal gyri, centered on the lateral occipitotemporal sulcus. The VWFA abuts the inferoposteromedial tumor margin. Arcuate fibers are seen to course between putative Wernicke's area and the VWFA. These results alerted the neurosurgeon that Wernicke's area, the VWFA, and the arcuate fasciculus were at risk along the posterior and inferomedial tumor margins.

naming test. However, these conclusions do not necessarily generalize to other language paradigms, analysis methods, patient populations, or surgical procedures (Binder, 2011a).

Finally, DTI tractography augments fMRI by visualizing models for major language-related long association tracts, including the superior longitudinal/arcuate fasciculi (SLF/AF) and the inferior occipitofrontal fasciculus (IOFF) (Bello et al., 2008; Pillai, 2010) (Fig. 4.14). Disruption of the SLF/AF can elicit phonemic paraphasias (frontotemporal fibers), speech apraxia (frontoparietal fibers) (Duffau et al., 2008), or conduction aphasia (Aralasmak et al., 2006). Disruption of the IOFF can elicit semantic paraphasias (Duffau et al., 2008). Additionally, in the past decade, a new dual-stream model for connectivity within the language network has emerged (Hickok and Poeppel, 2007; Saur et al., 2008, 2010). The SLF and AF constitute the dorsal stream, connecting the posterior superior temporal lobe with the inferior parietal lobule and premotor frontal cortex. The extreme capsule constitutes the ventral stream, connecting middle portions of the temporal lobe to ventrolateral prefrontal cortex, apparently also accompanied by fibers of the IOFF. The dorsal stream is hypothesized to mediate phonologic processing, while the ventral stream is hypothesized to mediate semantic processing. This model significantly modifies classic assumptions, and is particularly relevant to resection of insular gliomas (Duffau et al., 2008, 2009).

Memory mapping

While many cognitive neuroscience studies have investigated memory encoding and retrieval using fMRI, memory fMRI is not yet well validated for clinical use (Binder et al., 2010; Pillai, 2010; Binder, 2011a). Interestingly, one promising approach uses fMRI language lateralization to predict postoperative verbal memory decline after temporal-lobe epilepsy surgery (Binder et al., 2008). In a study of 60 patients who underwent left anterior temporal lobectomy, postoperative verbal memory declined in over 30%. Stronger left lateralization on a semantic decision vs tone decision task predicted a greater degree of postoperative verbal memory decline, especially in conjunction with preoperative verbal memory performance and age at seizure onset. Surprisingly, invasive measures of memory and language lateralization using the Wada test failed to add additional predictive power over these noninvasive measures. Therefore, using this methodology, language fMRI may play a valuable role in assessing the risk of both language and memory deficits following left temporal lobectomy for epilepsy (Binder, 2011b).

Impact of presurgical fMRI

Controlled trials to prove that fMRI improves patient outcome are extremely difficult to accomplish. Several studies have demonstrated that fMRI significantly alters surgical decision making, sometimes allowing a more aggressive approach to management, more aggressive resection, reduced surgical time, or a smaller craniotomy (Lee et al., 1999; Medina et al., 2005; Roessler et al., 2005; Petrella et al., 2006; Pillai, 2010). Several studies have also indicated that fMRI may predict the risk of postoperative deficits, based on the proximity between the lesion and activating eloquent cortex (Krainik et al., 2003; Håberg et al., 2004; Krishnan et al., 2004). For example, in a study of 54 patients undergoing surgery near the motor strip, a lesion-to-activation distance of less than 5 mm was associated with a higher risk of neurologic deterioration (Krishnan et al., 2004). The authors recommended ECS mapping for a lesion-to-activation distance less than 10 mm and suggested that complete resection is safe if the lesion-to-activation distance exceeds 10 mm. Similarly, a study of 25 patients with lesions near motor or language cortex concluded that a lesion-to-activation distance of greater than 10 mm reduced the risk of postoperative deficit (Håberg et al., 2004). While these observations are reasonable, precise criteria for safety are not generally available. fMRI and DTI tractography complement but do not replace sound surgical judgment and experience.

Pitfalls in clinical fMRI

Safe and appropriate application of fMRI to individual patients requires attention to several methodologic pitfalls. Of particular importance is that disease pathology can disrupt the mechanisms of neurometabolic and neurovascular coupling that give rise to the BOLD fMRI signal. Mass effect, tumor infiltration, vascular steal phenomenon, or proximal arterial stenosis can cause atypical activation patterns related to abnormal neurovascular coupling or functional reorganization. Disrupted neurovascular coupling can attenuate the BOLD response, while vascular steal can invert it (paradoxic response). Both phenomena can lead to false-negative results (Holodny et al., 2000; Krings et al., 2002a; Lehéricy et al., 2002; Liu et al., 2005; Fierstra and Mikulis, 2011). The integrity of neurovascular coupling can be evaluated using BOLD to test global cerebral vasodilatory capacity in response to CO_2 challenge, either using a breath-hold paradigm, or a device to precisely control $p\text{CO}_2$ and O_2 (Fierstra and Mikulis, 2011). Other important issues for clinical fMRI include appropriate interpretation of statistical thresholding, appropriate selection of task paradigms, and methods to optimize reproducibility and reliability.

RESTING-STATE fMRI (rsfMRI) AND FUNCTIONAL CONNECTIVITY

Resting-state neural activity

Much neuroscience and functional neuroimaging has focused on stimulus–response patterns of brain activation. This perspective emphasizes interaction of the organism with the external world through auditory, visual, and somatosensory input, on the one hand, and motor/speech output, on the other (Raichle, 2010). In the context of task-based fMRI, the focus is on relative changes in neural activity between a baseline condition and an activation condition. However, more recently, much attention has turned to intrinsic activity occurring continuously during the so-called baseline resting state itself. Several considerations suggest that activations represent relatively small ripples in a larger sea of ongoing resting-state activity (Raichle and Mintun, 2006; Raichle, 2010). First, neuroenergetics supports this view: since focal neural activation increases energy expenditure only slightly over a high level of baseline brain energy metabolism, the baseline resting state accounts for the great majority of all neural activity. For example, at rest the brain accounts for 20% of total body energy consumption while accounting for only 2% of total body weight (Attwell and Laughlin, 2001). Thus, the level of baseline brain energy consumption is extraordinarily high, and most of it is attributable to ongoing intrinsic neural activity (Attwell and Laughlin, 2001). In contrast, intense primary visual stimulation induces only small increases in local oxidative energy metabolism, ranging between approximately 5% (Fox et al., 1988) and 15% (Lin et al., 2010), depending on precise stimulus conditions. Moreover, increases in energy demand induced by higher cognitive tasks are even smaller. For example, various language-related tasks increase local CBF by 5% or less (Petersen et al., 1988; Raichle, 2010) Assuming a typical ratio for $n = \%\Delta CBF/\%\Delta CMRO_2$ of at least 2, these tasks increase local energy consumption by less than 2.5%. Second, primary thalamocortical afferents account for a surprisingly small fraction of all synapses: the great majority of axon terminals arise from nonprimary (e.g., corticocortical, thalamocortical, and striatocortical) connections that support resting-state activity. For example, as mentioned earlier, only 5% of axon terminals in primary visual cortex (V1) arise from the lateral geniculate nucleus in the cat (Peters and Payne, 1993). Surprisingly, most neural activity within primary visual cortex is intrinsic; extrinsic visual stimuli induce only small modulations of this ongoing intrinsic activity (Fiser et al., 2004). Third, ongoing electroencephalogram activity reflects underlying neural processing, even during sleep and anesthesia. Finally, PET and fMRI consistently demonstrate activity decreases (deactivations)

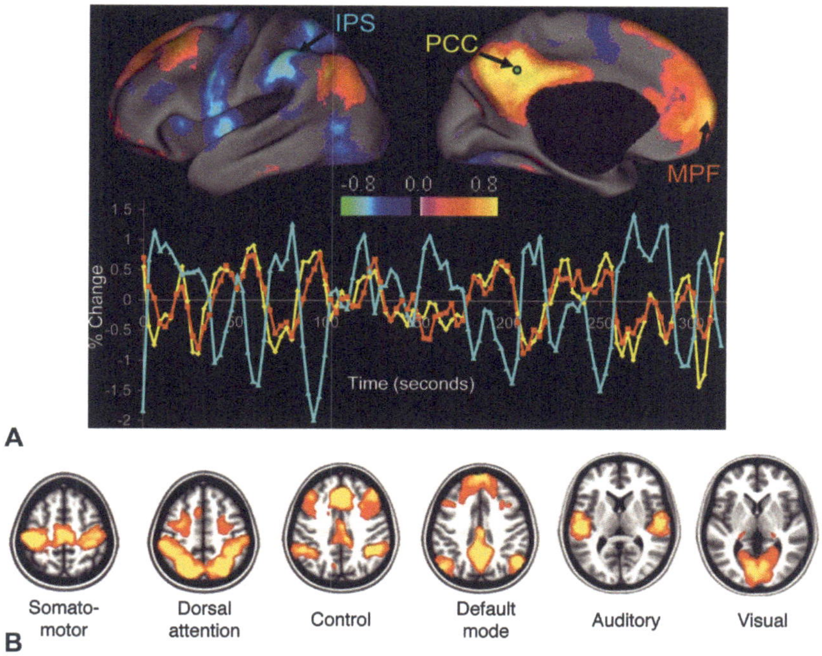

Fig. 4.15. Examples of resting-state functional magnetic resonance imaging. (**A**) A seed voxel was placed in the posterior cingulate cortex/precuneus (PCC) (green disk). The time course of the seed voxel was correlated with all other brain voxels and maps of the correlation coefficients are displayed on partially inflated brain surfaces. Red-yellow areas indicate positive correlations, while blue-turquoise areas indicate negative correlations (anticorrelations). Correlated regions encompass the default-mode network (DMN), including PCC, medial prefrontal cortex (MPF), and lateral parietal cortex. Anticorrelated regions include intraparietal sulcus (IPS), frontal eye fields, and middle temporal region. The time course for the seed voxel, shown in yellow, is clearly correlated with the time course of a voxel in the MPF (orange), and negatively correlated with a voxel in IPS (turquoise). Anticorrelations in these two resting-state networks mirror their opposite behavior during task activation: task-induced activations in regions outside the DMN, such as the blue regions here, routinely cause deactivation of the DMN. (Reproduced with permission from Fox et al., 2005, copyright (2005) National Academy of Sciences, USA.) (**B**) Example of six spatially coherent resting-state networks: somatomotor, dorsal attention, executive control, default mode, auditory, and visual. Each map shows all brain voxels that are positively correlated with one small seed region placed within the network. Similar patterns of intrinsic activity may be derived without the need for seed regions using independent component analysis. (Modified from Raichle, 2010, with permission.)

in certain brain regions when shifting from a resting baseline condition to a cognitive task. These regions are apparently active by default during the resting state, representing the so-called default-mode network (Binder et al., 1999; Raichle et al., 2001; Greicius et al., 2003), and they are downregulated when resources are redistributed to other cognitive networks (Fig. 4.15). Together, these factors suggest that ongoing intrinsic activity accounts for the majority of all neural activity.

The resting-state BOLD signal

How can one tease out the spatiotemporal structure of resting-state neural activity? Remarkably, regions of temporally correlated spontaneous low-frequency ($\approx$ 0.01–0.1 Hz) fluctuations in the BOLD signal define reproducible coherent networks in the brain (Fig. 4.15). Many of these resting-state networks encompass brain regions that are known or suspected to participate in particular types of cognitive processing, including somatomotor, visual, auditory, attention, executive, salience, language, episodic memory, and default-mode processing (Fox and Raichle, 2007) (Fig. 4.15). The strength of correlation between different brain regions defines their functional connectivity. The neurophysiologic origins of the low-frequency BOLD fluctuations are incompletely understood, but the BOLD fluctuations correlate with low-frequency components of local field potentials that collectively are called slow cortical potentials (Raichle, 2010).

The rsfMRI experiment and its analysis

The subject is usually asked to simply lie still in the scanner without falling asleep, either with eyes closed or with visual fixation on a crosshair, while T_2^*-weighted BOLD images are continuously acquired over a period of minutes. While unconstrained mental activity probably modulates the resting-state signal, most of it is more intrinsic, since similar connectivity patterns persist during rest, task performance, sleep, and anesthesia (Fox and Raichle, 2007).

There are currently two main approaches to the analysis of rsfMRI data (Fox and Raichle, 2007). In one, the correlation between the BOLD signal time course in a small seed region is correlated with the BOLD signal time course in each of the other voxels throughout the brain (Fig. 4.15). The correlation coefficients map the functional connectivity to the seed region of interest (Biswal et al., 1995). A hierarchic clustering analysis offers a more comprehensive view of network organization: first, a correlation matrix is computed from the pairwise correlations among a large collection of seed regions. Then, a graph-theoretic hierarchic clustering algorithm segregates seed voxels into clusters based on their connectivities, and produces a hierarchic tree or topologic map to describe the overall cluster connectivities (Salvador et al., 2005). The second major approach to rsfMRI analysis is independent component analysis, which extracts multiple spatiotemporally coherent components that are maximally statistically independent (Damoiseaux et al., 2006; Smith et al., 2009). An advantage of independent component analysis is that it is entirely data-driven, automated, without the need for seed regions. A disadvantage is that results may vary with the number of components generated, and putative cognition-related components must be distinguished from noise-related components.

Applications of rsfMRI

The rsfMRI literature is growing exponentially, with a doubling time of about 2 years – like task-based fMRI, rsfMRI is having an enormous impact on many fields of cognitive neuroscience (Snyder and Raichle, 2012). Translational clinical applications are also emerging, though further studies will be required to assess their reliability and applicability to individual patients, rather than groups (Matthews et al., 2006; Fox and Greicius, 2010; Lee et al., 2013). For example, resting-state studies show promise for presurgical motor (Liu et al., 2009; Zhang et al., 2009) and language (Tie et al., 2014) mapping, especially when volitional task performance is difficult (such as patients with neurologic deficits) or impossible (such as younger children). Several groups have identified the epileptogenic zone in candidates for epilepsy surgery by its increased functional connectivity to other brain regions (Bettus et al., 2010; Stufflebeam et al., 2011; Zhang et al., 2011). Several studies have found altered patterns of resting-state connectivity in patients with Alzheimer disease and mild cognitive impairment compared with normal controls and patients with behavioral variant frontotemporal dementia, suggesting that rsfMRI may play a role in the diagnosis of dementias (Supekar et al., 2008; Zhou et al., 2010; Chen et al., 2011; Dai et al., 2012; Koch et al., 2012). Other potential clinical applications include: (1) evaluation of patients with actual or apparent alterations of consciousness (Vanhaudenhuyse et al., 2010); (2) identification of patients with neuropsychiatric disorders, including schizophrenia (Shen et al., 2010; Bassett et al., 2012), major depressive disorder (Craddock et al., 2009), attention deficit/hyperactivity disorder (Zhu et al., 2008), and autism spectrum disorder (Anderson et al., 2011); and (3) evaluation of cognitive network development in normal and premature infants (Doria et al., 2010; Smyser et al., 2010; Fransson et al., 2011).

CONCLUSION

Since its first observation in 1991 (Belliveau et al., 1991), fMRI has rapidly become a major tool in laboratories and hospitals throughout the world. A majority of fMRI studies are performed in the fields of basic and applied neuroscience research. Task-based presurgical functional brain mapping is by far the most established and widely used clinical application. Translational clinical applications continue to develop. rsfMRI represents an important paradigm shift, focusing attention on functional connectivity within intrinsic cognitive networks. This chapter has reviewed physiologic, biophysical, and methodologic principles that underlie both task-based and rsfMRI, regardless of its particular area of application. These principles inform a nuanced interpretation of the BOLD fMRI signal, along with its neurophysiologic significance and pitfalls. Illustrative examples have highlighted the value of integrated clinical fMRI and DTI tractography to guide presurgical planning and intraoperative neuronavigation. Several promising clinical applications of rsfMRI have been noted. Future developments in high-field magnet design, coil design, pulse sequence design, experimental design, analysis methodologies, and multimodal integration will continue to improve the power of fMRI to explore the workings of the brain in health and disease.

References

Akgören N, Dalgaard P, Lauritzen M (1996). Cerebral blood flow increases evoked by electrical stimulation of rat cerebellar cortex: relation to excitatory synaptic activity and nitric oxide synthesis. Brain Res 710: 204–214.

Anderson JS, Nielsen JA, Froehlich AL et al. (2011). Functional connectivity magnetic resonance imaging classification of autism. Brain 134: 3742–3754.

Aralasmak A, Ulmer JL, Kocak M et al. (2006). Association, commissural, and projection pathways and their functional deficit reported in literature. J Comput Assist Tomogr 30: 695–715.

Attwell D, Laughlin SB (2001). An energy budget for signaling in the grey matter of the brain. J Cereb Blood Flow Metab 21: 1133–1145.

Attwell D, Buchan AM, Charpak S et al. (2010). Glial and neuronal control of brain blood flow. Nature 468: 232–243.

Baron JC, Rougemont D, Soussaline F et al. (1984). Local interrelationships of cerebral oxygen consumption and glucose utilization in normal subjects and in ischemic stroke patients: a positron tomography study. J Cereb Blood Flow Metab 4: 140–149.

Barros LF (2013). Metabolic signaling by lactate in the brain. Trends Neurosci 36: 396–404.

Barros LF, Deitmer JW (2010). Glucose and lactate supply to the synapse. Brain Res Rev 63: 149–159.

Bassett DS, Nelson BG, Mueller BA et al. (2012). Altered resting state complexity in schizophrenia. Neuroimage 59: 2196–2207.

Beckmann CF, Jenkinson M, Smith SM (2003). General multilevel linear modeling for group analysis in FMRI. Neuroimage 20: 1052–1063.

Belliveau JW, Kennedy DN, McKinstry RC et al. (1991). Functional mapping of the human visual cortex by magnetic resonance imaging. Science 254: 716–719.

Bello L, Gambini A, Castellano A et al. (2008). Motor and language DTI fiber tracking combined with intraoperative subcortical mapping for surgical removal of gliomas. Neuroimage 39: 369–382.

Benjamini Y, Hochberg Y (1995). Controlling the false discovery rate: a practical and powerful approach to multiple testing. J Roy Stat Soc B 57: 289–300.

Benson RR, FitzGerald DB, LeSueur LL et al. (1999). Language dominance determined by whole brain functional MRI in patients with brain lesions. Neurology 52: 798–809.

Berg JM, Tymoczko JL, Stryer L et al. (2012). Biochemistry. 7th edn. W. H. Freeman, New York.

Berman JI, Berger MS, Chung SW et al. (2007). Accuracy of diffusion tensor magnetic resonance imaging tractography assessed using intraoperative subcortical stimulation mapping and magnetic source imaging. J Neurosurg 107: 488–494.

Bettus G, Bartolomei F, Confort-Gouny S et al. (2010). Role of resting state functional connectivity MRI in presurgical investigation of mesial temporal lobe epilepsy. J Neurol Neurosurg Psychiatry 81: 1147–1154.

Bélanger M, Allaman I, Magistretti PJ (2011). Brain energy metabolism: focus on astrocyte-neuron metabolic cooperation. Cell Metab 14: 724–738.

Binder JR (2011a). fMRI of language systems: methods and applications. In: SH Faro, FB Mohamed, M Law (Eds.), Functional Neuroradiology: Principles and Clinical Applications, Springer, New York, pp. 393–417.

Binder JR (2011b). Functional MRI is a valid noninvasive alternative to Wada testing. Epilepsy Behav 20: 214–222.

Binder JR, Swanson SJ, Hammeke TA et al. (1996). Determination of language dominance using functional MRI: a comparison with the Wada test. Neurology 46: 978–984.

Binder JR, Frost JA, Hammeke TA et al. (1997). Human brain language areas identified by functional magnetic resonance imaging. J Neurosci 17: 353–362.

Binder JR, Frost JA, Hammeke TA et al. (1999). Conceptual processing during the conscious resting state. A functional MRI study. J Cogn Neurosci 11: 80–95.

Binder JR, Sabsevitz DS, Swanson SJ et al. (2008). Use of preoperative functional MRI to predict verbal memory decline after temporal lobe epilepsy surgery. Epilepsia 49: 1377–1394.

Binder JR, Desai RH, Graves WW et al. (2009). Where is the semantic system? A critical review and meta-analysis of 120 functional neuroimaging studies. Cereb Cortex 19: 2767–2796.

Binder JR, Swanson SJ, Sabsevitz DS et al. (2010). A comparison of two fMRI methods for predicting verbal memory decline after left temporal lobectomy: language lateralization versus hippocampal activation asymmetry. Epilepsia 51: 618–626.

Biswal B, Yetkin FZ, Haughton VM et al. (1995). Functional connectivity in the motor cortex of resting human brain using echo-planar MRI. Magn Reson Med 34: 537–541.

Bittar RG, Olivier A, Sadikot AF et al. (1999). Presurgical motor and somatosensory cortex mapping with functional magnetic resonance imaging and positron emission tomography. J Neurosurg 91: 915–921.

Bittner CX, Valdebenito R, Ruminot I et al. (2011). Fast and reversible stimulation of astrocytic glycolysis by K^+ and a delayed and persistent effect of glutamate. J Neurosci 31: 4709–4713.

Bobholz JA, Rao SM, Saykin AJ et al. (2007). Clinical use of functional magnetic resonance imaging: reflections on the new CPT codes. Neuropsychol Rev 17: 189–191.

Bookheimer S (2007). Pre-surgical language mapping with functional magnetic resonance imaging. Neuropsychol Rev 17: 145–155.

Bouzier-Sore A-K, Pellerin L (2013). Unraveling the complex metabolic nature of astrocytes. Front Cell Neurosci 7: 179.

Boxerman JL, Bandettini PA, Kwong KK et al. (1995a). The intravascular contribution to fMRI signal change: Monte Carlo modeling and diffusion-weighted studies in vivo. Magn Reson Med 34: 4–10.

Boxerman JL, Hamberg LM, Rosen BR et al. (1995b). MR contrast due to intravascular magnetic susceptibility perturbations. Magn Reson Med 34: 555–566.

Boynton GM, Engel SA, Glover GH et al. (1996). Linear systems analysis of functional magnetic resonance imaging in human V1. J Neurosci 16: 4207–4221.

Bushong EA, Martone ME, Jones YZ et al. (2002). Protoplasmic astrocytes in CA1 stratum radiatum occupy separate anatomical domains. J Neurosci 22: 183–192.

Buxton RB (2009). Introduction to functional magnetic resonance imaging. Cambridge University Press, Cambridge.

Buxton RB (2010). Interpreting oxygenation-based neuroimaging signals: the importance and the challenge of understanding brain oxygen metabolism. Front Neuroenergetics 2: 8.

Buxton RB, Uludağ K, Dubowitz DJ et al. (2004). Modeling the hemodynamic response to brain activation. Neuroimage 23: S220–S233.

Cauli B, Tong X-K, Rancillac A et al. (2004). Cortical GABA interneurons in neurovascular coupling: relays for subcortical vasoactive pathways. J Neurosci 24: 8940–8949.

Chen G, Ward BD, Xie C et al. (2011). Classification of Alzheimer disease, mild cognitive impairment, and normal cognitive status with large-scale network analysis based on resting-state functional MR imaging. Radiology 259: 213–221.

Chih C-P, Roberts Jr EL (2003). Energy substrates for neurons during neural activity: a critical review of the astrocyte-neuron lactate shuttle hypothesis. J Cereb Blood Flow Metab 23: 1263–1281.

Cholet N, Seylaz J, Lacombe P et al. (1997). Local uncoupling of the cerebrovascular and metabolic responses to somatosensory stimulation after neuronal nitric oxide synthase inhibition. J Cereb Blood Flow Metab 17: 1191–1201.

Chuquet J, Quilichini P, Nimchinsky EA et al. (2010). Predominant enhancement of glucose uptake in astrocytes versus neurons during activation of the somatosensory cortex. J Neurosci 30: 15298–15303.

Coenen VA, Krings T, Axer H et al. (2003). Intraoperative three-dimensional visualization of the pyramidal tract in a neuronavigation system (PTV) reliably predicts true position of principal motor pathways. Surg Neurol 60: 381–390.

Craddock RC, Holtzheimer PE, Hu XP et al. (2009). Disease state prediction from resting state functional connectivity. Magn Reson Med 62: 1619–1628.

Dai Z, Yan C, Wang Z et al. (2012). Discriminative analysis of early Alzheimer's disease using multi-modal imaging and multi-level characterization with multi-classifier (M3). Neuroimage 59: 2187–2195.

Damoiseaux JS, Rombouts SARB et al. (2006). Consistent resting-state networks across healthy subjects. Proc Natl Acad Sci U S A 103: 13848–13853.

Davis TL, Kwong KK, Weisskoff RM et al. (1998). Calibrated functional MRI: mapping the dynamics of oxidative metabolism. Proc Natl Acad Sci U S A 95: 1834–1839.

Devor A, Dunn AK, Andermann ML et al. (2003). Coupling of total hemoglobin concentration, oxygenation, and neural activity in rat somatosensory cortex. Neuron 39: 353–359.

Devor A, Sakadzic S, Saisan PA et al. (2011). "Overshoot" of O_2 is required to maintain baseline tissue oxygenation at locations distal to blood vessels. J Neurosci 31: 13676–13681.

Dienel GA, Cruz NF (2004). Nutrition during brain activation: does cell-to-cell lactate shuttling contribute significantly to sweet and sour food for thought? Neurochem Int 45: 321–351.

Doria V, Beckmann CF, Arichi T et al. (2010). Emergence of resting state networks in the preterm human brain. Proc Natl Acad Sci U S A 107: 20015–20020.

Drake CT, Iadecola C (2007). The role of neuronal signaling in controlling cerebral blood flow. Brain Lang 102: 141–152.

Dronkers NF, Wilkins DP, Van Valin Jr RD et al. (2004). Lesion analysis of the brain areas involved in language comprehension. Cognition 92: 145–177.

Duffau H, Gatignol P, Mandonnet E et al. (2008). Intraoperative subcortical stimulation mapping of language pathways in a consecutive series of 115 patients with grade II glioma in the left dominant hemisphere. J Neurosurg 109: 461–471.

Duffau H, Moritz-Gasser S, Gatignol P (2009). Functional outcome after language mapping for insular World Health Organization grade II gliomas in the dominant hemisphere: experience with 24 patients. Neurosurg Focus 27: E7.

Dunning HS, Wolff HG (1937). The relative vascularity of various parts of the central and peripheral nervous system of the cat and its relation to function. J Comp Neurol 67: 433–450.

Duvernoy HM, Delon S, Vannson JL (1981). Cortical blood vessels of the human brain. Brain Res Bull 7: 519–579.

Enager P, Piilgaard H, Offenhauser N et al. (2009). Pathway-specific variations in neurovascular and neurometabolic coupling in rat primary somatosensory cortex. J Cereb Blood Flow Metab 29: 976–986.

Escartin C, Rouach N (2013). Astroglial networking contributes to neurometabolic coupling. Front Neuroenergetics 5: 4.

Fierstra J, Mikulis DJ (2011). Neurovascular uncoupling in functional MR imaging. In: SH Faro, FB Mohamed, M Law (Eds.), Functional Neuroradiology, Springer, New York, pp. 345–353.

Figley CR (2011). Lactate transport and metabolism in the human brain: implications for the astrocyte-neuron lactate shuttle hypothesis. J Neurosci 31: 4768–4770.

Filosa JA, Bonev AD, Straub SV et al. (2006). Local potassium signaling couples neuronal activity to vasodilation in the brain. Nat Neurosci 9: 1397–1403.

Fiser J, Chiu C, Weliky M (2004). Small modulation of ongoing cortical dynamics by sensory input during natural vision. Nature 431: 573–578.

FitzGerald DB, Cosgrove GR, Ronner S et al. (1997). Location of language in the cortex: a comparison between functional MR imaging and electrocortical stimulation. AJNR Am J Neuroradiol 18: 1529–1539.

Forman SD, Cohen JD, Fitzgerald M et al. (1995). Improved assessment of significant activation in functional magnetic resonance imaging (fMRI): use of a cluster-size threshold. Magn Reson Med 33: 636–647.

Fox MD, Greicius M (2010). Clinical applications of resting state functional connectivity. Front Syst Neurosci 4: 19.

Fox PT, Raichle ME (1986). Focal physiological uncoupling of cerebral blood flow and oxidative metabolism during somatosensory stimulation in human subjects. Proc Natl Acad Sci U S A 83: 1140–1144.

Fox MD, Raichle ME (2007). Spontaneous fluctuations in brain activity observed with functional magnetic resonance imaging. Nat Rev Neurosci 8: 700–711.

Fox PT, Raichle ME, Mintun MA et al. (1988). Nonoxidative glucose consumption during focal physiologic neural activity. Science 241: 462–464.

Fox MD, Snyder AZ, Vincent JL et al. (2005). The human brain is intrinsically organized into dynamic, anticorrelated functional networks. Proc Natl Acad Sci U S A 102: 9673–9678.

Fransson P, Aden U, Blennow M et al. (2011). The functional architecture of the infant brain as revealed by resting-state fMRI. Cereb Cortex 21: 145–154.

Friston KJ, Jezzard P, Turner R (1994). Analysis of functional MRI time-series. Hum Brain Mapp 1: 153–171.

Friston KJ, Fletcher P, Josephs O et al. (1998). Event-related fMRI: characterizing differential responses, Neuroimage 7: 30–40.

Friston KJ, Ashburner JT, Kiebel SJ et al. (Eds.), (2007). Statistical Parametric Mapping: The Analysis of Functional Brain Images, Academic Press, London.

Genoud C, Quairiaux C, Steiner P et al. (2006). Plasticity of astrocytic coverage and glutamate transporter expression in adult mouse cortex. PLoS Biol 4: e343.

Geschwind N (1971). Current concepts: aphasia. N Engl J Med 284: 654–656.

Goebel R (2007). Localization of brain activity using functional magnetic resonance imaging. In: C Stippich (Ed.), Clinical functional MRI, Springer-Verlag, Berlin, Heidelberg, pp. 9–51.

Goense JBM, Logothetis NK (2008). Neurophysiology of the BOLD fMRI signal in awake monkeys. Curr Biol 18: 631–640.

Greicius MD, Krasnow B, Reiss AL et al. (2003). Functional connectivity in the resting brain: a network analysis of the default mode hypothesis. Proc Natl Acad Sci U S A 100: 253–258.

Grubb RL, Raichle ME, Eichling JO et al. (1974). The effects of changes in $PaCO_2$ on cerebral blood volume, blood flow, and vascular mean transit time. Stroke 5: 630–639.

Håberg A, Kvistad KA, Unsgård G et al. (2004). Preoperative blood oxygen level-dependent functional magnetic resonance imaging in patients with primary brain tumors: clinical application and outcome. Neurosurgery 54: 902–914.

Halassa MM, Fellin T, Takano H et al. (2007). Synaptic islands defined by the territory of a single astrocyte. J Neurosci 27: 6473–6477.

Hertz L, Peng L, Dienel GA (2007). Energy metabolism in astrocytes: high rate of oxidative metabolism and spatiotemporal dependence on glycolysis/glycogenolysis. J Cereb Blood Flow Metab 27: 219–249.

Hickok G, Poeppel D (2007). The cortical organization of speech processing. Nat Rev Neurosci 8: 393–402.

Hirsch J, Ruge MI, Kim KH et al. (2000). An integrated functional magnetic resonance imaging procedure for preoperative mapping of cortical areas associated with tactile, motor, language, and visual functions. Neurosurgery 47: 711–721.

Hoffmeyer HW, Enager P, Thomsen KJ et al. (2007). Nonlinear neurovascular coupling in rat sensory cortex by activation of transcallosal fibers. J Cereb Blood Flow Metab 27: 575–587.

Holodny AI, Schulder M, Liu WC et al. (2000). The effect of brain tumors on BOLD functional MR imaging activation in the adjacent motor cortex: implications for image-guided neurosurgery. AJNR Am J Neuroradiol 21: 1415–1422.

Howarth C, Gleeson P, Attwell D (2012). Updated energy budgets for neural computation in the neocortex and cerebellum. J Cereb Blood Flow Metab 32: 1222–1232.

Huettel SA, Song AW, McCarthy G (2009). Functional magnetic resonance imaging, 2nd edn. Sinauer, Sunderland.

Humphrey AL, Hendrickson AE (1983). Background and stimulus-induced patterns of high metabolic activity in the visual cortex (area 17) of the squirrel and macaque monkey. J Neurosci 3: 345–358.

Hyder F, Patel AB, Gjedde A et al. (2006). Neuronal-glial glucose oxidation and glutamatergic-GABAergic function. J Cereb Blood Flow Metab 26: 865–877.

Iadecola C, Nedergaard M (2007). Glial regulation of the cerebral microvasculature. Nat Neurosci 10: 1369–1376.

Iadecola C, Yang G, Ebner TJ et al. (1997). Local and propagated vascular responses evoked by focal synaptic activity in cerebellar cortex. J Neurophysiol 78: 651–659.

Janecek JK, Swanson SJ, Sabsevitz DS et al. (2013). Language lateralization by fMRI and Wada testing in 229 patients with epilepsy: rates and predictors of discordance. Epilepsia 54: 314–322.

Kasischke KA, Lambert EM, Panepento B et al. (2011). Two-photon NADH imaging exposes boundaries of oxygen diffusion in cortical vascular supply regions. J Cereb Blood Flow Metab 31: 68–81.

Klein B, Kuschinsky W, Schröck H et al. (1986). Interdependency of local capillary density, blood flow, and metabolism in rat brains. Am J Physiol 251: H1333–H1340.

Koch W, Teipel S, Mueller S et al. (2012). Diagnostic power of default mode network resting state fMRI in the detection of Alzheimer's disease. Neurobiol Aging 33: 466–478.

Krainik A, Lehéricy S, Duffau H et al. (2001). Role of the supplementary motor area in motor deficit following medial frontal lobe surgery. Neurology 57: 871–878.

Krainik A, Lehéricy S, Duffau H et al. (2003). Postoperative speech disorder after medial frontal surgery: role of the supplementary motor area. Neurology 60: 587–594.

Krings T, Buchbinder BR, Butler WE et al. (1997). Functional magnetic resonance imaging and transcranial magnetic stimulation: complementary approaches in the evaluation of cortical motor function. Neurology 48: 1406–1416.

Krings T, Foltys H, Reinges MH et al. (2001). Navigated transcranial magnetic stimulation for presurgical planning – correlation with functional MRI. Minim Invasive Neurosurg 44: 234–239.

Krings T, Reinges MHT, Willmes K et al. (2002a). Factors related to the magnitude of T2* MR signal changes during functional imaging. Neuroradiology 44: 459–466.

Krings T, Schreckenberger M, Rohde V et al. (2002b). Functional MRI and 18 F FDG-positron emission tomography for presurgical planning: comparison with electrical cortical stimulation. Acta Neurochir 144: 889–899. discussion899.

Krishnan R, Raabe A, Hattingen E et al. (2004). Functional magnetic resonance imaging-integrated neuronavigation: correlation between lesion-to-motor cortex distance and outcome. Neurosurgery 55: 904–914.

Kwong KK, Belliveau JW, Chesler DA et al. (1992). Dynamic magnetic resonance imaging of human brain activity during primary sensory stimulation. Proc Natl Acad Sci U S A 89: 5675–5679.

Lauritzen M (2001). Relationship of spikes, synaptic activity, and local changes of cerebral blood flow. J Cereb Blood Flow Metab 21: 1367–1383.

Lauritzen M, Mathiesen C, Schaefer K et al. (2012). Neuronal inhibition and excitation, and the dichotomic control of brain hemodynamic and oxygen responses. Neuroimage 62: 1040–1050.

Lee CC, Ward HA, Sharbrough FW et al. (1999). Assessment of functional MR imaging in neurosurgical planning. AJNR Am J Neuroradiol 20: 1511–1519.

Lee MH, Smyser CD, Shimony JS (2013). Resting-state fMRI: a review of methods and clinical applications. AJNR Am J Neuroradiol 34: 1866–1872.

Lehéricy S, Duffau H, Cornu P et al. (2000). Correspondence between functional magnetic resonance imaging somatotopy and individual brain anatomy of the central region: comparison with intraoperative stimulation in patients with brain tumors. J Neurosurg 92: 589–598.

Lehéricy S, Biondi A, Sourour N et al. (2002). Arteriovenous brain malformations: is functional MR imaging reliable for studying language reorganization in patients? Initial observations. Radiology 223: 672–682.

Lin A-L, Fox PT, Hardies J et al. (2010). Nonlinear coupling between cerebral blood flow, oxygen consumption, and ATP production in human visual cortex. Proc Natl Acad Sci U S A 107: 8446–8451.

Lindauer U, Megow D, Matsuda H et al. (1999). Nitric oxide: a modulator, but not a mediator, of neurovascular coupling in rat somatosensory cortex. Am J Physiol 277: H799–H811.

Lindauer U, Leithner C, Kaasch H et al. (2010). Neurovascular coupling in rat brain operates independent of hemoglobin deoxygenation. J Cereb Blood Flow Metab 30: 757–768.

Liu W-C, Feldman SC, Schulder M et al. (2005). The effect of tumour type and distance on activation in the motor cortex. Neuroradiology 47: 813–819.

Liu H, Buckner RL, Talukdar T et al. (2009). Task-free presurgical mapping using functional magnetic resonance imaging intrinsic activity. J Neurosurg 111: 746–754.

Loaiza A, Porras OH, Barros LF (2003). Glutamate triggers rapid glucose transport stimulation in astrocytes as evidenced by real-time confocal microscopy. J Neurosci 23: 7337–7342.

Logothetis NK, Pauls J, Augath M et al. (2001). Neurophysiological investigation of the basis of the fMRI signal. Nature 412: 150–157.

Malonek D, Grinvald A (1996). Interactions between electrical activity and cortical microcirculation revealed by imaging spectroscopy: implications for functional brain mapping. Science 272: 551–554.

Mangia S, Simpson IA, Vannucci SJ et al. (2009). The in vivo neuron-to-astrocyte lactate shuttle in human brain: evidence from modeling of measured lactate levels during visual stimulation. J Neurochem 109: 55–62.

Mathiesen C, Caesar K, Thomsen K et al. (2011). Activity-dependent increases in local oxygen consumption correlate with postsynaptic currents in the mouse cerebellum in vivo. J Neurosci 31: 18327–18337.

Matthews PM, Honey GD, Bullmore ET (2006). Applications of fMRI in translational medicine and clinical practice. Nat Rev Neurosci 7: 732–744.

Medina LS, Bernal B, Dunoyer C et al. (2005). Seizure disorders: functional MR imaging for diagnostic evaluation and surgical treatment – prospective study. Radiology 236: 247–253.

Menon RS, Ogawa S, Hu X et al. (1995). BOLD based functional MRI at 4 Tesla includes a capillary bed contribution: echo-planar imaging correlates with previous optical imaging using intrinsic signals. Magn Reson Med 33: 453–459.

Mintun MA, Lundstrom BN, Snyder AZ et al. (2001). Blood flow and oxygen delivery to human brain during functional activity: theoretical modeling and experimental data. Proc Natl Acad Sci U S A 98: 6859–6864.

Mukamel R, Gelbard H, Arieli A et al. (2005). Coupling between neuronal firing, field potentials, and fMRI in human auditory cortex. Science 309: 951–954.

Nedergaard M, Ransom B, Goldman SA (2003). New roles for astrocytes: redefining the functional architecture of the brain. Trends Neurosci 26: 523–530.

Nehlig A, Wittendorp-Rechenmann E, Lam CD (2004). Selective uptake of [^{14}C]2-deoxyglucose by neurons and astrocytes: high-resolution microautoradiographic imaging by cellular ^{14}C-trajectography combined with immunohistochemistry. J Cereb Blood Flow Metab 24: 1004–1014.

Offenhauser N, Thomsen K, Caesar K et al. (2005). Activity-induced tissue oxygenation changes in rat cerebellar cortex: interplay of postsynaptic activation and blood flow. J Physiol (Lond) 565: 279–294.

Ogawa S, Lee TM, Nayak AS et al. (1990). Oxygenation-sensitive contrast in magnetic resonance image of rodent brain at high magnetic fields. Magn Reson Med 14: 68–78.

Ogawa S, Tank DW, Menon R et al. (1992). Intrinsic signal changes accompanying sensory stimulation: functional brain mapping with magnetic resonance imaging. Proc Natl Acad Sci U S A 89: 5951–5955.

Ogawa S, Menon RS, Tank DW et al. (1993). Functional brain mapping by blood oxygenation level-dependent contrast magnetic resonance imaging. A comparison of signal characteristics with a biophysical model. Biophys J 64: 803–812.

Ojemann GA (1991). Cortical organization of language. J Neurosci 11: 2281–2287.

Pellerin L, Magistretti PJ (1994). Glutamate uptake into astrocytes stimulates aerobic glycolysis: a mechanism coupling neuronal activity to glucose utilization. Proc Natl Acad Sci U S A 91: 10625–10629.

Peters A, Payne BR (1993). Numerical relationships between geniculocortical afferents and pyramidal cell modules in cat primary visual cortex. Cereb Cortex 3: 69–78.

Petersen SE, Fox PT, Posner MI et al. (1988). Positron emission tomographic studies of the cortical anatomy of single-word processing. Nature 331: 585–589.

Petrella JR, Shah LM, Harris KM et al. (2006). Preoperative functional MR imaging localization of language and motor areas: effect on therapeutic decision making in patients with potentially resectable brain tumors 1. Radiology 240: 793–802.

Pillai JJ (2010). The evolution of clinical functional imaging during the past 2 decades and its current impact on neurosurgical planning. AJNR Am J Neuroradiol 31: 219–225.

Poldrack RA, Mumford JA, Nichols TE (2011). Handbook of Functional MRI Data Analysis, Cambridge University Press, Cambridge.

Pouratian N, Bookheimer SY, Rex DE et al. (2002). Utility of preoperative functional magnetic resonance imaging for identifying language cortices in patients with vascular malformations. J Neurosurg 97: 21–32.

Pouratian N, Bookheimer SY, Rubino G et al. (2003). Category-specific naming deficit identified by intraoperative stimulation mapping and postoperative neuropsychological testing. Case report J Neurosurg 99: 170–176.

Powers WJ, Hirsch IB, Cryer PE (1996). Effect of stepped hypoglycemia on regional cerebral blood flow response to physiological brain activation. Am J Physiol 270: H554–H559.

Pujol J, Conesa G, Deus J, López-Obarrio L et al. (1998). Clinical application of functional magnetic resonance imaging in presurgical identification of the central sulcus. J Neurosurg 88: 863–869.

Raichle ME (2010). Two views of brain function. Trends Cogn Sci (Regul Ed) 14: 180–190.

Raichle ME, Mintun MA (2006). Brain work and brain imaging. Annu Rev Neurosci 29: 449–476.

Raichle ME, Grubb RL, Gado MH et al. (1976). Correlation between regional cerebral blood flow and oxidative metabolism. In vivo studies in man. Arch Neurol 33: 523–526.

Raichle ME, MacLeod AM, Snyder AZ et al. (2001). A default mode of brain function. Proc Natl Acad Sci U S A 98: 676–682.

Rancillac A, Rossier J, Guille M et al. (2006). Glutamatergic control of microvascular tone by distinct GABA neurons in the cerebellum. J Neurosci 26: 6997–7006.

Reinges MHT, Krings T, Meyer PT et al. (2004). Preoperative mapping of cortical motor function: prospective comparison of functional magnetic resonance imaging and [15O]-H2O-positron emission tomography in the same co-ordinate system. Nucl Med Commun 25: 987–997.

Roessler K, Donat M, Lanzenberger R et al. (2005). Evaluation of preoperative high magnetic field motor functional MRI (3 Tesla) in glioma patients by navigated electrocortical stimulation and postoperative outcome. J Neurol Neurosurg Psychiatry 76: 1152–1157.

Rosen BR, Savoy RL (2012). fMRI at 20: has it changed the world? Neuroimage 62: 1316–1324.

Roux FE, Boulanouar K, Ranjeva JP et al. (1999). Cortical intraoperative stimulation in brain tumors as a tool to evaluate spatial data from motor functional MRI. Invest Radiol 34: 225–229.

Roux F-E, Boulanouar K, Lotterie J-A et al. (2003). Language functional magnetic resonance imaging in preoperative assessment of language areas: correlation with direct cortical stimulation. Neurosurgery 52: 1335–1347.

Roy CS, Sherrington CS (1890). On the regulation of the blood-supply of the brain. J Physiol (Lond) 11: 85–108.

Ruminot I, Gutiérrez R, Peña-Münzenmayer G et al. (2011). NBCe1 mediates the acute stimulation of astrocytic glycolysis by extracellular K^+. J Neurosci 31: 14264–14271.

Rutten GJM, Ramsey NF, Van Rijen PC et al. (2002). Development of a functional magnetic resonance imaging protocol for intraoperative localization of critical temporoparietal language areas. Ann Neurol 51: 350–360.

Sabsevitz DS, Swanson SJ, Hammeke TA et al. (2003). Use of preoperative functional neuroimaging to predict language deficits from epilepsy surgery. Neurology 60: 1788–1792.

Salvador R, Suckling J, Coleman MR et al. (2005). Neurophysiological architecture of functional magnetic resonance images of human brain. Cereb Cortex 15: 1332–1342.

Saur D, Kreher BW, Schnell S et al. (2008). Ventral and dorsal pathways for language. Proc Natl Acad Sci U S A 105: 18035–18040.

Saur D, Schelter B, Schnell S et al. (2010). Combining functional and anatomical connectivity reveals brain networks for auditory language comprehension. Neuroimage 49: 3187–3197.

Schwartz WJ, Smith CB, Davidsen L et al. (1979). Metabolic mapping of functional activity in the hypothalamoneurohypophysial system of the rat. Science 205: 723–725.

Shen H, Wang L, Liu Y et al. (2010). Discriminative analysis of resting-state functional connectivity patterns of schizophrenia using low dimensional embedding of fMRI. Neuroimage 49: 3110–3121.

Sheth SA, Nemoto M, Guiou M et al. (2004). Linear and nonlinear relationships between neuronal activity, oxygen metabolism, and hemodynamic responses. Neuron 42: 347–355.

Sibson NR, Mason GF, Shen J et al. (2001). In vivo (13)C NMR measurement of neurotransmitter glutamate cycling, anaplerosis and TCA cycle flux in rat brain during [2-(13) C]glucose infusion. J Neurochem 76: 975–989.

Simpson IA, Carruthers A, Vannucci SJ (2007). Supply and demand in cerebral energy metabolism: the role of nutrient transporters. J Cereb Blood Flow Metab 27: 1766–1791.

Smith SM, Jenkinson M, Woolrich MW et al. (2004). Advances in functional and structural MR image analysis and implementation as FSL. Neuroimage 23: S208–S219.

Smith SM, Fox PT, Miller KL et al. (2009). Correspondence of the brain's functional architecture during activation and rest. Proc Natl Acad Sci U S A 106: 13040–13045.

Smyser CD, Inder TE, Shimony JS et al. (2010). Longitudinal analysis of neural network development in preterm infants. Cereb Cortex 20: 2852–2862.

Snyder AZ, Raichle ME (2012). A brief history of the resting state: the Washington University perspective. Neuroimage 62: 902–910.

Sokoloff L (1999). Energetics of functional activation in neural tissues. Neurochem Res 24: 321–329.

Stippich C, Blatow M, Krakow K (2007). Presurgical functional MRI in patients with brain tumors. In: C Stippich (Ed.), Clinical Functional MRI, Springer-Verlag, Berlin, pp. 87–148.

Stufflebeam SM, Liu H, Sepulcre J et al. (2011). Localization of focal epileptic discharges using functional connectivity magnetic resonance imaging. J Neurosurg 114: 1693–1697.

Supekar K, Menon V, Rubin D et al. (2008). Network analysis of intrinsic functional brain connectivity in Alzheimer's disease. PLoS Comput Biol 4: e1000100.

Takano T, Tian G-F, Peng W et al. (2006). Astrocyte-mediated control of cerebral blood flow. Nat Neurosci 9: 260–267.

Thulborn KR, Waterton JC, Matthews PM et al. (1982). Oxygenation dependence of the transverse relaxation time of water protons in whole blood at high field. Biochim Biophys Acta 714: 265–270.

Tie Y, Rigolo L, Norton IH et al. (2014). Defining language networks from resting-state fMRI for surgical planning – a feasibility study. Hum Brain Mapp 35: 1018–1030.

Vanhaudenhuyse A, Noirhomme Q, Tshibanda LJ-F et al. (2010). Default network connectivity reflects the level of consciousness in non-communicative brain-damaged patients. Brain 133: 161–171.

Vigneau M, Beaucousin V, Hervé PY et al. (2006). Meta-analyzing left hemisphere language areas: Phonology, semantics, and sentence processing. Neuroimage 30: 1414–1432.

Wang X, Lou N, Xu Q et al. (2006). Astrocytic Ca^{2+} signaling evoked by sensory stimulation in vivo. Nat Neurosci 9: 816–823.

Woermann FG, Jokeit H, Luerding R et al. (2003). Language lateralization by Wada test and fMRI in 100 patients with epilepsy. Neurology 61: 699–701.

Wolf T, Lindauer U, Villringer A et al. (1997). Excessive oxygen or glucose supply does not alter the blood flow response to somatosensory stimulation or spreading depression in rats. Brain Res 761: 290–299.

Woolsey TA, Rovainen CM, Cox SB et al. (1996). Neuronal units linked to microvascular modules in cerebral cortex: response elements for imaging the brain. Cereb Cortex 6: 647–660.

Worsley KJ (2007). Random field theory. In: KJ Friston, JT Ashburner, SJ Kiebel et al. (Eds.), Statistical Parametric Mapping: The Analysis of Functional Brain Images, Academic Press, London, pp. 232–236.

Worsley KJ, Evans AC, Marrett S et al. (1992). A three-dimensional statistical analysis for CBF activation studies in human brain. J Cereb Blood Flow Metab 12: 900–918.

Wu J-S, Zhou L-F, Tang W-J et al. (2007). Clinical evaluation and follow-up outcome of diffusion tensor imaging-based functional neuronavigation: a prospective, controlled study in patients with gliomas involving pyramidal tracts. Neurosurgery 61: 935–948.

Yablonskiy DA, Haacke EM (1994). Theory of NMR signal behavior in magnetically inhomogeneous tissues: the static dephasing regime. Magn Reson Med 32: 749–763.

Yang G, Zhang Y, Ross ME et al. (2003). Attenuation of activity-induced increases in cerebellar blood flow in mice lacking neuronal nitric oxide synthase. Am J Physiol Heart Circ Physiol 285: H298–H304.

Yetkin FZ, Mueller WM, Morris GL et al. (1997). Functional MR activation correlated with intraoperative cortical mapping. AJNR Am J Neuroradiol 18: 1311–1315.

Zhang D, Johnston JM, Fox MD et al. (2009). Preoperative sensorimotor mapping in brain tumor patients using spontaneous fluctuations in neuronal activity imaged with functional magnetic resonance imaging: initial experience. Neurosurgery 65: 226–236.

Zhang X, Tokoglu F, Negishi M et al. (2011). Social network theory applied to resting-state fMRI connectivity data in the identification of epilepsy networks with iterative feature selection. J Neurosci Methods 199: 129–139.

Zheng D, LaMantia A-S, Purves D (1991). Specialized vascularization of the primate visual cortex. J Neurosci 11: 2622–2629.

Zhou J, Greicius MD, Gennatas ED et al. (2010). Divergent network connectivity changes in behavioural variant frontotemporal dementia and Alzheimer's disease. Brain 133: 1352–1367.

Zhu C-Z, Zang Y-F, Cao Q-J et al. (2008). Fisher discriminative analysis of resting-state brain function for attention-deficit/hyperactivity disorder. Neuroimage 40: 110–120.

Zonta M, Angulo MC, Gobbo S et al. (2003). Neuron-to-astrocyte signaling is central to the dynamic control of brain microcirculation. Nat Neurosci 6: 43–50.

Handbook of Clinical Neurology, Vol. 135 (3rd series)
Neuroimaging, Part I
J.C. Masdeu and R.G. González, Editors

Chapter 5

Clinical magnetic resonance spectroscopy of the central nervous system

EVA-MARIA RATAI* AND R. GILBERTO GONZÁLEZ
Division of Neuroradiology, Department of Radiology, Massachusetts General Hospital and Harvard Medical School, and Athinoula A. Martinos Center for Biomedical Imaging, Boston, MA, USA

Abstract

Proton magnetic resonance spectroscopy (1H MRS) is a noninvasive imaging technique that can easily be added to the conventional magnetic resonance (MR) imaging sequences. Using MRS one can directly compare spectra from pathologic or abnormal tissue and normal tissue. Metabolic changes arising from pathology that can be visualized by MRS may not be apparent from anatomy that can be visualized by conventional MR imaging. In addition, metabolic changes may precede anatomic changes. Thus, MRS is used for diagnostics, to observe disease progression, monitor therapeutic treatments, and to understand the pathogenesis of diseases. MRS may have an important impact on patient management. The purpose of this chapter is to provide practical guidance in the clinical application of MRS of the brain. This chapter provides an overview of MRS-detectable metabolites and their significance. In addition some specific current clinical applications of MRS will be discussed, including brain tumors, inborn errors of metabolism, leukodystrophies, ischemia, epilepsy, and neurodegenerative diseases. The chapter concludes with technical considerations and challenges of clinical MRS.

INTRODUCTION

Conventional magnetic resonance imaging (MRI) provides detailed anatomic information and has become a crucial tool in the assessment of central nervous system (CNS) disorders. However, structural MRI typically provides very little physiologic information. The ability of magnetic resonance spectroscopy (MRS) to probe tissue biochemistry is a powerful tool that complements the information obtained by conventional MRI. The purpose of this chapter is to provide practical guidance in the clinical application of MRS of the brain. The focus is on proton MRS (^{1}H MRS) because it is the method that is widely available clinically.

^{1}H MRS is a noninvasive imaging technique that can easily be added to the conventional MRI sequences and is able to measure metabolism in the brain. Metabolic changes arising from pathology that can be visualized by MRS may not be apparent from anatomy. In addition, metabolic changes often precede anatomic changes. Thus, MRS is used for diagnostics, to observe disease progression, monitor therapeutic treatments, and to understand the pathogenesis of diseases.

This chapter covers the biochemical pattern of ^{1}H MRS, including the debatable metabolites and their significance as biomarkers, followed by a review of some current clinical applications of MRS. The clinical applications have been divided into three classes based on practical considerations: (1) MRS applications in which the interpretation of the MR spectrum is of value in individual patients, such as brain tumors or inborn errors of metabolism; (2) neurologic diseases in which the changes in the MRS spectrum are occasionally large enough that they may useful for clinical management in some individual patients; and (3) MRS applications in which MRS is most meaningful in assessing groups of patients or possibly individual patients who have serial MRS

*Correspondence to: Eva-Maria Ratai, Building 149, 13th Street, Room 2301, Charlestown MA 02129, USA. Tel: +1-617-726-1744, Fax: +1-617-726-7422, E-mail: ratai@nmr.mgh.harvard.edu

studies. In these cases, the MR spectrum is abnormal, but the change is more subtle, and may not be reliably appreciated by the radiologist because the change may fall within the range of normal variation between individuals. The chapter concludes with technical considerations and challenges of MRS.

BIOCHEMICAL PATTERN BY MAGNETIC RESONANCE SPECTROSCOPY

^{1}H MRS offers the unique ability to measure metabolite levels in a noninvasive manner. The resonances seen in the brain by ^{1}H MRS are typically low-weight molecules (Fig. 5.1). In the normal brain, the most prominent peak arises from *N*-acetylaspartate (NAA) at 2.0 ppm. The other major peaks include creatine (Cr)/phosphocreatine (PCr), as well as choline (Cho)-containing compounds, which are observed at 3.0 and 3.2 ppm, respectively. MR spectra acquired with short echo times (TE) are characterized by additional resonances from myo-inositol (mI) at ~3.5 ppm (observed as multiplet), and glutamate (Glu)/glutamine (Gln) at ~2.4 ppm (also observed as multiplet) and lipids between 0.9 and 1.3 ppm. Under normal conditions, one should not be able to observe lactate as lactate concentration is very low in the adult brain. Lactate resonance (observed as a doublet) occurs at 1.3 ppm.

N-acetyl aspartate

In the normal brain, the most prominent spectral peak originates from the *N*-acetyl group of NAA assigned at 2.02 ppm. NAA is a free amino acid present in the brain at relatively high concentrations (Govindaraju et al., 2000). It is localized primarily in the central and peripheral nervous system (Miyake et al., 1981; Birken and Oldendorf, 1989). Its function is not fully understood, but it is believed to act as an osmolyte, a storage form of aspartate, and a precursor of *N*-acetyl aspartylglutamate, as well as having a variety of other functions (Birken and Oldendorf, 1989; Tsai and Coyle, 1995). NAA within the adult brain is found almost exclusively in neurons, and serves as a marker of neuronal density and viability (Moffett et al., 1991; Simmons et al., 1991; Urenjak et al., 1992, 1993). In addition, in the developing brain, NAA can be found in the oligodendrocyte type 2 astrocyte progenitor cells. NAA is decreased in almost every neurodegenerative disease due to either neuronal loss (Cheng et al., 1997, 2002) or neuronal dysfunction. For example, recovery of NAA levels has been observed with incomplete reversible ischemia (Brulatout et al., 1996) and brain injury (De Stefano et al., 1995). Interestingly, increased NAA levels have been observed with Canavan's disease, an inherited disorder in which NAA is not broken down and accumulates to toxic concentrations (Grodd et al., 1991; Tsai and Coyle, 1995).

Creatine

The Cr peak at 3.03 ppm is composed of resonances from Cr and from PCr, a high-energy reservoir for adenosine triphosphate (ATP) generation. Collectively, Cr and PCr are referred to as tCr (total Cr) or simply Cr. Since Cr serves as a marker for energy-dependent

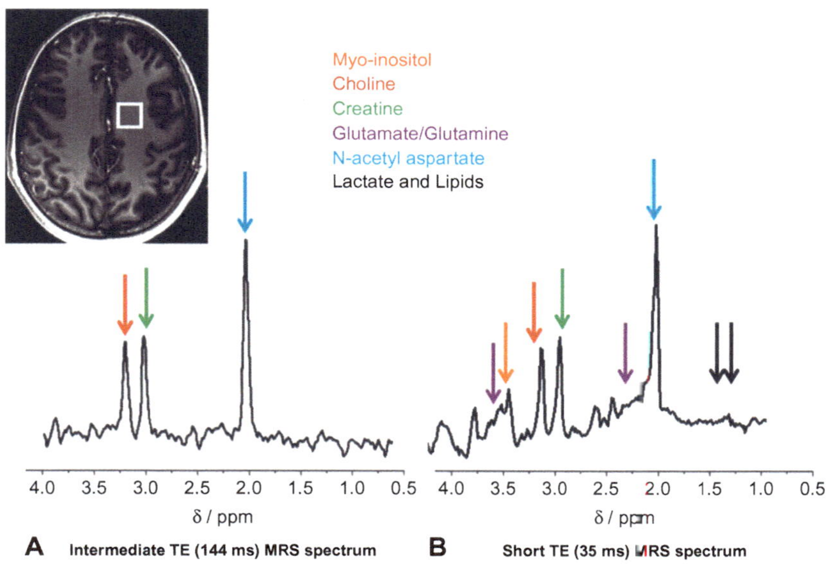

Fig. 5.1. Magnetic resonance spectroscopy (MRS) of white matter in a normal brain. (**A**) Intermediate echo time (TE) spectra of 135–144 ms have less baseline distortion and are easy to process and analyze but show fewer metabolites than short TE spectra. (**B**) Short TE demonstrates peaks attributable to more metabolites, including lipids and macromolecules, glutamine and glutamate, and myo-inositol.

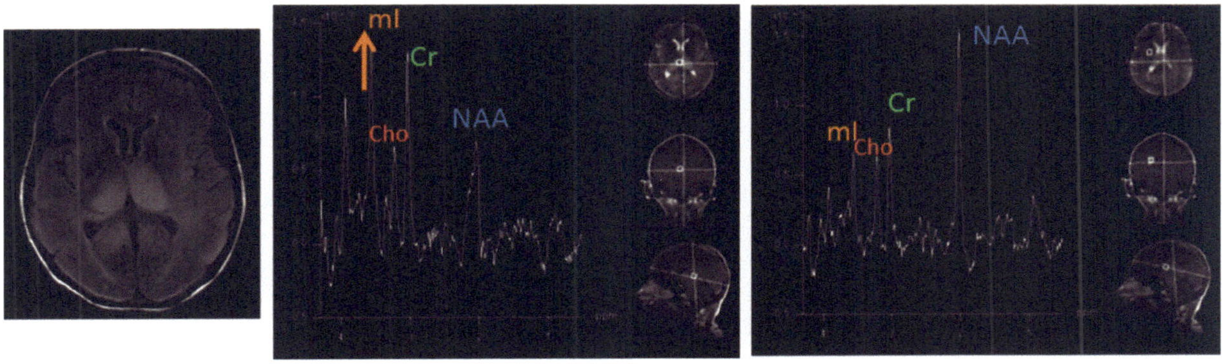

Fig. 5.2. Magnetic resonance spectroscopy of a low-grade tumor. Myo-inositol levels may have implications in the grading of cerebral astrocytomas, as its concentration is high in low-grade gliomas (left). A spectrum from the normal-appearing white matter is also shown (right). mI, myo-inositol; Cho, choline; Cr, creatine; NAA, *N*-acetyl aspartate.

systems in cells, it tends to be low in diseases associated with low metabolism, such as in necrosis and infarctions. However, Cr and PCr are in equilibrium and thus the Cr peak remains stable in size despite bioenergetic abnormalities that occur with many pathologies or with age (Saunders et al., 1999). Consequently, the Cr resonance is often used as an internal standard. However, changes in Cr have been reported in tumors (Ishimaru et al., 2001; Murphy et al., 2002; Howe et al., 2003), stroke (Saunders, 2000) and neuroAIDS (Chang et al., 2002; Ratai et al., 2011).

Choline

The Cho resonance arises from signals of several soluble components that resonate at 3.2 ppm. This resonance contains contributions primarily from glycerophosphocholine, phosphocholine, and Cho. Changes in Cho resonance are commonly seen with diseases that have alterations in membrane turnover and processes that are accompanied by hypercellularity. Neoplasms, leukodystrophies, and multiple sclerosis (MS) result in a substantial increase in MRS-visible Cho (Blusztajn and Wurtman, 1983; Matthews et al., 1991; Brenner et al., 1993; Chang et al., 1995; Miller et al., 1996; Lin et al., 1999). It is increased in primary and secondary brain tumors, with higher Cho/Cr ratios found in malignant tumors (Bendszus et al., 2000). Elevated Cho has also been seen in developing brain (Kreis et al., 1993; Holshouser et al., 1997), and in inflammatory and gliotic processes (Menon et al., 1992; Chong et al., 1993; Barker et al., 1995; Meyerhoff et al., 1999).

Myo-inositol

MRS obtained with short TE (e.g., 35 ms) offers the possibility of visualizing additional resonances, particularly those produced by compounds having short relaxation times, such as mI. mI has its most prominent peaks at 3.5 and 3.6 ppm. The function of mI is not fully understood, although it is believed to be an essential requirement for cell growth, an osmolyte, and a storage source of glucose (Ross, 1991). mI is primarily located in glia and an increase in mI is commonly thought to be a marker of gliosis (Brand et al., 1993). The identification of mI can be important in the evaluation of brain tumors. This metabolite is usually decreased in high-grade primary brain tumors and elevated in low-grade gliomas (Fig. 5.2) (Castillo et al., 2000; Howe et al., 2003; Majos et al., 2004). Elevated mI levels have been associated with Alzheimer's disease (Miller et al., 1993; Shonk et al., 1995), acquired immunodeficiency syndrome (AIDS) dementia, other neurodegenerative diseases, and brain injury (Ross et al., 1998). In addition, elevated mI has been reported in newborns (Holshouser et al., 1997). Reduced mI is observed in hepatic encephalopathy (Lee et al., 1999).

Glycine

The resonance of glycine (Gly) overlaps with those of mI; however, Gly can be unambiguously detected with the choice of longer TEs due to the cancellation of the inositol multiplet (Fig. 5.3). Gly is an amino acid that acts as an inhibitory neurotransmitter and antioxidant and is distributed throughout the CNS. High concentrations of Gly are observed in high-grade gliomas compared to low-grade gliomas (Hattingen et al., 2009; Davies et al., 2010) and in patients with hyperglycinemia (Heindel et al., 1993).

Lactate

Under normal conditions, the lactate concentration is very low in the adult brain. Lactate is produced by anaerobic metabolism and has been detected in stroke patients

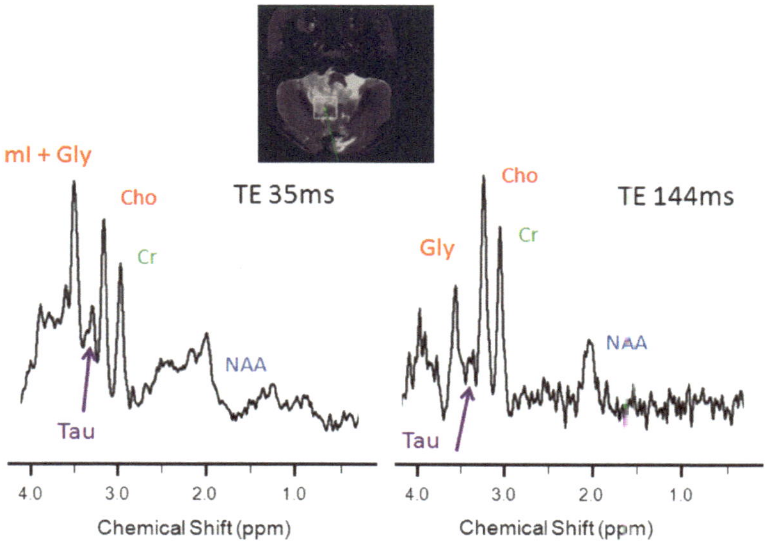

Fig. 5.3. The resonance of glycine (Gly) overlaps with those of myo-inositol (mI); however, Gly can be unambiguously detected with the choice of longer echo times (TE) due to the cancellation of the inositol multiplet. High concentrations of Gly are observed in high-grade gliomas such as in this medulloblastoma. In addition, elevated taurine (at 3.4 ppm) can be detected in this tumor. Cho, choline; Cr, creatine; NAA, *N*-acetyl aspartate.

(Bruhn et al., 1989; Henriksen et al., 1992; Graham et al., 1993) during hypoxia (Kreis et al., 1996), mitochondrial diseases (Cross et al., 1993; Mathews et al., 1993; Castillo et al., 1995), seizures (Breiter et al., 1994), and in the first hours after birth (Barkovich et al., 2001).

The presence of lactate in brain tumors has received a great deal of attention. Accelerated anaerobic glycolysis occurs in highly cellular and metabolically active tumors which have begun to outgrow their blood supply. Consequently, the presence of lactate may indicate a high level of malignancy (Meyerand et al., 1999; Opstad et al., 2007). It has been observed that regions containing lactate correspond to areas of increased cerebral blood volume in brain perfusion studies and thus may serve as an indicator of angiogenesis, another feature typical of highly malignant brain tumors (Hartmann et al., 2003).

This resonance (observed as a doublet) occurs at 1.32 ppm and may be masked by the spectra contribution of lipids. Confirmation of the presence of lactate can be achieved by obtaining MRS with intermediate TE of 136–144 ms, which results in inversion of the lactate doublet below the baseline and long TE of 270–288 ms, when lactate is once more phased up, but the lipid peaks are considerably decreased due to T2 effects. At higher field strength we suggest a TE of 270–288 ms; this technical adjustment at 3T is necessary, because at higher field strengths, lactate may show reduced or absent signal intensity at a TE of 144 ms (Lange et al., 2006).

Lipids

Lipids resonate between 0.8 and 1.5 ppm and may obscure the presence of lactate. Mobile lipids are generally found in necrosis and, as such, are indicators of high-grade malignancies, both primary brain tumors and metastases (Kuesel et al., 1994, 1996) or radiation necrosis. Lipids may also be present in the spectra due to contamination by subcutaneous fat and fat from marrow of the skull. Due to their short T2 relaxation time their presence is most obvious at short TE (~35 ms) and is typically not detectable at long TEs. However, lipids could still be detected at 288 ms in patients with carnitine/acylcarnitine translocase deficiency, a metabolic disorder in which long-chain fatty acids cannot be metabolized (Fig. 5.4).

Glutamate and glutamine

Glu is the major excitatory neurotransmitter of the brain, although it has other important metabolic functions (Ross, 1991; Westergaard et al., 1995; Govindaraju et al., 2000). Excess of Glu surrounding neural cells can be toxic and can eventually result in neuronal death. Cerebral Glu concentration is reported to be increased in cerebral ischemia (Glodzik-Sobanska et al., 2006), hepatic encephalopathy (Chamuleau et al., 1991), and Rett's syndrome (Pan et al., 1996); Glu is also high in some tumors, such as meningiomas (Opstad et al., 2003). Gln is a precursor and storage form of Glu and

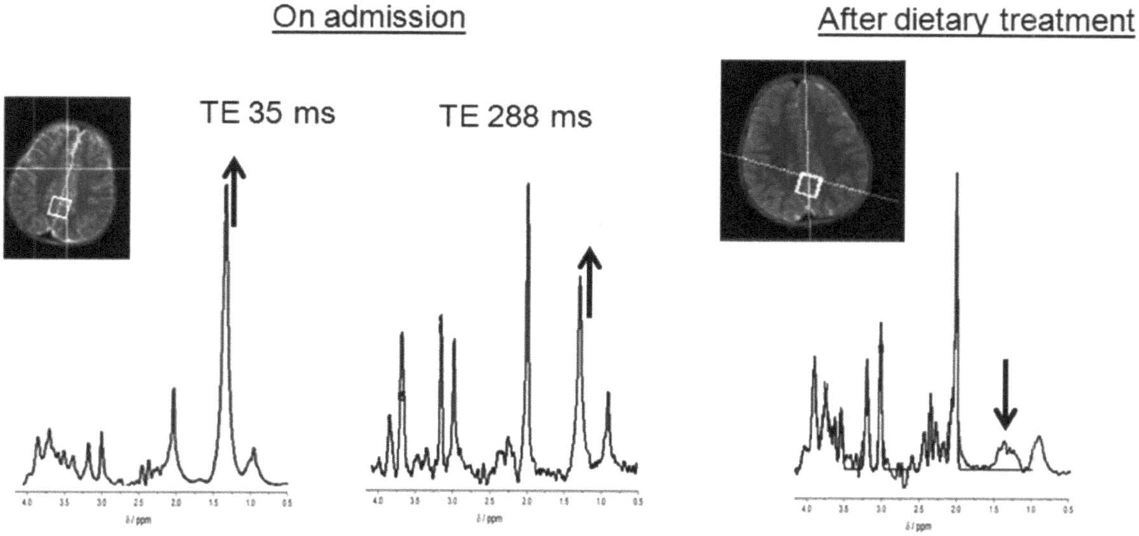

Fig. 5.4. Carnitine/acylcarnitine translocase deficiency causes significant elevation of long-chain fatty acids. Magnetic resonance spectra of a 9-month-old boy with normal fetal and birth history, as well as normal development until ~ 3 weeks prior to admission. Patient developed an acute gastroenteritis and multiorgan failure with encephalopathy, liver and renal failure, cardiac rhythm abnormalities, and elevated pancreatic enzymes. Magnetic resonance spectroscopy spectra showed elevated lipid peaks even at long echo time (TE) of 288 ms. Dietary treatment (portagen formula) resulted in normalization of lipid peaks and clinical improvement after ~ 1 year.

is primarily located in astrocytes. Glu and Gln have strongly coupled spin systems that give rise to complex spectra (Wilman and Allen, 1995; Wilman et al., 1995). Since Gln and Glu are structurally very similar it is very difficult to separate their resonances at low field strength, and therefore the sum of Glu and Gln is commonly referred to as Glx. The peaks of interest resonate between 2.1–2.5 and 2.75 ppm. At higher field strengths (7 T) Glu and Gln can be separated.

In some neurodegenerative diseases Glx and Glu are often decreased (Griffith et al., 2008; Shiino et al., 2012). Decreased tissue density could simply reflect neuronal loss, in addition to decreased production by degenerating neurons, because MRS is not able to differentiate intra- from extracellular metabolite changes.

γ-Aminobutyric acid (GABA)

GABA is an amino acid and an inhibitory neurotransmitter. GABA concentrations in the brain are close to the detection limits of *in vivo* MRS. In addition, the GABA resonances overlap considerably with contributions from other more abundant metabolites, in particular, Cr. However, the invention of specialized MRS techniques, such as selective editing techniques (Rothman et al., 1993; Mullins et al., 2014), localized two-dimensional chemical shift methods (Thomas et al., 2001), or multi quantum filtering methods (Keltner et al., 1997), has enhanced the ability to detect and measure GABA (Puts and Edden, 2012). MRS studies have found reduced or abnormal GABA concentrations in several neuropsychiatric disorders, including epilepsy, anxiety disorders, major depression, and drug addiction (Chang et al., 2003; Rowland et al., 2012; Simpson et al., 2012).

Amino acids

Alanine (Ala) is a nonessential amino acid that resonates at 1.5 ppm. Ala has been found to be elevated in some meningiomas (Jungling et al., 1993; Howe et al., 2003). Valine is an essential amino acid necessary for protein synthesis. The spectrum consists of two doublets from the two methyl protons that overlap with resonances of leucine and isoleucine in the range of 0.95–1.05 ppm. Hypervalinemia and branched-chain ketonuria are some of the diseases in which valine levels become elevated (Holmes et al., 1997). Increased concentrations have also been observed in brain abscesses (Kim et al., 1997).

Taurine is another nonessential amino acid that is synthesized within in the brain and can be chiefly obtained from food. It is involved in osmoregulation. Concentrations are high at the time of birth and decrease with age to 1.5 mM. Medulloblastomas have high taurine concentrations (Fig. 5.3) (Kovanlikaya et al., 2005). The spectrum consists of two triplets at 3.25 and

3.42 ppm and, since these resonances overlap with the resonances from mI and Cho, selective irradiation technique or double-quantum filter are necessary to better resolve the resonances (Rothman et al., 1984; Hardy and Norwood, 1998).

CLINICAL APPLICATIONS OF MAGNETIC RESONANCE SPECTROSCOPY

MRS applications in which the interpretation of the MR spectrum is of value in individual patients

Brain tumors

The evaluation of brain tumors is one of the areas where MRS has significantly impacted patient management. However, one has to keep in mind that information provided by MRS is complementary to the imaging data and needs to be interpreted in light of other imaging data.

MRS can provide information on some key clinical questions, including:

1. diagnosis (differentiate neoplasm from MRI mimics) and tumor grading
2. distinguishing primary CNS neoplasm from metastasis
3. therapeutic planning (biopsy guidance and radiosurgery)
4. prognosis
5. therapeutic response and tumor progression (radiation necrosis versus recurrent tumor and pseudonormalization versus true response to antiangiogenic treatment).

A few examples of each of these clinical applications follow.

Diagnosis

Neoplastic tissue generally exhibits elevated Cho and decreased NAA (Howe et al., 2003) and an increase in the Cho/NAA ratio is typically correlated with tumor malignancy (Fig. 5.5). The Cho/NAA ratio has often been used to distinguish brain neoplasm from nonneoplastic

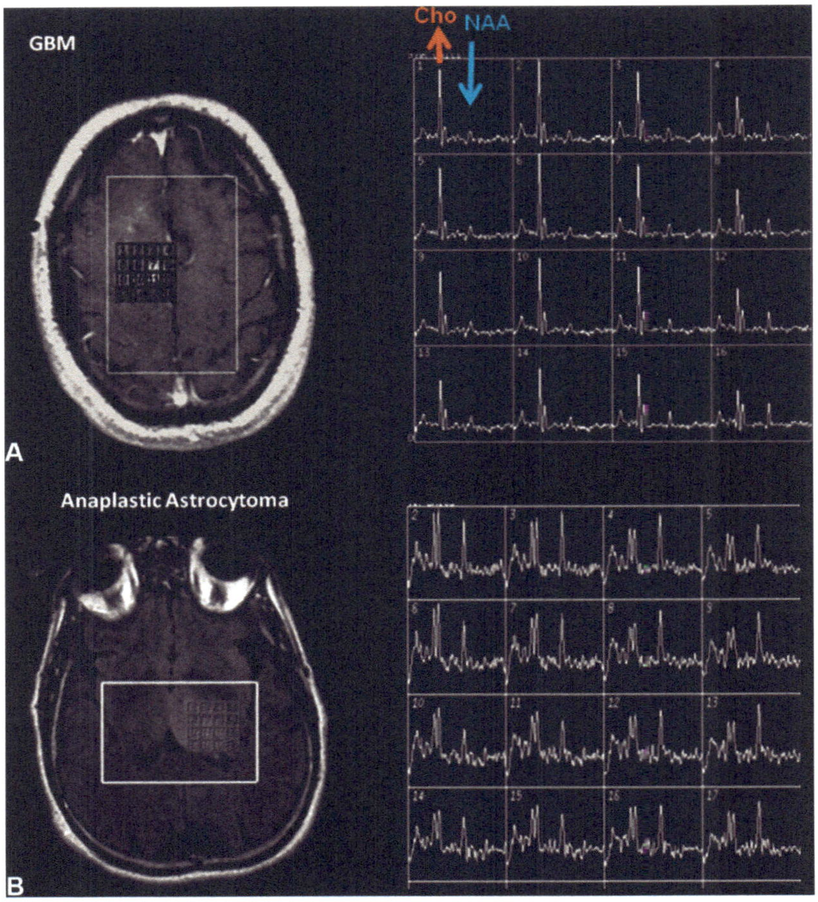

Fig. 5.5. Higher levels of choline (Cho)/*N*-acetyl aspartate (NAA) can be seen in high-grade glioma compared to anaplastic astrocytoma. GBM, glioblastoma multiforme.

brain masses. High-grade gliomas have high Cho and low or absent NAA: the Cho/NAA ratio is typically correlated with tumor malignancy. Also elevated lactate and lipids are typically seen with high-grade neoplasms and are associated with poor survival (Opstad et al., 2007). By contrast, mI resonance is elevated in lower-grade gliomas compared to high-grade gliomas (Fig. 5.2).

However, low-grade tumors as well as tumefactive demyelinating lesions as seen in MS are both characterized by moderate elevations in Cho. Here other functional MRI techniques such as perfusion-weighted MRI can aid in the correct diagnosis (Law et al., 2003; Law, 2005).

On the other hand, other nonneoplastic lesions can easily be discriminated from neoplastic lesions; abscesses only demonstrate cytosolic amino acids while NAA, Cho, and Cr are absent (Kim et al., 1997). Untreated primitive neuroectodermal tumors in pediatric patients have elevated taurine concentration (Kovanlikaya et al., 2005). High concentrations of Gly are often observed in high-grade pediatric tumors (Davies et al., 2010). Meningiomas are characterized by low mI, Cr, and NAA, and in some instances the presence of Ala (Gill et al., 1990; Howe et al., 2003).

In the last decade, pattern recognition algorithms have been used to develop classifiers for automatic brain tumor diagnosis. Several multicenter studies have been able to aid in the diagnosis of tumor cell types and grade (Garcia-Gomez et al., 2009). A meta-analysis concluded that the accuracy of MRS for characterizing brain tumors is promising (Hollingworth et al., 2006). One large study on 176 patients demonstrated a statistically significant increase in diagnostic accuracy for indeterminate brain lesions from 55%, based on MRI alone, to 71% after analysis of MRI and MRS (Moller-Hartmann et al., 2002). Furthermore, information extracted from ^{1}H MRS significantly improved the radiologists' MRI-based characterization of grade IV tumors (glioblastomas, metastases, medulloblastomas, and lymphomas) and also of the less malignant glial tumors (Julia-Sape et al., 2012).

Distinguishing primary CNS neoplasm from metastasis

Discriminating glioblastoma from metastasis is typically challenging as both tumor types exhibit very similar spectroscopic patterns. However, Law et al. (2003) demonstrated that the gradient of decline in the Cho levels extending from the mass can be used to suggest primary tumor or metastasis. The decline in Cho is more gradual in most gliomas – starting from the tumor mass out to normal-appearing brain – due to the infiltrative nature of glioblastomas, whereas the decline in Cho is typically more abrupt with metastasis.

Therapeutic planning

Pathology is still the gold standard for the diagnosis of cancer and a biopsy is required to confirm the nature of the tumor whenever possible. Prior to stereotactic biopsy, two-dimensional (2D) or, better, 3D magnetic resonance spectroscopic imaging (MRSI) can help determine the most malignant part of a tumor to image-guide biopsy of an infiltrative or heterogeneously enhancing mass (Fig. 5.6).

Identifying regions of more aggressive phenotype within a heterogeneous tumor can help plan radiotherapy. In fact, there are indications that boosting these regions can improve the effectiveness of treatment. Einstein et al. (2012) demonstrated in a prospective phase II trial that MRS-targeted gamma-knife stereotactic radiosurgery is feasible and resulted in higher patient survival compared to historic controls.

Prognosis

Most recently, MRS was used to identify molecular subtypes of gliomas with enzyme isocitrate dehydrogenase (IDH) mutations (Choi et al., 2012). Patients with IDH1 gene mutations survive about twice as long as patients with wild-type IDH1 gliomas (Parsons et al., 2008). Mutations in the IDH lead to the accumulation of the metabolite 2-hydroxyglutarate, which can be detected by spectral editing and 2D correlation MRS (Andronesi et al., 2012b). Thus, MRS can be used to predict cancer outcome and patient survival (Fig. 5.7).

Therapeutic response and tumor progression

Typical management for high-grade tumors, such as glioblastoma multiforme (GBMs), includes resection to the greatest clinically feasible degree, followed by high-energy radiation therapy to include the peritumoral regions surrounding the resection margins. It is not uncommon for patients to return with an enhancing mass near the resection site due to the infiltrative nature of glioblastomas. The critical question is whether this mass is recurrent tumor or radiation necrosis, or something else.

Radiation change and tumor recurrence look the same on conventional MR images but they are different metabolically, thus MRS has been shown to be useful in differentiating radiation change from brain tumor recurrence (Taylor et al., 1996; Kamada et al., 1997; Kinoshita et al., 1997; Preul et al., 1998; Pivawer et al., 2007). In radiation necrosis, there is typically a slight elevation of Cho and often the presence of the lipid resonance,

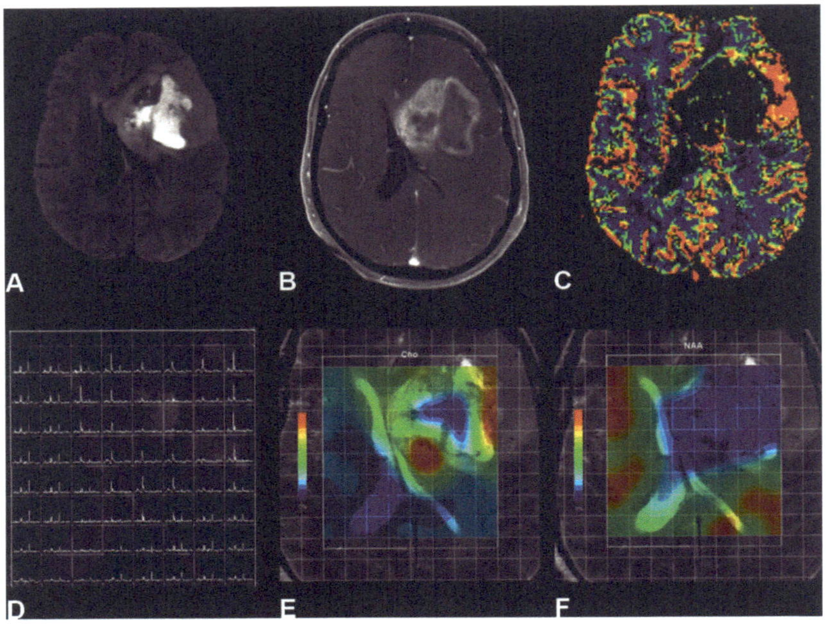

Fig. 5.6. Image guide biopsy. Three-dimensional magnetic resonance spectroscopic imaging (MRSI) can help determine the most malignant part of a heterogeneously enhancing tumor. (**A**) T2-weighted image, (**B**) Postcontrast T1-weighted image, (**C**) Perfusion MR imaging, based on dynamic susceptibility contrast, showing the relative cerebral blood volume of the tumor. (**D**) MRSI. (**E**) Metabolic image of choline (Cho: intensities displayed are proportional to particular metabolite signal strength, here Cho). (**F**) Metabolic image of *N*-acetyl aspartate (NAA). Biopsy in regions of high Cho and low NAA revealed glioblastoma with oligodendroglioma components. (Courtesy of Otto Rapalino.)

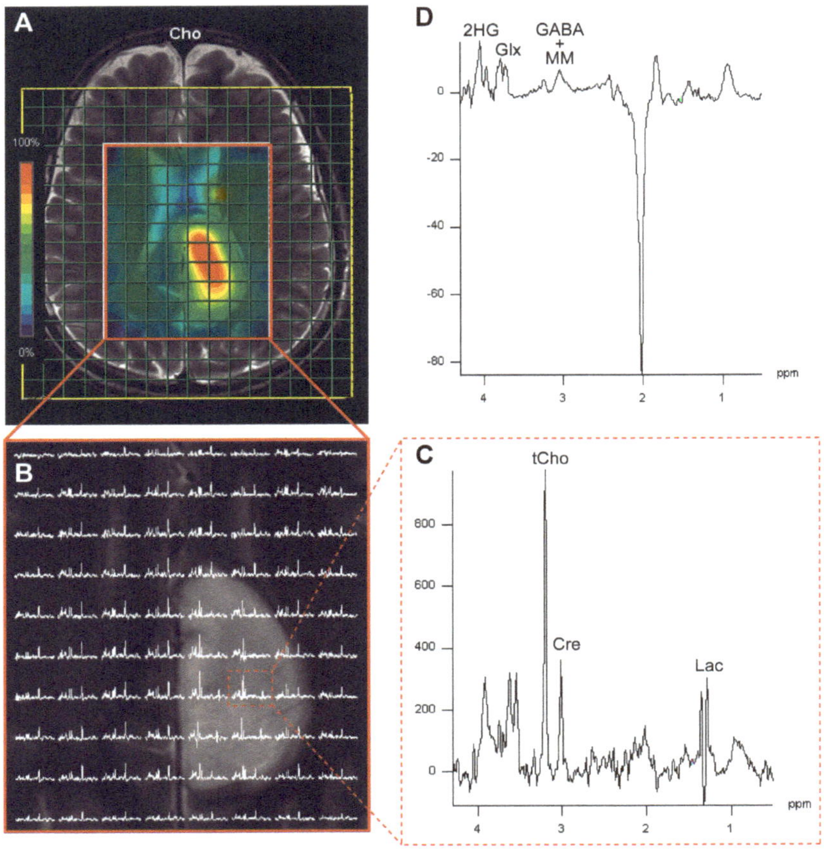

Fig. 5.7. Magnetic resonance spectroscopic imaging (MRSI) of a patient with preoperative glioblastoma multiforme (GBM) shows elevated choline (Cho: **A–C**). Spectral editing MRS (**D**) reveals 2-hydroxyglutarate (2HG in panel **D**). This patient proved to have an R132G isocitrate dehydrogenase (IDH) mutation. GABA, gamma-aminobutyric acid; Glx, glutamate/glutamine; MM, macromolecules; tCho, total choline; Cre, creatine; Lac, lactate. (Courtesy of Ovidiu Andronesi: Andronesi et al., 2012b.)

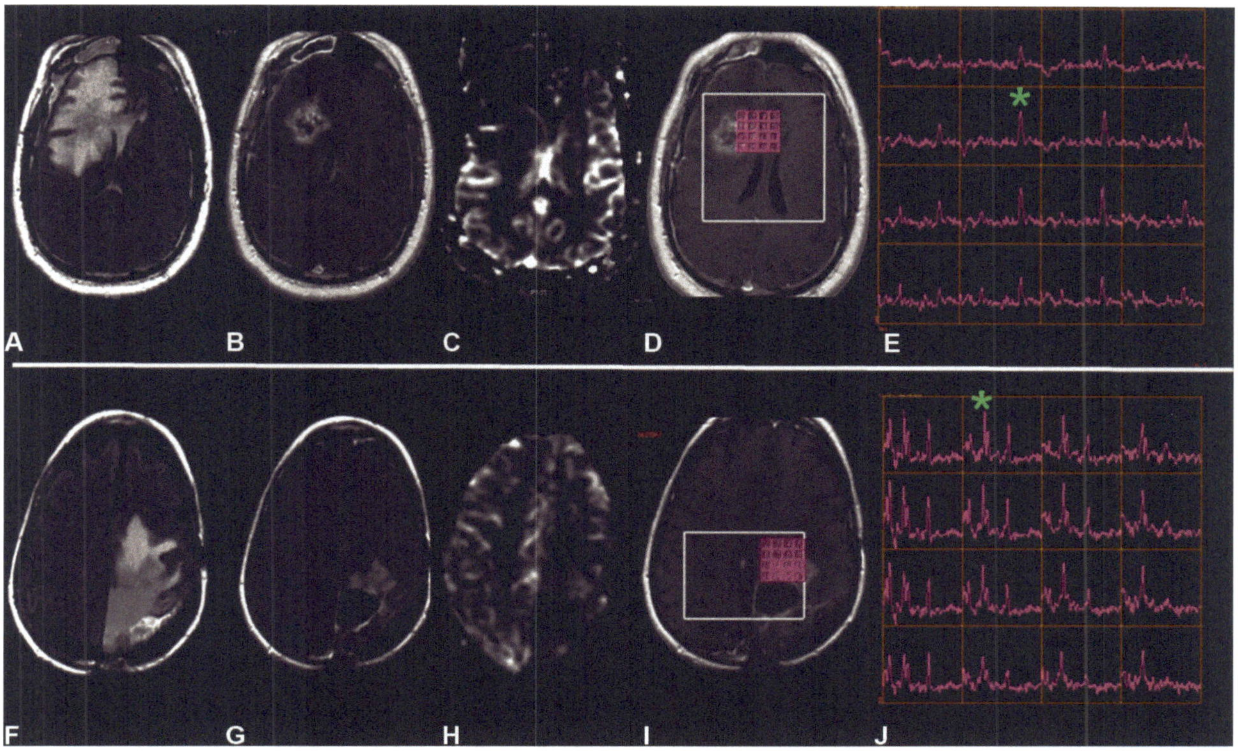

Fig. 5.8. Radiation necrosis (top) vs tumor recurrence (bottom). Top: The patient is status postresection of an esthesioneuroblastoma. He received high-dose radiation to the region of the right frontal lobe. Follow-up imaging revealed an irregularly enhancing focus (**B**) in the right frontal lobe with surrounding fluid-attenuated inversion recovery (FLAIR) hyperintensity (**A**). Perfusion magnetic resonance imaging (MRI) (**C**) revealed low cerebral blood volume (CBV) in the right frontal region. Magnetic resonance spectroscopy (MRS) (**D** and **E**) demonstrated a high lipid resonance (green star) consistent with necrosis. Follow-up imaging obtained multiple times over the subsequent 2 years demonstrated a gradual resolution of the enhancement and tissue loss.

Bottom: A left parietal glioblastoma multiforme was resected, and this was followed by high-dose radiation targeted to the region surrounding the resection cavity. FLAIR MRI (**F**) demonstrates abnormal signal extending from the resection cavity. Postcontrast T1-weighted images (**G**) demonstrated enhancement immediately anterior to the resection cavity. Perfusion MRI (**H**) demonstrates high CBV in this region. MRS (**I** and **J**) of this region demonstrates high levels of choline (green star), consistent with recurrent tumor. (Adapted from Ratai and Gonzalez, 2009.)

while recurrent tumor is characterized by high Cho levels (Fig. 5.8) (Ratai and Gonzalez, 2009). However, elevated lipids have also been detected in GBMs and radiation leads to inflammatory processes in which Cho also becomes elevated. A study at 3 T showed that the ratio of Cho at the biopsy site to Cr of the contralateral site is a good marker to distinguish between radiation necrosis and recurrent tumor (Rabinov et al., 2002).

In GBM patients treated with bevacizumab or other vascular endothelial growth factor-targeting agents, it can be challenging to distinguish actual tumor response to therapy from blood–tumor barrier improvement with decreased contrast leakage. Diminished contrast enhancement commonly seen on standard posttreatment MRI may not always correspond with reduction of viable tumor, a phenomenon called "pseudo-response" (Gerstner et al., 2010). MRS may potentially be useful in assessing response to antiangiogenic treatment. A recent multicenter trial by the Radiation Therapy Oncology Group and the American College of Radiology Imaging Network demonstrated that treatment of bevacizumab in combination with cytotoxic agents resulted in transient increases of NAA/Cho in enhancing tumor regions at 2 weeks posttreatment in patients with recurrent GBM. The increase in NAA/Cho at 2 weeks was uniform in all subjects, regardless of their overall survival status. However, subsequent increases in NAA/Cho levels in the tumor at 8 weeks posttreatment were associated with 6-month progression-free survival (Ratai et al., 2013) (Fig. 5.9). In a different study, increases in NAA/Cho levels at 8 weeks after tumor treatment with AZD2171 (cediranib) predicted accurately 6-month overall survival (Kim et al., 2011). These studies suggest that changes in NAA/Cho may potentially be useful as an imaging biomarker in assessing response to antiangiogenic treatment.

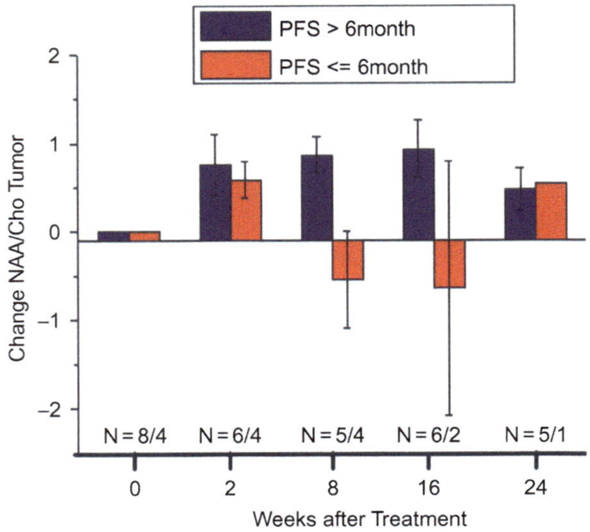

Fig. 5.9. Changes in *N*-acetyl aspartate (NAA)/choline (Cho) from baseline in tumor voxels grouped by progression-free survivors (PFS) at 6 months (PFS > 6 months) and those with tumor progression at 6 months (PFS $\leq$ 6 months). Error bars represent standard error of the mean. Numbers of patients are noted on the bottom. Note that higher NAA/Cho levels in weeks 8 and 16 predict lack of progression at 6 months. (Adapted from Ratai et al., 2013.)

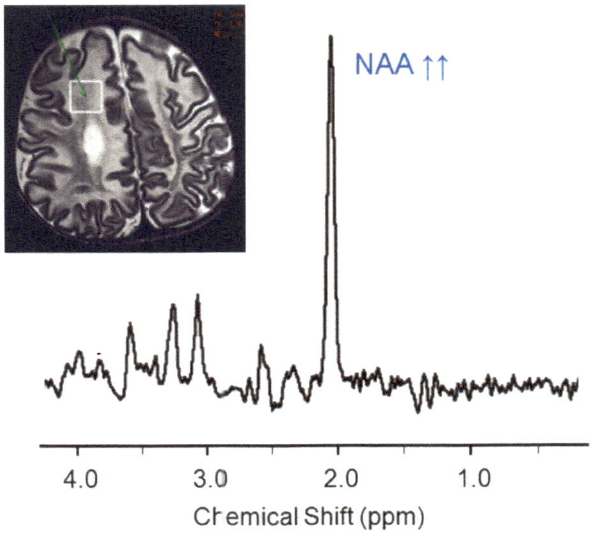

Fig. 5.10. Magnetic resonance spectrum of a 4-year-old boy with Canavan disease. Mutation in the enzyme aspartoacylase (ASPA) results in the inability to catabolize NAA, which is highly increased in the white matter.

Pediatric disorders

MRS is valuable in the identification of pediatric brain disorders that are due to inborn errors of metabolism. These include the leukodystrophies, mitochondrial disorders, and enzyme defects that cause an absence or accumulation of metabolites. Furthermore, MRS has been proven helpful in the assessment of hypoxic-ischemic injuries in the pediatric population.

Inborn errors of metabolism

Many diseases have specific biomarkers which aid in the diagnoses of their respective disorders; for example, phenylalanine in phenylketonuria (Leuzzi et al., 2000, 2007), high concentrations of Gly in nonketotic hyperglycinemia (Heindel et al., 1993; Gabis et al., 2001; Suzuki et al., 2001; Huisman et al., 2002) and the presence of branched-chain amino acids and oxo acids in maple syrup urine disease (Heindel et al., 1995). Significantly increased NAA levels have been observed in Canavan's disease, an inherited disorder in which NAA is not broken down and accumulates to toxic concentrations (Grodd et al., 1991; Tsai and Coyle, 1995) (Fig. 5.10).

Cr is synthesized mainly in the liver and pancreas by the action of L-arginine-glycine amidinotransferase (AGAT) and guanidinoacetate methyltransferase (GAMT). Two inherited enzymatic defects (abnormal AGAT or GAMT) and one inherited defect in Cr transport (SLC6A8) have been characterized that result in a deficiency of cerebral Cr (Nasrallah et al., 2010), which can be detected with MRS. The Cr synthesis defects can be treated with daily oral supplementation of Cr monohydrate (Fig. 5.11), while patients with the transporter defect do not benefit from Cr therapy.

Leukoencephalopathies

X-linked adrenoleukodystrophy is a peroxisomal disorder characterized by accumulation of very-long-chain fatty acids in the CNS, adrenal cortex, and testes. In children, X-linked adrenoleukodystrophy may manifest as rapidly progressive inflammatory demyelination (Moser et al., 2001). Although it is not possible to predict phenotype by mutation analysis or biochemical assays, MRSI is able to identify impending or early stages of degeneration in normal-appearing white matter (Kruse et al., 1994; Eichler et al., 2002). Demyelinating leukodystrophies are generally characterized by increases in Cho and mI and a reduction in NAA – in severe cases lactate can be detected. Follow-up studies are of extreme importance to monitor disease progression in terms of gliosis, demyelination, and axonal damage to determine the prognosis and subsequent choice of therapy. Single-voxel MRS and multivoxel MRSI at high field have revealed extensive neurochemical changes in childhood (Oz et al., 2005) and adult (Ratai et al., 2008) adrenoleukodystrophy.

Hereditary disorders that do not show demyelination but rather hypomyelination have come to increasing attention (Steenweg et al., 2010). The MR spectra of

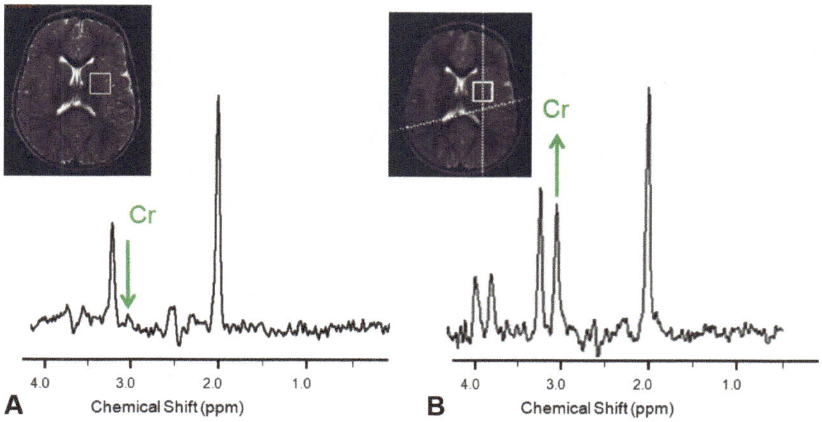

Fig. 5.11. Magnetic resonance spectrum of a 2.5-year-old child with creatine (Cr) deficiency before and after 3 months of supplementation of creatine monohydrate.

patients with ^{4}H-syndrome, a rare form of hypomyelinating leukodystrophy, reveal low Cho/Cr and NAA/Cr, while a prominent mI peak can be observed (Wolf et al., 2005; Outteryck et al., 2010). Low Cho levels are indicative of hypomyelination due to decreased membrane synthesis and turnover. In Pelizaeus–Merzbacher disease, another hypomyelinating disorder, there have been discrepant reports on metabolite abnormalities detected by MRS. In part, these findings may be explained by the concurrent pathophysiologic processes of hypomyelination, gliosis, and neuronal loss over time (Cecil, 2006). Many other hypomyelinating disorders exist; however, only about 50% of the patients with evidence of hypomyelination on MRI come to a definitive diagnosis. Yet, specific MRI and MRS features can be pathognomonic and lead to diagnosis (Ratai et al., 2012).

Hypoxic ischemia

Hypoxic-ischemic injury continues to be a major cause of perinatal mortality and morbidity (Rutherford et al., 1995) and MRS has emerged as a potential biomarker for outcome. Many publications show that the presence of lactate is predictive of adverse outcome (Zarifi et al., 2002; Kadri et al., 2003; Khong et al., 2004; da Silva et al., 2006; Zhu et al., 2008). NAA and Cho are also predictive of unfavorable outcome of severely asphyxiated term neonates (Boichot et al., 2006). Experimental data indicate that excitatory amino acids, particularly Glu, play a critical role in the mediation of hypoxic neuronal injury (Hill, 1991). Higher Glx levels are correlated with severity of hypoxic-ischemic injury by Sarnat criteria (Groenendaal et al., 2001). Furthermore, Zhu et al. (2008) showed that the alpha-Glx peak at 3.8 ppm is predictive of poor outcome. A recent meta-analysis showed increased lactate and decreased NAA as the best predictor of adverse outcome (Thayyil et al., 2010). Hypothermia is the standard-of-care neuroprotective treatment for perinatal asphyxia and MRS can be used as a means to assess treatment efficacy (Azzopardi et al., 2009). ^{1}H MRS can provide valuable prognostic information in the case of near drowning. A spectroscopic prognosis index (including diminished cerebral NAA, Cr, and mI and the appearance of lactate) distinguished between good and poor outcome (Kreis et al., 1996).

Infections

Brain infections need to be treated immediately and thus require a prompt diagnosis. Laboratory testing can be time consuming and may delay therapy. MRS is useful to distinguish abscesses from other ring-enhancing lesions. Pyogenic abscesses are characterized by the presence of cytosolic amino acids, such as valine, Ala, leucine, lactate, acetate, and succinate in the spectrum, while NAA, Cho, and Cr are absent (Kim et al., 1997). Furthermore, parasitic cysts show succinate and acetate in the absence of amino acids (Jayakumar et al., 2004) and tuberculous abscesses show only lactate and lipid signals (at 0.9 and 1.3 ppm), devoid of cytosolic amino acids (Oz et al., 2014).

Neurologic diseases in which changes in the MRS spectrum are occasionally large enough to be useful for clinical management

Epilepsy

Epilepsy is a common neurologic disorder characterized by seizures which may have variable etiologies, including neoplasms, cortical dysplasia, or metabolic disorders. MRS is indicated for screening for metabolic disorders that may present with seizures, such as mitochondrial disorders, and for the characterization of masses

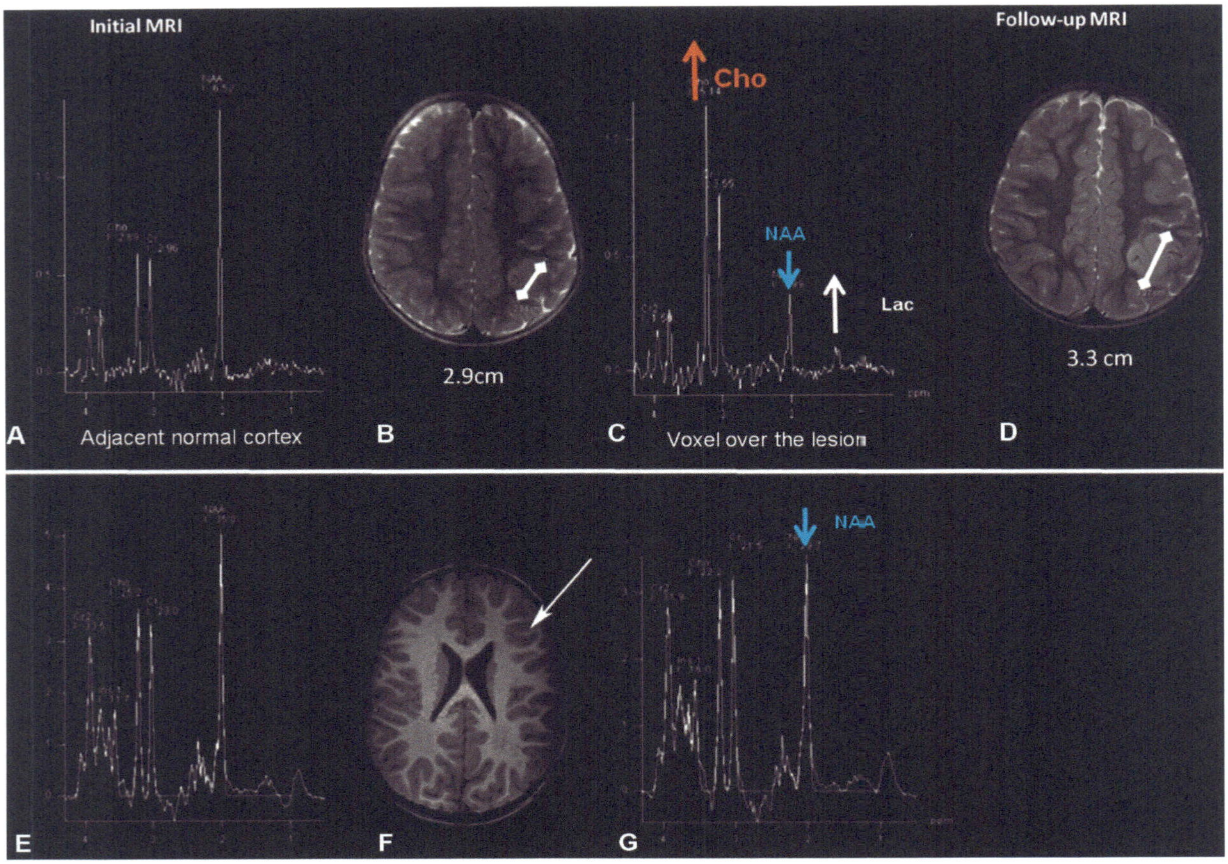

Fig. 5.12. Magnetic resonance spectroscopy (MRS) of a neoplasm (top) vs a focal cortical dysplasia (bottom).

Top: MRS raises concern for a neoplasm rather than a focal cortical dysplasia. Magnetic resonance imaging (MRI: **B**) and MRS (**A** and **C**) in a 7-year-old developmentally normal boy who presents with sudden onset of right face and arm twitching; electroencephalogram (EEG) shows left parietal slowing and spikes. Axial T2 images show a lesion which is largely isointense to gray matter and that expands the involved left parietal cortex (**B**). Single-voxel MRS performed at echo time (TE) 288 at 3 T shows elevation in the choline (Cho) and decrease in *N*-acetylaspartate (NAA: **C**) compared to adjacent normal cortex (**A**) that raised concern for neoplasia; a small lactate (Lac) peak was also seen over the lesion (**C**). The lesion was followed closely and comparison between the presentation MRI and a follow-up MRI several months later showed interval increase in size (**D**). The lesion was resected and pathology showed an angiocentric astrocytoma. (Adapted from Caruso et al., 2013.)

Bottom: MRI (**F**) and MRS (**E** and **G**) were performed for evaluation of a 2-year-old boy with focal seizure semiology consisting of right head turn and eye deviation and staring, that evolved to tonic seizures with bilateral arm raising. EEG showed nearly continuous spikes with slow-wave discharges in the left frontal region F3/Fp1. Axial reformats from an MPRAGE show asymmetric sulcation and fullness of the left middle frontal gyrus that raised concern for focal cortical dysplasia versus neoplasm. MRS at TE 35 over the lesion (**G**) compared to MRS obtained over the contralateral normal right middle frontal gyrus (**E**) shows reduced NAA/Cr but no elevation in choline. These findings are thought to favor dysplasia rather than neoplasia. The patient became medically refractory over the course of the next 2 years, underwent resection of the left middle frontal gyral lesion, and pathology confirmed a type IIB focal cortical dysplasia. (Adapted from Caruso et al., 2013.)

detected by conventional MRI as neoplasm versus dysplasia (Fig. 5.12).

During a seizure, the metabolic demands exceed the supply of oxygen and nutrients to the portion of the brain that is undergoing the enhanced electric activity. Under these circumstances, metabolic changes can be detected by MRS, including the production of lactate (Matthews et al., 1990; Cendes et al., 1997b), and, if prolonged, the reduction of NAA, and an increase in Cho. These abnormalities can still be observed some time after seizure activity ceases.

By far the most common clinical scenario for the use of MRS is temporal-lobe epilepsy (TLE) to help localize the source of the seizures. A large proportion of TLE patients do not respond to medications; however, surgical approaches can be curative. Identifying the correct side for resection is critical. A variety of methods have been used in attempts to identify the abnormal side in patients with TLE, including electroencephalography, Wada testing, single-photon emission computed tomography, or positron emission tomography. The imaging findings on MRI include hyperintensity of the medial temporal lobe and/or shrinkage of the hippocampal formation. However, many cases can be negative on MRI.

MRS also can contribute to the decision-making process (Cendes et al., 1993, 1997a; Hetherington et al., 1995; Achten et al., 1997, 1998; Cohen-Gadol et al., 2004; Kuzniecky, 2004). Typically, findings on MRS, when present, include a reduction of NAA and an increase of Cho in the abnormal side as compared to the contralateral side. It has been demonstrated that both medial temporal regions are abnormal in patients with TLE. After resection of the correct side, the metabolic abnormalities in the contralateral temporal lobe have been observed to revert to normal after a few months.

Ischemia

Ischemia and hypoxic injury to the brain are major causes of morbidity and mortality worldwide. Ischemia is caused by the occlusion of a cerebral blood vessel. If the occlusion is severe, oxygen and metabolite flow will be greatly altered and the brain will switch to anaerobic energy production. This will result in a change in the MR spectrum, most notably the addition of lactate, the product of anaerobic respiration (Gillard et al., 1996; Saunders, 2000). This increase is usually accompanied by a decrease in NAA (Graham et al., 1992; Demougeot et al., 2004).

Like ischemia, a cardiac arrest produces a cessation of blood flow into the brain. Despite their clear differences in mechanism, the metabolite changes observed on a spectrum are largely the same. When someone is found after a cardiac arrest of undetermined duration, MRS can be employed to determine the length of time of the arrest. As the time of arrest increases, the level of hypoxic injury increases. This will present as a persistent elevation of lactate and reduction of NAA on the MR spectrum (Welch et al., 1992; Fischer et al., 1995; Higuchi et al., 1997; Keltner et al., 1998; Krep et al., 2003; Wartenberg et al., 2004; Kano et al., 2006). With more prolonged arrest, significant metabolic abnormalities can be observed by MRS despite the re-establishment of normal blood flow to the brain.

MRS applications in which MRS is most meaningful in assessing groups patients or individuals with serial MRS studies

Neurodegenerative diseases

Neurodegenerative diseases such as Alzheimer's disease, Parkinson's disease, Huntington's disease, amyotrophic lateral sclerosis, and MS are characterized by injury to, and ultimately loss of, neurons. Thus, the characteristic features of neurodegenerative diseases include a decrease in neuronal marker NAA and, in some cases, elevation of glial markers mI and Cho.

Alzheimer's disease is the most common neurodegenerative disease. Individuals with mild cognitive impairment and presymptomatic Alzheimer's disease already demonstrate reduction in NAA/Cr and elevation of mI/Cr and Cho/Cr. The reduction in NAA parallels symptom severity (Adalsteinsson et al., 2000; Kantarci et al., 2000, 2008). This suggests that MRS may be a valuable spectroscopic biomarker either alone or in combination with volumetric measurements (Kantarci et al., 2009) in predicting future development of dementia and monitoring early disease progression for preventive therapies (Kantarci, 2007).

In Parkinson's disease, the primary insult is to the substantia nigra, but this structure is typically too small to be probed effectively by MRS in a clinical setting. A comprehensive review of MRS studies in Parkinson's disease showed a small decrease (5%) in the NAA level in the lentiform nucleus compared with controls (Firbank et al., 2002). More prominent changes on the MR spectrum have been observed in the other parkinsonian syndromes. Decline in NAA in the striatum and the lentiform nucleus has been reported in progressive supranuclear palsy, multiple system atrophy and corticobasal degeneration (Davie et al., 1995; Federico et al., 1997; Tedeschi et al., 1997; Firbank et al., 2002).

MRS studies of patients with Huntington's disease have demonstrated decreased NAA and increased Cho in the basal ganglia and in the cortex of patients who are symptomatic (Jenkins et al., 1993; Harms et al., 1997; Hoang et al., 1998). There have been reports of increased lactate in certain regions of the brain. As more effective therapies are developed, MRS may be useful in monitoring their efficacy, e.g., MRS has been used to demonstrate increased cortical NAA/Cho and NAA/Cr ratios after successful bilateral subthalamic nucleus stimulation (Llumiguano et al., 2008).

Amyotrophic lateral sclerosis is a rapidly progressive neurodegenerative disease characterized by upper and lower motor neuron dysfunction in the brain, spinal cord, and motor cortex. As would be expected, the motor strip has maximal changes in NAA (Pioro et al., 1994; Jones et al., 1995; Gredal et al., 1997), but additional cortical areas, including the sensory strip, also demonstrate a decrease in this metabolite.

MS is a heterogeneous and complex autoimmune disease that is characterized by inflammation, demyelination, and axon degeneration in the CNS. MRS changes that occur during the development of an acute MS plaque include elevation of Cho and a decline in

NAA (Arnold et al., 1990, 1992, 1994; Miller et al., 1991; Davie et al., 1994; Husted et al., 1994; Ferguson et al., 1997; Trapp et al., 1998; Narayana, 2005; Gonzalez-Toledo et al., 2006; Tartaglia and Arnold, 2006; De Stefano and Filippi, 2007). These changes reflect the inflammatory process and the resulting neuronal injury. After the acute phase these metabolic changes can return to normal. However, MRS of a chronic plaque, especially if sufficient injury has resulted, may reveal a permanent decline in NAA along with a persistent Cho elevation. Interestingly, in patients with long-standing MS, NAA may also be reduced in normal-appearing white matter (Fu et al., 1998; De Stefano et al., 1998; Miller et al., 2003).

MS has traditionally been viewed as an inflammatory demyelinating white-matter disease of the CNS. However, recent pathology and MRI studies have shown lesions in the gray matter as well (Mainero et al., 2009). MRS studies of whole-brain NAA demonstrated that the loss in NAA cannot be explained by white-matter involvement alone, leading to a conclusion of extensive gray-matter involvement even in a relatively early stage of the disease (Inglese et al., 2004).

The first reports on the use of MRS in neuroAIDS were published in the early 1990s. These early studies demonstrated significantly reduced levels of NAA in the brains of these patients (Jarvik et al., 1993; Meyerhoff et al., 1993; Chong et al., 1993). Subsequently it was shown that earlier in the disease elevations of Cho (Tracey et al., 1996) and mI (Ernst and Chang, 2004; Sacktor et al., 2005) preceded a decrease in NAA. These findings of elevated Cho and mI suggested that a cerebral inflammatory process occurred before neuronal injury and that neuronal injury occurred after the inflammatory process had persisted for some time. ^{1}H MR spectroscopy has been used in studies on the effects of drugs. With antiretroviral therapy, the reversal of the metabolic abnormalities has been reported (Chang et al., 1999).

Psychiatric diseases

Technologic advances in MRS in recent years have expanded the potential to measure neurotransmitters such as Glu, Gln, and GABA that may be altered in patients with psychiatric disorders (Keshavan et al., 2000; Stanley et al., 2000; Puts and Edden, 2012; Mullins et al., 2014). In particular, Glu and GABA have been shown to be decreased in schizophrenia and some mood disorders. Unmedicated adults with obsessive compulsive disorder may have decreased GABA levels (Simpson et al., 2012). These studies suggest altered neurotransmission. MRS has also been used to detect alterations in NAA (in bipolar disorder and anxiety disorders), Cho (in schizophrenia, mood disorders, bipolar disorder), and changes in energy consumption and production through alterations in Cr concentration (in schizophrenia and obsessive compulsive disorder). In addition, recovery of normal metabolite levels with treatments has been monitored with MRS (Bertolino et al., 2001; Braus et al., 2001).

Traumatic brain injury

Nearly 2 million traumatic brain injuries occur in the USA each year, making it the leading cause of death and disability in children and young adults (Collins, 1990). MRS is not routinely used in the acute setting of head injuries. However, during the recovery period following traumatic brain injury, the NAA/Cr ratio can be used to predict clinical outcome (Brooks et al., 2000; Nakabayashi et al., 2007). A global decline of the neuronal marker NAA was reported using whole-brain NAA quantification (Cohen et al., 2007). In addition, patients with poorer outcomes had elevated mean Cho postinjury – suggesting active inflammation – compared to patients with better outcomes (Brooks et al., 2000; Schuhmann et al., 2003; Govindaraju et al., 2004; Hunter et al., 2005). Lactate also may have predictive value in determining the outcome in pediatric head injury (Ashwal et al., 2000; Barkovich et al., 2001; Kadri et al., 2003). In adult traumatic brain injury this predictive ability may be lacking; some reports indicate changes in lactate in this group, while others reported conflicting observations (Garnett et al., 2000a, b, 2001).

TECHNICAL CONSIDERATIONS AND PITFALLS

In order to effectively interpret MRS data, knowledge of data acquisition and analysis is essential. Thus, the chapter concludes with technical considerations and challenges of MRS.

Data acquisition

Localization techniques

The two standard localization methods include point resolved spectroscopy (PRESS) (Bottomley, 1987) and stimulated echo acquisition mode (STEAM). STEAM is able to utilize very short TEs: however, the stimulated echo signal has half the amplitude of the primary echo signal. Recently, more specialized pulse sequences have been integrated on the clinical MR scanners, including MEGA-PRESS (Mescher et al., 1998) or semi-LASER (Oz and Tkac, 2011).

Basically, two methods exist to obtain the spatially localized metabolic information *in vivo*:

1. Single-voxel spectroscopy uses selective excitation pulses to localize a voxel of typically 3–8 cm^3 in the brain. Single-voxel spectroscopy has the advantage of higher signal-to-noise ratio (SNR) and typically shorter acquisition times (~3 minutes).
2. MRSI can be obtained in two or three dimensions, resulting in individual voxel sizes of typically 0.5–3 cm^3. MRSI allows one to collect the spectral information from a volume consisting of many voxels. MRSI is preferred for clinical studies, where it is indicated to obtain metabolic information of a large and heterogeneous lesion, e.g., in tumors. Additionally, spectral information from control regions may be obtained simultaneously. However, the main limitation of MRSI is the lengthy acquisition time, especially with 3D data acquisition (>8 minutes).

A number of fast MRSI experiments have been presented to reduce data acquisition duration. Some improvement can be achieved by acquiring data by reduced *k*-space sampling (Maudsley et al., 1994; Kuehn, 1996). Fast MRSI sequences have evolved from concepts related to spatial encoding using gradient switching during acquisition (Mansfield, 1984; Guilfoyle et al., 1989; Webb et al., 1989; Posse et al., 1995). Spiral trajectories in *k*-space allow fast encoding of spatial information. A recent study showed that clinical 3D MRS images can be acquired four times faster with spiral protocols than with the elliptical phase-encoding protocol at a high spatial resolution of 1 cm^3 in 2.5 minutes (Andronesi et al., 2012a).

Acquisition parameters

As with MRI, the choice of TE and repetition time (TR) can have considerable effects on the appearance of the information obtained in a proton MRS study.

Echo time

MR spectra obtained with shorter TEs (<35 ms) allow the detection of more metabolites, including Glx and mI (Fig. 15.1B). Spectra obtained with intermediate TEs (135–144 ms) depict a reduced number of metabolites (Fig. 15.1A). However, spectra are easier to process and analyze due to the relatively flat baseline. In addition, lactate (1.3 ppm) and Ala (1.5 ppm) doublets are inverted, therefore allowing better differentiation between these metabolites and lipids/macromolecules. Spectra obtained at long TEs of 270–288 ms have the advantage that typically no lipid contamination is present, lactate is once more phased up, but the SNR is considerably decreased due to T2 effects. At 3 T a TE of 270–288 ms is warranted, as lactate may be missed at intermediate TEs (Lange et al., 2006).

Spin-lattice relaxation time (T1)

Spin-lattice relaxation times for selected resonances at 1.5 T vary between 1100 and 1700 ms (Frahm et al., 1989) and are becoming longer at higher field strengths. Ideally, one has to wait three times T1 (3×1500 ms = 4500 ms) to gain approximately 95% of the original magnetization. With longer TR (>3 seconds), the SNR and the quantification improve. A long TR, however, results in a long exam time. Therefore, typical TRs for clinical MRS experiments lie between 1000 and3000 ms and should not be altered once chosen.

Voxel location and chemical shift artifact

It is well known that the volume of interest (VOI) selection pulse will always excite spins outside the targeted VOI, resulting in: (1) chemical shift displacement error; (2) spatial nonuniformity of radiofrequency excitation; and (3) contamination with subcutaneous lipid signal from tissues outside the region of interest. This limits the VOI placement, MRS voxels cannot be placed in close proximity to the skull, and with increasing field strength these issues are becoming more and more severe. However, outer volume saturation pulses can be applied to address the geometric limits (Tran et al., 2000). To compensate for radiofrequency inhomogeneity, adiabatic pulses can be implemented (Garwood et al., 1989; Andronesi et al., 2010). Recently, a 3D MRS imaging technique with low-power adiabatic pulses and fast spiral acquisition was implemented (Andronesi et al., 2012a), resulting in high-resolution, high-SNR MRS data.

Signal-to-noise ratio

MRS suffers from inherently low SNR, resulting in MRSI with low spatial resolution or long acquisition times. MRS SNR can be improved significantly by using higher magnetic field strengths. In general, MRS is preferred at 3 T over 1.5 T. Physics predicts a linear increase in signal with field strength, if T1 and T2 relaxation times, coil and system losses and radiofrequency penetration effects do not change significantly. However, shorter T2 and T2* relaxation times adversely affect SNR and resolution at higher field. But the increased chemical shift range at 3 T and 7 T results in greater separation of the resonance peaks, and consequently, allows for better quantification of those metabolites that generally overlap with others such as Glu and Gln (Tkac et al., 2001).

Multichannel receiver coils such as 32-channel brain improve the SNR in MRS. Moreover, a recent study demonstrated that size-optimized multichannel array coils (for neonates, 6 months old, 1 year old, 4 years old, and 7 years old) provided significant sensitivity gains for pediatric brain imaging at 3 T (Keil et al., 2011).

Shimming

Shimming is a procedure to maximize B_0 homogeneity. A homogeneous static magnetic field B_0 is essential for the acquisition of high-quality spectroscopy data, as spectral resolution and symmetric line shape are critical for reliable metabolite quantification. B_0 inhomogeneities result primarily from susceptibility differences between air and tissue and are scaled with the field strength. On most commercial scanners, shimming routines are readily available and are typically performed by generating a B_0 field map (Schneider and Glover, 1991; Webb and Macovski, 1991; Kanayama et al., 1996; Hetherington et al., 2006). Rapid imaging techniques such as echo-planar imaging or spiral imaging are often used to minimize scan time (Reese et al., 1995; Gruetter and Tkac, 2000). All MRI scanners have at least three coils available for shimming, namely the linear x, y, and z gradient coils for imaging. At higher field strengths $\geq$ 3 T, higher-order shimming routines, e.g., second-order shim coils ($z_2, x_2 - y_2, x_y, x_z$, and y_z) are necessary for improved performance.

Motion correction

Motion artifact and patient cooperation often limit the feasibility of MRI and MRS; especially for children between 2 months and 7 years of age sedation must often be used. However, anesthesia carries risks to patients, thus the search for motion correction techniques. Using image-based navigators, it is possible to correct motion in structural imaging and single-voxel spectroscopy prospectively (Keating et al., 2010; Hess et al., 2011).

Data analysis

The area under the peak in the MR spectrum is proportional to the concentration of the metabolite (more precisely, its proton equivalent) weighted by T1 and T2 relation depending on TR or TE, respectively. To date, automated parametric spectral analysis methods have been implemented that seek to determine the optimum parameters that enable some functions (so-called model functions) to best describe the data. These model functions are based on prior information. Fortunately, considerable information on the observable metabolites and their spectral characteristics are available (Govindaraju et al., 2000). Parametric modeling based on *a priori* spectral information has been made reasonably robust (Provencher, 1993; Stanley et al., 1995; Soher et al., 1998; Slotboom et al., 1998; Young et al., 1998a, b). Currently, the most commonly used MRS analysis programs are MRUI (Naressi et al., 2001) and LCModel (Provencher, 1993). The quality of a fit should be carefully assessed by examining the residual signal and the Cramer-Rao lower bounds. Additionally, the macromolecule contributions in short TE spectra should be taken into account during the fitting procedure (Oz et al., 2014).

The easiest quantification method is to employ metabolite ratios, such as NAA/Cr or Cho/NAA. Ratios reported using Cr as an internal standard are often based on the assumption that the Cr concentration does not change during the disease process, an assumption which is sometimes, but not always, true. "Absolute quantification" of brain metabolites by MRS is more difficult to obtain. Metabolite concentrations are generally expressed in institutional units or units of mmol/kg. Methods used for absolute quantification include: (1) phantom replacement techniques (Alger et al., 1993; Michaelis et al., 1993; Soher et al., 1996; Jacobs et al., 2001); (2) water signal as a reference using a second MR spectrum in which the water is unsuppressed (Barker et al., 1993; Christiansen et al., 1993); and (3) the use of an external reference (Tofts and Wray, 1988; Hennig et al., 1992).

For 2D or 3D MRSI data acquisition, the resulting data can be displayed as a grid of many voxels, as individual voxels, or as metabolite maps in which the intensities displayed in the image are proportional to particular metabolite signal strength. However, one has to be careful in interpreting the color maps as they can introduce artifacts, which may lead to misinterpretation, and one must always inspect the raw data (the spectra) themselves.

Data interpretation

To ensure that a ^{1}H MR spectrum is clinically interpretable, we would like to provide a simple checklist with minimum technical requirements. The summary of technical factors that ensure that MRS is clinically interpretable is as follows:

- spectrum SNR $>$ 3
- spectral resolution: full width at half maximum of metabolites $<$0.1 ppm
- line shape symmetric
- water suppression $>$98%
- no lipid contamination from the scalp
- understanding of other possible artifacts, such as chemical shift artifact, ghosting, patient motion, eddy currents
- regular quality assurance on phantoms.

Details on these technical criteria can be found in a comprehensive review by Kreis (2004).

In conclusion, the ability of MRS to probe tissue biochemistry is a powerful tool that may add important clinical information to that obtained by conventional MRI. Because of the inherently low signal in MRS, biologic changes have to be large to be reliably detected by this method in individuals. This may be true in several diseases, including brain tumors, hypoxia-ischemia, metabolic disorders, and others described in this chapter. To be clinically useful, MRS requires careful attention to the technical issues related to acquiring clinical quality spectra. With high-quality MR spectra, this method can help significantly in the care of many patients.

References

Achten E, Boon P, Van De Kerckhove T et al. (1997). Value of single-voxel proton MR spectroscopy in temporal lobe epilepsy. AJNR Am J Neuroradiol 18: 1131–1139.

Achten E, Santens P, Boon P et al. (1998). Single-voxel proton MR spectroscopy and positron emission tomography for lateralization of refractory temporal lobe epilepsy. AJNR Am J Neuroradiol 19: 1–8.

Adalsteinsson E, Sullivan EV, Kleinhans N et al. (2000). Longitudinal decline of the neuronal marker N-acetyl aspartate in Alzheimer's disease. Lancet 355: 1696–1697.

Alger JR, Symko SC, Bizzi A et al. (1993). Absolute quantitation of short TE brain 1H-MR spectra and spectroscopic imaging data. J Comput Assist Tomogr 17: 191–199.

Andronesi OC, Ramadan S, Mountford CE et al. (2010). Low-power adiabatic sequences for in vivo localized two-dimensional chemical shift correlated MR spectroscopy. Magn Reson Med 64: 1542–1556.

Andronesi OC, Gagoski BA, Sorensen AG (2012a). Neurologic 3D MR spectroscopic imaging with low-power adiabatic pulses and fast spiral acquisition. Radiology 262: 647–661.

Andronesi OC, Kim GS, Gerstner E et al. (2012b). Detection of 2-hydroxyglutarate in IDH-mutated glioma patients by in vivo spectral-editing and 2D correlation magnetic resonance spectroscopy. Sci Transl Med 4: 116ra4.

Arnold DL, Matthews PM, Francis G et al. (1990). Proton magnetic resonance spectroscopy of human brain in vivo in the evaluation of multiple sclerosis: assessment of the load of disease. Magn Reson Med 14: 154–159.

Arnold DL, Matthews PM, Francis GS et al. (1992). Proton magnetic resonance spectroscopic imaging for metabolic characterization of demyelinating plaques. Ann Neurol 31: 235–241.

Arnold DL, Riess GT, Matthews PM et al. (1994). Use of proton magnetic resonance spectroscopy for monitoring disease progression in multiple sclerosis. Ann Neurol 36: 76–82.

Ashwal S, Holshouser BA, Shu SK et al. (2000). Predictive value of proton magnetic resonance spectroscopy in pediatric closed head injury. Pediatr Neurol 23: 114–125.

Azzopardi DV, Strohm B, Edwards AD et al. (2009). Moderate hypothermia to treat perinatal asphyxial encephalopathy. N Engl J Med 361: 1349–1358.

Barker PB, Soher BJ, Blackband SJ et al. (1993). Quantitation of proton NMR spectra of the human brain using tissue water as an internal concentration reference. NMR Biomed 6: 89–94.

Barker PB, Lee RR, Mcarthur JC (1995). AIDS dementia complex: evaluation with proton MR spectroscopic imaging. Radiology 195: 58–64.

Barkovich AJ, Westmark KD, Bedi HS et al. (2001). Proton spectroscopy and diffusion imaging on the first day of life after perinatal asphyxia: preliminary report. AJNR Am J Neuroradiol 22: 1786–1794.

Bendszus M, Warmuth-Metz M, Klein R et al. (2000). MR spectroscopy in gliomatosis cerebri. AJNR Am J Neuroradiol 21: 375–380.

Bertolino A, Callicott JH, Mattay VS et al. (2001). The effect of treatment with antipsychotic drugs on brain N-acetylaspartate measures in patients with schizophrenia. Biol Psychiatry 49: 39–46.

Birken DL, Oldendorf WH (1989). N-acetyl-L-aspartic acid: a literature review of a compound prominent in 1H-NMR spectroscopic studies of brain. Neurosci Biobehav Rev 13: 23–31.

Blusztajn JK, Wurtman RJ (1983). Choline and cholinergic neurons. Science 221: 614–620.

Boichot C, Walker PM, Durand C et al. (2006). Term neonate prognoses after perinatal asphyxia: contributions of MR imaging, MR spectroscopy, relaxation times, and apparent diffusion coefficients. Radiology 239: 839–848.

Bottomley PA (1987). Spatial localization in NMR spectroscopy in vivo. Ann N Y Acad Sci 508: 333–348.

Brand A, Richter-Landsberg C, Leibfritz D (1993). Multinuclear NMR studies on the energy metabolism of glial and neuronal cells. Dev Neurosci 15: 289–298.

Braus DF, Ende G, Weber-Fahr W et al. (2001). Favorable effect on neuronal viability in the anterior cingulate gyrus due to long-term treatment with atypical antipsychotics: an MRSI study. Pharmacopsychiatry 34: 251–253.

Breiter SN, Arroyo S, Mathews VP et al. (1994). Proton MR spectroscopy in patients with seizure disorders. AJNR Am J Neuroradiol 15: 373–384.

Brenner RE, Munro PM, Williams SC et al. (1993). The proton NMR spectrum in acute EAE: the significance of the change in the Cho:Cr ratio. Magn Reson Med 29: 737–745.

Brooks WM, Stidley CA, Petropoulos H et al. (2000). Metabolic and cognitive response to human traumatic brain injury: a quantitative proton magnetic resonance study. J Neurotrauma 17: 629–640.

Bruhn H, Frahm J, Gyngell ML et al. (1989). Cerebral metabolism in man after acute stroke: new observations using localized proton NMR spectroscopy. Magn Reson Med 9: 126–131.

Brulatout S, Meric P, Loubinoux I et al. (1996). A one-dimensional (proton and phosphorus) and two-dimensional (proton) in vivo NMR spectroscopic study of reversible global cerebral ischemia. J Neurochem 66: 2491–2499.

Caruso PA, Johnson J, Thibert R et al. (2013). The use of magnetic resonance spectroscopy in the evaluation of epilepsy. Neuroimaging Clin N Am 23: 407–424.

Castillo M, Kwock L, Green C (1995). MELAS syndrome: imaging and proton MR spectroscopic findings. AJNR Am J Neuroradiol 16: 233–239.

Castillo M, Smith JK, Kwock L (2000). Correlation of myo-inositol levels and grading of cerebral astrocytomas. AJNR Am J Neuroradiol 21: 1645–1649.

Cecil KM (2006). MR spectroscopy of metabolic disorders. Neuroimaging Clin N Am 16: 87–116. viii.

Cendes F, Andermann F, Gloor P et al. (1993). MRI volumetric measurement of amygdala and hippocampus in temporal lobe epilepsy. Neurology 43: 719–725.

Cendes F, Andermann F, Dubeau F et al. (1997a). Normalization of neuronal metabolic dysfunction after surgery for temporal lobe epilepsy. Evidence from proton MR spectroscopic imaging. Neurology 49: 1525–1533.

Cendes F, Stanley JA, Dubeau F et al. (1997b). Proton magnetic resonance spectroscopic imaging for discrimination of absence and complex partial seizures. Ann Neurol 41: 74–81.

Chamuleau RA, Bosman DK, Bovee WM et al. (1991). What the clinician can learn from MR glutamine/glutamate assays. NMR Biomed 4: 103–108.

Chang L, Mcbride D, Miller BL et al. (1995). Localized in vivo 1H magnetic resonance spectroscopy and in vitro analyses of heterogeneous brain tumors. J Neuroimaging 5: 157–163.

Chang L, Ernst T, Leonido-Yee M et al. (1999). Highly active antiretroviral therapy reverses brain metabolite abnormalities in mild HIV dementia. Neurology 53: 782–789.

Chang L, Ernst T, Witt MD et al. (2002). Relationships among brain metabolites, cognitive function, and viral loads in antiretroviral-naive HIV patients. Neuroimage 17: 1638–1648.

Chang L, Cloak CC, Ernst T (2003). Magnetic resonance spectroscopy studies of GABA in neuropsychiatric disorders. J Clin Psychiatry 64 (Suppl 3): 7–14.

Cheng LL, Ma MJ, Becerra L et al. (1997). Quantitative neuropathology by high resolution magic angle spinning proton magnetic resonance spectroscopy. Proc Natl Acad Sci U S A 94: 6408–6413.

Cheng LL, Newell K, Mallory AE et al. (2002). Quantification of neurons in Alzheimer and control brains with ex vivo high resolution magic angle spinning proton magnetic resonance spectroscopy and stereology. Magn Reson Imaging 20: 527–533.

Choi C, Ganji SK, Deberardinis RJ et al. (2012). 2-hydroxyglutarate detection by magnetic resonance spectroscopy in IDH-mutated patients with gliomas. Nat Med 18: 624–629.

Chong WK, Sweeney B, Wilkinson ID et al. (1993). Proton spectroscopy of the brain in HIV infection: correlation with clinical, immunologic, and MR imaging findings. Radiology 188: 119–124.

Christiansen P, Henriksen O, Stubgaard M et al. (1993). In vivo quantification of brain metabolites by 1H-MRS using water as an internal standard. Magn Reson Imaging 11: 107–118.

Cohen BA, Inglese M, Rusinek H et al. (2007). Proton MR spectroscopy and MRI-volumetry in mild traumatic brain injury. AJNR Am J Neuroradiol 28: 907–913.

Cohen-Gadol AA, Pan JW, Kim JH et al. (2004). Mesial temporal lobe epilepsy: a proton magnetic resonance spectroscopy study and a histopathological analysis. J Neurosurg 101: 613–620.

Collins JG (1990). Types of injuries by selected characteristics. Vital Health Stat 10: 1–68.

Cross JH, Gadian DG, Connelly A et al. (1993). Proton magnetic resonance spectroscopy studies in lactic acidosis and mitochondrial disorders. J Inherit Metab Dis 16: 800–811.

Da Silva LF, Hoefel Filho JR, Anes M et al. (2006). Prognostic value of 1H-MRS in neonatal encephalopathy. Pediatr Neurol 34: 360–366.

Davie CA, Hawkins CP, Barker GJ et al. (1994). Serial proton magnetic resonance spectroscopy in acute multiple sclerosis lesions. Brain 117 (Pt 1): 49–58.

Davie CA, Wenning GK, Barker GJ et al. (1995). Differentiation of multiple system atrophy from idiopathic Parkinson's disease using proton magnetic resonance spectroscopy. Ann Neurol 37: 204–210.

Davies NP, Wilson M, Natarajan K et al. (2010). Non-invasive detection of glycine as a biomarker of malignancy in childhood brain tumours using in-vivo 1H MRS at 1.5 tesla confirmed by ex-vivo high-resolution magic-angle spinning NMR. NMR Biomed 23: 80–87.

De Stefano N, Filippi M (2007). MR spectroscopy in multiple sclerosis. J Neuroimaging 17 (Suppl 1): 31S–35S.

De Stefano N, Matthews PM, Arnold DL (1995). Reversible decreases in N-acetylaspartate after acute brain injury. Magn Reson Med 34: 721–727.

De Stefano N, Matthews PM, Fu L et al. (1998). Axonal damage correlates with disability in patients with relapsing-remitting multiple sclerosis. Results of a longitudinal magnetic resonance spectroscopy study. Brain 121 (Pt 8): 1469–1477.

Demougeot C, Marie C, Giroud M et al. (2004). N-acetylaspartate: a literature review of animal research on brain ischaemia. J Neurochem 90: 776–783.

Eichler FS, Barker PB, Cox C et al. (2002). Proton MR spectroscopic imaging predicts lesion progression on MRI in X-linked adrenoleukodystrophy. Neurology 58: 901–907.

Einstein DB, Wessels B, Bangert B et al. (2012). Phase II trial of radiosurgery to magnetic resonance spectroscopy-defined high-risk tumor volumes in patients with glioblastoma multiforme. Int J Radiat Oncol Biol Phys 84: 668–674.

Ernst T, Chang L (2004). Effect of aging on brain metabolism in antiretroviral-naive HIV patients. AIDS 18 (Suppl 1): S61–S67.

Federico F, Simone IL, Lucivero V et al. (1997). Proton magnetic resonance spectroscopy in Parkinson's disease and progressive supranuclear palsy. J Neurol Neurosurg Psychiatry 62: 239–242.

Ferguson B, Matyszak MK, Esiri MM et al. (1997). Axonal damage in acute multiple sclerosis lesions. Brain 120 (Pt 3): 393–399.

Firbank MJ, Harrison RM, O'brien JT (2002). A comprehensive review of proton magnetic resonance spectroscopy studies in dementia and Parkinson's disease. Dement Geriatr Cogn Disord 14: 64–76.

Fischer M, Bockhorst K, Hoehn-Berlage M et al. (1995). Imaging of the apparent diffusion coefficient for the evaluation of cerebral metabolic recovery after cardiac arrest. Magn Reson Imaging 13: 781–790.

Frahm J, Bruhn H, Gyngell ML et al. (1989). Localized proton NMR spectroscopy in different regions of the human brain in vivo. Relaxation times and concentrations of cerebral metabolites. Magn Reson Med 11: 47–63.

Fu L, Matthews PM, De Stefano N et al. (1998). Imaging axonal damage of normal-appearing white matter in multiple sclerosis. Brain 121 (Pt 1): 103–113.

Gabis L, Parton P, Roche P et al. (2001). In vivo 1H magnetic resonance spectroscopic measurement of brain glycine levels in nonketotic hyperglycinemia. J Neuroimaging 11: 209–211.

Garcia-Gomez JM, Luts J, Julia-Sape M et al. (2009). Multiproject-multicenter evaluation of automatic brain tumor classification by magnetic resonance spectroscopy. MAGMA 22: 5–18.

Garnett MR, Blamire AM, Corkill RG et al. (2000a). Early proton magnetic resonance spectroscopy in normal-appearing brain correlates with outcome in patients following traumatic brain injury. Brain 123 (Pt 10): 2046–2054.

Garnett MR, Blamire AM, Rajagopalan B et al. (2000b). Evidence for cellular damage in normal-appearing white matter correlates with injury severity in patients following traumatic brain injury: a magnetic resonance spectroscopy study. Brain 123 (Pt 7): 1403–1409.

Garnett MR, Corkill RG, Blamire AM et al. (2001). Altered cellular metabolism following traumatic brain injury: a magnetic resonance spectroscopy study. J Neurotrauma 18: 231–240.

Garwood M, Uğurbil K, Rath AR et al. (1989). Magnetic resonance imaging with adiabatic pulses using a single surface coil for RF transmission and signal detection. Magn Reson Med 9: 25–34.

Gerstner ER, Frosch MP, Batchelor TT (2010). Diffusion magnetic resonance imaging detects pathologically confirmed, nonenhancing tumor progression in a patient with recurrent glioblastoma receiving bevacizumab. J Clin Oncol 28: e91–e93.

Gill SS, Thomas DG, van Bruggen N et al. (1990). Proton MR spectroscopy of intracranial tumours: in vivo and in vitro studies. J Comput Assist Tomogr 14: 497–504.

Gillard JH, Barker PB, van Zijl PC et al. (1996). Proton MR spectroscopy in acute middle cerebral artery stroke. AJNR Am J Neuroradiol 17: 873–886.

Glodzik-Sobanska L, Slowik A, Mchugh P et al. (2006). Single voxel proton magnetic resonance spectroscopy in post-stroke depression. Psychiatry Res 148: 111–120.

Gonzalez-Toledo E, Kelley RE, Minagar A (2006). Role of magnetic resonance spectroscopy in diagnosis and management of multiple sclerosis. Neurol Res 28: 280–283.

Govindaraju V, Young K, Maudsley AA (2000). Proton NMR chemical shifts and coupling constants for brain metabolites. NMR Biomed 13: 129–153.

Govindaraju V, Gauger GE, Manley GT et al. (2004). Volumetric proton spectroscopic imaging of mild traumatic brain injury. AJNR Am J Neuroradiol 25: 730–737.

Graham GD, Blamire AM, Howseman AM et al. (1992). Proton magnetic resonance spectroscopy of cerebral lactate and other metabolites in stroke patients. Stroke 23: 333–340.

Graham GD, Blamire AM, Rothman DL et al. (1993). Early temporal variation of cerebral metabolites after human stroke. A proton magnetic resonance spectroscopy study. Stroke 24: 1891–1896.

Gredal O, Rosenbaum S, Topp S et al. (1997). Quantification of brain metabolites in amyotrophic lateral sclerosis by localized proton magnetic resonance spectroscopy. Neurology 48: 878–881.

Griffith HR, Den Hollander JA, Okonkwo OC (2008). Brain metabolism differs in Alzheimer's disease and Parkinson's disease dementia. Alzheimers Dement 4: 421–427.

Grodd W, Krageloh-Mann I, Klose U et al. (1991). Metabolic and destructive brain disorders in children: findings with localized proton MR spectroscopy. Radiology 181: 173–181.

Groenendaal F, Roelants-van Rijn AM, van Der Grond J et al. (2001). Glutamate in cerebral tissue of asphyxiated neonates during the first week of life demonstrated in vivo using proton magnetic resonance spectroscopy. Biol Neonate 79: 254–257.

Gruetter R, Tkac I (2000). Field mapping without reference scan using asymmetric echo-planar techniques. Magn Reson Med 43: 319–323.

Guilfoyle DN, Blamire A, Chapman B et al. (1989). PEEP–a rapid chemical-shift imaging method. Magn Reson Med 10: 282–287.

Hardy DL, Norwood TJ (1998). Spectral editing technique for the in vitro and in vivo detection of taurine. J Magn Reson 133: 70–78.

Harms L, Meierkord H, Timm G et al. (1997). Decreased N-acetyl-aspartate/choline ratio and increased lactate in the frontal lobe of patients with Huntington's disease: a proton magnetic resonance spectroscopy study. J Neurol Neurosurg Psychiatry 62: 27–30.

Hartmann M, Heiland S, Harting I et al. (2003). Distinguishing of primary cerebral lymphoma from high-grade glioma with perfusion-weighted magnetic resonance imaging. Neurosci Lett 338: 119–122.

Hattingen E, Lanfermann H, Quick J et al. (2009). 1H MR spectroscopic imaging with short and long echo time to discriminate glycine in glial tumours. MAGMA 22: 33–41.

Heindel W, Kugel H, Roth B (1993). Noninvasive detection of increased glycine content by proton MR spectroscopy in the brains of two infants with nonketotic hyperglycinemia. AJNR Am J Neuroradiol 14: 629–635.

Heindel W, Kugel H, Wendel U et al. (1995). Proton magnetic resonance spectroscopy reflects metabolic decompensation in maple syrup urine disease. Pediatr Radiol 25: 296–299.

Hennig J, Pfister H, Ernst T et al. (1992). Direct absolute quantification of metabolites in the human brain with in vivo localized proton spectroscopy. NMR Biomed 5: 193–199.

Henriksen O, Gideon P, Sperling B et al. (1992). Cerebral lactate production and blood flow in acute stroke. J Magn Reson Imaging 2: 511–517.

Hess AT, Tisdall MD, Andronesi OC et al. (2011). Real-time motion and B0 corrected single voxel spectroscopy using volumetric navigators. Magn Reson Med 66: 314–323.

Hetherington H, Kuzniecky R, Pan J et al. (1995). Proton nuclear magnetic resonance spectroscopic imaging of human temporal lobe epilepsy at 4.1 T. Ann Neurol 38: 396–404.

Hetherington HP, Chu WJ, Gonen O et al. (2006). Robust fully automated shimming of the human brain for high-field 1H spectroscopic imaging. Magn Reson Med 56: 26–33.

Higuchi T, Graham SH, Fernandez EJ et al. (1997). Effects of severe global ischemia on N-acetylaspartate and other metabolites in the rat brain. Magn Reson Med 37: 851–857.

Hill A (1991). Current concepts of hypoxic-ischemic cerebral injury in the term newborn. Pediatr Neurol 7: 317–325.

Hoang TQ, Bluml S, Dubowitz DJ et al. (1998). Quantitative proton-decoupled 31P MRS and 1H MRS in the evaluation of Huntington's and Parkinson's diseases. Neurology 50: 1033–1040.

Hollingworth W, Medina LS, Lenkinski RE et al. (2006). A systematic literature review of magnetic resonance spectroscopy for the characterization of brain tumors. AJNR Am J Neuroradiol 27: 1404–1411.

Holmes E, Foxall PJ, Spraul M et al. (1997). 750 MHz 1H NMR spectroscopy characterisation of the complex metabolic pattern of urine from patients with inborn errors of metabolism: 2-hydroxyglutaric aciduria and maple syrup urine disease. J Pharm Biomed Anal 15: 1647–1659.

Holshouser BA, Ashwal S, Luh GY et al. (1997). Proton MR spectroscopy after acute central nervous system injury: outcome prediction in neonates, infants, and children. Radiology 202: 487–496.

Howe FA, Barton SJ, Cudlip SA et al. (2003). Metabolic profiles of human brain tumors using quantitative in vivo 1H magnetic resonance spectroscopy. Magn Reson Med 49: 223–232.

Huisman TA, Thiel T, Steinmann B et al. (2002). Proton magnetic resonance spectroscopy of the brain of a neonate with nonketotic hyperglycinemia: in vivo-in vitro (ex vivo) correlation. Eur Radiol 12: 858–861.

Hunter JV, Thornton RJ, Wang ZJ et al. (2005). Late proton MR spectroscopy in children after traumatic brain injury: correlation with cognitive outcomes. AJNR Am J Neuroradiol 26: 482–488.

Husted CA, Goodin DS, Hugg JW et al. (1994). Biochemical alterations in multiple sclerosis lesions and normal-appearing white matter detected by in vivo 31P and 1H spectroscopic imaging. Ann Neurol 36: 157–165.

Inglese M, Ge Y, Filippi M et al. (2004). Indirect evidence for early widespread gray matter involvement in relapsing-remitting multiple sclerosis. Neuroimage 21: 1825–1829.

Ishimaru H, Morikawa M, Iwanaga S et al. (2001). Differentiation between high-grade glioma and metastatic brain tumor using single-voxel proton MR spectroscopy. Eur Radiol 11: 1784–1791.

Jacobs MA, Horska A, van Zijl PC et al. (2001). Quantitative proton MR spectroscopic imaging of normal human cerebellum and brain stem. Magn Reson Med 46: 699–705.

Jarvik JG, Lenkinski RE, Grossman RI et al. (1993). Proton MR spectroscopy of HIV-infected patients: characterization of abnormalities with imaging and clinical correlation. Radiology 186: 739–744.

Jayakumar PN, Chandrashekar HS, Srikanth SG et al. (2004). MRI and in vivo proton MR spectroscopy in a racemose cysticercal cyst of the brain. Neuroradiology 46: 72–74.

Jenkins BG, Koroshetz WJ, Beal MF et al. (1993). Evidence for impairment of energy metabolism in vivo in Huntington's disease using localized 1H NMR spectroscopy. Neurology 43 2689–2695.

Jones AP, Gunawardena WJ, Coutinho CM et al. (1995). Preliminary results of proton magnetic resonance spectroscopy in motor neurone disease (amytrophic lateral sclerosis). J Neurol Sci 129 (Suppl): 85–89.

Julia-Sape M, Coronel I, Majos C et al. (2012). Prospective diagnostic performance evaluation of single-voxel 1H MRS for typing and grading of brain tumours. NMR Biomed 25: 661–673.

Jungling FD, Wakhloo AK, Hennig J (1993). In vivo proton spectroscopy of meningioma after preoperative embolization. Magn Reson Med 30: 155–160.

Kadri M, Shu S, Holshouser B et al. (2003). Proton magnetic resonance spectroscopy improves outcome prediction in perinatal CNS insults. J Perinatol 23: 181–185.

Kamada K, Houkin K, Abe H et al. (1997). Differentiation of cerebral radiation necrosis from tumor recurrence by proton magnetic resonance spectroscopy. Neurol Med Chir (Tokyo) 37: 250–256.

Kanayama S, Kuhara S, Satoh K (1996). In vivo rapid magnetic field measurement and shimming using single scan differential phase mapping. Magn Reson Med 36: 637–642.

Kano H, Houkin K, Harada K et al. (2006). Neuronal cell injury in patients after cardiopulmonary resuscitation: evaluation by diffusion-weighted imaging and magnetic resonance spectroscopy. Neurosurg Rev 29: 88–92.

Kantarci K (2007). 1H magnetic resonance spectroscopy in dementia. Br J Radiol 80 (Spec No 2): S146–S152.

Kantarci K, Jack Jr CR, Xu YC et al. (2000). Regional metabolic patterns in mild cognitive impairment and Alzheimer's disease: a 1H MRS study. Neurology 55: 210–217.

Kantarci K, Knopman DS, Dickson DW et al. (2008). Alzheimer disease: postmortem neuropathologic correlates of antemortem 1H MR spectroscopy metabolite measurements. Radiology 248: 210–220.

Kantarci K, Weigand SD, Przybelski SA et al. (2009). Risk of dementia in MCI: combined effect of cerebrovascular disease, volumetric MRI, and 1H MRS. Neurology 72: 1519–1525.

Keating B, Deng W, Roddey JC et al. (2010). Prospective motion correction for single-voxel 1H MR spectroscopy. Magn Reson Med 64: 672–679.

Keil B, Alagappan V, Mareyam A et al. (2011). Size-optimized 32-channel brain arrays for 3 T pediatric imaging. Magn Reson Med 66: 1777–1787.

Keltner JR, Wald LL, Frederick BD et al. (1997). In vivo detection of GABA in human brain using a localized double-quantum filter technique. Magn Reson Med 37: 366–371.

Keltner JR, Wald LL, Ledden PJ et al. (1998). A localized double-quantum filter for the in vivo detection of brain glucose. Magn Reson Med 39: 651–656.

Keshavan MS, Stanley JA, Pettegrew JW (2000). Magnetic resonance spectroscopy in schizophrenia: methodological issues and findings–part II. Biol Psychiatry 48: 369–380.

Khong PL, Tse C, Wong IY et al. (2004). Diffusion-weighted imaging and proton magnetic resonance spectroscopy in perinatal hypoxic-ischemic encephalopathy: association with neuromotor outcome at 18 months of age. J Child Neurol 19: 872–881.

Kim SH, Chang KH, Song IC et al. (1997). Brain abscess and brain tumor: discrimination with in vivo H-1 MR spectroscopy. Radiology 204: 239–245.

Kim H, Catana C, Ratai EM et al. (2011). Serial magnetic resonance spectroscopy reveals a direct metabolic effect of cediranib in glioblastoma. Cancer Res 71: 3745–3752.

Kinoshita K, Tada E, Matsumoto K et al. (1997). Proton MR spectroscopy of delayed cerebral radiation in monkeys and humans after brachytherapy. AJNR Am J Neuroradiol 18: 1753–1761.

Kovanlikaya A, Panigrahy A, Krieger MD et al. (2005). Untreated pediatric primitive neuroectodermal tumor in vivo: quantitation of taurine with MR spectroscopy. Radiology 236: 1020–1025.

Kreis R (2004). Issues of spectral quality in clinical 1H-magnetic resonance spectroscopy and a gallery of artifacts. NMR Biomed 17: 361–381.

Kreis R, Ernst T, Ross BD (1993). Development of the human brain: in vivo quantification of metabolite and water content with proton magnetic resonance spectroscopy. Magn Reson Med 30: 424–437.

Kreis R, Arcinue E, Ernst T et al. (1996). Hypoxic encephalopathy after near-drowning studied by quantitative 1H-magnetic resonance spectroscopy. J Clin Invest 97: 1142–1154.

Krep H, Bottiger BW, Bock C et al. (2003). Time course of circulatory and metabolic recovery of cat brain after cardiac arrest assessed by perfusion- and diffusion-weighted imaging and MR-spectroscopy. Resuscitation 58: 337–348.

Kruse B, Hanefeld F, Holzbach U et al. (1994). Proton spectroscopy in patients with Leigh's disease and mitochondrial enzyme deficiency. Dev Med Child Neurol 36: 839–843.

kuehn B (1996). Fast proton spectroscopic imaging employing k-space weighing achieved by variable repetition times. Magn Reson Med 35: 457–464.

Kuesel AC, Donnelly SM, Halliday W et al. (1994). Mobile lipids and metabolic heterogeneity of brain tumours as detectable by ex vivo 1H MR spectroscopy. NMR Biomed 7: 172–180.

Kuesel AC, Briere KM, Halliday WC et al. (1996). Mobile lipid accumulation in necrotic tissue of high grade astrocytomas. Anticancer Res 16: 1485–1489.

Kuzniecky R (2004). Clinical applications of MR spectroscopy in epilepsy. Neuroimaging Clin N Am 14: 507–516.

Lange T, Dydak U, Roberts TP et al. (2006). Pitfalls in lactate measurements at 3T. AJNR Am J Neuroradiol 27: 895–901.

Law M (2005). Perfusion and MRS for brain tumor diagnosis. In: H Edelman, Zlatkin, JV Crues (Eds.), Clinical Magnetic Resonance Imaging, 3rd edn Elsevier, Amsterdam.

Law M, Yang S, Wang H et al. (2003). Glioma grading: sensitivity, specificity, and predictive values of perfusion MR imaging and proton MR spectroscopic imaging compared with conventional MR imaging. AJNR Am J Neuroradiol 24: 1989–1998.

Lee JH, Seo DW, Lee YS et al. (1999). Proton magnetic resonance spectroscopy (1H-MRS) findings for the brain in patients with liver cirrhosis reflect the hepatic functional reserve. Am J Gastroenterol 94: 2206–2213.

Leuzzi V, Bianchi MC, Tosetti M et al. (2000). Clinical significance of brain phenylalanine concentration assessed by in vivo proton magnetic resonance spectroscopy in phenylketonuria. J Inherit Metab Dis 23: 563–570.

Leuzzi V, Tosetti M, Montanaro D et al. (2007). The pathogenesis of the white matter abnormalities in phenylketonuria. A multimodal 3.0 tesla MRI and magnetic resonance spectroscopy (1H MRS) study. J Inherit Metab Dis 30: 209–216.

Lin A, Bluml S, Mamelak AN (1999). Efficacy of proton magnetic resonance spectroscopy in clinical decision making for patients with suspected malignant brain tumors. J Neurooncol 45: 69–81.

Llumiguano C, Kovacs N, Usprung Z et al. (2008). 1H-MRS experiences after bilateral DBS of the STN in Parkinson's disease. Parkinsonism Relat Disord 14 (3): 229–232.

Mainero C, Benner T, Radding A et al. (2009). In vivo imaging of cortical pathology in multiple sclerosis using ultra-high field MRI. Neurology 73: 941–948.

Majos C, Julia-Sape M, Alonso J et al. (2004). Brain tumor classification by proton MR spectroscopy: comparison of diagnostic accuracy at short and long TE. AJNR Am J Neuroradiol 25: 1696–1704.

Mansfield P (1984). Spatial mapping of the chemical shift in NMR. Magn Reson Med 1: 370–386.

Mathews PM, Andermann F, Silver K et al. (1993). Proton MR spectroscopic characterization of differences in regional brain metabolic abnormalities in mitochondrial encephalomyopathies. Neurology 43: 2484–2490.

Matthews PM, Andermann F, Arnold DL (1990). A proton magnetic resonance spectroscopy study of focal epilepsy in humans. Neurology 40: 985–989.

Matthews PM, Francis G, Antel J et al. (1991). Proton magnetic resonance spectroscopy for metabolic characterization of plaques in multiple sclerosis. Neurology 41: 1251–1256.

Maudsley AA, Matson GB, Hugg JW et al. (1994). Reduced phase encoding in spectroscopic imaging. Magn Reson Med 31: 645–651.

Menon DK, Ainsworth JG, Cox IJ et al. (1992). Proton MR spectroscopy of the brain in AIDS dementia complex. J Comput Assist Tomogr 16: 538–542.

Mescher M, Merkle H, Kirsch J et al. (1998). Simultaneous in vivo spectral editing and water suppression. NMR Biomed 11: 266–272.

Meyerand ME, Pipas JM, Mamourian A et al. (1999). Classification of biopsy-confirmed brain tumors using single-voxel MR spectroscopy. AJNR Am J Neuroradiol 20: 117–123.

Meyerhoff DJ, Mackay S, Bachman L et al. (1993). Reduced brain N-acetylaspartate suggests neuronal loss in cognitively impaired human immunodeficiency virus-seropositive individuals: in vivo 1H magnetic resonance spectroscopic imaging. Neurology 43: 509–515.

Meyerhoff DJ, Bloomer C, Cardenas V et al. (1999). Elevated subcortical choline metabolites in cognitively and clinically asymptomatic HIV+ patients. Neurology 52: 995–1003.

Michaelis T, Merboldt KD, Bruhn H et al. (1993). Absolute concentrations of metabolites in the adult human brain in vivo: quantification of localized proton MR spectra. Radiology 187: 219–227.

Miller DH, Austin SJ, Connelly A et al. (1991). Proton magnetic resonance spectroscopy of an acute and chronic lesion in multiple sclerosis. Lancet 337: 58–59.

Miller BL, Moats RA, Shonk T et al. (1993). Alzheimer disease: depiction of increased cerebral myo-inositol with proton MR spectroscopy. Radiology 187: 433–437.

Miller BL, Chang L, Booth R et al. (1996). In vivo 1H MRS choline: correlation with in vitro chemistry/histology. Life Sci 58: 1929–1935.

Miller DH, Thompson AJ, Filippi M (2003). Magnetic resonance studies of abnormalities in the normal appearing white matter and grey matter in multiple sclerosis. J Neurol 250: 1407–1419.

Miyake M, Kakimoto Y, Sorimachi M (1981). A gas chromatographic method for the determination of N-acetyl-L-aspartic acid, N-acetyl-alpha-aspartylglutamic acid and beta-citryl-L-glutamic acid and their distributions in the brain and other organs of various species of animals. J Neurochem 36: 804–810.

Moffett JR, Namboodiri MA, Cangro CB et al. (1991). Immunohistochemical localization of N-acetylaspartate in rat brain. Neuroreport 2: 131–134.

Moller-Hartmann W, Herminghaus S, Krings T et al. (2002). Clinical application of proton magnetic resonance spectroscopy in the diagnosis of intracranial mass lesions. Neuroradiology 44: 371–381.

Moser H, Smith K, Watkins P et al. (2001). X-linked adrenoleukodystrophy. McGraw Hill, New York.

Mullins PG, Mcgonigle DJ, O'gorman RL et al. (2014). Current practice in the use of MEGA-PRESS spectroscopy for the detection of GABA. Neuroimage 86: 43–52.

Murphy M, Loosemore A, Clifton AG et al. (2002). The contribution of proton magnetic resonance spectroscopy (1H MRS) to clinical brain tumour diagnosis. Br J Neurosurg 16: 329–334.

Nakabayashi M, Suzaki S, Tomita H (2007). Neural injury and recovery near cortical contusions: a clinical magnetic resonance spectroscopy study. J Neurosurg 106: 370–377.

Narayana PA (2005). Magnetic resonance spectroscopy in the monitoring of multiple sclerosis. J Neuroimaging 15: 46S–57S.

Naressi A, Couturier C, Castang I et al. (2001). Java-based graphical user interface for MRUI, a software package for quantitation of in vivo/medical magnetic resonance spectroscopy signals. Comput Biol Med 31: 269–286.

Nasrallah F, Feki M, Kaabachi N (2010). Creatine and creatine deficiency syndromes: biochemical and clinical aspects. Pediatr Neurol 42: 163–171.

Opstad KS, Provencher SW, Bell BA et al. (2003). Detection of elevated glutathione in meningiomas by quantitative in vivo 1H MRS. Magn Reson Med 49: 632–637.

Opstad KS, Ladroue C, Bell BA et al. (2007). Linear discriminant analysis of brain tumour (1)H MR spectra: a comparison of classification using whole spectra versus metabolite quantification. NMR Biomed 20: 763–770.

Outteryck O, Devos D, Jissendi P et al. (2010). 4H syndrome: a rare cause of leukodystrophy. J Neurol 257: 1759–1761.

Oz G, Tkac I (2011). Short-echo, single-shot, full-intensity proton magnetic resonance spectroscopy for neurochemical profiling at 4 T: validation in the cerebellum and brainstem. Magn Reson Med 65: 901–910.

Oz G, Tkac I, Charnas LR et al. (2005). Assessment of adrenoleukodystrophy lesions by high field MRS in nonsedated pediatric patients. Neurology 64: 434–441.

Oz G, Alger JR, Parker GB et al. (2014). Clinical proton MR spectroscopy in central nervous system disorders. Radiology 270: 658–679.

Pan JW, Mason GF, Pohost GM et al. (1996). Spectroscopic imaging of human brain glutamate by water-suppressed J-refocused coherence transfer at 4.1 T. Magn Reson Med 36: 7–12.

Parsons DW, Jones S, Zhang X et al. (2008). An integrated genomic analysis of human glioblastoma multiforme. Science 321: 1807–1812.

Pioro EP, Antel JP, Cashman NR et al. (1994). Detection of cortical neuron loss in motor neuron disease by proton magnetic resonance spectroscopic imaging in vivo. Neurology 44: 1933–1938.

Pivawer G, Law M, Zagzag D (2007). Perfusion MR imaging and proton MR spectroscopic imaging in differentiating necrotizing cerebritis from glioblastoma multiforme. Magn Reson Imaging 25: 238–243.

Posse S, Tedeschi G, Risinger R et al. (1995). High speed 1H spectroscopic imaging in human brain by echo planar spatial-spectral encoding. Magn Reson Med 33: 34–40.

Preul MC, Leblanc R, Caramanos Z et al. (1998). Magnetic resonance spectroscopy guided brain tumor resection: differentiation between recurrent glioma and radiation change in two diagnostically difficult cases. Can J Neurol Sci 25: 13–22.

Provencher SW (1993). Estimation of metabolite concentrations from localized in vivo proton NMR spectra. Magn Reson Med 30: 672–679.

Puts NA, Edden RA (2012). In vivo magnetic resonance spectroscopy of GABA: a methodological review. Prog Nucl Magn Reson Spectrosc 60: 29–41.

Rabinov JD, Lee PL, Barker FG et al. (2002). In vivo 3-T MR spectroscopy in the distinction of recurrent glioma versus radiation effects: initial experience. Radiology 225: 871–879.

Ratai EM, Gonzalez RG (2009). Magnetic resonance spectroscopy and the biochemical basis of neurologic disease. In: SW Atlas (Ed.), Magnetic resonance imaging of the brain and spine. Vol. 2. Lippincott Williams & Wilkins, Philadelphia.

Ratai E, Kok T, Wiggins C et al. (2008). Seven-Tesla proton magnetic resonance spectroscopic imaging in adult X-linked adrenoleukodystrophy. Arch Neurol 65: 1488–1494.

Ratai EM, Annamalai L, Burdo T et al. (2011). Brain creatine elevation and N-Acetylaspartate reduction indicates neuronal dysfunction in the setting of enhanced glial energy metabolism in a macaque model of neuroAIDS. Magn Reson Med 66: 625–634.

Ratai EM, Caruso P, Eichler F (2012). Advances in MR imaging of leukodystrophies. In: P Bright (Ed.), Neuroimaging – clinical applications, Available online at: http://www.intechopen.com/books/neuroimaging-clinical-applications/advances-in-mr-imaging-of-leukodystrophies (accessed 20 May 2015).

Ratai E-M, Zhang Z, Snyder BS et al. (2013). Magnetic resonance spectroscopy as an early indicator of response to anti-angiogenic therapy in patients with recurrent glioblastoma: ACRIN 6677 / RTOG 0625. Neuro Oncol 15: 936–944.

Reese TG, Davis TL, Weisskoff RM (1995). Automated shimming at 1.5 T using echo-planar image frequency maps. J Magn Reson Imaging 5: 739–745.

Ross BD (1991). Biochemical considerations in 1H spectroscopy. Glutamate and glutamine; myo-inositol and related metabolites. NMR Biomed 4: 59–63.

Ross BD, Bluml S, Cowan R et al. (1998). In vivo MR spectroscopy of human dementia. Neuroimaging Clin N Am 8: 809–822.

Rothman DL, Behar KL, Hetherington HP et al. (1984). Homonuclear 1H double-resonance difference spectroscopy of the rat brain in vivo. Proc Natl Acad Sci U S A 81: 6330–6334.

Rothman DL, Petroff OA, Behar KL et al. (1993). Localized 1H NMR measurements of gamma-aminobutyric acid in human brain in vivo. Proc Natl Acad Sci U S A 90: 5662–5666.

Rowland LM, Kontson K, West J et al. (2012). In vivo measurements of glutamate, GABA, and NAAG in schizophrenia. Schizophr Bull 39 (5): 1096–10410.1093/schbul/sbs092.

Rutherford MA, Pennock JM, Schwieso JE et al. (1995). Hypoxic ischaemic encephalopathy: early magnetic resonance imaging findings and their evolution. Neuropediatrics 26: 183–191.

Sacktor N, Skolasky RL, Ernst T et al. (2005). A multicenter study of two magnetic resonance spectroscopy techniques in individuals with HIV dementia. J Magn Reson Imaging 21: 325–333.

Saunders DE (2000). MR spectroscopy in stroke. Br Med Bull 56: 334–345.

Saunders DE, Howe FA, van Den Boogaart A et al. (1999). Aging of the adult human brain: in vivo quantitation of metabolite content with proton magnetic resonance spectroscopy. J Magn Reson Imaging 9: 711–716.

Schneider E, Glover G (1991). Rapid in vivo proton shimming. Magn Reson Med 18: 335–347.

Schuhmann MU, Stiller D, Skardelly M et al. (2003). Metabolic changes in the vicinity of brain contusions: a proton magnetic resonance spectroscopy and histology study. J Neurotrauma 20: 725–743.

Shonk TK, Moats RA, Gifford P et al. (1995). Probable Alzheimer disease: diagnosis with proton MR spectroscopy. Radiology 195: 65–72.

Shiino A, Watanabe T, Shirakashi Y et al. (2012). The profile of hippocampal metabolites differs between Alzheimer's disease and subcortical ischemic vascular dementia, as measured by proton magnetic resonance spectroscopy. J Cereb Blood Flow Metab 32: 805–815.

Simmons ML, Frondoza CG, Coyle JT (1991). Immunocytochemical localization of N-acetyl-aspartate with monoclonal antibodies. Neuroscience 45: 37–45.

Simpson HB, Shungu DC, Bender Jr J et al. (2012). Investigation of cortical glutamate-glutamine and gamma-aminobutyric acid in obsessive-compulsive disorder by proton magnetic resonance spectroscopy. Neuropsychopharmacology 37: 2684–2692.

Slotboom J, Boesch C, Kreis R (1998). Versatile frequency domain fitting using time domain models and prior knowledge. Magn Reson Med 39: 899–911.

Soher BJ, van Zijl PC, Duyn JH et al. (1996). Quantitative proton MR spectroscopic imaging of the human brain. Magn Reson Med 35: 356–363.

Soher BJ, Young K, Govindaraju V et al. (1998). Automated spectral analysis III: application to in vivo proton MR spectroscopy and spectroscopic imaging. Magn Reson Med 40: 822–831.

Stanley JA, Drost DJ, Williamson PC et al. (1995). The use of a priori knowledge to quantify short echo in vivo 1H MR spectra. Magn Reson Med 34: 17–24.

Stanley JA, Pettegrew JW, Keshavan MS (2000). Magnetic resonance spectroscopy in schizophrenia: methodological issues and findings–part I. Biol Psychiatry 48: 357–368.

Steenweg ME, Vanderver A, Blaser S et al. (2010). Magnetic resonance imaging pattern recognition in hypomyelinating disorders. Brain 133: 2971–2982.

Suzuki Y, Ueda H, Toribe Y (2001). Proton MR spectroscopy of nonketotic hyperglycinemia. No To Hattatsu 33: 422–425.

Tartaglia MC, Arnold DL (2006). The role of MRS and fMRI in multiple sclerosis. Adv Neurol 98: 185–202.

Taylor JS, Langston JW, Reddick WE et al. (1996). Clinical value of proton magnetic resonance spectroscopy for differentiating recurrent or residual brain tumor from delayed cerebral necrosis. Int J Radiat Oncol Biol Phys 36: 1251–1261.

Tedeschi G, Litvan I, Bonavita S et al. (1997). Proton magnetic resonance spectroscopic imaging in progressive supranuclear palsy, Parkinson's disease and corticobasal degeneration. Brain 120 (Pt 9): 1541–1552.

Thayyil S, Chandrasekaran M, Taylor A et al. (2010). Cerebral magnetic resonance biomarkers in neonatal encephalopathy: a meta-analysis. Pediatrics 125: e382–e395.

Thomas MA, Yue K, Binesh N et al. (2001). Localized two-dimensional shift correlated MR spectroscopy of human brain. Magn Reson Med 46: 58–67.

Tkac I, Andersen P, Adriany G et al. (2001). In vivo 1H NMR spectroscopy of the human brain at 7 T. Magn Reson Med 46: 451–456.

Tofts PS, Wray S (1988). A critical assessment of methods of measuring metabolite concentrations by NMR spectroscopy. NMR Biomed 1: 1–10.

Tracey I, Carr CA, Guimaraes AR et al. (1996). Brain choline-containing compounds are elevated in HIV-positive patients before the onset of AIDS dementia complex: a proton magnetic resonance spectroscopic study. Neurology 46: 783–788.

Tran TK, Vigneron DB, Sailasuta N et al. (2000). Very selective suppression pulses for clinical MRSI studies of brain and prostate cancer. Magn Reson Med 43: 23–33.

Trapp BD, Peterson J, Ransohoff RM et al. (1998). Axonal transection in the lesions of multiple sclerosis. N Engl J Med 338: 278–285.

Tsai G, Coyle JT (1995). N-acetylaspartate in neuropsychiatric disorders. Prog Neurobiol 46: 531–540.

Urenjak J, Williams SR, Gadian DG et al. (1992). Specific expression of N-acetylaspartate in neurons, oligodendrocyte-type-2 astrocyte progenitors, and immature oligodendrocytes in vitro. J Neurochem 59: 55–61.

Urenjak J, Williams SR, Gadian DG et al. (1993). Proton nuclear magnetic resonance spectroscopy unambiguously identifies different neural cell types. J Neurosci 13: 981–989.

Wartenberg KE, Patsalides A, Yepes MS (2004). Is magnetic resonance spectroscopy superior to conventional diagnostic tools in hypoxic-ischemic encephalopathy? J Neuroimaging 14: 180–186.

Webb P, Macovski A (1991). Rapid, fully automatic, arbitrary-volume in vivo shimming. Magn Reson Med 20: 113–122.

Webb P, Spielman D, Macovski A (1989). A fast spectroscopic imaging method using a blipped phase encode gradient. Magn Reson Med 12: 306–315.

Welch KM, Levine SR, Martin G et al. (1992). Magnetic resonance spectroscopy in cerebral ischemia. Neurol Clin 10: 1–29.

Westergaard N, Sonnewald U, Schousboe A (1995). Metabolic trafficking between neurons and astrocytes: the glutamate/glutamine cycle revisited. Dev Neurosci 17: 203–211.

Wilman AH, Allen PS (1995). The response of the strongly coupled AB system of citrate to typical 1H MRS localization sequences. J Magn Reson B 107: 25–33.

Wilman AH, Astridge M, Snyder RE et al. (1995). Same-scan acquisition of both edited J-coupled multiplets and singlet resonances of uncoupled spins for proton MRS. J Magn Reson B 109: 202–205.

Wolf NI, Harting I, Boltshauser E et al. (2005). Leukoencephalopathy with ataxia, hypodontia, and hypomyelination. Neurology 64: 1461–1464.

Young K, Govindaraju V, Soher BJ et al. (1998a). Automated spectral analysis I: formation of a priori information by spectral simulation Magn Reson Med 40: 812–815.

Young K, Soher BJ, Maudsley AA (1998b). Automated spectral analysis II: application of wavelet shrinkage for characterization of non-parameterized signals. Magn Reson Med 40: 816–821.

Zarifi MK, Astrakas LG, Poussaint TY et al. (2002). Prediction of adverse outcome with cerebral lactate level and apparent diffusion coefficient in infants with perinatal asphyxia. Radiology 225: 859–870.

Zhu W, Zhong W, Qi J et al. (2008). Proton magnetic resonance spectroscopy in neonates with hypoxic-ischemic injury and its prognostic value. Transl Res 152: 225–232.

Handbook of Clinical Neurology, Vol. 135 (3rd series)
Neuroimaging, Part I
J.C. Masdeu and R.G. González, Editors

Chapter 6

Brain perfusion: computed tomography and magnetic resonance techniques

WILLIAM A. COPEN*, MICHAEL H. LEV, AND OTTO RAPALINO
Division of Neuroradiology, Department of Radiology, Massachusetts General Hospital and Harvard Medical School, Boston, MA, USA

Abstract

Cerebral perfusion imaging provides assessment of regional microvascular hemodynamics in the living brain, enabling *in vivo* measurement of a variety of different hemodynamic parameters. Perfusion imaging techniques that are used in the clinical setting usually rely upon X-ray computed tomography (CT) or magnetic resonance imaging (MRI). This chapter reviews CT- and MRI-based perfusion imaging techniques, with attention to image acquisition, clinically relevant aspects of image postprocessing, and fundamental differences between CT- and MRI-based techniques. Correlations with cerebrovascular physiology and potential clinical applications of perfusion imaging are reviewed, focusing upon the two major classes of neurologic disease in which perfusion imaging is most often performed: primary perfusion disorders (including ischemic stroke, transient ischemic attack, and reperfusion syndrome), and brain tumors.

INTRODUCTION

Perfusion can be defined as the process in which blood is forced to flow through a network of microscopic vessels within biologic tissue, allowing exchange of oxygen and other molecules across semipermeable microvascular walls. Accordingly, brain perfusion imaging techniques are those that allow measurement of regional hemodynamic conditions in very small blood vessels, unlike the larger vessels that are evaluated in angiographic imaging techniques. In the clinical setting, brain perfusion imaging is usually performed using either X-ray computed tomography (CT) or magnetic resonance imaging (MRI).

Because the small size of the vessels that are studied with perfusion imaging makes it impossible to visualize them directly, CT and MR perfusion imaging techniques involve aggregating information obtained from all of the vessels within a single volume element of the brain, or voxel. This information affects the appearance of a single picture element, or pixel, in so-called "source images" images, which are acquired using special techniques on a standard clinical CT or MR scanner. The perfusion source images then undergo computation postprocessing, to yield "maps" of various different regional hemodynamic parameters. It is these perfusion maps that undergo visual interpretation.

This chapter begins by discussing briefly how CT and MR perfusion source images are most often acquired. Subsequently, the algorithms used to produce the most common types of perfusion maps are presented, along with a brief review of potential uses of these maps in two classes of disease: primary cerebral perfusion disorders (including ischemic stroke, transient ischemic attack, and reperfusion syndrome), and brain tumors.

IMAGE ACQUISITION

CT perfusion imaging

In CT perfusion imaging, CT images of the head are acquired repeatedly, every 1–3 seconds, typically over the course of a scan lasting between approximately 40 seconds and 2 minutes (Hamberg et al., 1996). As

*Correspondence to: William A. Copen, MD, Massachusetts General Hospital, Neuroradiology GRB-273A, 55 Fruit Street, Boston MA 02114, USA. E-mail: wcopen@partners.org

images are being acquired, a bolus of a standard iodine-based X-ray contrast agent is injected into a peripheral intravenous catheter. The quality of the perfusion maps that are ultimately generated is optimized by achievement of high-contrast agent concentrations, which are obtained by using a mechanical power injector to inject at rates of up to 5–10 cc/s. A large-caliber intravenous catheter is preferred for such high-flow injections. When smaller-caliber intravenous catheters with higher resistance are used, the pressures required to maintain the desired flow may be sufficient to cause catheter fracture and embolization. Therefore, lower flow rates are sometimes used, with a resulting degradation of image quality, if large-bore intravenous access cannot be achieved. Longer catheters such as peripherally inserted central catheters (PICC lines) are not generally usable for perfusion imaging, unless they have been specifically designed for high-flow injection.

After the contrast agent bolus has traveled from its peripheral vein through the pulmonary circulation, it ultimately arrives in the systemic circulation, and some of it passes through the vessels of the brain. The iodine-based contrast agents used for CT perfusion imaging cannot pass through the intact blood–brain barrier, and the bolus exits rapidly from most parts of the brain several seconds after it has arrived. Therefore, the X-ray attenuation of each voxel of brain tissue transiently increases, and then decreases again, as the contrast agent passes through the blood vessels within it (Fig. 6.1).

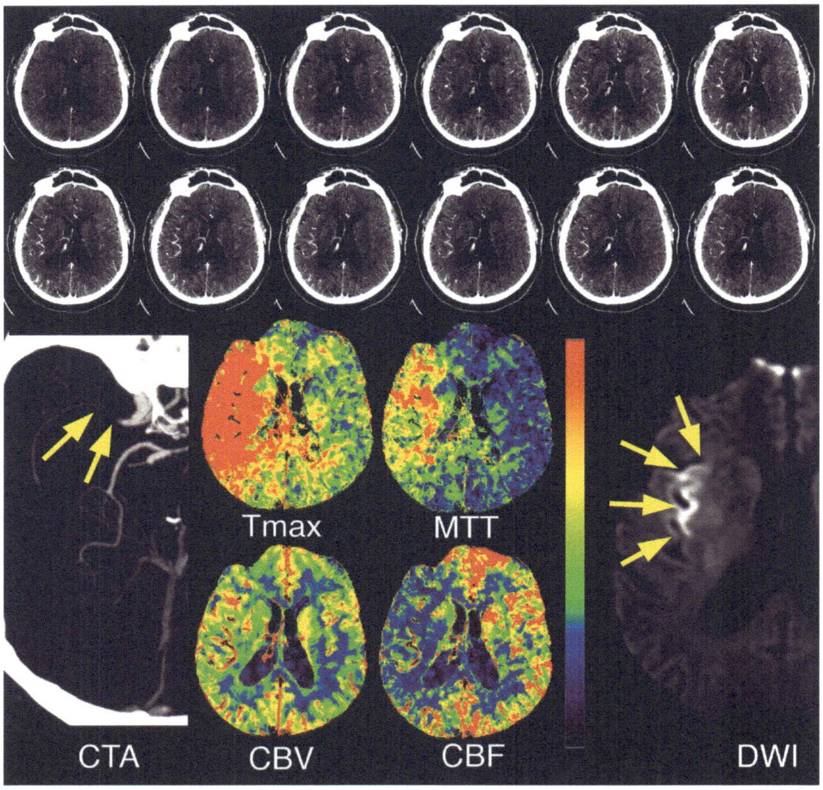

Fig. 6.1. Computed tomography (CT) perfusion imaging in cerebral perfusion disorders. A 53-year-old man with atrial fibrillation presented 1 hour after acute onset of left hemiparesis and dysarthria. A CT angiography (CTA) examination (lower left) showed filling defects in the proximal right middle cerebral artery (MCA) stem (arrows), and in several distal branches of that vessel, consistent with acute emboli. CT perfusion imaging was performed by acquiring axial images every 3 seconds, during and after injection of an intravenous contrast bolus. Selected consecutive CT perfusion source images (top two rows of the figure) show contrast arriving earlier in the left MCA territory than in the right MCA territory. This is apparent in a map of regional contrast arrival time (T_{max}), one of four perfusion maps derived from the source images by postprocessing software. Contrast opacification also appears to linger for a longer time in the right MCA territory, which corresponds to transit time elevation seen in the mean transit time (MTT) map. A map of cerebral blood volume (CBV) shows mild CBV elevation in the right MCA territory, reflecting expected vasodilation in the setting of a reduction in perfusion pressure. Such vasodilation sometimes preserves regional blood flow when perfusion pressure is reduced, but in this case a cerebral blood flow (CBF) map shows that CBF is reduced in most of the right MCA territory. A diffusion-weighted magnetic resonance image (DWI) obtained immediately after this scan shows that, so far, only a small cortical infarct has developed, limited to the insula and temporal operculum.

For each of the many time points at which a CT image is obtained, the instantaneous concentration of contrast material within each voxel may be calculated by subtracting from the X-ray attenuation or "density" of the tissue its density in the earliest-acquired "baseline" images, which were acquired before the contrast bolus arrived. These concentration measurements at various time points are combined to yield a "concentration-versus-time curve," C_t for each voxel. Mathematical analysis of C_t for each voxel by postprocessing software, which will be discussed in greater detail below, yields measurements of various hemodynamic parameters, which are then represented in the corresponding image pixel in postprocessed perfusion maps.

In CT perfusion imaging, the absolute serum concentration of the contrast agent is difficult to determine quantitatively. This is because, although the quantity of contrast material is known, the volume of distribution of blood into which it has been mixed cannot be known. Although some CT postprocessing algorithms attempt to calculate absolute serum concentrations, measurements derived from these methods may under- or overestimate absolute hemodynamic values by a factor of three or more (Nabavi et al., 1999; Wintermark et al., 2001). Therefore, more accurate measurements may be obtained by presuming that C_t measurements are relative ones.

MR perfusion imaging

In the clinical setting, MR perfusion is almost always performed using contrast agent-based techniques that are very similar to those used in CT perfusion imaging, i.e., dynamic acquisition of images during bolus injection of a contrast agent, followed by computation and analysis of a C_t function. Most of this chapter will be devoted to these bolus-tracking techniques. However, it will be worthwhile considering briefly MR perfusion techniques that do not involve injection of an exogenous contrast agent. This is usually accomplished using an arterial spin labeling (ASL) pulse sequence (Edelman et al., 1994). In ASL, the hydrogen nuclei ("spins") of water molecules within flowing blood are used as an endogenous contrast agent. ASL pulse sequences include a radiofrequency pulse that acts upon these spins as they pass through arteries in the neck, effectively "labeling" the spins. After waiting for several seconds, a period of time called the postlabeling delay, images of the brain are acquired. By mathematically subtracting these postlabeling images to images that have been acquired without use of the labeling pulse, the distribution of labeled spins throughout the brain can be measured. This produces a map of regional cerebral blood flow (rCBF), which is also delay-weighted, in that regions with delayed spin arrival appear to have lower blood flow.

Although ASL is a promising technique that is increasingly prevalent in the clinical setting, MR perfusion imaging is much more commonly performed using dynamic susceptibility contrast (DSC) imaging. DSC relies upon tracking a bolus of an intravenously injected exogenous contrast agent, using principles similar to those used for CT perfusion imaging (Villringer et al., 1988; Rosen et al., 1990). In the case of DSC, the contrast agent employed is a standard gadolinium-based MRI contrast agent, rather than the iodine-based CT agents that are used for CT.

DSC is performed using an echo-planar pulse sequence, which enables imaging a large part of the brain very rapidly. Images are acquired every 1–2 seconds, before, during, and after intravenous injection of the contrast agent, during a scan that lasts approximately 1–2 minutes (Fig. 6.2). Like those produced by CT perfusion imaging, quality of perfusion maps derived from DSC is generally improved by relatively rapid injection of the contrast agent. However, because of the much greater signal-to-noise ratio achieved by DSC (see below), injection rate is somewhat less critical than it is for CT perfusion imaging. Rates over 5 cc/s are generally unnecessary, and may even be undesirable.

DSC is so named because it relies upon gadolinium-based contrast agents' magnetic susceptibility, rather than their effects upon T1 relaxivity, which are exploited for conventional contrast-enhanced MRI. When placed within an external magnetic field, such as that within an MRI scanner, gadolinium ions exhibit the property of magnetic susceptibility, meaning that they cause a local intensification of field strength. When a susceptibility-sensitive pulse sequence is run, gadolinium ions' susceptibility effect causes a loss of signal intensity, so that nearby tissue appears hypointense or "dark" in MR images. Like CT contrast agents, gadolinium-based contrast agents are too large to pass through the intact blood–brain barrier. Therefore, just as CT contrast agents cause a transient increase in X-ray attenuation as they pass through the cerebral vasculature, MRI contrast agents cause a transient decrease in signal intensity as they pass through the brain.

At any time point following the arrival of the contrast bolus, signal intensity in an image pixel can be compared to that obtained in precontrast baseline images, and the degree of signal loss can be converted to a measurement of gadolinium concentration in the corresponding brain voxel at that instant. Just as in CT perfusion imaging, these serial concentration measurements are assembled into a concentration-versus-time curve C_t for each voxel.

Whereas CT perfusion imaging is commonly used only in evaluating known or suspected primary

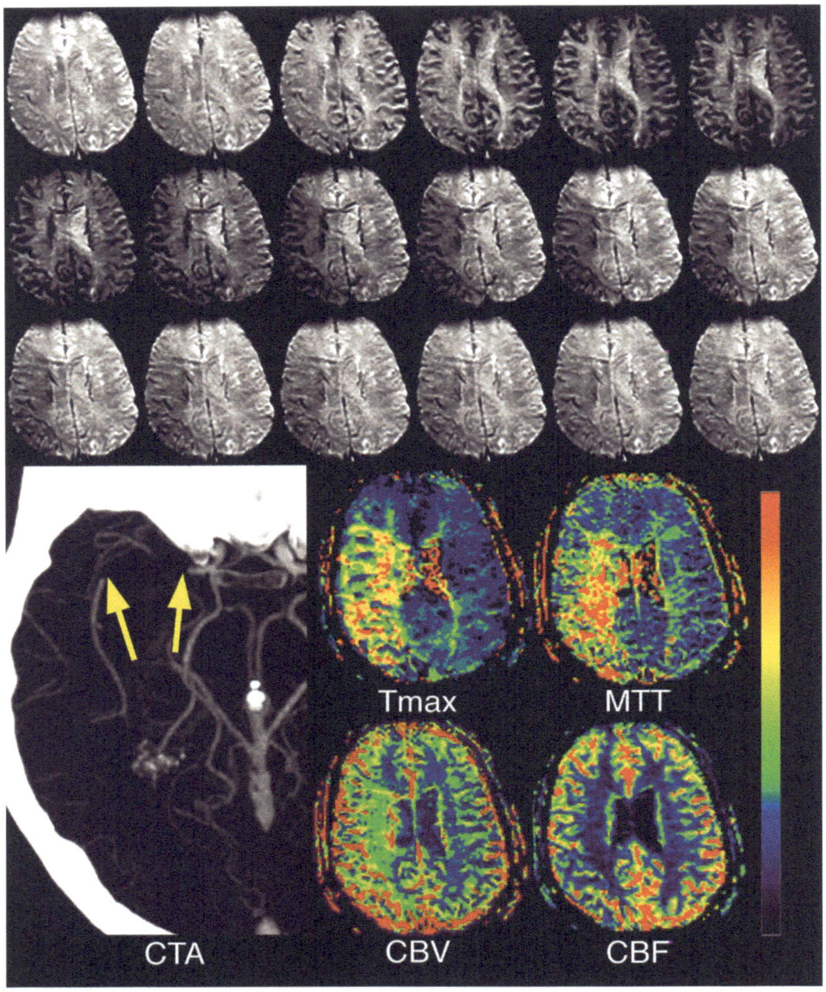

Fig. 6.2. Magnetic resonance (MR) perfusion imaging in cerebral perfusion disorders. A 56-year-old man presented following an episode of transient left-sided weakness and dysarthria that had resolved by the time of imaging. A computed tomography angiography (CTA) examination (lower left) showed a filling defect in the proximal right middle cerebral artery (MCA) stem (arrows), consistent with acute embolic occlusion. MR perfusion imaging was performed by acquiring axial images every 1.5 seconds before, during, and after injection of an intravenous contrast bolus. Selected consecutive MR perfusion source images (top three rows of the figure) show contrast arriving earlier in the left MCA territory than in the right MCA territory, resulting in an earlier drop in signal intensity. This is confirmed by a map of regional contrast arrival time (T_{max}). Contrast also appears to linger for a longer time in the right MCA territory, reflected by mean transit time (MTT) elevation. A map of cerebral blood volume (CBV) shows CBV consistent with expected vasodilation in right MCA territory. In this patient, unlike the patient in Figure 6.1, this autoregulatory response is sufficient to maintain normal cerebral blood flow (CBF) in the visualized portions of the MCA territory, and no abnormality is evident in the CBF map. Diffusion-weighted images (not shown) demonstrated a small infarct in the posterior putamen, with no infarct visible at the level of these images.

perfusion disorders, MR perfusion imaging is commonly used in both primary perfusion disorders, and in evaluation of brain tumors and other intracranial pathology. Therefore, MR postprocessing algorithms sometimes must be capable of yielding accurate results when the blood–brain barrier is disrupted, and contrast material leaks out of the blood vessels and accumulates in the brain's interstitial space. This accumulation may cause either spurious underestimation of instantaneous intravascular contrast concentrations due to T1 effects, or overestimation of concentration due to susceptibility effects. These effects increase progressively during the course of a perfusion scan. While they have little effect upon measurements of CBF (see below), they may cause marked errors in the estimation of cerebral blood volume (CBV) within enhancing lesions.

The effects of contrast leakage upon MR perfusion measurements of CBV may be reduced by the use of additional postprocessing algorithms that seek to correct for contrast leakage, typically using a curve-fitting approach (Bjornerud et al., 2011). Although leakage correction algorithms can improve the accuracy and clinical utility of MR perfusion images (Boxerman et al., 2006; Emblem et al., 2011), they may also introduce artifacts of their own when contrast leakage is not present. For this reason, when regions of blood–brain barrier breakdown are present (as evidenced by enhancing lesions in post-contrast T1-weighted images), it is preferable to produce both leakage-corrected and nonleakage-corrected CBV maps, and to review the former in regions of contrast enhancement, and the latter in regions where there is no enhancement.

Like those used for CT perfusion postprocessing, some MR perfusion postprocessing algorithms attempt to develop absolute measurements of contrast concentration, in order to allow absolute quantification of various hemodynamic parameters. However, as is the case with CT perfusion imaging, these estimations may overestimate or underestimate the actual measurements by a factor of three or more, and relative measurements are more reliable (Hagen et al., 1999; Lin et al., 1999).

CT and MR perfusion image acquisition techniques: a practical comparison

Perhaps the most important advantage of CT perfusion imaging, compared to MR perfusion imaging, is that CT scanners are much more widely available than MR scanners in most parts of the world. One 2008 study reported that, in the USA, 94% of hospital emergency departments had round-the-clock access to CT scanners, with a technologist on site at all times. In comparison, only 13% of American emergency departments had access to an MR scanner with a technologist always on site (Ginde et al., 2008).

Besides the greater availability of scanners, CT perfusion imaging offers other logistic advantages. It is easier and faster to move acutely ill patients into and out of CT scanners than MR scanners, and unstable patients may be more readily monitored during a CT scan than during an MR scan. Whereas all patients may undergo CT perfusion imaging if their renal function is sufficient and they are not allergic to iodinated contrast agents, claustrophobic patients and those with some metallic surgical implants or other metal in their bodies may be unable to undergo MR scanning, and confirmation of a patient's eligibility for MRI may be difficult to achieve quickly in the acute setting.

Although both CT and MR perfusion scans work by quantifying local concentrations of an injected contrast agent as it passes through the brain, they rely on entirely different physical properties to do so. The CT approach of relying upon X-ray absorption results in images that are extremely noisy, compared to MR perfusion images. The passage of a contrast bolus through a white-matter voxel typically results in X-ray attenuations increasing by approximately 1–2 Hounsfield units over the baseline, whereas random noise causes fluctuations of similar magnitude from time point to time point. In comparison, the passage of a gadolinium-based contrast agent through the brain in an MR perfusion scan typically results in a peak signal drop of approximately 50%.

CT and MR perfusion postprocessing algorithms are based upon identical principles, as both produce the same types of hemodynamic maps from C_t data. However, in order to produce interpretable perfusion maps from relatively noisy data, CT postprocessing algorithms usually incorporate spatial smoothing algorithms that sacrifice spatial resolution for improved signal-to-noise ratio. CT algorithms also may make use of temporal smoothing, and may incorporate model-based constraints or other algorithmic modifications to help them extract hemodynamic information from noisy data. As most manufacturers of CT perfusion postprocessing software consider their algorithms to be protected trade secrets, and the details of their operation are seldom fully revealed, this may potentially conceal deficiencies in their accuracy.

In comparison, MR perfusion postprocessing algorithms can be simpler, as they work with data that are considerably less noisy, and therefore smoothing and other noise-reducing features are unnecessary or less important. The algorithms used in MR postprocessing software are usually revealed fully, which facilitates easier critical analysis and testing.

Unfortunately, the greater signal-to-noise ratio that is afforded by DSC perfusion imaging is accompanied by two significant disadvantages, compared to CT perfusion imaging. First, DSC's reliance upon susceptibility effects means that large vessels "bloom" in DSC source images, making them seem larger in postprocessed perfusion maps than they truly are. This obscures nearby brain parenchyma, making it particularly difficult to evaluate parts of the brain that are near the surface.

Second, whereas CT perfusion images are equally sensitive to contrast material in blood vessels of all sizes, when MR perfusion imaging is performed using gradient-echo DSC imaging (as is most often the case), its concentration measurements are disproportionately influenced by gadolinium in relatively large vessels that measure more than approximately 5 microns in diameter (Boxerman et al., 1995). As a result, their perfusion maps inaccurately emphasize hemodynamic conditions that exist in those larger vessels.

It is also possible to perform DSC perfusion imaging using a spin-echo echo-planar pulse sequence. Also this results in contrast concentration measurements that are closer to uniform across all vessel sizes; spin-echo DSC perfusion still disproportionately emphasizes the contribution of gadolinium in vessels close to approximately 5 microns in diameter, relative to that in larger or smaller vessels. Spin-echo DSC was once more performed more commonly in the clinical setting, but because of spin-echo sequences' lesser overall sensitivity to susceptibility effects, particularly at lower magnetic field strengths, they were usually performed with injection of a double dose of a gadolinium-based contrast agent. Higher doses of gadolinium have become disfavored in light of concerns regarding gadolinium-induced nephrogenic systemic fibrosis.

Some DSC pulse sequences are able to acquire both gradient-echo and spin-echo perfusion data during a single perfusion scan, with a single bolus of contrast material (Donahue et al., 2000). By simultaneously providing concentration measurements with two different vessel-size selectivity profiles, which can be compared with one another, it is possible to derive elementary assessments of microvascular architecture. For example, it appears that the disordered angiogenic process that occurs in some aggressive brain tumors results in a less nutritionally efficient pattern of vascular arborization, with a relative abundance of larger blood vessels that do not directly participate in oxygen exchange, and fewer gas-permeable capillaries. An increase in the relative abundance of smaller vessels in response to antiangiogenic therapy may suggest a favorable response to treatment, and a more favorable clinical prognosis (Emblem et al., 2013).

HEMODYNAMIC PARAMETERS COMMONLY MEASURED WITH PERFUSION IMAGING: CALCULATION METHODS AND INTERPRETATION IN CEREBRAL PERFUSION DISORDERS

Cerebral blood volume

Definition

CBV is defined as the volume occupied by intravascular blood within a particular quantity of brain tissue. Classically, CBV was measured in mL of blood per 100 g of brain tissue. However, CT and MR perfusion imaging techniques provide measurements of the volume of blood within the volume occupied by each image voxel. Such measurements may be expressed in terms of a percentage. For example, in normal gray matter and white matter, approximately 4–6% and 1–3% of tissue volume is occupied by blood, respectively (Yamaguchi et al., 1986; Leenders et al., 1990; Hatazawa et al., 1995). If it is assumed that the densities of blood, brain tissue, and water are all the same, then these percentages are interchangeable, with measurements expressed in mL of blood per 100 g of tissue. As the CBV measurements produced by CT and MR perfusion algorithms are generally relative, and not absolute, the choice of units is not critical.

CBV calculation

Under idealized conditions, it is possible to calculate relative regional CBV in each brain voxel simply by summing the contrast concentrations measured at each time point during the scan, i.e., calculating the area under C_t. For example, if the area under C_t in one voxel is twice that of another voxel, then CBV in the first voxel is twice the CBV in the second voxel.

Unfortunately, the idealized conditions that are necessary for this method to produce perfectly accurate CBV measurements are not present in real perfusion scans, and this may lead to significant errors in measurement, particularly for scans with short durations (Deipolyi et al., 2012). The duration of a CT or MR perfusion scan is limited practically by patient comfort, clinical expediency, and, in the case of CT perfusion imaging, the principle of limiting ionizing radiation exposure. These considerations may result in a scan's being too short to sample the entire passage of the contrast bolus in some parts of the brain. This is most likely to occur in the setting of cerebral perfusion disease, which often results in greatly prolonged transit of the bolus through the brain (Bartolini, 1981; Kikuchi et al., 2002; Calamante et al., 2000, 2003; Chiu et al., 2012).

A typical MR perfusion contrast injection lasts at least 5 seconds, and the larger quantities of contrast material required for CT perfusion imaging may take more than 10 seconds to inject (Murphy et al., 2006). The average time required for the bolus to travel from the arm to the brain may be more than 35 seconds, if the bolus must travel via stenotic vessels and/or collateral perfusion pathways (Bartolini, 1981; Kikuchi et al., 2002; Chiu et al., 2012), and some parts of the bolus arrive far later (Calamante et al., 2000, 2003).

Short perfusion scans may cause CBV measurement errors even if they are longer than the transit time of the contrast bolus through the brain, because of the phenomenon of recirculation. After the contrast agent passes through brain, it returns to the heart via systemic veins and passes through the pulmonary circulation, and then parts of the bolus recirculate back to the brain. Multiple recirculation passes through the brain may occur during a single perfusion scan, with the first recirculation pass generally beginning even before the first pass of the contrast agent is complete. Therefore, the C_t measured in any voxel actually reflects the summation of multiple passes of the contrast agent.

This poses a technical challenge for the postprocessing algorithms that are used to calculate CBV. Calculation of CBV by integration of C_t is accurate only if the same number of passes of the bolus are recorded in every part of the brain. However, if bolus arrival in one part of the brain is delayed, and/or transit of the bolus through that part of the brain is slowed, fewer passes of the bolus will be recorded in that region, and its CBV will be erroneously underestimated.

One proposed solution to this problem is to mathematically extract from C_t the theoretic C_t curve that would exist, if only the first pass of the contrast bolus were detectable. However, this method is difficult to implement, because no particular mathematic model is known to describe accurately the first pass of a contrast bolus under all physiologic conditions. Consequently, first-pass fitting methods currently are seldom used in the clinical setting.

More commonly, perfusion postprocessing algorithms simply ignore the multiple-pass problem, and calculate regional CBV by integrating C_t over the entire duration of the scan. Strictly speaking, this method is perfectly accurate only for a scan of infinite duration. However, the magnitude of the truncation artifact decreases as scan duration increases, and relatively long scans lasting approximately 2 minutes may be long enough to produce reasonably accurate CBV measurements, even in patients with perfusion disease (Deipolyi et al., 2012).

Some CT perfusion postprocessing programs use algorithms other than integration of C_t to compute CBV. For example, one manufacturer computes CBV by integrating the tissue response function R_t, which is introduced in the next section, rather than C_t (GE Healthcare, 2011). This particular algorithm appears to be similarly prone to truncation artifacts as simple integration of C_t. The vulnerability of other CT postprocessing algorithms to truncation artifacts may be difficult to assess without empiric testing, as those algorithms' details are often withheld by their manufacturers.

CBV IN CEREBRAL PERFUSION DISORDERS

In response to a fall in regional perfusion pressure, such as that which occurs in brain tissue supplied by a stenotic or occluded artery, the walls of precapillary resistance vessels relax, resulting in vasodilation and capillary recruitment. This autoregulatory response reduces vascular resistance, and, depending upon the severity of the drop in perfusion pressure, it may or may not be sufficient to prevent a fall in blood flow (Powers, 1991).

Autoregulatory vasodilation results in an increase in regional CBV, which may be visible in CBV maps, and therefore may provide evidence of reduced perfusion pressure. However, when evaluating CBV maps to assess whether or not autoregulatory vasodilation is present, several important pitfalls must be considered. First, reductions in regional perfusion pressure are usually accompanied by delayed bolus arrival, and are almost always accompanied by prolonged vascular transit time. As discussed above, these two conditions may contribute to underestimation of CBV in affected tissue, particularly when scan duration is short, and this may make it difficult or impossible to appreciate vasodilation in CBV maps. Second, the increases in CBV that occur with autoregulatory vasodilation are relatively small, and may be difficult to appreciate in CT or MR perfusion maps, which are relatively noisy.

Third, even if autoregulatory vasodilation is present and appreciable in CBV maps, this does not necessarily imply that there is an ongoing reduction in regional perfusion pressure. In perfusion disorders, it is common for perfusion pressure to be restored to normal levels in tissue where it previously has been decreased. This may occur, for example, if systemic blood pressure rises, or when an arterial embolus disintegrates spontaneously or is therapeutically removed. Perfusion pressure also may be therapeutically restored by arterial stenting, or by endarterectomy.

Following restoration of previously reduced cerebral perfusion pressure, blood vessels in the affected tissue often remain dilated for some time, even though vasodilation is no longer necessary for preservation of blood flow. Therefore, when CBV maps do provide evidence of vasodilation, inspection of other perfusion maps, particularly CBF maps, is necessary in order to determine whether there is an ongoing reduction in perfusion pressure, versus a recent reduction that has resolved.

It has been hypothesized that, at extremely low perfusion pressures, CBV may fall to below-normal levels, despite maximum vascular relaxation. This could occur because intravascular pressure is insufficient to hold vessel walls open ("microvascular collapse"), or because slowly moving blood simply clots within vessels. Although both of these phenomena could theoretically result in low CBV, the incidence of CBV reduction has not been thoroughly studied, and it is not clear how often CBV falls (Powers, 1991).

Some authors have proposed that regions in which CBV appears decreased may be presumed to represent tissue that has undergone irreversible ischemic damage, i.e., the so-called "infarct core." However, CBV maps, like other perfusion maps, demonstrate only the instantaneous hemodynamic conditions in the brain at the time of imaging. CBV maps cannot identify the metabolic changes that result from a sufficiently prolonged period of reduced blood flow, and that eventually become irreversible. Indeed, consistent with the experimental observation that vasodilation occurs in response to reduced perfusion pressure, and often following restoration of perfusion pressure in previously ischemic tissue, CBV appears to be elevated, not reduced, in the majority of infarcts (Deipolyi et al., 2012).

Cerebral blood flow

Definition

CBF is defined as the volume of blood that passes through a specific quantity of brain tissue during a particular period of time. Classically, CBF is measured in units of mL of blood per 100 g of tissue per minute. CT and MR perfusion techniques measure the quantity of blood that flows through a particular volume of brain tissue, i.e., a voxel, rather than a particular mass. Nevertheless, if it is assumed that blood, water, and brain tissue all have the same mass density, then CBF units incorporating masses of brain tissue may be interchanged with those incorporating volumes of brain tissue. As with CBV, CBF measurements obtained using CT and MR perfusion techniques are relative, not absolute, and therefore the choice of units is not critical.

CBF calculation

CBF reflects the rate at which blood, and therefore contrast material, is delivered into an image voxel. Accordingly, a rough estimation of CBF in a voxel may be obtained by simply inspecting the slope of the initial increase in C_t that occurs when the contrast bolus arrives, with a steeper slope suggesting greater CBF. Indeed, under certain conditions that do not usually exist in CT or MR perfusion imaging, accurate CBF measurements theoretically may be obtained by simply measuring this slope (Kwong et al., 2011). In practice, however, the temporal resolution achieved by CT and MR perfusion scans is not sufficient for this technique to work accurately, and CBF measurements instead must be calculated using a mathematic algorithm called deconvolution (Østergaard et al., 1996a, b).

In a theoretic, idealized perfusion scan, the entire contrast bolus would be delivered during a single instant in time, directly into a distal artery with branches that supply blood to several tissue voxels. If this could be achieved, then the C_t observed in each of those voxels would reflect the amount of the instantaneously delivered contrast bolus that remains in that voxel at each time point following its arrival. The contrast concentration in each voxel would be highest immediately upon the arrival of the bolus, with a subsequent gradual decrease of C_t reflecting the amount of initially delivered contrast material still remaining in the voxel, as it is gradually washed out. The C_t that would be observed if this idealized experiment could be performed is called the tissue response function, or R_t. The initial peak value of R_t is a measurement of CBF. If the peak value of R_t in one voxel is twice the peak value in a different voxel, then the first voxel has twice the CBF of the second.

In real perfusion scans, the bolus of contrast material cannot be delivered into brain voxels in a single instant, and is instead injected into a peripheral vein over several seconds. Although the bolus is usually injected at a constant rate, it must travel through the systemic veins, into the right heart, through the pulmonary circulation, and through the left heart, before it reaches the brain. During this trip, the bolus experiences considerable dispersion. Its arrival in the brain is gradual, with its concentration increasing over a few seconds. After the concentration peaks, it declines somewhat gradually, over perhaps 10 seconds.

The function reflecting contrast concentration in an artery supplying the brain, as opposed to tissue concentration, is called the arterial input function, which may be abbreviated as AIF, or A_t. The shape of A_t is determined by numerous complex factors, including the quantity and rate of contrast injection, the patient's size and vascular anatomy, stenotic or occlusive arterial lesions, and moment-to-moment changes in cardiac output. These factors are too complex to allow for *a priori* estimation of A_t, so it must be measured directly during the course of perfusion postprocessing. In order to do this, several arterial pixels are identified, and the contrast concentrations in all of these pixels are averaged together at every time point, yielding a measured A_t. Typically, a single A_t is measured and used for perfusion calculations involving the entire brain.

As discussed above, CBF is measured by noting the peak value of the tissue response function R_t. R_t is a technique-invariant attribute of a patient's physiologic state at a particular moment in time, and it is not altered by, for example, variations in contrast injection rate. However, R_t cannot be observed directly, because it is not possible to inject the entire contrast bolus into every voxel during a single instant. Instead, R_t must be calculated, using a mathematic algorithm called deconvolution.

Mathematically speaking, the observed concentration function C_t is the convolution of two other functions, A_t and R_t. Because C_t and A_t can be observed, the unobservable R_t can be derived from the other two functions, using deconvolution. Various deconvolution algorithms exist. One of the most frequently used in CT and MR perfusion imaging is singular value decomposition (SVD).

The SVD deconvolution algorithm has the benefit of being model-independent, and applicable in a wide variety of physiologic conditions. Also, compared to CBV calculation, calculation of CBF using SVD deconvolution is relatively reliable, even with short scan durations. Provided that scans last long enough to sample most of the initial arrival of the contrast agent, truncation of C_t by moderately short scans appears to have little artifactual effect upon CBF calculations derived from SVD.

However, R_t functions derived using SVD, and therefore the CBF maps that they produce, are affected by several other artifacts that are important to consider. Among the most important of these are underestimation of CBF due to bolus arrival delay, and bolus dispersion. Both of these artifacts result from the assumption, usually made in CBF calculations, that a single AIF can be used to perform deconvolution in all parts of the brain. In reality, delivery of the contrast bolus to different parts of the brain occurs at different times and rates, particularly in the setting of a perfusion disorder, and a single AIF is not perfectly accurate in all parts of the brain.

Frequently, arrival of the contrast bolus is delayed, relative to its arrival in the arteries from which the AIF is derived, in regions of the brain that are perfused via stenotic arteries and/or circuitous collateral pathways. In these regions, C_t is shifted later in time, relative to the A_t that is used for deconvolution. This temporal shift should have no effect on deconvolution or CBF calculation. However, SVD and some related deconvolution algorithms erroneously underestimate CBF when bolus arrival is delayed.

Many modern postprocessing programs now eliminate this problem in one of two ways. Some programs simply attempt to detect the bolus arrival times in each pixel's A_t and C_t, and then artificially shift one of the two curves so that the arrival times are the same in both. The other common solution is to use a modified version of the SVD deconvolution algorithm that simply does not suffer from delay-related underestimation of CBF (Wu et al., 2003).

Underestimation of CBF due to bolus dispersion is a more difficult technical problem to solve. In brain tissue that is perfused via stenotic arteries and/or collateral pathways, there is not only a delay in the initial arrival of the contrast bolus, but also a widening of A_t, relative to the A_t that is measured in normal-appearing arteries, and is usually used for deconvolution in all parts of the brain. This bolus dispersion also results in underestimation of rCBF.

Some have proposed addressing the bolus dispersion problem by performing deconvolution in each part of the brain using a "local A_t," derived from measurements in nearby arteries, rather than using a single "global A_t" for deconvolution in all parts of the brain (Calamante et al., 2004; Lorenz et al., 2006a, b). While this approach is sound in theory, in practice it is seldom employed, because in most parts of the brain it is difficult to locate and sample the small arteries that contribute to the local A_t. In most perfusion postprocessing software, underestimation of CBF due to bolus dispersion is simply not addressed.

CBF IN CEREBRAL PERFUSION DISORDERS

In cerebral perfusion disorders, CBF is the hemodynamic parameter that is most directly related to both tissue viability and patients' neurologic status. CBF reflects the rate of arrival of blood in brain tissue, and therefore the rate of delivery of oxygen and glucose, which are required for neuronal transmission and cellular survival.

The effects of changes in perfusion pressure upon CBF, and those of CBF reductions upon neuronal function and tissue survival, have been well established by numerous experiments that were performed decades ago. As discussed above, mild reductions in regional perfusion pressure that do not exceed the cerebral vasculature's autoregulatory reserve do not cause any decrement in CBF. Larger reductions in perfusion pressure do cause CBF to fall, with greater reductions in perfusion pressure resulting in lower levels of CBF (Powers, 1991).

A very mild reduction of CBF causes no impairment of electric function, and therefore has no clinically observable effect. However, if CBF falls below a physiologic "electric function threshold," neuronal transmission ceases, and a neurologic deficit may be observed clinically. If CBF does not fall too far below this threshold, cellular membrane integrity is preserved, and brain tissue can survive indefinitely in this condition, with no threat to its viability. In the 1970s, researcher Lyndsay Symon and his colleagues coined the term "ischemic penumbra" to describe this condition, in which electric function is impaired by low CBF, but tissue viability is not threatened (Symon, 2007). In current usage, however, this original definition "ischemic penumbra" is seldom used. Instead, the term is used with a wide variety of conflicting definitions, none of which has gained consensus acceptance. Indeed, many papers use "ischemic penumbra" to refer to tissue that is not necessarily ischemic, and it has become common to use the term without offering any definition at all.

More severe reductions in CBF do threaten tissue viability, and will ultimately result in permanent infarction. One of the most critically important discoveries of research on brain ischemia is the observation that ischemic injury becomes irreversible after a period of time whose length is inversely related to the severity of the ischemia. Brain tissue may survive a complete cessation of CBF for only a few minutes, whereas a more moderate CBF reduction may persist for hours before its effects become permanent.

This relationship between CBF, time, and tissue survival forms the basis of much of current acute stroke therapeutic strategy. It implies that, in some acute stroke patients, there is a portion of the brain in which CBF is reduced sufficiently to cause permanent infarction, but in which permanent infarction has not yet occurred. Presumably, this underperfused tissue could be saved by therapeutic manipulations that increase blood flow. The most definitive of these would be arterial recanalization therapies, such as intravenous or intra-arterial administration of thrombolytic medications, mechanical clot removal, rapid endarterectomy, and stenting. However, CBF is also increased by manipulations that increase cerebral perfusion pressure without achieving arterial recanalization. The simplest and most widely available of these is pharmacologically induced hypertension. Other proposed methods for increasing CBF without achieving arterial recanalization include external counterpulsation (Han and Wong, 2008) and partial aortic occlusion (Shuaib et al., 2011; Schellinger et al., 2013).

In theory, the need for and efficacy of such therapies could be assessed by reviewing CBF maps. For example, if an acute stroke patient's perfusion maps showed no regions with below-normal CBF, it might be concluded that therapeutic elevation of the patient's blood pressure above its current level is not immediately necessary to preserve tissue survival (although a subsequent worsening of arterial stenosis could change this assessment). Alternatively, if a large region with reduced CBF were to be discovered, this would not necessarily confirm that the CBF reduction was severe enough to threaten tissue viability, or even to impair electric function. Indeed, perfusion imaging alone could not determine whether or not the affected tissue had already undergone irreversible infarction before the time of imaging. Nevertheless, some of this information could potentially be filled in by clinical examination and other imaging modalities, and a relatively aggressive approach to acute stroke treatment might suggest attempting to preserve normal CBF in still-viable brain tissue, perhaps as a temporizing measure, until arterial recanalization occurs spontaneously or as a result of recanalization therapy.

By identifying when reperfusion occurs, CBF maps could potentially help in the care of ischemic stroke patients in another way: limitation of reperfusion injury. Even without therapeutic recanalization therapy, reperfusion occurs spontaneously in approximately 16% of patients within 8 hours of stroke onset (Rubin et al., 1999), 33% within 48 hours (Hakim et al., 1987), and 42–60% within a week (Jorgensen et al., 1994; Bowler et al., 1998). As discussed above, autoregulatory vasodilation may persist unnecessarily for some time following restoration of normal perfusion pressure to previously ischemic tissue. This state of hyperperfusion may cause additional injury to stroke patients' brains, by aggravating vasogenic edema, increasing the risk of hemorrhagic transformation, and possibly free radical-mediated mechanisms. Current stroke treatment guidelines generally suggest allowing stroke patients' systemic blood pressure to remain high, in order to preserve blood flow to threatened tissue that might otherwise undergo infarction. However, when reperfusion has already occurred, high blood pressure may worsen reperfusion-related injury, and aggressive lowering of blood pressure might be a worthwhile therapeutic goal. CBF maps potentially could be used to document reperfusion.

Although previous research has established theoretic basis for such uses of CBF maps in acute stroke care, CBF maps are seldom mentioned in the clinical stroke imaging literature. Some studies have shown that lower levels of CBF are correlated with greater likelihood of being part of the infarct core, as putatively identified by diffusion-weighted MRI. However, like other perfusion maps, CBF maps cannot be used to identify the infarct core, because the state of irreversible infarction is a metabolic one that reflects the cumulative effects of CBF reduction that have occurred prior to the time of imaging. Perfusion imaging cannot determine for how long CBF deficits have existed prior to imaging, how they have fluctuated during that time, or what the CBF thresholds of viability may be in different parts of a particular patient's brain.

Mean transit time (MTT)

Definition

MTT is the average period of time that blood, or an element of blood such as a single red blood cell, spends within the blood vessels in a particular part of the brain. MTT is measured in seconds, and is typically on the order of 6 seconds in normal brain tissue (Mihara et al., 2003). In the setting of reduced perfusion pressure, decreased blood flow, and vasodilation, MTT may increase to 10–20 seconds (Carrera et al., 2011).

Calculation of MTT

The relationship between CBV, CBF, and MTT is a simple one, described by the central volume principle (Stewart, 1894):

$$CBV = CBF \times MTT$$

Most perfusion postprocessing software calculates MTT by first calculating CBV and CBF, and then dividing the former by the latter. When this is the case, artifactual errors in CBV and CBF maps such as those described above may be propagated to MTT maps. For example, short perfusion scans may cause underestimation of CBV, and this in turn may lead to underestimation of MTT. Also, to the extent that deconvolution algorithms erroneously underestimate CBF because of bolus arrival delay or bolus dispersion, this error will also be manifested as an overestimation of MTT.

MTT in cerebral perfusion disorders

MTT maps are mentioned much more frequently than CBV or CBF maps in the clinical neuroimaging literature, and are much more commonly used in clinical image interpretation. This is probably because MTT maps are simply easier to interpret. Because CBV and CBF are several times higher in gray matter than in white matter, there is considerable heterogeneity in CBV and CBF maps, and this can make identification of lesions more difficult. However, normal gray matter and white matter have very similar MTTs. As a result, MTT maps present a relatively homogeneous background appearance, against which regions of abnormal MTT prolongation are relatively easy to identify.

In acute stroke imaging research, regions of abnormal MTT prolongation are sometimes described as representing tissue that is at risk of infarction, and some clinical trials have offered experimental thrombolytic therapy to acute stroke patients only if their MTT maps showed large abnormalities.

This use of MTT maps is partially consistent with cerebrovascular physiology. In cerebral perfusion disorders, MTT prolongation reflects autoregulatory vasodilation that is a response to a recent or ongoing reduction in cerebral perfusion pressure. When MTT prolongation is seen in the presence of normal or reduced CBF, the reduction in perfusion pressure is likely ongoing, and therefore the affected tissue is, in a sense, at risk. However, MTT prolongation per se does not threaten the viability of brain tissue. Indeed, quite the opposite is true: MTT prolongation is protective. By allowing additional time for oxygen to diffuse out of brain capillaries in underperfused tissue, MTT prolongation enables an increase in the fraction of available oxygen that the brain is able to extract from blood. This has the effect of preserving oxidative metabolism when CBF is low (Powers, 1991).

From a practical perspective, inspection of MTT maps alone cannot assess the adequacy or even the necessity of the cerebrovascular autoregulatory response to a reduction in perfusion pressure. If MTT is prolonged but CBF is normal, the affected tissue presumably could remain in this condition indefinitely with no threat to its viability and without appearance of a clinical deficit, assuming that systemic blood pressure does not fall, collateral vessels remain patent, and no new vascular event occurs. However, if MTT is prolonged but CBF is low, this condition might or might not result in a clinical deficit and a potential threat to tissue viability, depending on the severity of the CBF decrement. The contrast between these conditions highlights the imprecision of reports that describe tissue with abnormal MTT as "hypoperfused." Such tissue may or may not be hypoperfused, depending upon whether or not CBF is low.

Time-to-peak of the tissue response function (T_{max})

Definition

The section on CBF, above, described how perfusion postprocessing algorithms use deconvolution to derive a tissue response function R_t from an observed AIF A_t, and an observed tissue concentration function C_t. The maximum amplitude of this function reflects CBF. Many perfusion postprocessing programs also calculate the time at which this maximum amplitude is reached, and produce maps of that parameter, which is often simply called "T_{max}." In theory, T_{max} is a pure measurement of arrival delay. It reflects the time that elapses between arrival of the contrast bolus in the artery that is used to derive A_t, and arrival in the voxel where T_{max} is measured.

Calculation of T_{max}

Postprocessing algorithms usually calculate T_{max} simply by performing the deconvolution operation described above, but producing maps of T_{max}, rather than CBF maps. T_{max} is unlike the other hemodynamic measurements discussed in this chapter because, although it is theoretically a continuously varying quantity, the T_{max} values that are calculated by postprocessing algorithms are usually quantized, in that they can only reflect the time point of the sample at which the maximum value of R_t was calculated. So, for example, a CT or MR perfusion scan in which images are obtained every 1.5 seconds will produce T_{max} maps with values of 0 seconds, 1.5 seconds, 3 seconds, etc., whereas if images are obtained every 2 seconds, the values in the T_{max} maps will be 0 seconds, 2 seconds, 4 seconds, etc.

Artifactual influences of factors other than actual bolus arrival delay upon T_{max} measurements are infrequently studied. One simulation study found that bolus dispersion and MTT also influenced T_{max} values (Calamante et al., 2010) and truncation artifacts introduced by short perfusion scans also may result in lower calculated values of T_{max}.

T_{MAX} IN CEREBRAL PERFUSION DISORDERS

T_{max} theoretically measures arrival delay, which has no direct effect upon tissue viability in cerebral perfusion disorders. Nevertheless, T_{max} maps are frequently cited in the stroke imaging literature, and have been used as an enrollment criterion in clinical trials of experimental thrombolytic therapies (Davis et al., 2008). This is probably because, like MTT, T_{max} values do not vary greatly in different parts of the brain under normal conditions, and this makes abnormalities relatively easy to detect in visual inspection of T_{max} maps.

Justification for the use of T_{max} maps as a surrogate for other, more physiologically significant hemodynamic parameters may be found in the principle that, in cerebral perfusion disorders, more severe perturbations of any one hemodynamic measurement tend to be associated with more severe perturbations of all other parameters. Statistically significant inverse correlations between T_{max} and CBF have been reported, indicating that tissue with prolonged T_{max} is more likely to be hypoperfused. However, correlation does not reflect interchangeability. An increasing number of reports inaccurately refer to tissue with prolonged T_{max} as "hypoperfused." Such tissue is not necessarily hypoperfused, and the degree of hypoperfusion cannot be inferred from the degree of T_{max} prolongation. For example, one study that used positron emission tomography measurement of CBF as a gold standard found that a T_{max} threshold of 5.5 seconds best identified tissue with CBF under a threshold value of 20 mL/100 g/s (Zaro-Weber et al., 2010). However, in that study, the actual CBF values measured in tissue with T_{max} values close to 5.5 seconds varied from approximately 0 to 65 mL/100 g/s, spanning essentially the entire range of possible CBF values in normally perfused and hypoperfused tissue.

PERFUSION IMAGING OF BRAIN TUMORS

Perfusion imaging is increasingly used in the diagnosis and imaging follow-up of intracranial neoplastic lesions. Although perfusion imaging of brain tumors is sometimes performed with ASL (Wolf et al., 2005; Lehmann et al., 2010; Canale et al., 2011), DSC remains the most commonly used perfusion technique in brain tumor imaging, as it is in MRI of primary perfusion disorders. In contrast to the wide variety of postprocessed perfusion maps that are typically generated when studying primary cerebral perfusion disorders, brain tumors are most commonly evaluated only in maps of regional CBV, which assess the overall degree of tumor vascularity. CBF maps are also used in brain tumor imaging, but less commonly. Perfusion imaging techniques provide information that is complementary to that derived from conventional MR images and other advanced imaging techniques (e.g., MR spectroscopy or nuclear medicine studies) and should not be interpreted in isolation. The most common clinical applications that benefit from the use of perfusion imaging include the initial characterization of intracranial mass lesions, guidance of diagnostic or therapeutic interventions, differentiation between recurrent tumor and treatment-related changes, and prediction of therapeutic responses or clinical outcome.

Characterization of intracranial mass lesions

There have been a large number of basic and clinical research studies supporting the use of MR perfusion, particularly DSC perfusion, for differentiation of high-grade versus low-grade glial tumoral lesions (Law et al., 2003; Hakyemez et al., 2005; Emblem et al., 2008); nonneoplastic pathologies versus malignant lesions (Fig. 6.3) (Law et al., 2004a; Pivawer et al., 2007; Hourani et al., 2008; Chiang et al., 2009; Liu et al., 2011; Floriano et al., 2013), as well as differentiation between high-grade gliomas and metastatic lesions (Bulakbasi et al., 2005; Hakyemez et al., 2006; Senturk et al., 2009; Young and Setayesh, 2009; Bendini et al., 2011). Multiple studies have documented a significant correlation between intratumoral vascular area and CBV values (Hu et al., 2012a). Low-grade neoplastic lesions without pathologic evidence of vascular proliferation do not show any significant increase of CBV, compared to the surrounding or contralateral brain parenchyma (Law et al., 2004b; Server et al., 2011a). High-grade tumors such as glioblastoma show marked CBV elevation (Fig. 6.4). Lymphoma and metastatic lesions typically demonstrate CBV values that are moderately elevated (Cotton et al., 2006; Rizzo et al., 2009; Blasel et al., 2013; Toh et al., 2013). Some benign intracranial tumors such as pilocytic astrocytomas may have high CBV due to high intratumoral vascularity that is not associated with mitotic activity or clinical aggressiveness (Cha, 2006; Poussaint and Rodriguez, 2006). Anaplastic astrocytomas often demonstrate lack of significant increase of rCBV values due to the absence of microvascular proliferation required for their pathologic definition based on the most recent World Health Organization (WHO) brain tumor classification system. rCBV values in nonenhancing T2-hyperintense regions surrounding the enhancing lesions (Law et al., 2002; Cha et al., 2007; Lehmann et al., 2012) are also useful for the differentiation between metastatic lesions and glioblastoma (Huang et al., 2010; Server et al., 2011b) (Figs 6.4 and 6.5).

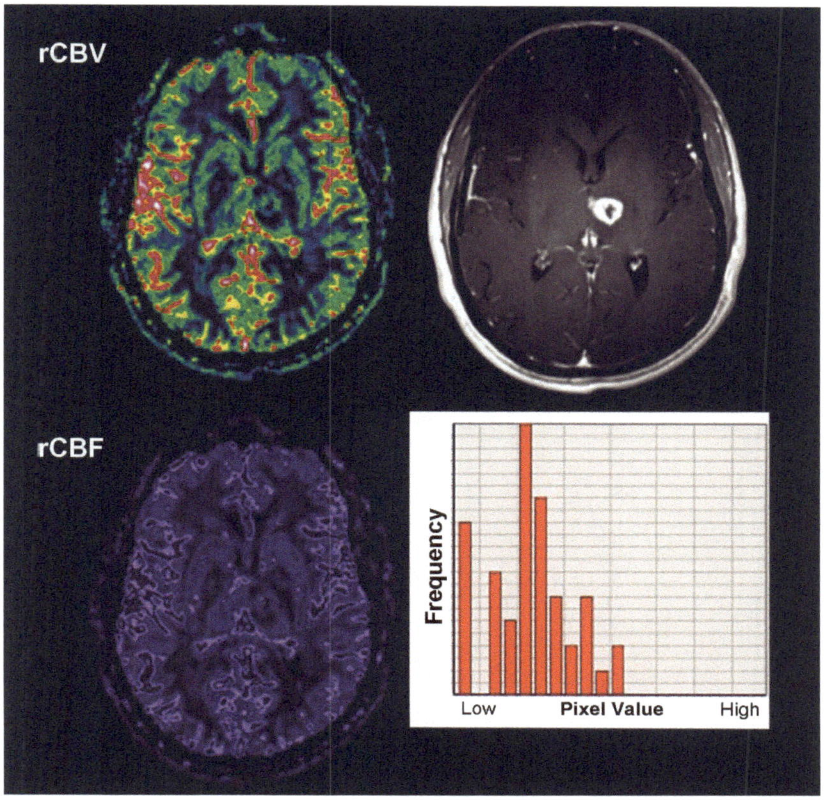

Fig. 6.3. Use of magnetic resonance perfusion imaging in distinguishing between cerebral perfusion disorders and brain tumors. A 28-year-old man presented 1 week after a single episode of transient lightheadedness, visual disturbance, and difficulty speaking. Postcontrast T1-weighted images (upper right) demonstrated a ring-enhancing left thalamic mass lesion whose appearance is suspicious for neoplasm. A leakage-corrected cerebral blood volume (CBV) map (upper left) and a histogram analysis of CBV within the lesion (lower right) showed no apparent CBV elevation. A cerebral blood flow (CBF) map (lower left) showed mildly decreased blood flow. These findings are suggestive of subacute infarction, a diagnosis that was ultimately confirmed by stereotactic biopsy.

Guidance of diagnostic or therapeutic procedures

MR perfusion imaging can be used to improve the accuracy of diagnostic biopsy by demonstrating regions with higher rCBV values that are more likely to represent areas of higher histopathologic grade or recurrent high-grade tumor, against a background of posttreatment changes. A similar approach can also be helpful in preprocedural planning before radiation treatment (Dhermain, 2010). MR perfusion may also be sensitive enough to detect early evidence of transformation into a higher tumoral grade in low-grade gliomas (Danchaivijitr et al., 2008).

Monitoring treatment-related changes, including pseudophenomena and radiation necrosis

Perfusion imaging can be used to increase the diagnostic accuracy of brain MR studies immediately after radiation treatment. Up to 30% of patients will develop transiently increased enhancement, T2 hyperintensity, or mass effect approximately 1–4 months after chemoradiation, resulting from a phenomenon called pseudoprogression (Brandsma and van den Bent, 2009; Clarke and Chang, 2009). Several studies have shown the important role of DSC MR perfusion in complementing conventional images in these diagnostically challenging cases (Vrabec et al., 2011; Baek et al., 2012; Hu et al., 2012b; Choi et al., 2013; Gahramanov et al., 2013; Suh et al., 2013; Young et al., 2013; Martinez-Martinez and Martinez-Bosch, 2014). Approximately 6 months to several years after chemoradiation of high-grade tumors, many patients develop areas of radiation necrosis that are difficult to differentiate from recurrent tumor based on conventional MR findings. MR perfusion imaging (including ASL and DSC) has been shown to be highly sensitive and specific for this differentiation (Weber et al., 2003; Barajas et al., 2009a, b; Thomassin-Naggara et al., 2010; Huang et al., 2011; Jain et al., 2011). Areas of radiation necrosis do not have increased

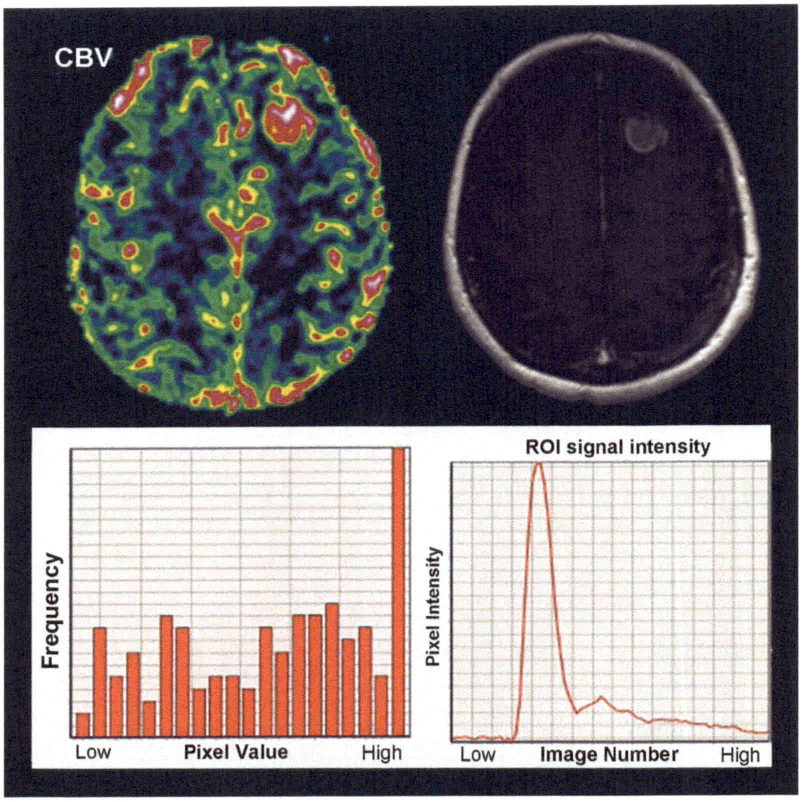

Fig. 6.4. Magnetic resonance (MR) perfusion imaging in primary brain tumors. A 71-year-old woman presented after her first seizure. Postcontrast T1-weighted MR images showed multiple enhancing brain lesions, the largest in the left frontal lobe (upper right). A leakage-corrected cerebral blood volume (CBV) map (upper left) and CBV histogram analysis (lower left) show markedly elevated CBV within the lesion. Sampling the C_t curve in the lesion (lower right) revealed return of contrast concentrations within the tumor almost to zero. These findings are suggestive of high-grade glioma, and the lesion was pathologically shown to be a glioblastoma.

CBV values, whereas recurrent high-grade tumors are likely to reflect the CBV profile of the original tumor (Sugahara et al., 2000; Bobek-Billewicz et al., 2010; Kim et al., 2010; Narang et al., 2011; Fink et al., 2012; Chung et al., 2013).

A different diagnostic problem is seen in patients who develop progressive tumoral involvement and are started on antiangiogenic treatment. These antiangiogenic agents "normalize" the blood–brain barrier within tumors and surrounding brain, resulting in marked decrease of enhancement, edema, and mass effect. This therapeutic effect affects the sensitivity of DSC MR perfusion in this setting (Pradel et al., 2003; Hygino da Cruz et al., 2011).

Several studies have suggested the potential role of DSC perfusion imaging in the prediction of therapeutic response to antiangiogenic therapies (Sawlani et al., 2010) and overall survival (independent of the histopathologic WHO tumoral grade) (Fuss et al., 2001; Law et al., 2006, 2008; Hirai et al., 2008; Bisdas et al., 2009; Emblem et al., 2011; Jiang et al., 2011; Fellah et al., 2013; Valles et al., 2013).

SUMMARY

CT- and MR-based perfusion imaging techniques provide measurements of a variety of different cerebral microvascular hemodynamic parameters that can be readily obtained in the clinical setting. In primary cerebral perfusion disorders, such as ischemic stroke, transient ischemic attack, and reperfusion syndrome, the complementary information contained in maps of regional CBV, blood flow, MTT, and arrival time enable more detailed understanding of the cerebral vasculature's responses to alterations in perfusion pressure, and potentially may help in the patient management in a variety of different ways. Perfusion imaging of brain tumors typically focuses on evaluation of CBV and blood flow, parameters that, when combined with conventional MR images, may help in initial

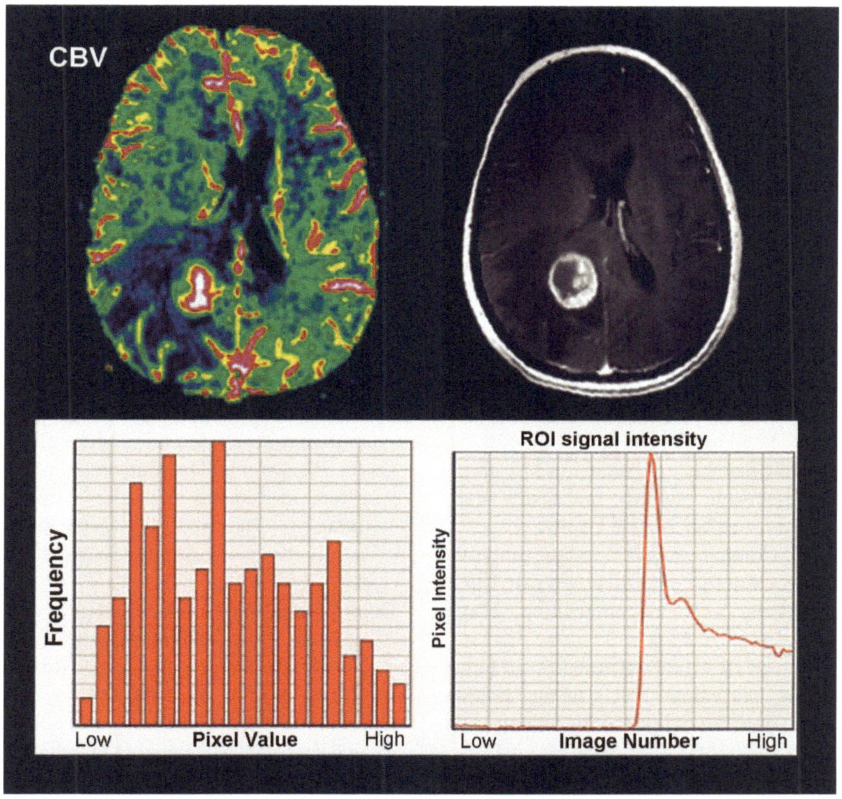

Fig. 6.5. Magnetic resonance (MR) perfusion imaging in metastatic disease. A 42-year-old woman presented with a headache of 1 week's duration. Postcontrast T1-weighted MR images showed a single enhancing mass lesion in the right parietal lobe (upper right). A leakage-corrected cerebral blood volume (CBV) map (upper left) and CBV histogram analysis (lower left) showed CBV to be elevated, though less so than in the lesion in Figure 6.4. In the lesion's C_t curve (lower right), contrast concentrations remain elevated, even in the latest images obtained. These findings are commonly found in brain metastases, and this lesion was found to reflect metastatic adenocarcinoma of the lung.

characterization of brain tumors, selection of optimal treatment strategies, and monitoring the effects of treatment.

References

Baek HJ, Kim HS, Kim N et al. (2012). Percent change of perfusion skewness and kurtosis: a potential imaging biomarker for early treatment response in patients with newly diagnosed glioblastomas. Radiology 264: 834–843.

Barajas RF, Chang JS, Sneed PK et al. (2009a). Distinguishing recurrent intra-axial metastatic tumor from radiation necrosis following gamma knife radiosurgery using dynamic susceptibility-weighted contrast-enhanced perfusion MR imaging. AJNR Am J Neuroradiol 30: 367–372.

Barajas RF, Chang JS, Segal MR et al. (2009b). Differentiation of recurrent glioblastoma multiforme from radiation necrosis after external beam radiation therapy with dynamic susceptibility-weighted contrast-enhanced perfusion MR imaging. Radiology 253: 486–496.

Bartolini A (1981). Regional arm-brain mean transit time in the diagnostic evaluation of patients with cerebral vascular disease. Stroke 12: 241–245.

Bendini M, Marton E, Feletti A et al. (2011). Primary and metastatic intraaxial brain tumors: prospective comparison of multivoxel 2D chemical-shift imaging (CSI) proton MR spectroscopy, perfusion MRI, and histopathological findings in a group of 159 patients. Acta Neurochir (Wien) 153: 403–412.

Bisdas S, Kirkpatrick M, Giglio P et al. (2009). Cerebral blood volume measurements by perfusion-weighted MR imaging in gliomas: ready for prime time in predicting short-term outcome and recurrent disease? AJNR Am J Neuroradiol 30: 681–688.

Bjornerud A, Sorensen AG, Mouridsen K et al. (2011). T1- and T2*-dominant extravasation correction in DSC-MRI: part I–theoretical considerations and implications for assessment of tumor hemodynamic properties. J Cereb Blood Flow Metab 31: 2041–2053.

Blasel S, Jurcoane A, BAHR O et al. (2013). MR perfusion in and around the contrast-enhancement of primary CNS lymphomas. J Neurooncol 114: 127–134.

Bobek-Billewicz B, Stasik-Pres G, Majchrzak H et al. (2010). Differentiation between brain tumor recurrence and radiation injury using perfusion, diffusion-weighted imaging and MR spectroscopy. Folia Neuropathol 48: 81–92.

Bowler JV, Wade JP, Jones BE et al. (1998). Natural history of the spontaneous reperfusion of human cerebral infarcts as assessed by 99mTc HMPAO SPECT. J Neurol Neurosurg Psychiatry 64: 90–97.
Boxerman JL, Hamberg LM, Rosen BR et al. (1995). MR contrast due to intravascular magnetic susceptibility perturbations. Magn Reson Med 34: 555–566.
Boxerman JL, Schmainda KM, Weisskoff RM (2006). Relative cerebral blood volume maps corrected for contrast agent extravasation significantly correlate with glioma tumor grade, whereas uncorrected maps do not. AJNR Am J Neuroradiol 27: 859–867.
Brandsma D, van den Bent MJ (2009). Pseudoprogression and pseudoresponse in the treatment of gliomas. Curr Opin Neurol 22: 633–638.
Bulakbasi N, Kocaoglu M, Farzaliyev A et al. (2005). Assessment of diagnostic accuracy of perfusion MR imaging in primary and metastatic solitary malignant brain tumors. AJNR Am J Neuroradiol 26: 2187–2199.
Calamante F, Gadian DG, Connelly A (2000). Delay and dispersion effects in dynamic susceptibility contrast MRI: simulations using singular value decomposition. Magn Reson Med 44: 466–473.
Calamante F, Yim PJ, Cebral JR (2003). Estimation of bolus dispersion effects in perfusion MRI using image-based computational fluid dynamics. Neuroimage 19: 341–353.
Calamante F, Morup M, Hansen LK (2004). Defining a local arterial input function for perfusion MRI using independent component analysis. Magn Reson Med 52: 789–797.
Calamante F, Christensen S, Desmond PM et al. (2010). The physiological significance of the time-to-maximum (T_{max}) parameter in perfusion MRI. Stroke 41: 1169–1174.
Canale S, Rodrigo S, Tourdias T et al. (2011). Grading of adults primitive glial neoplasms using arterial spin-labeled perfusion MR imaging. J Neuroradiol 38: 207–213.
Carrera E, Jones PS, Iglesias S et al. (2011). The vascular mean transit time: a surrogate for the penumbra flow threshold? J Cereb Blood Flow Metab 31: 1027–1035.
Cha S (2006). Dynamic susceptibility-weighted contrast-enhanced perfusion MR imaging in pediatric patients. Neuroimaging Clin N Am 16: 137–147. ix.
Cha S, Lupo JM, Chen MH et al. (2007). Differentiation of glioblastoma multiforme and single brain metastasis by peak height and percentage of signal intensity recovery derived from dynamic susceptibility-weighted contrast-enhanced perfusion MR imaging. AJNR Am J Neuroradiol 28: 1078–1084.
Chiang IC, Hsieh TJ, Chiu ML et al. (2009). Distinction between pyogenic brain abscess and necrotic brain tumour using 3-tesla MR spectroscopy, diffusion and perfusion imaging. Br J Radiol 82: 813–820.
Chiu FY, Kao YH, Teng MM et al. (2012). Validation and absolute quantification of MR perfusion compared with CT perfusion in patients with unilateral cerebral arterial stenosis. Eur J Radiol 81: 4087–4093.
Choi YJ, Kim HS, Jahng GH et al. (2013). Pseudoprogression in patients with glioblastoma: added value of arterial spin labeling to dynamic susceptibility contrast perfusion MR imaging. Acta Radiol 54: 448–454.
Chung WJ, Kim HS, Kim N et al. (2013). Recurrent glioblastoma: optimum area under the curve method derived from dynamic contrast-enhanced T1-weighted perfusion MR imaging. Radiology 269: 561–568.
Clarke JL, Chang S (2009). Pseudoprogression and pseudoresponse: challenges in brain tumor imaging. Curr Neurol Neurosci Rep 9: 241–246.
Cotton F, Ongolo-Zogo P, Louis-Tisserand G et al. (2006). Diffusion and perfusion MR imaging in cerebral lymphomas. J Neuroradiol 33: 220–228.
Danchaivijitr N, Waldman AD, Tozer DJ et al. (2008). Low-grade gliomas: do changes in rCBV measurements at longitudinal perfusion-weighted MR imaging predict malignant transformation? Radiology 247: 170–178.
Davis SM, Donnan GA, Parsons MW et al. (2008). Effects of alteplase beyond 3 h after stroke in the Echoplanar Imaging Thrombolytic Evaluation Trial (EPITHET): a placebo-controlled randomised trial. Lancet Neurol 7: 209–309.
Deipolyi AR, Wu O, Macklin EA et al. (2012). Reliability of cerebral blood volume maps as a substitute for diffusion-weighted imaging in acute ischemic stroke. J Magn Reson Imaging 36: 1083–1087.
Dhermain F (2010). Role of perfusion, vascular permeability and anatomic MR imaging in radiation therapy for gliomas. Bull Cancer 97: 753–758.
Donahue KM, Krouwer HG, Rand SD et al. (2000). Utility of simultaneously acquired gradient-echo and spin-echo cerebral blood volume and morphology maps in brain tumor patients. Mag Reson Med 43: 845–853.
Edelman RR, Siewert B, Darby DG et al. (1994). Qualitative mapping of cerebral blood flow and functional localization with echo-planar MR imaging and signal targeting with alternating radio frequency. Radiology 192: 513–520.
Emblem KE, Zoellner FG, Tennoe B et al. (2008). Predictive modeling in glioma grading from MR perfusion images using support vector machines. Magn Reson Med 60: 945–952.
Emblem KE, Bjornerud A, Mouridsen K et al. (2011). T(1)- and T(2)(*)-dominant extravasation correction in DSC-MRI: part II-predicting patient outcome after a single dose of cediranib in recurrent glioblastoma patients. J Cereb Blood Flow Metab 31: 2054–2064.
Emblem KE, Mouridsen K, Bjornerud A et al. (2013). Vessel architectural imaging identifies cancer patient responders to anti-angiogenic therapy. Nat Med 19: 1178–1183.
Fellah S, Caudal D, De Paula AM et al. (2013). Multimodal MR imaging (diffusion, perfusion, and spectroscopy): is it possible to distinguish oligodendroglial tumor grade and 1p/19q codeletion in the pretherapeutic diagnosis? AJNR Am J Neuroradiol 34: 1326–1333.
Fink JR, Carr RB, Matsusue E et al. (2012). Comparison of 3 Tesla proton MR spectroscopy, MR perfusion and MR diffusion for distinguishing glioma recurrence from posttreatment effects. J Magn Reson Imaging 35: 56–63.

Floriano VH, Torres US, Spotti AR et al. (2013). The role of dynamic susceptibility contrast-enhanced perfusion MR imaging in differentiating between infectious and neoplastic focal brain lesions: results from a cohort of 100 consecutive patients. PLoS One 8: e81509.

Fuss M, Wenz F, Essig M et al. (2001). Tumor angiogenesis of low-grade astrocytomas measured by dynamic susceptibility contrast-enhanced MRI (DSC-MRI) is predictive of local tumor control after radiation therapy. Int J Radiat Oncol Biol Phys 51: 478–482.

Gahramanov S, Muldoon LL, Varallyay CG et al. (2013). Pseudoprogression of glioblastoma after chemo- and radiation therapy: diagnosis by using dynamic susceptibility-weighted contrast-enhanced perfusion MR imaging with ferumoxytol versus gadoteridol and correlation with survival. Radiology 266: 842–852.

Ginde AA, Foianini A, Renner DM et al. (2008). Availability and quality of computed tomography and magnetic resonance imaging equipment in U.S. emergency departments. Acad Emerg Med 15: 780–783.

Hagen T, Bartylla K, Piepgras U (1999). Correlation of regional cerebral blood flow measured by stable xenon CT and perfusion MRI. J Comput Assist Tomogr 23: 257–264.

Hakim AM, Pokrupa RP, Villanueva J et al. (1987). The effect of spontaneous reperfusion on metabolic function in early human cerebral infarcts. Ann Neurol 21: 279–289.

Hakyemez B, Erdogan C, Ercan I et al. (2005). High-grade and low-grade gliomas: differentiation by using perfusion MR imaging. Clin Radiol 60: 493–502.

Hakyemez B, Erdogan C, Bolca N et al. (2006). Evaluation of different cerebral mass lesions by perfusion-weighted MR imaging. J Magn Reson Imaging 24: 817–824.

Hamberg LM, Hunter GJ, Halpern EF et al. (1996). Quantitative high-resolution measurement of cerebrovascular physiology with slip-ring CT. AJNR Am J Neuroradiol 17: 639–650.

Han JH, Wong KS (2008). Is counterpulsation a potential therapy for ischemic stroke? Cerebrovasc Dis 26: 97–105.

Hatazawa J, Fujita H, Kanno I et al. (1995). Regional cerebral blood flow, blood volume, oxygen extraction fraction, and oxygen utilization rate in normal volunteers measured by the autoradiographic technique and the single breath inhalation method. Ann Nucl Med 9: 15–21.

Hirai T, Murakami R, Nakamura H et al. (2008). Prognostic value of perfusion MR imaging of high-grade astrocytomas: long-term follow-up study. AJNR Am J Neuroradiol 29: 1505–1510.

Hourani R, Brant LJ, Rizk T et al. (2008). Can proton MR spectroscopic and perfusion imaging differentiate between neoplastic and nonneoplastic brain lesions in adults? AJNR Am J Neuroradiol 29: 366–372.

Hu LS, Eschbacher JM, Dueck AC et al. (2012a). Correlations between perfusion MR imaging cerebral blood volume, microvessel quantification, and clinical outcome using stereotactic analysis in recurrent high-grade glioma. AJNR Am J Neuroradiol 33: 69–76.

Hu LS, Eschbacher JM, Heiserman JE et al. (2012b). Reevaluating the imaging definition of tumor progression: perfusion MRI quantifies recurrent glioblastoma tumor fraction, pseudoprogression, and radiation necrosis to predict survival. Neuro Oncol 14: 919–930.

Huang BY, Kwock L, Castillo M et al. (2010). Association of choline levels and tumor perfusion in brain metastases assessed with proton MR spectroscopy and dynamic susceptibility contrast-enhanced perfusion weighted MRI. Technol Cancer Res Treat 9: 327–337.

Huang J, Wang AM, Shetty A et al. (2011). Differentiation between intra-axial metastatic tumor progression and radiation injury following fractionated radiation therapy or stereotactic radiosurgery using MR spectroscopy, perfusion MR imaging or volume progression modeling. Magn Reson Imaging 29: 993–1001.

Hygino Da Cruz Jr LC, Rodriguez I, Domingues RC et al. (2011). Pseudoprogression and pseudoresponse: imaging challenges in the assessment of posttreatment glioma. AJNR Am J Neuroradiol 32: 1978–1985.

Jain R, Narang J, Gutierrez J et al. (2011). Correlation of immunohistologic and perfusion vascular parameters with MR contrast enhancement using image-guided biopsy specimens in gliomas. Acad Radiol 18: 955–962.

Jiang Z, Le Bas JF, Grand S et al. (2011). Prognostic value of perfusion MR imaging in patients with oligodendroglioma: a survival study. J Neuroradiol 38: 53–61.

Jorgensen HS, Sperling B, Nakayama H et al. (1994). Spontaneous reperfusion of cerebral infarcts in patients with acute stroke. Incidence, time course, and clinical outcome in the Copenhagen Stroke Study. Arch Neurol 51: 865–873.

Kikuchi K, Murase K, Miki H et al. (2002). Quantitative evaluation of mean transit times obtained with dynamic susceptibility contrast-enhanced MR imaging and with (133)Xe SPECT in occlusive cerebrovascular disease. AJR Am J Roentgenol 179: 229–235.

Kim HS, Kim JH, Kim SH et al. (2010). Posttreatment high-grade glioma: usefulness of peak height position with semi-quantitative MR perfusion histogram analysis in an entire contrast-enhanced lesion for predicting volume fraction of recurrence. Radiology 256: 906–915.

Kwong KK, Reese TG, Nelissen K et al. (2011). Early time points perfusion imaging. Neuroimage 54: 1070–1082.

Law M, Cha S, Knopp EA et al. (2002). High-grade gliomas and solitary metastases: differentiation by using perfusion and proton spectroscopic MR imaging. Radiology 222: 715–721.

Law M, Yang S, Wang H et al. (2003). Glioma grading: sensitivity, specificity, and predictive values of perfusion MR imaging and proton MR spectroscopic imaging compared with conventional MR imaging. AJNR Am J Neuroradiol 24: 1989–1998.

Law M, Hamburger M, Johnson G et al. (2004a). Differentiating surgical from non-surgical lesions using perfusion MR imaging and proton MR spectroscopic imaging. Technol Cancer Res Treat 3: 557–565.

Law M, Yang S, Babb JS et al. (2004b). Comparison of cerebral blood volume and vascular permeability from dynamic susceptibility contrast-enhanced perfusion MR imaging with glioma grade. AJNR Am J Neuroradiol 25: 746–755.

Law M, Oh S, Babb JS et al. (2006). Low-grade gliomas: dynamic susceptibility-weighted contrast-enhanced perfusion MR imaging–prediction of patient clinical response. Radiology 238: 658–667.

Law M, Young RJ, Babb JS et al. (2008). Gliomas: predicting time to progression or survival with cerebral blood volume measurements at dynamic susceptibility-weighted contrast-enhanced perfusion MR imaging. Radiology 247: 490–498.

Leenders KL, Perani D, Lammertsma AA et al. (1990). Cerebral blood flow, blood volume and oxygen utilization. Normal values and effect of age. Brain 113: 27–47.

Lehmann P, Monet P, De Marco G et al. (2010). A comparative study of perfusion measurement in brain tumours at 3 Tesla MR: arterial spin labeling versus dynamic susceptibility contrast-enhanced MRI. Eur Neurol 64: 21–26.

Lehmann P, Saliou G, De Marco G et al. (2012). Cerebral peritumoral oedema study: does a single dynamic MR sequence assessing perfusion and permeability can help to differentiate glioblastoma from metastasis? Eur J Radiol 81: 522–527.

Lin W, Celik A, Paczynski RP (1999). Regional cerebral blood volume: a comparison of the dynamic imaging and the steady state methods. J Magn Reson Imaging 9: 44–52.

Liu X, Kolar B, Tian W et al. (2011). MR perfusion-weighted imaging may help in differentiating between nonenhancing gliomas and nonneoplastic lesions in the cervicomedullary junction. J Magn Reson Imaging 34: 196–202.

Lorenz C, Benner T, Chen PJ et al. (2006a). Automated perfusion-weighted MRI using localized arterial input functions. J Magn Reson Imaging 24: 1133–1139.

Lorenz C, Benner T, Lopez CJ et al. (2006b). Effect of using local arterial input functions on cerebral blood flow estimation. J Magn Reson Imaging 24: 57–65.

Martinez-Martinez A, Martinez-Bosch J (2014). Perfusion magnetic resonance imaging for high grade astrocytomas: can cerebral blood volume, peak height, and percentage of signal intensity recovery distinguish between progression and pseudoprogression? Radiologia 56: 35–43.

Mihara F, Kuwabara Y, Tanaka A et al. (2003). Reliability of mean transit time obtained using perfusion-weighted MR imaging; comparison with positron emission tomography. Magn Reson Imaging 21: 33–39.

Murphy BD, Fox AJ, Lee DH et al. (2006). Identification of penumbra and infarct in acute ischemic stroke using computed tomography perfusion-derived blood flow and blood volume measurements. Stroke 37: 1771–1777.

Nabavi DG, Cenic A, Dool J et al. (1999). Quantitative assessment of cerebral hemodynamics using CT: stability, accuracy, and precision studies in dogs. J Comput Assist Tomogr 23: 506–515.

Narang J, Jain R, Arbab AS et al. (2011). Differentiating treatment-induced necrosis from recurrent/progressive brain tumor using nonmodel-based semiquantitative indices derived from dynamic contrast-enhanced T1-weighted MR perfusion. Neuro Oncol 13: 1037–1046.

Østergaard L, Sorensen AG, Kwong KK et al. (1996a). High resolution measurement of cerebral blood flow using intravascular tracer bolus passages. Part II: Experimental comparison and preliminary results. Magn Reson Med 36: 726–736.

Østergaard L, Weisskoff RM, Chesler DA et al. (1996b). High resolution measurement of cerebral blood flow using intravascular tracer bolus passages. Part I: Mathematical approach and statistical analysis. Magn Reson Med 36: 715–725.

Pivawer G, Law M, Zagzag D (2007). Perfusion MR imaging and proton MR spectroscopic imaging in differentiating necrotizing cerebritis from glioblastoma multiforme. Magn Reson Imaging 25: 238–243.

Poussaint TY, Rodriguez D (2006). Advanced neuroimaging of pediatric brain tumors: MR diffusion, MR perfusion, and MR spectroscopy. Neuroimaging Clin N Am 16: 169–192. ix.

Powers WJ (1991). Cerebral hemodynamics in ischemic cerebrovascular disease. Ann Neurol 29: 231–240.

Pradel C, Siauve N, Bruneteau G et al. (2003). Reduced capillary perfusion and permeability in human tumour xenografts treated with the VEGF signalling inhibitor ZD4190: an in vivo assessment using dynamic MR imaging and macromolecular contrast media. Magn Reson Imaging 21: 845–851.

Ge Healthcare (2011). CT Perfusion 4D User Guide, 2nd edn. GE Healthcare Publications, Buc, France.

Rizzo L, Crasto SG, Moruno PG et al. (2009). Role of diffusion- and perfusion-weighted MR imaging for brain tumour characterisation. Radiol Med 114: 645–659.

Rosen BR, Belliveau JW, Vevea JM et al. (1990). Perfusion imaging with NMR contrast agents. Magn Reson Med 14: 249–265.

Rubin G, Firlik AD, Levy EI et al. (1999). Xenon-enhanced computed tomography cerebral blood flow measurements in acute cerebral ischemia: review of 56 cases. J Stroke Cerebrovasc Dis 8 404–411.

Sawlani RN, Raizer J, Horowitz SW et al. (2010). Glioblastoma: a method for predicting response to antiangiogenic chemotherapy by using MR perfusion imaging – pilot study. Radiology 255: 622–628.

Schellinger PD, Shuaib A, Kohrmann M et al. (2013). Reduced mortality and severe disability rates in the SENTIS trial. AJNR Am J Neuroradiol 34: 2312–2316.

Senturk S, Oguz KK, Cila A (2009). Dynamic contrast-enhanced susceptibility-weighted perfusion imaging of intracranial tumors: a study using a 3 T MR scanner. Diagn Interv Radiol 15: 3–12.

Server A, Graff BA, Orheim TE et al. (2011a). Measurements of diagnostic examination performance and correlation analysis using microvascular leakage, cerebral blood volume, and blood flow derived from 3 T dynamic susceptibility-weighted contrast-enhanced perfusion MR imaging in glial tumor grading. Neuroradiology 53: 435–447.

Server A, Orheim TE, Graff BA et al. (2011b). Diagnostic examination performance by using microvascular leakage, cerebral blood volume, and blood flow derived from 3-T dynamic susceptibility-weighted contrast-enhanced perfusion MR imaging in the differentiation of glioblastoma multiforme and brain metastasis. Neuroradiology 53: 319–330.

Shuaib A, Bornstein NM, Diener HC et al. (2011). Partial aortic occlusion for cerebral perfusion augmentation: safety and efficacy of NeuroFlo in Acute Ischemic Stroke trial. Stroke 42: 1680–1690.

Stewart GN (1894). Researches on the circulation time in organs and on the influences which affect it, Parts I-III. J Physiol (Lond) 15: 1–89.

Sugahara T, Korogi Y, Tomiguchi S et al. (2000). Posttherapeutic intraaxial brain tumor: the value of perfusion-sensitive contrast-enhanced MR imaging for differentiating tumor recurrence from nonneoplastic contrast-enhancing tissue. AJNR Am J Neuroradiol 21: 901–909.

Suh CH, Kim HS, Choi YJ et al. (2013). Prediction of pseudoprogression in patients with glioblastomas using the initial and final area under the curves ratio derived from dynamic contrast-enhanced T1-weighted perfusion MR imaging. AJNR Am J Neuroradiol 34: 2278–2286.

Symon L (2007). The ischemic penumbra – the beginning. In: GA Donnan, JC Baron, SM Davis et al. (Eds.), The Ischemic Penumbra: Pathophysiology, Imaging and Therapy. Informa Healthcare, New York.

Thomassin-Naggara I, Balvay D, Cuenod CA et al. (2010). Dynamic contrast-enhanced MR imaging to assess physiologic variations of myometrial perfusion. Eur Radiol 20: 984–994.

Toh CH, Wei KC, Chang CN et al. (2013). Differentiation of primary central nervous system lymphomas and glioblastomas: comparisons of diagnostic performance of dynamic susceptibility contrast-enhanced perfusion MR imaging without and with contrast-leakage correction. AJNR Am J Neuroradiol 34: 1145–1149.

Valles FE, Perez-Valles CL, Regalado S et al. (2013). Combined diffusion and perfusion MR imaging as biomarkers of prognosis in immunocompetent patients with primary central nervous system lymphoma. AJNR Am J Neuroradiol 34: 35–40.

Villringer A, Rosen BR, Belliveau JW et al. (1988). Dynamic imaging with lanthanide chelates in normal brain: contrast due to magnetic susceptibility effects. Magn Reson Med 6: 164–174.

Vrabec M, Van Cauter S, Himmelreich U et al. (2011). MR perfusion and diffusion imaging in the follow-up of recurrent glioblastoma treated with dendritic cell immunotherapy: a pilot study. Neuroradiology 53: 721–731.

Weber MA, Lichy MP, Thilmann C et al. (2003). Monitoring of irradiated brain metastases using MR perfusion imaging and 1H MR spectroscopy. Radiologe 43: 388–395.

Wintermark M, Thiran JP, Maeder P et al. (2001). Simultaneous measurement of regional cerebral blood flow by perfusion CT and stable xenon CT: a validation study. AJNR Am J Neuroradiol 22: 905–914.

Wolf RL, Wang J, Wang S et al. (2005). Grading of CNS neoplasms using continuous arterial spin labeled perfusion MR imaging at 3 Tesla. J Magn Reson Imaging 22: 475–482.

Wu O, Østergaard L, Weisskoff RM et al. (2003). Tracer arrival timing-insensitive technique for estimating flow in MR perfusion-weighted imaging using singular value decomposition with a block-circulant deconvolution matrix. Magn Reson Med 50: 164–174.

Yamaguchi T, Kanno I, Uemura K et al. (1986). Reduction in regional cerebral metabolic rate of oxygen during human aging. Stroke 17: 1220–1228.

Young GS, Setayesh K (2009). Spin-echo echo-planar perfusion MR imaging in the differential diagnosis of solitary enhancing brain lesions: distinguishing solitary metastases from primary glioma. AJNR Am J Neuroradiol 30: 575–577.

Young RJ, Gupta A, Shah AD et al. (2013). MRI perfusion in determining pseudoprogression in patients with glioblastoma. Clin Imaging 37: 41–49.

Zaro-Weber O, Moeller-Hartmann W, Heiss WD et al. (2010). Maps of time to maximum and time to peak for mismatch definition in clinical stroke studies validated with positron emission tomography. Stroke 41: 2817–2821.

Handbook of Clinical Neurology, Vol. 135 (3rd series)
Neuroimaging, Part I
J.C. Masdeu and R.G. González, Editors

Chapter 7

Magnetic resonance angiography: physical principles and applications

ANDREW J.M. KIRULUTA[1,2]* AND R. GILBERTO GONZÁLEZ[1]

[1]*Department of Radiology, Massachusetts General Hospital, Boston, MA, USA*

[2]*Department of Biophysics, Harvard University, Cambridge, MA, USA*

Abstract

Magnetic resonance angiography (MRA) is the visualization of hemodynamic flow using imaging techniques that discriminate flowing spins in blood from those in stationary tissue. There are two classes of MRA methods based on whether the magnetic resonance imaging signal in flowing blood is derived from the amplitude of the moving spins, the time-of-flight methods, or is based on the phase accumulated by these flowing spins, as in phase contrast methods. Each method has particular advantages and limitations as an angiographic imaging technique, as evidenced in their application space. Here we discuss the physics of MRA for both classes of imaging techniques, including contrast-enhanced approaches and the recent rapid expansion of the techniques to fast acquisition and processing techniques using parallel imaging coils as well as their application in high-field MR systems such as 3 T and 7 T.

INTRODUCTION

Clinical applications of magnetic resonance angiography (MRA) are rapidly expanding with improvements in magnetic resonance imaging (MRI) hardware performance and the increasing concerns for repeated ionization exposure from X-ray-based computed tomographic angiography (CTA) (Brenner and Hall, 2007). There are two classes of MRA methods based on whether the MRI signal of flowing blood is derived from the amplitude of the moving spins, the time-of-flight (TOF) methods (Wehrli et al., 1985; Dixon et al., 1986; Nishimura et al., 1987), or is based on the phase accumulated by these flowing spins, as in phase contrast (PC) methods (Wedeen et al., 1985; Dumoulin and Hart, 1986). Each method has particular advantages and limitations as an angiographic imaging technique, as evidenced in their application space. Here we present the physics of MRA for both classes of imaging, including contrast-enhanced approaches and the recent rapid expansion of the techniques to fast acquisition and processing techniques as well as their application in high-field MR systems such as 3 T and 7 T.

TIME-OF-FLIGHT METHODS

TOF in MRI is based on the idea that T1 of flowing water is effectively shorter than T1 of stationary water (Suryan, 1959). The difference could be attributed to the fact that, when stationary, the spins would be saturated by the radiofrequency excitation but when flowing, fresh spins with full magnetization would replace the stationary spins, thereby increasing the signal. The concept of spin saturation is key to understanding TOF methods and we shall return to it in more detail later. Early spin-echo multislice MR images of the neck showed signal void (black pixels) in the region of blood vessels, as shown in Figure 7.1 (Axel, 1984). Understanding this phenomenon is the basis of exploiting this artifact to create TOF MRA. Consider a multislice imaging experiment with a spin-echo sequence as depicted in Figure 7.2. Blood flowing through the vessel is not

*Correspondence to: Andrew J.M. Kiruluta, Massachusetts General Hospital, 55 Fruit St, Ellison 229D, Boston MA 02114, USA. Tel: +1-617-724-6536, E-mail: kiruluta@physics.harvard.edu

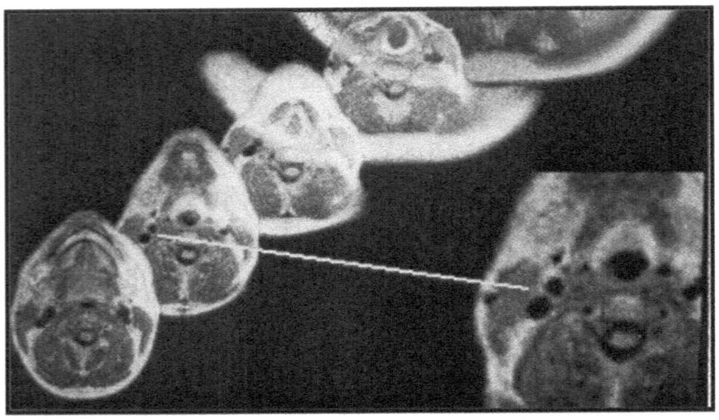

Fig. 7.1. Early multislice spin-echo axial images of the neck, showing areas of signal voids where vessels are located. Flowing spins were not refocused by the spin echo as they had moved out of the slice region by the time of application of the 180° pulse.

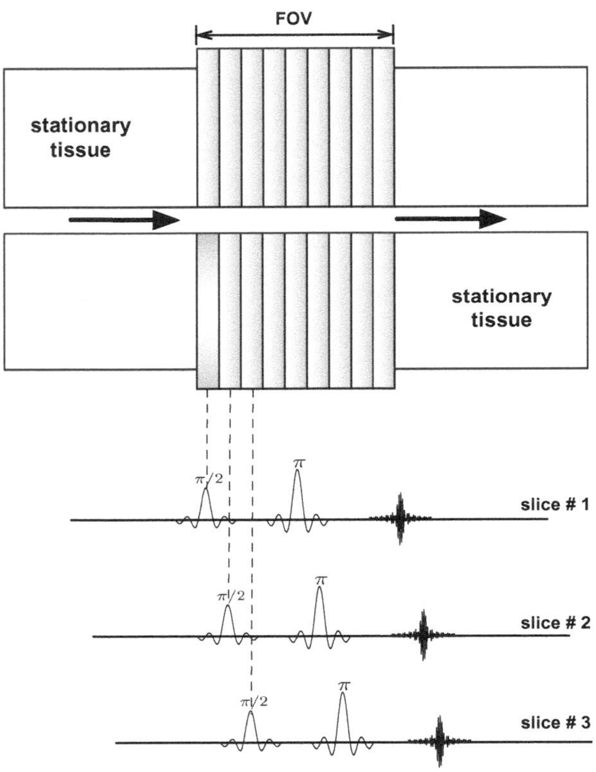

Fig. 7.2. Multislice spin-echo imaging through a volume in which blood is flowing as shown. As shown, flowing spins are not refocused by the 180° pulse for a given slice, since they have moved on to the successive slice by the time of the refocusing pulse. FOV, field of view.

refocused since, by the time the 180° pulse is applied, the segment of blood for a given slice has moved on to a subsequent slice segment. As a result this lack of refocusing of the blood in the vessel results in a much lower signal intensity for regions in the blood vessel, resulting in a black blood image. TOF MRA reverses this contrast such that blood appears bright while stationary tissue is dark. To accomplish this, we will exploit the artifactual signal changes caused by flowing blood to depict vessel lumen since the T1 of flowing spins is effectively shorter than T1 of stationary spins. As well, we will prepare the spins so as to suppress signal from stationary tissues or venous flow using the concept of spin saturation (Dumoulin et al., 1989).

Consider a train of pulses in a gradient echo sequence, as shown in Figure 7.3. We assume here that the repetition time (TR) of the sequence is much shorter than T1 of stationary tissue (TR << T1). Initially, the magnetization is allowed to reach steady state such that the bulk magnetization of the sample is M_0, as shown in Figure 7.3. The first α pulse tips a fraction of this magnetization into the transverse plane, where it starts to dephase in the interval τ, while the longitudinal magnetization component grows along the z-axis. Since TR << T1, the next 90° excitation tips a much smaller magnetization from the longitudinal to the transverse axis. A subsequent excitation at the next interval will result in a much smaller magnetization tipped into the transverse plane. By repeating this train of excitation in the same interval, at some point there will not be any magnetization along the longitudinal axis to tip into the transverse plane, as the sample has not had enough time to recover its magnetization. The sample is then said to be saturated.

Let us combine the idea of spin saturation with the fact that moving spins have a shorter T1 than stationary spins to construct images based on the concept of TOF. Consider a single-slice excitation with a blood vessel passing perpendicular to the slice orientation, as shown in Figure 7.4. The stationary spins in the selected slice are saturated by a gradient echo sequence with TR << T1, while fresh spins washed in by blood are unsaturated and hence yield an MR signal when their magnetization is tipped into the transverse plane, which results in signal enhancement for all vessel orthogonal to this slice orientation. An example of such a TOF imaging experiment is show in Figure 7.4, with an axial slice through the head showing enhancement of the carotid tree with relatively weak signal coming from the stationary surrounding tissue.

To track the vessels through a 3D volume, consider the arterial and venous vasculature shown in Figure 7.5. Presaturation can be set up as shown to visualize either the arterial or venous flow at the expense of the other counterflow and stationary tissue. For example, to visualize just the arterial flow, a saturation band is set up in the upper region, as demarcated in the rectangular region in Figure 7.5, to saturate both the outflowing venous blood as well as the stationary tissue in the indicated slice region. Similarly, we can obtain images of venous enhancement

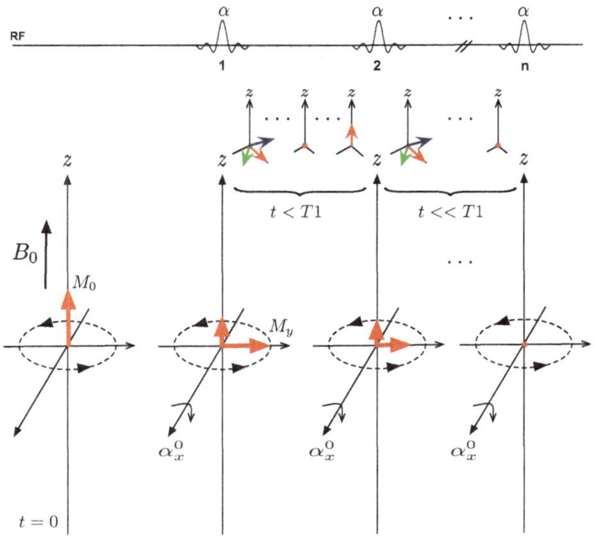

Fig. 7.3. Concept of spin saturation. Initially, the sample is in steady state with its full magnetization M_0 along the longitudinal z-axis. The sample is then excited with a small flip angle pulse 1 applied on the x-axis, which rotates a fraction of the magnetization into the transverse plane (on to the y-axis), where it starts to precess and the various frequency components disperse, as shown in the inset between points 1 and 2. Applying another excitation pulse 2 at a time less than the T_1 of the sample tips, a smaller fraction of the magnetization component since the sample is not fully recovered to its initial steady-state condition and hence both the transverse and longitudinal components are significantly smaller than in the previous excitation phase. If the excitation is repeated at intervals much shorter than the T_1 of the sample, then the sample is said to be saturated, since no steady-state magnetization is allowed to build up along the z-axis, as shown on the nth excitation step, and hence no transverse magnetization component is available either. RF, radiofrequency.

by saturating signal from both the arterial vessels as well as static tissue by selecting a saturation region, as shown by the bottom rectangle in Figure 7.5.

The imaging volume can be collected as a multislice (2D), single-slab (3D), or multislab acquisition, as shown in Figure 7.6.

Once the volume of data is collected, whether as a 2D stack of slices or slabs, it is arranged as shown in Figure 7.7. The slices or slabs are stacked to make a 3D volume and the projections around this volume generated by picking out pixels with the maximum intensity when viewed from a given direction. The next projection is then generated in another direction rotated by 1° from the previous direction by again selecting pixels with the maximum intensity when the volume is viewed from that direction. The process is repeated 360° around the volume. If we imagine that the vessel that transverse this volume is in a shape of a Y as shown, then the corresponding projections from this scheme are as shown

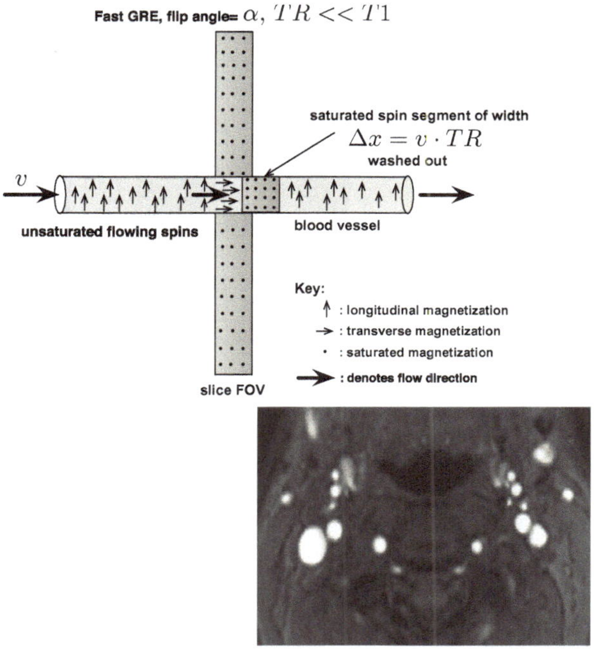

Fig. 7.4. A slice is selected and saturated by using a very short repetition time gradient echo sequence such that repetition time (TR) $<< T_1$. All the stationary spins are saturated while the inflow of fresh spins through the blood vessel is unaffected by the repetitive excitation since on average they experience a single excitation that tips them in the transverse plane. As a result, blood signal appears much brighter than the surrounding stationary tissue. GRE, gradient recalled echo; FOV, field of view.

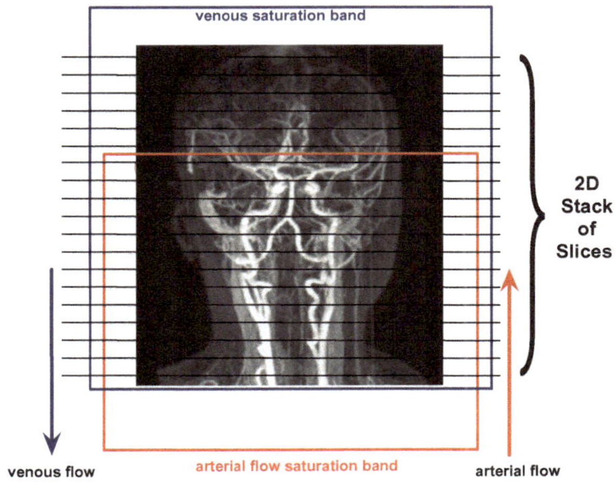

Fig. 7.5. An example of selective flow suppression. Either venous or arterial enhancement can be imaged by an appropriate choice of saturation region. For example, for arterial enhancement without venous flow contamination, a saturation region is set up as shown to saturate all blood returning to the heart, so that all unsaturated spins are from the arterial inflow into the imaging volume. Thus both the venous and stationary tissue are saturated and only the arterial vasculature is visible. Similarly, we can image venous enhancement by selecting a saturation band, as shown in the figure.

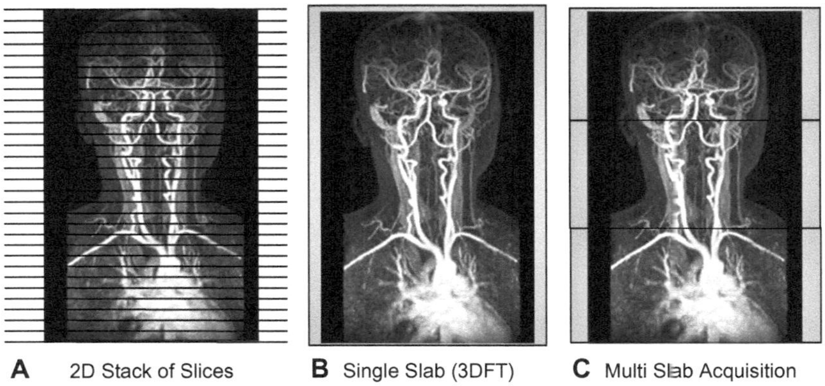

Fig. 7.6. Various approaches for breaking up the imaging volume, as in multislice 2D acquisition, single-slab 3D (3DFT), or multi-slab acquisition.

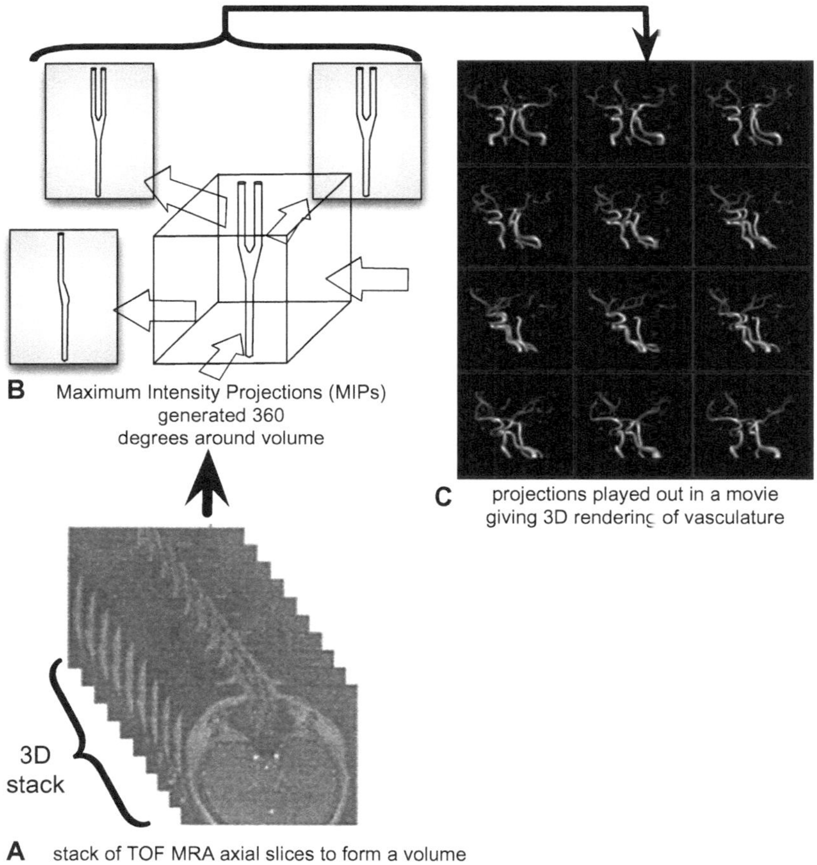

Fig. 7.7. Principle of maximum-intensity projection (MIP), consisting of stacking up slices to make a volume and then generating projections of that volume when viewed from all around the volume. The projections are generated by preserving only the pixels with the maximum intensity when viewed from a given direction. The highest-intensity pixels should correspond to flowing spins from a time-of-flight (TOF) magnetic resonance angiography (MRA) acquisition. The projections are acquired at 1° increments 360° around the sample, and the resulting projections played out in a movie (**C**), giving the impression of a 3D rendering of the vasculature.

since the spins in the flowing blood will correspond to the maximum signal for each projection. By displaying the derived projections in a repetitive movie, it gives the viewer the impression of a 3D rendering of the vessels in the volume. This is the method of maximum-intensity projection, as illustrated in Figure 7.7B and C for a carotid MRA study. In this case, the imaging volume is segmented into 2D slices. Alternatively, the volume could also be segmented as a 3D volume using a 3D gradient recalled echo sequence.

The advantage of 2D TOF MRA is that it achieves good stationary to blood flow contrast, high sensitivity to flow with minimal saturation effects of blood vessels, in addition to shorter scan times afforded by multi-slice acquisition strategies. However, the small volume selected by each slice does present a number of challenges. 2D TOF MRA tends to have poor signal-to-noise ratio (SNR) and poor in-plane flow sensitivity, as blood in vessels lying in plane is saturated just like stationary tissue and there is high sensitivity to short T1 species in stationary tissue.

To overcome some of the shortcomings of 2D MRA, the region is imaged as a 3D volume with phase encoding along the slice direction. 3D TOF MRA results in higher resolution with slice thicknesses limited only by the number of phase-encoding steps, higher SNR than 2D methods and, due to the use of lower slab selection gradient amplitudes, 3D methods result in fewer phase artifacts than 2D methods (Fig. 7.8).

The challenge with 3D TOF MRA is the ease with which blood signal is saturated in vessels with slow flow, particularly if the imaging volume is large. In addition, this method still suffers from the problems of relatively poor background suppression and of short T1 tissue being mistaken for blood vessels.

BACKGROUND TISSUE SUPPRESSION

A major objective of MRA is to obtain high contrast between the vasculature and the background tissue. For example, in 3D TOF, vascular contrast is limited by the necessity to use small flip angle excitation pulses in order to minimize the saturation of spin flowing into the slab. However, the use of a small flip angle limits the degree of background tissue suppression. Edelman et al. (1992) have proposed the use of magnetization transfer (MT) effects to reduce the signal from stationary brain tissue. MT refers to the exchange of magnetization between two pools of protons: those in bulk water, found in tissue cellular structures, and those associated with large macromolecular structures such as proteins. Protons in bulk water are freely mobile and as such have relatively long T2 relaxation time (>10 ms) and are thus easily imaged with MRI. On the other hand, protons bound to macromolecules have restricted motion, very short T2 relaxation time (<200 μs), and are therefore inaccessible to image in an MRI experiment. However, these two proton pools are interconnected via relaxation pathways such as chemical exchange and dipolar interaction, so that the relaxation in one pool influences the relaxation in the other pool.

In the frequency domain shown in Figure 7.9, the bound protons with short T2 relaxation times are characterized by a very broad frequency distribution, whilst the free protons resonate over a much narrower frequency range. The MT effect can be observed by selectively irradiating the magnetization spins of the bound proton pool by applying a high-power, narrow-bandwidth radiofrequency pulse 1–2 kHz away from the free-water resonance. This pulse saturates the bound pool by virtue of its broad frequency distribution but has little effect on the free-water resonance. This saturation is then transferred to the coupled free-water protons, thereby decreasing the signal intensity in the stationary tissue of the image. Since different tissues have different macromolecular compositions, MT provides a novel contrast mechanism on its own merit (Balaban and Ceckler, 1992). With application to MRA, blood has low concentration of macromolecules and therefore demonstrates only a small MT effect. This results in MT effectively

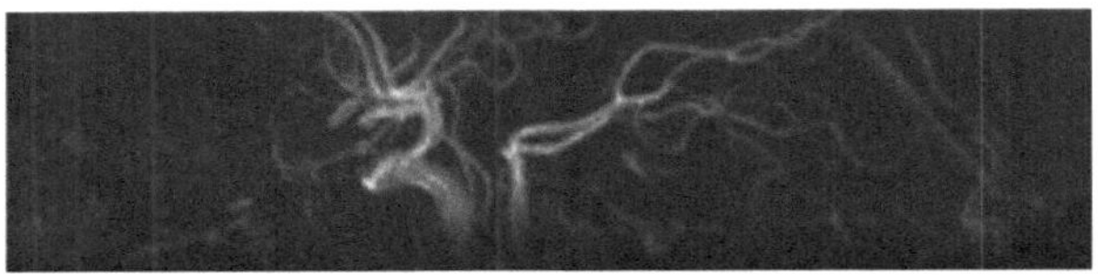

Fig. 7.8. 3D time-of-flight (TOF) magnetic resonance angiography (MRA) depiction of circle of Willis with repetition time (TR)/echo time (TE) = 40/4.7 ms, 64 partitions, 48-mm slabs, 0.75 mm per partition, 25° flip angle, 256 × 256, 18 cm field of view.

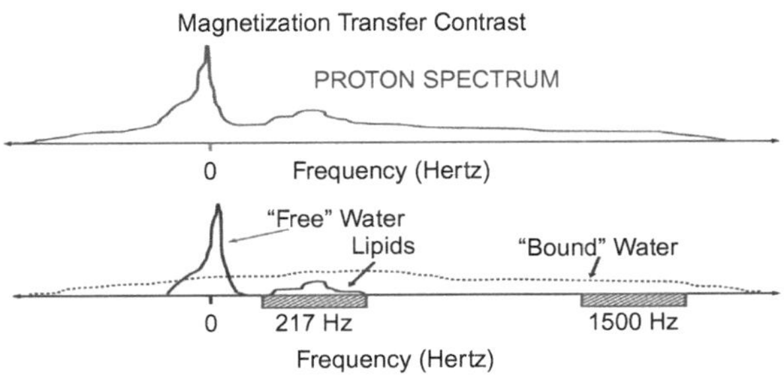

Fig. 7.9. Broad spectrum from the spectral extent of proton resonance ranging from free water to those bound in macromolecular pools. A magnetization transfer (MT) pulse can be crafted to excite only the bound proton pools in the macromolecules. MT effect then transfers the magnetization to the free proton pools via chemical exchange or dipolar interactions.

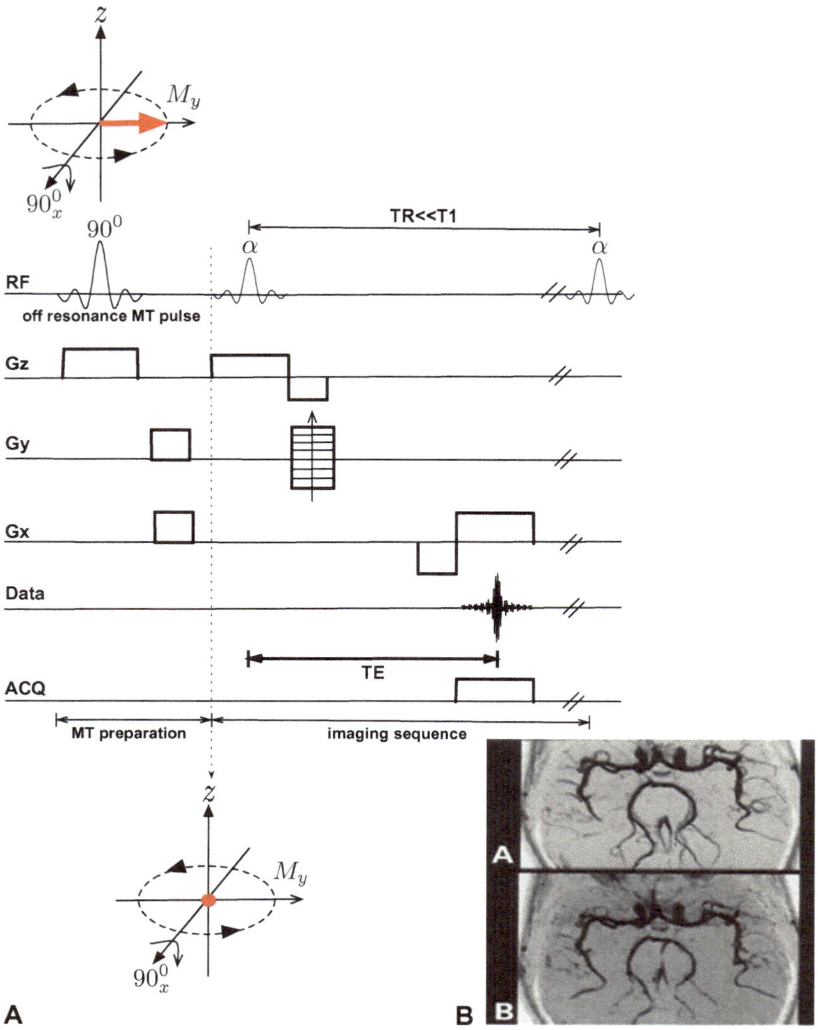

A B

Fig. 7.10. Magnetization transfer (MT) preparation at the beginning of a small flip angle gradient recalled echo (GRE) sequence for a magnetic resonance angiography acquisition. The initial MT 90° pulse is tuned off resonance to excite bound water and through dipolar and chemical exchange, the magnetization is transferred to the free proton in the surface layer around the macromolecules. The magnetization is then spoiled and immediately a fast GRE sequence with repetition time (TR) < < T1 is used to image inflow of fresh unsaturated spins from the blood. Image A was acquired with a magnetization transfer contrast pulse, while image B was acquired without. The improved stationary suppression in A is clearly discernible with improved visualization of the posterior arteries and branches of the middle cerebral arteries. RF, radiofrequency; ACQ, acquisition.

reducing the background signal intensity and improving the conspicuity of small vessels, such as in Figure 7.10.

The choice of off-resonance MT frequency represents a trade-off between adequate background suppression through MT effects and the desire not to saturate the free water of the blood pool. The MT is often applied as a prepulse structure at the beginning of the MRA sequence, as shown in Figure 7.10B. The signal of the macromolecules and the resulting coupling to the free water are destroyed immediately by the dephasing large gradients on the other two encoding axes. Immediately after that, a small flip angle GRE sequence to acquire the MRA is played out.

CONTRAST-ENHANCED TOF MRA

The TOF methods discussed thus far did not involve contrast injection but relied solely on the intrinsic T1 of blood and of tissue. These are the so-called noncontrast-enhanced MRA techniques. Contrast-enhanced (CE) MRA uses T1 shortening agents such as gadolinium to further increase the contrast between blood and tissue in a TOF MRA study. Gadolinium-based contrast agent is administered by hand or via a power injector to deliver a dose of 0.03 mmol/kg of tissue in 25–30 seconds. The gadolinium then increases the T1-weighted signal of the vasculature by markedly decreasing the T1 relaxation time of the blood. CE MRA has revolutionalized the imaging of vessels with MR as a first line of investigation of the vasculature tree.

There are effectively three strategies in CE MRA based on the stages of imaging as contrast washes through the vasculature. One approach is a conventional "flow arrest" or single phase in which the imaging is very fast and freezes the flow of contrast in vessels in a very fast acquisition, as shown in Figure 7.11. This is the most widely used CE MRA technique and demonstrates vascular anatomy with high spatial resolution ($1.2 \times 0.6 \times 0.8$ mm^3 in Fig. 7.11), but contrast timing is required and fast acquisitions (TR/TE 3.5/1.2 ms, where TE is echo time) are typically collected in two to three breath holds.

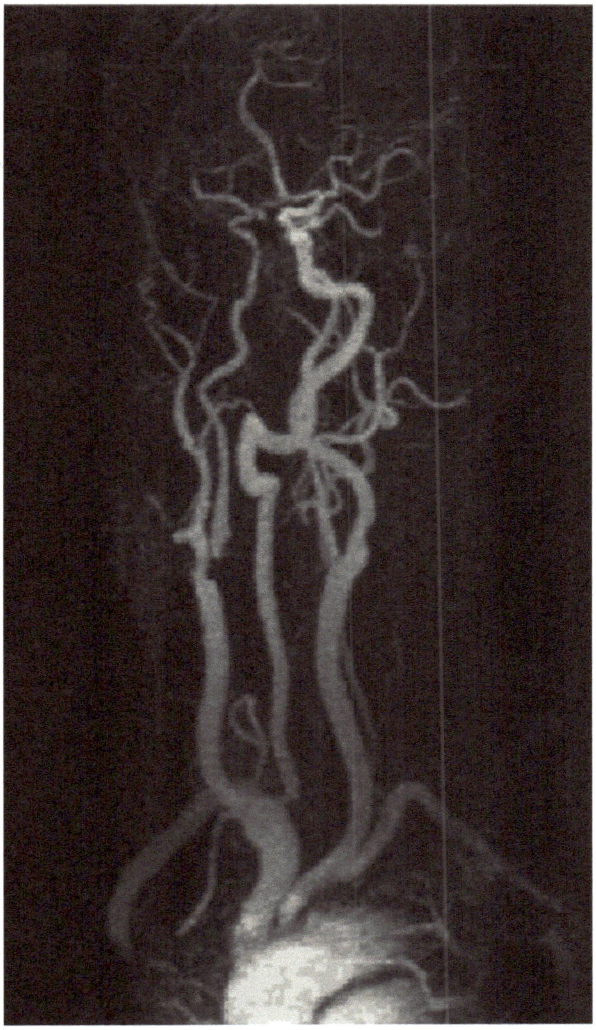

Fig. 7.11. Conventional "flow arrest" contrast-enhanced magnetic resonance angiogram image of the vascular tree feeding the head. 20 cc of gadolinium-based contrast agent is administered at the rate of 2 cc per second. Data collection is triggered by monitoring the signal in a plane that intersects the aortic arch. As soon as the signal peaks indicating the arrival of contrast, data collection begins. In this example, a fast low flip angle gradient recalled echo sequence is used with repetition time (TR)/echo time (TE) = 3.5/1.2 ms. Flip angle = 25°, 512 readout resolution with 80 partitions of thickness 0.8 mm for an overall resolution of $1.2 \times 0.6 \times 0.8$ mm^3.

Time-resolved CE MRA

An alternative approach is to image all phases of contrast washing into the arterial vasculature, signal arterial peak and finally arrival into the venous vasculature and peak signal to wash out. This approach requires visualization of all stages of vessel enhancements, which requires very fast imaging capabilities. Because contrast is collected over all cycles, no bolus timing is required. It is especially useful for high-flow lesions such as shunts and dissections. When contrast is injected, a period of delay time specific to the patient must be allowed before it shows up in the arterial vasculature. Very often this period is determined by monitoring the signal strength in a plane that intersects the aortic arch next to the heart. When the signal intensity peaks, it indicates that contrast is now being pushed through the aorta and hence arterial monitoring can begin. This is the so-called fluoro-triggering approach. As shown in Figure 7.12, for absolutely no venous signal contamination, the acquisition should be limited to the arterial phase only. Unfortunately, this can be as short as 5 seconds. Compounding the challenge is the resultant restriction in the number of phase encodes that can be collected in such a short time window, thus limiting the spatial resolution. The solution to avoiding venous contamination is to refer back to the concepts of *k*-space discussed in Chapter 2.

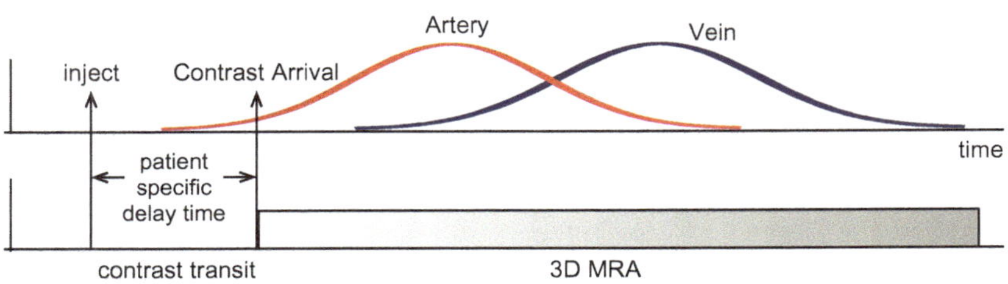

Fig. 7.12. Contrast injected in the arm of a patient will be delayed prior to its peaking in the arterial vasculature. A 3D contrast-enhanced magnetic resonance angiogram can then be collected over the volume of interest.

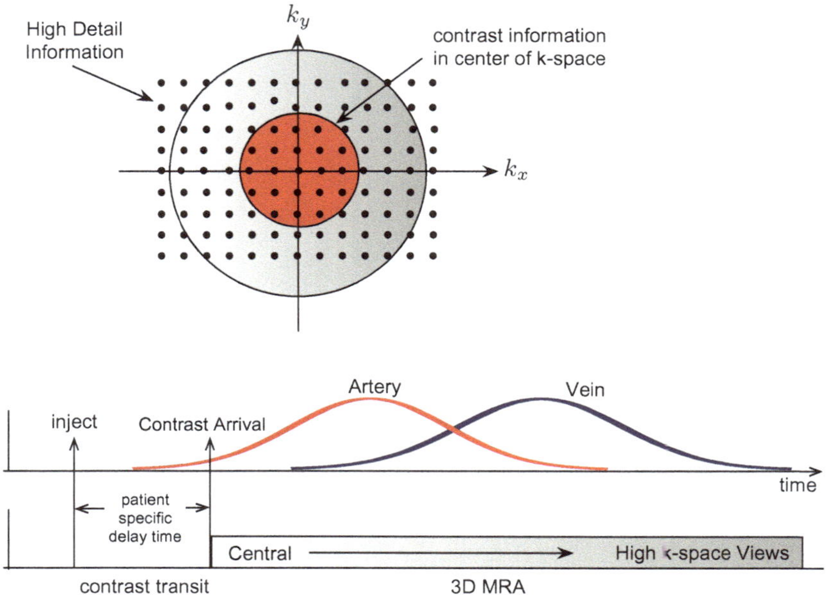

Fig. 7.13. The center of *k*-space contains contrast information while the outer regions determine the overall resolution of the image. Illustration of the concept of centric view ordering where the center of *k*-space, which contains contrast information, is collected during the earlier uncontaminated phase of arterial filling while the high-frequency components of *k*-space are collected much later. MRA, magnetic resonance angiography.

The center of *k*-space is where the contrast information is located. The reason for collecting data further out in *k*-space is driven by the need for high-resolution information, as shown in Figure 7.13. Hence, the concept of "centric ordering" is based on collecting the center of *k*-space during the time when contrast is only in the arterial phase and then collecting the high *k*-space frequencies later when data are potentially contaminated with the venous enhancement, but since these frequencies do not contribute to contrast, it does not matter. This centric ordering data collection approach, when combined with multichannel acquisition and parallel imaging techniques, covered in Chapter 2, provides the necessary means of generating dynamic MRA for all stages of contrast filling and draining of blood vessels.

Moving-table CE MRA methods

Newer approaches follow contrast by moving the imaging table to the field of view (FOV) where contrast is located. These are the moving-table methods. They use the same parallel imaging acquisition techniques to acquire *k*-space very quickly but move the FOV of the imaging volume to follow contrast following fluoro triggering. The tracking of contrast can be in multisegmented acquisition, as shown in Figure 7.14A, or in the future, in a single dynamic acquisition as the table is moved, as shown in Figure 7.14B.

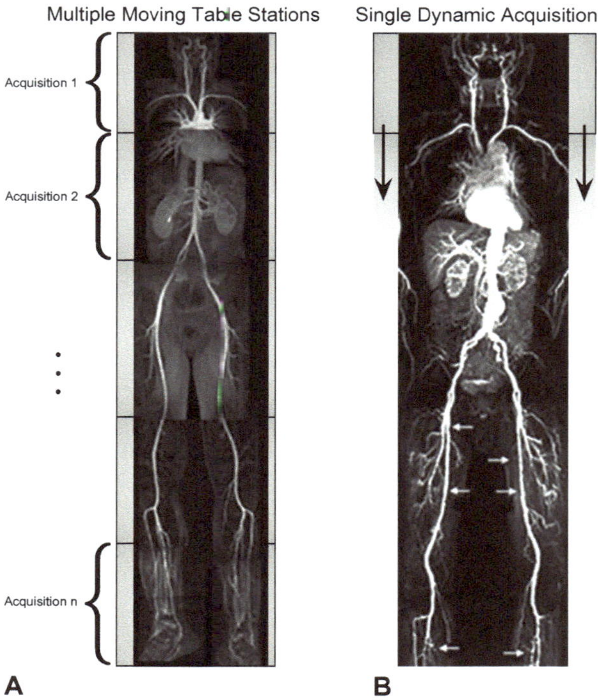

Fig. 7.14. Moving-table methods of tracking contrast filling and draining phases in the vasculature using either a segmented approach (**A**) or in a proposed single continuous sweep of the table in a single dynamic acquisition, as shown in (**B**).

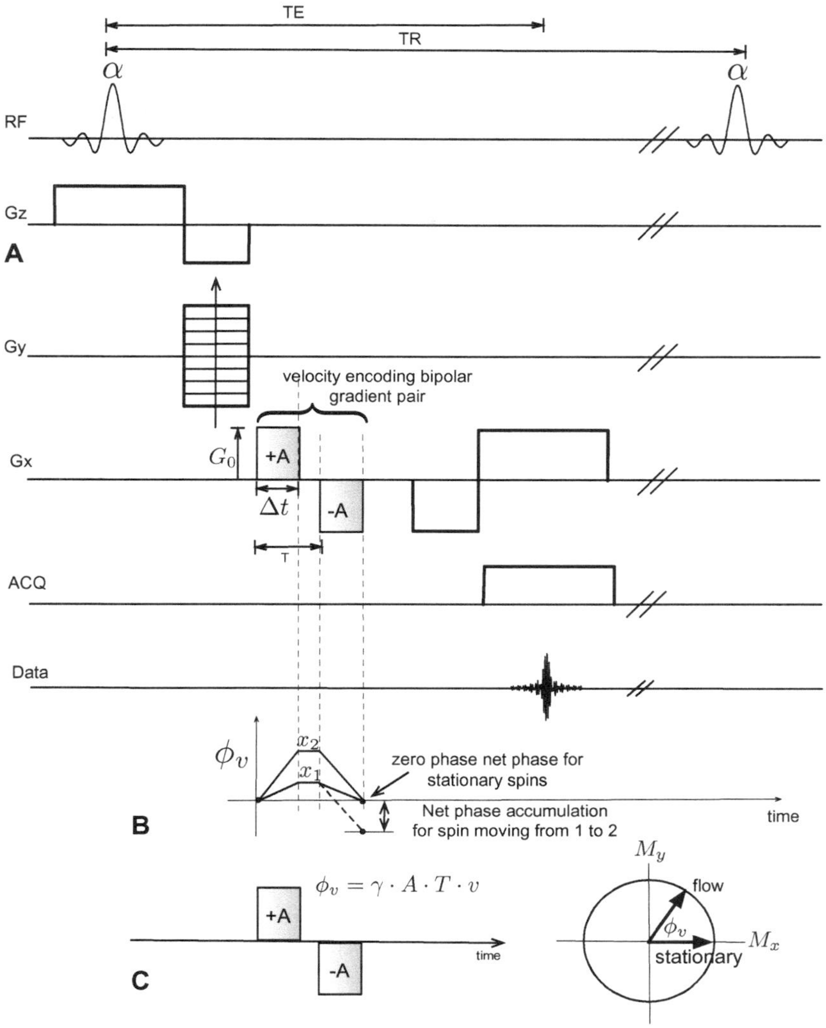

Fig. 7.15. (**A**) Velocity-encoding gradient echo sequence applied along the x-axis. The total area is zero, resulting in zero-phase accumulation by static spins, while spins moving along the x direction experience unequal fractions of the positive and negative lobes proportional to their velocity, resulting in a phase accrual proportional to their velocity, as shown in (**B**). Stationary spins at two different positions x_1 and x_2 acquire no net phase from the bipolar gradient but spins that move from one position to the other during this gradient accumulate a net phase, shown in (**B**). TE, echo time; TR, repetition time; RF, radiofrequency; ACQ, acquisition.

PHASE CONTRAST MRA

The previous methods were all based on the TOF concept, in which the MR signal intensity is related directly to flow. In PC MR, the velocity of flow is encoded in the phase of the MR signal, providing a mechanism of not only visualizing flow but also the ability to quantify it. Consider a simple flow-encoding gradient echo sequence (Fig. 7.15), consisting of a bipolar gradient pair along the x-axis, as shown in Figure 7.15. The total area of this bipolar pair is zero, so that stationary spins will experience first the positive lobe and then the negative lobe, which effectively cancels the accumulated phase. However, spins moving in the direction of the applied gradient (x in this case) will experience unequal fractions of the positive lobe and negative lobes, resulting in a residue accumulated phase that is carried by those spins. The resulting phase is proportional to the velocity of the moving spins and can be calculated as illustrated in Figure 7.15C, where A is the area of velocity-encoding lobe while τ is the temporal spacing between the two lobes and γ is the gyromagnetic constant for protons, all of which are known, and hence the velocity of the spins can be directly calculated from this relationship, as shown.

Two images are required to complete the calculation. First, the velocity-sensitive sequence in Figure 7.15 is used to generate velocity-encoded phase images for a specific direction, as discussed. Then another sequence with velocity-compensated gradients on all axes is used to generate phase images in the same FOV as in the first sequence. This last set of phase maps serves as the reference for flow-compensated images.

The two sets of data are then subtracted from each other to generate a relative phase map for which each intensity is proportional to the velocity of the spins in that voxel. Using the phase/velocity relationship given in Figure 7.15, the velocity for each phase in a given voxel can be determined. Now, we know that phase cycles over a range $-\pi \leq \phi \leq \pi$ and thus to avoid aliasing or wraparound, we need to map the maximum expected velocity to $\pm\pi$. This maximum velocity, denoted as V_{enc}, is an *a priori* determination, so that if it is too large relative to the maximum velocity of flow measured, we lose velocity resolution since we map the available range of phases to rather larger than required velocities. Similarly, if we underestimate V_{enc} to be lower than the maximum velocity of flow, then we will get wraparound of all velocity values larger than V_{enc} to lower phase values, resulting in errors in our measurements (Fig. 7.16).

An example of using PC MRA is shown in Figure 7.17, where it is shown that, in addition to a flow phase image, this approach allows the quantification of flow, unlike TOF MRA, which provides only qualitative information on flow.

Like TOF MRA, PC MRA volumes can be segmented into 2D multislice or 3D acquisitions. Unlike TOF MRA, PC MRA does not rely on T1 saturation effects but only on the phase accumulated by moving spins and hence provides superior background suppression of stationary spins. It is extremely sensitive to slow flow but motion is imaged in one direction at a time, corresponding to the gradient axis of the velocity-encoding bipolar pair that is applied. As well, two separate acquisitions are required to characterize motion: one is a motion-compensated acquisition while the other has the bipolar gradient pair for motion sensitization. In case of a 3D acquisition, four images are required, including one flow-compensated image plus three velocity-encoded phase maps corresponding to the three orthogonal directions *x*, *y*, and *z*. 3D PC MRAs are thus very time consuming. In summary, PC MRA requires more time to acquire images but can result in high resolution and fewer flow-related artifacts, and is the only method capable of providing a quantitative measurement of flow.

HIGH-FIELD TOF MRA

Contrast-enhanced TOF MRA is used routinely to clinically evaluate a large number of cerebrovascular diseases, such as aneurysm and arteriovenous malformations, but has difficulty at more subtle microvascular diseases at conventional field strength MRI due to SNR limits on resolution. The pathophysiologies leading up to many neurovascular diseases are thought to include hypoperfusion, vascular insult, and/or chaotic vessel growth (Fisher et al., 2005; Betts et al., 2006). Thus MRA methods depicting finer vascular detail may be useful in assessing these pathologies. Currently, the

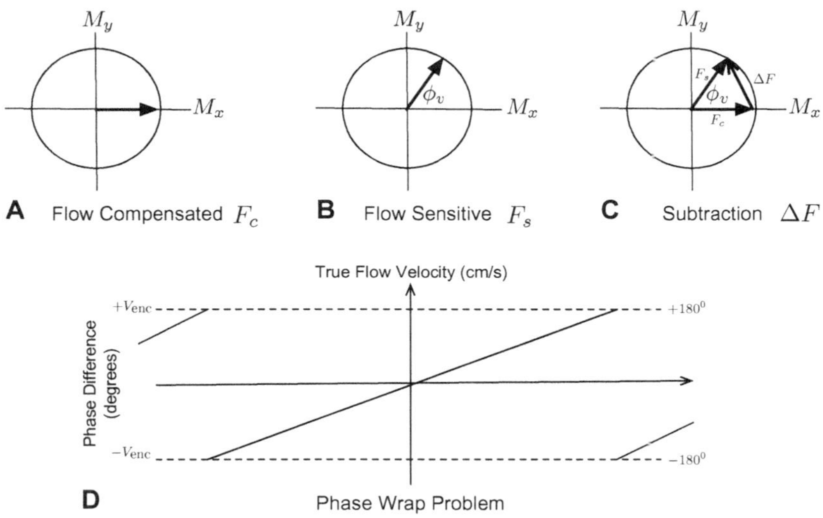

Fig. 7.16. (**A**) Flow-compensated images are collected in one sequence while flow-sensitized images are collected in another and the corresponding phase maps from these two sequences are subtracted to generate the relative phase due to flow in a given direction. Calculation of the respective velocity for a given phase value is determined by mapping the expected maximum velocity to $\pm\pi$.

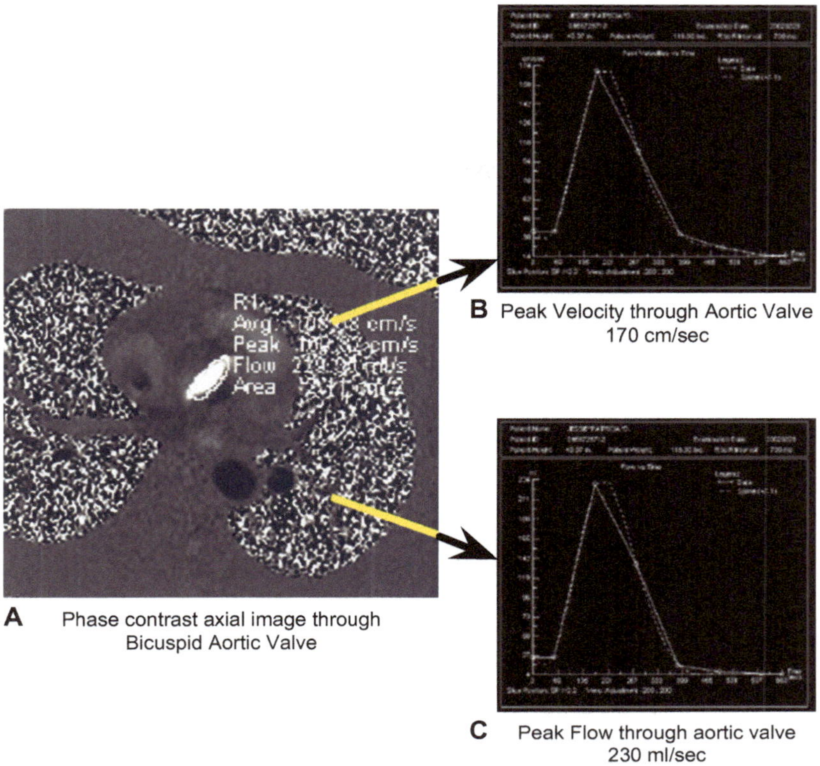

Fig. 7.17. (**A**) Use of phase contrast magnetic resonance angiography to quantify blood flow characteristics in evaluating bicuspid aortic valve stenosis. Both the peak velocity (**B**) and the peak flow (**C**) are easily determined from the phase measurements.

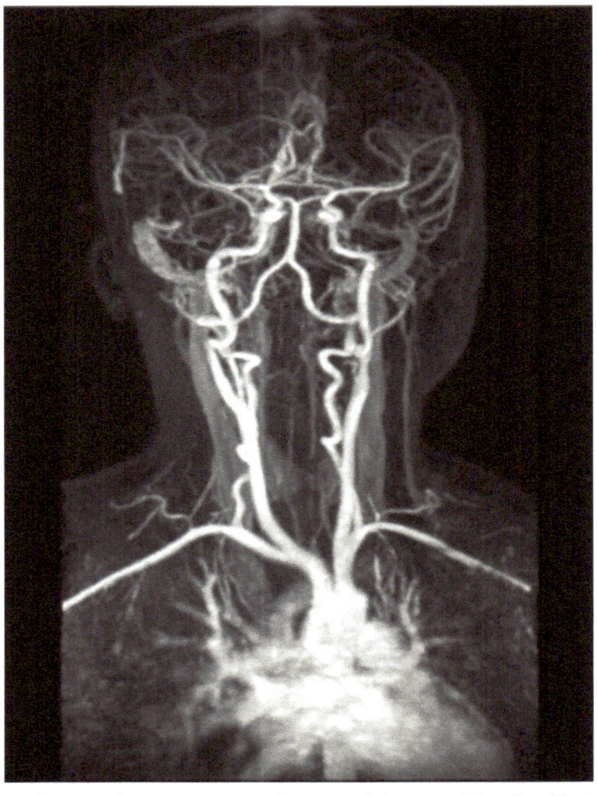

Fig. 7.18. 3 T 3D contrast-enhanced magnetic resonance angiogram of the carotid and calf arteries showing detailed microvasculature in the head, 110 slices of thickness 1.4 mm with resolution of 320×320, repetition time/echo time = 5.3/1.4 ms.

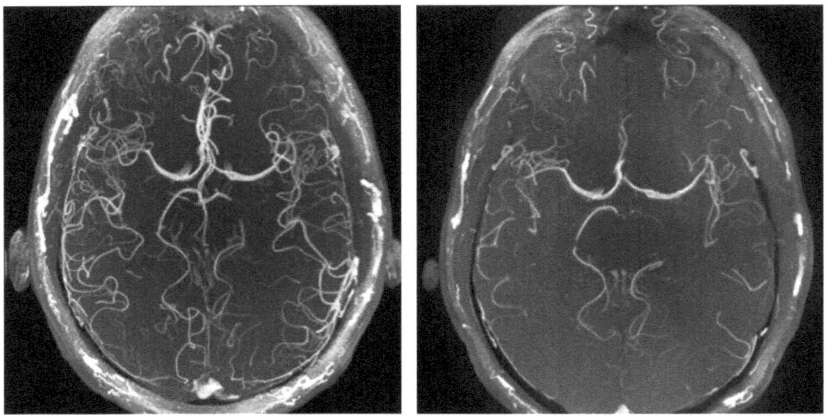

Fig. 7.19. 7 T 3D time-of-flight magnetic resonance angiography maximum-intensity projection images of the cerebral arteries showing detailed microvasculature in the head. (**A**) 96 slices of thickness 0.2 mm with resolution of 870 × 960, repetition time (TR)/echo time (TE) = 20/4 ms. (**B**) 178 slices of thickness 0.3 mm with resolution of 580 × 640, TR/TE = 20/4.9 ms. Note the fine detail of the anterior perforating substance, including the lenticulostriate arteries arising from the proximal middle cerebral arteries. (Courtesy of Jason Johnson, MD, and Jonathan Polimeni, MD, MGH.)

standard technique to visualize the small cerebral arteries is to use contrast-enhanced digital subtraction angiography, an invasive procedure with a risk of serious, although rare, side effects and considerable radiation dose to the patient (Kaufmann et al., 2007). Another routine clinical tool is computed tomography angiography of the cerebral arteries, providing superior spatial resolution compared to MRA but with high doses of iodinated contrast agents (Johnson et al., 2013). Recent developments in ultrahigh-field MRI systems (such as 7 T systems) enable assessment of the cerebral arteries with a spatial resolution previously not achievable with standard 1.5 T or even 3 T MRI scanners (Morze et al., 2007).

For example, at 3 T, the T1 of tissue is longer than at 1.5 T and hence the use of CE MRA further reduces the T1 of blood to the extent that the difference in contrast between blood and stationary tissue is much greater. The result is much better background tissue suppression and conspicuity of small vessels, as demonstrated in Figure 7.18. This phenomenon is amplified at 7 T imaging, as shown in Figure 7.19.

CONCLUSIONS

TOF MRA is the easiest technique to implement and is much more robust relative to PC MRA. Combined with gadolinium-based contrast agents, it has become an extremely valuable tool in the depiction of vascular structures. The combination of 3T scanners with parallel imaging has revolutionized both 2D and 3D CE MRA. By contrast, PC MRA requires more time to acquire more images and, although it can result in relatively high-resolution images, the technique is more prone to flow-related artifacts. However, it is the only MRA technique that results in quantitative measurement of flow for hemodynamic analysis in lieu of invasive methods.

References

Axel L (1984). Blood flow effects in magnetic resonace. AJR 143: 1157–1166.

Balaban RS, Ceckler TI (1992). Magnetisation transfer contrast in magnetic resonance imaging. Magn Reson Q 8: 116–137.

Betts J, Jaros E, Perry RH et al. (2006). Molecular neuropathology of MELAS: level of heteroplasmy in individual neurones and evidence of extensive vascular involvement. Neuropathol Appl Neurobiol 32: 359–373.

Brenner DJ, Hall EJ (2007). Computed tomography – an increasing source of radiation exposure. N Engl J Med 357: 2277–2284.

Dixon WT, Du LN, Faul DD et al. (1986). Projection angiograms of blood labeled by adiabatic fast passage. Magn Res Med 3: 454.

Dumoulin CL, Hart HR (1986). Magnetic resonance angiography. Radiology 161: 717.

Dumoulin CL, Cline HE, Souza SP et al. (1989). Three-dimensional time-of-flight magnetic resonance angiography using spin saturation. Magn Res Med 11: 35–46.

Edelman RR, Ahn SS, Chien D et al. (1992). Improved time-of-flight MR angiography of the brain with magnetization transfer contrast. Radiology 184: 395–399.

Fisher I, Gagner JP, Law M et al. (2005). Angiogenesis in gliomas: biology and molecular pathophysiology. Brain Pathol 15: 297–310.

Johnson JM, Reed MS, Burbank HN et al. (2013). Quality of extracranial carotid evaluation with 256-slice computed tomography. Am J Neuroradiol 34: 1626–1631.

Kaufmann TJ, Huston J, Mandrekar JN et al. (2007). Complications of diagnostic cerebral angiography:

evaluation of 19 826 consecutive patients. Radiology 243: 812–819.

Morze von C, Xu D, Purcell DD et al. (2007). Intracranial time-of-flight MR angiography at 7 T with comparison to 3 T. J Magn Reson Imaging 26: 900–904.

Nishimura DG, Macovski A, Pauly J et al. (1987). MR angiography by selective inversion recovery. Magn Res Med 4: 193.

Suryan G (1959). Nuclear resonance in flowing liquids. Proc Indian Acad Sci 33: 1652–1653.

Wedeen VJ, Meuli RA, Edelman RR et al. (1985). Projective imaging of pulsatile flow with magnetic resonance. Science 230: 949.

Wehrli FW, Shimakawa A, MacFall JR et al. (1985). MR imaging of venous and arterial flow by a selective saturation-recovery spin echo (SSRSE) method. J Comput Assist Tomo 9: 537.

Handbook of Clinical Neurology, Vol. 135 (3rd series)
Neuroimaging, Part I
J.C. Masdeu and R.G. González, Editors

Chapter 8

Diagnostic angiography of the cerebrospinal vasculature

JAMES D. RABINOV*, THABELE M. LESLIE-MAZWI, AND JOSHUA A. HIRSCH
Neurointerventional Service, Massachusetts General Hospital, Boston, MA, USA

Abstract

Diagnostic catheter angiography remains the gold standard for evaluation of vascular lesions of the brain, head and neck, and spine. It is often combined with cross-sectional and functional imaging to provide a complete anatomic and physiologic workup of patients. Such data are combined with clinical information to help make treatment decisions. This chapter describes the specific techniques for arterial access and catheter navigation of the cerebrospinal vasculature. Discussion of patient positioning, injection rates, and basic anatomy of arterial and venous systems is included. Finally, important safety issues related to contrast allergy, renal failure, and complications are considered.

INTRODUCTION

The first report of X-ray angiography of blood vessels was from Vienna in 1896 (Haschek and Lindenthal, 1896). E. Haschek and O.T. Lindenthal obtained X-rays of blood vessels by injecting a mixture of petroleum, quicklime, and mercuric sulfide into the hand of a cadaver. Antonio Egas Moniz, a Portuguese neurologist, is credited with the practical development of cerebral angiography. With cadaver and animal studies using strontium bromide and sodium iodide, he identified the branching pattern of intracranial arteries. In 1927 he performed the first angiogram in a living human patient with his pupil, Almeida Lima (Krayenbühl, 1977). Fortuitously, the first venographic image was made in 1931, when a delay in exposure timing after arterial injection demonstrated the venous anatomy. In the 1930s direct carotid puncture replaced surgical cut-down (Moniz, 1934), and organic iodinated contrast media was developed. The first direct puncture of the vertebral artery was done in 1956 (Sheldon, 1956).

Transfemoral angiography was developed as a safer mode of arterial access, and the neurosurgeon Gazi Yasargil used this technique extensively in the 1950s and 1960s (Dagi, 2001). The development of nonionic iso-osmolar iodonated contrast media and the advent of digital subtraction angiography in the 1980s have made diagnostic cerebral angiography the gold standard for vascular evaluation of the brain and spine. In recent years rotational angiography and flat panel detector technology have improved spatial and temporal resolution while limiting radiation dose.

INDICATIONS FOR CEREBRAL ANGIOGRAPHY

Current advances in computed tomography (CT) and magnetic resonance imaging (MRI) have produced techniques for evaluating cerebral vasculature. These noninvasive methods form the initial diagnosis and triage phase for patients. For example, CT and MRI serve as primary imaging modalities in the evaluation of acute stroke patients to identify large-vessel occlusion, estimate stroke tissue injury, and look for hemorrhage (Gonzalez et al., 2013). CT angiography is also effective as a diagnostic and triage method for both intracerebral hemorrhage (Delgado Almandoz et al., 2010) and subarachnoid hemorrhage (Hoh et al., 2004), but there are limitations related to inherent temporal and spatial factors of these techniques.

Diagnostic cerebral angiography has become a focused tool for delineating vascular disease processes identified or raised as a differential diagnosis on CT or MRI studies. Catheter-based angiography provides

*Correspondence to: James D. Rabinov, M.D., Interventional Neuroradiology/Gray 241, Massachusetts General Hospital, 55 Fruit Street, Boston MA 02114, USA. Tel: +1-617-726-1767, Fax: +1-617-726-3089, E-mail: jrabinov@mgh.harvard.edu

a very high spatial resolution (200–300 μm) with excellent temporal resolution (1–6 frames per second), making it invaluable in assessing primary neurovascular disease. Diagnostic cerebral angiography has the highest sensitivity and specificity for vascular pathology. Indications include evaluation of both intracranial hemorrhagic and ischemic disease. It provides the best characterization of intracranial aneurysms, arteriovenous malformations (AVMs), dural arteriovenous fistulas, acute ischemic stroke, cerebral vasculopathies, and cerebral vasospasm.

Diagnostic angiography can be followed by primary endovascular therapy for many of the vascular diseases listed above. It is also an important surveillance method after coil embolization of aneurysm, radiosurgical treatment of brain AVM, or medical therapy for vasculitis. Such angiographic information can guide further treatment plans for patients. Even in patients for whom treatment is not done, it can be a useful method for determining progression or resolution of disease.

There is also a role for angiography in combined treatment modality or to assess immediate postsurgical results. It may be performed in the operating suite using mobile or embedded C-arm technology. Intraoperative angiography is most often used during surgery for clipping of intracranial aneurysms or resection of AVMs. It allows immediate assessment of the surgical results, facilitating operative modifications that may be necessary before closure of the craniotomy. During aneurysm surgery, up to 34% of cases undergo clip adjustment as a result of intraoperative angiography findings (Origitano et al., 1999). Radiolucent surgical equipment (head holder, operating table) is helpful, but not essential.

PREPROCEDURE EVALUATION OF PATIENTS

Neurologic assessment, evaluation of laboratory results, electrocardiogram, and chest radiograph are parts of a baseline medical evaluation before angiography. It is important to review noninvasive imaging to understand native vascular anatomy and focus the cerebral angiographic procedure to answer the specific clinical question. Informed consent is an important standard of care in all situations. Explanation should be given to patients of standard risks of approximately 2–3%, including stroke, bleeding, blood vessel injury, infection, contrast or medication allergy, renal failure, radiation change, and approval of conscious sedation. For pediatric patients or those not competent for consent, a parent, family member, or legal guardian should be involved.

ANESTHESIA AND CONSCIOUS SEDATION

Many diagnostic cerebral angiograms can be performed with local anesthesia at the puncture site using 8–10 mL of 1% lidocaine. Moderate sedation, typically using midazolam and fentanyl, is useful to promote the patient's comfort and therefore reduce patient motion (Baris et al., 2001). Excessive sedation, however, should be avoided because it can make detection of intraprocedural neurologic change more challenging. Moreover, in a small minority of patients, there can be paradoxic agitation (Thurston et al., 1996; Mancuso et al., 2004). Thus, reversal agents such as naloxone and flumazenil should be readily available when using conscious sedation. Patients who are unlikely to tolerate moderate sedation (usually because of comorbidities) are monitored by an anesthesiologist, and these patients can be managed with deep sedation and laryngeal mask airway or tracheal intubation at their discretion.

ANGIOGRAPHIC TECHNIQUE

Vascular access

The first step in catheter-based angiography of the cerebral vessels is safe arterial access. This is most typically accomplished through a transfemoral route. The common femoral artery is punctured adjacent to the femoral head (Fig. 8.1). The location of the puncture site is important because it allows effective compression of the arteriotomy site after the procedure. A puncture location too low (in the superficial femoral artery) risks inadequate postprocedural compression because of the absence of a firm structure to compress against, and a puncture too high (above the inguinal ligament) risks retroperitoneal hematoma formation. Transfemoral angiography is usually performed with a sheath but can be accomplished without one. By convention, the right groin is the site of access unless extenuating circumstances (e.g., previous right iliofemoral surgery, right iliofemoral atherosclerotic occlusion) are present, in which case the left groin is used.

The artery may be located by manual palpation for the femoral pulse and the underlying femoral head or, if location by palpation is difficult, with ultrasound guidance. Arterial access is done using a variation of the Seldinger technique (Seldinger, 2013) with single-wall arterial puncture. It is typically accomplished using a micropuncture kit, and then an 0.038 J tip guidewire is used to facilitate insertion of a sheath.

If femoral access is not an option because of the patient's anatomy or comorbid disease, alternative routes of access may be used. One approach is to catheterize the radial artery (Levy et al., 2002). This should be

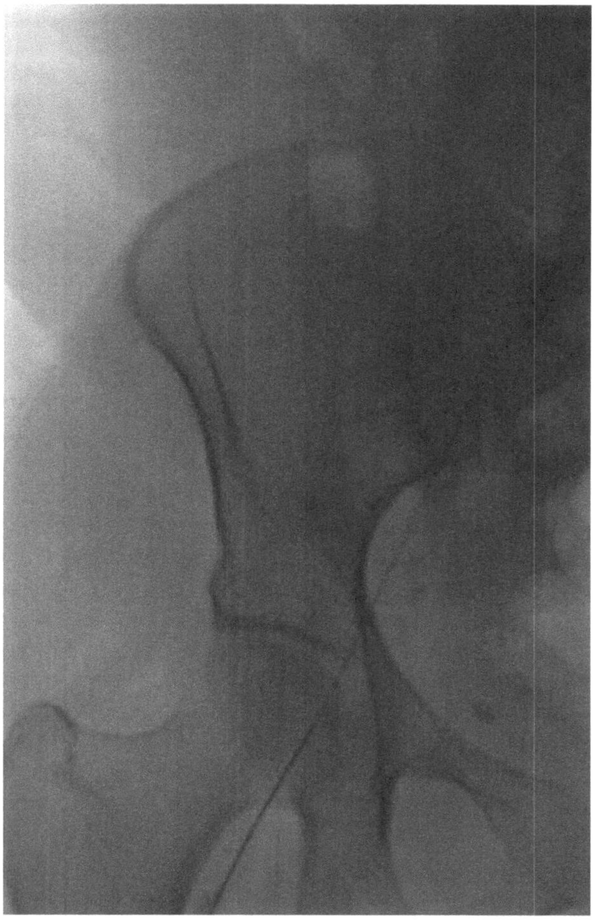

Fig. 8.1. Ideal positioning for arterial access through the common femoral arteriotomy. The needle and microwire mark the typical course of the superficial femoral artery, common femoral artery, and external iliac artery. Note that the arteriotomy site is positioned to allow compression of the artery against the underlying medial femoral head once the sheath is removed.

preceded by an Allen test to ensure adequate collateral circulation to the hand from the ulnar artery. Data suggest poor collateral circulation in the hand is sometimes present in patients, and if it is noted with the Allen test, it is a reason to proceed with caution (Benit et al., 1996). The technique of access resembles the transfemoral approach, with placement of a 4 or 5 French (Fr) sheath. A spasmolytic medication (e.g., calcium-channel blocker) infused through the radial sheath is often required to prevent reactive spasm and possible thrombosis of the radial artery.

A second alternative is a brachial artery approach (Uchino, 1988; Hildick-Smith et al., 1998), but because this artery is the sole vascular supply to the distal upper extremity, the consequence of access complications must be considered. The advantages of the radial and brachial approaches include avoiding the risk of retroperitoneal hemorrhage and the need for bed rest associated with femoral artery puncture. In addition, an upper-extremity approach may be useful for access to subclavian artery branches when vessel tortuosity or atherosclerosis prohibits a femoral approach. When an upper-extremity approach is necessary, a brachial artery access provides a better opportunity for compression after the procedure compared to the axillary artery.

Sheath and catheter principles

The presence of a sheath allows rapid catheter exchange and decreases the risk of intraprocedural bleeding at the puncture site by minimizing trauma to the arteriotomy (Moran et al., 2001). Typically, a short sheath (10–13 cm) is used, though in the presence of significant iliofemoral tortuosity or atherosclerosis, sheath lengths up to 25 cm may be useful. Sheath diameters are measured where 1 Fr = 0.33 mm. The range of sheath sizes is from 4 to 9 F for cerebral angiography, and the typical sheath size for diagnostic angiography is 5 Fr. It is important to note that the size refers to the inner diameter of the sheath and therefore determines what size catheter or device can be placed through the sheath. The outer diameter is approximately 1.5–2 Fr larger than the listed size and reflects the diameter of the actual arteriotomy.

Diagnostic catheters are inserted through the sheath. A wide range of catheters are available, with a variety of distal tip shapes to accommodate variations in vascular anatomy. Less distal catheter curvature is typically required in younger patients because of their more linear vasculature. In patients with markedly tortuous vessels, a reverse-curve catheter is required to access vessels arising from the aortic arch.

Diagnostic catheters are typically advanced over a hydrophilic guidewire. The guidewire allows nontraumatic navigation of the catheter by keeping the catheter tip away from the wall of the vessel and therefore preventing dissection. A sufficient length of wire should protrude from the distal tip of the catheter to provide support for catheter advancement and to maximize the flexibility of the wire. If the distal wire protrudes only a short distance from the catheter tip, the exposed wire segment becomes exceedingly stiff and risks injury to the vessel. While catheters are measured in Fr, wire measurements are in thousandths of an inch (for example, a 0.038 wire is 0.038 inches in diameter).

Manual compression of the femoral artery is commonly done at the close of a procedure, but patients need to lie flat for 5–6 hours. Closure devices may be considered for early mobilization of patients following angiography. There is a variety of devices which have evolved over the last decade with improved safety profiles

(Applegate et al., 2003; Fischer et al., 2004; Nikolsky et al., 2004; Fields et al., 2010).

Vessel selection

A cerebral angiogram should always be planned before the procedure. In general, it is easiest to begin with the right common carotid artery, then the left common carotid followed by the left vertebral artery (in left vertebral artery-dominant patients) to constitute a three-vessel cerebral arteriogram. The intradural right vertebral artery can often be visualized through the injection of the left vertebral artery, with the reverse being true in right vertebral artery-dominant patients. If the patient's tolerance or cooperation is a concern, it is helpful to begin with the vessel of interest, because the procedure might need to be terminated early. All catheter navigation should be accomplished under direct fluoroscopic visualization. Discussion of individual vessel selection follows.

Right common carotid artery

An angled-tip hydrophilic wire is advanced through the angled-tip diagnostic catheter that has been positioned in the descending thoracic aorta. The wire is advanced gently over the aortic arch, ensuring the tip of the wire is pointed around the curve of the arch to avoid disrupting potential atherosclerotic plaque at the great vessel origins. The tip of the wire is positioned in the ascending aorta proximal to the expected origin of the brachiocephalic artery. The diagnostic catheter is advanced over the stationary hydrophilic wire, again ensuring that the tip of the catheter is angled to follow the curvature of the aortic arch. Once the catheter nears the wire tip, the wire is brought back into the catheter. The catheter is gently pulled back while the tip is rotated clockwise to point peripherally in order to engage the brachiocephalic origin.

Once the diagnostic catheter is well seated in the vessel origin, the hydrophilic wire is advanced gently out of the catheter, with the tip oriented anteromedially to engage the right common carotid origin (the subclavian artery arises posterolaterally). The hydrophilic wire is advanced into the distal right common carotid artery, proximal to the carotid bifurcation (usually at the C4–5 disc level). It is helpful to look for calcified plaque at the carotid bifurcation to prevent the wire from crossing the bifurcation. The diagnostic catheter is then advanced over the wire. If there is tortuosity, one can obtain a roadmap image to facilitate arterial navigation.

The wire should be removed slowly to make sure that a vacuum pressure does not create bubbles and the catheter does not change in position. One allows a small amount of back bleeding, watching for bubbles or thrombus, and then the catheter is flushed with heparinized saline (Markus et al., 1993). A gentle hand puff of contrast should be used to confirm good catheter position and antegrade flow before injecting contrast for angiography.

Left common carotid artery

From the brachiocephalic origin, the catheter tip is pulled back under direct fluoroscopic visualization until the catheter engages the left common carotid origin. Make sure to orient the catheter tip superiorly as it approaches the aortic arch. The hydrophilic wire can then be advanced into the common carotid artery proximal to the expected location of the carotid bifurcation and the diagnostic catheter can be advanced over the stationary wire.

If the catheter immediately engages the left subclavian artery, the left common carotid and brachiocephalic arteries might have a common origin (i.e., bovine configuration). In this scenario, gentle puffs of contrast as the catheter is drawn down the brachiocephalic artery can identify the origin and course of the left common carotid artery, and roadmap angiography can facilitate selective catheterization.

In older patients with a tortuous origin of a bovine left common carotid artery or those with a type III aortic arch, a reverse-angled catheter such as the Simmons II catheter can be extremely helpful.

Right and left vertebral artery

In general, the dominant vertebral artery should be catheterized to assess the posterior circulation. By using an appropriate injection rate, adequate reflux into the contralateral vertebral artery can be achieved to assess the intradural segment and the origin of the posterior inferior cerebellar artery. During angiography, the diagnostic catheter is advanced over the hydrophilic wire into the proximal subclavian artery. Gentle puffs of contrast identify the vertebral origin, and roadmap angiography is obtained. The hydrophilic wire is gently advanced under roadmap guidance into the distal cervical vertebral artery, taking care to orient the tip laterally when possible to avoid inadvertently engaging and injuring potential spinal arterial origins. The tip should be advanced into the distal cervical segment just proximal to the lateral turn at C2. This allows satisfactory purchase to facilitate smooth delivery of the catheter into the vertebral artery. The tip of the catheter should also be oriented laterally to avoid inadvertently engaging potential spinal arterial origins.

The wire should be removed slowly to prevent vacuum formation and support catheter stability. One allows a small amount of backflow of blood before clearing with heparinized saline. A gentle hand puff of contrast should be used to confirm good catheter position and antegrade flow. Intracranial outflow should also be assessed to avoid full-volume injections into vertebral arteries that terminate in the posterior inferior cerebellar arteries or that have hypoplastic intradural segments.

If there is significant atherosclerotic narrowing at the vertebral arterial origin, or if significant vertebral artery tortuosity exists, subclavian angiography should be performed instead of vertebral artery selection. Good intracranial opacification can be achieved from a catheter position in the subclavian artery using an arm blood pressure cuff inflated to a pressure above systolic arterial pressure. This impedes distal flow and increases reflux into the vertebral circulation. To accomplish this, the catheter should be positioned just distal to the apex of the subclavian artery, with the tip oriented inferiorly to avoid catheter kickback into subclavian branches.

Catheter position

The aim of good catheter tip position is to minimize wall shear stress and thus the risk of iatrogenic dissection. The catheter tip's position is ideally assessed on biplane angiography with a gentle puff of contrast. Gently rotate the catheter tip with gentle puffs to correct position. Aim to place the catheter tip in a position that is parallel to the lumen. With the catheter in good position, one can see it move with the cardiac cycle.

The common carotid artery is large enough to accommodate minor deviations in the catheter tip, and iatrogenic common carotid dissection is uncommon. Direction of the catheter tip posteromedially can facilitate preferential contrast opacification of the internal carotid circulation.

The internal and external carotid arteries are more vulnerable to catheter-induced vasospasm and iatrogenic dissection than the common carotid artery. Positioning of the catheter in a straight segment of artery with the tip oriented along the line of blood flow helps to minimize trauma to the vessel.

In the vertebral arteries, the catheter tip should be positioned laterally to avoid inadvertent injection into spinal arteries that, if present, arise from the medial wall. In tortuous vertebral arteries in which only the origin can be engaged, a hand injection or power injection with a gradual 1-second rise produces better posterior circulation opacification than a subclavian angiogram with an inflated blood pressure cuff.

CEREBRAL ANGIOGRAPHIC IMAGING

Cerebral angiography is best accomplished with biplane imaging equipment, in contrast to the monoplane traditionally used in peripheral angiography. Digital subtraction angiography is used, and image contrast and brightness should be adjusted to semitransparency of the vessels for optimal viewing. Images should be inspected after each acquisition to guide whether further views are necessary.

Interpretation should focus on vascular course and caliber, presence of vessel occlusion and collateral supply, contrast transit delay (indicating hemodynamically significant stenosis), aneurysm, and early venous opacification (arteriovenous shunting). The parenchymal phase should be assessed for defects that could signal a distal branch occlusion. Normally, early venous structures begin to opacify at 4–5 seconds after injection of contrast material into the carotid artery, and the complete cerebral venous system is opacified in 7–8 seconds. Delays or accelerations of these times suggest pathology that needs to be identified.

Five typical angiographic views are used (Fig. 8.2):

1. Townes view: cranial–caudal angulation aligns the petrous ridges with the superior orbital rim. This view is used for assessing the posterior circulation, effectively looking down upon it.
2. Caldwell view: caudal–cranial angulation aligns the petrous ridges with the inferior orbital rim to improve evaluation of the carotid siphon. The supraclinoid internal carotid artery is foreshortened in this view.
3. Posteroanterior view: petrous ridges are placed in the lower one-third of the orbits. This view is employed for assessing the anterior circulation, and it is the standard initial view.
4. Waters view: caudal–cranial angulation at 35–45° from the skull base may be used for both anterior and posterior circulations, depending on the region of interest.
5. Lateral view: a direct lateral view is the goal, with the external acoustic meatus aligned on both sides and the floors of the left and right anterior cranial fossae overlapping. The regional focus is different depending on whether the anterior circulation or the posterior circulation is being imaged.

In addition to these views, a number of obliquities are used depending on the patient and the vessel of interest. The biplane is usually positioned orthogonally to characterize the vessel segment of interest.

Contrast agents

A variety of different contrast agents are available for use in catheter-based angiography. Currently available iodinated contrast media can be divided into four classes with regard to their chemical structure: ionic monomers,

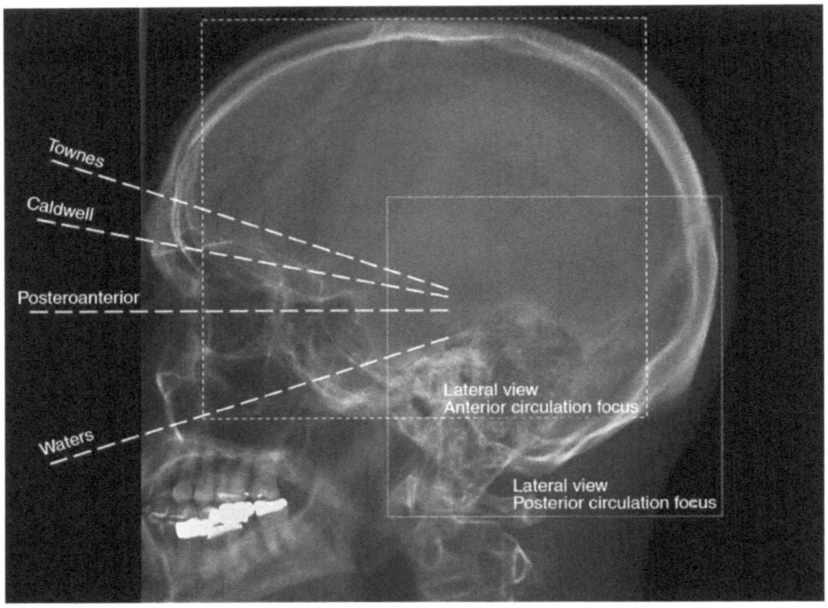

Fig. 8.2. Schematic image to demonstrate typical angiographic views. The four dashed lines represent the plane of imaging for the typical labeled views described in the text (note that the path of the imaging beam is from posterior to anterior). The fifth view, a lateral view, demonstrates variable focus if the anterior or posterior circulation is being evaluated, as illustrated by the boxes superimposed on the image. From Chandra et al. (2014).

ionic dimers, nonionic monomers, and nonionic dimers. The most important properties of these various agents are their viscosity, osmolality, solubility, hydrophilicity, and electric charge. The low-osmolar agents are less concentrated than conventional agents (600–850 mOsmol/kg versus 1500–1800 mOsmol/kg) but still are more concentrated than plasma. The iso-osmolar agents represent the more recent additions to the market. Low- and iso-osmolality contrast media are more comfortable for the patient and potentially cause less hemodynamic disruption and renal compromise than the conventional agents (Barrett et al., 1992a, b; Barrett and Carlisle, 1993; Katholi et al., 1993; Rosovsky et al., 1996). However, these newer contrast media are significantly more expensive, which limits their widespread adoption.

Radiocontrast media can lead to acute kidney injury that begins soon after administration and is usually reversible. The nephrotoxic properties of these agents vary, and nonionic contrast agents are associated with a relatively decreased incidence of renal injury. The primary benefit of nonionic contrast agents in preventing renal dysfunction is seen in high-risk patients (e.g., serum creatinine $\geq$1.5 mg/dL or a glomerular filtration rate <60 mL/min per 1.73 m^2), particularly if the patient has diabetes (though the risk may still be as high as 25%). Therefore, these agents should be used instead of ionic high-osmolal agents in patients at risk. Additionally, contrast for hand injections can be diluted with saline to a 50:50 ratio to minimize its concentration.

Optimal therapy to prevent contrast-induced acute kidney failure is best managed with intravenous (IV) sodium bicarbonate infusion, started 1 hour before and continued for 6 hours after the procedure (Merten et al., 2004; Ozcan et al., 2007). It may also include oral *N*-acetylcysteine (Mucomyst), usually dosed at 600–1200 mg twice daily for four dosages (two dosages before and two after the procedure) and may be preferable in patients with congestive heart failure. Patients with normal kidney function are at little risk, and few precautions are necessary other than avoiding volume depletion. In patients with near-normal kidney function, contrast doses up to 700 mL at iodine concentrations up to 300 mg/mL can be tolerated. For diagnostic cases that are anticipated to require many vessel injections (e.g., cerebrospinal angiogram) the total volume of contrast used should be monitored throughout the procedure to prevent excessive contrast administration.

Patients on oral antihyperglycemic medications such as metformin are at risk of lactic acidosis and resulting renal injury. It is recommended that a patient refrain from such medications for 24 hours pre- and 48 hours postprocedure (Wiholm and Myrhed, 1993; Lalau and Race, 2001).

Patients who have a confirmed or suspected allergic reaction to previous contrast exposure may still undergo cerebral angiography safely (Delaney et al., 2006). However, they need to receive preprocedural medications. A typical protocol involves prednisone 50 mg by mouth

(PO) every 8 hours for three dosages, ending 1 hour before the procedure, and diphenhydramine 50 mg PO with ranitidine 150 mg PO 1 hour before the procedure, which helps to reduce the incidence of allergic reactions through mast cell stabilization and blockade of histamine receptors. In emergency patients where premedication is not possible, hydrocortisone 200 mg IV stat and repeated every 4 hours during the procedure is recommended. A thorough discussion of this specific risk should be initiated with the patient or the patient's health care proxy before the procedure and informed consent should be obtained.

Catheter injection rates

An appropriate injection rate (Table 8.1) opacifies only the circulation of interest without excessive wall shear stress from the contrast jet or catheter tip kickback, both of which can result in an iatrogenic dissection. Higher rates and/or volumes of contrast may be required in larger than average vessels to delineate the angioarchitecture in arteriovenous shunts. One may intentionally inject more than standard if the goal is to assess collateral circulation around the circle of Willis for treatment considerations of a therapeutic vessel occlusion. Similarly, lower injection rates should be used in the setting of occluded distal vessels or a ruptured aneurysm. Typical filming frame rates are 3 frames per second for the arterial phase and 1 frame per second in the venous phase. Higher frame rates (6–10 frames per second) may be required to clearly assess high flow shunts. Overall, 10–12 seconds of imaging allows sufficient assessment of the arterial, parenchymal, and venous phases of the vasculature.

Table 8.1

Standard injection rates for cerebral and spinal angiography

Vessel	Power injection rates
Aortic arch	20 mL/s × 25 mL total
Common carotid artery, cervical	3–4 mL/s × 6 mL total
Common carotid artery, cranial	7–10 mL/s × 10–12 mL total
Internal carotid artery, cranial	4–6 mL/s × 6–8 mL total
External carotid artery, cranial	2–3 mL/s × 6–8 mL total
Subclavian artery	6–7 mL/s × 12–14 mL total
Vertebral artery	3–5 mL/s × 8–10 mL total
Spinal segmental artery	1–2 mL/s × 3–6 mL total
Internal iliac artery	3–4 mL/s × 6–8 mL total

CERVICAL AND CRANIAL ANGIOGRAPHIC ANATOMY

The images in Figures 8.3–8.6 provide a basic map of cervical and intracranial angiographic anatomy.

SPINAL ANGIOGRAPHY

Indications

Spinal angiography is a highly detailed evaluation of the vascular supply and venous outflow of the spinal cord, vertebrae, and surrounding soft tissue. It can be considered for evaluation of patients with suspected primary vascular lesions, including dural arteriovenous fistulas, spinal cord AVMs, juvenile AVMs, perimedullary AV fistulas, and epidural AV fistulas (Spetzler et al., 2002). It is also commonly done to evaluate patients with spinal vertebral masses. Orthopedists and neurosurgeons considering patients with spinal cord compression may request identification of native spinal artery supply for surgical approach. For example, in cases of cervical chordoma which involve a vertebral artery, one must evaluate vertebral artery dominance and collateral flow to the brain as well as spinal cord supply. It can also be helpful as the initial phase of preoperative embolization in patients with vascular tumors such as renal cell or thyroid metastases. Intradural vascular tumors such as hemangioblastomas may be assessed and managed in a similar way but with the awareness that spinal arteries are often involved.

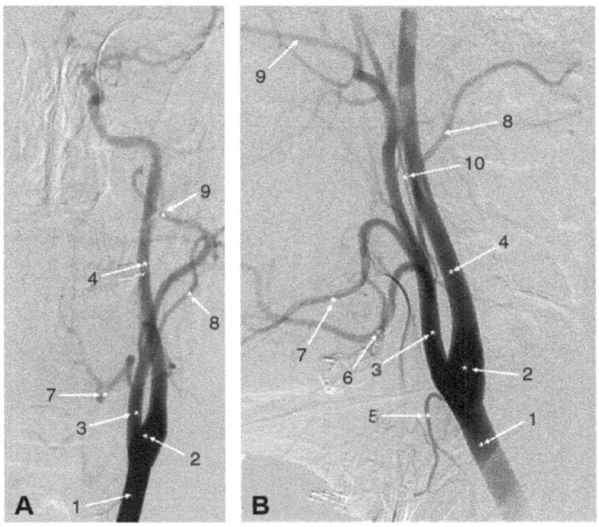

Fig. 8.3. Left common carotid artery injection, cervical views, posteroanterior (**A**) and lateral (**B**): 1, common carotid artery; 2, carotid bulb; 3, external carotid artery; 4, internal carotid artery; 5, superior thyroid artery; 6, lingual artery; 7, facial artery; 8, occipital artery; 9, internal maxillary artery; 10, ascending pharyngeal artery. From Chandra et al. (2014).

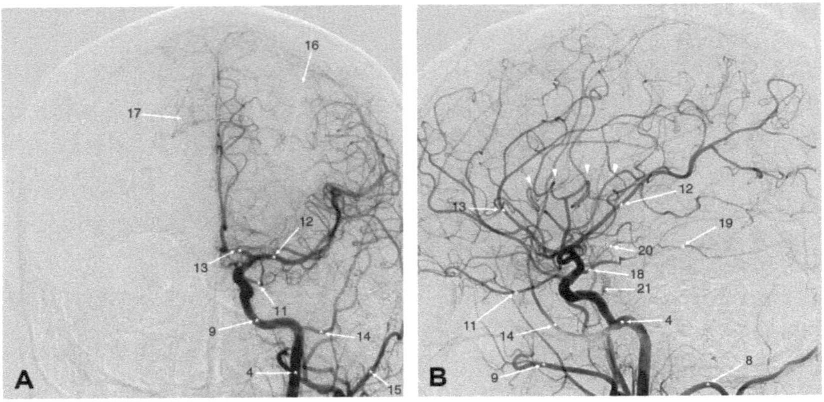

Fig. 8.4. (**A**) Left common carotid artery injection, posteroanterior view, cranial: 4, internal carotid artery; 9, internal maxillary artery; 11, ophthalmic artery; 12, middle cerebral artery; 13, anterior cerebral artery; 14, middle meningeal artery; 15, superficial temporal artery; 16, angiographic watershed between the anterior and middle cerebral arterial territories; 17, contralateral anterior cerebral artery opacification illustrating the presence of an anterior communicating artery with cross-filling. (**B**) Left common carotid artery injection, lateral view, cranial: 4, internal carotid artery; 8, occipital artery; 9, internal maxillary artery; 11, ophthalmic artery; 12, middle cerebral artery (arrowheads represent the M2–M3 junction over the Sylvian fissure); 13, anterior cerebral artery; 14, middle meningeal artery; 18, posterior communicating artery; 19, posterior cerebral artery (faint opacification due to wash-in of unopacified blood); 20, anterior choroidal artery; 21, pituitary blush from branches of the meningohypophyseal trunk. From Chandra et al. (2014).

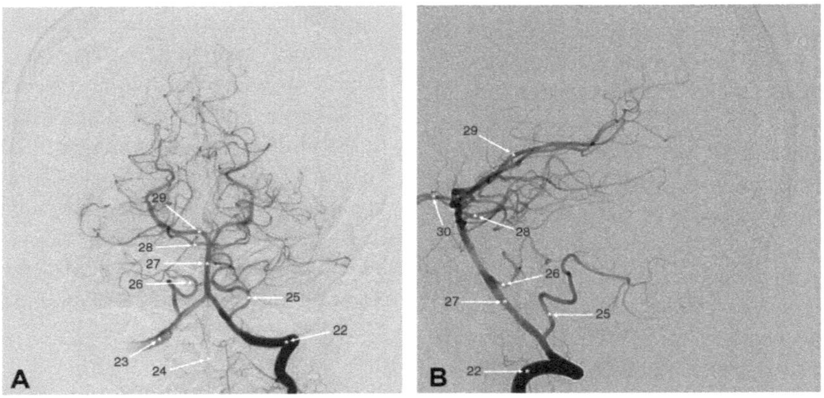

Fig. 8.5. (**A**) Left vertebral artery injection, Townes view, cranial: 22, vertebral artery, left; 23, vertebral artery, right; 24, anterior spinal axis supply arising from the right vertebral artery; 25, left posterior inferior cerebellar artery; 26, right anterior inferior cerebellar artery; 27, basilar artery; 28, right superior cerebellar artery; 29, right posterior cerebral artery. (**B**) Left vertebral artery injection, lateral view, cranial: 22, vertebral artery, left; 25, posterior inferior cerebellar artery, left; 26, anterior inferior cerebellar artery, right; 27, basilar artery; 28, right superior cerebellar artery; 29, right posterior cerebral artery; 30, posterior communicating arteries. From Chandra et al. (2014).

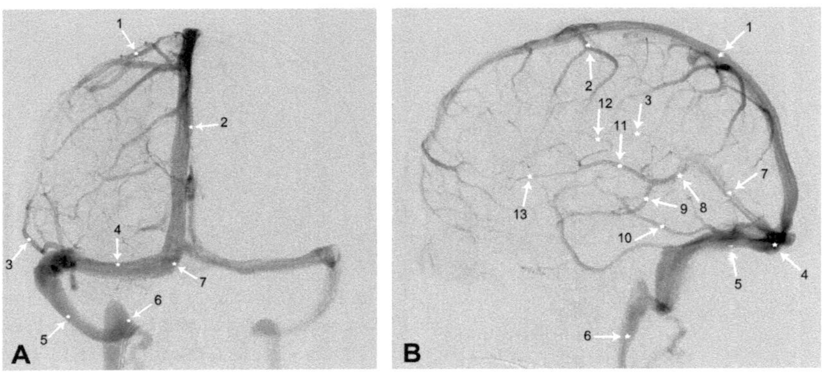

Fig. 8.6. (**A**) Cranial venous anatomy, anteroposterior view: 1, vein of Trolard; 2, superior sagittal sinus; 3, vein of Labbe; 4, right transverse sinus; 5, right sigmoid sinus; 6, right jugular bulb; 7, torcular herophili. (**B**) Cranial venous anatomy, lateral view: 1, superior sagittal sinus; 2, vein of Trolard; 3, inferior sagittal sinus; 4, torcular heophili; 5, sigmoid sinus; 6, jugular vein; 7, straight sinus; 8, vein of Galen; 9, basal vein of Rosenthal; 10, vein of Labbe; 11, internal cerebral vein; 12, thalamostriate vein; 13, septal vein.

Routine spine imaging with CT or MRI is generally part of patient workup in the progression toward spinal angiography. Contrast-enhanced studies are done in the setting of tumors. Vascular etiologies are usually considered when serpiginous signal voids are identified in the parenchymal, intradural, epidural paraspinal locations on MRI. Noninvasive vascular imaging of the spine can be useful, and gadolinium-enhanced magnetic resonance angiography techniques can provide important diagnostic testing (Lindenholz et al., 2014). Finally, with diffuse, juvenile spinal AVMs, cross-sectional imaging of the bony and soft tissues has a role in treatment planning.

Technique

Preprocedure planning is the first step in structuring a spinal angiogram. For spinal vascular malformation workup it is important to study the entire cerebrospinal axis. This includes bilateral carotid, vertebral, and subclavian angiograms for cervicocranial vascular evaluation. For the spine itself, thoracic segmental arteries starting at T3 or T4 down are paired down to the lumbar arteries at L4 or L5 depending on individual anatomy. There is significant variation in location of the level of spinal vascular supply depending on which were preserved and which regressed during fetal development. Medial sacral artery and internal iliac arteries complete the evaluation of the sacrum and coccyx.

In other circumstances, such as tumor evaluation, one can tailor the extent of each study. A focused exam for tumor evaluation might include the segmental arteries of an involved vertebra plus several levels above and below to evaluate collateral supply. One should also extend the levels included until one identifies anterior spinal artery supply. This may affect how one chooses to make a treatment plan of embolization, and surgeons rely on such data to preserve spinal arterial supply.

In either case spinal angiography is most often done under general anesthesia as the length of the procedure and detailed anatomy are optimized. Patients who are undergoing surveillance studies after treatment of spinal vascular lesions may undergo angiography tailored to the specific lesion and may be considered for conscious sedation.

During the procedure there are specific points which distinguish it from cerebral angiography. Once a femoral artery sheath is placed, it is important to count vertebral levels in the cervical, thoracic, and lumbar spine. This allows accurate nomenclature which must be reported in the angiographic procedure note.

Catheters used in spinal angiography include a spectrum of curvatures to enable access to these small branches arising from the aorta. Catheters including Cobra 2, Simmons I or II, or Mickelson can be considered for different segments of the aorta as pedicles arise at different angles.

Technique of catheter position is important. One should rotate the catheter tip until it is posteriorly pointed. Thoracic segmental arteries are located inferior to the bony pedicle of a vertebra on the right and left sides. For access to a segmental artery one uses a blank mask fluoroscopic technique to engage a segmental branch and test with a small puff of contrast. Injection rates are typically 2 mL/second for a total of 4 mL. It is important to have the imaging centered and not rotated. This can be a valuable quality measure when trying to identify anterior spinal and posterior spinal arteries. For subsequent levels one employs a fluoroscopic blank mask and pulls the catheter down and around the previous branch. The catheter is then advanced cephalad and rotated back to a similar angle under the next bony pedicle to find an adjacent segmental or lumbar artery. One generally ascends one side of the aorta and then descends the other side. An important point is that some of these small branches may be difficult to access because of similar or small size than the catheter itself. Tortuosity, aortic pulsatility, atherosclerosis, or abdominal aortic aneurysm can be other causes of difficulty for stable catheter position. Hand injection angiograms may be necessary for parts of a spinal angiogram. Finally, the median sacral artery and the ipsilateral internal iliac can be studied by making a Waltman loop. These combined techniques are efficient for time, radiation dose, and contrast usage during spinal angiography.

Spinal angiographic imaging

During fetal development there is paired arterial supply to the spinal cord from each vertebral body level. Subsequently, many branches regress because of redundancy. In the child and adult, spinal supply is divided into two general categories (Lasjaunias et al., 2002). The midline anterior spinal supply is referred to as radiculomedullary arteries. The most consistent anterior spinal artery branches of the cervical region include the distal vertebral artery just below the vertebrobasilar junction and the artery of the cervical enlargement from the mid to lower cervical spine. In the thoracic spine the artery of Adamkiewicz (1882), which supplies the conus, arises from T9–L1 in 90% of patients (Fig. 8.7A). The dorsal arterial supply to the spinal cord is formed by a radiculopial network of small posterior spinal arteries. These branches arise from a paramedian set of vessels and are variable in number and location (Fig. 8.7B).

Most spinal cord vascular malformations occur in the thoracic spine as the bulk of the cord is there. In the presence of an AV shunt, venous outflow may be compromised. This increased venous volume and pressure can

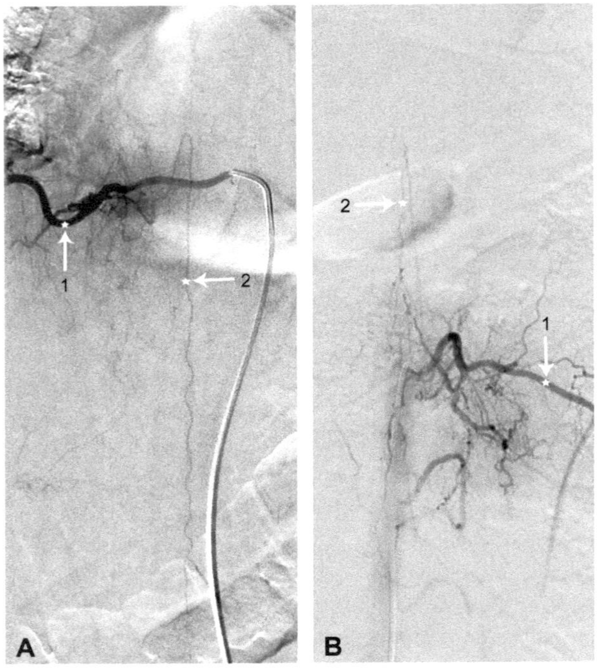

Fig. 8.7. (**A**) Thoracic spinal angiogram: 1, thoracic segmental artery; 2, anterior spinal artery. (**B**) Thoracic spinal angiogram: 1, thoracic segmental artery; 2, posterior spinal artery.

result in a delay in the transit time. It is important to assess this transit time as a secondary finding which may support the diagnosis of a high-flow vascular shunt.

PROCEDURAL PRECAUTIONS FOR CEREBRAL AND SPINAL ANGIOGRAPHY

Precautions must be taken before and during angiography to minimize the risk of cerebral embolism and stroke. Syringes filled with contrast or heparinized saline should be inspected for air bubbles before injection. Bubbles can be removed by introducing a small column of air into the syringe and tipping the syringe so that the column travels along the wall, removing adherent microbubbles. Whenever syringes are connected to the diagnostic catheter or stopcocks, the connection should be meticulously checked for introduction of bubbles. Before injection, hold the syringe vertically and tap the connection to allow any bubbles to rise to the plunger.

In many centers a continuous-flush system using heparinized saline is maintained through the catheter during the procedure. This keeps the catheter lumen free of stagnant blood, preventing potential thrombus formation and embolism. Continuous infusion is mandatory for any therapeutic intervention, but syringe injections alone can be used for diagnostic studies.

When a continuous heparinized saline flush line is not being used, the wire should be removed within 60 seconds of its introduction and the catheter should be double-flushed. A double-flush technique ensures that the catheter lumen is free of thrombus or air. This should be performed every time the wire is removed from the catheter. The wire within the catheter promotes stagnant blood within the lumen that can lead to thrombus formation. Moreover, rapid removal of a wire from the catheter can lead to negative pressure, which can draw air into the lumen. In the double-flush technique, a 10-mL syringe partially filled with heparinized saline is connected to the diagnostic catheter, and the contents of the catheter are aspirated into the syringe. This is followed by connecting a second 10-mL syringe with heparinized saline, partially aspirating to ensure free-flowing blood, and then anterograde flushing to clear the dead space within the catheter.

COMPLICATIONS OF CEREBRAL AND SPINAL ANGIOGRAPHY

A thorough understanding of the hazards inherent in cerebral and spinal angiography is essential to effectively weigh benefit and risk and to ensure informed consent from the patient. Overall complications at high-volume centers are approximately 3%. Complications can be divided into neurologic and nonneurologic.

Neurologic complications

Stroke is one of the most serious complications of cerebral angiography. Ischemic cerebral events can result from thromboembolism or air embolism from the catheter or guidewire. Prolonged attempts at selecting vessels or at catheterizing small-caliber vessels with relatively large catheters will result in slow flow or occlusive hemodynamic conditions that predispose to clot formation. Atherosclerotic plaque disruption and vessel dissection are other sources of cerebral emboli and vessel occlusion.

The reported rate of neurologic complications up to 72 hours after cerebral angiography is highly variable, with ranges from 0.06% to 6.8% (Mani and Eisenberg, 1978; Hankey et al., 1990; Heiserman et al., 1994; Young et al., 1996; Cloft et al., 1999; Willinsky et al., 2003). The true rate of neurologic complications from diagnostic procedures is likely closer to the figure reported by Willinsky et al. (2003), at 1.3%. In a large prospective analysis of 2899 studies from a single institution, transient (<24 hours), reversible (>24 hours to <7 days), and permanent (>7 days) neurologic complications were seen in 0.7%, 0.2%, and 0.5% of cases, respectively. In the same series, age (>55 years), cardiovascular disease, and fluoroscopic time (>10 minutes) were significantly associated with more common neurologic complications.

Though the overall neurologic complication rates can approximate 1%, this is likely to be the proverbial tip of the iceberg of a much larger incidence of cerebral embolization, most of which may be clinically silent with a bedside examination but perhaps not with a neuropsychologic battery, which may be more sensitive to subtle cognitive changes. Dagirmanjian and coworkers (1993) have shown that, on average, more than 70 microembolic events are detected on Doppler sonography per patient during cerebral angiography, without clinical deficits. The incidence of clinically silent T2-weighted or diffusion-weighted abnormalities on MRI following diagnostic or interventional cerebral angiography procedures may be as high as 26% (Bendszus et al., 1999).

Specific risks to spinal arterial vasculature resulting in spinal cord infarct are rare. Dissection or a segmental or lumbar artery from access or contrast injection is rare and can be accommodated by spinal collateral supply.

Patients considered for angiography who are anticoagulated with warfarin for conditions such as atrial fibrillation can undergo angiography, as described here. One should consult with the patient's Cardiology service for consideration of temporarily stopping the medication or using enoxaparin bridge. This can be held on the day of the procedure and then warfarin can be restarted before discharge. The development of relatively safe arterial closure devices for the access site has decreased some of these concerns.

Special consideration should be given to inpatients undergoing multiple cerebral angiograms within a short time frame (e.g., vasospasm patients secondary to aneurysmal subarachnoid hemorrhage receiving repeat intra-arterial cerebral vasodilator therapy or balloon angioplasty). These patients are exposed to heparin on multiple occasions and can develop heparin-induced thrombocytopenia. The first presentation of heparin-induced thrombocytopenia may be cerebrovascular thromboembolism during angiography (Lewis et al., 2001). Based on our experience, patients who return for a third cerebral angiogram within the same admission are given heparin-free saline infusions and flushes. They are usually administered either low-dose Argatroban infusion or saline alone.

Other, less commonly reported neurologic complications include transient cortical blindness (Saigal et al., 2004) and transient global amnesia (Yildiz et al., 2003). In both, the management is expectant after noninvasive imaging has excluded structural causes.

Nonneurologic complications

The most common nonneurologic complication of cerebral angiography by way of the femoral artery is groin hematoma. The series of Willinsky et al. (2003) reported a hematoma rate of 0.4%. Identified risk factors for femoral puncture site complications include age older than 75 years, female gender, hypertension, diabetes mellitus, obesity, location of puncture site, sheath size, duration of the procedure, and use of antithrombotic drugs. The most dangerous subset are patients with retroperitoneal hematomas which can result in significant blood loss leading to cardiovascular compromise. On occasion, these hematomas are complicated by pseudoaneurysm. Left alone, these lesions can enlarge and cause substantial discomfort in the groin and significant blood loss or infection.

Dissections can occur in major vessels during catheter navigation. Most of these can be managed with stopping the procedure and careful neurologic evaluation. In the case of nonocclusive dissection and the absence of neurologic deficit, one can consider short-term treatment with aspirin. In the circumstance of cold foot after angiography, one must evaluate with pulse check with palpation or Doppler ultrasound evaluation of the affected leg and foot. If there is significant pain and poor perfusion of the limb, one must consider the possibility of endovascular or open surgical management.

Severe allergic reaction to medication or iodinated contrast should be managed as medical emergency. All medical personnel involved in the procedure should be familiar with the location of emergency equipment and code cart in the department and be aware of hospital respiratory code team contacts. Assessment with verbal responses of a patient, blood pressure, and electrocardiogram monitoring are important clinical data. Treatment with oxygen, IV fluids, epinephrine, and airway management should be considered in appropriate circumstances.

References

Adamkiewicz A (1882). Die Blutgafabe des menschlichen Ruckenmarkes. II. Die Gefasse der Ruckenmarksoberflache. Mathematisch-natureissenschaftliche Klasse. Sitzungsberiche der Akademie der Wissenschaften Wien 101–130.

Applegate RJ, Rankin KM, Little WC et al. (2003). Restick following initial Angioseal use. Catheter Cardiovasc Interv 58: 181–184.

Baris S, Karakaya D, Aykent R et al. (2001). Comparison of midazolam with or without fentanyl for conscious sedation and hemodynamics in coronary angiography. Can J Cardiol 17: 277–281.

Barrett BJ, Carlisle EJ (1993). Metaanalysis of the relative nephrotoxicity of high- and low-osmolality iodinated contrast media. Radiology 188: 171–178.

Barrett BJ, Parfrey PS, McDonald JR et al. (1992a). Nonionic low-osmolality versus ionic high-osmolality contrast material for intravenous use in patients perceived to be at high risk: randomized trial. Radiology 183: 105–110.

Barrett BJ, Parfrey PS, Vavasour HM et al. (1992b). A comparison of nonionic, low-osmolality radiocontrast agents with ionic, high-osmolality agents during cardiac catheterization. N Engl J Med 326: 431–436.

Bendszus M, Koltzenburg M, Burger R et al. (1999). Silent embolism in diagnostic cerebral angiography and neurointerventional procedures: a prospective study. Lancet 354: 1594–1597.

Benit E, Vranckx P, Jaspers L et al. (1996). Frequency of a positive modified Allen's test in 1,000 consecutive patients undergoing cardiac catheterization. Cathet Cardiovasc Diagn 38: 352–354.

Chandra RV, Leslie-Mazwi TM, Oh DC et al. (2014). Arteriographic Evaluation of Cerebrovascular Disease. In: JC Stanley, FJ Veith, TW Wakefield (Eds.), Current Therapy in Vascular and Endovascular Surgery. Elsevier, Philadelphia, pp. 13–18.

Cloft HJ, Joseph GJ, Dion JE (1999). Risk of cerebral angiography in patients with subarachnoid hemorrhage, cerebral aneurysm, and arteriovenous malformation: a meta-analysis. Stroke 30: 317–320.

Dagi T (2001). Neurosurgery and the introduction of cerebral angiography. Neurosurg Clin N Am 12: 145–153.

Dagirmanjian A, Davis DA, Rothfus WE et al. (1993). Silent cerebral microemboli occurring during carotid angiography: frequency as determined with Doppler sonography. AJR Am J Roentgenol 161: 1037–1040.

Delaney A, Carter A, Fisher M (2006). The prevention of anaphylactoid reactions to iodinated radiological contrast media: a systematic review. BMC Med Imaging 6: 2.

Delgado Almandoz JE, Yoo AJ, Stone MJ et al. (2010). The spot sign score in primary intracerebral hemorrhage identifies patients at highest risk of in-hospital mortality and poor outcome among survivors. Stroke 41: 54–60.

Fields JD, Liu KC, Lee DS et al. (2010). Femoral artery complications associated with the Mynx closure device. AJNR Am J Neuroradiol 31: 1737–1740.

Fischer TH, Connolly R, Thatte HS et al. (2004). Comparison of structural and hemostatic properties of the poly-*N*-acetyl glucosamine Syvek patch with products containing chitosan. Microsc Res Tech 63: 168–174.

Gonzalez RG, Copen WA, Schaefer PW et al. (2013). The Massachusetts General Hospital acute stroke imaging algorithm: an experience and evidence based approach. J Neurointerv Surg 5 (Suppl 1): i7–i12.

Hankey GJ, Warlow CP, Molyneux AJ (1990). Complications of cerebral angiography for patients with mild carotid territory ischaemia being considered for carotid endarterectomy. J Neurol Neurosurg Psychiatry 53: 542–548.

Haschek E, Lindenthal O (1896). Ein Beitrag zur Praktischen Verwerthung der Photographie nach Röntgen. Wien Klin Wochenschr 9: 63–64.

Heiserman JE, Dean BL, Hodak JA et al. (1994). Neurologic complications of cerebral angiography. Am J Neuroradiol 15: 1401–1407.

Hildick-Smith DJR, Ludman PF, Lowe MD et al. (1998). Comparison of radial versus brachial approaches for diagnostic coronary angiography when the femoral approach is contraindicated. Am J Cardiol 81: 770–772.

Hoh BL, Cheung AC, Rabinov JD et al. (2004). Results of a prospective protocol of computed tomographic angiography in place of catheter angiography as the only diagnostic and pretreatment planning study for cerebral aneurysms by a combined neurovascular team. Neurosurgery 54: 1329–1342.

Katholi RE, Taylor GJ, Woods WT et al. (1993). Nephrotoxicity of nonionic low-osmolality versus ionic high-osmolality contrast media: a prospective double-blind randomized comparison in human beings. Radiology 186: 183–187.

Krayenbühl H (1977). History of cerebral angiography and its development since Egaz Moniz. In: Comissao Executiva das Comemoracoes do Centenario do Nascimento do Prof, Egas Moniz, Lisbon, pp. 63–74.

Lalau JD, Race JM (2001). Lactic acidosis in metformin therapy: searching for a link with metformin in reports of 'metformin-associated lactic acidosis'. Diabetes Obes Metabol 3: 195–201.

Lasjaunias P, Berenstein A, Ter Brugge K (2002). Clinical vascular anatomy and variations. Springer, New York.

Levy EI, Boulos AS, Fessler RD et al. (2002). Transradial cerebral angiography: an alternative route. Neurosurgery 51: 335–342.

Lewis BE, Wallis DE, Berkowitz SD et al. (2001). Argatroban anticoagulant therapy in patients with heparin-induced thrombocytopenia. Circulation 103: 1838–1843.

Lindenholz A, Terbrugge KG, van Dijk JM et al. (2014). The accuracy and utility of contrast-enhanced MR angiography for localization of spinal dural arteriovenous fistulas: the Toronto experience. Eur Radiol 24: 2885–2894.

Mancuso CE, Tanzi MG, Gabay M (2004). Paradoxical reactions to benzodiazepines: literature review and treatment options. Pharmacotherapy 24: 1177–1185.

Mani RL, Eisenberg RL (1978). Complications of catheter cerebral arteriography: analysis of 5,000 procedures. III. Assessment of arteries injected, contrast medium used, duration of procedure, and age of patient. AJR Am J Roentgenol 131: 871–874.

Markus H, Israel D, Brown MM et al. (1993). Microscopic air embolism during cerebral angiography and strategies for its avoidance. Lancet 341: 784–787.

Merten GJ, Burgess WP Gray LV et al. (2004). Prevention of contrast-induced nephropathy with sodium bicarbonate: a randomized controlled trial. JAMA 291: 2328–2334.

Moniz E (1934). L'angiographie cérébrale. Masson, Paris.

Moran CJ, Milburn JM, Cross 3rd DT et al. (2001). Randomized controlled trial of sheaths in diagnostic neuroangiography. Radiology 218: 183–187.

Nikolsky E, Mehran R, Halkin A et al. (2004). Vascular complications associated with arteriotomy closure devices in patients undergoing percutaneous coronary procedures: a meta-analysis. J Am Coll Cardiol 44: 1200–1209.

Origitano TC, Schwartz K, Anderson D et al. (1999). Optimal clip application and intraoperative angiography for intracranial aneurysms. Surg Neurol 51: 117–128.

Ozcan EE, Guneri S, Akdeniz B et al. (2007). Sodium bicarbonate, *N*-acetylcysteine, and saline for prevention of radiocontrast-induced nephropathy. A comparison of 3 regimens for protecting contrast-induced nephropathy in patients undergoing coronary procedures. A single-center prospective controlled trial. Am Heart J 154: 539–544.

Rosovsky MA, Rusinek H, Berenstein A et al. (1996). High-dose administration of nonionic contrast media: a retrospective review. Radiology 200: 119–122.

Saigal G, Bhatia R, Bhatia S et al. (2004). MR findings of cortical blindness following cerebral angiography: is this entity related to posterior reversible leukoencephalopathy? Am J Neuroradiol 25: 252–256.

Seldinger SI (2013). Catheter replacement of the needle in percutaneous arteriography: a new technique. Acta Radiol 39: 368–376.

Sheldon P (1956). A special needle for percutaneous vertebral angiography. Br J Radiol 29: 231–232.

Spetzler RF, Detwiler PW, Riina HA et al. (2002). Modified classification of spinal cord vascular lesions. J Neurosurg Spine 96: 145–156.

Thurston TA, Williams CGA, Foshee SL (1996). Reversal of a paradoxical reaction to midazolam with flumazenil. Anesth Analg 83: 192.

Uchino A (1988). Selective catheterization of the brachiocephalic arteries via the right brachial artery. Neuroradiology 30: 524–527.

Wiholm BE, Myrhed M (1993). Metformin-associated lactic acidosis in Sweden 1977–1991. Eur J Clin Pharmacol 44: 589–591.

Willinsky RA, Taylor SM, Terbrugge K et al. (2003). Neurologic complications of cerebral angiography: prospective analysis of 2,899 procedures and review of the literature. Radiology 227: 522–528.

Yildiz A, Yencilek E, Apaydin FD et al. (2003). Transient partial amnesia complicating cardiac and peripheral arteriography with nonionic contrast medium. Eur Radiol 13 (Suppl 4): L113–L115.

Young B, Moore WS, Robertson JT et al. (1996). An analysis of perioperative surgical mortality and morbidity in the asymptomatic carotid atherosclerosis study. Stroke 27: 2216–2224.

Handbook of Clinical Neurology, Vol. 135 (3rd series)
Neuroimaging, Part I
J.C. Masdeu and R.G. González, Editors

Chapter 9

Neurosonology and noninvasive imaging of the carotid arteries

RAFFAELLA PIZZOLATO AND JAVIER M. ROMERO*
Department of Neuroradiology, Massachusetts General Hospital, Harvard Medical School, Boston, MA, USA

Abstract

In this chapter, we review imaging of the extracranial carotid arteries and the indications for noninvasive carotid artery evaluation, measuring the degree of arterial stenosis and plaque morphology. We also analyze the types of noninvasive imaging, including carotid duplex ultrasound, transcranial Doppler, magnetic resonance angiography, and computer tomography angiography. We look at each of these modalities, briefly discussing techniques, benefits, limitations, and sources of error. Furthermore, we discuss the apparent accuracy and the need for multimodality imaging. Finally, an imaging algorithm for the evaluation of the extracranial carotid arteries is proposed, which is in routine use at our hospital.

CAROTID DUPLEX ULTRASONOGRAPHY

Justification for use

Carotid duplex ultrasound (DUS) is an excellent screening exam for asymptomatic patients with high risk of cerebrovascular disease (Patel et al., 2002; Peterson et al., 2005b). On the other hand neurologically symptomatic patients should be evaluated with magnetic resonance imaging (MRI)/magnetic resonance angiography (MRA) or computed tomography angiography (CTA) to assess cranial-cervical vasculature and brain parenchyma status because they are more accurate than DUS (Lev et al., 2001; Patel et al., 2002; U-King-Im et al., 2004a, b, c). Patients may be evaluated with DUS when medical therapy is decided and periodic follow-up is required. MRA with gadolinium and CTA both have a better discriminatory power compared with DUS in diagnosing 70–99% of stenoses and are more sensitive and specific tests than digital subtraction angiography (DSA) in the evaluation of carotid artery stenosis (Barnett et al., 1998; Josephson et al., 2004; Jauch et al., 2013).

Cerebrovascular disease is the third most common cause of death and one of the leading causes of adult disability in the USA (Murray and Lopez, 1997a, b). The annual direct and indirect cost of stroke in the USA in 2008 was $34.3 and future total costs of care for stroke are predicted to increase to $143.0 billion in 2030 (Writing Group Members et al., 2012).

Different pathologies are involved in anterior circulation stroke, and 20% of all cases are caused by carotid artery atherosclerosis (Sacco, 2001). Carotid bifurcation and the proximal 2 cm of the origin of the internal carotid artery (ICA) are mostly affected by atherosclerosis process (Grant et al., 1989). The pathogenic substrate of stroke due to carotid pathology is a plaque that causes hemodynamic effects due to area reduction and a complicated structure and surface, eventually creating emboli and occlusion. The North American Carotid Endarterectomy Trail (NASCET) (Barnett et al., 1998) and the European Carotid Surgery Trial (ECST) (1998) (Rothwell et al., 2003) reported significant benefit of surgical intervention vs medical treatment in symptomatic patients with severe (>70%) carotid stenosis. The benefit of the intervention was also showed in asymptomatic patients with severe carotid stenosis by the Asymptomatic Carotid Surgery Studies (1995) (Executive Committee for the Asymptomatic Carotid Atherosclerosis Study, 1995) and the Asymptomatic Carotid Surgery Trial (2004) (Halliday et al., 2004). However, the benefit of revascularization is less clear in asymptomatic patients with 50–70% ICA stenosis.

*Correspondence to: Javier M. Romero, M.D., Department of Neuroradiology, Massachusetts General Hospital, Harvard Medical School, Gray Building 254, 55 Fruit Street, Boston MA 02114, USA. E-mail: JMROMERO@mgh.harvard.edu

Table 9.1

Clinical indication for noninvasive carotid imaging

Transient ischemic attack
Ischemic stroke
Carotid bruits
Preoperative evaluation of coronary artery bypass graft or aortic valve replacement
Follow-up after carotid endarterectomy or carotid stenting

Surgical approaches to carotid stenosis included carotid endarterectomy (CEA) and stenting (CAS). On the basis of these results, the identification of the severity of ICA stenosis plays a pivotal role in defining which patients may benefit from carotid artery revascularization.

Noninvasive imaging of ICA is indicated in several clinical settings (Table 9.1), such as patients with transient ischemic attacks (TIAs) or ischemic strokes, asymptomatic patients with cervical carotid bruits, and as a preoperative evaluation prior to coronary artery bypass graft surgery (Suematsu et al., 2000), aortic valve replacement, and follow-up after CEA or CAS.

All patients who have experienced TIAs should be evaluated for carotid stenosis due to the significantly increased risk of stroke in the months following a TIA. There is an 11% overall stroke risk at 90 days for patients who have TIA. This risk exceeds 25% if there is a more than 70% ipsilateral carotid stenosis (Romero et al., 2005) (Fig. 9.1). Also, patients with acute stroke should undergo carotid imaging due to elevated proportion of embolic strokes originating from the carotid arteries (20–30%) (Aaslid et al., 1982). Also, carotid DUS is indicated in patients with carotid bruits, since they have over four times the risk of TIA, over twice the risk of stroke, and an increased risk of death from stroke compared with patients without carotid bruits (Pickett et al., 2010).

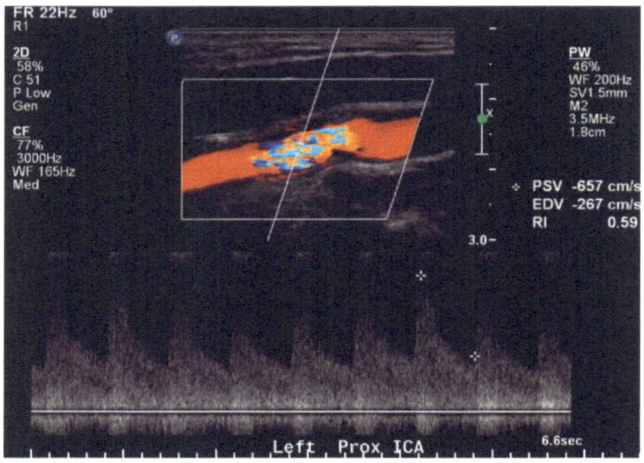

Fig. 9.1. Carotid duplex ultrasound, demonstrating a severe left internal carotid artery stenosis. Spectral broadening is noted.

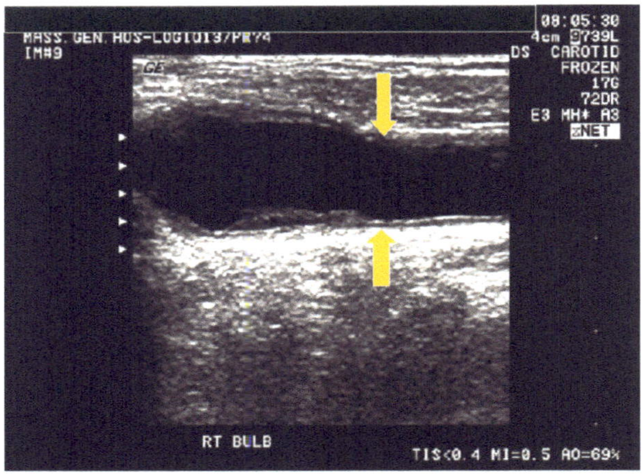

Fig. 9.2. Longitudinal carotid ultrasound, B-mode of the carotid artery, demonstrating postsurgical intima-hyperplasia.

Candidates to coronary artery bypass graft or aortic valve replacement who are 60 years or older or those presenting with a minimum of two cardiovascular risk factors should undergo carotid evaluation to reduce the risk of perioperative stroke (Bishop et al., 1986; Kliewer et al., 2000).

DUS is also useful for follow-up after carotid intervention for the detection of neointimal hyperplasia or restenosis (Fig. 9.2). The risk of restenosis has been shown to be similar after both CEA and CAS (Lal et al., 2012). Neointimal hyperplasia is a stable condition, usually peaking 3 months after surgery, and followed by a regression (Zubilewicz et al., 2001); restenosis after revascularization results from vessel trauma with subsequent neointimal hyperplasia, which occurs within 24 months of the postoperative period or *de novo* neoatherosclerosis thereafter (Lal et al., 2007).

Technique

A standard carotid DUS consists of a bilateral examination of the common carotid arteries (CCA), ICA, external carotid arteries (ECA) and the vertebral arteries (VA). Multiple ultrasound parameters are investigated to evaluate carotid artery characteristics and composition, such as Doppler blood flow velocity criteria and the presence of plaque on gray-scale and/or color DUS images.

Gray-scale images of CCA and ICA are obtained in transverse and longitudinal planes, while the ECA and VA are studied only in longitudinal planes. These images allow the identification of plaque location and composition (i.e., homogeneous, heterogeneous, calcific). Separately, B-mode imaging is conducted to study the arterial wall thickness, providing images of the wall itself. In severe disease, cross-sectional B-mode images, together with color flow images, are more difficult to generate because of shadowing and other artifacts. Therefore, in these cases the hemodynamic criteria prevail.

Arterial narrowing leads to locally increased velocities. Spectral Doppler waveforms are gained with a defined technique: the waveforms should be obtained by placing the cursor in the longitudinal view of the artery with the cursor placed in the center of the stream of flow, the "flow jet" (Fig. 9.3). The recommended Doppler angle is between 40° and 60° in order to align the cursor parallel to the vessel wall; a correct Doppler angle is required to calculate the peak systolic velocity (PSV). Nine standardized sites are imaged: the proximal, middle, and distal CCA; the proximal, middle, and distal ICA; the proximal ECA, and the proximal and middle VA. Each vessel has a characteristic normal waveform pattern based on the vascular bed distal to the artery (Table 9.2).

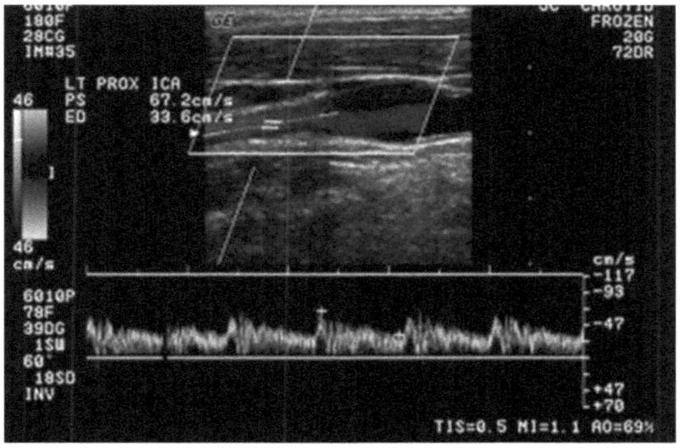

Fig. 9.3. Carotid artery duplex ultrasound, demonstrating normal velocities of the internal carotid artery.

Table 9.2

Typical waveform patterns for carotid duplex ultrasonography (DUS)

Vessel	Normal carotid DUS waveform patterns
ICA	Low-resistance waveform with continuous forward flow throughout diastole
ECA	High-resistance waveform with a sharp systolic upstroke and decreased diastolic flow
CCA	Sharp systolic upstroke as well as continuous flow throughout the diastole
VA	Low-resistance waveform with continuous forward flow in the diastole

CCA, common carotid arteries; ECA, external carotid arteries; ICA, internal carotid arteries; VA, vertebral arteries.

The American College of Radiology, the American Institute of Ultrasound in Medicine, and the Society of Radiologists in Ultrasound (Radiology Accountable Care Organizations, 2012) suggest recording blood flow velocity measurements at proximal and mid or distal CCA (generally 2–3 cm below the bifurcation), proximal ECA, two sites in the ICA, and VA. As a result of NASCET, percent stenosis has become the widely accepted parameter, categorized in broad ranges of severity (i.e., 50–69% and 70–99%), and a significant plaque stenosis is defined as ≥70%. If significant stenosis is detected, spectra should be sampled within and distal to each stenosis, with the highest velocity determined and recorded.

Since the velocity values that are used to define percent stenosis categories are not always uniform, each laboratory needs to develop internally validated Doppler criteria. We use the guidelines set out in Table 9.3 in our laboratory to determine the degree of carotid artery stenosis.

Gray-scale and color flow imaging and spectral Doppler provide the necessary tools to determine the severity of carotid stenosis and avoid misinterpretation. Although results vary greatly between laboratories and operators, the sensitivity and specificity for detection or exclusion of 70% stenosis of the ICA are 85–90% compared with conventional angiography (Brott et al., 2011).

Postrevascularized ICA evaluation

DUS is a reproducible, affordable, noninvasive method that can be used to assess for restenosis during the follow-up after carotid revascularization for the detection of restenosis. Different studies indicated that restenosis following CAS was higher than following CEA (Eckstein et al., 2008; Bonati et al., 2009; Arquizan et al., 2011), although the Carotid Revascularization Endarterectomy versus Stenting Trial (CREST) reported similar restenosis frequency in 2 years of follow-up (Lal et al., 2012) (Table 9.4). Given these results, DUS may have a significant role in the follow-up of CAS patients. Conventional carotid artery DUS velocity criteria are thought to be less accurate in patients who have undergone CAS (Lal et al., 2004). Several studies were carried out to establish sonographic cut-off criteria for the diagnosis of different degrees of carotid in-stent restenosis, using PSV, end-diastolic velocity, and ICA:CCA PSV ratio. PSV is the most accurate criterion of in-stent restenosis. In fact, it increases according to the increment of the stenosis (Grant et al., 2000). A PSV value of 300–350 cm/s may be used as threshold criterion of high-grade restenosis (Levy et al., 2005; Peterson et al., 2005a; Stanziale et al., 2005;

Table 9.3

Guidelines for determining degree of vessel stenosis in carotid duplex ultrasonography

Degree of stenosis	Peak systolic velocity (cm/s)	Approx. % degree of stenosis	Luminal diameter (mm)	Other indirect signs (TCD, assumes NL ECAs)
NL	<150	<50%	>3	
Mild	150–200	50–60%	2.5–3	
Moderate	200–300	60–70%	2–2.5	Normal distal ICA waveforms
Severe	300–400	70–80%	1–2 mm	Reversal flow ipsilateral ACA (TCD) Tardus parvus waveforms in the distal ICA
Critical	>400	80–90%	0.7–1	Reversal flow ophthalmic artery (TCD) Tardus parvus waveforms in the distal ICA Velocities falling off
	Falling off	>90%	<0.7	MRA shows absent distal ICA signal (slow flow vs occlusion), consider CTA

ACA, anterior cerebral artery A1 segment; CTA, computed tomography angiography; ECA, external carotid artery; ICA, internal carotid artery; MRA, magnetic resonance angiography; NL, normal; TCD, transcranial Doppler ultrasonography.
Courtesy of Neurovascular Laboratory, Massachusetts General Hospital, Boston, MA, USA.

Table 9.4

Frequency of restenosis ≥70% or occlusion

		CAVATAS (#)	EVA-3S (#)	SPACE (#)	CREST (#)
Number of patients evaluated	CAS	200	242	541	1086
	CEA	213	265	522	1105
Restenosis rate	CAS	21.07% in 1 year 30.7% in 5 years	3.3% in 3 years	11.1% in 2 years	6% in 2 years
	CEA	7.5% in 1 year 10.5% in 5 years	2.8% in 3 years	4.6% in 2 years	6.3% in 2 years
	p-value	/	0.44	0.0007	0.58

CAS, carotid stenting; CAVATAS, Carotid and Vertebral Artery Transluminal Angioplasty Study; CEA, carotid endarterectomy; CREST, Carotid Revascularization Endarterectomy versus Stenting Trial; EVA-3S, Endarterectomy Versus Angioplasty in Patients with Symptomatic Severe Carotid Stenosis; SPACE, Stent-Protected Angioplasty versus Carotid Endarterectomy.
Reproduced from Pizzolato et al. (2014).

Armstrong et al., 2007; Chahwan et al., 2007; Chi et al., 2007; AbuRahma et al., 2008; Cumbie et al., 2008; Lal et al., 2008; Setacci et al., 2008; Zhou et al., 2008; Heck, 2009; Pizzolato et al., 2014) (Fig. 9.4).

According to the existing literature and guidelines, DUS may be performed at 1 month and 6 months and annually after CAS or CEA (Brott et al., 2011). The evaluation of the revascularized carotid artery should be focused on the areas of surgical incision and clamping. For instance, after CEA DUS evaluation should be concentrated on the near carotid wall, which is usually the area of carotid artery incision, and special attention should be paid to the distal portion of ICA, where a clamp is usually placed and intraoperative inspection is often limited. If the results of DUS are inconclusive, CTA is required. Different results with either of these techniques should be confirmed by DSA (Goldman et al., 2006).

Principal indications for sequential carotid artery studies

DUS is a reliable, noninvasive, and economic tool for long-term follow-up of patients at high risk for atheromatous disease of the carotid arteries and postsurgical complications (Fig. 9.5).

The guidelines to justify sequential carotid artery imaging are synthesized in Table 9.5.

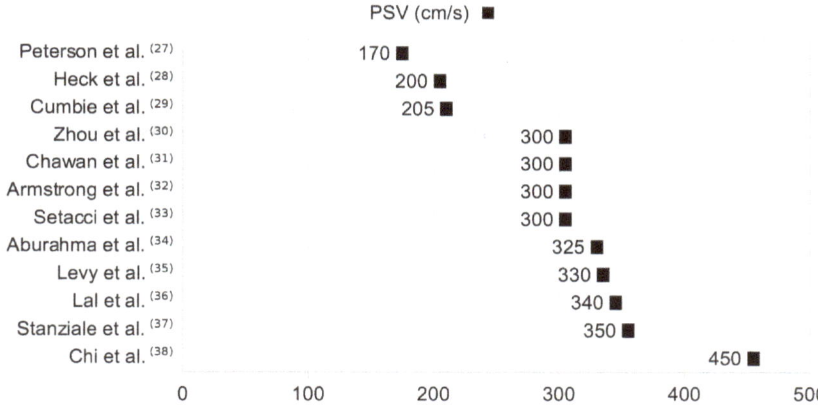

Fig. 9.4. Peak systolic velocity (PSV) thresholds of multiple specified studies. This demonstrates a cluster of velocities in the 300–320 cm/s range in lesions with confirmed ≥70%.

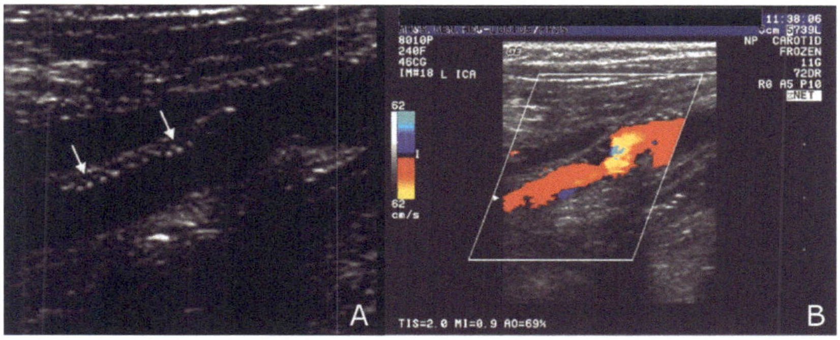

Fig. 9.5. (**A**) B-mode carotid artery ultrasound shows Dacron patch of the left internal carotid artery status post carotid endarterectomy. (**B**) Color flow images demonstrate restenosis.

Table 9.5

Clinical indications for sequential noninvasive carotid imaging

Assessing for progression of carotid artery stenosis due to atheromatous disease
Monitoring the revascularized carotid for evidence of intimal hyperplasia or recurrent atheromatous disease
Evaluating dissected carotid arteries for evidence of progression or resolution of occlusive process

Intima-media thickness

Carotid intima-media thickness (IMT) is an indicator of early atherosclerosis and it is correlated to increased vascular risk (Griffin et al., 2009; Finn et al., 2010; Mauriello et al., 2010). B-mode imaging may be used to determine both the carotid intimal and medial thickness. The advantages to using carotid DUS are that it is an easily reproducible, economic, and reliable method in measuring IMT (Fig. 9.6). The normal measurements of the IMT at different age ranges are shown in Table 9.6.

As reported by Juonala et al. (2008), when adjustments for risk factors and carotid diameter are taken into account, there is no significant difference between the IMT of healthy men and that of healthy women. In 2007, Lorenz et al. carried out a meta-analysis on 37 197 patients followed up for a mean of 5.5 years to investigate the role of IMT measured by DUS in predicting future cardiovascular events. For an absolute carotid IMT increase of 0.1 mm, the future risk of myocardial infarction increases by 10–15%, and the stroke risk increases by 13–18%. Also, recent studies have showed positive correlations between reduction of IMT achieved by lipid-modifying drugs and the risk for cardiovascular events (Crouse et al., 2007; Peters et al., 2011).

Plaque characterization

The degree of carotid stenosis is the most widely accepted predictor of stroke risk, but other imaging features are becoming recognized as significant factors in the identification of the vulnerable plaque. This term is used to describe atherosclerotic plaques with a high risk of causing neurologic symptoms. A number of

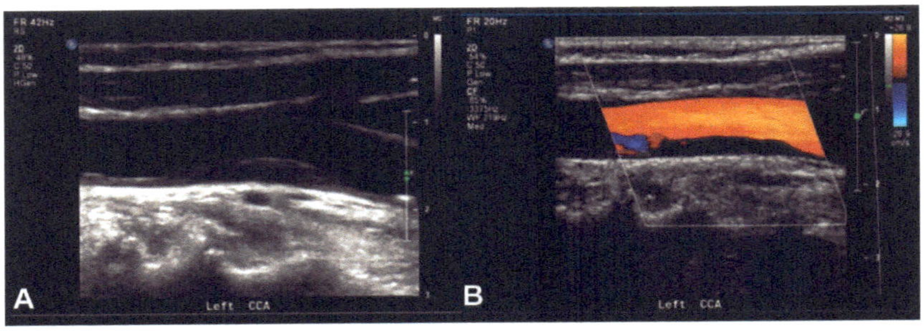

Fig. 9.6. (**A**) B-mode in the longitudinal axis demonstrating a segment of intima-media thickening, which is prominent in the distal wall. (**B**) Color flow of the internal carotid artery, demonstrating the degree of stenosis.

Table 9.6

Reference limits for duplex ultrasound measurement of intimal/medial thickness (IMT) in healthy patients

	Carotid IMT (mm)	
Age/sex	Lower limit	Upper limit
Women		
24 years	0.411	0.698
27 years	0.420	0.719
30 years	0.430	0.742
33 years	0.440	0.765
36 years	0.451	0.789
39 years	0.462	0.814
Men		
24 years	0.411	0.734
27 years	0.422	0.760
30 years	0.433	0.787
33 years	0.444	0.816
36 years	0.456	0.846
39 years	0.469	0.878

Adapted from Juonala et al. (2008).

noninvasive diagnostics, including ultrasound, CTA, and MRA, exist to date and allow characterization of plaque composition, such as active inflammation, thin cap with a large lipid core, plaque ulceration, intraplaque hemorrhage, and vasa vasorum neovascularization (Fig. 9.7).

The accuracy of ultrasound in detecting plaque components shows a large variability. An unstable plaque may be characterized by a lipid core and is likely to rupture into the lumen if the fibrous cap attenuates. Good correlation has been demonstrated with homogeneous hypoechoic plaque and the presence of the lipid core (Gronholdt et al., 1998) (Fig. 9.8). Although a thin fibrous cap and plaque enhancement have a strong relationship with symptoms, these findings are difficult to evaluate with ultrasound. Also, the identification of plaque heterogeneity predicted fibrous cap thickness and the location of the lipid core with sensitivities of 77% and 74% and specificities of 22% and 17%, respectively (Sztajzel et al., 2005). The presence of an irregular border and/or heterogeneity predicts the presence of an intraplaque hemorrhage (AbuRahma, 2002).

Contrast-enhanced ultrasound provides images of the adventitial vasa vasorum and intraplaque neovascularization as a hallmark of acute inflammation in carotid lesions. This technique uses contrast agent microspheres as intravascular tracers (Vicenzini et al., 2007; Staub et al., 2009), but the short microsphere half-life *in vivo*, low resolution, and poor reproducibility limit its use for the detection of carotid neovascularization. Enhancement of the vasa vasorum overlying carotid plaque can be appreciated by CTA and it has been correlated with acute neurologic symptoms in patients with $\geq$70% carotid stenosis (Romero et al., 2009).

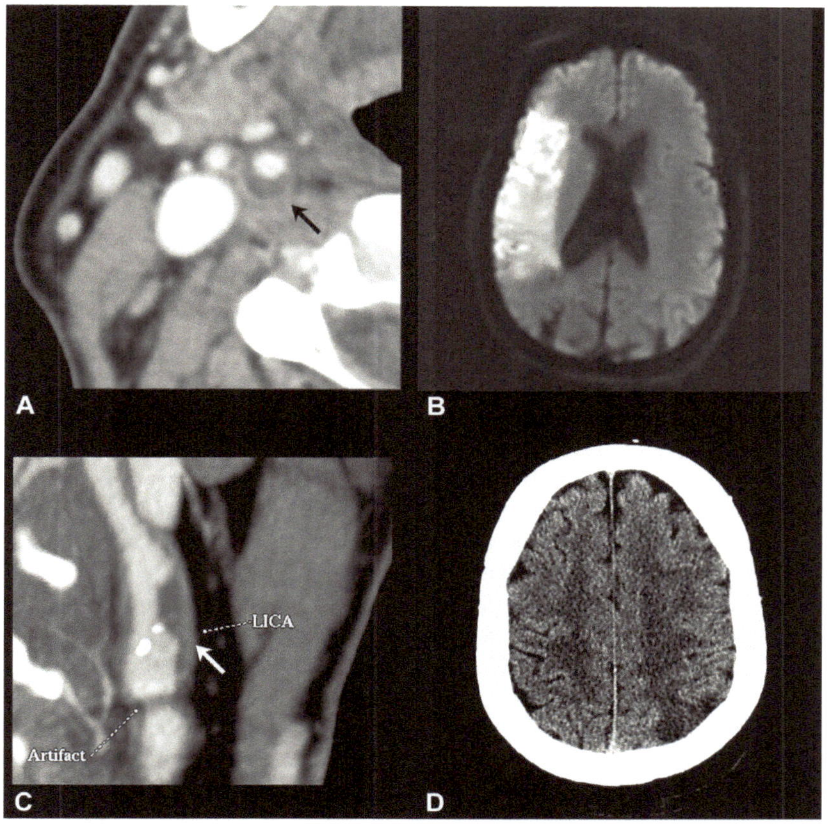

Fig. 9.7. (**A**) Patient 1: axial computed tomography (CT) angiography of the neck demonstrates enhancement of the adventitial vasa vasorum of the proximal right internal carotid artery (black arrow). (**B**) Axial diffusion magnetic resonance imaging demonstrates restricted water diffusion of the right middle cerebral artery territory, representing an acute infarct. (**C**) Patient 2: parasagittal CT angiography of the neck demonstrates enhancement of the adventitial vasa vasorum of the proximal left internal carotid artery (LICA: white arrow). (**D**) Axial noncontrast CT of the head demonstrates a subacute infarction of the left upper parietal lobule.

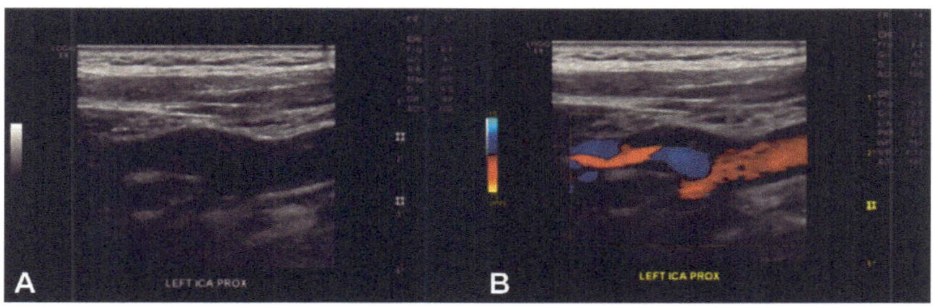

Fig. 9.8. (**A**) B-mode and (**B**) color flow of the left internal carotid artery demonstrating a hypoechoic plaque.

Limitations

Technical pitfalls

A number of technical pitfalls may limit the value of ultrasound examination, such as choosing the correct probe and selecting appropriate imaging parameters (color gain, pulse repetition frequency (PRF), filters, speckle reduction software). The choice of an appropriate transducer is made according to the patient body habitus. Generally a 7–9 MHz probe is used; a 5 MHz probe is more appropriate in patients with a large body habitus or deep vessels, while a 10–12 MHz probe is indicated in case of very superficial vessels. A correct angle of insonation is also important when performing and interpreting carotid ultrasound, and it has to be parallel to the vessel wall. The recommended DUS angle should not exceed 60°, as measurements are likely to be inaccurate. An exception is insonating tortuous vessels that may require an angle of 0°. Moreover, the color gain should be adjusted carefully, as excessive color gain results in overestimation of residual lumen and may overshadow an intimal flap in case of carotid dissection. To enable the detection of highly reduced blood flow velocity, the color gain should be increased as high as possible, while PRF should be reduced. In case of pseudo-occlusion (hairline lumen), pseudonormalization is observed and PRF between 10 and 40 is indicated. A PRF below 10 results in excess color artifact, while a PRF above 40 diminishes all low-level flow and images could be misinterpreted as a true occlusion.

Two types of artifact are also common. Reverberation artifact is caused by sound bouncing between multiple structures that are strong specular reflectors, such as the near wall of the carotid artery and a high-impedance carotid plaque or a calcified nodule. When the transducer is above the high-impedance object, the ultrasound pulse will reflect back and forth several times between the object and the carotid wall. This gives rise to echoes that appear on the gray-scale images as a series of lines within the carotid lumen, causing inaccurate detection of the vessel wall.

Mirror-image artifact is detected in carotid artery stenosis when strongly reflecting plaques on the vessel wall distant from the transducer head are insonated obliquely. In this case, the echoes from the oblique structure are received later than those from perpendicular structures and they may be interpreted as deeper than the true surface. This artifact may be easily discovered by changing the angle of insonation.

Anatomic limitations

Carotid DUS is limited in its ability to evaluate the entire ICA and CCA. The distal ICA, defined as the ICA at the skull base, and the CCA origin are evaluated with MRA or CTA. However, changes in the proximal ICA and distal CCA waveforms can provide clues about the presence of stenosis that cannot be directly visualized. High-resistance waveforms with sharp systolic upstrokes are suggestive of a more distal stenosis of the ICA, likely in the intracranial portion. On the contrary, delayed systolic upstrokes and low PSV noted throughout the course of the ICA are suggestive of more proximal stenosis, whether at the ICA origin, in the bulb or more proximal CCA. Again, delayed systolic upstrokes and low PSV recorded in the course of CCA indicate a more proximal stenosis, either of the aorta or at the CCA origin.

Variants of origin, caliber, course (tortuosity, coiling, or kinking), and bifurcation (spatial position, absence of carotid bulb) may be other potential pitfalls.

Interpretation pitfalls

ICA versus ECA

During interpretation it is essential to identify the ICA and ECA correctly. There are four anatomic and waveform patterns that help distinguish the ECA from the ICA. First, unlike ICA, ECA has visible branches and responds to a temporal tap. Secondly, as previously discussed, the ECA will demonstrate high-resistance waveforms while the ICA demonstrates low-resistance waveforms.

Sometimes the waveform patterns are unreliable. When an ICA is occluded or demonstrates very slow flow consistent with a pseudo-occlusion, flow in the ipsilateral ECA may also demonstrate hemodynamic changes. It is not uncommon for the ECA to show an increased diastolic flow and lower resistance; this is referred to as internalization of the ECA. This phenomenon is secondary to creation of spontaneous compensatory shunts such as internal maxillary artery–ophthalmic artery–distal ICA anastomosis (Fig. 9.9). These waveform alterations could also be caused by dilatation of ECA branches. These abnormalities are usually identified with chronic critical stenosis or complete occlusion of the ICA. Transcranial Doppler (TCD) may be used to detect retrograde flow within the ophthalmic artery and to indirectly prove the presence of severe ICA disease (Reynolds et al., 2002).

Heavy calcified plaque

Heavily calcified plaques are characterized by zones of acoustic shadowing that obscure the arterial wall as well as the arterial lumen, impeding Doppler measurements. This limitation is of great importance when a calcified plaque extends more than 1 cm down the course of the vessel. In fact, distal Doppler measurements are not reliable to infer the degree of proximal stenosis in these cases. MRA and dual-energy CTA with calcium removal are useful to characterize these plaques.

Tandem lesions

Rarely, although the B-mode imaging visualizes a severe arterial stenosis, the velocities and spectral flow configurations appear normal or slightly abnormal. This can occur in case of tandem lesions in the carotid artery. These are defined as two separate stenoses occurring at least 3 cm apart, determining a severe stenosis. The second stenosis, located downstream from the insonated lesion, causes dampening of the PSV in the vascular segment between the two lesions. This phenomenon is secondary to increased pulse pressure between the two lesions, which eliminates the pressure gradient distal

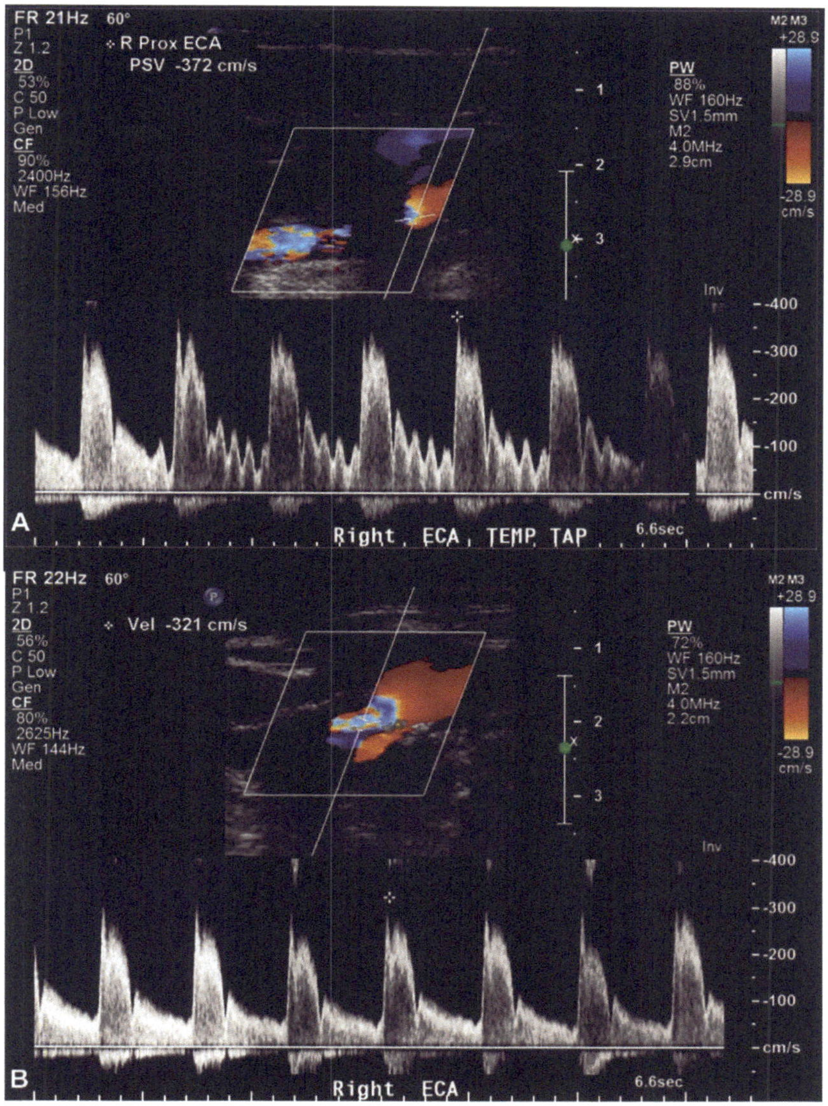

Fig. 9.9. Color duplex ultrasound of the right external carotid artery (ECA) demonstrating an internalized ECA secondary to occlusion of the internal carotid artery.

to the initial lesion. This hemodynamic effect is caused by the stenosis with the greatest narrowing (Rouleau et al., 1999; Romero et al., 2002). When tandem lesions are suspected, CTA, contrast-enhanced MRA, or conventional angiography of the neck should be performed for a definitive diagnosis.

Occlusion versus pseudo-occlusion

Vessel occlusion is characterized by lack of signal or Doppler shift within the vessel lumen. However, very slow flow may not be detected during routine DUS examination, and a pseudo-occlusion (hairline lumen) must be considered. Carotid DUS displays a sensitivity of 80–90% for detecting hairline lumens when correct parameters are used, such as maximum level of color gain and reduced PRF (Furst et al., 1999).

When DUS imaging raises the suspicion for ICA or CCA pseudo-occlusion with DUS, CTA may be required for a definitive diagnosis (Lev et al., 2003), although conventional catheter angiography remains the more definitive study (Romero et al., 2002, 2005) (Fig. 9.10).

Velocities falling off

Typically, PSVs in a vessel increase as the lumen of the vessel decreases according to the increase of the pressure gradient. The phenomenon of "velocities falling off" or pseudonormalization is referred to the sudden decrease in velocity in vessels with a stenosis of >90%

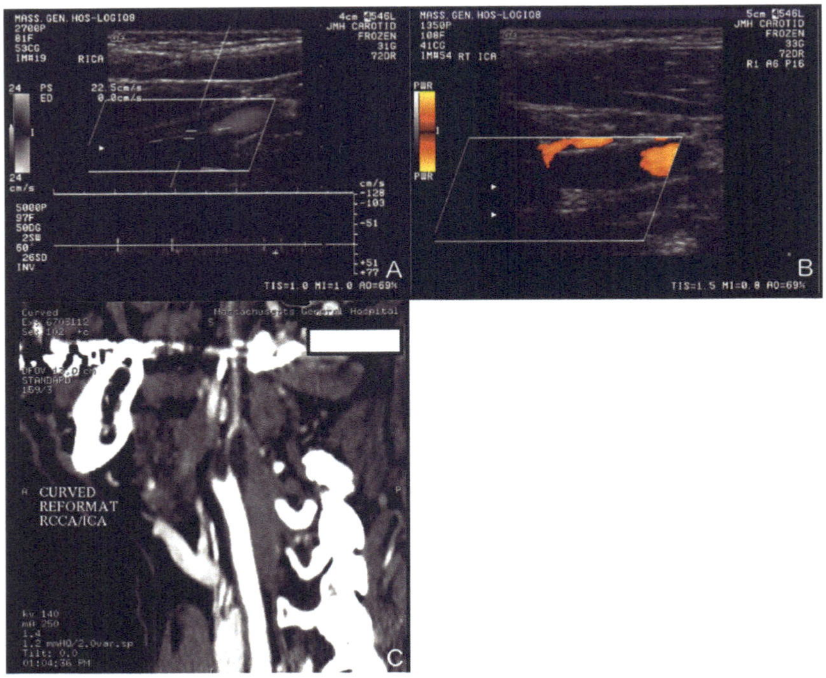

Fig. 9.10. (**A**) Color duplex ultrasound of the right internal carotid artery (RICA) with absence of color flow. (**B**) Power Doppler demonstrates no flow in the RICA. (**C**) Computed tomography angiography of the neck demonstrates a hairline lumen of the internal carotid artery, secondary to critical stenosis.

(typically a <0.7 mm residual lumen diameter). It results in a decrease in PSV into a range associated with a less severe stenosis or absence of stenosis. This is problematic when velocities alone are considered in a description of vessels, determining an inaccurate description or oversight of vessel stenosis. To avoid this kind of error, other factors must be considered as indicators of pseudonormalization:

- turbulent flow
- decrease in the resistance index
- spectral broadening found in the presence of "normal" velocities
- dampening of the distal vessel waveform
- pinpoint residual lumen on color flow images in either the longitudinal or transverse plane.

Additionally, TCD ultrasonography detects a retrograde flow direction in the ophthalmic artery in case of severe stenosis or occlusion of the ipsilateral CCA or ICA, so it may be used to identify pseudonormalization. CTA or conventional arteriography is required to definitely establish the degree of stenosis.

Contralateral carotid artery stenosis

Velocities in the ICA and/or CCA can sometimes be falsely elevated in the absence of significant carotid artery stenosis. This can occur if there is a severe stenosis or occlusion of the contralateral ICA and/or CCA, resulting in increased (collateral) blood flow through the patent carotid artery (Henderson et al., 2000). This phenomenon is a reflection of compensatory collateral flow in the contralateral vessel in order to supply the cerebral hemisphere with the diseased vessel via the circle of Willis (Kluytmans et al., 1999). Collateral flow should be suspected when elevated velocities are noted, but no lesion is noted on B-mode and color Doppler. Thus, PSVs alone can lead to overestimation of the degree of stenosis in these cases (Fig. 9.11).

Carotid artery dissection

Carotid artery dissection (CAD) has been increasingly recognized as a cause of stroke, particularly in young people. Incidence rates of spontaneous CAD have been reported to be approximately 2.6–2.9 per 100 000 (Lee et al., 2006). CAD is an important risk factor for embolic stroke, since luminal stenosis and the release of thrombogenic factors by the injured vessel promote thrombus formation. Other symptoms caused by local dissection effects are neck pain, Horner's syndrome, and cranial nerve palsies (Thanvi, 2005).

The etiopathogenesis of CAD is not fully understood. Trauma is a common cause, but also heritable connective disorders (Marfan's syndrome, Ehlers–Danlos syndrome, etc.) may predispose to CAD (Fig. 9.12).

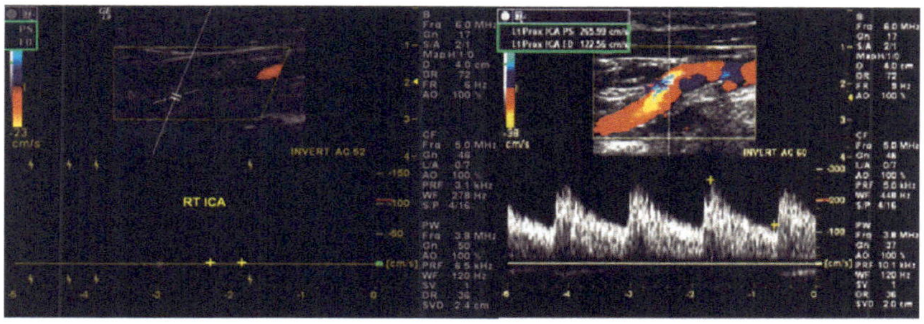

Fig. 9.11. (**A**) (Left) Color Doppler ultrasound demonstrates a right internal carotid artery occlusion with (**B**) (Right) pseudo-elevation of the contralateral internal carotid artery, which shows normal lumen on color flow images.

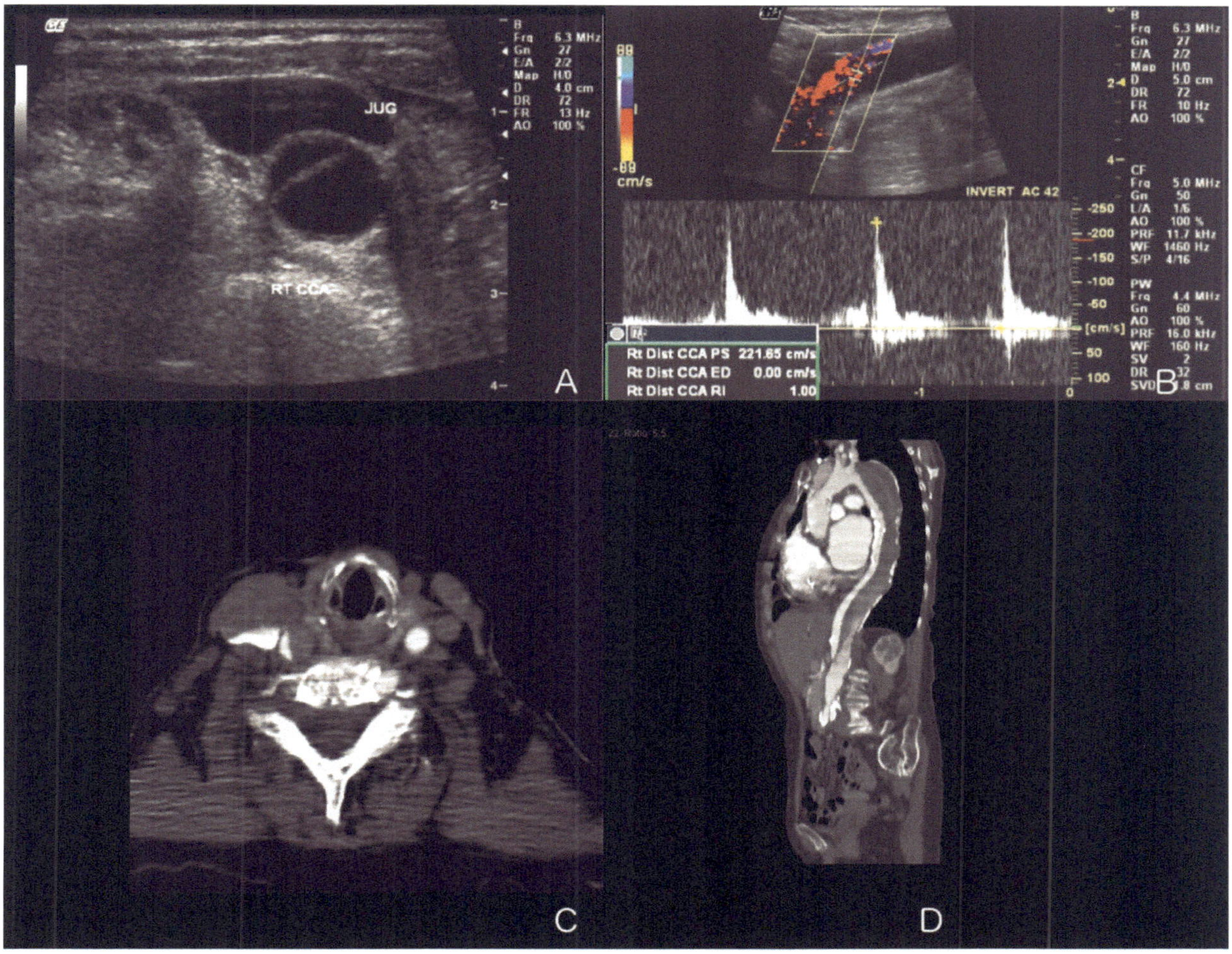

Fig. 9.12. (**A**) B-mode in transverse of the right common carotid artery (CCA), showing a CCA flap representing a dissection. (**B**) High-resistance waveforms are noted, likely representing a significant stenosis. (**C** and **D**) Computed tomography of the neck and chest, demonstrating an extensive dissection of the carotid arteries and aorta.

Traumatic dissections differ from spontaneous dissections by location (more commonly involving the CCA, rather than the ICA), appearance (more commonly resulting in complete occlusion), and outcome (more often failing to resolve) (Provenzale, 1995).

Spontaneous ICA dissection usually occurs at the supraclinoid segment of the ICA, which is distal to and likely out of the anatomic scope of DUS. For these cases an evaluation of the entire course of the ICA with MRA or CTA is recommended. MRA plays an important role in the diagnosis of spontaneous dissection. MRI findings are typically a periarterial rim of intramural hematoma, which initially is hyperintense on T1-weighted images and later on T2-weighted images, surrounding either a normal or narrowed flow void (Provenzale, 1995).

Traumatic CAD occurs mostly after motor vehicle accidents or other mechanisms that cause stretching of the carotid arteries. This category of dissection may likely be evaluated by DUS, given that the trauma is usually at the level of the exposed cervical segment.

DUS has a diagnostic sensitivity of >90% in identifying CAD (Thanvi, 2005). Continuous-wave Doppler velocimetry, standard duplex scanning, and color Doppler flow imaging have all been used in the diagnosis of carotid dissections. B-mode may give morphologic information about the endothelial flap, likely representing the dissection lesion; hemodynamic significance may be determined via pulsed-wave Doppler. While imaging a carotid dissection in the longitudinal plane, the false lumen created by the entry of blood into the vessel wall should be insonated; unless occluded by thrombus, flow in the lumen will demonstrate high-resistance flow. Different signs can help in the diagnosis of CAD. The most frequent direct sign in the B-scan is tapering ICA lumen. Indirect signs, such as a mirror image artifact, are detected in carotid artery stenosis when strongly reflecting plaques on the vessel wall distant from the transducer head were insonated obliquely. Occasionally the ICA may appear normal; however, an increase in the resistance of the waveform should alert one to the possibility of dissection (Sturzenegger et al., 1995).

Sublclavian steal syndrome

Subclavian steal syndrome (SSS) is a condition secondary to an occlusion in the proximal subclavian artery which leads to upper-extremity blood supply to be derived by reversal of flow within the ipsilateral VA. Symptoms of SSS include vertigo during arm exertion and hand or arm pain, and numbness or weakness in the arm involved due to hypoperfusion. Also, patients exhibit marked differences in blood pressure between the left and right arms (typically >20 mmHg). Retrograde flow in the VA is the classic hallmark of this syndrome, which can be divided into four types on the basis of characteristic waveform changes. Each waveform is defined by the ratio of the flow velocity at the mid-systolic notch to the flow velocity at the end diastole. The greater the ratio, the more advanced is the steal phenomenon (Kliewer et al., 2000). Type I steal is characterized by a mild notch between systolic peaks, type II steal demonstrates a more pronounced systolic notch, while a type III steal shows a systolic notch extending to or slightly below baseline. In the most severe steal (type IV), flow in the ipsilateral VA is completely retrograde.

Changes in the waveforms of the subclavian artery may also be suggestive of subclavian stenosis. A healthy subclavian artery demonstrates triphasic flow, with end-systolic flow in the retrograde direction before returning to the forward direction in diastole. In case of a stenosis >50% in the subclavian artery, waveforms are generally monophasic, occurring only above baseline. Additionally, in a subclavian artery with a segment of >50% stenosis, multiple insonations along the course of the vessel will reveal that the area of stenosis displays velocities at least double of those velocities in the healthy proximal-vessel segment. However, DUS cannot reliably image the proximal intrathoracic subclavian artery; the visualization of VA may also be difficult in obese patients and requires skilled technicians (Wu et al., 2005).

TRANSCRANIAL DOPPLER

TCD is a noninvasive ultrasonography technique that was introduced over 30 years ago (Aaslid et al., 1982). TCD is considered effective in the detection of stenosis, occlusion of basal cerebral arteries such as middle cerebral artery (MCA), ICA siphon, and vertebrobasilar system. Its accuracy is less than that of CTA and MRA for steno-occlusive disease, with a TCD sensitivity and specificity ranging from 55% to 90% and from 90% to 95%, respectively (Jauch et al., 2013). However, TCD can reliably rule out intracranial stenosis according to the findings of the Stroke Outcomes and Neuroimaging of Intracranial Atherosclerosis trial. For arteries with 50–99% stenoses that were angiographically confirmed (the "gold standard"), TCD was able to positively predict 55% of these lesions, but was able to rule out 83% of vessels that had <80% stenosis (Feldmann et al., 2007). TCD can also be used to detect vasospasm in subarachnoid hmorrhage (SAH), microembolic signals, which are seen with extracranial or cardiac sources of embolism, and to evaluate the cerebrovascular reserve (CVR).

Technique

TCD is a noninvasive ultrasonography technology that involves the use of a low-frequency (≤2 MHz) transducer probe to insonate basal cerebral arteries through cranial bone windows. It is based on pulsed-wave Doppler measurement of cerebral blood flow velocity (CBF-V) and vessel pulsatility, and it combines two-dimensional gray-scale imaging with real-time Doppler, providing a color-coded representation of CBF-V. It is relatively inexpensive and repeatable, allowing bedside monitoring of CBF-V. However, the usefulness of TCD is limited in 10–20% of patients with poor bony windows (Naqvi et al., 2013), and its overall accuracy is dependent on the experience of the technician, the interpreter, and the patient's vascular anatomy. For posterior-circulation stroke, TCD is not as accurate; CTA, MRA, or a conventional angiography is required.

In a full TCD examination, a bilateral examination of the anterior cerebral arteries, MCAs, and posterior cerebral arteries, as well as the intracranial and extracranial VAs, proximal basilar artery, and ophthalmic arteries, and carotid siphon region is performed (Table 9.7). The target artery is insonated by selecting an appropriate acoustic window, probe angle, and sample volume depth. The artery is recognized through flow direction, resistance (pulsatility), and velocity, in addition to waveform changes induced by dynamic maneuvers such as proximal carotid artery compression and artery tapping over bony landmarks (Nicoletto and Burkman, 2009a).

The velocities (Table 9.8) and direction of flow and waveform characteristics determine the presence and degree of hemodynamically significant vessel stenosis. Mean flow velocity is a central parameter in TCD and it may be influenced by a number of physiologic factors (Table 9.9). Flow should be oriented toward the probe when insonating the MCA and ophthalmic arteries, and oriented away from the probe when insonating the anterior and posterior cerebral arteries. The direction of flow may vary when insonating the carotid siphon region, basilar artery, and VAs. Waveforms of high resistance are typically found in the ophthalmic arteries, whereas low-resistance waveform may be found throughout the rest of the intracranial vasculature.

TCD in the diagnosis of subarachnoid hemorrhage vasospasm

Cerebral vasospasm is the delayed narrowing of large capacitance intracranial arteries following SAH, often associated with radiographic or clinical evidence of diminished perfusion in the distal territory of the affected arteries (Rigamonti et al., 2008). Vasospasm contributes to high levels of mortality and morbidity. It may evolve anywhere between the third and the seventh day following the initial hemorrhage in the neural parenchyma. Evaluation of vasospasm is one of the most common uses of TCD. Although conventional angiography may be considered the "gold standard" in vasospasm diagnosis, it should not be used in frequent monitoring due to its invasive nature, radiation exposure, and increased risk of cerebral ischemia (Aaslid et al., 1984). Therefore, since the TCD is noninvasive and can be applied frequently both pre- and postoperatively, it has a great potential for monitoring and guiding the therapy of SAH patients. Also, it can detect the development of vasospasm days before it can become clinically apparent (days 2–5 following SAH onset). However, since TCD provides only vessel flow velocity, it does not provide any direct sign of decreased tissue perfusion.

Vasospasm is characterized by an increase in mean CBF-V above the upper limit for a patient's age (Table 9.10 describes the normal mean CBF-V). In detail, MCA velocities >120 cm/s are considered suggestive of vasospasm, with velocities above 200 cm/s considered a critical vasospasm (Aaslid et al., 1984). In addition, vasospasm can be represented by an increased mean blood flow velocity within a 5–10 mm segment, usually by

Table 9.7

Guidelines for transcranial Doppler vessel insonation

Vessel	Depths (mm)	Flow direction in reference to probe	Window	Optimal boost setting
MCA	45–65	Toward	Middle transtemporal	Medium
ACA	65–75	Away	Middle transtemporal	Medium
PCA	65–75	Away	Posterior transtemporal	Medium
OphA	45 to approximately 65	Toward	Transorbital	Low
Siphon	Approximately 65–75	Either	Transorbital	Medium
Vertebral				
Extracranial	45–55	Away	Suboccipital	Low
Intracranial	60–75	Away	Transforaminal	Medium
Basilar	80–120	Away	Transforaminal	Medium

ACA, anterior cerebral artery; MCA, middle cerebral artery; OphA, ophthalmic artery; PCA, posterior cerebral artery.
Reproduced from Standard guidelines for vascular insonation by transcranial Doppler ultrasound, adapted from the guidelines of the Neurovascular Laboratory of Massachusetts General Hospital, Boston (unpublished).

Table 9.8

Guide to determining vessel stenosis based on insonated vessel velocity

	Velocity of pulse wave (cm/s)	
Degree of stenosis	Anterior	Vertebral and basilar
"Gray zone"		80–100
Mild	120–160	101–150
Moderate	161–200	150–180
Severe	>200	>180

Table 9.9

Factors influencing the mean flow velocity (MFV)

Factor	Change in MFV
Age	Increases up to 6–10 years of age then decrease
Sex	Higher MFV in women than men
Pregnancy	Decreased in the third trimester
$P\text{CO}_2$	Increases with increasing $P\text{CO}_2$
Mean arterial pressure	Increases with increasing mean arterial pressure
Hematocrit	Increases with decreasing hematocrit

Adapted from Naqvi et al. (2013).

Table 9.10

Normal reference for carotid blood flow velocities (cm/s) in different age groups

	20–40 years	41–60 years
Common carotid artery		
Peak systolic	96	75
End diastolic	23	21
Internal carotid artery		
Peak systolic	65	61
End diastolic	27	25
Vertebral artery		
Peak systolic	49	48
End diastolic	17	17

Adapted from Babikian et al. (2003).

>30 cm/s compared with the asymptomatic side (Nicoletto and Burkman, 2009b). The Lindegaard ratio can be used to differentiate hyperdynamic flow from vasospasm and is defined as the ratio of MCA flow velocity to extracranial ICA flow velocity (Lindegaard et al., 1989). In the context of a high mean flow velocity, a Lindegaard ratio <3 indicates hyperdynamic flow and >3 indicates vasospasm (Aaslid et al., 1984). TCD is most reliable in diagnosing vasospasm of the M1 segment, followed by the basilar and VAs, while it is not reliable for diagnosis of anterior cerebral artery (A2) vasospasm (Naqvi et al., 2013).

TCD in the detection of cerebral embolism

Cerebral ischemia is frequently attributed to emboli that originate in the cardiac chambers and at stenotic lesions along the aortic arch and carotid arteries. Some of these strokes occur without warning symptoms. In patients with symptomatic carotid stenosis greater than 50–70%, CEA reduces ipsilateral stroke risk by about 75% (Rothwell, 2004) and is generally accepted as being cost-effective. However, the situation in patients with asymptomatic carotid stenosis is less clear. Screening for asymptomatic carotid stenosis as well as CEA has been suggested as a prevention strategy (King et al., 2011). The presence of emboli distal to a high-grade asymptomatic ICA stenosis identifies patients at higher risk of first-ever stroke (King and Markus, 2009). TCD is a valuable technique in the detection of emboli via the continuous monitoring of the Doppler spectrum of the intracranial arteries, most often MCA. The identification of emboli particles is possible because of their emission of high-intensity transient signal (HITS) during their course through the MCA (Sliwka et al., 1995). Signal intensity is dependent on embolus size and composition; however, because intensity depends on multiple factors, no conclusion about embolus nature may be detected from the signal intensity alone. Signals are unidirectional and occur randomly throughout the cardiac cycle; for this reason HITS detection is most often undertaken over a period of 1 hour. The prognostic value of the detection of HITS by TCD in patients with asymptomatic carotid stenosis was shown in the Asymptomatic Carotid Emboli Study, a prospective, multicenter observational study (Markus et al., 2010). The investigators evaluated patients with $\geq$70% asymptomatic carotid stenosis for the presence of HITS with consecutive 1-hour TCD recordings of the ipsilateral MCA. They concluded that TCD detection of HITS could identify groups of patients with asymptomatic carotid stenosis who are at significantly low (no HITS detected) or high (HITS detected) risk of future stroke. Consequently, assessment of the presence of embolic signals on TCD might be useful in the selection of patients with asymptomatic carotid stenosis who are likely to benefit from CEA (Markus et al., 2010).

Cerebrovascular reserve

CVR or cerebral vascular reactivity is a measure of the homeostatic mechanism that minimizes deviation of the cerebral blood flow when there is an increase of partial pressure of blood CO_2 (P_{CO_2}). This autoregulation acts through vasomotor effectors that control cerebrovascular resistance in order to regulate sudden changes of local metabolism to changes in blood pressure, hydration, and pulse pressure. The aim of this physiologic system is to maintain an adequate blood flow to all areas of the brain. M1 segment of MCA has a constant diameter during increase of P_{CO_2}, which facilitates accurate measurement of any changes of blood velocity. A reactive vasodilatation of the arterioles distal to the M1 segment follows an increase of P_{CO_2}. This phenomenon decreases the intraluminal pressure within this vasculature, which consequently increases the blood flow and flow velocity though the MCA. This change can be monitored by TCD as an increase of PSV of the MCA. It can be studied also by other modalities, including CT perfusion, positron emission tomography (PET), single-photon emission computed tomography (SPECT), and xenon CT blood flow. Among all these techniques, TCD has the advantage of being noninvasive and relatively inexpensive, and has been used widely to assess cerebral vasoreactivity (Ringelstein et al., 1988; Aaslid et al., 1989, 1991; Dahl et al., 1992; Markus and Harrison, 1992; Silvestrini et al., 1996; White and Markus, 1997; Gahn et al., 1999; Markus and Cullinane, 2001; Diehl, 2002). CVR with TCD usually can be assessed by measuring the change in CBF-V of the MCA occurring in response to a vasodilatory stimulus such as CO_2 inhalation at 6%, 8%, or 10%, or acetazolamide administration. The breath-holding maneuver or Valsalva maneuver can also be used as an alternative and simple method for studying cerebral hemodynamics.

CVR is impaired in patients with a long-standing stenosis of the ICA, MCA, or a cardiac disease (Ringelstein et al., 1988), as the microcirculation is already vasodilated in an attempt to improve impaired cerebral blood flow (Ringelstein et al., 1988). This determines an increased risk of border-zone infarcts with an odds ratio of 14.4 (Markus and Cullinane, 2001). CVR was demonstrated to improve in the ipsilateral MCA following CEA due to the restoration of blood flow and cerebrovascular tone (Vriens et al., 2001). Improved collateral blood supply to the contralateral cerebral hemisphere via the circle of Willis leads to improved CVR in both cerebral hemispheres (Vriens et al., 2001). Nevertheless, the presence of asymptomatic HITS signals on TCD is likely to be a stronger predictor of stroke than exhausted CVR in patients with asymptomatic carotid stenosis (Markus and Cullinane, 2001). CVR can be further lost after stroke or SAH, or can be decreased by medications, diabetes mellitus (Fülesdi et al., 1997), and amyloid angiopathy.

CT ANGIOGRAPHY

CTA has several advantages over DUS and MRA for carotid imaging. In fact, CTA has a higher spatial resolution and quicker acquisition times than the other techniques, providing more accurate and detailed vascular anatomy. It is less susceptible to artifacts than MRA because – like DSA – it is a digital subtraction technique that relies on intraluminal contrast rather than signal changes attributable to alterations in blood flow. Also, artifacts due to patient motion are less common due to its faster scan. In addition, CT is a more widely available imaging technique than MRI. The development of multidetector CT has made CTA a feasible imaging modality for the evaluation of intracranial and extracranial vasculature in the emergency department.

Technique

Unenhanced CT of the head and cervical spine, as well as multidetector CTA, were performed with 16- or 64-section scanners (LightSpeed; GE Healthcare). The unenhanced axial CT examinations were performed with the following parameters: tube voltage, 120–140 kVp; tube current, 170 mA; and section thickness, 1.25 mm (for the cervical spine), 5 mm (for the standard head algorithm), or 2.5 mm (for the head bone algorithm). Multidetector CTA was performed by scanning from either the superior orbital rim to the aortic arch (neck) or from the vertex to the aortic arch (head and neck) by using the following parameters: pitch, 0.5; collimation, 1.25 mm; maximal tube current, 350 mA; tube charge, 120 kVp; and field of view, 22 cm. A dose of 80–100 mL of nonionic contrast material was administered by using a power injector (ACIST Medical Systems, Eden Prairie, MN) at a rate of 4–5 mL/s in an antecubital vein either with a fixed 25-second delay between the onset of contrast material injection and the start of scanning, or with Smart-Prep (GE Healthcare), a semiautomatic contrast bolus-triggering technique. Standard maximum-intensity projection images of the major cervical arterial structures were created by the three-dimensional laboratory.

Safety

CTA is a noninvasive to minimally invasive procedure. The major safety concerns are the administration of intravenous nonionic iodinated contrast material and the exposure of the patient to ionizing radiation. The intravenous administration of ionic iodinated contrast material in patients with stroke has been demonstrated to be generally safe (Shrier et al., 1997). Nonionic contrast material has been demonstrated to have higher safety and tolerability than ionic contrast (Christiansen, 2005). Also, it has been demonstrated, both clinically and experimentally within laboratory experiments, to not worsen the symptoms of stroke or to enlarge brain infarction volumes (Romero, 2005). Recent publications have evaluated the utility of decreasing the volume of the contrast material and peak kilovoltage (kVp) required to achieve diagnostic-quality images in order to reduce the risks of nephrotoxicity, allergic reaction, and radiation-induced skin changes. Bahner and colleagues (2005) demonstrated improved signal-to-noise ratio of the intracranial vasculature with 80 kVp compared to 120 kVp despite an increased image noise at 80 kVp. Multiphasic intravenous injection methods with decreased contrast material volume for uniform prolonged vascular enhancement at CTA have also been experimented in an effort to reduce nephrotoxicity without deteriorating vessel enhancement (Bae et al., 2000).

The number of CT studies in the USA and Europe has exponentially increased over the last 20 years, determining an increase of medical radiation dose of about seven times since the 1980s (Thurston, 2010). CT scanning accounts for approximately 15% of radiologic examinations but represents the most important source of medical radiation exposure, accounting for up to 70% of the radiation dose delivered (Linton et al., 2003). Also, as the applications for medical imaging continue to increase and the population ages, it will be incumbent on radiologists and clinicians to work together to minimize the population dose. An appropriate selection of patients who will benefit from CTA, and using imaging modalities that do not use ionizing radiation, such as DUS and MRI, when feasible, can enable this goal to be achieved. For patients undergoing CTA, optimization of CT parameters will allow image acquisition with a lower radiation dose. A recent study has shown that reducing the kVp from 120 to 100 and reducing the mA from 235 to 140 lead to a dose reduction of 62% while still producing source images and three-dimensional (3D) reconstructions of diagnostic quality (Lira et al., 2014). Additional studies are indicated to determine how much the dose can be reduced before the image quality suffers.

CTA in the assessment of major vessel occlusion

CTA demonstrates excellent sensitivity and specificity in the assessment of stenosis or occlusion (Fig. 9.13). Using comparison with the conventional angiogram for the

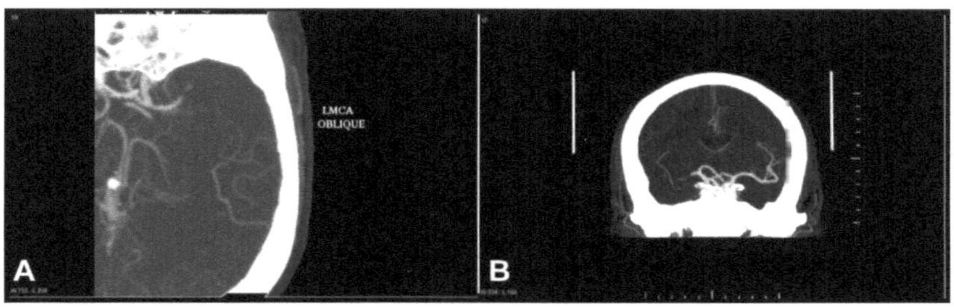

Fig. 9.13. (**A**) Axial collapsed maximal-intensity projection (MIP) of the head demonstrates an occlusion of the proximal left middle cerebral artery. (**B**) Coronal MIP of the head demonstrates a right M1 occlusion.

detection of large-vessel occlusion, Lev and colleagues (2001) demonstrated CTA sensitivity and specificity of 98.4% and 98.1%, with an accuracy of 99%. CTA is also the imaging technique of choice in the case of tortuous carotid, severe calcification, short neck, and high bifurcation (Corti et al., 1998). Novel postprocessing algorithms have improved the visualization of stented carotid arteries, which has traditionally been a weakness of CTA-source images (SI) evaluation. Furthermore, CTA-SI is significantly more sensitive and specific in the detection of basilar artery patency compared to TCD in patients with clinical symptoms of basilar ischemia. In fact, it not only allows the detection of the site of occlusion/stenosis, but also provides information on the length of the occlusion and collateral pathways (Brandt et al., 1999). Also, a small review compared CTA and TCD in the evaluation of MCA stenosis, and found that abnormal TCD results are highly suggestive of MCA stenosis. However, normal TCD findings do not exclude MCA stenosis, especially in patients with distal M1 or M2 branch disease.

A systematic review of the literature showed excellent accuracy of CTA in the differentiation between hairline residual lumen from total ICA with sensitivity and specificity of 97% (95% confidence interval (CI), 93–99%) and 99% (95% CI, 98–100%), respectively (Lev et al., 2003) (Fig. 9.14).

CTA-SI is a useful tool in the early detection of infarct combined with noncontrast CT (Ezzeddine et al., 2002). Moreover, it improves overall accuracy in infarct localization (40%, $p < 0.001$), vascular territory determination (28%, $p = 0.003$), vessel occlusion identification (38%, $p < 0.001$), Trial of Org 10172 in Acute Stroke Treatment (TOAST) classification (18%, $p = 0.039$), and Oxfordshire Community Stroke Project classification (32%, $p < 0.001$) (Ezzeddine et al., 2002). These results highlight the potential use of CTA-SI in the triage of patients with clinical stroke.

Several reports demonstrated a similar accuracy in the evaluation of suspected steno-occlusive diseases of the major intracranial arteries between CTA-SI combined with MRA and DSA (Hirai et al., 2002). In addition, good agreement between CTA and DSA in the evaluation of carotid stenosis has been demonstrated (Josephson et al., 2004). Using a 70% cutoff value for stenosis, CTA and DSA were in agreement in 78 of 81% vessels (96%; 95% CI, 90–99%). CTA was 100% sensitive and 63% specific (95% CI, 25–88%), and the negative predictive value of CTA demonstrating <70% stenosis was 100% (Josephson et al., 2004).

Limitations and interpretation pitfalls

Practical limitations of CTA are primarily related to:

- adverse reaction to contrast material administration (contrast material allergy, nephrotoxicity, osmotic load causing cardiorespiratory challenge, contrast material extravasation)
- radiation exposure
- need for large-gauge intravenous access
- time required to make formalized 3D renderings
- time required to evaluate numerous images.

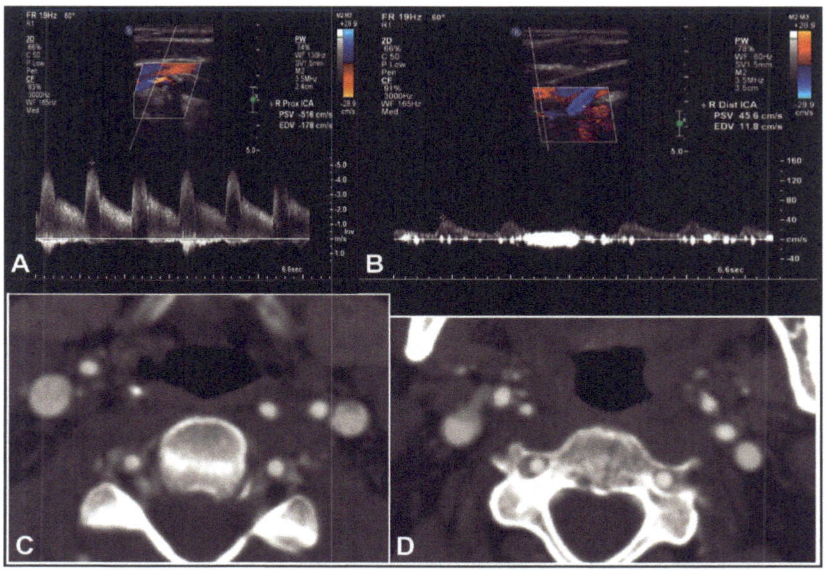

Fig. 9.14. (**A**) Color duplex ultrasound demonstrates extremely elevated velocities representing a critical stenosis of the right internal carotid artery (RICA). (**B**) Damped waveforms in the distal portion of the vessel represent velocities falling off. (**C** and **D**) Computed tomography angiography of the neck shows a punctate or hairline lumen of the RICA.

CTA has also significant difficulty in demonstrating distal-branch occlusion, compared to conventional angiogram. Smaller, M3, branch occlusions are a common source of error on CTA-SI; on the other hand, several studies have demonstrated that these abnormalities are still more readily detected with CTA than with other noninvasive modalities (Shrier et al., 1997).

MAGNETIC RESONANCE ANGIOGRAPHY

MRA is a safe and high-resolution imaging technique for carotid artery stenosis. Also it does not expose the patient to radiation and can be performed with or without a contrast agent, offering the advantage of adding concurrent brain imaging to the examination. The literature reports excellent and robust sensitivities and specificities of DUS, MRA, and CTA in distinguishing $<70\%$ and $>70\%$ ICA stenosis (Randoux et al., 2001; Patel et al., 2002; Remonda et al., 2002; Josephson et al., 2004; Romero et al., 2005). Two-dimensional time-of-flight (2D TOF) MRA is frequently used to evaluate carotid vasculature; however, it is suboptimal for evaluation of the great-vessel origins (Romero et al., 2005). Therefore, contrast-enhanced MRA (CE-MRA) appears to be the most accurate noninvasive modality and is considered by some the noninvasive gold standard for assessing ICA narrowing (Remonda et al., 2002; Borisch et al., 2003; Romero et al., 2005; Maldonado, 2007).

Since MR is relatively time-consuming, more costly than, and not as accessible as DUS or CTA in some centers, it is not the imaging of choice. Multimodality evaluation of carotid artery disease can be accurate enough to replace DSA; therefore two noninvasive techniques in combination, with a third one performed if the first two disagree, appear to improve accuracy over a single technique (Patel et al., 2002). In patients where DUS and CE-MRA are discordant, CTA is an appropriate troubleshooter.

Technique

Two noncontrast MRA techniques are used to evaluate carotid vasculature: TOF or phase contrast flow-sensitive imaging, which can be either a 2D or 3D volumetric acquisition (Fig. 9.15). Both these methods have the advantage of avoiding the administration of contrast agents, which are best avoided in patients with poor kidney function; however, there are issues with the diagnostic quality of this technique, particularly in the setting of pulsation artifact (e.g., from the aorta), diminutive vessels, or in the setting of slow flow. Also these sequences are vulnerable to signal-intensity drop-out

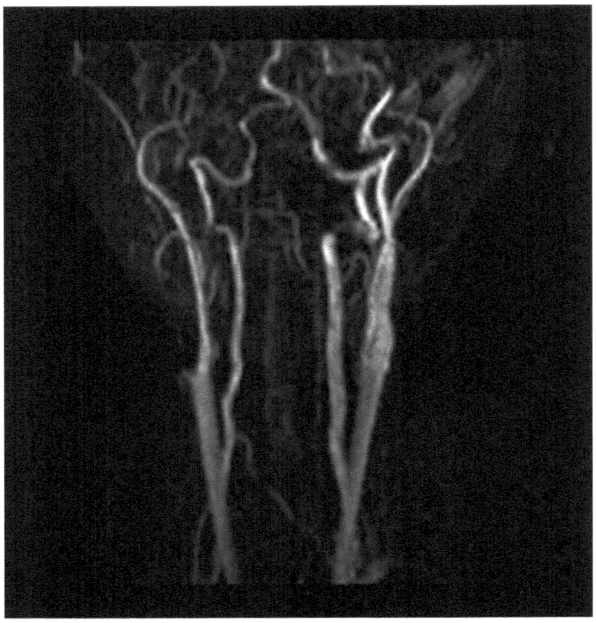

Fig. 9.15. Two-dimensional time-of-flight magnetic resonance angiography of the neck.

(or flow-void) artifacts in the stenotic vascular segments, and this can cause issues with distinguishing near from total occlusion (Mustert et al., 1998; Nederkoorn et al., 2002).

CE-MRA uses the intravenous injection of gadolinium, which improves contrast between the vessel lumen and adjacent soft tissues, helping to overcome the limitations seen with unenhanced MRA. In addition, the time of the examination is considerably shorter with CE-MRA compared to the 2D and 3D-TOF MRAs, thus decreasing motion artifacts. However, it also adds to the cost and complexity of imaging (Leclerc et al., 1999; Carr et al., 2001; Yang et al., 2005). CE-MRA is increasingly used for evaluation of the carotid and VA due to high sensitivity and specificity compared with DSA. CE-MRA is an attractive imaging option, when used as a complementary modality to DUS, by enhancing the already high sensitivity/specificity (U-King-Im et al., 2004b) and cost-effectiveness of DUS (U-King-Im et al., 2004a). CE-MRA appears to be superior to 2D-TOF MRA in visualizing long-segment carotid artery morphology and anatomy (Timaran et al., 2007) as well as airline occlusion, dissection (Fig. 9.16), or tandem lesions (Romero et al., 2005; Yang et al., 2005) (Fig. 9.17). However, CE-MRA does not offer significant advantages over 2D-TOF MRA for screening and identification of patients with $\geq 70\%$ ICA stenosis (Babiarz et al., 2009).

Contrast-enhanced and unenhanced MRA acquisitions can be viewed as a series of images or

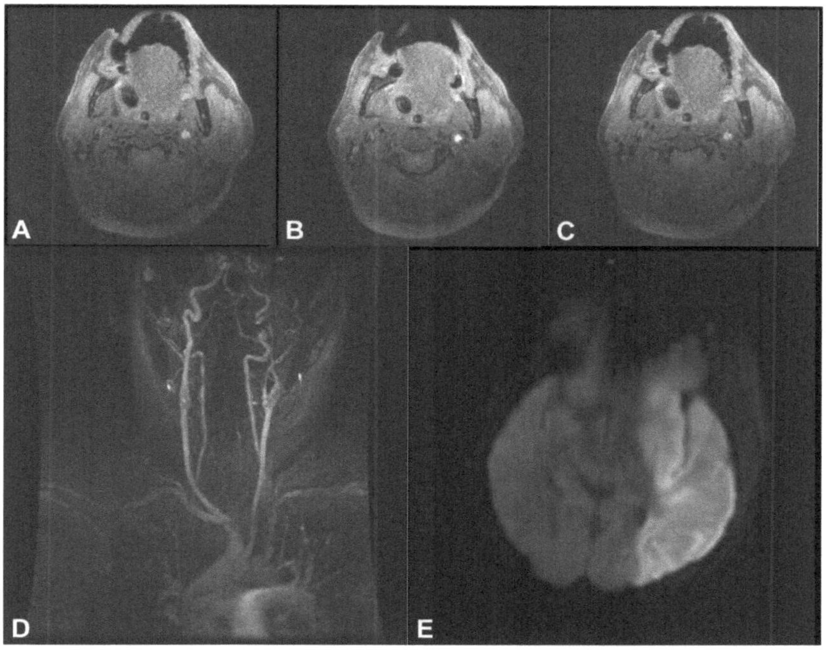

Fig. 9.16. (**A–C**) Axial fat-saturated T1-weighted magnetic resonance imaging (MRI) of the neck shows a hyperintense lesion in the left internal carotid artery (ICA), likely representing the intramural clot of the dissection. (**D**) There is focal loss of contrast-related enhancement of the left ICA, with a string sign secondary to the dissection. (**E**) Diffusion-weighted MRI demonstrates an extensive infarction of the left middle cerebral artery territory.

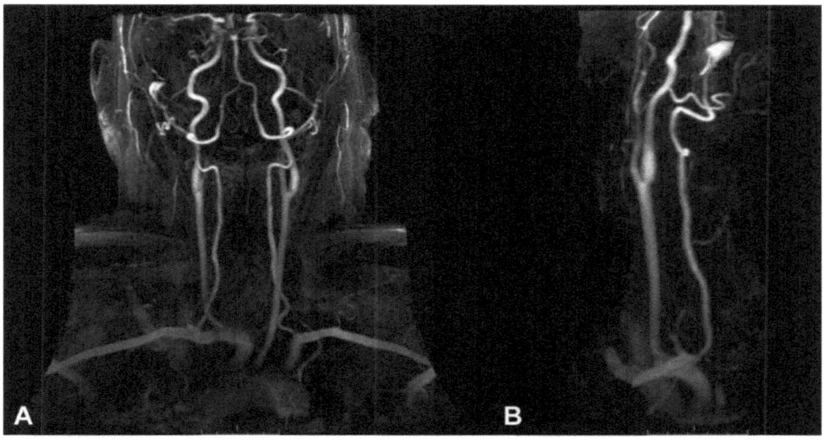

Fig. 9.17. Contrast-enhanced magnetic resonance angiography of the neck.

reconstructed in a variety of maximal-intensity projection (MIP) formats. Lesion detection is typically maximized using a combined review of "raw" data and MIP reformations. Several different methods have been used for measuring the degree of stenosis –NASCET, ECST, and minimal residual lumen size. When comparing these methods for CE-MRA and DSA, the NASCET criteria are performed most consistently between the examinations and therefore is the standard method of assessing CE-MRA images (U-King-Im et al., 2004c).

Safety

The major safety issues related to MRA include contraindications to gadolinium-based contrast materials and general MRI issues, including metallic foreign bodies, claustrophobia, and patient issues related to remaining motionless during the imaging procedure. Contraindications to gadolinium-based contrast materials include a history of anaphylactic reaction upon prior administration and renal failure. The concern for patients with poor renal function is a reaction called nephrogenic systemic fibrosis, which is exclusively seen in patients with glomerular filtration rate <15 mL/min/1.73 m^2. At our institution, patients in acute or chronic renal insufficiency with glomerular filtration rate <30 mL/min/1.73 m^2 must receive clearance from nephrology before receiving gadolinium-based contrast materials. In these cases, the diagnostic information must be considered essential and not available from noncontrast-enhanced MRI.

Limitations and interpretation pitfalls

In all MRI, patient motion (including swallowing and vessel pulsation) and flow-related signal drop-out in regions of turbulence or vortex flow can degrade image quality. Although CE-MRA may improve flow-related enhancement, turbulence, and susceptibility effects from motion, subclavian steal (and other high-flow shunts), metallic stents and metal continue to be a limiting factors in the assessment of carotid artery stenosis (Fig. 9.18).

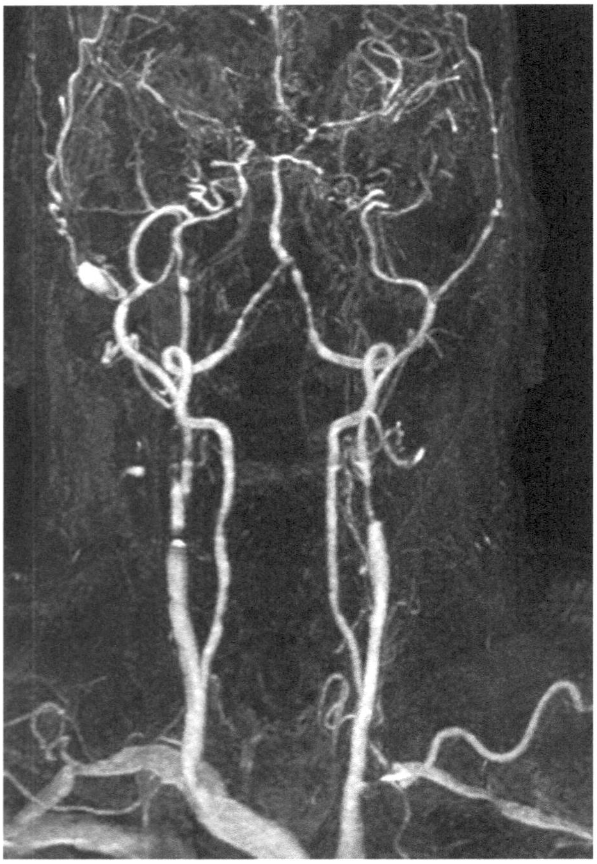

Fig. 9.18. Gadolinium-enhanced magnetic resonance angiography of the neck demonstrating multiple areas of loss of signal in the proximal and distal margins of the bilateral internal carotid artery stents. This is likely artifact secondary to susceptibility blooming.

Overestimation of stenosis and drop-out artifacts

Pitfalls in MRA evaluation of extracranial carotid disease include overestimation of stenosis and inability to discriminate between subtotal and complete arterial occlusion.

TOF-MRA, because it is dependent on the flow of freshly magnetized blood into the volume being imaged, is highly susceptible to conditions that disrupt laminar flow. Also, it is unreliable for distinguishing complete occlusion and hairline lumen because of signal-intensity drop-out artifacts. Vascular areas of signal-intensity drop-out are found in approximately 15% of all 2D-TOF MRA studies. The presence of these signal intensity drop-outs is highly correlated with severe (>70%) ICA stenosis. Another artifact that decreases the accuracy of TOF-MRA is "in-plane" flow-related signal drop-out, which occurs with tortuous vessels that are not perpendicular to the imaging plane.

Overestimation of carotid artery narrowing on CE-MRA can result from the dephasing artifacts along the margin of the lumen (which become exaggerated in areas of tight narrowing), the signal-intensity threshold used to create the MIPs, and the section thickness causing partial volume-averaging effect (Randoux et al., 2001; Cosottini et al., 2003; Babiarz et al., 2007) (Fig. 9.19).

Subclavian steal

Several studies have shown the effectiveness of MRA for diagnosis of SSS (Turjman et al., 1992; Flynn et al., 1993; Van Grimberge et al., 2000). Several MRA techniques are able to demonstrate the retrograde flow in the VA. These include 2D-TOF MRI with a selective presaturation pulse applied first above and then below the volume of interest. Moreover, phase-contrast MRI can be useful to detect reversal of flow, but there are issues related to susceptibility or aliasing effects. 3D CE-MRA is now commonly used to evaluate the proximal aortic arch vessels and the VAs. However, while this technique can be used to evaluate the anatomy of the VAs and to assess stenosis and occlusion, it cannot reliably be used to directly determine flow direction (Wu et al., 2005). CE-MRA can accurately demonstrate the anatomic relationships of the vascular structures in association with the flow reversal visible on 2D-TOF MRA (Van Grimberge et al., 2000).

Stent

Metallic-related artifacts related to the stent can hamper the use of MRA, despite improvement in stent design, stent materials, and MRI parameters. Knowledge of

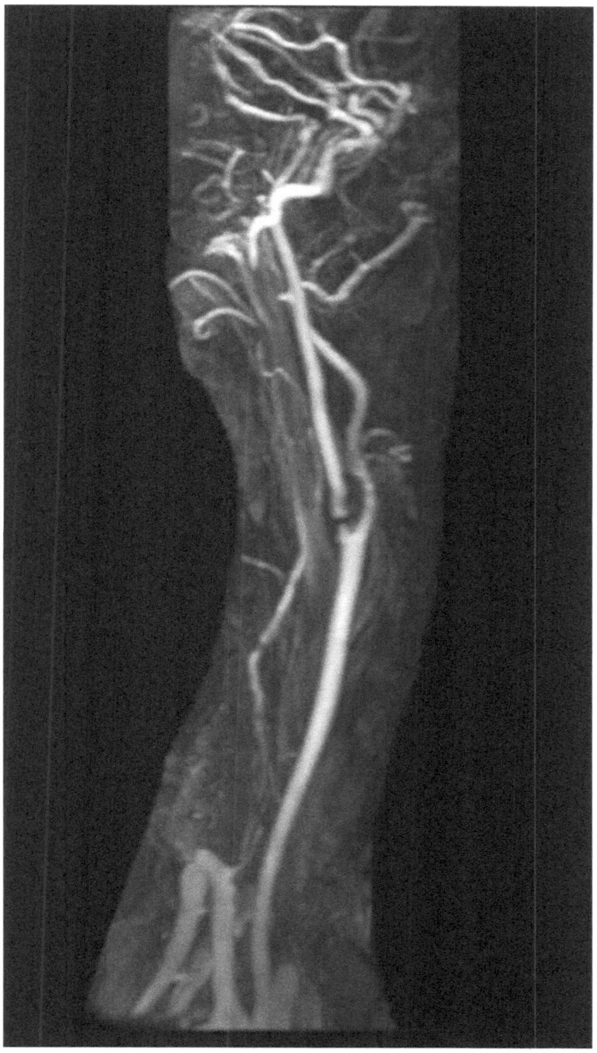

Fig. 9.19. Severe stenosis of the proximal internal carotid artery, with intravoxel dephasing (signal loss) secondary to the critical lesion.

the degree of signal intensity reduction and artificial lumen narrowing within vascular stents is essential to differentiate between artifact and stenosis. Stent geometry, the relative orientation to the magnetic field, and alloy composition influence signal intensity alteration within the stent lumen (Lenhart et al., 2000). Thus far, nitinol- and tantalum-based stents have shown the least artifacts in both *in vitro* and *in vivo* experiments (Schürmann et al., 1999; Klemm et al., 2000; Meyer et al., 2000). Moreover, the commercially available platinum-based balloon-expandable stents allow assessment of luminal patency on CE-MRA using standard sequences. Stent-induced artifacts resulting in luminal narrowing do not reach a degree that would be considered hemodynamically significant (Hagspiel et al., 2005). However, CTA and DUS are to be preferred to MRA for surveillance of carotid in-stent restenosis (Goldman et al., 2006).

Metal

Local magnetic field inhomogeneity caused by metal can degrade the image quality of MRA. Attention is necessary in evaluating MRA because the recorded signal is based on flow characteristics and does not display necessarily "true" anatomy. Dephasing artifacts related to local magnetic field inhomogeneity can cause signal intensity that can mimic either focal flow or occlusion. If the reconstructed MR angiograms show arterial stenosis, the source images must be viewed (Kuta et al., 1995). The source images may show less stenosis than the MIP. When a discrepancy is identified between the source images and the MIP reconstructions, it is recommended to analyze the patient history, and comparison examinations should be performed to evaluate for artifact-causing material such as vascular clips, bullet fragments, or shunt tube joints.

FUTURE OF IMAGING

Current imaging research is focused on developing new techniques that may lead to earlier and more specific diagnosis, and will enable individualized patient-centered diagnosis and therapy. Also, these techniques may help in detecting morphologic features of carotid atheroma, which might add further prognostic information to luminal stenosis. Recent advancement in MR involves the incorporation of higher-field strengths. Imaging at 7 T affords advantages in signal-to-noise ratio and image contrast and resolution; however, these benefits require the realization of proper coils to capture the images, and it is currently used in research studies (Metcalf et al., 2010). MRI at 7 T for brain imaging has demonstrated relevant diagnostic benefits for brain tumors, cerebral malformations, Parkinson's disease, and multiple sclerosis. In 2012, Madai et al. investigated the role of ultrahigh-field MRI at 7 T for stroke imaging in comparison with imaging at 3 T. They demonstrated that 7 T imaging for stroke provides improved spatial resolution, which helps to reveal more anatomic details and pathophysiologic characteristics of the ischemic lesions and peri-infarct alterations as well as vessel morphology. 7 T TOF MRA allows the detection of much finer vessel branches, such as the lenticulostriate arteries. Moreover, it can be helpful in identifying aneurysms smaller than 3 mm, which may not always be detected with TOF MRA at lower field strength (Moser et al., 2011). However, MR at 7 T has several limitations. It requires longer acquisition times and is really susceptible to motion (T2 imaging), and this problem needs to be solved before clinical use (Madai et al., 2012). As for patient safety and comfort, it has been reported that 7 T is correlated with increased number of side effects (i.e., vertigo and anxiety) than 1.5 T, although 7 T is tolerated by the majority of subjects (Theysohn et al., 2007) (Fig. 9.20).

Another promising imaging technique is PET combined with CT or MRI. ^{18}F-fluorodeoxyglucose (FDG) is a PET contrast agent that competes with glucose for uptake into metabolically active cells, where it accumulates in proportion to metabolic activity. Rudd (2002)

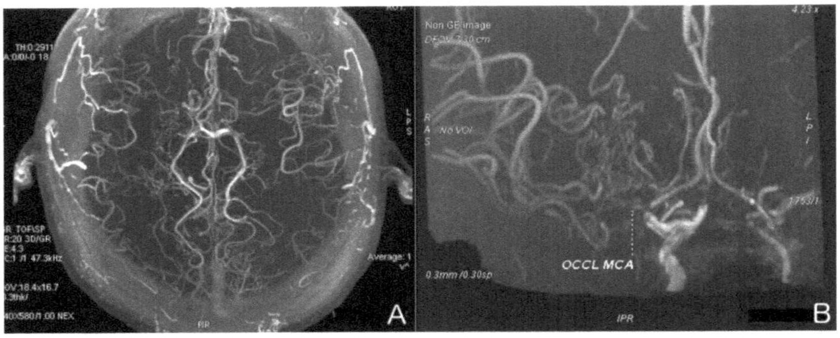

Fig. 9.20. (**A, B**) Three-dimensional time-of-flight magnetic resonance angiography of the brain, with a 7 T scanner in a patient with moyamoya. Multiple anastomosis and neovascularization are noted.

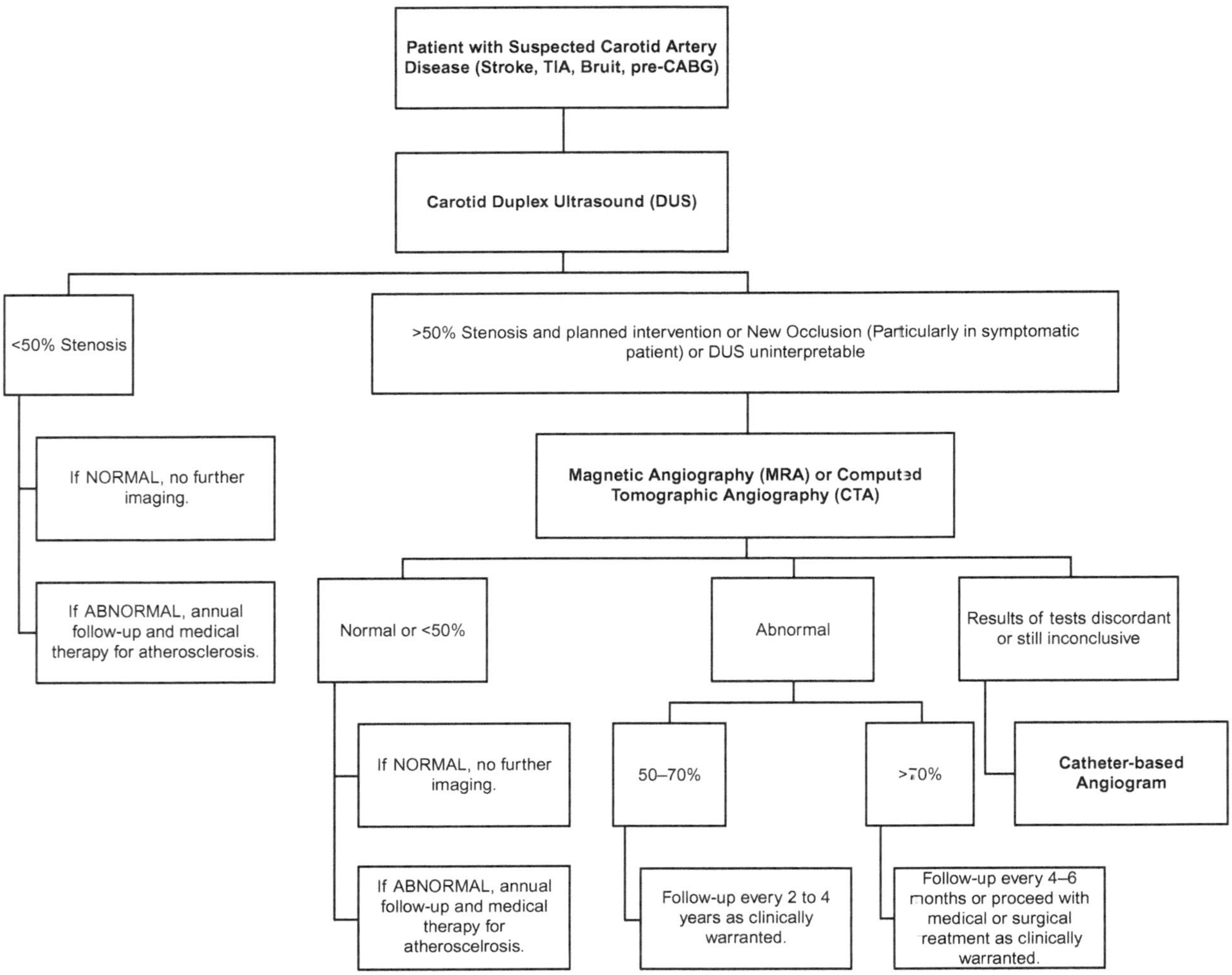

Fig. 9.21. Imaging flow chart for carotid disease. TIA, transient ischemic attack; CABG, coronary artery bypass graft.

demonstrated that ^{18}FDG accumulates within carotid-artery atherosclerotic plaques analyzed with PET/CT, with significantly higher uptake in symptomatic lesions than in contralateral asymptomatic arteries. Furthermore, they noted that the degree of arterial ^{18}FDG uptake is associated with high blood levels of several systemic inflammatory biomarkers, including those from the matrix metalloproteinase family, and strong trends among both the interleukin group and C-reactive protein (Rudd et al., 2009). Combined use of FDG-PET with MRI is also possible to provide both structural and metabolic information about the plaque status (Davies et al., 2005). Tahara et al. (2006) highlighted the ability of ^{18}F-FDG-PET to monitor the therapeutic effect of statins on the stabilization of vulnerable atherosclerotic plaques, which are of potential use in future antiatheroma drug trials.

Ultrahigh-field MRI and PET combined with CT or MRI and now robust enough for clinical practice, but further clinical data, possibly through large randomized controlled trials, are needed before they can be routinely implemented and accepted in clinical practice.

CONCLUSION

Over recent years, noninvasive imaging of the carotid arteries has improved significantly. DUS and CTA or MRA each measures different biologic variables. Initial imaging of the carotid artery is with high-quality DUS. If abnormal, MRA or CTA may be helpful in adding further information in the diagnosis and in planning the appropriate therapeutic strategies. In our experience, if the findings based on two noninvasive tests (any combination of DUS, MRA, or CTA) are contradictory or inconclusive, DSA is required for a definitive diagnosis (Fig. 9.21).

In conclusion, the combined use of these noninvasive techniques and the avoidance of the above-described imaging pitfalls have enabled achievement of high diagnostics quality and cost-efficiency in the diagnosis of carotid artery disease.

References

Aaslid R, Markwalder TM, Nornes H (1982). Noninvasive transcranial Doppler ultrasound recording of flow velocity in basal cerebral arteries. J Neurosurg 57: 769–774.

Aaslid R, Huber P, Nornes H (1984). Evaluation of cerebrovascular spasm with transcranial Doppler ultrasound. J Neurosurg 60: 37–41.

Aaslid R, Lindegaard KF, Sorteberg W et al. (1989). Cerebral autoregulation dynamics in humans. Stroke 20: 45–52.

Aaslid R, Newell DW, Stooss R et al. (1991). Assessment of cerebral autoregulation dynamics from simultaneous arterial and venous transcranial Doppler recordings in humans. Stroke 22: 1148–1154.

AbuRahma AF (2002). Carotid plaque ultrasonic heterogeneity and severity of stenosis. Stroke 33: 1772–1775.

AbuRahma AF, Abu-Halimah S, Bensenhaver J et al. (2008). Optimal carotid duplex velocity criteria for defining the severity of carotid in-stent restenosis. J Vasc Surg 48: 589–594.

Armstrong PA, Bandyk DF, Johnson BL et al. (2007). Duplex scan surveillance after carotid angioplasty and stenting: a rational definition of stent stenosis. J Vasc Surg 46: 460–466.

Arquizan C, Trinquart L, Touboul PJ et al. (2011). Restenosis is more frequent after carotid stenting than after endarterectomy: the EVA-3S study. Stroke 42: 1015–1020.

Babiarz L, Astor B, Mohamed M et al. (2007). Comparison of gadolinium-enhanced cardiovascular magnetic resonance angiography with high-resolution black blood cardiovascular magnetic resonance for assessing carotid artery stenosis. J Cardiovasc Magn Reson 9: 63–70.

Babiarz LS, Romero JM, Murphy EK et al. (2009). Contrast-enhanced MR angiography is not more accurate than unenhanced 2D time-of-flight MR angiography for determining $>=70\%$ internal carotid artery stenosis. Am J Neuroradiol 30: 761–768.

Babikian VL, Wechsler LR, Higashida RT (2003). Ultrasound images of cerebrovascular disease. In: VL Babikian, LR Wechsler, RT Higashida (Eds.), Imaging Cerebrovascular Disease, Butterworth Heinemann, Philadelphia, pp. 3–35.

Bae KT, Tran HQ, Heiken JP (2000). Multiphasic injection method for uniform prolonged vascular enhancement at CT angiography: pharmacokinetic analysis and experimental porcine model. Radiology 216: 872–880.

Bahner ML, Bengel A, Brix G et al. (2005). Improved vascular opacification in cerebral computed tomography angiography with 80 kVp. Invest Radiol 40: 229–234.

Barnett HJM, Taylor DW, Eliasziw M et al. (1998). Benefit of carotid endarterectomy in patients with symptomatic moderate or severe stenosis. N Engl J Med 339: 1415–1425.

Bishop CC, Powell S, Rutt D et al. (1986). Transcranial Doppler measurement of middle cerebral artery blood flow velocity: a validation study. Stroke 17: 913–915.

Bonati LH, Ederle J, McCabe DJ et al. (2009). Long-term risk of carotid restenosis in patients randomly assigned to endovascular treatment or endarterectomy in the Carotid and Vertebral Artery Transluminal Angioplasty Study (CAVATAS): long-term follow-up of a randomised trial. Lancet Neurol 8: 908–917.

Borisch I, Horn M, Butz B et al. (2003). Preoperative evaluation of carotid artery stenosis: comparison of contrast-enhanced MR angiography and duplex sonography with digital subtraction angiography. AJNR Am J Neuroradiol 24: 1117–1122.

Brandt T, Knauth M, Wildermuth S et al. (1999). CT angiography and Doppler sonography for emergency assessment in acute basilar artery ischemia. Stroke 30: 606–612.

Brott TG, Halperin JL, Abbara S et al. (2011). 2011 ASA/ACCF/AHA/AANN/AANS/ACR/ASNR/CNS/SAIP/SCAI/SIR/SNIS/SVM/SVS Guideline on the management of patients with extracranial carotid and vertebral artery disease. J Am Coll Cardiol 57: e16–e94.

Carr JC, Shaibani A, Russell E et al. (2001). Contrast-enhanced magnetic resonance angiography of the carotid circulation. Top Magn Reson Imaging 12: 349–357.

Chahwan S, Miller MT, Pigott JP et al. (2007). Carotid artery velocity characteristics after carotid artery angioplasty and stenting. J Vasc Surg 45: 523–526.

Chi Y-W, White CJ, Woods TC et al. (2007). Ultrasound velocity criteria for carotid in-stent restenosis. Cathet Cardiovasc Interv 69: 349–354.

Christiansen C (2005). X-ray contrast media – an overview. Toxicology 209: 185–187.

Corti R, Ferrari C, Roberti M et al. (1998). Spiral computed tomography: a novel diagnostic approach for investigation of the extracranial cerebral arteries and its complementary role in duplex ultrasonography. Circulation 98: 984–989.

Cosottini M, Pingitore A, Puglioli M et al. (2003). Contrast-enhanced three-dimensional magnetic resonance angiography of atherosclerotic internal carotid stenosis as the noninvasive imaging modality in revascularization decision making. Stroke 34: 660–664.

Crouse III JR, Raichlen JS, Riley WA et al. (2007). Effect of rosuvastatin on progression of carotid intima-media thickness in low-risk individuals with subclinical atherosclerosis. JAMA 297: 1344–1353.

Cumbie T, Rosero EB, Valentine RJ et al. (2008). Utility and accuracy of duplex ultrasonography in evaluating in-stent restenosis after carotid stenting. Am J Surg 196: 623–628.

Dahl A, Lindegaard KF, Russell D et al. (1992). A comparison of transcranial Doppler and cerebral blood flow studies to assess cerebral vasoreactivity. Stroke 23: 15–19.

Davies JR, Rudd JHF, Fryer TD et al. (2005). Identification of culprit lesions after transient ischemic attack by combined ^{18}F fluorodeoxyglucose positron-emission tomography and high-resolution magnetic resonance imaging. Stroke 36: 2642–2647.

Diehl RR (2002). Cerebral autoregulation studies in clinical practice. Eur J Ultrasound 16: 31–36.

Eckstein HH, Ringleb P, Allenberg JR et al. (2008). Results of the Stent-Protected Angioplasty versus Carotid Endarterectomy (SPACE) study to treat symptomatic stenoses at 2 years: a multinational, prospective, randomised trial. Lancet Neurol 7: 893–902.

Executive Committee for the Asymptomatic Carotid Atherosclerosis Study (1995). Endarterectomy for asymptomatic carotid artery stenosis. JAMA 273 (18): 1421–1428.

Ezzeddine MA, Lev MH, McDonald CT et al. (2002). CT angiography with whole brain perfused blood volume imaging: added clinical value in the assessment of acute stroke. Stroke 33: 959–966.

Feldmann E, Wilterdink JL, Kosinski A et al. (2007). The Stroke Outcomes and Neuroimaging of Intracranial Atherosclerosis (SONIA) trial. Neurology 68: 2099–2106.

Finn AV, Kolodgie FD, Virmani R (2010). Correlation between carotid intimal/medial thickness and atherosclerosis: a point of view from pathology. Arterioscler Thromb Vasc Biol 30: 177–181.

Flynn PD, Delany DJ, Gray HH (1993). Magnetic resonance angiography in subclavian steal syndrome. Br Heart J 70: 193–194.

Fülesdi B, Limburg M, Bereczki D et al. (1997). Impairment of cerebrovascular reactivity in long-term type 1 diabetes. Diabetes 46: 1840–1845.

Furst G, Saleh A, Wenserski F et al. (1999). Reliability and validity of noninvasive imaging of internal carotid artery pseudo-occlusion. Stroke 30: 1444–1449.

Gahn G, Richter A, Bourquain H et al. (1999). Cerebrovascular reserve before and after vertebral artery angioplasty. AJNR Am J Neuroradiol 20: 785–786.

Goldman CK, Morshedi-Meibodi A, White CJ et al. (2006). Surveillance imaging for carotid in-stent restenosis. Cathet Cardiovasc Interv 67: 302–308.

Grant EG, Tessler FN, Perrella RR (1989). Clinical Doppler imaging. AJR Am J Roentgenol 152: 707–717.

Grant EG, Duerinckx AJ, Saden El SM et al. (2000). Ability to use duplex US to quantify internal carotid arterial stenoses: fact or fiction? Radiology 214: 247–252.

Griffin M, Nicolaides A, Tyllis T et al. (2009). Carotid and femoral arterial wall changes and the prevalence of clinical cardiovascular disease. Vasc Med 14: 227–232.

Gronholdt MLM, Nordestgaard BG, Wiebe BM et al. (1998). Echo-lucency of computerized ultrasound images of carotid atherosclerotic plaques are associated with increased levels of triglyceride-rich lipoproteins as well as increased plaque lipid content. Circulation 97: 34–40.

Hagspiel KD, Leung DA, Nandalur KR et al. (2005). Contrast-enhanced MR angiography at 1.5 T after implantation of platinum stents: in vitro and in vivo comparison with conventional stent designs. Am J Roentgenol 184: 288–294.

Halliday A, Mansfield A, Marro J et al. (2004). MRC Asymptomatic Carotid Surgery Trial (ACST) Collaborative Group. Prevention of disabling and fatal strokes by successful carotid endarterectomy in patients without recent neurological symptoms: randomised controlled trial. Lancet 363 (9420): 1491–1502.

Heck D (2009). Incidence and time course of carotid in-stent restenosis in a consecutive series of 295 patients. J NeuroInterv Surg 1: 44–47.

Henderson RD, Steinman DA, Eliasziw M et al. (2000). Effect of contralateral carotid artery stenosis on carotid ultrasound velocity measurements. Stroke 31: 2636–2640.

Hirai T, Korogi Y, Ono K et al. (2002). Prospective evaluation of suspected stenoocclusive disease of the intracranial artery: combined MR angiography and CT angiography compared with digital subtraction angiography. AJNR Am J Neuroradiol 23: 93–101.

Jauch EC, Saver JL, Adams HP et al. (2013). Guidelines for the early management of patients with acute ischemic stroke: a guideline for healthcare professionals from the American Heart Association/American Stroke Association. Stroke 44: 870–947.

Josephson SA, Bryant SO, Mak HK et al. (2004). Evaluation of carotid stenosis using CT angiography in the initial evaluation of stroke and TIA. Neurology 63: 457–460.

Juonala M, Kahonen M, Laitinen T et al. (2008). Effect of age and sex on carotid intima-media thickness, elasticity and brachial endothelial function in healthy adults: the Cardiovascular Risk in Young Finns Study. Eur Heart J 29: 1198–1206.

King A, Markus HS (2009). Doppler embolic signals in cerebrovascular disease and prediction of stroke risk: a systematic review and meta-analysis. Stroke 40: 3711–3717.

King A, Serena J, Bornstein NM et al. (2011). Does impaired cerebrovascular reactivity predict stroke risk in asymptomatic carotid stenosis? A prospective substudy of the asymptomatic carotid emboli study. Stroke 42: 1550–1555.

Klemm T, Duda S, Machann J et al. (2000). MR imaging in the presence of vascular stents: a systematic assessment of artifacts for various stent orientations, sequence types, and field strengths. J Magn Reson Imaging 12: 606–615.

Kliewer MA, Hertzberg BS, Kim DH et al. (2000). Vertebral artery Doppler waveform changes indicating subclavian steal physiology. AJR Am J Roentgenol 174: 815–819.

Kluytmans M, van der Grond J, van Everdingen KJ et al. (1999). Cerebral hemodynamics in relation to patterns of collateral flow. Stroke 30: 1432–1439.

Kuta AJ, Smoker WR, Cole TJ et al. (1995). MR angiography artifact due to metal joint of ventriculoperitoneal shunt mimicking severe carotid stenosis. J Magn Reson Imaging 5: 125–126.

Lal BK, Hobson II RW, Goldstein J et al. (2004). Carotid artery stenting: is there a need to revise ultrasound velocity criteria? J Vasc Surg 39: 58–66.

Lal BK, Kaperonis EA, Cuadra S et al. (2007). Patterns of in-stent restenosis after carotid artery stenting: classification and implications for long-term outcome. J Vasc Surg 46: 833–840.

Lal BK, Hobson II RW, Tofighi B et al. (2008). Duplex ultrasound velocity criteria for the stented carotid artery. J Vasc Surg 47: 63–73.

Lal BK, Beach KW, Roubin GS et al. (2012). Restenosis after carotid artery stenting and endarterectomy: a secondary analysis of CREST, a randomised controlled trial. Lancet Neurol [online] 11: 755–763.

Leclerc X, Gauvrit JY, Nicol L et al. (1999). Contrast-enhanced MR angiography of the craniocervical vessels: a review. Neuroradiology 41: 867–874.

Lee VH, Brown RD, Mandrekar JN et al. (2006). Incidence and outcome of cervical artery dissection: a population-based study. Neurology 67: 1809–1812.

Lenhart M, Völk M, Manke C et al. (2000). Stent appearance at contrast-enhanced MR angiography: in vitro examination with 14 stents. Radiology 217: 173–178.

Lev MH, Farkas J, Rodriguez VR et al. (2001). CT angiography in the rapid triage of patients with hyperacute stroke to intraarterial thrombolysis: accuracy in the detection of large vessel thrombus. J Comput Assist Tomogr 25: 520–528.

Lev MH, Romero JM, Goodman DNF et al. (2003). Total occlusion versus hairline residual lumen of the internal carotid arteries: accuracy of single section helical CT angiography. AJNR Am J Neuroradiol 24: 1123–1129.

Levy EI, Hanel RA, Lau T et al. (2005). Frequency and management of recurrent stenosis after carotid artery stent implantation. J Neurosurg 102: 29–37.

Lindegaard KF, Nornes H, Bakke SJ et al. (1989). Cerebral vasospasm diagnosis by means of angiography and blood velocity measurements. Acta Neurochir 100: 12–24.

Linton OW, Mettler FANational Council on Radiation Protection and Measurements (2003). National conference on dose reduction in CT, with an emphasis on pediatric patients. AJR 321–329.

Lira DA, Romero JM, Gonzalez RG et al. (2014). Application of different acquisition techniques for radiation dose lowering on neck CTA studies. In: RSNA 99th Annual Meeting, Available online at: http://www.rsna.org/.

Lorenz MW, Markus HS, Bots ML et al. (2007). Prediction of clinical cardiovascular events with carotid intima-media thickness: a systematic review and meta-analysis. Circulation 115: 459–467.

Madai VI, Samson-Himmelstjerna von FC, Bauer M et al. (2012). Ultrahigh-field MRI in human ischemic stroke – a 7 Tesla study. PLoS One 7: e37631.

Maldonado TS (2007). What are current preprocedure imaging requirements for carotid artery stenting and carotid endarterectomy: have magnetic resonance angiography and computed tomographic angiography made a difference? Semin Vasc Surg 20: 205–215.

Markus H, Cullinane M (2001). Severely impaired cerebrovascular reactivity predicts stroke and TIA risk in patients with carotid artery stenosis and occlusion. Brain 124: 457–467.

Markus HS, Harrison MJ (1992). Estimation of cerebrovascular reactivity using transcranial Doppler, including the use of breath-holding as the vasodilatory stimulus. Stroke 23: 668–673.

Markus HS, King A, Shipley M et al. (2010). Asymptomatic embolisation for prediction of stroke in the Asymptomatic Carotid Emboli Study (ACES): a prospective observational study. Lancet Neurol 9: 663–671.

Mauriello A, Sangiorgi GM, Virmani R et al. (2010). A pathobiologic link between risk factors profile and morphological markers of carotid instability. Atherosclerosis 208: 572–580.

Metcalf M, Xu D, Okuda DT et al. (2010). High-resolution phased-array MRI of the human brain at 7 Tesla: initial experience in multiple sclerosis patients. J Neuroimaging 20: 141–147.

Meyer JM, Buecker A, Schuermann K et al. (2000). MR evaluation of stent patency: in vitro test of 22 metallic stents and the possibility of determining their patency by MR angiography. Invest Radiol 35: 739–746.

Moser E, Stahlberg F, Ladd ME et al. (2011). 7-T MR-from research to clinical applications? NMR Biomed 25: 695–716.

Murray CJ, Lopez AD (1997a). Global mortality, disability, and the contribution of risk factors: Global Burden of Disease Study. Lancet 349: 1436–1442.

Murray CJL, Lopez AD (1997b). Mortality by cause for eight regions of the world: Global Burden of Disease Study. Lancet 349: 1269–1276.

Mustert BR, Williams DM, Prince MR (1998). In vitro model of arterial stenosis: correlation of MR signal dephasing and trans-stenotic pressure gradients. Magn Reson Imaging 16: 301–310.

Naqvi J, Yap KH, Ahmad G et al. (2013). Transcranial Doppler ultrasound: a review of the physical principles and major applications in critical care. Int J Vasc Med 2013: 1–13.

Nederkoorn PJ, van der Graaf Y, Eikelboom BC et al. (2002). Time-of-flight MR angiography of carotid artery stenosis: does a flow void represent severe stenosis? AJNR Am J Neuroradiol 23: 1779–1784.

Nicoletto HA, Burkman MH (2009a). Transcranial Doppler series part II: performing a transcranial Doppler. Am J Electroneurodiagnostic Technol 49: 14–27.

Nicoletto HA, Burkman MH (2009b). Transcranial Doppler series part III: interpretation. Am J Electroneurodiagnostic Technol 49: 244–259.

Patel SG, Collie DA, Wardlaw JM et al. (2002). Outcome, observer reliability, and patient preferences if CTA, MRA, or Doppler ultrasound were used, individually or together, instead of digital subtraction angiography before carotid endarterectomy. J Neurol Neurosurg Psychiatr 73: 21–28.

Peters SA, Ruijter HMD, Bots ML (2011). Attenuation of rate of change in carotid intima-media thickness by lipid-modifying drugs: impact on clinical outcomes. Am J Cardiovasc Drugs 11: 253–263.

Peterson BG, Longo GM, Kibbe MR et al. (2005a). Duplex ultrasound remains a reliable test even after carotid stenting. Ann Vasc Surg 19: 793–797.

Peterson BG, Longo GM, Kibbe MR et al. (2005b). Duplex ultrasound remains a reliable test even after carotid stenting. Ann Vasc Surg 19: 793–797.

Pickett CA, Jackson JL, Hemann BA et al. (2010). Carotid bruits and cerebrovascular disease risk: a meta-analysis. Stroke 41: 2295–2302.

Pizzolato R, Hirsch JA, Romero JM (2014). Imaging challenges of carotid artery in-stent restenosis. J NeuroInterv Surg 1: 32–41.

Provenzale JM (1995). Dissection of the internal carotid and vertebral arteries: imaging features. AJR Am J Roentgenol 165: 1099–1104.

Radiology Accountable Care Organizations (2012). ACR–AIUM–SRU Practice guideline for the performance of an ultrasound examination of the extracranial cerebrovascular system. J Ultrasound Med 31: 145–154. pp. 1–5.

Randomised trial of endarterectomy for recently symptomatic carotid stenosis: final results of the MRC European Carotid Surgery Trial (1998). Lancet 351: 1379–1387.

Randoux B, Marro B, Koskas F et al. (2001). Carotid artery stenosis: prospective comparison of CT, three-dimensional gadolinium-enhanced MR, and conventional angiography. Radiology 220: 179–185.

Remonda L, Senn P, Barth A et al. (2002). Contrast-enhanced 3D MR angiography of the carotid artery: comparison with conventional digital subtraction angiography. AJNR Am J Neuroradiol 23: 213–219.

Reynolds PS, Greenberg JP, Lien LM et al. (2002). Ophthalmic artery flow direction on color flow duplex imaging is highly specific for severe carotid stenosis. J Neuroimaging 12: 5–8.

Rigamonti A, Ackery A, Baker AJ (2008). Transcranial Doppler monitoring in subarachnoid hemorrhage: a critical tool in critical care. Can J Anaesth 55: 112–123.

Ringelstein EB, Sievers C, Ecker S et al. (1988). Noninvasive assessment of CO_2-induced cerebral vasomotor response in normal individuals and patients with internal carotid artery occlusions. Stroke 19: 963–969.

Romero JM (2005). CT angiography source image evaluation for stroke. Semin Ultrasound CT MRI 26: 387–393.

Romero JM, Lev MH, Chan S-T et al. (2002). US of neurovascular occlusive disease: interpretive pearls and pitfalls. Radiographics 22: 1165–1176.

Romero JM, Ackerman RH, Dault NA et al. (2005). Noninvasive evaluation of carotid artery stenosis: indications, strategies, and accuracy. Neuroimaging Clin N Am 15: 351–365.

Romero JM, Babiarz LS, Forero NP et al. (2009). Arterial wall enhancement overlying carotid plaque on CT angiography correlates with symptoms in patients with high grade stenosis. Stroke 40: 1894–1896.

Rothwell PM (2004). Carotid endarterectomy for asymptomatic carotid stenosis: asymptomatic carotid surgery trial. Stroke 35: 2425–2427.

Rothwell PM, Eliasziw M, Gutnikov SA et al. (2003). Analysis of pooled data from the randomised controlled trials of endarterectomy for symptomatic carotid stenosis. Lancet 361: 107–116.

Rouleau PA, Huston J, Gilbertson J et al. (1999). Carotid artery tandem lesions: frequency of angiographic detection and consequences for endarterectomy. AJNR Am J Neuroradiol 20: 621–625.

Rudd JHF (2002). Imaging atherosclerotic plaque inflammation with [18 F]-fluorodeoxyglucose positron emission tomography. Circulation 105: 2708–2711.

Rudd JHF, Myers KS, Bansilal S et al. (2009). Relationships among regional arterial inflammation, calcification, risk factors, and biomarkers: a prospective fluorodeoxyglucose positron-emission tomography/computed tomography imaging study. Circ Cardiovasc Imaging 2: 107–115.

Sacco RL (2001). Clinical practice. Extracranial carotid stenosis. N Engl J Med 345: 1113–1118.

Schürmann K, Vorwerk D, Bücker A et al. (1999). Magnetic resonance angiography of nonferromagnetic iliac artery stents and stent-grafts: a comparative study in sheep. Cardiovasc Intervent Radiol 22: 394–402.

Setacci C, Chisci E, Setacci F et al. (2008). Grading carotid intrastent restenosis: a 6-year follow-up study. Stroke 39: 1189–1196.

Shrier DA, Tanaka H, Numaguchi Y et al. (1997). CT angiography in the evaluation of acute stroke. AJNR Am J Neuroradiol 18: 1011–1020.

Silvestrini M, Troisi E, Matteis M et al. (1996). Transcranial Doppler assessment of cerebrovascular reactivity in symptomatic and asymptomatic severe carotid stenosis. Stroke 27: 1970–1973.

Sliwka U, Job FP, Wissuwa D et al. (1995). Occurrence of transcranial Doppler high-intensity transient signals in patients with potential cardiac sources of embolism. A prospective study. Stroke 26: 2067–2070.

Stanziale SF, Wholey MH, Boules TN et al. (2005). Determining in-stent stenosis of carotid arteries by duplex ultrasound criteria. J Endovasc Ther 12: 346–353.

Staub D, Patel MB, Tibrewala A et al. (2009). Vasa vasorum and plaque neovascularization on contrast-enhanced carotid ultrasound imaging correlates with cardiovascular disease and past cardiovascular events. Stroke 41: 41–47.

Sturzenegger M, Mattle HP, Rivoir A et al. (1995). Ultrasound findings in carotid artery dissection analysis of 43 Patients. Neurology 45: 691–698.

Suematsu Y, Nakano K, Sasako Y et al. (2000). Strategies for CABG patients with carotid artery disease and perioperative neurological complications. Heart Vessels 15: 129–134.

Sztajzel R, Momjian S, Momjian-Mayor I et al. (2005). Stratified gray-scale median analysis and color mapping of the carotid plaque: correlation with endarterectomy specimen histology of 28 patients. Stroke 36: 741–745.

Tahara N, Kai H, Ishibashi M et al. (2006). Simvastatin attenuates plaque inflammation. J Am Coll Cardiol 48: 1825–1831.

Thanvi B (2005). Carotid and vertebral artery dissection syndromes. Postgrad Med J 81: 383–388.

Theysohn JM, Maderwald S, Kraff O et al. (2007). Subjective acceptance of 7 Tesla MRI for human imaging. Magn Reson Mater Phy 21: 63–72.

Thurston J (2010). NCRP Report No. 160: Ionizing radiation exposure of the population of the United States. Phys Med Biol 55 (20): 6327.

Timaran CH, Rosero EB, Valentine RJ et al. (2007). Accuracy and utility of three-dimensional contrast-enhanced magnetic resonance angiography in planning carotid stenting. J Vasc Surg 46: 257–264.

Turjman F, Tournut P, Baldy-Porcher C et al. (1992). Demonstration of subclavian steal by MR angiography. J Comput Assist Tomogr 16: 756–759.

U-King-Im JM, Hollingworth W, Trivedi RA et al. (2004a). Contrast-enhanced MR angiography vs intra-arterial digital subtraction angiography for carotid imaging: activity-based cost analysis. Eur Radiol 14: 730–735.

U-King-Im JM, Trivedi RA, Graves MJ et al. (2004b). Contrast-enhanced MR angiography for carotid disease: diagnostic and potential clinical impact. Neurology 62: 1282–1290.

U-King-Im JMKS, Trivedi RA, Cross JJ et al. (2004c). Measuring carotid stenosis on contrast-enhanced magnetic resonance angiography: diagnostic performance and reproducibility of 3 different methods. Stroke 35: 2083–2088.

Van Grimberge F, Dymarkowski S, Budts W et al. (2000). Role of magnetic resonance in the diagnosis of subclavian steal syndrome. J Magn Reson Imaging 12: 339–342.

Vicenzini E, Giannoni MF, Puccinelli F et al. (2007). Detection of carotid adventitial vasa vasorum and plaque vascularization with ultrasound cadence contrast pulse sequencing technique and echo-contrast agent. Stroke 38: 2841–2843.

Vriens EM, Wieneke GH, Hillen B et al. (2001). Flow redistribution in the major cerebral arteries after carotid endarterectomy: a study with transcranial Doppler scan. YMVA 33: 139–147.

White RP, Markus HS (1997). Impaired dynamic cerebral autoregulation in carotid artery stenosis. Stroke 28: 1340–1344.

Writing Group Members, Roger VL, Go AS et al. (2012). Heart disease and stroke statistics – 2012 update: a report from the American Heart Association. Circulation 125: e2–e220.

Wu C, Zhang J, Ladner CJ et al. (2005). Subclavian steal syndrome: diagnosis with perfusion metrics from contrast-enhanced MR angiographic bolus-timing examination – initial experience. Radiology 235: 927–933.

Yang CW, Carr JC, Futterer SF et al. (2005). Contrast-enhanced MR angiography of the carotid and vertebrobasilar circulations. AJNR Am J Neuroradiol 26: 2095–2101.

Zhou W, Felkai DD, Evans M et al. (2008). Ultrasound criteria for severe in-stent restenosis following carotid artery stenting. J Vasc Surg 47: 74–80.

Zubilewicz T, Wronski J, Bourriez A et al. (2001). Injury in vascular surgery – the intimal hyperplastic response. Med Sci Monit 7: 316.

Handbook of Clinical Neurology, Vol. 135 (3rd series)
Neuroimaging, Part I
J.C. Masdeu and R.G. González, Editors

Chapter 10

Myelography: modern technique and indications

STUART R. POMERANTZ*
Department of Neuroradiology, Massachusetts General Hospital, Boston, MA, USA

Abstract

Myelography describes the instillation of intrathecal contrast media for the imaging evaluation of spinal canal pathology. The technique has evolved with the use of progressively less toxic contrast agents over its 90-year history and the inclusion of advanced image acquisition technology, including both computed tomography (CT) and magnetic resonance imaging (MRI), in addition to plain radiographic projections. The use of myelography for routine evaluation of spinal disease has diminished greatly due to the advent of MRI which has superior soft-tissue contrast and is relatively non-invasive. However, it is still a critical technique for conventional indications, such as spinal stenosis, when MRI is contraindicated or nondiagnostic. It is also recognized as the study of choice for brachial plexus injury, radiation therapy treatment planning, and cerebrospinal fluid (CSF) leak. Modern myelographic procedural technique and a discussion of how it contributes to these current indications will be reviewed in this chapter.

INTRODUCTION

Myelography is the technique of instilling intrathecal contrast media for the imaging evaluation of the spinal canal and its contents for all manner of spinal pathology. The procedure has evolved greatly over its 90-year history, with the development of progressively less toxic contrast agents and the addition to basic radiographic projections of advanced image acquisition technology, including both computed tomography (CT) and magnetic resonance imaging (MRI). Though the phenomenal soft-tissue contrast and relative noninvasiveness of MRI have greatly reduced the role for routine myelographic evaluation of spinal disease, myelography is still a critical technique for evaluating conventional indications, such as spinal stenosis when MRI is contraindicated or nondiagnostic. Moreover, it is recognized as the study of choice for a number of key investigations, including brachial plexus injury, radiation therapy treatment planning, and cerebrospinal fluid (CSF) leak. Modern myelographic procedural technique and a discussion of how it contributes to these current indications will be reviewed in this chapter.

HISTORIC OVERVIEW

Contrast agents

In the early 1920s, the introduction of air into the subarachnoid space for the X-ray evaluation of spinal tumors was first described and shortly followed by the use of radiopaque contrast agents. The positive-contrast technique provided much higher-quality diagnostic information and continues to be our practice today. However, unlike our modern water-soluble contrast agents, the technique, first described by Sicard and Forestier, utilized an oil-based agent, lipiodol, which was slow to absorb, fragmented into globules, and was associated with prolonged pain, acute inflammation, and severe complications, such as chronic adhesive arachnoiditis (Hoeffner et al., 2012). In the 1930s, the presurgical evaluation of ruptured discs and sciatica increased the accepted indications for the procedure. To decrease the associated downsides, it became common practice to dependently collect and drain the injected oil at the conclusion of the procedure. The less viscous contrast agent iophendylate (Pantopaque) was introduced in the 1940s, though issues with nonabsorption and arachnoiditis

*Correspondence to: Stuart R. Pomerantz, MD, MGH Neuroradiology, 55 Fruit Street, Gray 2 B 275, Boston MA 02114, USA. Tel: +1-617-726-8320, E-mail: SPOMERANTZ@PARTNERS.ORG

persisted. Iodinated water-soluble contrast agents, such as methiodal (Abrodil), meglumine iothalamate (Conray), and meglumine iocarmate (Dimer X) became available over the ensuing decades; however, their ionic neurotoxicity was still highly associated with acute and chronic side effects, such as muscle spasm and seizures. Moreover, the serious risk of arachnoiditis persisted until the first nonionic water-soluble contrast medium metrizamide (Amipaque) became available in the 1970s, which significantly reduced this complication. The water-soluble nonionic agents we use today, such as iohexol (Omnipaque) and iopamidol (Isovue), are even less toxic, with an extremely low risk of seizure complications. The most prominent side effect of the modern contrast agents remains headache (Sandow and Donnal, 2005).

Imaging technology

Fluoroscopic guidance for contrast instillation followed by plain radiographic diagnostic examination had been the mainstay of myelography until the 1970s. Then the addition of CT imaging (myelo-CT) added the benefits of cross-sectional imaging to the evaluation of spinal cord and nerve root pathology and is now routine part of myelographic evaluation (Di Chiro and Schellinger, 1976). In the 1980s, the compelling advantages of spinal imaging with MRI, including its noninvasive character, lack of ionizing radiation, and superior soft-tissue characterization, superseded much of the indications for myelography and myelo-CT (Larsson et al., 1989). However, contraindications to MRI have safeguarded the necessity of myelo-CT in the imaging armamentarium. Additionally, advances in CT technology, such as dual-energy CT and new techniques such as dynamic CT myelography, have enlarged the clinical utility of myelo-CT. The continued complementary role of myelo-CT in both common and less common but critical indications will be discussed and illustrated further below.

MYELOGRAPHY – SAFE AND EFFECTIVE TECHNIQUE

Preparation

Up-to-date standard practice guidelines for the performance of myelography and cisternography (evaluation of the posterior fossa and skull base structures) are available from the American College of Radiology (ASNR–SPR 2013). Prior to the procedure, it is essential that the patient's clinical history and any prior imaging be thoroughly reviewed for any contraindications and relative risks. The three main areas of concern are allergic reactions to contrast media, contrast-induced seizures, and hemorrhage.

Allergic reactions

Adverse reactions to administration of iodinated contrast material can range from mild symptoms such as hives and facial swelling to moderate and life-threatening anaphylactoid responses, including severe bronchospasm and hypotension. If a patient has a history of mild-to-moderate reaction, an oral steroid preparation (50 mg prednisone PO 13, 7, and 1 hour prior to the procedure) can be prophylactic (Namasivayam et al., 2006). Premedication does not completely eliminate the risk of a repeat event, however, so the additive benefit of myelographic evaluation should be weighed against the risks of a severe reaction (Hagan, 2004).

Seizure

Though the latest generation of nonionic, water-soluble contrast agents have a significantly reduced risk of inducing seizures with myelography (Klein et al., 2004), certain classes of medications are known to lower the seizure threshold (Fedutes and Ansani, 2003). These primarily consist of antipsychotic, muscle relaxant, and antidepressant drugs from the phenothiazine, monoamine oxidase inhibitors, and tricyclic classes. It is customary to discontinue these medications 48 hours before and 24–48 hours after the procedure when possible. Of note, the risk of seizure has been found to be higher with cervical myelography compared to lumbar evaluation (Klein et al., 2004).

Hemorrhage

In order to reduce hemorrhagic complications, particularly spinal cord compression from spinal hematoma formation, anticoagulant therapies should be discontinued for an appropriate time prior to the procedure. The period of time varies per medication and their different modes of action, such as platelet inhibition or disruption of the coagulation cascade. Moreover any combination of medications is likely to increase the risk further (Layton et al., 2006). A safe approach, which may include assessing laboratory values prior to the procedure, can be guided by consensus guidelines, such as those of the Society of Interventional Radiology (Table 10.1) (Patel et al., 2012). Additionally, for patients with known hematologic disorders, a recent platelet count greater than 50 000 and international normalized ratio (INR) of less than 1.5 should be confirmed. Elective myelography should be delayed until coagulation status has normalized. If emergent, transfusion of platelets can be used to correct thrombocytopenia and administration of fresh frozen plasma and vitamin K can address elevated INR levels.

Table 10.1

Guidelines for coagulation status management prior to myelography (Layton et al., 2006; Patel et al., 2012)

Medication	Time to withhold	Lab value to check prior to procedure
Warfarin (Coumadin)	4–5 days	International normalized ratio < 1.5
Thienopyridines: clopidogrel (Plavix), ticlopidine (Ticlid)	7–10 days	–
Intravenous heparin	2–4 hours	Partial thromboplastin time < 35
Low-molecular-weight heparin	Therapeutic 24 hours, prophylactic 12 hours	–
Aspirin/nonsteroidal anti-inflammatory drugs	–	–

A general principle is that alterations to a patient's medication regimen should be done in conjunction with the prescribing physician as some medications such as antipsychotics may need to be tapered gradually.

Procedural approach

Before beginning the procedure, pertinent prior imaging should be reviewed to identify the optimal level for needle placement, taking into account conus level, spinal curvature, postsurgical anatomy, and hardware. The patient is placed in a prone position on the procedural table and an appropriate level identified under fluoroscopy and marked with a felt-tip pen. For lumbar puncture, the L2/3 level is preferred, as it allows needle passage safely below the conus and above the most common levels of spinal stenosis. A pillow or soft cushion placed under the abdomen will flex the back and open up the spinous processes to ease access. After the lower back is cleansed and sterilely draped, superficial and deep local anesthesia is performed with 1–2% lidocaine buffered 9:1 with 4.2% sodium bicarbonate to reduce discomfort (Ruegg et al., 2009). In younger patients, a median interspinous approach is usually possible and tends to be less painful by avoiding the paraspinal musculature (Fig. 10.1A, B). In patients with advanced spinal degeneration, interspinous osteoarthritis (Baastrup's disease) may obstruct the midline approach. In these cases, an oblique interlaminar approach can be used, and this is facilitated by a combination of caudal and oblique angulation of the image intensifier to "open up" a needle path on fluoroscopy (Fig. 10.1C) (Williams, 2014).

The choice of spinal needle is based on a balanced consideration of ease of performing the procedure and risk of postprocedural postdural puncture headache from continued CSF leakage. Larger needles with a beveled cutting tip (Quincke-type, 20–22 gauge) are more easily steered and have sufficient stiffness to navigate thick ligamentous tissue and tight osseous spaces encountered in advanced spinal degeneration (Fig. 10.2A). However, studies have demonstrated that the rate of postprocedural postdural puncture headache can be reduced approximately fourfold to 5–12% by selecting finer needles in the 24–27-gauge range (Evans et al., 2000). Moreover, use of needles with non-cutting "pencil-point" tips, such as Whitacre and Sprotte types, also may further reduce headache risk (Fig. 10.2B) (Quaynor et al., 1995; Strupp et al., 2001).

Proper intrathecal needle positioning is initially confirmed by observing CSF return and dependent layering of injected contrast material away from the needle tip on cross-table fluoroscopic views, if available. After further contrast injection of 1–2 mL, anteroposterior fluoroscopic views should be checked to distinguish the expected intrathecal subarachnoid appearance of the contrast column from epidural and subdural injection patterns (Fig. 10.3). Water-soluble nonionic iodinated contrast in concentrations of 180–300 mg iodine/mL are used, with higher concentrations preferable for thoracic or cervical myelography and cisternography. The increased density compensates for dilution when tilting the patient Trendelenburg to document the advance of contrast cephalad from the site of lumbar instillation. Though an instilled volume containing up to 3 grams of iodine is felt to be safe with regard to seizure risk,

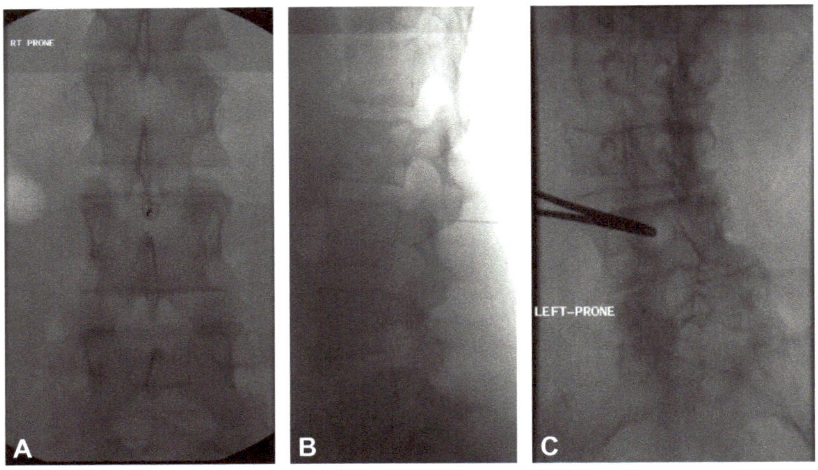

Fig. 10.1. Different approaches to lumbar puncture. The median interspinous approach, optimal in younger patients with less spinal degeneration, is achieved by aligning the spinous processes centrally on the anteroposterior fluoroscopic view and caudally angulating the image intensifier (II) to create an enlarged "down the barrel" path (**A**), through which the course of the needle can be followed into the spinal canal on lateral views (**B**). The oblique interlaminar approach (**C**) is preferable when disc height loss and interspinous osteoarthritis narrow or obliterate interspinous space. Caudal angulation with approximately 20° lateral obliquity opens the ovoid path under the arch formed by the inferior border of the ipsilateral lamina (marker).

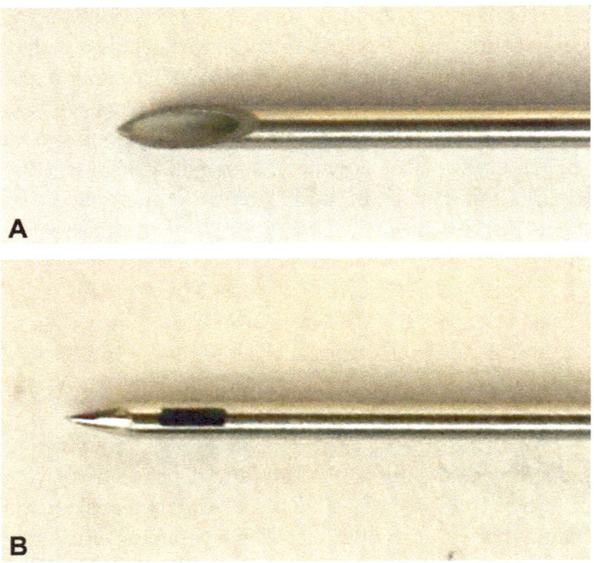

Fig. 10.2. Types of spinal needle tip. Quincke needle with cutting tip (**A**) is easy to introduce through the skin and the beveled edge allows "steering" around osseous obstacles. Needles with noncutting, pencil-point tips, such as on the Whitacre spinal needle pictured here (**B**), reduce the risk of postdural puncture headache, likely by causing less gaping of cut dural fibers. An introducer needle is necessary, as well as a relatively direct path into the spinal canal for successful use of such needles.

typically lower total amounts in the 5–10 cc range are found to be sufficient for myelo-CT and help prevent excessively dense layering on myelo-CT images. If severe spinal stenosis results in obstruction to caudal flow of contrast material, the patient can be placed in a seated position with the back flexed forward. This maneuver reduces encroachment upon the spinal canal from ligamentum flavum infolding and thus often allows passage of contrast below the stenosis prior to CT imaging (Fig. 10.4).

A cervical puncture site may be considered if the lumbar approach is precluded due to local wound infection, recent postoperative state, low-lying conus, myelomeningocele, severe spinal stenosis, osseous fusion, or other technical factors blocking access (Fig. 10.5A). Additionally, a spinal tumor that completely obstructs the flow of CSF is a contraindication for lumbar puncture below, as it poses the risk for spinal "coning" or impaction of the spinal cord due to alteration of the CSF pressure across the level of obstruction (Hollis et al., 1986). To reduce the risk of the cervical approach, preprocedural MRI should be obtained to confirm sufficient CSF space dorsal to the cord at the C1–2 level without obstruction along the needle course by degenerative stenosis, low-lying tonsils, posterior positioned vertebral arteries, or low posterior-inferior-cerebellar artery loops (Fig. 10.5B). The lateral C1–2 approach is most easily performed with the patient in the prone position and the needle directed to the posterior one-third of the spinal canal on a true lateral projection (Fig. 10.5C). Additionally, it is imperative to confirm proper subarachnoid needle tip positioning by observing free flow of CSF from the needle hub prior to injecting contrast in order to avoid catastrophic cord injury from intramedullary injection (Orrison et al., 1983).

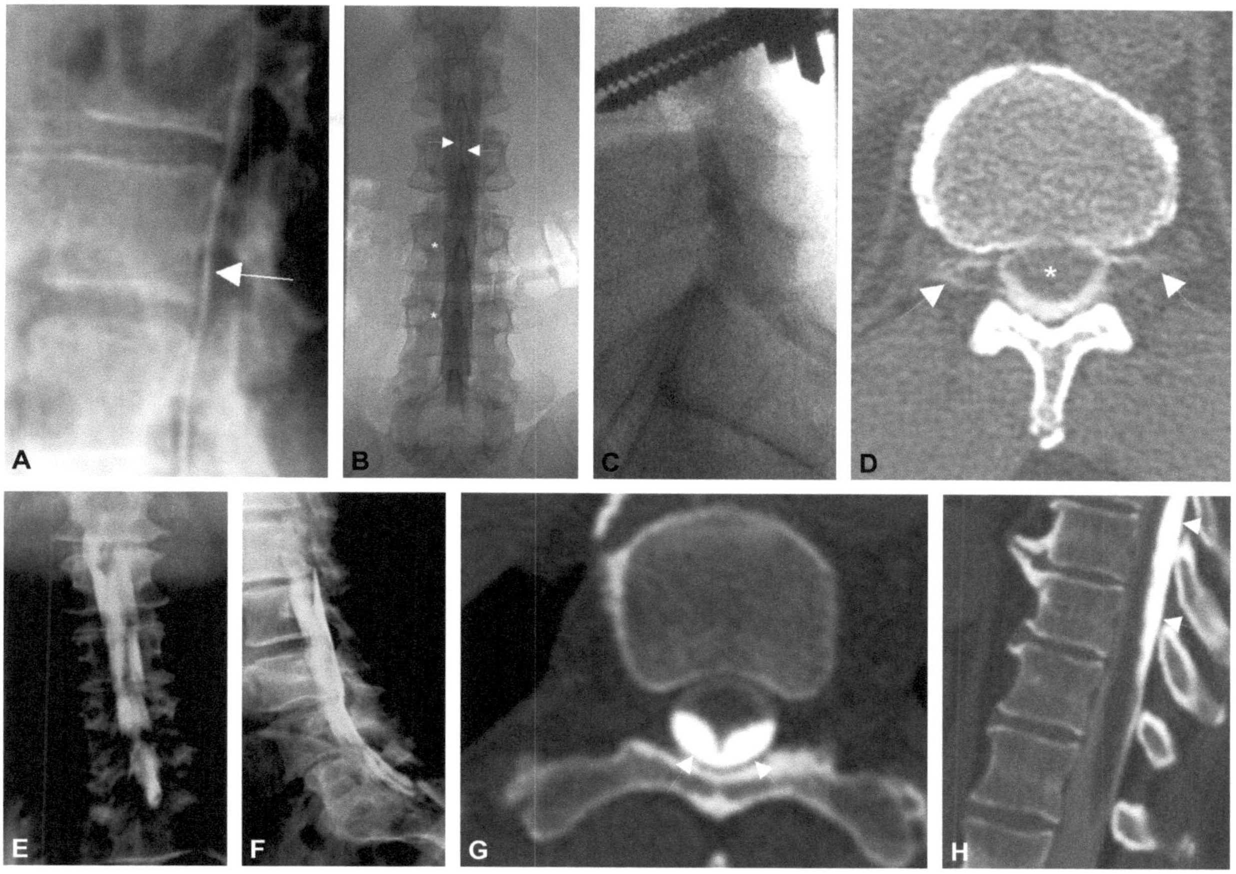

Fig. 10.3. Confirmation of successful intrathecal subarachnoid contrast injection. Initial trace contrast injection on cross-table lateral views should demonstrate flow of the contrast away from the needle tip with thin layering on the dependent ventral aspect of the spinal canal (**A**, arrow). After further contrast instillation, the anteroposterior (AP) view becomes helpful for establishing the proper intrathecal pattern (**B**). Signs of proper intrathecal contrast placement include homogeneous opacification across the width of the spinal canal, filling of nerve root sleeves in a "Christmas tree" pattern (asterisks) and linear cauda equina nerve root-filling defects (arrows). A key sign of an unwanted epidural-injection collection of contrast in the dorsal epidural fat pad (**C**), confirmed on subsequent computed tomography (CT) imaging (**D**), where lack of opacification of the thecal sac is seen (asterisk) and contrast delineation of the circumferential epidural space and epineurial sheaths noted (arrows). An intrathecal yet subdural contrast injection is also to be avoided, yet harder to prospectively identify on fluoroscopic imaging, where there may be mixed subarachnoid and subdural opacification, creating inhomogeneous opacification with irregular contours of the contrast column on AP (**E**) and lateral views (**F**). However, subdural compartment injection is characteristic on axial CT imaging (**G**) and sagittal reformatted views (**H**) with lentiform undiluted hyperdense contrast opacification along the inner dural margin identified (arrows).

CT image acquisition and postprocessing

After successful intrathecal instillation of contrast, the patient is transported immediately to the CT suite for thin-section high-resolution imaging (0.5–0.625 mm thick slices) (Fig. 10.6). In the interests of time and to reduce radiation exposure, the radiographic series obtained in the fluoroscopy suite are no longer routinely acquired given the superior diagnostic quality of CT. The patient should be rolled several times immediate prior to scanning to avoid dense contrast layering, which can obscure intrathecal detail. If CSF leak is suspected, delayed imaging should be performed to capture slow leaks not visible on initial imaging.

Postprocessing techniques are extremely beneficial to interpretation and include routine sagittal and coronal multiplanar reformatting in bone and soft-tissue reconstruction algorithms performed at the scanner console, with additional obliquities obtained using 3D imaging software as necessary (Fig. 10.7). In the setting of a severely scoliotic spine, curved planar reformatting can "unwind" the tortuous spinal canal and its contents into long confluent views rather than coursing in and out of plane (Fig. 10.8) (Yoshioka et al., 2006). Dual-energy CT acquisition enables high-energy virtual monoenergetic reconstruction and other metal artifact reduction techniques, which can dramatically improve streak

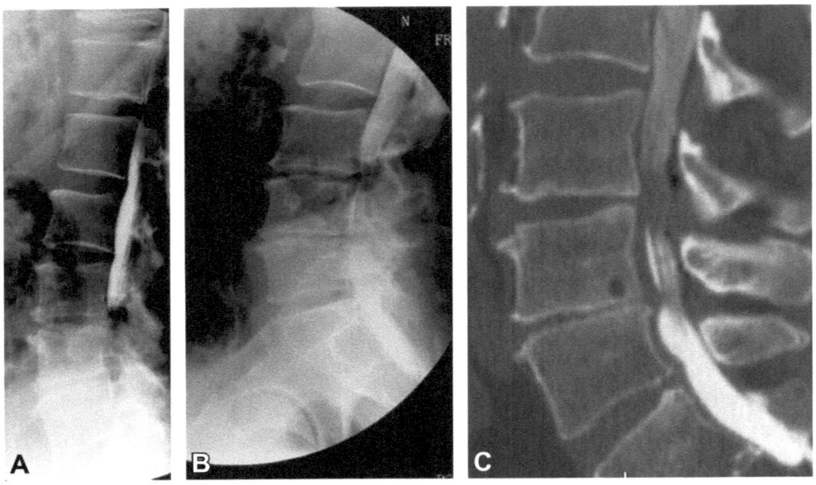

Fig. 10.4. Flexion maneuver enabling contrast flow across severely stenotic spinal level. Lateral fluoroscopic view demonstrating complete subarachnoid block at the L3–4 level with the patient in prone positioning (**A**). With the patient in the seated position, flexing the back forward enlarges the spinal canal diameter by stretching out the infolded ligamentum flavum. Repeat fluoroscopic confirms caudal flow (**B**), allowing successful subsequent myelo-computed tomography (CT) where the extent of stenosis at L3–4 is defined as well as characterizing additional degrees of stenosis at more caudal levels (**C**, sagittal reformatted CT view).

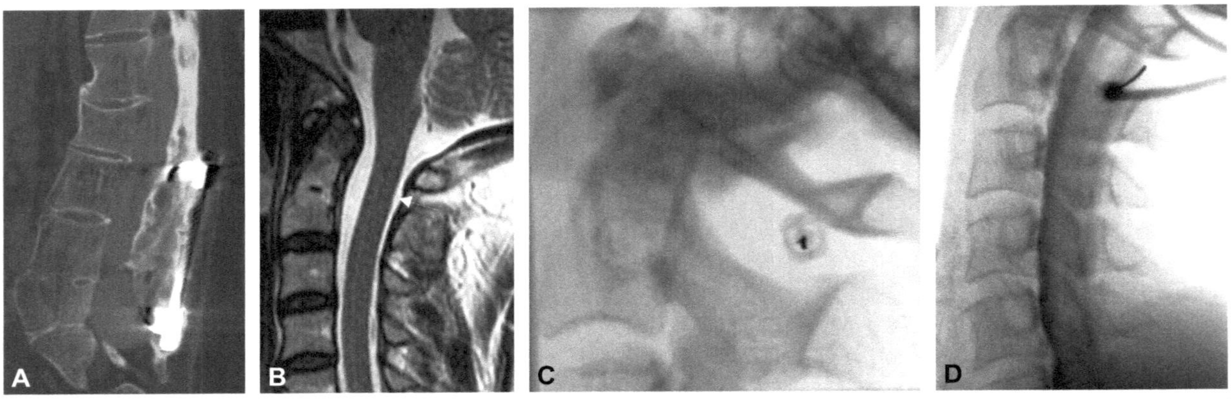

Fig. 10.5. Lateral C1–2 puncture. Prior lumbar decompression surgery with thick osseous fusion mass and spinal rods, visualized on sagittal computed tomography (CT) reformatted image (**A**), precludes lumbar approach for dural puncture. Sufficient cerebrospinal fluid (CSF) space dorsal to the cord is confirmed on sagittal T-weighted image from preprocedural magnetic resonance imaging (**B**, arrow) and an absence of obstructing tonsillar ectopia or vascular loops. The needle is positioned on a true lateral cervical fluoroscopic view directed to the posterior one-third of the spinal canal (**C**), with free flow of contrast observed on fluoroscopic views (**D**) only after CSF flow needle hub confirmed extramedullary positioning of the needle tip.

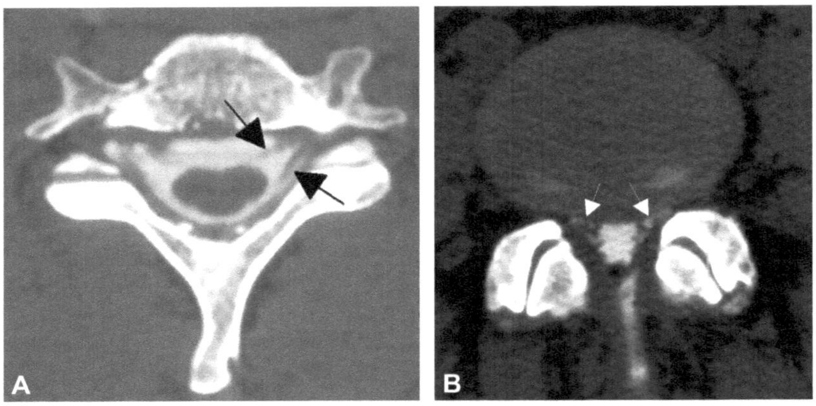

Fig. 10.6. High-resolution computed tomography (CT) myelography. Thin-section (0.5–0.625 mm) slice reconstruction enables depiction of exquisite anatomic detail, such as the delineation of the normal course of distinct ventral and dorsal nerve roots from the cervical cord to the neuroforamina on axial CT images (**A**, arrows) and encroachment of descending nerve roots in the lumbar subarticular zones (**B**, arrows).

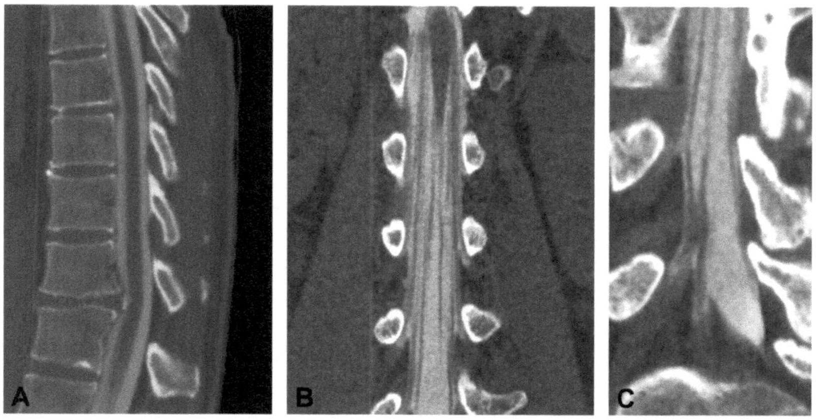

Fig. 10.7. Multiplanar reformatting of myelo-computed tomography source images. Thin-section acquisition enables routine sagittal (**A**) and coronal reformatting as well as additional obliquities using 3D imaging software to show normal anatomy optimally, such as the cauda equina arising off the conus medullaris in a vertically obliqued coronal view (**B**) or the derangement of the descending nerve roots in the subarticular zone on a laterally obliqued coronal view (**C**).

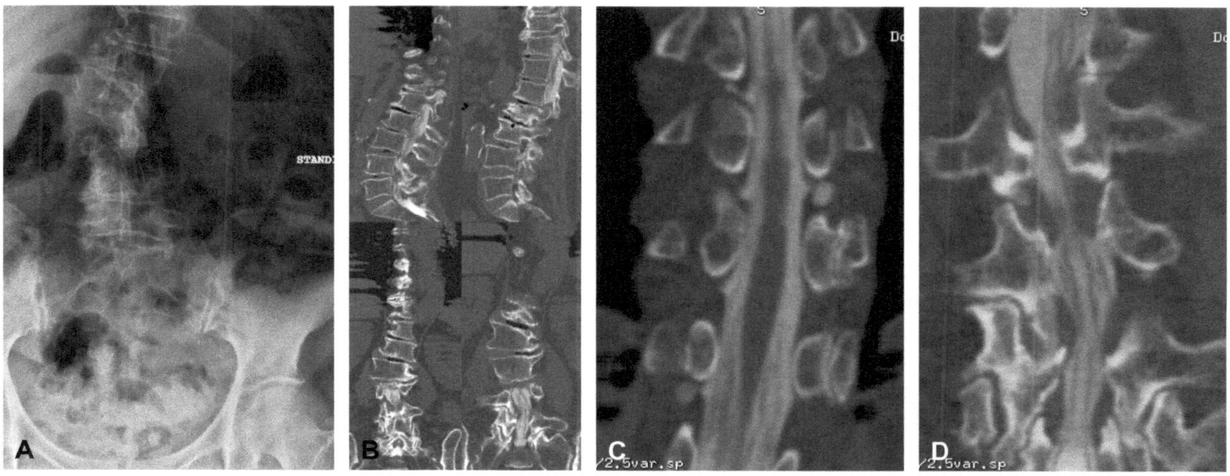

Fig. 10.8. Curved-planar reformatting for myelo-computed tomography of scoliotic spines. A severely scoliotic spine, as seen on plain radiography (**A**), results in cumbersome interpretation on standard reformatting due to the course of the spinal canal in and out of sagittal and coronal planes (**B**). Curved-planar reformatting can be performed in seconds by quickly tracing the course of the spinal canal in 3D software, available at the scanner console or in standalone applications to "unwind" the spine into long-segment views that aid in efficient interpretation (**C, D**).

artifacts in the setting of surgical hardware or bullet fragments (Fig. 10.9) (Guggenberger et al., 2012).

MODERN MYELOGRAPHY INDICATIONS

Spinal stenosis

The relative disadvantages of myelography compared to MRI for evaluating neck and back pain are well recognized, including the risks of a percutaneous invasive procedure, reactions to contrast media, as well as exposure to ionizing radiation (Janssen et al., 2011). Moreover, systematic review and meta-analysis of the literature demonstrate relatively poor accuracy of conventional myelography compared with CT, and especially MRI, for diagnosis of spinal stenosis (Modic et al., 1986; Kent et al., 1992; Miller and Krauss, 2003; de Schepper et al., 2013). However, MR is less accurate than CT for distinguishing bony osteophytes from soft-tissue components of spinal canal stenosis, such as disc herniation, fibrotic bulging, and ligamentous hypertrophy (Dorenbeck et al., 2004). The combination of exquisite osseous detail and the accurate assessment of spinal canal stenosis without blooming from magnetic susceptibility, CSF pulsation artifact, or motion degradation still leads many to rely on myelo-CT in preoperative planning, especially if MRI is contraindicated, in the presence of extensive pre-existing metallic hardware, or when there is strong clinical suspicion of nerve root compression, even after negative, ambiguous, or technically suboptimal MRI (Song et al., 2009; Eadsforth et al., 2012).

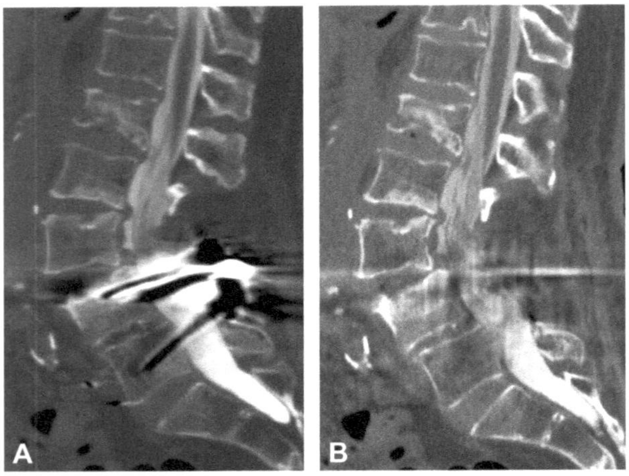

Fig. 10.9. Metallic hardware artifact reduction with dual-energy computed tomography (DECT). (**A**) Image reconstruction at DECT mid-range virtual-monochromatic energy level of 65 kEv, similar to a routine single-energy scan of 120 kVp, is severely degraded by bright and dark streaks from spinal rods and pedicular screws, which obscure the spinal canal, vertebrae, and dorsal paraspinal soft tissues. (**B**) Higher-energy reconstruction at 100 kEv with metal artifact reduction option dramatically improves visualization in all regions.

Additionally, images acquired during the fluoroscopic portion of the myelogram procedure can reflect functional aspects to spinal stenosis that may not be apparent on MRI. For example, the delayed passage of contrast across a severely narrowed level can be observed dynamically at myelography but be underestimated even on subsequent myelo-CT. Myelographic image acquisition in the upright position can be useful to document increased disc bulging, spondylolisthesis, and resultant nerve root encroachment compared to recumbent CT and MR positioning, especially in patients whose radiculopathy symptoms develop during standing or walking (Fig. 10.10) (Ido et al., 2002).

Cervical nerve root avulsion in brachial plexus injury

Brachial plexus injury can arise in the adolescent and adult population, most typically from motorcycle and bicycle accidents, and in the young pediatric population, most often related to perinatal trauma (Tseng and Tseng, 1997; Moran et al., 2005). Conventional myelography and myelo-CT can play a critical role in determining the level and extent of cervical nerve injury root injury in the case of suspected brachial plexus injury (Carvalho et al., 1997). Tearing of the dural sheath with cervical root avulsion can heal with development of a pseudomeningocele. This finding appears on myelographic imaging as a lateral outpouching of contrast extending from the thecal sac and foramen into the

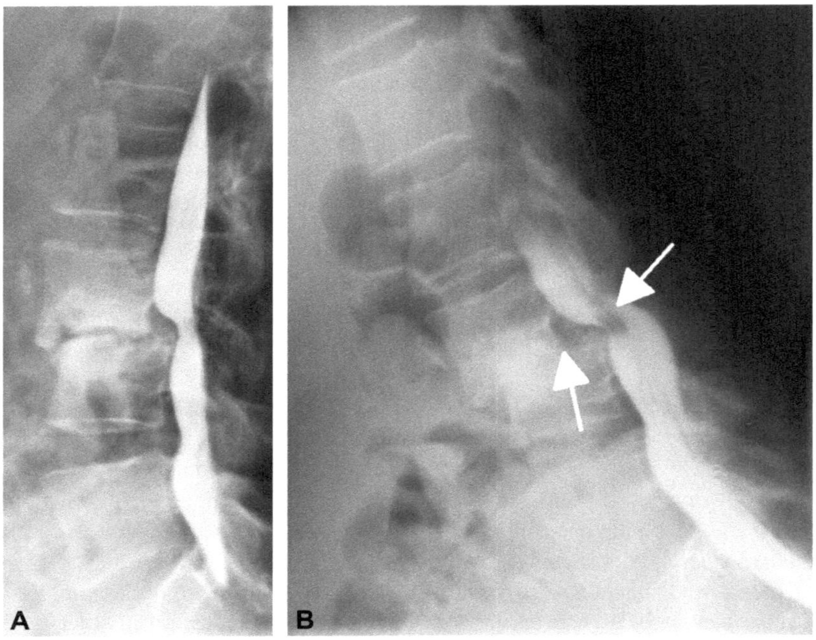

Fig. 10.10. Recumbent versus standing myelography. When comparing prone conventional myelographic images (**A**) with standing images obtained in flexion (**B**), dynamic changes, including markedly increased spondylolisthesis with resultant narrowing of the opacified thecal sac and crowding of the nerve root filling defects, are noted (arrows).

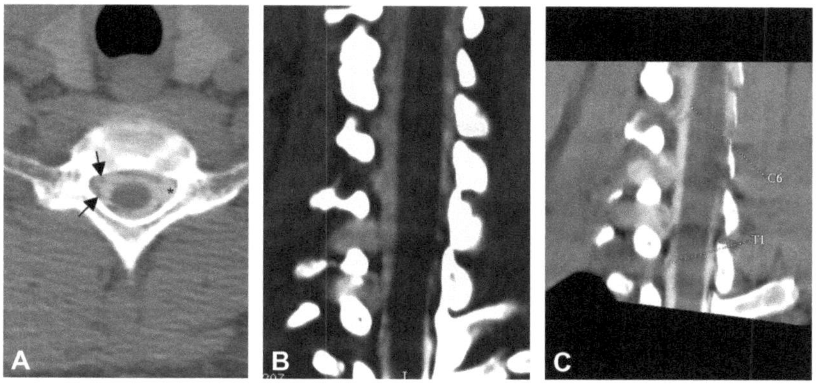

Fig. 10.11. Cervical nerve root avulsion in brachial plexus injury. High-resolution axial myelo-computed tomography image (**A**) demonstrates a left-sided pseudomeningocele (asterisk) at the C7–T1 level in this 36-year-old male with left brachial plexopathy after a motorcycle accident. The C8 nerve roots are well delineated on the right (arrows), but absent on the left. In a 20-year-old woman with pseudomeningocele formation at the right C6–7 and C7–T1 levels after a car accident, the presence of nerve roots at adjacent normal levels and the absence of intact nerve roots at affected levels are not well distinguished on a standard multiplanar view (**B**), but very conspicuous on thick-slab minimum-intensity projection views (**C**).

paraspinal region. Myelo-CT demonstrates opacification of pseuodomeningoceles as well as providing high-resolution delineation of ventral and dorsal nerve roots and their absence or reduced number if avulsed (Fig. 10.11A) (Steens et al., 2011).

Optimal myelo-CT evaluation of the nerve roots benefits from complementing thin-section axial views with reformatting in an oblique coronal plane tilted to the plane of the nerve roots (Yamazaki et al., 2007). Minimum-intensity projections can also dramatically increase conspicuity of intact nerve roots. In this readily available 3D technique, lower pixel density values from the nerve root filling defects are projected on to the image plane preferentially over immediately adjacent higher-density contrast-opacified regions, rather than volume-averaging them as in standard multiplanar reformatting. Thus thicker slabs can be utilized to capture the oblique course of the nerve roots over a longer distance at each level (Fig. 10.11B, C). A pitfall in early diagnosis, however, is the presence of a blood clot occupying the site of avulsion, preventing delineation of the expanded nerve root sheath; thus, waiting several weeks prior to myelography can increase sensitivity of the exam.

Radiation therapy treatment planning

An emerging indication for myelo-CT is aiding in the radiation therapy treatment planning for skull base, spinal, and paraspinal tumors. After surgical resection and for treating tumor recurrence, local control with high-dose radiotherapy can be effective. However, paraspinal tumors with low radiosensitivity, such as chordomas and sarcomas, show poor local control with conventional radiation at doses less than 60 Gy, whereas dose limits for the spinal cord range between 45 and 50 Gy (Delaney et al., 2014). Thus the target dose is limited by the radiation tolerance of the spinal cord, nerves, and surrounding viscera. This remains true even with relatively recent techniques such as proton beam therapy, which enable reductions in the dose delivered to nontarget tissue.

Myelo-CT enables precise delineation of spinal cord contours distinct from tumor and surrounding normal soft-tissue and osseous anatomy (Uhl et al., 2011). This results in increased confidence in the safe use of higher target doses to increase the chance of therapeutic benefit while limiting the risk of radiation-induced myelitis/myelopathy and other treatment complications. Compared to MRI, CT offers higher spatial resolution, better characterization of bone, and shorter imaging times, allowing greater coverage and less motion artifact (Fig. 10.12). The benefit of myelo-CT is particularly compelling in the presence of surgical hardware. Postsurgical stabilization is often achieved with metallic constructs, including fusion plates, pedicular screws, spinal rods, and/or vertebrectomy spacers, which have a preferentially deleterious effect on MR over CT imaging.

CSF leak

Spontaneous intracranial hypotension (SIH) is an often debilitating syndrome arising from spinal CSF leaks. It involves mostly young and middle-aged adults, is female-predominant, and the most typical manifestation is daily persistent orthostatic headaches, but is often accompanied by a variety of other symptoms, including nausea, dizziness, and tinnitus. Brain imaging characteristically reveals diffuse pachymeningeal enhancement but other associated findings include subdural hygroma collections and "brain sagging," with low-lying cerebellar tonsils, flattening of the ventral pons, and inferior displacement of the optic chiasm (Fig. 10.13A–C)

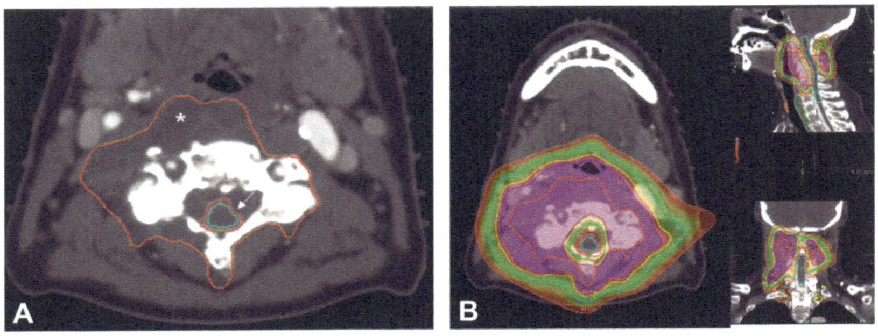

Fig. 10.12. Computed tomography (CT) myelography in a 71-year-old female for proton beam radiation therapy for C3–C5 cervical-level chordoma. CT images were acquired using "double-contrast" technique following both intrathecal and intravenous iodinated contrast administration. Axial CT image (**A**) with contour lines delineating spinal cord (blue) and intraspinal and paraspinal tumor extent (red). Myelographic contrast material provides positive contrast around circumferential tumor extension around cervical spinal cord, identifying areas of contour deformity from tumor mass effect (arrow) and intravenous contrast provides excellent conspicuity of hypoenhancing tumor insinuating through enhancing paraspinal musculature (asterisk). Dose distribution maps for maximizing target dose to the areas of tumor involvement while limiting the risk of radiation-injury to the cord are plotted on triplanar reformatted images (**B**). (Courtesy of Dr. Norbert J. Liebsch, Department of Radiation Oncology, Massachusetts General Hospital.)

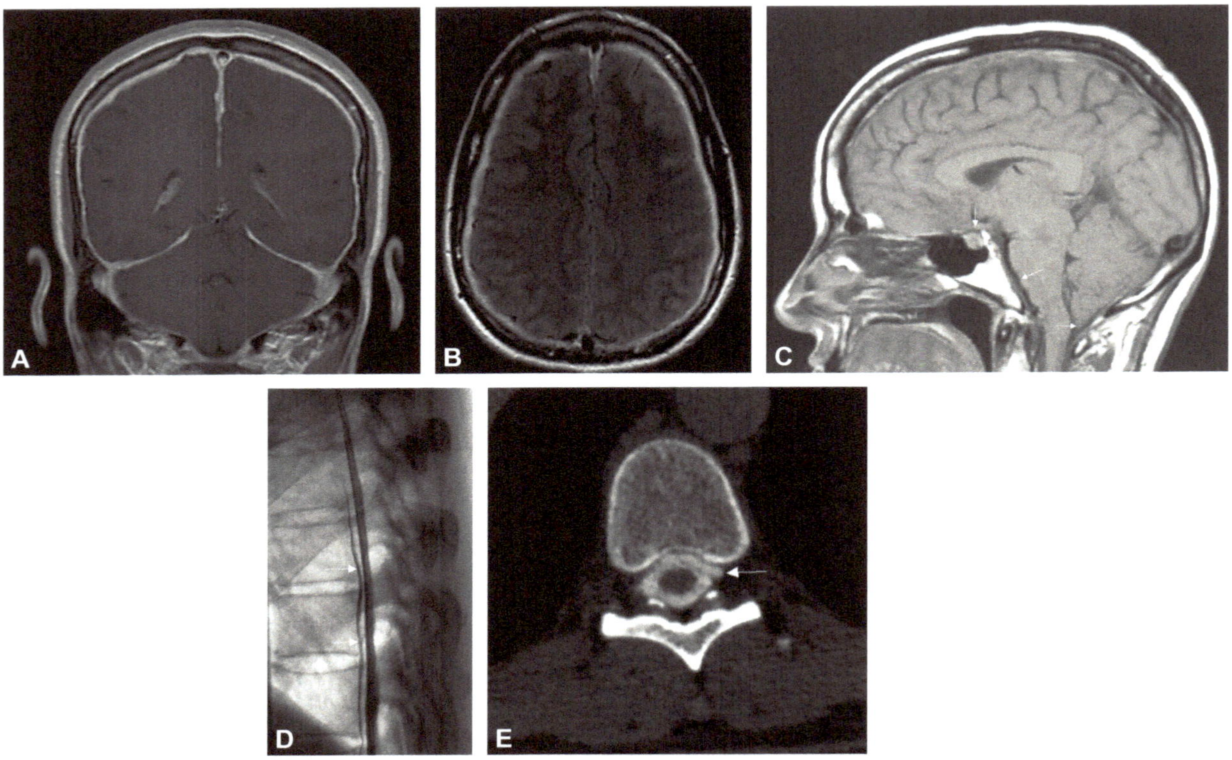

Fig. 10.13. Brain magnetic resonance imaging and myelographic findings of spontaneous intracranial hypotension due to epidural cerebrospinal fluid leak. A 48-year-old woman with intractable positional headaches demonstrates characteristic imaging features on MRI of the brain, including (**A**) diffuse pachymeningeal enhancement on gadolinium-enhanced T1-weighted coronal imaging, (**B**) hyperintense subdural hygromas on axial fluid attenuation inversion recovery (FLAIR) imaging, and (**C**) signs of "brain sagging" on sagittal T1-weighted imaging, including low-lying cerebellar tonsils, flattening of the ventral pons, and inferior displacement of the optic chiasm (arrows). Rapid contrast leakage into the lower thoracic ventral epidural space is detected on fluoroscopic views when tilting the patient Trendelenburg after lumbar instillation (**D**, arrow) and confirmed on myelo-computed tomography imaging, where a ventral extrathecal contrast collection opacifies (**E**, arrow).

(Schievink, 2008). A low opening pressure ($\leq$6 cm H_2O) on lumbar puncture may be measured and empiric epidural blood patching (EBP) can result in successful resolution of symptoms if a trial of conservative measures fails (Amoozegar et al., 2013). These clinical and imaging features are highly suggestive of CSF leak in a patient with SIH syndrome, but more definitive diagnosis is achieved with demonstration of extrathecal CSF collections on spinal imaging (Fig. 10.13). When patients have persistent symptoms despite EBP, the imaging identification of the focal site of leakage becomes more important to guide additional percutaneous or surgical therapy, including targeted EBP, fibrin glue injections, or surgical repair, including ligation of suspect meningeal diverticula or primary dural closure if a defect is found (Schievink et al., 1994; Schievink, 2008; Wendl et al., 2012).

Imaging findings related to CSF leaks on myelo-CT include frank leakage into extrathecal CSF collections or associated anatomic derangements which may predispose to CSF leak. It is important to note focal dilatations of the cervicothoracic nerve root sleeves, known as spinal meningeal diverticula (Fig. 10.14), even if not seen to demonstrate frank leakage on myelography, as they can be the effective target of directed EBP or fibrin glue deposition or surgical exploration (Khosla and Wippold, 2002; Schievink et al., 2008). Thoracic osteophytes are another recognized cause of CSF leaks (Hasiloglu et al., 2012). They can result in dural tears despite being remarkably subtle on MR and CT imaging (Fig. 10.15).

If initial myelo-CT does not demonstrate CSF leakage, delayed imaging up to 4 hours from injection can increase sensitivity for slow leaks. Conversely, the spread of extrathecal contrast material may be so rapid and extensive by the time the patient is transferred from the myelography suite to the CT scanner that confident identification of a focal source of CSF leakage is impossible. This situation is especially challenging if there are numerous widely spread diverticula or osteophytes in question. In this situation, dynamic myelo-CT can provide the temporal and spatial resolution necessary to localize such rapid CSF leaks. In this technique, the injection of contrast material occurs with the patient already on the CT table. Myelo-CT scan acquisition is obtained both during and immediately following contrast instillation. Additional acquisitions are obtained rapidly in succession, with the patient quickly turned from prone to supine and bilateral decubitus positions as necessary (Luetmer and Mokri, 2003). Careful analysis of the multiphasic acquisition will ideally capture the initial localized leakage at the site of leakage before extensive spread occurs. Given the additional procedural time and radiation exposure with this technique, it should be utilized in those patients predicted most likely to have fast CSF leaks based on previous imaging. According to the retrospective review and algorithm proposed by Luetmer et al. (2012), the primary predictor of a fast leak are those SIH syndrome patients already demonstrated to have extensive spinal extra-arachnoid fluid collections (epidural or subdural) on MRI (Fig. 10.16).

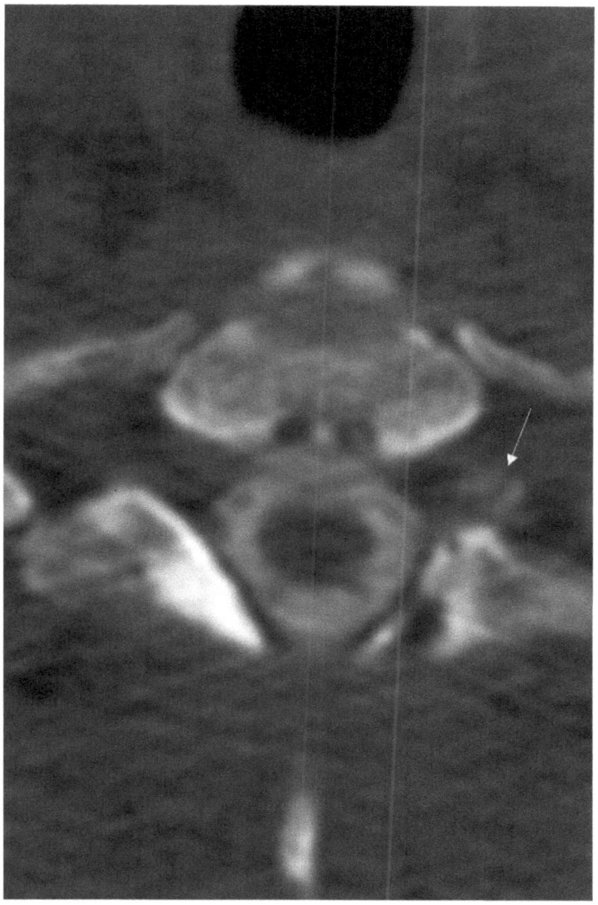

Fig. 10.14. Spinal meningeal diverticula in spontaneous intracranial hypotension syndrome. A 33-year-old female with disabling positional headache, diffuse pachymeningeal enhancement on brain magnetic resonance imaging, and low opening pressure of 2 cm H_2O on lumbar puncture had computed tomography myelogram performed which demonstrated focal asymmetric contrast opacification of a left C7–T1 meningeal diverticulum (arrow). Surgical exploration with placement of fibrin glue over the ectatic dura resulted in symptomatic improvement.

When patients with the syndrome of intracranial hypotension fail to demonstrate either a focal or extensive site of extrathecal CSF spread on MRI or CT of the spine or skull base, MRI after intrathecal gadolinium instillation (MR myelography) can provide increased

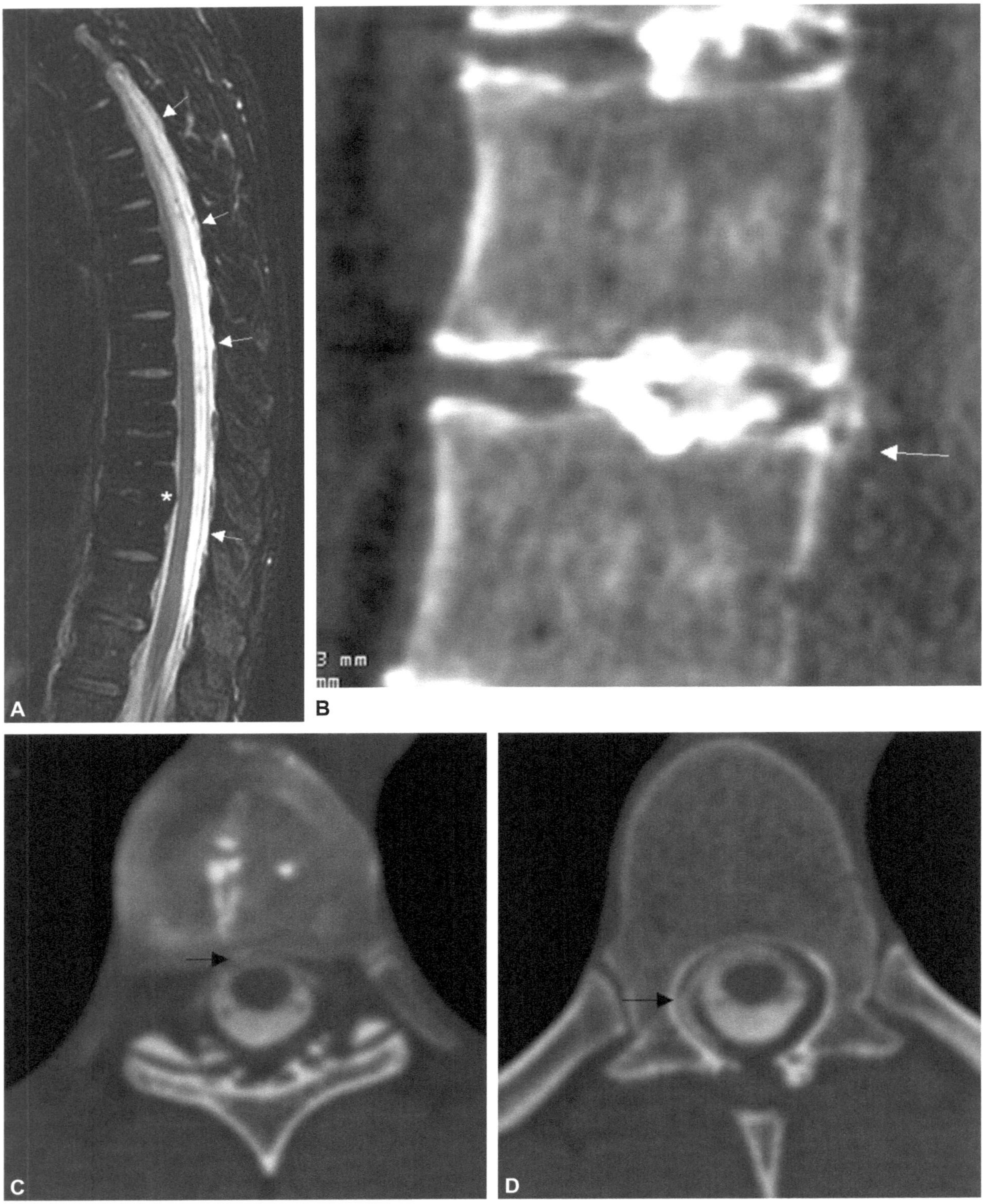

Fig. 10.15. Epidural cerebrospinal fluid (CSF) leak due to thoracic osteophyte. Extensive epidural fluid collection is identified on fat-saturated sagittal T2-weighted imaging of the spine (**A**, arrows) with barely perceptible T10–11 posterior osteophyte (**A**, asterisk) projecting into the spinal canal, much better visualized on sagittal routine computed tomography (CT) sagittal reformatted image (**B**, arrow). Localized epidural accumulation during CT myelography at sight of osteophyte confirms source of CSF leakage (**C** and **D**, arrows).

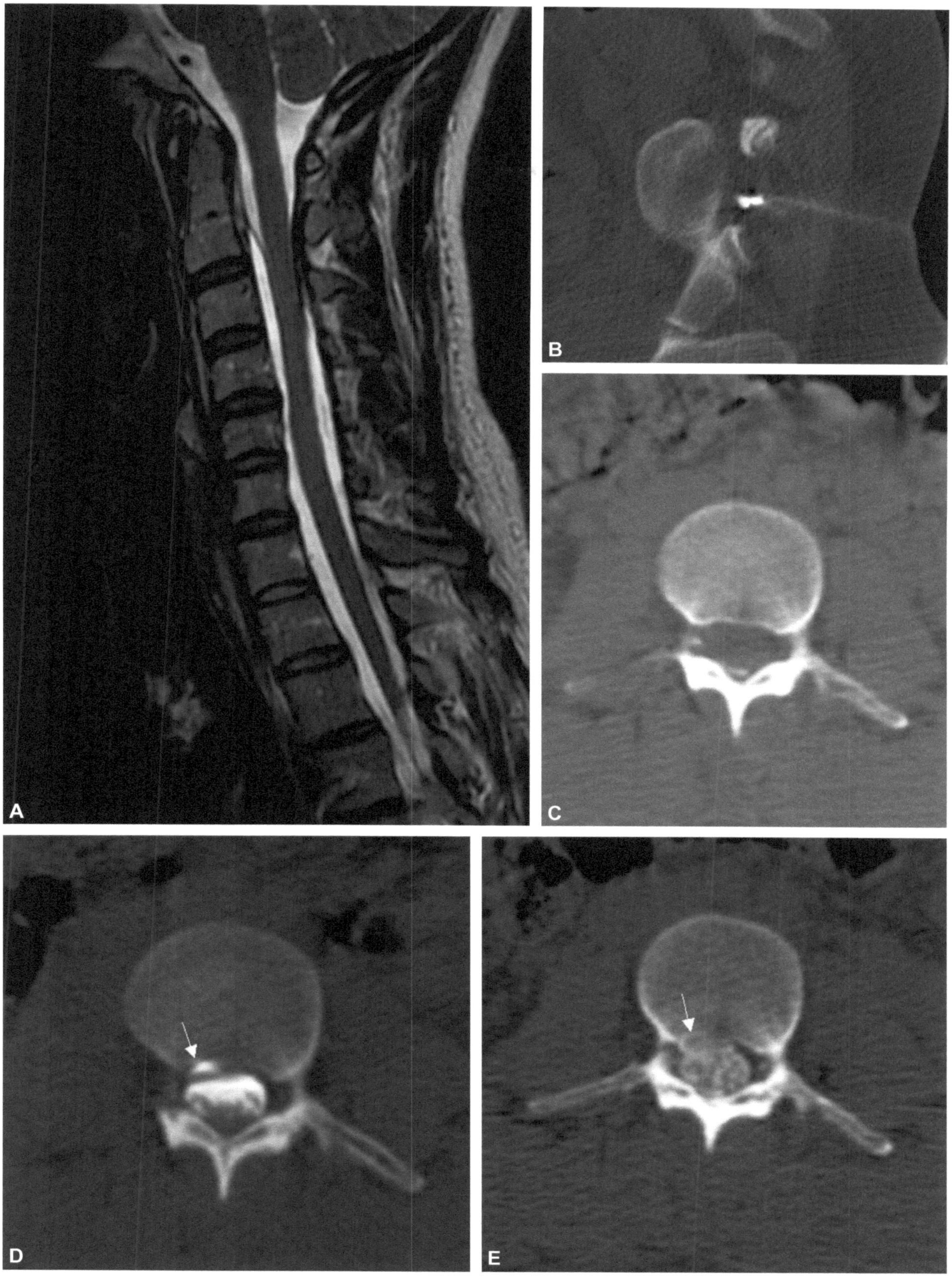

Fig. 10.16. Dynamic computed tomography (CT) myelography for rapid cerebrospinal fluid leak. (**A**) Long epidural fluid collections demonstrated on magnetic resonance imaging suggest the likelihood of rapid extensive opacification of epidural space during conventional fluoroscopic contrast instillation, obscuring the focal site of leakage by time of standard myelo-CT. Dynamic CT myelography performed with contrast instillation on the CT table (**B**) allows rapid enough serial imaging to capture early localized leakage (**D** and **E**, arrows) at a site that did not initially demonstrate leakage on first post-injection scan (**C**).

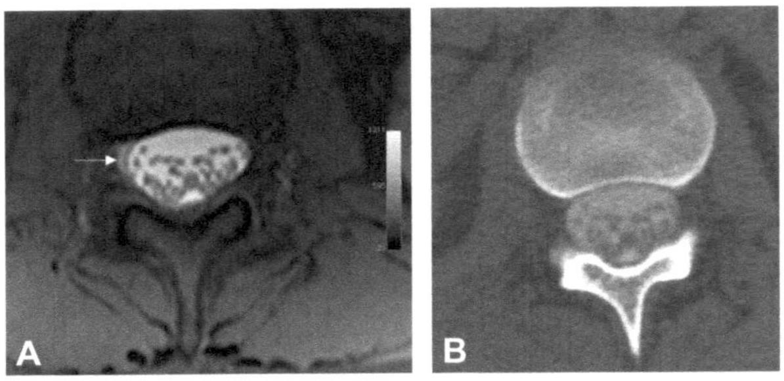

Fig. 10.17. Magnetic resonance myelography with intrathecal gadolinium for localization of slow cerebrospinal fluid leak. Following intrathecal gadolinium instillation via lumbar puncture, axial T1-weighted images demonstrated localized contrast collection in right T12–L1 epidural space (**A**, arrow), which was not visualized on prior myelo-computed tomography (**B**).

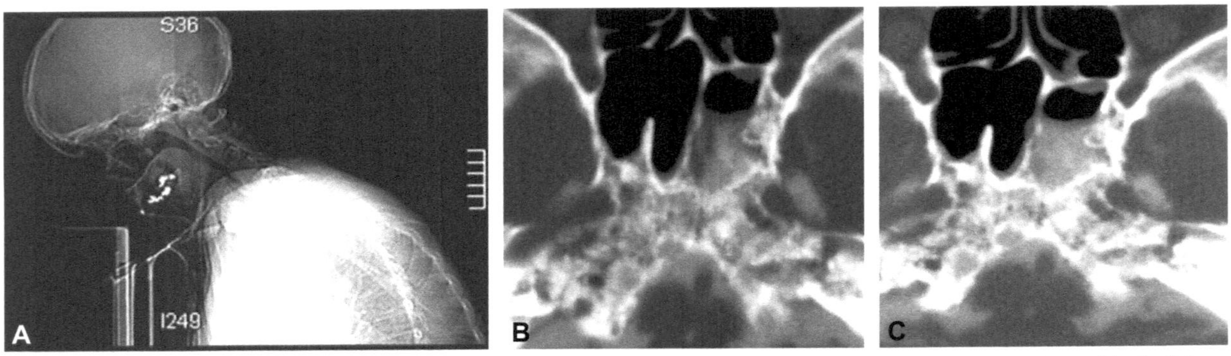

Fig. 10.18. Computed tomography cisternogram for cerebrospinal fluid rhinorrhea. Serial imaging of patient with skull-base radiation osteitis in prone positioning with downward tilt of the head (**A**) to induce symptomatic nasal fluid drainage demonstrates opacification of irregular osseous defect through basisphenoid with progressive contrast leakage into the sphenoid sinus (**B** and **C**).

sensitivity (Fig. 10.17) (Akbar et al., 2012; Starling et al., 2013). Though intrathecal administration of gadolinium is still considered off-label use, there are increasing reports of its safe administration at appropriate concentrations and its effectiveness in identifying otherwise occult CSF leaks in SIH syndrome patients (Zeng et al., 1999; Algin and Turkbey, 2013; Papadopoulou et al., 2013).

Another category of patients with presumed CSF leak are those with CSF rhinorrhea or otorrhea. Radionuclide cisternography with scintigraphic imaging and pledget analysis and contrast-enhanced CT cisternography are often used to identify skull-base sites of leakage. Noncontrast high-resolution skull-base CT may show highly suggestive focal defects arising from trauma, surgery (sinus or mastoid disease or skull-base tumors), or congenital defects such as an encephalocele (Lloyd et al., 2008). CT cisternogram images are reviewed for frank dense extracranial contrast pooling near focal defects or fracture lines or more subtle areas of soft-tissue density increased over baseline CT (Fig. 10.18) (Stone et al., 1999).

CONCLUSION

Though myelography is a technique whose safety has progressed greatly over its 90-year history, its role in the workup of spinal disease has been largely supplanted by MRI. Nonetheless, not every patient can obtain MRI and there are a number of indications for which myelography in combination with postmyelography CT is complementary to MRI, if not the study of choice. Proper procedural preparation and technique for both contrast instillation and image acquisition are essential to patient safety and optimal diagnostic quality, including dynamic fluoroscopic and CT image acquisition techniques not possible with conventional MRI. Advanced image acquisition such as dual-energy myelo-CT and 3D postprocessing capabilities can help overcome hardware-related artifacts and provide optimal conspicuity of complex anatomy. Thus, myelography continues to play a role in the preoperative evaluation of spinal stenosis, particularly when MRI is contraindicated or nondiagnostic, and is recognized as a key investigatory technique in the evalution of brachial plexus injury, radiation therapy treatment planning, and CSF leak.

References

ASNR–SPR Practice Guideline for the Performance of Myelography and Cisternography Res. 9-2013. www.acr.org/~/media/ACR/Documents/PGTS/guidelines/Myelography.pdf. Published 2014. (accessed August 2014).

Akbar JJ, Luetmer PH, Schwartz KM et al. (2012). The role of MR myelography with intrathecal gadolinium in localization of spinal CSF leaks in patients with spontaneous intracranial hypotension. AJNR Am J Neuroradiol 33: 535–540.

Algin O, Turkbey B (2013). Intrathecal gadolinium-enhanced MR cisternography: a comprehensive review. AJNR Am J Neuroradiol 34: 14–22.

Amoozegar F, Guglielmin D, Hu W et al. (2013). Spontaneous intracranial hypotension: recommendations for management. Can J Neurol Sci 40: 144–157.

Carvalho GA, Nikkhah G, Matthies C et al. (1997). Diagnosis of root avulsions in traumatic brachial plexus injuries: value of computerized tomography myelography and magnetic resonance imaging. J Neurosurg 86: 69–76.

Delaney TF, Liebsch NJ, Pedlow FX et al. (2014). Long-term results of phase II study of high dose photon/proton radiotherapy in the management of spine chordomas, chondrosarcomas, and other sarcomas. J Surg Oncol 110: 115–122.

de Schepper EI, Overdevest GM, Suri P et al. (2013). Diagnosis of lumbar spinal stenosis: an updated systematic review of the accuracy of diagnostic tests. Spine (Phila Pa 1976) 38: E469–E481.

di Chiro G, Schellinger D (1976). Computed tomography of spinal cord after lumbar intrathecal introduction of metrizamide (computer-assisted myelography). Radiology 120: 101–104.

Dorenbeck U, Schreyer AG, Schlaier J et al. (2004). Degenerative diseases of the cervical spine: comparison of a multiecho data image combination sequence with a magnetisation transfer saturation pulse and cervical myelography and CT. Neuroradiology 46: 306–309.

Eadsforth T, Niven S, Barrett C (2012). The utility of myelography in lumbar canal stenosis. Br J Neurosurg 26: 578–579.

Evans RW, Armon C, Frohman EM et al. (2000). Assessment: prevention of post-lumbar puncture headaches: report of the therapeutics and technology assessment subcommittee of the American Academy of Neurology. Neurology 55: 909–914.

Fedutes BA, Ansani NT (2003). Seizure potential of concomitant medications and radiographic contrast media agents. Ann Pharmacother 37: 1506–1510.

Guggenberger R, Winklhofer S, Osterhoff G et al. (2012). Metallic artefact reduction with monoenergetic dual-energy CT: systematic ex vivo evaluation of posterior spinal fusion implants from various vendors and different spine levels. Eur Radiol 22: 2357–2364.

Hagan JB (2004). Anaphylactoid and adverse reactions to radiocontrast agents. Immunol Allergy Clin North Am 24: vii–viii.

Hasiloglu ZI, Abuzayed B, Imal AE et al. (2012). Spontaneous intracranial hypotension due to intradural thoracic osteophyte with superimposed disc herniation: report of two cases. Eur Spine J 21: S383–S386.

Hoeffner EG, Mukherji SK, Srinivasan A et al. (2012). Neuroradiology back to the future: spine imaging. AJNR Am J Neuroradiol 33: 999–1006.

Hollis PH, Malis LI, Zappulla RA (1986). Neurological deterioration after lumbar puncture below complete spinal subarachnoid block. J Neurosurg 64: 253–256.

Ido K, Shiode H, Sakamoto A et al. (2002). The validity of upright myelography for diagnosing lumbar disc herniation. Clin Neurol Neurosurg 104: 30–35.

Janssen M, Nabih A, Moussa W et al. (2011). Evaluation of diagnosis techniques used for spinal injury related back pain. Pain Res Treat 2011: 478798.

Kent DL, Haynor DR, Larson EB et al. (1992). Diagnosis of lumbar spinal stenosis in adults: a metaanalysis of the accuracy of CT, MR, and myelography. AJR Am J Roentgenol 158: 1135–1144.

Khosla A, Wippold 2nd FJ (2002). CT myelography and MR imaging of extramedullary cysts of the spinal canal in adult and pediatric patients. AJR Am J Roentgenol 178: 201–207.

Klein KM, Shiratori K, Knake S et al. (2004). Status epilepticus and seizures induced by iopamidol myelography. Seizure 13: 196–199.

Larsson EM, Holtas S, Cronqvist S et al. (1989). Comparison of myelography, CT myelography and magnetic resonance imaging in cervical spondylosis and disk herniation. Pre- and postoperative findings. Acta Radiol 30: 233–239.

Layton KF, Kallmes DF, Horlocker TT (2006). Recommendations for anticoagulated patients undergoing image-guided spinal procedures. AJNR Am J Neuroradiol 27: 468–470.

Lloyd KM, Delgaudio JM, Hudgins PA (2008). Imaging of skull base cerebrospinal fluid leaks in adults. Radiology 248: 725–736.

Luetmer PH, Mokri B (2003). Dynamic CT myelography: a technique for localizing high-flow spinal cerebrospinal fluid leaks. AJNR Am J Neuroradiol 24: 1711–1714.

Luetmer PH, Schwartz KM, Eckel LJ et al. (2012). When should I do dynamic CT myelography? Predicting fast spinal CSF leaks in patients with spontaneous intracranial hypotension. AJNR Am J Neuroradiol 33: 690–694.

Miller GM, Krauss WE (2003). Myelography: still the gold standard. AJNR Am J Neuroradiol 24: 298.

Modic MT, Masaryk T, Boumphrey F et al. (1986). Lumbar herniated disk disease and canal stenosis: prospective evaluation by surface coil MR, CT, and myelography. AJR Am J Roentgenol 147: 757–765.

Moran SL, Steinmann SP, Shin AY (2005). Adult brachial plexus injuries: mechanism, patterns of injury, and physical diagnosis. Hand Clin 21: 13–24.

Namasivayam S, Kalra MK, Torres WE et al. (2006). Adverse reactions to intravenous iodinated contrast media: a primer for radiologists. Emerg Radiol 12: 210–215.

Orrison WW, Sackett JF, Amundsen P (1983). Lateral C1-2 puncture for cervical myelography. Part II: Recognition of improper injection of contrast material. Radiology 146: 395–400.

Papadopoulou A, Ahlhelm FJ, Ulmer S et al. (2013). Detection of cerebrospinal fluid leaks by intrathecal contrast-enhanced magnetic resonance myelography. JAMA Neurol 70: 1576–1577.

Patel IJ, Davidson JC, Nikolic B et al. (2012). Consensus guidelines for periprocedural management of coagulation status and hemostasis risk in percutaneous image-guided interventions. J Vasc Interv Radiol 23: 727–736.

Quaynor H, Tronstad A, Heldaas O (1995). Frequency and severity of headache after lumbar myelography using a 25-gauge pencil-point (Whitacre) spinal needle. Neuroradiology 37: 553–556.

Ruegg TA, Curran CR, Lamb T (2009). Use of buffered lidocaine in bone marrow biopsies: a randomized, controlled trial. Oncol Nurs Forum 36: 52–60.

Sandow BA, Donnal JF (2005). Myelography complications and current practice patterns. AJR Am J Roentgenol 185: 768–771.

Schievink WI (2008). Spontaneous spinal cerebrospinal fluid leaks. Cephalalgia 28: 1345–1356.

Schievink WI, Reimer R, Folger WN (1994). Surgical treatment of spontaneous intracranial hypotension associated with a spinal arachnoid diverticulum. Case report. J Neurosurg 80: 736–739.

Schievink WI, Maya MM, Louy C et al. (2008). Diagnostic criteria for spontaneous spinal CSF leaks and intracranial hypotension. AJNR Am J Neuroradiol 29: 853–856.

Song KJ, Choi BW, Kim GH et al. (2009). Clinical usefulness of CT-myelogram comparing with the MRI in degenerative cervical spinal disorders: is CTM still useful for primary diagnostic tool? J Spinal Disord Tech 22: 353–357.

Starling A, Hernandez F, Hoxworth JM et al. (2013). Sensitivity of MRI of the spine compared with CT myelography in orthostatic headache with CSF leak. Neurology 81: 1789–1792.

Steens SC, Pondaag W, Malessy MJ et al. (2011). Obstetric brachial plexus lesions: CT myelography. Radiology 259: 508–515.

Stone JA, Castillo M, Neelon B et al. (1999). Evaluation of CSF leaks: high-resolution CT compared with contrast-enhanced CT and radionuclide cisternography. AJNR Am J Neuroradiol 20: 706–712.

Strupp M, Schueler O, Straube A et al. (2001). "Atraumatic" Sprotte needle reduces the incidence of post-lumbar puncture headaches. Neurology 57: 2310–2312.

Tseng SH, Tseng WS (1997). Acute hydrocephalus after iotrolan lumbar myelography. Neuroradiology 39: 863–864.

Uhl M, Sterzing F, Habl G et al. (2011). CT-myelography for high-dose irradiation of spinal and paraspinal tumors with helical tomotherapy: revival of an old tool. Strahlenther Onkol 187: 416–420.

Wendl CM, Schambach F, Zimmer C et al. (2012). CT myelography for the planning and guidance of targeted epidural blood patches in patients with persistent spinal CSF leakage. AJNR Am J Neuroradiol 33: 541–544.

Williams MT (2014). The oblique interlaminar approach for fluoroscopy-guided lumbar puncture: Keep the eye opened! Diagn Interv Imaging 95: 629–632.

Yamazaki H, Doi K, Hattori Y et al. (2007). Computerized tomography myelography with coronal and oblique coronal view for diagnosis of nerve root avulsion in brachial plexus injury. J Brachial Plex Peripher Nerve Inj 2: 16.

Yoshioka N, Hayashi N, Akahane M et al. (2006). Bezier surface reformation: an original visualization technique of cervical nerve roots on myelographic CT. Radiat Med 24: 600–604.

Zeng Q, Xiong L, Jinkins JR et al. (1999). Intrathecal gadolinium-enhanced MR myelography and cisternography: a pilot study in human patients. AJR Am J Roentgenol 173: 1109–1115.

Handbook of Clinical Neurology, Vol. 135 (3rd series)
Neuroimaging, Part I
J.C. Masdeu and R.G. González, Editors

Chapter 11

Positron Emission Tomography

KATHERINE LAMEKA[1]*, MICHAEL D. FARWELL[2], AND MASANORI ICHISE[3]

[1]*Department of Radiology, Tufts University, Boston and Department of Radiology, Baystate Medical Center, Springfield, MA, USA*

[2]*Department of Radiology, Perelman School of Medicine of the University of Pennsylvania, Philadelphia, PA, USA*

[3]*Molecular Neuroimaging Program, Molecular Imaging Center, National Institute of Radiological Sciences, Anagawa, Inage, Chiba, Japan*

Abstract

Positron emission tomography (PET) is a minimally invasive imaging procedure with a wide range of clinical and research applications. PET allows for the three-dimensional mapping of administered positron-emitting radiopharmaceuticals such as ^{18}F-fluorodeoxyglucose (for imaging glucose metabolism). PET enables the study of biologic function in both health and disease, in contrast to magnetic resonance imaging (MRI) and computed tomography (CT), that are more suited to study a body's morphologic changes, although functional MRI can also be used to study certain brain functions by measuring blood flow changes during task performance. This chapter first provides an overview of the basic physics principles and instrumentation behind PET methodology, with an introduction to the merits of merging functional PET imaging with anatomic CT or MRI imaging. We then focus on clinical neurologic disorders, and reference research on relevant PET radiopharmaceuticals when applicable. We then provide an overview of PET scan interpretation and findings in several specific neurologic disorders such as dementias, epilepsy, movement disorders, infection, cerebrovascular disorders, and brain tumors.

INTRODUCTION

Positron emission tomography (PET) is an excellent noninvasive imaging procedure with a wide range of clinical and research applications in the evaluation of the pathophysiology of many brain disorders, such as neurodegenerative disorders, infection, epilepsy, seizures, psychiatric disorders, and brain tumors, as well as in the study of neurophysiology of the normal brain. PET is a highly sensitive imaging technique allowing for the three-dimensional mapping of positron-emitting radiopharmaceuticals administered in miniscule (µg) quantities without causing any significant physiologic or pharmacologic effects. PET is thus often referred to as a functional or molecular imaging tool that enables the study of biologic function in both health and disease, in contrast to magnetic resonance imaging (MRI) and computed tomography (CT), that are more suited to study a body's morphologic changes, although functional MRI can also be used to study certain brain functions by measuring blood flow changes during task performance. After its introduction in the early 1970s, PET was initially considered to be a powerful research tool for the evaluation of physiologic phenomena, including cerebral blood flow using $^{15}O\text{-}H_2O$. In 1976, however, based on the work of Sokoloff and colleagues, ^{18}F-fluorodeoxyglucose (FDG) was developed to study the glucose metabolism of the brain, which greatly expanded the scope of PET (Sokoloff et al., 1977; Reivich et al., 1979; Raichle, 2001). FDG PET is currently a widely used clinically approved tool in neurology, cardiology, and oncology. Many other PET radiopharmaceuticals, including those that target neuroreceptor systems such as the dopamine and serotonin systems, have also been developed and are widely used in

*Correspondence to: Katherine Lameka, MD, Radiology and Imaging, Inc., Baystate Medical Center, 759 Chestnut Street, Springfield MA 01199, USA. Tel: +1-413-794-3333, E-mail: klameka@yahoo.com

brain research. PET also allows detection of β-amyloid plaques (neuritic plaques) typically found in the brains of patients with Alzheimer's disease (AD). In 2012, ^{18}F-amyvid (a β-amyloid radiopharmaceutical) was approved for clinical use in the USA. Although PET was initially developed as a single modality, PET/CT systems that allow merging of physiologic PET images and detailed morphologic CT images are now widely used to enhance the unique physiologic capabilities of PET. Furthermore, PET/MRI systems are also emerging as a clinical tool that takes advantage of the excellent soft-tissue discriminatory capability of MRI. This chapter highlights the physics and instrumentation of PET imaging systems together with some specific clinical and research uses of PET imaging.

PET PHYSICS AND INSTRUMENTATION

In PET imaging, radiopharmaceuticals labeled with positron-emitting radioisotopes such as ^{11}C and ^{18}F are administered. The positron emission decay process is characterized by the conversion of a proton into a neutron with emission of a positron, the positively charged antiparticle of the electron, and a neutrino, a chargeless and almost massless particle that does not interact with matter. When an emitted positron unites with a nearby electron in an annihilation event, a pair of two photons (γ-rays) are produced, each with an energy of 511 keV, which travel in equal and (nearly) opposite directions (Fig. 11.1). PET scanners are equipped with coincidence γ-ray detectors to detect these pairs of photons as they hit opposing detectors at approximately the same time.

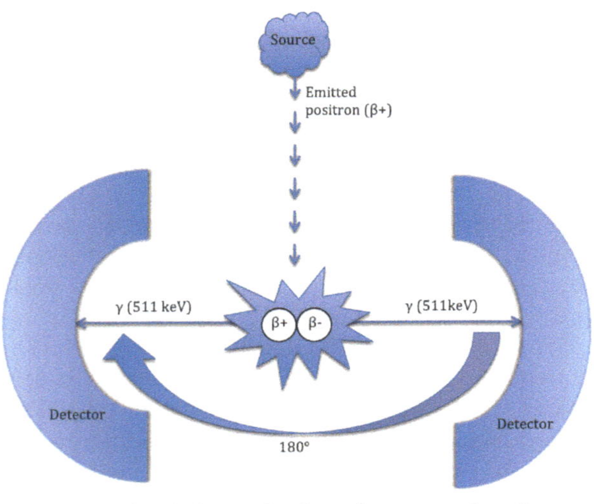

Fig. 11.1. After being emitted, positrons travel a distance before combining with an electron in an annihilation event. This results in the production of two antiparallel 511 keV photons which strike opposing detectors within a coincidence time window.

The coincidence-resolving time window between detectors is typically 4–5 nanoseconds, although new state-of-the-art PET scanners utilizing time-of-flight coincidence circuitry have a time resolution close to 500 picoseconds (Spanoudaki and Levin, 2010). When two photons are detected in opposed detectors within the coincidence time window, a coincidence event is recorded, and the positron annihilation is assumed to have occurred somewhere along the line of response (LOR) connecting the two detectors. However, annihilation events do not always generate a detectable coincidence event, either because one of the two γ-rays is absorbed or because it is simply not detected (the detector is not 100% efficient); these single photons actually make up the vast majority of the total count rate. However, approximately 97% of single photons are eliminated by the coincidence window. This electronic collimation is one of the primary advantages to PET imaging over single-photon emission computed tomography (SPECT), which requires a physical collimator that absorbs a large fraction of the incident photons; PET is thus about two orders of magnitude more sensitive than SPECT (Rahmim and Zaidi, 2008).

Although single unpaired photons are easily excluded by the coincidence window, additional processes occur in PET imaging which degrade image contrast. The first is termed *randoms*, which occurs when single photons from two different annihilations are detected in coincidence. In whole-body PET imaging the randoms rate sometimes exceeds the true coincidence rate; however in brain imaging the randoms rate seldom exceeds 25% of the true rate (Zanzonico, 2004). The second process is *scatter*, in which one or both photons from an annihilation event are deflected from their normal path but retain enough energy to be accepted by the detection system. Both of these processes cause the coincidence event to be assigned to the wrong LOR, thereby misrepresenting the true activity distribution within the field of view. Thus, various algorithms and techniques are employed during data processing to correct for randoms and scatter.

Several additional corrections are required during data processing in order to generate a final image. Correcting for *dead time*, a count rate-dependent phenomenon by which the detector is paralyzed and stops recording counts, and for varying sensitivity among detectors, is relatively straightforward for brain imaging. For accurate quantitative results, one of the most important corrections to the acquired PET image is the attenuation correction. This correction is necessary because photons released from the center of the brain are attenuated to a greater extent than photons released from the periphery; without attenuation correction, the intensity in the center of the brain is decreased by

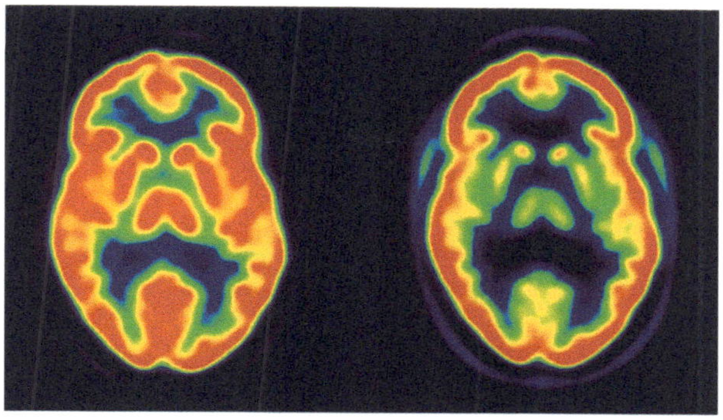

Fig. 11.2. Transaxial ^{18}F-fluorodeoxyglucose positron emission tomography images of a normal brain with attenuation correction (left image) and without attenuation correction (right image).

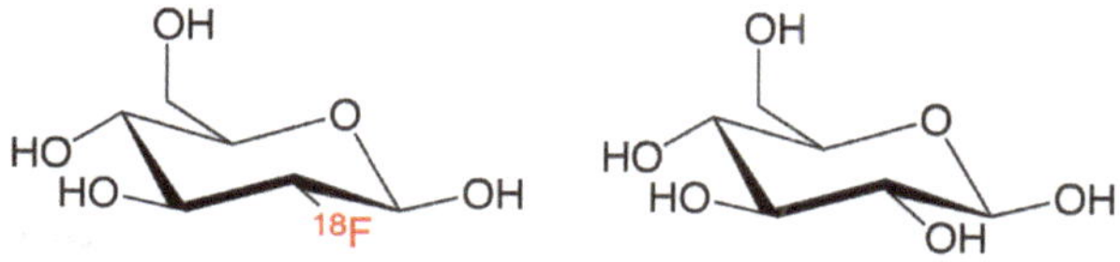

Fig. 11.3. The chemical structure of ^{18}F-fluorodeoxyglucose (FDG) (left) is very similar to glucose (right); in FDG the 2' hydroxyl group has been replaced by ^{18}F.

approximately 50% (Fig. 11.2). Attenuation correction of PET data is simpler than correction of SPECT data because, in contrast to SPECT, the probability of detection is uniform at each point along an LOR. The correction factor depends only on the total thickness and density of tissue along the LOR. Patient-specific attenuation measurements can be obtained from a transmission scan, using either an external radioisotope source or an X-ray tube mounted on the PET scanner or, more recently, an attenuation map from a CT scan obtained by hybrid PET/CT scanners.

Spatial resolution of PET images is limited by several factors. The first is the distance that the positron travels from its site of origin to its point of annihilation. This distance is dependent on its initial kinetic energy, which varies over a spectrum but is generally related to the emitting radioisotope. Typical positron ranges in tissue are 2.3 mm (^{18}F), 3.9 mm (^{11}C), 5.1 mm (^{13}N), and 8.0 mm (^{15}O) (Evans, 1972). When the initial kinetic energy of a positron has almost been lost, the probability of an annihilation reaction with an electron becomes very high. Because both energy and momentum must be conserved in the reaction, two photons are emitted with 511 keV of energy that are traveling in opposite directions, 180°, of each other. However, the positron is often not completely at rest but has a small residual momentum at the time of annihilation. This produces a small change in the observed colinearity, with the accuracy being $180° \pm 0.25°$ (Berko and Hereford, 1956). This deviation in photon direction is the second factor that limits scanner resolution. While these physical effects place a fundamental limit on the spatial resolution that can be achieved with PET, contributions from the size and design of the PET detectors further degrade the spatial resolution. Modern PET scanners are typically able to achieve a spatial resolution of about 4–6 mm, of which physical effects (positron range and photon noncolinearity) contribute about 2 mm (Townsend, 2004).

Preparation of PET imaging agents requires the generation of short-lived radioactive isotopes at a cyclotron facility via bombardment of a target with a beam of protons. The most commonly administered PET radionuclide is ^{18}F, which is used for the production of FDG (Fig. 11.3). This isotope is generated when ^{18}O-enriched water is employed as a target for high-energy protons. The half-life of ^{18}F is 110 minutes, which enables the imaging facility to use an off-site cyclotron radiopharmacy with a delivery time of up to several hours; for comparison, ^{11}C, ^{13}N, and ^{15}O require an on-site radiopharmacy because of their very short half-lives (20, 10, and 2 minutes, respectively) (Esser, 2009).

The radiation exposure dose to the patient is an important consideration in PET imaging. The radiopharmaceutical transfers energy to tissue via ionizing events from the emitted positrons as well as the annihilation γ radiation. However, the radiation dose from the radiopharmaceutical is only one component of the total radiation dose to the patient from a PET scan. Because the current generation of hybrid PET/CT scanners incorporates a diagnostic CT scanner to generate attenuation maps and also provide detailed anatomic information (Fig. 11.4), the radiation exposure dose from the CT component of the scan must be added to the radiation exposure dose from the administered radiopharmaceutical. For example, the effective radiation dose to the brain from a 10 mCi dose of FDG is 4 mSv (urinary bladder wall = 59 mSv, whole body = 6 mSv) while the multidetector CT adds an additional 20 mSv (this dose depends on the radiographic technique, the CT scanner model, and the patient) (Huang et al., 2009). In general, the radiation exposure dose from the CT examination is higher than the radiation exposure dose from the administered radiopharmaceutical.

A basic imaging protocol for ^{18}F-FDG PET requires no the patient to fast for at least six hours prior to injection time and avoid insulin. After injection of radiopharmaceutical, the patient is asked to sit in a quiet uptake room for approximately 40–50 minutes with the eyes closed. The patient is asked to refrain from speaking since that may cause specific areas of the brain to demonstrate artifactual variation in glucose metabolism and cause a false-positive or a false-negative examination.

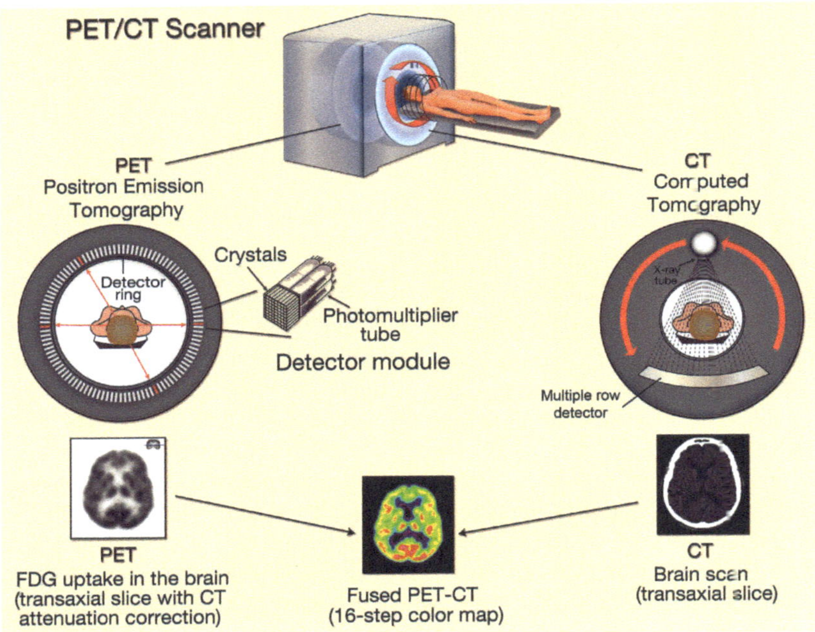

Fig. 11.4. Typical multimodality positron emission tomography (PET)/computed tomography (CT) imaging system combining a state-of-the-art PET scanner, for molecular imaging, with a multiple-detector-row CT scanner, for anatomic imaging. The software and hardware are optimized to acquire complementary information from a patient bed moving through both scanners. For the CT component of the scan, lasting seconds, the table moves uninterrupted while a continuous volume is acquired in spiral scan mode. For PET images, the bed moves in incremental steps based on the PET detectors' field-of-view (typically 16.2 cm) with each acquisition typically taking 3–6 minutes. The PET detector ring is shown with a multicrystal scintillation detector and photomultiplier tubes. The electronics and detector localize annihilation-photon absorption to a single crystal. FDG, ^{18}F-fluorodeoxyglucose. (Reproduced with permission from Esser, 2009.)

EMERGING PET SYSTEMS

Although CT and MRI are excellent tools for evaluation of structural abnormalities of the brain, the addition of PET as a hybrid PET/CT offers the benefit of functional imaging. For example, while CT and MRI provide anatomic information, they do not usually distinguish between malignant and benign tissue. This is particularly significant when assessing response of tumor to treatment. Anatomic imaging has limits in the delineation of tumor extension when tumor-bearing structures have unchanged anatomy or when tumor and normal tissues have similar density, similar magnetic properties, or similar contrast enhancement (Nestle et al., 2009). The additional value of hybrid PET/CT is that PET and CT scans are obtained in the same scanner in one imaging session with the patient in the same position, allowing for the use of the CT scan component for attenuation correction of the PET scan. Patient motion between CT and PET scanning can result in an inaccurate CT attenuation map as well as misregistration of the two image datasets; however, image misregistration can be easily corrected by using image coregistration software programs.

Although CT and MRI both provide excellent anatomic information, MRI is more capable of distinguishing different soft-tissue components. Furthermore, MRI can also provide functional information such as tissue perfusion as well as information on brain activation after performing a task (functional MRI). Recent developments in hybrid PET/MRI scanners attempt to take advantage of MRI's unique capabilities merged into PET's superb functional imaging capabilities. However, the combination of the two technologies has been initially problematic. Some problems in early investigations included interactions between the two systems in the form of electromagnetic interference (EMI), leading to artifacts and signal-to-noise reduction in the PET or MR images. Subsequently, MR-compatible PET scanners were developed based on fiberoptic coupling of the scintillator and the photodetectors, in which only the scintillator material is actually placed inside the MR scanner. The optical fibers then transmit the scintillation photons out of the main magnetic field, to the photomultiplier tubes and PET electronics that reside in the fringe field. This approach has been found to reduce EMI interaction between the two imaging systems (Slates et al., 1999). Other potential solutions that permit PET detectors to be compatible with the MR magnetic field include replacement of photomultiplier technology with magnetic field Y-insensitive avalanche photodiodes or silicon photomultipliers (Catana et al., 2006;

Varrone et al., 2009). Siemens recently introduced a PET/MRI scanner that is capable of concurrent dynamic PET and MRI scanning; this allows the MRI information to be used for dynamic motion correction during PET data acquisition. Other advantages of PET/MRI systems include the possibility of correcting the partial volume error in PET images by using MRI-based tissue segmentation (Meltzer et al., 1996), as well as reduced radiation exposure by not using CT, which is particularly beneficial in the pediatric population (Garibotto et al., 2013). Although MRI's functional and anatomic capabilities are expected to further enhance unique PET imaging potentials, the use of MRI instead of CT for accurate attenuation correction of PET images needs to be fully developed.

Another concept currently under development is dual tracer PET and SPECT imaging. This may be beneficial in instances when the physiologic functions studied depend on each other (e.g., perfusion and metabolism), hence requiring simultaneous assessment under identical conditions. This approach can greatly reduce quantification errors associated with physical factors that can change between acquisitions, such as anatomic alignment or a change in the attenuation map as a function of time (Fakhri, 2012). Chapman et al. (2012) explored simultaneous and sequential SPECT/PET imaging in studies that included ^{99m}Tc-MAA/^{18}F-NaF and ^{99m}Tc-Pentetate/^{18}F-NaF. Although down-scatter and cross-talk from the 511 keV photons emitted by the PET radiopharmaceutical interfered with obtaining useful SPECT information, the authors suggested an alternative strategy that consists of performing sequential SPECT and PET studies in hybrid SPECT/PET/CT scanners (Chapman et al., 2012).

PET SCAN INTERPRETATION

Currently, two brain PET examinations, ^{18}F-FDG (glucose metabolism) and ^{18}F-amyvid (β-amyloid imaging) are approved for clinical use in the USA.

Normal ^{18}F-FDG brain PET appearance

The most metabolically active areas of the brain include the cortical gray matter, especially the primary visual cortex, motor cortex, and the subcortical gray matter of the basal ganglia and thalamus. In the normal adult, the cerebellum demonstrates slightly less glucose metabolism relative to the supratentorial cortical structures (Fig. 11.5A) (Silverman, 2004). As a person ages, there is progressive dilation of the sulci and fissures as well as a gradual and progressive decrease in the metabolic activity throughout the gray and white matter. CT and MRI are useful in discriminating areas of ^{18}F-FDG activity that are decreased due to anatomic reasons (such as encephalomalacia or severe atrophy) from regions of ^{18}F-FDG activity that are decreased in an otherwise morphologically unremarkable brain (Fig. 11.5B). It is of note that there are some age-related changes in the normal

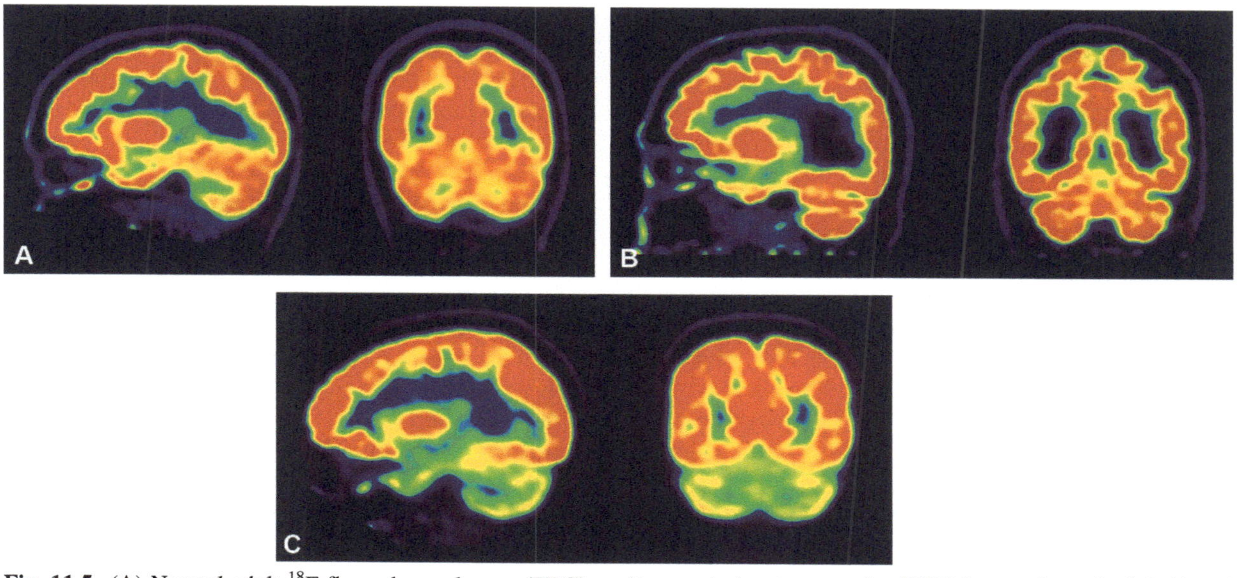

Fig. 11.5. (**A**) Normal adult ^{18}F-fluorodeoxyglucose (FDG) positron emission tomography (PET) images in sagittal (left) and coronal (right) planes. FDG activity in the cerebellum is slightly less than the FDG activity in cerebral cortex. (**B**) FDG PET images from an adult with cerebral atrophy in sagittal (left) and coronal (right) planes. FDG activity in the cerebellum is very similar to the FDG activity in cerebral cortex. Note the widened sulci and enlarged lateral ventricles from the patient's cerebral atrophy. (**C**) Normal FDG PET images from a 6-year-old girl in sagittal (left) and coronal (right) planes. FDG activity in the cerebellum is significantly decreased compared to cerebral cortex.

pattern of brain glucose metabolism. For example, cerebral glucose metabolism is relatively much higher compared with the cerebellar glucose metabolism in children, particularly those younger than age 6 (Fig. 11.5C) (Chugani et al., 1987). With age, this relative difference in glucose metabolism between the cerebral and cerebellar cortices becomes less marked. The knowledge of these normal variations of ^{18}F-FDG brain activity is important in interpreting ^{18}F-FDG brain PET scans. Visual interpretation of ^{18}F-FDG brain PET scans by experienced readers is common practice; however, quantitative approaches can also be employed to aid and complement the visual interpretation.

Quantification of regional glucose metabolism with ^{18}F-FDG PET is feasible. However, absolute glucose metabolism measurements require dynamic PET imaging with concurrent arterial blood sampling, which is a laborious and invasive procedure that is typically only used in selected research studies (Toyama et al., 2004). Alternatively, a measure of the degree of ^{18}F-FDG uptake is commonly determined by calculating the standardized uptake value (SUV), which is a popular method to assess differences in tumor grade as well as to monitor tumor response to treatment (Lucignani et al., 2004). The most commonly used definition of SUV is the ratio of regional ^{18}F-FDG radioactivity concentration (mCi/mL) to whole-body ^{18}F-FDG radioactivity concentration (injected ^{18}F-FDG dose administered divided by the weight of the patient in grams) (Kim et al., 1994). However, the SUV is a relative quantification measurement and has several limitations. Factors that affect SUV include weight and body composition, glucose level at the time of injection, physical activity of the patient prior to the examination, as well as extravasation or infiltration during injection. Therefore, it has been suggested that the SUV should be used as a guideline rather than an absolute value. Another relative quantitative measurement often used for ^{18}F-FDG brain PET is the ratio of regional ^{18}F-FDG activity to that of a reference region that is assumed to be normal (such as the cerebellar cortex in neurodegenerative disorders). In addition, there are several software applications that allow relative quantitative analysis of ^{18}F-FDG brain PET data. For example, SPM (Kiebel and Friston, 2004) allows voxel-wise comparative analyses with a normative database.

Finally, in research brain PET imaging studies, particularly with regard to imaging various neuroreceptors, dynamic PET or PET/CT image data acquisition is performed following the radiopharmaceutical injection. With appropriate radiopharmaceuticals that bind to neuroreceptors/transporters, dynamically acquired PET data with or without blood data can be mathematically modeled to quantify the density of target binding sites (Ichise, 2009). Examples of such quantitative images are shown in Figure 11.9 (see below: β-amyloid imaging; Becker et al., 2013) and Figure 11.12 (see below: serotonin transporter imaging; Ichise et al., 2003), described later in this chapter.

CLINICAL APPLICATIONS

Clinical applications of brain PET are highlighted in this section, which focuses on the use of ^{18}F-FDG (glucose metabolism) and ^{18}F-amyvid (β-amyloid imaging), as these radiopharmaceuticals are clinically approved, as well as other investigational radiopharmaceuticals.

Dementias

With modern medical advances, the life expectancy of the population has increased, with an accompanying increase in the prevalence of dementias. Among the various causes of dementia, Alzheimer's dementia (AD) accounts for approximately two-thirds of cases, followed by other dementias, such as diffuse Lewy-body disease (DLBD) and ischemic vascular dementia. Not infrequently dementias may have mixed causes, consisting of a combination of two or more dementia conditions, such as AD and vascular dementia. The earlier the diagnosis of a particular dementia can be made, the more effective treatment strategies and earlier prognostic counseling can be employed. The evaluation of dementias often presents with a diagnostic dilemma in patients who do not have a classic presentation of a particular entity. In such instances, PET imaging can play an important role (Van Heertum and Tikofsky, 2003).

Alzheimer's disease

In AD, PET imaging classically demonstrates a pattern of symmetric diminished regional glucose metabolism in the posterior temporoparietal cortices bilaterally as well as the anterior and mesial temporal lobes (Fig. 11.6A). The sensorimotor cortex and the gray matter of the subcortical structures and cerebellum are typically spared. However, the patterns of hypometabolism can often demonstrate a significant amount of asymmetry (Fig. 11.6B). The combined use of MRI or CT in conjunction with PET is useful in identifying areas of atrophy from hypometabolic brain regions.

A good correlation has been made between the degree of regional asymmetric hypometabolism and the clinically observed behavioral and cognitive deficits (Van Heertum, 2009). PET imaging has also been used in conjunction with biomarkers to predict future risk of developing the disease. For example, an abnormal apolipoprotein E (APOE) protein called APOE-ϵ4 has been implicated in some cases of AD, and studies have shown that it is likely that such individuals are at a greater risk of developing AD (Mayeux, 2006). Various studies have shown that those individuals who are homozygous for

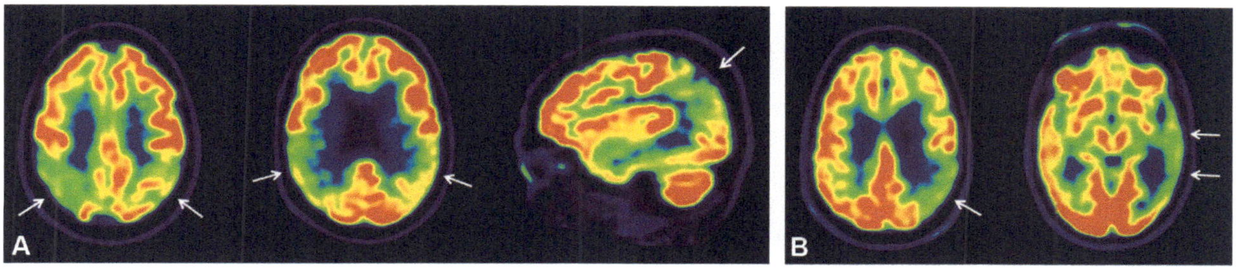

Fig. 11.6. (**A**) ^{18}F-Fluorodeoxyglucose (FDG) positron emission tomography (PET) images from a patient with Alzheimer's disease. Arrows indicate regions of diminished metabolism in the bilateral parietal and temporal lobes, with sparing of the sensorimotor strip. (**B**) FDG PET images from a patient with Alzheimer's disease. Imaging findings are often asymmetric, as demonstrated in this case. Arrows indicate regions of diminished metabolism in the left parietal and temporal lobes, with sparing of the sensorimotor strip.

the APOE-ϵ4 allele and demonstrate bilateral posterior parietal and temporal-lobe hypometabolic deficits are significantly more likely to progress to AD than individuals who are APOE-ϵ4-positive and PET-negative (Small et al., 2000; Reiman, 2007).

Frontotemporal dementia

Frontotemporal dementia (FTD) differs from AD in both clinical and imaging aspects. Clinically, FTD patients tend to present with mood and behavioral changes, which may include obsessive behavior and language difficulties. Many patients lose their inhibitions and exhibit antisocial behavior. However, as the severity of the disease progresses, symptoms may not be easily distinguishable from AD. On PET imaging, FTD demonstrates hypometabolism predominantly in the frontal and anterior temporal lobes (Fig. 11.7). As in AD, asymmetry in glucose metabolism can often be observed. In contrast to AD, the posterior cingulate gyrus tends to be preserved in FTD patients, but is commonly hypometabolic in AD patients (Ishii et al., 1998).

Diffuse Lewy-body dementia

DLBD is a neurologic disorder characterized by the presence of α-synuclein cytoplasmic inclusions (Lewy bodies) throughout the brain (Lippa et al., 2007). The clinical presentation consists of a "classic" triad of parkinsonism, visual hallucinations, and cognitive decline (Kramer and Schulz-Schaeffer, 2007). Unlike AD, DLBD may require treatment with dopaminergic compounds, but, like AD, it is usually treated with cholinesterase inhibitors and compounds that target specific disturbances, such as antidepressants, anxiolytics, or antipsychotics. However, prognosis differs and therefore it is important to distinguish between these entities (Weisman and McKeith, 2007). The main distinguishing features between AD and DLBD are the degree of hypometabolism in the parietal regions, which may be much more profound in DLBD than in AD, and extension of hypometabolism to the occipital cortex, which is more common in DLBD, especially if there is involvement of the primary visual cortex (Fig. 11.8) (Colloby and O'Brien, 2004). Furthermore, while in AD the posterior cingulate gyrus is uniformly involved, in DLBD it is spared ("cingulate island sign"). Therefore, the combination of visual hallucinations and involvement of the primary visual cortex on PET is very suggestive of DLBD (Ishii et al., 2004). In patients with DLBD, the anterior portions of the temporal lobes are usually not involved to the same degree as in AD patients. Of note, an FDG PET scan may also be helpful in distinguishing

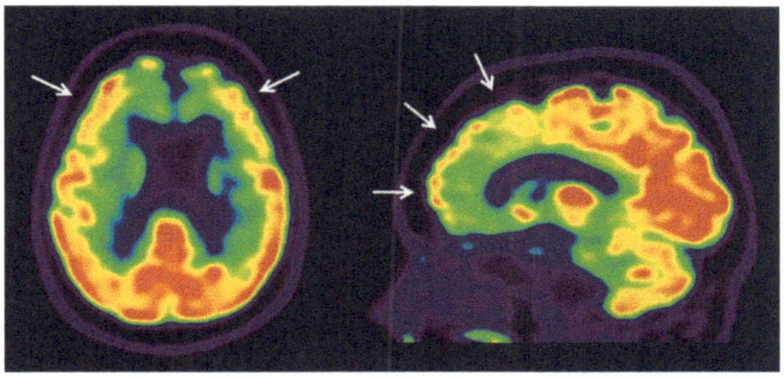

Fig. 11.7. ^{18}F-Fluorodeoxyglucose positron emission tomography images from a patient with frontotemporal dementia. Arrows indicate regions of diminished metabolism in the bilateral frontal and temporal lobes.

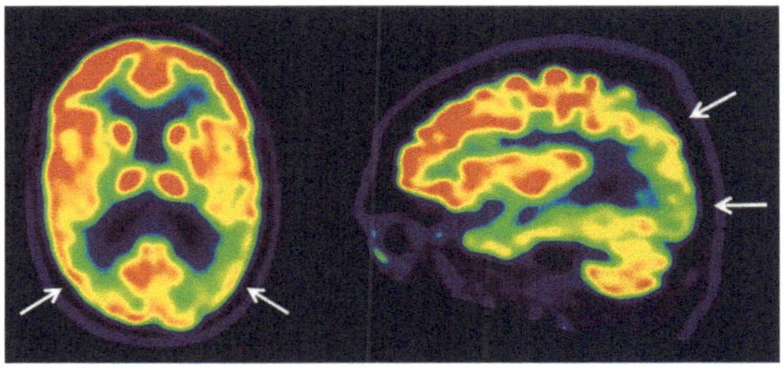

Fig. 11.8. ^{18}F-Fluorodeoxyglucose positron emission tomography images from a patient with diffuse Lewy body disease. Arrows indicate regions of diminished metabolism in the bilateral parietal and occipital lobes.

other forms of dementia, including Creutzfeldt–Jakob disease, corticobasal degeneration, and ischemic vascular dementia (Van Heertum et al., 2001).

More recently, there has been development of presynaptic dopamine imaging radiopharmaceuticals, such as ^{18}F-fluorodopa (FDOPA), for assessing dopamine synthesis capacity (which will be further discussed in the section on movement disorders, below), dopamine transporter imaging radiopharmaceuticals, including ^{11}C-methylphenidate and ^{11}C-PE2I, and vesicular monoamine transporter imaging radiopharmaceuticals such as ^{11}C-DTBZ and ^{18}F-FP-DTBZ. These radiopharmaceuticals allow evaluation of the integrity of the dopaminergic neurons and therefore are very useful for further distinguishing DLBD from AD. DLBD patients typically demonstrate abnormal presynaptic dopamine imaging, whereas AD patients are similar to age-matched normal control subjects (Walker et al., 2002). At present, these dopaminergic radiopharmaceuticals are not approved for clinical use in the USA. However, a SPECT dopamine transporter radiopharmaceutical, ^{123}I-FP-CIT (DaTscan), was approved by the Food and Drug Administration (FDA) in 2012 for clinical use in the USA; DaTscan was approved in Europe in 2000.

Amyloid imaging

Advances have recently been made in the development of β-amyloid-avid PET imaging radiopharmaceuticals. An optimal radiopharmaceutical for β-amyloid detection should rapidly penetrate the blood–brain barrier, have a high binding affinity for β-amyloid protein, and be able to quantify *in vivo* the amount of amyloid protein present (Cai et al., 2007). Several radiopharmaceuticals have been investigated, including 2-(4-methylamino) phenyl-6-hydroxy-benzothiazole (^{11}C-labeled BTA) (a.k.a. "Pittsburgh compound B," or PIB), 1-(1-[6[(2-fluoroethyl)(methyl)(amino)]-2-naphthyl]-ethylidene malonitrile (FDDNP) (Shoghi-Jadid et al., 2002; Klunk et al., 2004; Wolk et al., 2012), and florbetapir.

Florbetapir (Amyvid) was approved by the FDA in April 2012 for clinical use in the detection of amyloid plaques in the USA, and was subsequently approved for use in the European Union in January 2013. At the time of this writing, January 2015, two other β-amyloid imaging compounds have been approved by the FDA, ^{18}F-florbetaben, and ^{18}F-flutemetamol. These compounds bind to aggregated extraneuronal β-amyloid fibrils in brains of patients with AD. The presence of brain β-amyloid deposition is one of the two pathologic hallmarks of AD, the other being the presence of neurofibrillary tangles as a result of twisted fibers of microtubules resulting from hyperphosporylation of *tau* protein. However, accumulation of β-amyloid is also found in brains of cognitively normal individuals over 60 years of age (12–50% of aged individuals with increasing frequency with advancing age) (Rowe and Villemagne, 2011). Positive β-amyloid PET imaging thus is not diagnostic of AD and the accuracy of amyloid imaging for AD appears age-dependent, being over 90% for patients under the age of 70 years, about 85% for patients in their 70s, and 75–80% for those over 80 years (Rowe and Villemagne, 2011). In clinical trials, Amyvid was well tolerated, with no serious adverse events (Wong et al., 2010). A negative Amyvid scan indicates sparse to no neuritic plaques and is inconsistent with a neuropathologic diagnosis of AD; therefore, a negative scan reduces the likelihood that a patient's cognitive impairment is due to AD. A positive Amyvid scan indicates moderate to frequent amyloid neuritic plaques; neuropathologic examination has shown this amount of amyloid neuritic plaque is present in patients with AD, but may also be present in patients with other types of neurologic conditions as well as older people with normal cognition (Fig. 11.9). Amyvid is an adjunct to other diagnostic evaluations (Amyvid, 2012)).

The Society of Nuclear Medicine and Molecular Imaging and the Alzheimer's Association have jointly developed criteria for the appropriate use of amyloid imaging PET radiopharmaceuticals (Johnson et al., 2013). They proposed the following indications for clinical use:

1. Patients with persistent or progressive unexplained mild cognitive impairment.
2. Patients satisfying core clinical criteria for possible AD because of unclear clinical

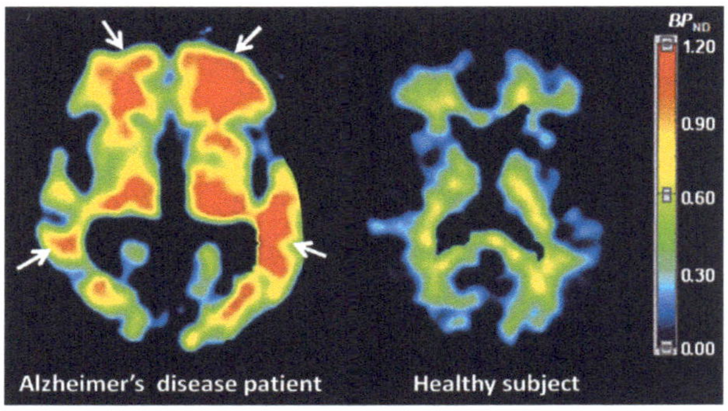

Fig. 11.9. Transaxial parametric images through a midthalamic level of an Alzheimer's patient (left) and a healthy subject (right) show voxel-wise binding potential (BP_{ND}) that is proportional to β-amyloid binding-site density, generated from 90 minutes dynamic positron emission tomography data acquired after an injection of ^{18}F-florbetaben. β-amyloid binding is seen in the frontotemporal cortices of the Alzheimer's patient's brain (arrows), with only mild nonspecific binding in the white matter and subcortical gray matter of the healthy subject's brain (right). No cortical β-amyloid binding is seen in the healthy subject's brain. (Reproduced from Becker et al., 2013.)

presentation, either an atypical clinical course or an etiologically mixed presentation.

3. Patients with progressive dementia and atypically early age of onset (usually defined as 65 years or less in age).

Amyloid imaging was suggested to be inappropriate in the following situations:

1. Patients with core clinical criteria for probable AD with typical age of onset.
2. To determine dementia severity.
3. based solely on a positive family history of dementia or presence of APOE-ϵ4.
4. Patients with a cognitive complaint that is unconfirmed on clinical examination.
5. In lieu of genotyping for suspected autosomal mutation carriers.
6. In asymptomatic individuals.
7. Nonmedical use (e.g., legal, insurance coverage, or employment screening).

Epilepsy

Another realm of neurology in which PET imaging is useful is in the evaluation of epilepsy. FDG PET is a clinically useful nuclear medicine imaging tool in the presurgical evaluation of epilepsy patients with medically refractory partial seizures. FDG PET is typically used in conjunction with other presurgical tests which include MRI, neuropsychologic tests, noninvasive video/electroencephalographic monitoring, and ictal and interictal perfusion SPECT using ^{99m}Tc-HMPAO or ^{99m}Tc-ECD.

Interictal PET detects regions of decreased glucose metabolism in the epileptogenic zone (Fig. 11.10). The sensitivity of interictal FDG PET for localization of the epileptogenic zone in more than 300 patients with temporal-lobe and extratemporal-lobe epilepsy studied at one institution was reported to be 85% (Won et al., 1999; Lee et al., 2006). In the same study, the sensitivities of ictal SPECT and MRI were 75% and 70%, respectively. Because FDG is taken up by the brain over a period of approximately 40 minutes after injection, ictal FDG PET is not useful for the localization of the epileptogenic zone.

Studies have suggested that combining ictal SPECT and interictal FDG PET can improve the accuracy of localization (Van Paesschen et al., 2007). The largest and most intense ictal hyperperfusion focus on ictal SPECT is usually considered the ictal onset zone, while the region of decreased glucose metabolism on FDG PET is considered to represent the epileptogenic zone. A drawback of ictal SPECT is poor temporal resolution due to the time it takes for the radiopharmaceutical to reach the brain and

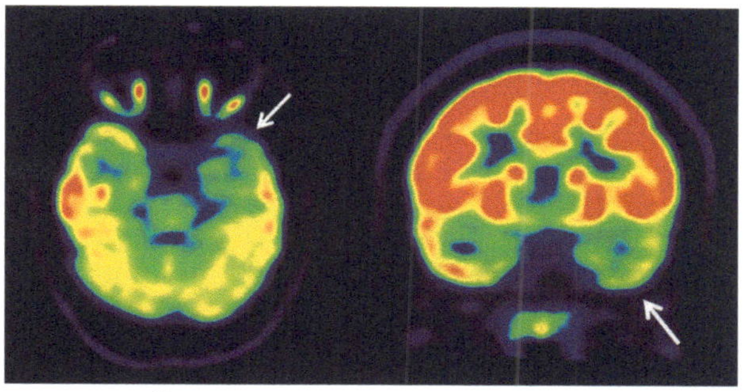

Fig. 11.10. ^{18}F-Fluorodeoxyglucose positron emission tomography images from a 12-year-old girl with medically refractory epilepsy. Transaxial (left) and coronal (right) planes are shown. These images were acquired in the interictal state, and demonstrate decreased metabolism in the mesial left temporal lobe, as indicated by the arrows. This finding is consistent with an epileptogenic focus in the mesial left temporal lobe.

become trapped in the brain after the intravenous injection. Ictal SPECT images therefore may reveal hyperperfusion both in the ictal onset zone and seizure propagation pathways, and the most intense perfusion focus on ictal SPECT may actually represent this seizure propagation (Dupont et al., 2006).

The region of hypometabolism on interictal FDG PET often exceeds the size of the anatomic region of seizure onset. These regions of decreased metabolism may also show changes over the course of the seizure history, where the extent of hypometabolism has been shown to positively correlate with seizure frequency (Benedek et al., 2006). A combined approach in which SPECT and PET images are analyzed together results in better definition of the epileptogenic onset zone (ictal SPECT), surround inhibition zones (ictal SPECT), and functional deficit (PET) in refractory partial epilepsy.

In addition to altered cerebral perfusion and glucose metabolism, the combined use of PET and SPECT has the potential to probe other pathophysiologic processes of epilepsy. For example, serotonin 1A receptors (5-HT1A) and γ-aminobutyric acid (GABA) receptors have been shown to be reduced in temporal lobe epilepsy using PET radiopharmaceuticals, ^{18}F-*trans*-4-fluoro-*N*-2[4- (2-methoxyphenyl)piperazin-1-yl]ethyl]-*N*-(2-pyridyl)-cyclohexanecarboxamide (^{18}F-FCWAY) and ^{11}C-flumazenil, that bind specifically to central 5-HT1A receptors and GABA receptors, respectively, providing additional information on the pathophysiology of epilepsy (Debets et al., 1997; Giovacchini et al., 2005). Another example is α-^{11}C-methyl-L-tryptophan (AMT), which has been used to detect the seizure focus in patients with epileptogenic tubers (Kagawa et al., 2005). AMT traces tryptophan metabolism via serotonin and/or kynurenine pathways and has been shown to pinpoint the epileptogenic focus in the interictal state by revealing a focus of increased AMT uptake (Kumar et al., 2011). However, the above-mentioned radiopharmaceuticals are investigational and not currently available for routine clinical use.

Movement disorders

PET imaging of the dopamine system has been used extensively in clinical research to evaluate patients with Parkinson's disease (PD) and other movement disorders, such as progressive supranuclear palsy (PSP) and multiple system atrophy (MSA). PD is the most common neurodegenerative cause of parkinsonism, followed by PSP and MSA (Jellinger, 1987). The accurate diagnosis of PD is important in deciding on the appropriate treatment, as well as for providing an indication of prognosis.

A number of PET radiopharmaceuticals have been developed for imaging of either presynaptic (D_1) or postsynaptic (D_2) components of the dopamine system (Jellinger, 1987). For example, ^{18}F-FDOPA, after intravenous injection, is converted by the aromatic amino acid decarboxylase (AADC) to ^{18}F-fluorodopamine, which becomes trapped within the presynaptic dopamine neuron (Brooks, 1998). FDOPA reflects AADC activity and is thus a marker for dopamine synthesis.

The reduction in striatal ^{18}F-FDOPA uptake has been shown to have two regional characteristics in PD: radiopharmaceutical uptake in the striatum contralateral to the clinically more affected side is reduced more than the ipsilateral side, and radiopharmaceutical uptake is reduced more in the putamen than in the caudate (Marek et al., 1996; Ichise et al., 1999; Seibyl, 2003). These findings are consistent with degeneration of nigrostriatal neurons, as shown by pathologic examination, which usually progresses asymmetrically. The ventrolateral substantia nigra projections to the putamen degenerate more severely than the ventromedial substantia nigra projections to the caudate (German et al., 1989; Fearnley and Lees, 1991). Dopamine neurons also degenerate in other parkinsonian syndromes, such as MSA and PSP, but have been shown to demonstrate less asymmetry than PD. PET imaging studies designed to evaluate the postsynaptic dopamine D_2 receptor have shown that striatal dopamine D_2 receptor binding is intact in PD, but it can be reduced in MSA and PSP and other movement disorders, such as Huntington's disease (Ichise et al., 1993; van Royen et al., 1993).

D_2 receptors may be upregulated in patients with untreated PD (Weiner, 2005), but may be normal or reduced in treated patients, especially in chronically treated patients (Brooks, 1998; Ichise et al., 1999). Therefore, by evaluating the status of D_2 receptors in patients with parkinsonism via postsynaptic scans, response to therapy with dopamine agonists can be predicted because these drugs require intact D_2 receptors to be effective (Schwarz et al., 1992). ^{18}F-FDG PET, ^{11}C-raclopride (RACLO) PET, and MRI can also be helpful in distinguishing these conditions, because there may be decreased striatal radiopharmaceutical uptake on FDG and RACLO PET in MSA but not in PD (Antonini et al., 1997), or increased signal in the putamen and pons on T2- or diffusion-weighted MR images in PSP but not in PD (Seppi et al., 2003). The clinical utility of these imaging techniques depends on their usefulness in changing the care of patients and/or reducing costs.

^{18}F-DOPA PET has also been used to determine the stage of dopaminergic degeneration in PD. It has been demonstrated that the decline of dopaminergic function starts in the dorsal caudal putamen contralateral to the clinically affected side and that the rate of degeneration in the caudate nucleus is slower than that of the putamen in early PD (Fearnley and Lees, 1991; Bruck et al., 2009; Loane and Politis, 2011).

In addition to dopamine receptors, alterations in the serotonin transporter (SERT) have also been described in PD as well as several other neuropsychiatric conditions, such as obsessive-compulsive disorder and severe depression. ^{11}C-3-amino-4-(2-dimethylaminomethyl-phenylsulfanyl)-benzonitrile (^{11}C-DASB) is a radiopharmaceutical for PET imaging that binds to presynaptic terminals expressing the serotonin transporter, thus providing a good measure of the integrity of serotonergic innervation (Fig. 11.11) (Ichise et al., 2003; Van Heertum, 2009). Preliminary human studies showed that the regional distribution of ^{11}C-DASB uptake was concordant with the known densities of SERT sites in the brain (Houle et al., 2000). Subsequently, a ^{11}C-DASB PET study with a larger sample size of 30 PD patients reported significant reductions in regional ^{11}C-DASB binding in striatal, brainstem, and cortical regions (Albin et al., 2008; Loane and Politis, 2011). The results have been strongly suggestive of a progressive, nonlinear serotonergic dysfunction in PD. However, ^{11}C-DASB and other serotonin transporter imaging radiopharmaceuticals are still under investigation.

Infection and inflammation

PET scanning has been useful in differentiating lymphoma from central nervous system infections, especially in human immunodeficiency virus (HIV)-positive patients. In this group of patients, a variety of infections as well as tumors can generate fevers and rapid mental status changes. In the HIV-positive patient, a diagnostic dilemma often arises when a space-occupying lesion is discovered on MRI, and rapid diagnosis is needed to institute the appropriate treatment.

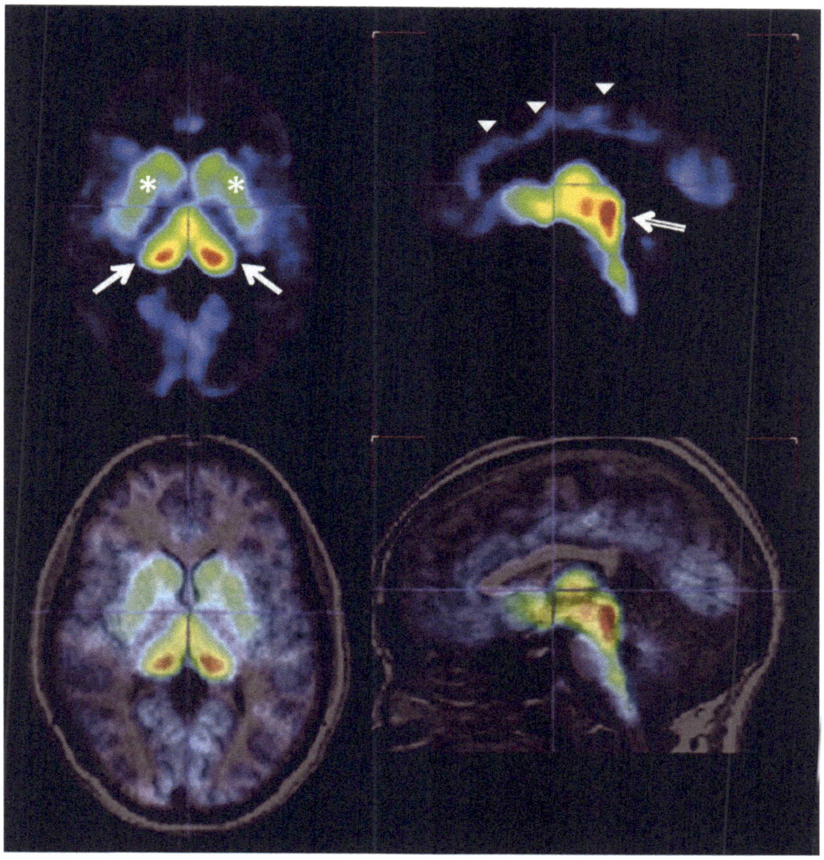

Fig. 11.11. Parametric images of brain serotonin transporter BP_{ND} modeled from 120 minutes dynamically acquired positron emission tomography (PET) data after an injection of ^{11}C-3-amino-4-(2-dimethylaminomethyl-phenylsulfanyl)-benzonitrile (^{11}C-DASB) in a healthy subject. Transaxial images at a midthalamic level (left) and mid-sagittal images (right) with PET only (top) and PET co-registered on to a magnetic resonance imaging scan (bottom) show high serotonin transporter densities in the posterior thalamus (solid arrow) and the raphe complex in the brainstem (hollow arrow) as well as moderate serotonin transporter binding in the striatum (asterisks) and mild binding in the limbic cortex (arrowhead). (Reproduced from Ichise et al., 2003.)

It has been suggested that empiric treatment with pyrimethamine and sulfadiazine should be initiated, and if there is no response after 2 weeks, a cerebral biopsy should be considered. However, because of a variety of adverse side effects and interactions with other medications, noninvasive testing is useful in determining which patients should receive empiric therapy versus cerebral biopsy early on in the course of disease (O'Doherty et al., 1997). PET imaging using FDG in this population has shown that highly metabolically active lymphomas demonstrate markedly increased FDG uptake (Fig. 11.12), while nonneoplastic lesions such as toxoplasmosis (Fig. 11.13) or syphilis gummas tend to be hypometabolic, although some infectious foci may be hypermetabolic and some lymphoma lesions may only be mildly hypermetabolic. In the latter situation, SPECT imaging with ^{201}Tl (thallium) may be of help because ^{201}Tl is a potassium analog that is transported into hypercellular tumors but not infectious foci (Hoffman et al., 1993).

Conversely, the more typical infectious processes such as bacterial abscesses or subdural empyemas tend to demonstrate varying degrees of glucose metabolism, some demonstrating photopenia while others demonstrating increased metabolism, particularly at the periphery. Although the mechanism of increased FDG uptake in abscesses is unclear, it is thought to be due to increased glucose metabolism associated with the inflammatory process and increased cellularity rather than disruption of the blood–brain barrier (Tsuyuguchi et al., 2003). The use of FDG PET/CT has been shown to be a useful adjunct to MRI in assessment of treatment response of brain abscesses (Park et al., 2011). Imaging with ^{11}C-methionine has also been shown to be useful in imaging abscesses (Ishii et al., 1993). In one case report, PET imaging with both FDG and ^{11}C-methionine demonstrated increased radiotracer uptake at the periphery of the lesions, but the study using ^{11}C-methionine demonstrated a greater

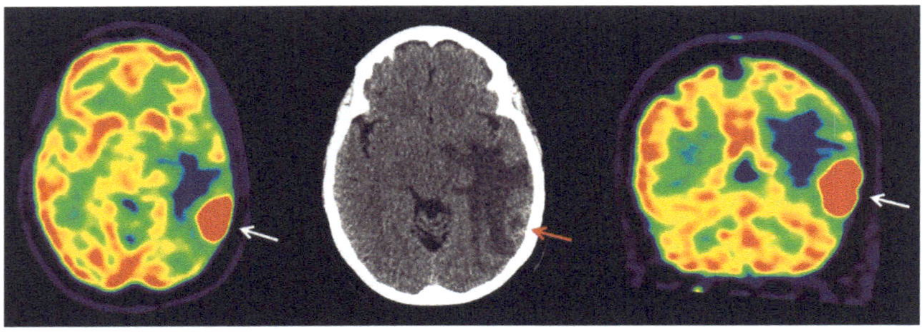

Fig. 11.12. ^{18}F-Fluorodeoxyglucose (FDG) positron emission tomography (PET) images from a 61-year-old woman with central nervous system lymphoma; transaxial PET and computed tomography (CT) images (left and middle) and a coronal PET image (right) are shown. The arrows indicate a markedly FDG-avid mass (standardized uptake value = 21) in the left temporal lobe which demonstrates increased density on CT images, with surrounding hypodensity/decreased FDG activity consistent with vasogenic edema.

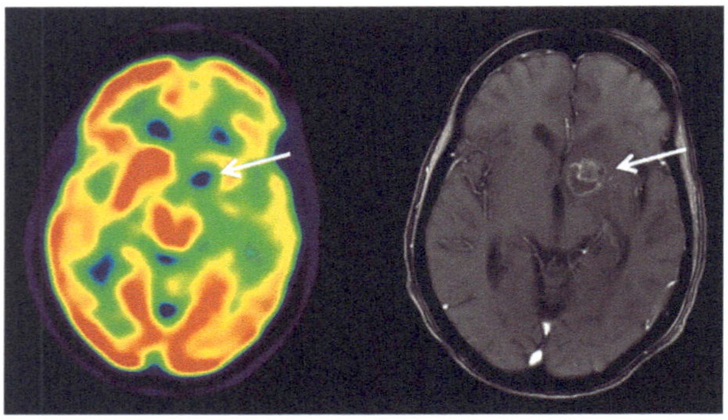

Fig. 11.13. Transaxial ^{18}F-fluorodeoxyglucose (FDG) positron emission tomography (left) and contrast-enhanced magnetic resonance imaging (right) images from a 62-year-old woman with human immunodeficiency virus and central nervous system toxoplasmosis. The arrows indicate an irregularly enhancing lesion near the left caudate head, which demonstrates very low FDG activity more suggestive of an infectious etiology rather than lymphoma. The diagnosis of toxoplasmosis was confirmed after the lesion responded to treatment.

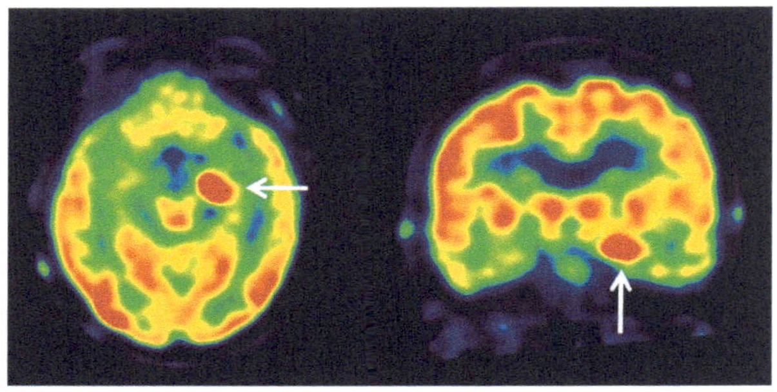

Fig. 11.14. Transaxial (left) and coronal (right) ^{18}F-fluorodeoxyglucose (FDG) positron emission tomography images in a 69-year-old woman with voltage-gated potassium channel antibody limbic encephalitis, syndrome of inappropriate antidiuretic hormone secretion (SIADH), sympathetic instability, and postural hypotension without clear underlying primary neoplasm. The arrows indicate a focus of increased FDG activity (standardized uptake value = 18.6) in the left amygdala consistent with active limbic encephalitis.

abscess-to-background ratio compared to FDG (Dethy et al., 1995). ^{11}C-Methionine imaging has also been shown to be useful in the imaging of pachymeningitis (Takahashi et al., 1996).

Several case reports have demonstrated the clinical utility of FDG PET in the evaluation of paraneoplastic encephalitis as compared with MRI. In many instances, unilateral or bilateral medial temporal hypermetabolism was discovered in the absence of abnormal enhancement on MRI (Fig. 11.14). Thus, it has been hypothesized that hypermetabolism on PET reflects different aspects or stages of inflammation that are not visible on contrast-enhanced MRI (Scheid et al., 2004). In several additional case reports, PET demonstrated bilateral hypermetabolism that extended beyond the abnormal lesions detected by contrast-enhanced MRI (Heiss et al., 1992). Some of the investigators suggested that the focal hypermetabolism on PET may represent seizure activity (Fakhoury et al., 1999), whereas others thought that the hypermetabolism may reflect an underlying inflammatory process (Provenzale et al., 1998; Kassubek et al., 2001). Acute disseminated encephalitis is another inflammatory process that can, in our experience, also show increased FDG activity in the acute setting (Fig. 11.15), although others have found decreased FDG activity (Tabata et al., 1990; Tan et al., 2004).

Cerebrovascular disease

Although CT, MRI, and functional MRI have largely replaced SPECT and PET for the evaluation of patients with acute stroke, PET imaging is still utilized in the determination of the oxygen extraction fraction in patients being considered for corrective surgery for carotid artery obstructive disease. The current standard of reference for measuring cerebral blood flow is PET

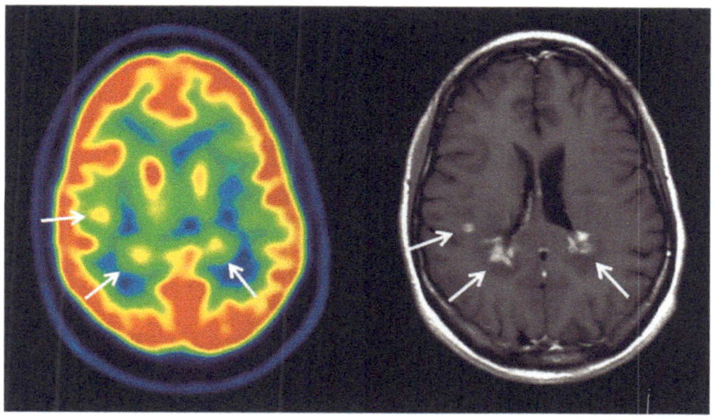

Fig. 11.15. Transaxial ^{18}F-fluorodeoxyglucose (FDG) positron emission tomography (left) and contrast-enhanced magnetic resonance imaging (right) images from a 34-year-old woman with acute disseminated encephalomyelitis (ADEM). The arrows indicate enhancing lesions in the posterior periventricular white matter and right parietal white matter which demonstrate increased FDG activity (standardized uptake value (SUV) = 6.3) relative to adjacent normal white matter (SUV = 2.7).

imaging with ^{15}O-labeled water, $H_2{}^{15}O$. In a recent study, strong correlations were found between MRI and PET cerebral blood flow indices (Vakil et al., 2013). In addition, there have been new radiopharmaceutical developments that may provide information unique to PET/SPECT on the pathophysiology of stroke. For example, cerebral cell death, specifically death of the "neurovascular unit," comprising the neuronal cell and associated endothelial and glial cells, is the major neuropathologic substrate in stroke. Therefore, information on the extent and dynamics of this cerebral cell death (apoptosis) as well as tissue hypoxia may be valuable for better diagnosis and monitoring of neuroprotective treatment for stroke patients. Hypoxia has been imaged using nitroimidazole-based radiopharmaceuticals such as ^{18}F-fluoromisonidazole (FMISO) and ^{18}F-fluoroazomycin-arabinoside (FAZA). The 2-nitroimidazole moiety acts as a bioreductive molecule that is trapped inside the cell constituents under hypoxic conditions (Bussink et al., 2010). Spratt et al. (2011) investigated the distribution of FMISO retention after induction of 2-hour temporary middle cerebral artery occlusion in rats utilizing a tritium-labeled tracer ^{3}H-FMISO. They concluded that FMISO retention occurs both within the ischemic penumbra and within the early infarct core. Most penumbral tissues show evidence of selective cellular injury (Spratt et al., 2011).

Brain tumors

Intracranial tumors are typically classified as either primary or metastatic. Of the primary brain tumors, gliomas constitute over 90% of tumors in the adult population and 60% of all brain tumors (Del Sole et al., 2001). FDG PET imaging of these tumors is based on glycolic activity of the tumor, with higher-grade tumors generally demonstrating higher glucose metabolism.

At present, the only agent approved for tumor imaging in the USA is FDG, which is typically used for defining extent of tumor and grade of malignancy, assessment of treatment response, and evaluation of radiation necrosis (Fig. 11.16) versus tumor recurrence (Fig. 11.17). Although FDG has been useful in imaging high-grade gliomas (Fig. 11.18), it has been shown to be less accurate in the detection of lower-grade tumors due to high background activity from normal brain glucose metabolism. However, low-grade tumors often demonstrate relatively decreased glucose metabolism when compared to normal brain (Di Chiro et al., 1982), and can be seen as photopenic defects superimposed on a background of normal glucose activity (Fig. 11.19).

The limitations of FDG for tumor evaluation have led to the development of novel PET imaging agents. Some of these developments stem from insights gained using MR spectroscopy, which is a technique that provides information on the concentration of specific intracellular metabolites, such as choline, creatine, phosphocreatine, *N*-acetyl aspartate, lactic acid, lipids, and triglycerides. Early reports of tumor analysis led to several conclusions. First, the concentration of choline-containing compounds is higher in brain tumor than in normal brain in most cases. Second, high-grade gliomas contain larger amounts of choline-containing compounds than do low-grade gliomas. Third, the concentration of choline-containing compounds in chronic radiation necrosis is less than in anaplastic tumors. Fourth, clinical improvement

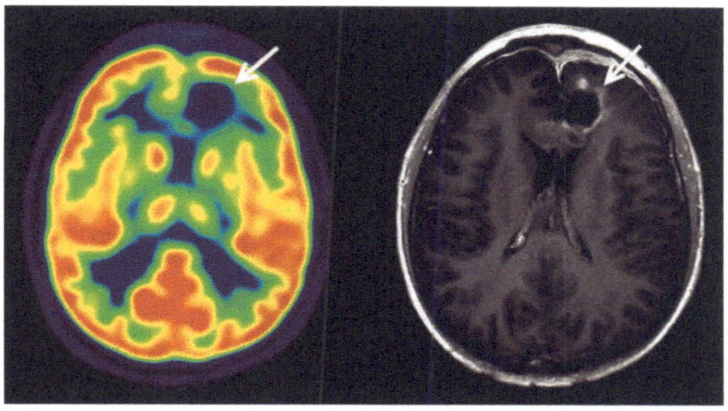

Fig. 11.16. Transaxial ^{18}F-fluorodeoxyglucose (FDG) (left) and contrast-enhanced magnetic resonance imaging (MRI) (right) images from a patient 6 months after resection of a glioblastoma multiforme (GBM) in the medial left frontal lobe. Ring enhancement on contrast-enhanced MRI images (arrow) raised concern for tumor recurrence, but lack of associated FDG activity on positron emission tomography images was consistent with radiation necrosis.

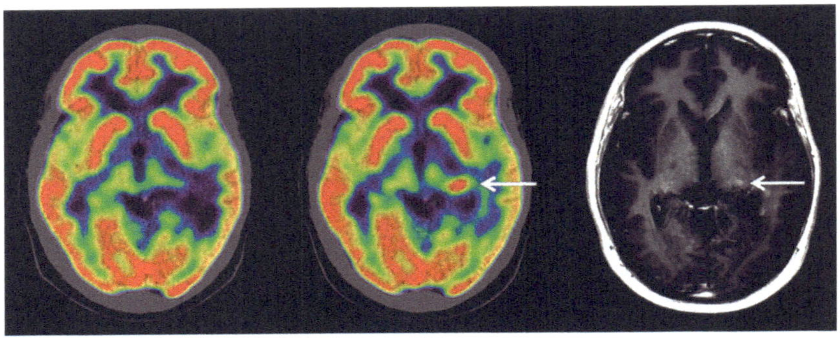

Fig. 11.17. A 43-year-old man 3 years after surgical resection/chemotherapy/radiation therapy for an anaplastic oligodendroglioma in the left medial temporal/thalamic region. Initial transaxial ^{18}F-fluorodeoxyglucose (FDG) positron emission tomography (PET) images demonstrate no abnormal FDG activity (left). Seven months later a follow-up FDG PET study (middle) reveals a new focus of FDG activity (standardized uptake value = 12) just posterior and lateral to the left thalamus (arrow), which corresponds to a focus of enhancement on contrast-enhanced magnetic resonance imaging (right).

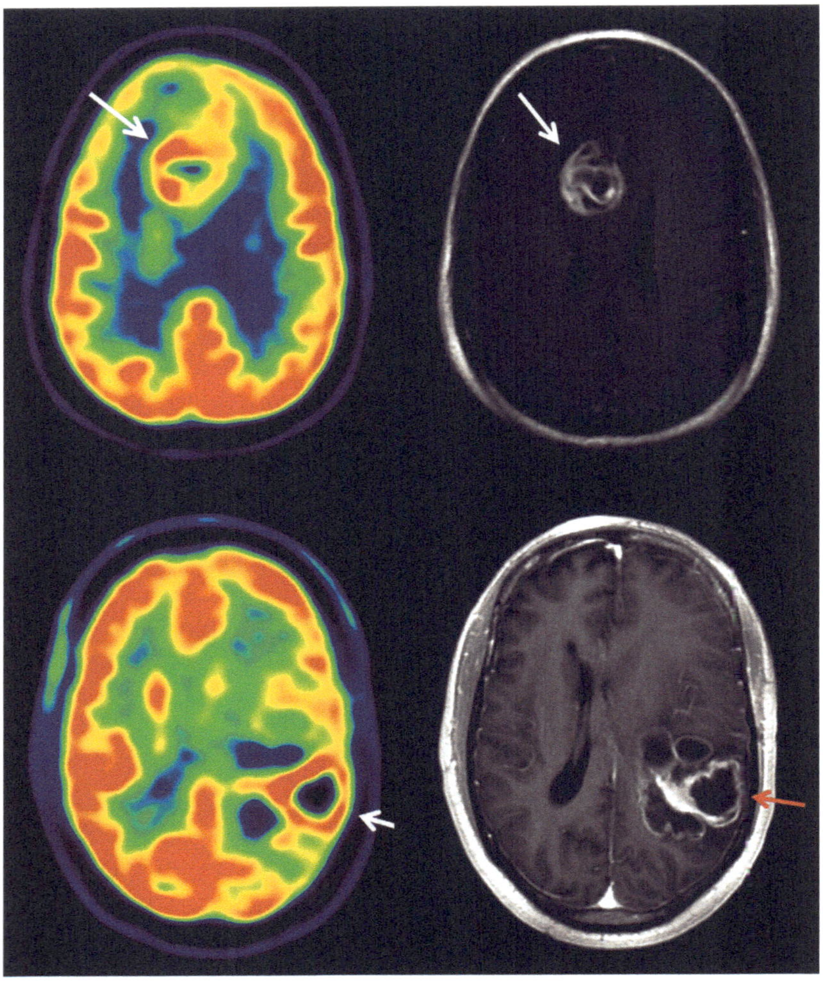

Fig. 11.18. Transaxial ^{18}F-fluorodeoxyglucose (FDG) positron emission tomography (PET) (upper left) and contrast-enhanced magnetic resonance imaging (MRI) (upper right) images from a 69-year-old man with a right frontal glioblastoma multiforme (GBM); the images demonstrate an FDG-avid mass (standardized uptake value (SUV) = 9.3) with central necrosis and heterogeneous enhancement, consistent with a high-grade neoplasm. Transaxial FDG PET and contrast-enhanced MRI images (lower left and right, respectively) from a 55-year-old man with a left parietal GBM; the images demonstrate an FDG-avid multicystic mass (SUV = 10) with central necrosis and peripheral enhancement, consistent with a high-grade neoplasm.

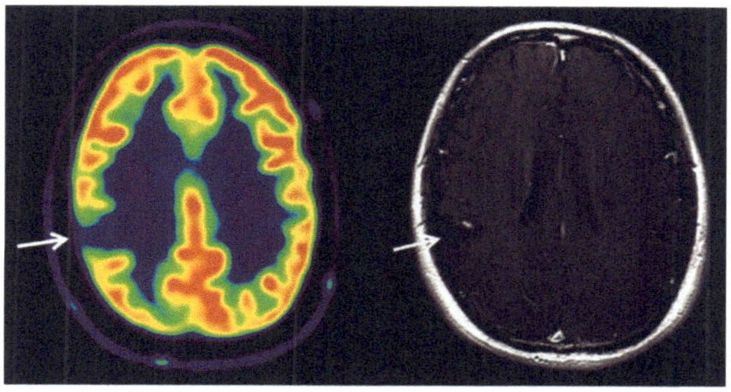

Fig. 11.19. Transaxial ^{18}F-fluorodeoxyglucose positron emission tomography (left) and contrast-enhanced magnetic resonance imaging (right) images from a 19-year-old man with a right parietal dysembryoplastic neuroepithelial tumor (DNET). The images demonstrate a nonenhancing cystic and solid hypometabolic mass, consistent with a low-grade neoplasm.

achieved by radiotherapy is followed by a reduction in the concentration of choline-containing compounds (Alger et al., 1990; Fulham et al., 1992).

Based on the above data, it has been postulated that rapidly proliferating tumors contain large amounts of membrane phospholipids, especially phosphatidylcholine. Hara et al. (1997) developed a direct method of measuring the rate of phospholipid synthesis in human brain tumors using ^{11}C-choline (CHO). They found that CHO PET demonstrates high uptake in malignant brain tumors and pituitary adenomas, surrounded by a background of very low radioactivity (Hara et al., 1997). ^{11}C-methionine (MET), an amino acid and a marker of protein synthesis, is also superior to FDG in properly delineating the border of brain tumors in PET imaging. This is because MET has very low background activity in the brain, whereas FDG activity in brain tumors is surrounded by significant background activity from normal brain tissue, which obscures the tumor border (Ogawa et al., 1991). Methionine is a naturally occurring essential amino acid that is crucial for the formation of proteins, and therefore MET provides a measure of the rate of protein synthesis. MET has been shown to have a higher accuracy than FDG at detecting low-grade tumors, and does not demonstrate the same degree of confounding uptake in the surrounding brain (Pirotte et al., 2004). MET PET has been evaluated to delineate target volumes for brain metastases and to investigate the extent to which tumor growth is measured by MRI versus MET PET. The authors concluded that tumor volumes defined by MRI and MET PET differ substantially, suggesting that MET PET may significantly improve the definition of target volumes in patients with brain metastases. Using MET PET/CT imaging, the biologic characterization of tissue can be combined with an accurate presentation of the anatomy (Matsuo et al., 2009).

Additionally, the use of MET and CHO in PET imaging of brain metastases has been correlated to histopathology findings from stereotactic biopsy. It has been found that CHO is promising for the imaging of brain metastases because of significantly higher lesion-to-normal brain tissue ratios in tumor tissue compared with MET, without evidence of lower specificity (Rottenburger et al., 2011). In a different study, CHO PET gave better images of brain tumors than did MET PET because the tumor-to-background ratio was higher with CHO PET (Hara et al., 1997).

Another radiopharmaceutical that is useful in brain tumor imaging is ^{18}F-fluorothymidine (FLT), a tracer for assessment of DNA synthesis and hence tumor cell proliferation. FLT is transported into the cell via human nucleoside transporters, and trapped intracellularly by the cytosolic enzyme thymidine kinase 1, which demonstrates increased activity during DNA synthesis. Thus, FLT trapping is related to *thymidine kinase 1* activity and to proliferation, enabling tumor proliferative activity to be monitored (Buck et al., 2002; Rasey et al., 2002; Bussink et al., 2010). Several investigations have demonstrated that FLT uptake often preceded changes in tumor volume delineated by CT, and may provide a means of early tumor response assessment that could inform treatment decisions (Menda et al., 2009; Troost et al., 2010).

In addition to its uses in the initial assessment of tumors, PET has been shown to be useful in follow-up assessment after treatment. Because of the significant inflammatory response after radiation treatment, it is typically suggested that follow-up PET imaging be performed at least 8 weeks after completion of treatment.

CONCLUSIONS

In summary, PET has many clinical and research applications in neuroimaging, and is a continually evolving field. At present, only two radiopharmaceuticals, FDG and Amyvid, are approved for routine clinical use in the USA. However, with a multitude of new imaging radiopharmaceuticals, as described in the chapter, PET will continue to expand and play a more integral role in the field of neurology and neurosurgery.

References

Albin R, Koeppe RA, Bohnen NI et al. (2008). Spared caudal brainstem SERT binding in early Parkinson's disease. J Cereb Blood Flow Metab 28: 441–444.

Alger JR, Frank JA, Bizzi A et al. (1990). Metabolism of human gliomas: assessment with H-1 MR spectroscopy and F-18 fluorodeoxyglucose PET. Radiology 177: 633–641.

Amyvid (2012). Highlights of prescribing information, Eli Lilly. Available online at: http://pi.lilly.com/us/amyvid-uspi.pdf (accessed 15 May 2015).

Antonini A, Leenders KL, Vontobel P et al. (1997). Complementary PET studies of striatal neuronal function in the differential diagnosis between multiple system atrophy and Parkinson's disease. Brain 120: 2187–2195.

Becker GA, Ichise M, Barthel H et al. (2013). PET quantification of ^{18}F-florbetaben binding to beta-amyloid deposits in human brains. J Nucl Med 54: 723–731.

Benedek K, Juhasz C, Chugani DC et al. (2006). Longitudinal changes in cortical glucose hypometabolism in children with intractable epilepsy. J Child Neurol 21: 26–31.

Berko S, Hereford FL (1956). Experimental studies of positron interactions in solids and liquids. Rev Mod Phys 28: 299–307.

Brooks DJ (1998). Positron emission tomography studies in movement disorders. Neurosurg Clin N Am 9: 263–282.

Bruck A, Aalto S, Rauhala E et al. (2009). A follow-up study on 6-[^{18}F]fluoro-L-dopa uptake in early Parkinson's disease shows nonlinear progression in the putamen. Mov Disord 24: 1009–1015.

Buck AK, Schirrmeister H, Hetzel M et al. (2002). 3-deoxy-3-[(18)F]fluorothymidine-positron emission tomography for noninvasive assessment of proliferation in pulmonary nodules. Cancer Res 62: 3331–3334.

Bussink J, van Herpen CM, Kaanders JH et al. (2010). PET-CT for response assessment and treatment adaptation in head and neck cancer. Lancet Oncol 11: 661–669.

Cai L, Innis RB, Pike VW (2007). Radioligand development for PET imaging of beta-amyloid (Abeta) – current status. Curr Med Chem 14: 19–52.

Catana C, Wu Y, Judenhofer MS et al. (2006). Simultaneous acquisition of multislice PET and MR images: initial results with a MR-compatible PET scanner. J Nucl Med 47: 1968–1976.

Chapman SE, Diener JM, Sasser TA et al. (2012). Dual tracer imaging of SPECT and PET probes in living mice using a sequential protocol. Am J Nucl Med Mol Imaging 2: 405–414.

Chugani HT, Phelps ME, Mazziotta JC (1987). Positron emission tomography study of human brain functional development. Ann Neurol 22: 487–497.

Colloby S, O'Brien J (2004). Functional imaging in Parkinson's disease and dementia with Lewy bodies. J Geriatr Psychiatry Neurol 17: 158–163.

Debets RM, Sadzot B, van Isselt JW et al. (1997). Is ^{11}C-flumazenil PET superior to ^{18}FDG PET and ^{123}I-iomazenil SPECT in presurgical evaluation of temporal lobe epilepsy? J Neurol Neurosurg Psychiatry 62: 141–150.

Del Sole A, Falini A, Ravasi L et al. (2001). Anatomical and biochemical investigation of primary brain tumours. Eur J Nucl Med 28: 1851–1872.

Dethy S, Manto M, Kentos A et al. (1995). PET findings in a brain-abscess associated with a silent atrial septal-defect. Clin Neurol Neurosurg 97: 349–353.

Di Chiro G, DeLaPaz RL, Brooks RA et al. (1982). Glucose utilization of cerebral gliomas measured by [^{18}F] fluorodeoxyglucose and positron emission tomography. Neurology 32: 1323–1329.

Dupont P, Van Paesschen W, Palmini A et al. (2006). Ictal perfusion patterns associated with single MRI-visible focal dysplastic lesions: implications for the noninvasive delineation of the epileptogenic zone. Epilepsia 47: 1550–1557.

Esser P (2009). PET physics and instrumentation. In: RL Van Heertum, RS Tikofsky, M Ichise (Eds.), Functional cerebral SPECT and PET imaging, 4th edn. Lippincott Williams and Wilkins, Philadelphia, pp. 23–33.

Evans RD (1972). The Atomic Nucleus. McGraw-Hill, New York.

Fakhoury T, Abou-Khalil B, Kessler RM (1999). Limbic encephalitis and hyperactive foci on PET scan. Seizure 8: 427–431.

Fakhri GE (2012). Ready for prime time? Dual tracer PET and SPECT imaging. Am J Nucl Med Mol Imaging 2: 415–417.

Fearnley JM, Lees AJ (1991). Ageing and Parkinson's disease: substantia nigra regional selectivity. Brain 114: 2283–2301.

Fulham MJ, Bizzi A, Dietz MJ et al. (1992). Mapping of brain tumor metabolites with proton MR spectroscopic imaging: clinical relevance. Radiology 185: 675–686.

Garibotto V, Heinzer S, Vulliemoz S et al. (2013). Clinical applications of hybrid PET/MRI in neuroimaging. Clin Nucl Med 38: e13–e18.

German DC, Manaye K, Smith WK et al. (1989). Midbrain dopaminergic cell loss in Parkinson's disease: computer visualization. Ann Neurol 26: 507–514.

Giovacchini G, Toczek MT, Bonwetsch R et al. (2005). 5-HT 1A receptors are reduced in temporal lobe epilepsy after partial-volume correction. J Nucl Med 46: 1128–1135.

Hara T, Kosaka N, Shinoura N et al. (1997). PET imaging of brain tumor with [methyl-^{11}C]choline. J Nucl Med 38: 842–847.

Heiss WD, Pawlik G, Holthoff V et al. (1992). PET correlates of normal and impaired memory functions. Cerebrovasc Brain Metab Rev 4: 1–27.

Hoffman JM, Waskin HA, Schifter T et al. (1993). FDG-PET in differentiating lymphoma from nonmalignant central nervous system lesions in patients with AIDS. J Nucl Med 34: 567–575.

Houle S, Ginovart N, Hussey D et al. (2000). Imaging the serotonin transporter with positron emission tomography: initial human studies with [^{11}C]DAPP and [^{11}C]DASB. Eur J Nucl Med 27: 1719–1722.

Huang B, Law MW, Khong PL (2009). Whole-body PET/CT scanning: estimation of radiation dose and cancer risk. Radiology 251: 166–174.

Ichise M (2009). Neuroreceptor imaging and kinetic modeling. In: RL Van Heertum, RS Tikofsky, M Ichise (Eds.), Functional Cerebral SPECT and PET Imaging, 4th edn. Lippincott Williams and Wilkins, Philadelphia, pp. 40–53.

Ichise M, Toyama H, Fornazzari L et al. (1993). Iodine-123-IBZM dopamine D2 receptor and technetium-99 m-HMPAO brain perfusion SPECT in the evaluation of patients with and subjects at risk for Huntington's disease. J Nucl Med 34: 1274–1281.

Ichise M, Kim YJ, Ballinger JR et al. (1999). SPECT imaging of pre- and postsynaptic dopaminergic alterations in L-dopa-untreated PD. Neurology 52: 1206–1214.

Ichise M, Liow JS, Lu JQ et al. (2003). Linearized reference tissue parametric imaging methods: application to [^{11}C] DASB positron emission tomography studies of the serotonin transporter in human brain. J Cereb Blood Flow Metab 23: 1096–1112.

Ishii K, Ogawa T, Hatazawa J et al. (1993). High L-methyl-[C-11]methionine uptake in brain-abscess – a PET study. J Comput Assist Tomogr 17: 660–661.

Ishii K, Sakamoto S, Sasaki M et al. (1998). Cerebral glucose metabolism in patients with frontotemporal dementia. J Nucl Med 39: 1875–1878.

Ishii K, Hosaka K, Mori T et al. (2004). Comparison of FDG-PET and IMP-SPECT in patients with dementia with Lewy bodies. Ann Nucl Med 18: 447–451.

Jellinger K (1987). The Pathology of Parkinsonism. In: CD Marsden, S Fahn (Eds.), Movement Disorders, Butterworth, London.

Johnson K, Minoshima S, Bohnen N et al. (2013). Appropriate use criteria for amyloid PET: A report of the Amyloid Imaging Task Force, the Society of Nuclear Medicine and Molecular Imaging, and the Alzheimer's Association. Alzheimer's & Dementia and Journal of Nuclear Medicine 9: e1–e16.

Kagawa K, Chugani DC, Asano E et al. (2005). Epilepsy surgery outcome in children with tuberous sclerosis complex evaluated with alpha-[^{11}C]methyl-L-tryptophan positron emission tomography (PET). J Child Neurol 20: 429–438.

Kassubek J, Juengling FD, Nitzsche EU et al. (2001). Limbic encephalitis investigated by ^{18}FDG-PET and 3D MRI. J Neuroimaging 11: 55–59.

Kiebel SJ, Friston KJ (2004). Statistical parametric mapping for event-related potentials (II): a hierarchical temporal model. Neuroimage 22: 503–520.

Kim CK, Gupta NC, Chandramouli B et al. (1994). Standardized uptake values of FDG – body-surface area correction is preferable to body-weight correction. J Nucl Med 35: 164–167.

Klunk WE, Engler H, Nordberg A et al. (2004). Imaging brain amyloid in Alzheimer's disease with Pittsburgh Compound-B. Ann Neurol 55: 306–319.

Kramer ML, Schulz-Schaeffer WJ (2007). Presynaptic alpha-synuclein aggregates, not Lewy bodies, cause neurodegeneration in dementia with Lewy bodies. J Neurosci 27: 1405–1410.

Kumar A, Asano E, Chugani HT (2011). alpha-[(1)(1)C]-methyl-L-tryptophan PET for tracer localization of epileptogenic brain regions: clinical studies. Biomark Med 5: 577–584.

Lee SK, Lee SY, Yun CH et al. (2006). Ictal SPECT in neocortical epilepsies: clinical usefulness and factors affecting the pattern of hyperperfusion. Neuroradiology 48: 678–684.

Lippa CF, Duda JE, Grossman M et al. (2007). DLB and PDD boundary issues: diagnosis, treatment, molecular pathology, and biomarkers. Neurology 68: 812–819.

Loane C, Politis M (2011). Positron emission tomography neuroimaging in Parkinson's disease. Am J Transl Res 3: 323–341.

Lucignani G, Paganelli G, Bombardieri E (2004). The use of standardized uptake values for assessing FDG uptake with PET in oncology: a clinical perspective. Nucl Med Commun 25: 651–656.

Marek KL, Seibyl JP, Zoghbi SS et al. (1996). [^{123}I] beta-CIT/SPECT imaging demonstrates bilateral loss of dopamine transporters in hemi-Parkinson's disease. Neurology 46: 231–237.

Matsuo M, Miwa K, Shinoda J et al. (2009). Target definition by C11-methionine-PET for the radiotherapy of brain metastases. Int J Radiat Oncol Biol Phys 74: 714–722.

Mayeux R (2006). Genetic epidemiology of Alzheimer disease. Alzheimer Dis Assoc Disord 20: S58–S62.

Meltzer CC, Zubieta JK, Links JM et al. (1996). MR-based correction of brain PET measurements for heterogeneous gray matter radioactivity distribution. J Cereb Blood Flow Metab 16: 650–658.

Menda Y, Ponto LLB, Dornfeld KJ et al. (2009). Kinetic analysis of 3'-deoxy-3'-(18)F-fluorothymidine ((18)F-FLT) in head and neck cancer patients before and early after initiation of chemoradiation therapy. J Nucl Med 50: 1028–1035.

Nestle U, Weber W, Hentschel M et al. (2009). Biological imaging in radiation therapy: role of positron emission tomography. Phys Med Biol 54: R1–R25.

O'Doherty MJ, Barrington SF, Campbell M et al. (1997). PET scanning and the human immunodeficiency virus-positive patient. J Nucl Med 38: 1575–1583.

Ogawa T, Kanno I, Shishido F et al. (1991). Clinical value of PET with ^{18}F-fluorodeoxyglucose and L-methyl-^{11}C-methionine for diagnosis of recurrent brain tumor and radiation injury. Acta Radiol 32: 197–202.

Park SH, Lee SW, Kang DH et al. (2011). The role of f-fluorodeoxyglucose positron emission tomography in the treatment of brain abscess. J Korean Neurosurg Soc 49: 278–283.

Pirotte B, Goldman S, Massager N et al. (2004). Comparison of ^{18}F-FDG and ^{11}C-methionine for PET-guided stereotactic brain biopsy of gliomas. J Nucl Med 45: 1293–1298.

Provenzale JM, Barboriak DP, Coleman RE (1998). Limbic encephalitis: comparison of FDG PET and MR imaging findings. AJR Am J Roentgenol 170: 1659–1660.

Rahmim A, Zaidi H (2008). PET versus SPECT: strengths, limitations and challenges. Nucl Med Commun 29: 193–207.

Raichle ME (2001). Functional neuroimaging: a historical and physiological perspective. In: A Cabeza, A Kingstone (Eds.), Handbook of Functional Neuroimaging of Cognition, MIT Press, Cambridge, MA.

Rasey JS, Grierson JR, Wiens LW et al. (2002). Validation of FLT uptake as a measure of thymidine kinase-1 activity in A549 carcinoma cells. J Nucl Med 43: 1210–1217.

Reiman EM (2007). Linking brain imaging and genomics in the study of Alzheimer's disease and aging. Ann N Y Acad Sci 1097: 94–113.

Reivich M, Kuhl D, Wolf A et al. (1979). The [^{18}F]fluorodeoxyglucose method for the measurement of local cerebral glucose utilization in man. Circ Res 44: 127–137.

Rottenburger C, Hentschel M, Kelly T et al. (2011). Comparison of C-11 methionine and C-11 choline for PET imaging of brain metastases: a prospective pilot study. Clin Nucl Med 36: 639–642.
Rowe CC, Villemagne VL (2011). Brain amyloid imaging. J Nucl Med 52: 1733–1740.
Scheid R, Lincke T, Voltz R et al. (2004). Serial ^{18}F-fluoro-2-deoxy-D-glucose positron emission tomography and magnetic resonance imaging of paraneoplastic limbic encephalitis. Arch Neurol 61: 1785–1789.
Schwarz J, Tatsch K, Arnold G et al. (1992). ^{123}I-iodobenzamide-SPECT predicts dopaminergic responsiveness in patients with de novo parkinsonism. Neurology 42: 556–561.
Seibyl JP (2003). Imaging studies in movement disorders. Semin Nucl Med 33: 105–113.
Seppi K, Schocke MF, Esterhammer R et al. (2003). Diffusion-weighted imaging discriminates progressive supranuclear palsy from PD, but not from the Parkinson variant of multiple system atrophy. Neurology 60: 922–927.
Shoghi-Jadid K, Small GW, Agdeppa ED et al. (2002). Localization of neurofibrillary tangles and beta-amyloid plaques in the brains of living patients with Alzheimer disease. Am J Geriatr Psychiatry 10: 24–35.
Silverman DH (2004). Brain 18 F-FDG PET in the diagnosis of neurodegenerative dementias: comparison with perfusion SPECT and with clinical evaluations lacking nuclear imaging. J Nucl Med 45: 594–607.
Slates RB, Farahani K, Shao Y et al. (1999). A study of artefacts in simultaneous PET and MR imaging using a prototype MR compatible PET scanner. Phys Med Biol 44: 2015–2027.
Small GW, Ercoli LM, Silverman DH et al. (2000). Cerebral metabolic and cognitive decline in persons at genetic risk for Alzheimer's disease. Proc Natl Acad Sci U S A 97: 6037–6042.
Sokoloff L, Reivich M, Kennedy C et al. (1977). The [^{14}C] deoxyglucose method for the measurement of local cerebral glucose utilization: theory, procedure, and normal values in the conscious and anesthetized albino rat. J Neurochem 28: 897–916.
Spanoudaki VC, Levin SC (2010). Photo-detectors for time of flight positron emission tomography (ToF-PET). Sensors (Basel) 10: 10484–10505.
Spratt NJ, Donnan GA, McLeod DD et al. (2011). 'Salvaged' stroke ischaemic penumbra shows significant injury: studies with the hypoxia tracer FMISO. J Cereb Blood Flow Metab 31: 934–943.
Tabata K, Shishido F, Uemura K et al. (1990). Positron emission tomography in acute disseminated encephalomyelitis: a case report. Kaku Igaku 27: 261–265.
Takahashi M, Sasajima T, Mineura K et al. (1996). Positron emission tomographic evaluation for frontal hypertrophic cranial pachymeningitis using ^{11}C-methyl-L-methionine. No Shinkei Geka 24: 287–293.
Tan HM, Chan LL, Chuah KL et al. (2004). Monophasic, solitary tumefactive demyelinating lesion: neuroimaging features and neuropathological diagnosis. Br J Radiol 77: 153–156.
Townsend DW (2004). Physical principles and technology of clinical PET imaging. Ann Acad Med Singapore 33: 133–145.
Toyama H, Ichise M, Liow JS et al. (2004). Absolute quantification of regional cerebral glucose utilization in mice by ^{18}F-FDG small animal PET scanning and 2-14C-DG autoradiography. J Nucl Med 45: 1398–1405.
Troost EG, Bussink J, Hoffmann AL et al. (2010). F-18-FLT PET/CT for early response monitoring and dose escalation in oropharyngeal tumors. J Nucl Med 51: 866–874.
Tsuyuguchi N, Sunada I, Ohata K et al. (2003). Evaluation of treatment effects in brain abscess with positron emission tomography: comparison of fluorine-18-fluorodeoxyglucose and carbon-11-methionine. Ann Nucl Med 17: 47–51.
Vakil P, Lee J, Mouannes-Srour J et al. (2013). Cerebrovascular occlusive disease: quantitative cerebral blood flow using dynamic susceptibility contrast MR imaging correlates with quantitative $H_2[^{15}O]$ PET. Radiology 266: 879–886.
Van Heertum RL (2009). Dementia: diagnosis of dementia. In: RL Van Heertum, RS Tikofsky, M Ichise (Eds.), Functional Cerebral SPECT and PET Imaging, 4th edn. Lippincott Williams and Wilkins, Philadelphia, pp. 81–95.
Van Heertum RL, Tikofsky RS (2003). Positron emission tomography and single-photon emission computed tomography brain imaging in the evaluation of dementia. Semin Nucl Med 33: 77–85.
Van Heertum R, Drocea C, Ichise M et al. (2001). Single photon emission CT and positron emission tomography in the evaluation of neurologic disease. Radiol Clin North Am 39: 1007–1033.
Van Paesschen W, Dupont P, Sunaert S et al. (2007). The use of SPECT and PET in routine clinical practice in epilepsy. Curr Opin Neurol 20: 194–202.
van Royen E, Verhoeff NF, Speelman JD et al. (1993). Multiple system atrophy and progressive supranuclear palsy. Diminished striatal D2 dopamine receptor activity demonstrated by ^{123}I-IBZM single photon emission computed tomography. Arch Neurol 50: 513–516.
Varrone A, Asenbaum S, Vander Borght T et al. (2009). EANM procedure guidelines for PET brain imaging using [^{18}F]FDG, version 2. Eur J Nucl Med Mol Imaging 36: 2103–2110.
Walker Z, Costa DC, Walker RW et al. (2002). Differentiation of dementia with Lewy bodies from Alzheimer's disease using a dopaminergic presynaptic ligand. J Neurol Neurosurg Psychiatry 73: 134–140.
Weiner MW (2005). Commentary on diagnosis of Alzheimer's disease: two decades of progress. Central role of technology in the treatment and prevention of Alzheimer's disease. Alzheimers Dement 1: 112–113.
Weisman D, McKeith I (2007). Dementia with Lewy bodies. Semin Neurol 27: 42–47.
Wolk DA, Zhang Z, Boudhar S et al. (2012). Amyloid imaging in Alzheimer's disease: comparison of florbetapir and Pittsburgh compound-B positron emission tomography. J Neurol Neurosurg Psychiatry 83: 923–926.

Won HJ, Chang KH, Cheon JE et al. (1999). Comparison of MR imaging with PET and ictal SPECT in 118 patients with intractable epilepsy. AJNR Am J Neuroradiol 20: 593–599.

Wong DF, Rosenberg PB, Zhou Y et al. (2010). In vivo imaging of amyloid deposition in Alzheimer disease using the radioligand 18 F-AV-45 (florbetapir [corrected] F 18). J Nucl Med 51: 913–920.

Zanzonico P (2004). Positron emission tomography: a review of basic principles, scanner design and performance, and current systems. Semin Nucl Med 34: 87–111.

Handbook of Clinical Neurology, Vol. 135 (3rd series)
Neuroimaging, Part I
J.C. Masdeu and R.G. González, Editors

Chapter 12

Positron emission tomography: ligand imaging

MATEEN MOGHBEL[1], ANDREW NEWBERG[2], AND ABASS ALAVI[3]*

[1]*Department of Radiology, Hospital of the University of Pennsylvania, Philadelphia, PA, USA*

[2]*Myrna Brind Center of Integrative Medicine, Thomas Jefferson University and Hospital, Philadelphia, PA, USA*

[3]*Division of Nuclear Medicine, Hospital of the University of Pennsylvania, Philadelphia, PA, USA*

Abstract

Since it was first used to image the brain in 1976, positron emission tomography (PET) has been utilized in a wide range of neurologic and psychiatric applications. From cerebral metabolism to receptor concentration, various PET imaging techniques involving a host of radiopharmaceuticals have provided insight into countless facets of both the normal and diseased brain. Although the majority of these radiopharmaceuticals are still limited to the realm of research, one PET ligand in particular has gained widespread clinical use: 18F-fluorodeoxyglucose, a radiolabeled analog of glucose, has become an exceedingly prevalent clinical tool for the measurement of metabolism in organs throughout the body, including the brain. In recent years, a number of novel PET ligands have also made it through the US Food and Drug Administration approval process and been used clinically. However, gaining approval is by no means the only challenge facing these radiopharmaceuticals. Traversing the blood–brain barrier is a formidable obstacle in drug delivery, and accurately modeling tracer kinetics and correcting for the partial-volume effect are among the difficult tasks that remain once the ligand reaches its intended target. Even so, the use of PET imaging in neurology and psychiatry can be expected to expand in the coming years as novel radiopharmaceuticals continue to be developed.

INTRODUCTION

Positron emission tomography (PET) has been utilized in the assessment of a wide range of physiologic and pathologic conditions, including those of the brain. These neurologic applications of PET have led to a series of critical findings that have furthered the understanding of a variety of disorders, including Alzheimer's disease and other dementias, Parkinson's disease and other movement disorders, cerebrovascular disease, head injury, brain tumors, and seizures. Furthermore, PET can inform the management of psychiatric conditions such as mood and anxiety disorders, attention deficit disorder, schizophrenia, and obsessive compulsive disorder (Fu and McGuire, 1999).

The most widely utilized radiopharmaceutical for clinical PET brain imaging is ^{18}F-fluorodeoxyglucose (^{18}F-FDG), which quantifies the rate of metabolism of glucose. However, there are myriad other tracers that have been developed over the past 40 years that explore many different molecular processes, including amino acid metabolism, blood flow, and neurotransmitter systems (Table 12.1). Radiotracers that label neurotransmitter systems in the brain may be of particular use in the study of psychiatric disorders. Radiotracers that bind the receptors of various neurotransmitter systems, such as serotonin, dopamine, and opiate, might aid in the delineation of the pathophysiologic processes of these neuropsychiatric disorders, as well as in the assessment of their diagnosis, prognosis, disease course, and drug

*Correspondence to: Abass Alavi, MD, PhD(Hon.), DSc(Hon.), Division of Nuclear Medicine, Department of Radiology, Hospital of the University of Pennsylvania, 3400 Spruce Street, Philadelphia PA 19104, USA. Tel: +1-215-662-3069, E-mail: abass.alavi@uphs.upenn.edu

Table 12.1

Partial list of radioligands used in neurologic positron emission tomography imaging

Compound	Application
$^{15}O-H_2O$	Blood flow
^{18}F-fluorodeoxyglucose	Glucose metabolism
$^{15}O-O_2$	Oxygen metabolism
^{11}C-L-methionine	Amino acid metabolism
^{11}C-raclopride, ^{11}C-methylspiperone	Dopamine receptor activity
6-^{18}F-fluoro-L-DOPA, 4-^{18}F-fluoro-*m*-tyrosine (fluorodopa)	Presynaptic dopaminergic system
^{11}C-WAY100635 and ^{18}F-altanserin	Serotonin receptor activity
^{11}C-(*N*,*N*-dimethyl-2-(2-amino-4-cyanophenylthio) benzylamine (DASB)	Serotonin transporter binding
^{11}C-carfentanil, ^{11}C-etorphine	Opiate receptor activity
^{11}C-flunitrazepam	Benzodiazepine receptor activity
^{11}C-scopolamine, ^{11}C-quinuclidinyl benzilate	Muscarinic cholinergic receptors
^{11}C-ephedrine, ^{18}F-fluorometaraminol	Adrenergic terminals
^{18}F-florbetapir, ^{11}C-Pittsburgh Compound B	Amyloid detection

effects (Gatley et al., 1989; Kopin, 1990; Sadzot et al., 1990; Kung, 1991; Maziere and Maziere, 1991; Abadie et al., 1992; Frost, 1992; Varastet et al., 1992). The following review will focus on the development and technical aspects of utilizing radioligands in brain PET imaging.

RADIOPHARMACEUTICAL BASICS

Early in the development of nuclear medicine, it was realized that positron-emitting radionuclides would allow for highly useful radiopharmaceuticals for brain imaging since the atoms would be isotopes of elements that naturally occur in the various organic molecules, such as glucose, amino acids, or neurotransmitters. Thus, radionuclides, such as carbon-11, fluorine-18, and nitrogen-13, would be useful in producing a vast number of tracers that could be used for studying body chemistry and function (Maziere and Maziere, 1991). Investigators from Brookhaven National Laboratory in collaboration with colleagues from the University of Pennsylvania were the first to synthesize ^{18}F-FDG that could be used for measuring regional cerebral glucose metabolism (Ido et al., 1978). The positron emitted by a decaying fluorine-18 atom travels several millimeters before annihilating to produce two 511-keV gamma rays that travel in opposite directions. Thus, PET has a theoretic limit of spatial resolution of 2–3 mm (compared to the resolution of single-photon emission computed tomography (SPECT), which is 8–10 mm) based upon the positron's mean path length before annihilation. Significant progress has been made in the design and manufacture of PET instruments that are capable of generating transaxial image reconstruction at close to the theoretic limit (Ter-Pogossian et al., 1975; Phelps et al., 1976; Alavi et al., 2002).

^{18}F-FDG, which is the most commonly utilized radiopharmaceutical for both research and clinical use, has a wide array of applications within neurology, ranging from the assessment of dementia and psychiatric illness to the study of the effects of various stimulatory phenomena on the central nervous system (Newberg et al., 1995, 2002). However, in addition to FDG, a number of novel radiotracers have been developed in recent years to study various neurophysiologic processes. Nevertheless, the number of studies that have attempted to discern normal variants and changes over time in the normal population has been limited.

When evaluating brain function, various technical factors – including the time elapsed between the injection of the tracer and scanning, the dosage of tracer administered, filtering and processing protocols, and test–retest variability – must be taken into consideration. Otherwise, variants of normal brain perfusion might be misinterpreted as artifacts on the scan. For instance, as the duration of time from the injection increases, the cerebral distribution of certain tracers may be altered, especially if they rapidly redistribute or bind to receptors reversibly. In the case of radiotracers with short half-lives, image acquisition must take place close to the time of injection. FDG, which has a half-life of 109 minutes, is typically injected 45–60 minutes prior to image acquisition. As a result of decay the quality of the PET image, as well as its sensitivity and specificity for the detection of abnormalities, is diminished if the scan takes place after this window of time. Similarly, the dosage of radiotracer that is injected can influence the image quality and, therefore, the diagnostic utility of the scan.

The filtering and processing of PET scans are of equal importance in the assessment of cerebral activity. PET imaging requires appropriate filtering, attenuation correction, correction for random events, single-photon detections, and dead time. Attenuation correction is particularly vital for properly visualizing and comparing activity in brain structures, especially deeper structures such as the thalamus or brainstem. Patient motion, such as head tilt, can often present problems during the interpretation of a PET scan. Significant head tilt can cause bilateral structures, such as the thalami, to appear asymmetric, especially when the patient's head is not in alignment with the scanner. The effects of head tilt and other forms of motion can be minimized with the use of equipment that holds the head in place, as well as software that is able to correct for motion artifacts. It is also easier for the patient to avoid movement if the image acquisition period is either shortened or split into shorter segments.

In spite of these various limitations, studies of cerebral metabolism, perfusion, and neurotransmitter systems have generally reported strong test–retest reliability along with limited variability (Ichise et al., 1997; Booij et al., 1998). In fact, most studies have found that repeat scans of healthy subjects yield values for regional activity and absolute activity that are within 5–10% of the initial measurement.

DEVELOPING RADIOPHARMACEUTICALS

The development of a novel PET ligand for human use entails collaboration between several disciplines, including radiochemistry, pharmacology, pathology, and clinical medicine. Usually, the initial issue is the determination of the new radiopharmaceutical's molecular target, which is selected based upon the pathophysiology of the disease process. For example, if the disease is Parkinson's, the dopaminergic system is a likely target since it is well established that dopamine plays a primary role in the disease process. The next step is determining what specific molecular target will be the focus of radiopharmaceutical development. Taking the Parkinson's example, pre- or postsynaptic receptors might be reasonable targets. Perhaps the research team decides on the dopamine transporter. The next step is then for the radiochemist and pharmacist to explore existing molecules or drugs that bind to the dopamine transporter. Once these are identified, radiolabeling must be attempted with a variety of isotopes that would be ideal for imaging.

The particular isotope to select depends on a variety of factors, including how long the isotope half-life should be, its gamma energy, whether it would be used for PET or SPECT imaging, and whether it has a chemistry that enables a good yield of the radiopharmaceutical. Several variations of both the isotopes and the molecule might be tried to determine the radiopharmaceutical with the best yield and imaging characteristics. However, it is important to verify that the radiopharmaceutical can bind to the receptor *in vitro* as well as *in vivo* and cross the blood–brain barrier. For a radiopharmaceutical to be useful in neuroimaging, it must be able to access its target neurons, and this necessitates the ability to cross the blood–brain barrier. To do so, they must be relatively small and moderately lipid-soluble (Waterhouse, 2003).

Since entry across the blood–brain barrier entails isolating the radiotracer from the blood plasma, it might be expected that the rate of entry would increase along with the lipophilicity of the radiotracer. However, this is only true to an extent, as excessive lipophilicity can cause a radiotracer to bind disproportionately to plasma proteins and limit the availability of free radiotracer for the brain. But ultimately, all of these issues still need to be tested in animals and humans *in vivo*.

It is important that the radiopharmaceutical has a high receptor affinity, as measured by its equilibrium dissociation constant (K_d), the concentration at which half of available receptors are bound by the drug. The binding affinity of PET ligands, which is the inverse of their dissociation constants, should be in the nanomolar range, since the concentration of receptor-binding sites in the brain is in the range of femtomolar to nanomolar per mg of tissue. Saturation and displacement binding assays can ensure that there is sufficient ligand binding to allow for adequate imaging results.

A radiopharmaceutical must also be designed to have a high specific radioactivity. Specific activity is a measure of the radioactivity of a radiotracer per unit mass. With regard to radiotracers developed for brain imaging, it is important that they possess a high specificity of radioactivity so that a smaller proportion of receptor-binding sites are occupied by the tracer. This allows for a smaller dose of radioactivity given for each scan, and, perhaps more importantly, prevents pharmacologic effects and saturation of binding sites. A tracer with which this has traditionally been an important issue is ^{11}C-carfentanil. Carfentanil itself is approximately 100 000 times stronger than morphine. If the specific activity of the ^{11}C-carfentanil is not high enough, too much nonradioactive or "cold" carfentanil is injected with each scan. This can result in subjects feeling morphine-like effects, such as dizziness, lightheadedness, or fatigue.

Developing a radiopharmaceutical also requires attention to the amount of metabolism of the compound in the body. Even if the radiopharmaceutical effectively crosses the blood–brain barrier and binds to its target with high affinity, if the body metabolizes it before reaching the brain, there will be no tracer that will be detected. A good example of this is ^{18}F-fluorodopa (FD). This is taken up into neurons and demonstrates dopamine production in the brain. However, when injected, it would be rapidly metabolized by the peripheral enzymes, dopa-decarboxylase and catachol-*O*-methyltransferase. In order to avoid this problem, prior to injection, subjects are given carbidopa and entacapone to block these enzymes in the periphery and allow a sufficient amount of the FD to enter the brain. In addition, a radiopharmaceutical may be metabolized to other compounds that can also enter the brain and bind to receptors. The inability to distinguish the radioactivity of these metabolites from that of the parent molecule constitutes a limitation that confounds the acquisition of accurate imaging data (Zoghbi et al., 2006). Thus, it is crucial that PET radiotracers are not excessively metabolized prior to image acquisition. Part of what mediates such metabolism is the position of the radioactive isotope in the molecule. It is of great importance to keep this in mind when developing the synthesis of a radiopharmaceutical, as a quickly metabolized molecule will be of limited use.

Other factors that are also important include the clearance rate from the blood and whether the radiopharmaceutical binds to plasma proteins. These factors affect the imaging protocol and how much radioactive signal gets into the brain and binds to the appropriate location. It is essential that the radiotracer binds to plasma proteins at a sufficiently low level, as these interactions limit the availability of ligands to diffuse out of the blood stream. Finally, whether or not the radiopharmaceutical binds reversibly and redistributes over time plays an important role in determining its usefulness and the imaging parameters. ^{18}F-FDG undergoes relatively mild redistribution and thus enables high-quality images to be obtained of the cerebral glucose metabolism. However, many receptor ligands that do not bind for a sufficient period of time during imaging will result in problematic images and quantitation.

PRECLINICAL EVALUATION OF RADIOPHARMACEUTICALS

Once a potential radiopharmaceutical is developed in the laboratory setting, it must go through a series of preclinical evaluations and then is ultimately tested in humans. The guidelines for nonclinical safety studies in humans was published by the US Food and Drug Administration (FDA) in 1997 (Guideline, 2009). The earliest stage of testing in humans involves studies that investigate drug safety. Compounds with the same physiologic targets as the pharmaceutical being tested can often guide evaluations of drug safety, as their pharmacologic effects are likely to be similar.

Assessments of drug safety in humans are also informed by animal studies. Mouse and rat studies using pharmaceuticals can often yield preliminary data not only on physiologic variables such as blood counts, electrolytes, cholesterol levels, liver function, and immune function, but also on adverse effects related to behavior, appetite, sleep, and activity. In the event that such side effects are observed in animal studies, investigators must be especially mindful of them in human trials and strive to minimize their risk of occurrence.

With regard to toxicology, animal studies are usually performed on both small and large animals, as well as nonhuman primates. If a suitable animal model has yet to be identified for a given disease process – a concern that has been raised in Alzheimer's disease – this step may not be performed. If appropriate, however, a pharmaceutical will generally be administered at varying doses to an animal, often at levels significantly exceeding those ultimately prescribed to humans. As the drug is administered in a regimen similar to what is intended for human use, measurements of serum concentration are made. In the case of radiopharmaceuticals designed for diagnostic purposes, animals are dosed with a single injection prior to scanning, then sacrificed to assess the physiologic effects of the molecule being tested. If the results of the various toxicology studies performed on animals indicate that a pharmaceutical could potentially be harmful to humans, testing may not even continue to human trials.

Over the course of animal studies, the subjects are regularly evaluated for eating and drinking habits, as well as morbidity and mortality. Similarly, observations of clinical signs are typically made on a daily basis for main study animals during the time that the radiopharmaceutical is expected to reside in the system. This window could be quite varied, since isotopes such as carbon-11 have a 20-minute half-life, while iodine-123 has a 13-hour half-life. However, since most positron emitters have relatively short half-lives, animal studies can generally be conducted over a relatively short period of time. Daily measurements of body weight are also logged for every animal, along with food intake for main study animals. Finally, blood samples are obtained at set intervals to measure the serum concentration of the drug in main study animals, while blood and urine samples are obtained at the conclusion of the study to check for abnormalities.

Following the study's conclusion, every main study animal undergoes a full necropsy, where organs are weighed and various tissues are assessed under a microscope. Studies involving large animals, such as dogs, involve comparable clinical and laboratory analysis postmortem. If any significant abnormalities are observed at this time, the FDA must be informed before proceeding to human trials. In this way, animal studies inform and guide the evaluation of safety during drug development for human patients.

ESTIMATING BIODISTRIBUTION AND PHARMACOKINETICS IN HUMANS

As is the case in most stages of drug development, pharmacologic studies in humans are preceded by animal models and estimates. In order to assess the pharmacologic effect of a radiopharmaceutical and evaluate any potential adverse effects, drug concentration and metabolism are studied via serum and tissue sampling. Urine and fecal samples are also informative in terms of drug concentration and clearance.

Since radiopharmaceuticals label a physiologically active molecule with a radioactive atom, their biodistribution can be assessed by detecting the radioactivity they emit using multiple time-point imaging. These evaluations of biodistribution can also inform dosimetry studies that deal with the exposure to radiation that patients receive following drug administration. Evaluations of potential toxicities and adverse reactions can be carried out using dose escalation studies, which systematically increase the dosage administered in set increments. A radiopharmaceutical may be administered in higher doses if these studies show that the compound is cleared more quickly in humans than in animals.

Once the safety risks associated with a radiopharmaceutical are shown in animal studies to be minor or negligible, phase I trials in humans are designed to discern the physiologic and pharmacologic effects of the compound, as well as its utility in visualizing its target through imaging. These preclinical studies are a necessary stepping stone to phase II and phase III trials, as well as investigational new drug applications.

THE INVESTIGATIONAL NEW DRUG PROCESS

Prior to commencing clinical trials in humans to evaluate novel drugs, including radiopharmaceuticals, the sponsors or investigators of the study must file an investigational new drug (IND) application with the FDA. The regulations and guidelines for this application process have been outlined not only by the FDA, by also by the Center for Drug Evaluation and Research and the Center for Biologics Evaluation and Research.

The IND application provides the FDA the opportunity to inspect preclinical data on a drug's safety prior to human trials. Although pharmaceutical companies are often very familiar with the IND application, the process can prove quite formidable for investigators in academic settings. As a result, the rights to pharmaceuticals are often acquired by larger corporations at this stage of development.

Following the filing of an IND, the FDA has a period of 30 days to examine the application and call for additional data before either replying with a nonobjection letter that allows investigators to begin phase I human trials or halting the development of the drug. Additional animal studies on toxicity and genotoxicity, as well as amendments to the study protocol, are commonly requested by the FDA during this period. If these requests are met and the FDA issues a nonobjection letter, the investigators may proceed to clinical trials.

Particularly when dealing with radiopharmaceuticals, it is valuable to consider whether an IND application is called for. A problem encountered frequently in the university setting is the "off-label" use of a particular radiopharmaceutical product in a research study. Studies performed on an approved radiopharmaceutical can warrant an IND, but may not require one under the following conditions:

- The pharmaceutical to be tested must already be approved by the FDA and lawfully marketed in the USA.
- The proposed study must not aim to support a novel indication for the pharmaceutical or justify a change in its marketing.
- The proposed study must not involve a route of administration, dose, or use that increases the safety risks of the pharmaceutical for human subjects.
- The protocol must be approved by the Institutional Review Board and follow standard regulations.

A study that meets these criteria is exempt from the IND application process. Such an exemption carries the advantage of permitting academic investigators without an interest in changing the indications or marketing of an existing pharmaceutical to carry out clinical studies without engaging in a lengthy application process with the FDA.

PHASE I STUDIES

The phase I evaluation of radiopharmaceuticals is a study that primarily measures safety. Safety in the context of radiopharmaceuticals relates to pharmacologic effects as well as radiation dose. Thus, one part of the phase I study involves measures of vital signs, laboratory values, and observation of any adverse events. But a phase I study also includes a more detailed measure of radioactive biodistribution and dosimetry. For radiopharmaceuticals, these assessments may only be necessary for 2–3 days after injection. Table 12.2 catalogs the laboratory values that are typically recorded in phase I studies. Measures of electrolytes, liver function, and complete blood counts are perhaps the most common, but the list will vary according to the findings of preclinical animal studies.

Evaluations of drug safety may also call for vital signs such as heart rate, blood pressure, respiratory rate, and oxygen saturation to be recorded. Especially when testing radiopharmaceuticals with potential effects on

Table 12.2

Laboratory values that may be assessed for safety studies

Cell blood count with differential
Electrolyte panel (blood urea nitrogen and creatinine)
Liver function tests
Urinalysis, routine
Urine toxicology screen
Thyroid function tests, including thyroid-stimulating hormone
Autoimmune screening panel
Cholesterol
Coagulation values (prothrombin time and partial thromboplastin time)
Pregnancy test (serum β-human chorionic gonadotropin)
Prolactin and cortisol levels
Follicle-stimulating hormone and leutinizing hormone

the heart, electrocardiography can prove informative over the period that the radiopharmaceutical remains in the system.

In addition to these laboratory values and clinical studies, a physical examination of the patient is necessary at set time points during the study. A full physical examination calls for the examination of the head and neck, heart, lungs, abdomen, extremities, and skin, as well as neurologic and musculoskeletal function. A review of systems that includes questions regarding a wide range of other issues, including gastrointestinal distress, disorientation, and sleep disturbances is also of great value.

BIODISTRIBUTION STUDIES IN HUMANS

It is also crucial to determine the biodistribution and dosimetry of radiopharmaceuticals in order to confirm their safety and also to assess for the maximum radioactive dose that may be given. The latter is important since higher doses provide better images, but also result in higher radioactive exposure to the patient. Thus, knowing the dosimetry will help determine a dose range that will be both safe and effective. In order to predict patients' exposure to radiation, radiotracer distribution throughout the body must be known at multiple time points and mathematic models must be used to calculate the uptake, retention, and clearance of the radiotracer.

Images of the whole body are typically acquired throughout the period in which radioactivity is expected to reside in the subject (Fig. 12.1). For carbon-11 compounds, this may only require 3–4 hours of imaging whereas with isotopes such as iodine-123, which has a 13-hour half-life, imaging may be required for several days. Ideally, the first image occurs at the time of injection so that the peak of the radioactivity can be adequately captured.

Images are then analyzed by placing regions of interest (ROIs) on each organ and calculating a time–activity curve. Time–activity curves are modeled using experimental data for a variety of organs such as the brain, heart, liver, bone marrow, and bladder. Special software

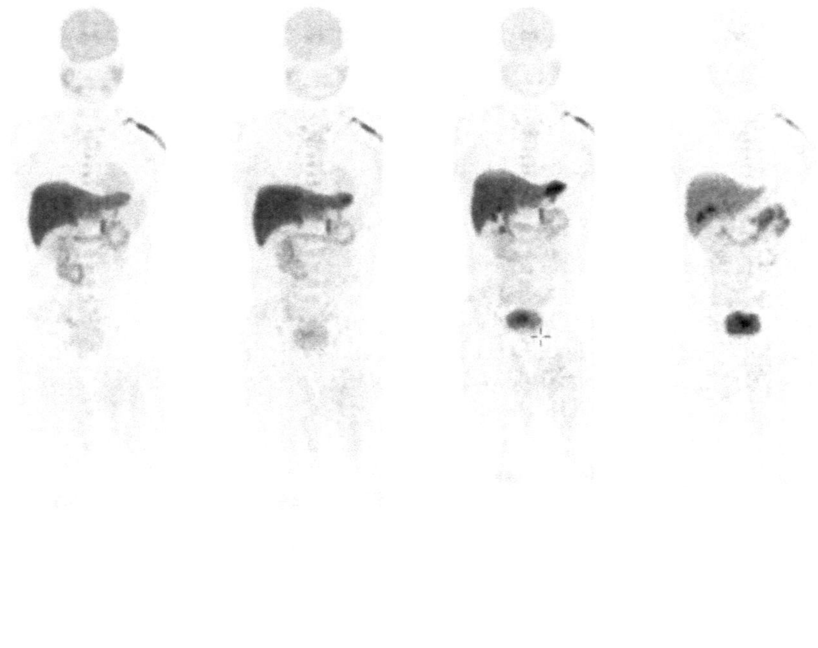

Fig. 12.1. Representative time points (left→right: starting at 0 minutes, 10 minutes, 20 minutes, 40 minutes postinjection) associated with the dosimetry evaluation of ^{11}C carfentanil. From Newberg et al. (2009).

Table 12.3

Comparison of the effective doses for selected positron emission tomography radiopharmaceuticals

Radiopharmaceutical	Effective dose equivalent (mSv/MBq)
^{18}F-FDG	0.030
^{18}F-NaF	0.023
^{18}F-fluorodopa	0.018
^{11}C-IMP	0.018
^{11}C-iomazenil	0.015
^{18}F-FPCIT	0.012
^{11}C-DASB	0.007
^{11}C-carfentanil	0.005

helps to estimate the absorbed doses based upon the data. The effective dose equivalent for the whole body can also be calculated in order to weigh the risk of low radiation exposures such as the procedures employed in diagnostic radiology (Table 12.3).

PHASE II STUDIES AND CLINICAL APPLICATIONS

The data that are collected on the safety, pharmacology, and toxicology of a pharmaceutical in phase I human trials should be submitted to the FDA prior to proceeding with further clinical studies. These data are typically used to support the protocols for phase II trials, which can be filed as amendments to the original IND. Phase II studies generally continue assessing patient safety, but more importantly, begin to evaluate the usefulness of the radiopharmaceutical for its potential indications in its intended patient population. Targeted study populations, which are larger than those of phase I trials, are examined and comparisons to clinical variables and other scan techniques are performed. Finally, if the phase II and III studies are successful, a new drug application is filed with the FDA so that it can be marketed commercially. Of course, many researchers never develop these radiopharmaceuticals for commercial use and continue to perform studies under an IND.

QUANTIFICATION OF RADIOLIGAND BRAIN IMAGING

Quantification of radiopharmaceutical scans of the brain can be performed using a number of methods that range from very simple to complex. Also, there is no clearly established standardized approach to quantifying radioligand images. Some of the methods use single scans while others require dynamic imaging over multiple time points along with the determination of serum concentrations.

One of the most traditional models is to perform quantification using a compartment analysis. A compartment is a physiologic or biochemical "space" with a radiotracer concentration that is assumed to be homogeneous. Typically, there are both three- and four-compartment models, with each compartment presumed to have its own tracer concentration along with the ability of the radiotracer to move back and forth between compartments at some rate constant. The four compartments that comprise the latter model include the plasma compartment, free compartment, specifically bound compartment, and nonspecifically bound compartment. The three-compartment model, on the other hand, combines the free and nonspecifically bound compartments, assuming that radiotracers in a free and nonspecifically bound state rapidly equilibrate in the brain. The transfer of radiotracers between compartments is determined by rate constants reflecting movement in and out of these compartments (Fig. 12.2). For PET imaging (Slifstein and Laruelle, 2001), concentrations within the arteries and capillaries can be considered one compartment. If this assumption is made, the rate constants k_1 and k_2, which represent the rate of influx and efflux across the blood–brain barrier, depend on both flow and permeability.

The classic approach to determining the various parameters for the compartmental models is to perform dynamic (or kinetic) imaging of the brain along with a dynamic determination of the serum concentration (usually based upon arterial blood sampling). However, it may not always be clear which compartment configuration is most appropriate in a given situation (Landaw and DiStefano, 1984). A more substantial problem with such models is the requirement of arterial line sampling, which is logistically complicated and frequently difficult on human subjects. To avoid needing arterial sampling, another approach, the reference tissue method, has been devised as an alternative. This can be very useful, but does not work for all radiopharmaceuticals. The reference tissue methods generally make assumptions regarding the concentration and rate constants across compartments that are determined by specific reference regions. These reference regions may include those that

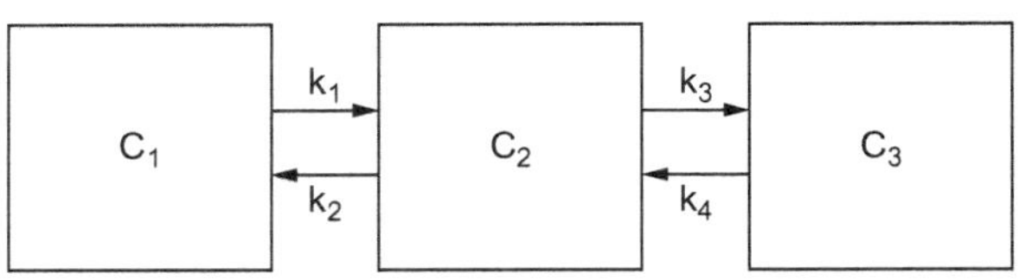

Fig. 12.2. Example of the three-compartment model for radiopharmaceutical kinetics.

have nonspecific binding or are in some equilibrium state which allows for easier calculations. For example, the simplified tissue reference model holds that radiotracer activity can be accurately estimated by fitting the data to a two-compartment model, assuming the kinetics of the specific binding compartment are rapid enough.

Another general approach has been to utilize graphic methods. Logan et al. (1990) put forward a model for reversible tracers in which the different variables are predicted on the basis of the slope of the nearly linear portion of the activity curve. This curve is in turn determined based upon the dynamic set of PET images with or without arterial sampling (if without, a reference region can be used).

The information derived from PET-based quantification is associated with the relationship between the brain and the radiopharmaceutical in equilibrium. However, the methods briefly described above do not necessitate a state of equilibrium in order to make their estimates. These approaches rely on mathematic modeling that predicts parameters in equilibrium despite fluctuating concentrations. On the other hand, there are also a number of simplified models that use measurements taken either at equilibrium or pseudoequilibrium. In single-bolus experiments, this form of modeling can be accomplished by determining equilibrium at the point where the concentration of the specific binding compartment transitions between a net influx and efflux. This has been termed the moment of peak equilibrium (Farde et al., 1989) or transient equilibrium (Ito et al., 1998). Another approach is to utilize the late scans obtained after a single-bolus injection of the radiopharmaceutical, at a point when clearance from the tissues is occurring at the same rate as in the plasma. This is known as transient or pseudoequilibrium (Carson et al., 1993). Another related approach is to administer the radiopharmaceutical as a constant infusion – sometimes following an initial bolus – allowing true equilibrium to be obtained and sustained. At these time points, ROIs between areas of specific and nonspecific binding can be utilized to quantify the activity in particular regions.

Ultimately, whatever approach is used, it is frequently important to compare the results to one or more other methods so as to confirm that the quantification is, in fact, as accurate as possible. However, each radiopharmaceutical can present different challenges and problems with each of these models. This makes true quantification of radioligand studies difficult.

NEUROTRANSMITTERS IN THE NORMAL BRAIN

Once all of the above issues are addressed with regard to performing and analyzing radioligands with PET, it becomes crucial to understand what the "normal" distribution is, and particularly how it relates to the life cycle. It is well known that the brain changes substantially throughout the life cycle, and therefore, an evaluation of these radioligands is essential so that they may be more effectively utilized for evaluating specific disorders. For example, studies of schizophrenia occur when patients are in their early adulthood while Parkinson's occurs late in life. Knowing how the dopamine system is different in normal subjects at different ages is necessary to accurately evaluate how the dopamine system is affected in these disorders.

The nigrostriatal dopaminergic pathways, which are closely related to Parkinson's disease as well as a range of extrapyramidal symptoms in the elderly, have been the subject of many PET imaging studies. *In vitro* studies have typically demonstrated a reduction in dopamine-2 receptor levels with age (Morgan et al., 1987; Rinne, 1987; Rinne et al., 1990). Neuroimaging studies measuring dopamine-1 receptor concentrations have been relatively less consistent, with some suggesting a decrease with age and others reporting no change or even an increase. However, an imaging study demonstrated significant declines in dopamine-1 receptor binding of approximately 7% per decade in both the striatum as well as several cortical areas (Wang et al., 1998).

A number of PET studies have indicated that the uptake of FD, a dopamine analog with affinity for dopamine-2 receptors, decreases with age (see Chapter 11, Fig. 11.14). Cordes et al. (1994) reported that FD uptake of elderly individuals (ages range from 70 to 80 years) was 21% lower than that of their grandchildren (ages range from 18 to 29 years). Previous reports from the same group showed similar reductions in FD uptake with age (Martin et al., 1989; Bhatt et al., 1991). It was suggested that this decline is related to the reduced levels of nigral dopaminergic neurons in the elderly, a hypothesis substantiated by the fact that the average annual decrease in FD uptake (0.35%) closely resembles that in nigral dopaminergic neurons (0.6%) (McGeer et al., 1977; Gibb and Lees, 1991). Several other studies have found similar results in both men and women with age-related decreases in binding of the dopamine-2 receptor (Inoue et al., 2001; Kaasinen et al., 2002). Earlier studies did not find a decrease in FD uptake with age (Sawle et al., 1990; Eidelberg et al., 1993).

This inconsistency may be the result of the small sample sizes of the studies or the methodologies employed for drawing ROIs. Vingerhoets et al. (1994) reported that ROIs spanning the entire striatum produced a significant relationship between FD uptake and age, whereas smaller ROIs did not. Numerous studies that visualized dopamine-2 receptors using ^{11}C-raclopride reported a decline in receptor density with age (Antonini and

Leenders, 1993; Rinne et al., 1993; Volkow et al., 1996). After 30 years of age, there was a 0.6% decline in raclopride binding per year. Another study also demonstrated that the decrease with age in dopamine-2 receptor binding occurs not only in the striatum, but in the extrastriatal regions as well (Kaasinen et al., 2000). Moreover, PET studies have shown that dopamine-1 receptor density falls with age (Suhara et al., 1991). The reuptake of dopamine at the synapse by the presynaptic terminal has also been visualized by PET radiotracers that bind dopamine transporters. One of these radiotracers, ^{11}C-nomifensine, demonstrated that dopamine transporters also decline in concentration with age (Tedroff et al., 1988).

The serotonergic system plays a crucial role in numerous neurologic functions, particularly the regulation of mood. The effect of age on this system has been the subject of many PET studies. One study of the serotonin reuptake receptors demonstrated a decline in binding of 9.6% per decade in the thalamus and 10.5% per decade in the midbrain (Yamamoto et al., 2002). Another study demonstrated a slightly lower rate of decline in women with age (Kuikka et al., 2001). It has also been reported that serotonin 1A receptor activity decreases by approximately 10% per decade in cortical regions excluding the medial temporal cortex (Tauscher et al., 2001). However, another report suggested that this finding is much more prominent in men and not significant in women (Meltzer et al., 2001). Comparable reductions have been found in the serotonin 2A receptor, with an overall 42% decline between the ages of 23 and 60 years (Baeken et al., 1998). However, a more recent study has reported a nonlinear decrease with age in activity in the serotonin 2A receptor with most of the decrease occurring through mid-life (Sheline et al., 2002). The decrease in serotonin 2A receptor binding remains significant even when corrected for age-related cerebral atrophy (Meltzer et al., 1998).

Relatively few PET studies have investigated age-related changes in other neurotransmitter systems. One PET study of benzodiazepine receptors demonstrated no significant decline in a small sample of subjects. A SPECT study measuring the vesicular acetylcholine transporter in healthy subjects 22–91 years of age demonstrated a decrease in binding of only 3.7% per decade (Kuhl et al., 1996). Several PET studies of the muscarinic cholinergic receptor ligand in healthy volunteers from 18 to 82 years old demonstrated a decrease of 45–50% over the age range (Dewey et al., 1990; Suhara et al., 1993; Lee et al., 1996). One study reported increased monoamine oxidase activity with increasing age (Fowler et al., 1997). Opiate receptor imaging can be performed by several different radiopharmaceuticals; the most common is ^{11}C-carfentanil, which specifically binds to the μ opiate receptor throughout the brain, including the cortex and subcortical structures (Fig. 12.3). However, changes related to age have not been reported.

Neutral amino acids traverse the blood–brain barrier with the help of a competitive carrier system. It is possible to visualize and measure the transport of these neutral amino acids across the blood–brain barrier by labeling them with positron-emitting isotopes. One such neutral amino acid (analog, ^{11}C-L-methionine, demonstrated higher transfer of this particular amino acid across the blood–brain barrier in children as compared to adults (O'Tuama et al., 1991). This finding suggests that, during developmental periods, the brain allows for a greater influx of amino acids. This finding also suggests that PET may have applications in evaluating inborn errors of metabolism. In adults, O'Tuama et al. (1988) used ^{11}C-L-methionine to investigate changes in amino acid transport associated with normal aging. The authors reported that amino acid transport declined with age, especially in the frontal lobes.

A limitation of the aforementioned technique is that the labeling of amino acids with positron emitters reduces the accuracy of the kinetic rate determinants determined using these compounds. However, ^{11}C-aminocyclohexanecarboxylate is not metabolized after crossing the blood–brain barrier, which simplifies the kinetic models applied to it. In a PET study using ^{11}C-aminocyclohexanecarboxylate, Koeppe et al. (1990) reported no significant decrease in uptake with age, a

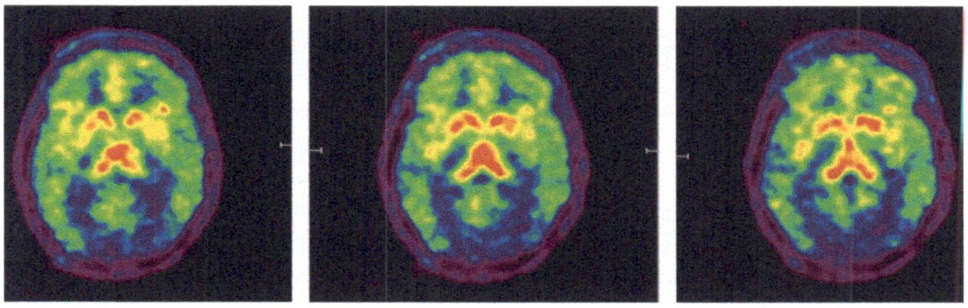

Fig. 12.3. ^{11}C-Carfentanil positron emission tomography brain scan in a healthy control subject showing uptake in the basal ganglia and thalamus, and much of the cortex. There is minimal uptake in the occipital lobe.

finding that may be a more accurate assessment of amino acid transport. Another study using L-(2-^{18}F)-fluorophenylalanine (^{18}F-Phe) substantiated this finding by similarly showing no significant decline in neuronal uptake with age (Ito et al., 1995). However, the authors did report that the rate constant for ^{18}F-Phe transport from the brain to the blood was positively correlated with age. This could be the result of reduced competition between ^{18}F-Phe and neutral amino acids, whose intracellular concentrations fall with age.

CONCLUSION

The applications of PET in psychiatric and neurologic disorders are highly diverse. At this time, the majority of these applications are still in the stage of research, but they have added insight to the pathophysiology of various diseases, allowed for the development of novel diagnostic criteria, and aided in the assessment of treatment response. In the coming years, it will be necessary to study the indications of the wide array of novel neurotransmitter ligands in psychiatric and neurologic disorders, allowing PET imaging to retain a critical role in their management and treatment.

References

Abadie P, Baron JC, Bisserbe JC et al. (1992). Central benzodiazepine receptors in human brain: estimation of regional B_{max} and KD values with positron emission tomography. Eur J Pharmacol 213: 107–115.

Alavi A, Surti K, Newberg A (2002). Preliminary report of performance of high resolution gadalinium orthosilicate (GSO)-based dedicated brain PET scanner. J Nucl Med 43: 296P.

Antonini A, Leenders KL (1993). Dopamine D2 receptors in normal human brain: effect of age measured by positron emission tomography (PET) and [11C]-raclopride. Ann N Y Acad Sci 695: 81–85.

Baeken C, D'haenen H, Flamen P et al. (1998). 123I-5-I-R91150, a new single-photon emission tomography ligand for 5-HT2A receptors: influence of age and gender in healthy subjects. Eur J Nucl Med 25: 1617–1622.

Bhatt MH, Snow BJ, Martin W et al. (1991). Positron emission tomography suggests that the rate of progression of idiopathic parkinsonism is slow. Ann Neurol 29: 673–677.

Booij J, Habraken JB, Bergmans P et al. (1998). Imaging of dopamine transporters with iodine-123-FP-CIT SPECT in healthy controls and patients with Parkinson's disease. J Nucl Med 39: 1879–1884.

Carson RE, Channing MA, Blasberg RG et al. (1993). Comparison of bolus and infusion methods for receptor quantitation: application to [18 F]cyclofoxy and positron emission tomography. J Cereb Blood Flow Metab 13: 24–42.

Cordes M, Snow BJ, Cooper S et al. (1994). Age-dependent decline of nigrostriatal dopaminergic function: a positron emission tomographic study of grandparents and their grandchildren. Ann Neurol 36: 667–670.

Dewey S, Volkow N, Logan J et al. (1990). Age-related decreases in muscarinic cholinergic receptor binding in the human brain measured with positron emission tomography (PET). J Neurosci Res 27: 569–575.

Eidelberg D, Takikawa S, Dhawan V et al. (1993). Striatal 18 F-dopa uptake: absence of an aging effect. J Cereb Blood Flow Metabol 13: 881–888.

Farde L, Eriksson L, Blomquist G et al. (1989). Kinetic analysis of central [11C] raclopride binding to D2-dopamine receptors studied by PET – a comparison to the equilibrium analysis. J Cereb Blood Flow Metabol 9: 696–708.

Fowler J, Volkow N, Wang G-J et al. (1997). Age-related increases in brain monoamine oxidase B in living healthy human subjects. Neurobiol Aging 18: 431–435.

Frost JJ (1992). Receptor imaging by positron emission tomography and single-photon emission computed tomography. Invest Radiol 27 S54–S58.

Fu CH, McGuire PK (1999). Functional neuroimaging in psychiatry. Philosophical Transactions of the Royal Society of London. Series B: Biological Sciences 354: 1359–1370.

Gatley S, DeGrado T, Kornguth M et al. (1989). Radiopharmaceuticals for positron emission tomography. Development of new, innovative tracers for measuring the rates of physiologic and biochemical processes. Acta Radiologica. Supplementum 374: 7–11.

Gibb W, Lees A (1991). Anatomy, pigmentation, ventral and dorsal subpopulations of the substantia nigra, and differential cell death in Parkinson's disease. J Neurol Neurosurg Psychiatry 54: 388–396.

Guideline IHT (2009). Guidance on nonclinical safety studies for the conduct of human clinical trials and marketing authorization for pharmaceuticals M3 (R2), International Conference on Harmonization, Geneva.

Ichise M, Ballinger JR, Vines D et al. (1997). Simplified quantification and reproducibility studies of dopamine D2-receptor binding with iodine-123-IBF SPECT in healthy subjects. J Nucl Med 38: 31–37.

Ido T, Wan CN, Casella V et al. (1978). Labeled 2-deoxy-D-glucose analogs. 18 F-labeled 2-deoxy-2-fluoro-D-glucose, 2-deoxy-2-fluoro-D-mannose and 14C-2-deoxy-2-fluoro-D-glucose. J Label Compd Radiopharm 14: 175–183.

Inoue M, Suhara T, Sudo Y et al. (2001). Age-related reduction of extrastriatal dopamine D2 receptor measured by PET. Life Sci 69: 1079–1084.

Ito H, Hatazawa J, Murakami M et al. (1995). Aging effect on neutral amino acid transport at the blood–brain barrier measured with L-[2-18 F]-fluorophenylalanine and PET. J Nucl Med 36: 1232–1237.

Ito H, Hietala J, Blomqvist G et al. (1998). Comparison of the transient equilibrium and continuous infusion method for quantitative PET analysis of [11C] raclopride binding. J Cereb Blood Flow Metabol 18: 941–950.

Kaasinen V, Vilkman H, Hietala J et al. (2000). Age-related dopamine D2/D3 receptor loss in extrastriatal regions of the human brain. Neurobiol Aging 21: 683–688.

Kaasinen V, Kemppainen N, Någren K et al. (2002). Age-related loss of extrastriatal dopamine D2-like receptors in women. J Neurochem 81: 1005–1010.

Koeppe RA, Mangner T, Betz AL et al. (1990). Use of [11C] Aminocyclohexane carboxylate for the measurement of amino acid uptake and distribution volume in human brain. J Cereb Blood Flow Metabol 10: 727–739.

Kopin I (1990). In-vivo quantitative imaging of catecholaminergic nerve terminals in brain and peripheral organs using positron emission tomography (PET). J Neural Transm 32: 19–27.

Kuhl DE, Minoshima S, Fessler JA et al. (1996). In vivo mapping of cholinergic terminals in normal aging, Alzheimer's disease, and Parkinson's disease. Ann Neurol 40: 399–410.

Kuikka JT, Tammela L, Bergström KA et al. (2001). Effects of ageing on serotonin transporters in healthy females. Eur J Nucl Med 28: 911–913.

Kung HF (1991). Overview of radiopharmaceuticals for diagnosis of central nervous disorders. Crit Rev Clin Lab Sci 28: 269–286.

Landaw E, DiStefano JJ (1984). Multiexponential, multicompartmental, and noncompartmental modeling. II Data analysis and statistical considerations. Am J Physiol 246: R665–R677.

Lee KS, Frey KA, Koeppe RA et al. (1996). In vivo quantification of cerebral muscarinic receptors in normal human aging using positron emission tomography and [11C] tropanyl benzilate. J Cereb Blood Flow Metabol 16: 303–310.

Logan J, Fowler JS, Volkow ND et al. (1990). Graphical analysis of reversible radioligand binding from time-activity measurements applied to [N-11C-methyl]-(-)-cocaine PET studies in human subjects. J Cereb Blood Flow Metabol 10: 740–747.

Martin W, Palmer M, Patlak C et al. (1989). Nigrostriatal function in humans studied with positron emission tomography. Ann Neurol 26: 535–542.

Maziere B, Maziere M (1991). Positron emission tomography studies of brain receptors. Fundam Clin Pharmacol 5: 61–91.

McGeer PL, McGeer EG, Suzuki JS (1977). Aging and extrapyramidal function. Arch Neurol 34: 33.

Meltzer CC, Smith G, Price JC et al. (1998). Reduced binding of [18 F] altanserin to serotonin type 2A receptors in aging: persistence of effect after partial volume correction. Brain Res 813: 167–171.

Meltzer CC, Drevets WC, Price JC et al. (2001). Gender-specific aging effects on the serotonin 1A receptor. Brain Res 895: 9–17.

Morgan DG, Marcusson JO, Nyberg P et al. (1987). Divergent changes in D-1 and D-2 dopamine binding sites in human brain during aging. Neurobiol Aging 8: 195–201.

Newberg A, Alavi A, Payer F (1995). Single photon emission computed tomography in Alzheimer's disease and related disorders. Neuroimaging Clin N Am 5: 103–123.

Newberg A, Alavi A, Reivich M (2002). Determination of regional cerebral function with FDG-PET imaging in neuropsychiatric disorders. Semin Nucl Med 2002: 13–34.

Newberg AB, Ray R, Scheuermann J et al. (2009). Dosimetry of 11C-carfentanil, a μ-opioid receptor imaging agent. Nuclear Medicine Communications 30: 314–318.

O'Tuama LA, Guilarte TR, Douglass KH et al. (1988). Assessment of [11C]-L-methionine transport into the human brain. J Cereb Blood Flow Metabol 8: 341–345.

O'Tuama LA, Phillips PC, Smith QR et al. (1991). L-methionine uptake by human cerebral cortex: maturation from infancy to old age. J Nucl Med 32: 16–22.

Phelps ME, Hoffman EJ, Mullani NA et al. (1976). Design considerations for a positron emission transaxial tomograph (PETT III), University of Pennsylvania, Philadelphia, Pennsylvania.

Rinne J (1987). Muscarinic and dopaminergic receptors in the aging human brain. Brain Res 404: 162–168.

Rinne JO, Lönnberg P, Marjamäki P (1990). Age-dependent decline in human brain dopamine D1 and D2 receptors. Brain Res 508: 349–352.

Rinne JO, Hietala J, Ruotsalainen U et al. (1993). Decrease in human striatal dopamine D2 receptor density with age: a PET study with [11C] raclopride. J Cereb Blood Flow Metabol 13: 310–314.

Sadzot B, Mayberg H, Frost J (1990). Detection and quantification of opiate receptors in man by positron emission tomography. Potential applications to the study of pain. Neurophysiologie Clinique/Clinical Neurophysiology 20: 323–334.

Sawle G, Colebatch J, Shah A et al. (1990). Striatal function in normal aging: implications for Parkinson's disease. Ann Neurol 28: 799–804.

Sheline YI, Mintun MA, Moerlein SM et al. (2002). Greater loss of 5-HT2A receptors in midlife than in late life. Am J Psychiatr 159: 430–435.

Slifstein M, Laruelle M (2001). Models and methods for derivation of in vivo neuroreceptor parameters with PET and SPECT reversible radiotracers. Nucl Med Biol 28: 595–608.

Suhara T, Fukuda H, Inoue O et al. (1991). Age-related changes in human D1 dopamine receptors measured by positron emission tomography. Psychopharmacology (Berl) 103: 41–45.

Suhara T, Inoue O, Kobayashi K et al. (1993). Age-related changes in human muscarinic acetylcholine receptors measured by positron emission tomography. Neurosci Lett 149: 225–228.

Tauscher J, Verhoeff N, Christensen BK et al. (2001). Serotonin 5-HT1A receptor binding potential declines with age as measured by [11C] WAY-100635 and PET. Neuropsychopharmacology 24: 522–530.

Tedroff J, Aquilonius SM, Hartvig P et al. (1988). Monoamine re-uptake sites in the human brain evaluated in vivo by means of 11C-nomifensine and positron emission tomography: the effects of age and Parkinson's disease. Acta Neurol Scand 77: 192–201.

Ter-Pogossian MM, Phelps ME, Hoffman EJ et al. (1975). A positron-emission transaxial tomograph for nuclear imaging (PETT). Radiology 114: 89–98.

Varastet M, Brouillet E, Chavoix C et al. (1992). In vivo visualization of central muscarinic receptors using [11C] quinuclidinyl benzilate and positron emission tomography in baboons. Eur J Pharmacol 213: 275–284.

Vingerhoets F, Snow B, Schulzer M et al. (1994). Reproducibility of fluorine-18-6-fluorodopa positron emission tomography in normal human subjects. J Nucl Med 35: 18–24.

Volkow ND, Wang G-J, Fowler JS et al. (1996). Measuring age-related changes in dopamine D2 receptors with 11C-raclopride and 18 F-N-methylspiroperidol. Psychiatr Res Neuroimaging 67: 11–16.

Wang Y, Chan GL, Holden JE et al. (1998). Age-dependent decline of dopamine D1 receptors in human brain: a PET study. Synapse 30: 56–61.

Waterhouse RN (2003). Determination of lipophilicity and its use as a predictor of blood–brain barrier penetration of molecular imaging agents. Mol Imaging Biol 5: 376–389.

Yamamoto M, Suhara T, Okubo Y et al. (2002). Age-related decline of serotonin transporters in living human brain of healthy males. Life Sci 71: 751–757.

Zoghbi SS, Shetty HU, Ichise M et al. (2006). PET imaging of the dopamine transporter with 18 F-FECNT: a polar radiometabolite confounds brain radioligand measurements. J Nucl Med 47: 520–527.

Handbook of Clinical Neurology, Vol. 135 (3rd series)
Neuroimaging, Part I
J.C. Masdeu and R.G. González, Editors

Chapter 13

Single-photon emission tomography

KAROLIEN GOFFIN AND KOEN VAN LAERE*
Division of Nuclear Medicine, University Hospital Leuven and KU Leuven, Leuven, Belgium

Abstract

Single-photon emission computed tomography (SPECT) is a functional nuclear imaging technique that allows visualization and quantification of different *in vivo* physiologic and pathologic features of brain neurobiology. It has been used for many years in diagnosis of several neurologic and psychiatric disorders. In this chapter, we discuss the current state-of-the-art of SPECT imaging of brain perfusion and dopamine transporter (DAT) imaging.

Brain perfusion SPECT imaging plays an important role in the localization of the seizure onset zone in patients with refractory epilepsy. In cerebrovascular disease, it can be useful in determining the cerebrovascular reserve. After traumatic brain injury, SPECT has shown perfusion abnormalities despite normal morphology. In the context of organ donation, the diagnosis of brain death can be made with high accuracy. In neurodegeneration, while amyloid or 18F-fluorodeoxyglucose positron emission tomography (FDG-PET) are the nuclear diagnostic tools of preference for early and differential diagnosis of dementia, perfusion SPECT imaging can be useful, albeit with slightly lower accuracy. SPECT imaging of the dopamine transporter system is widely available in Europe and Asia, but since recently also in the USA, and has been accepted as an important diagnostic tool in the early and differential diagnosis of parkinsonism in patients with unclear clinical features. The combination of perfusion SPECT (or FDG-PET) and DAT imaging provides differential diagnosis between idiopathic Parkinson's disease, Parkinson-plus syndromes, dementia with Lewy bodies, and essential tremor.

INTRODUCTION

Single-photon emission computed tomography (SPECT) is a functional nuclear imaging technique that allows visualization of different *in vivo* physiologic and pathologic features of brain neurobiology. SPECT imaging is based on the detection of a photon in a dedicated gamma-camera. This photon is emitted by a single-photon-emitting radionuclide during its radioactive decay. After conversion of the gamma-ray energy into light in the gamma-camera crystal, the light photons are converted into an electric pulse containing information on place and energy of the incident ray. The resulting distribution of such interactions, acquired over a circular orbit around the subject, is then digitized and reconstructed into tomographic images. For SPECT imaging, technetium-99 m (^{99m}Tc) and iodine-123 (^{123}I) are mainly used as radionuclides. These radionuclides can be incorporated into a multitude of different radioligands that allow visualization and quantification of brain function, such as perfusion, or specific proteins and targets, such as receptors, transporters, or pathologic brain inclusions. Noninvasive imaging of the brain with SPECT has obtained an important role in the diagnostic workup of several neurologic and psychiatric disorders that will be highlighted below.

BRAIN PERFUSION

Tracers

For imaging of brain perfusion with SPECT, the two commonly used tracers are ^{99m}Tc-hexamethylene propylene amine (^{99m}Tc-HMPAO) (Neirinckx et al., 1987)

*Correspondence to: Prof. Dr. Koen Van Laere, Division of Nuclear Medicine – E901, UZ Leuven, Herestraat 49, 3000 Leuven. Tel: +00-32-16-34-37-15, E-mail: Koen.vanlaere@uzleuven.be and ^{99m}Tc-ethyl cysteinate dimer (^{99m}Tc-ECD) (Oku et al., 1997). These lipophilic amines rapidly cross the blood–brain barrier (around 85% of brain uptake on the first pass). Once inside the brain, they form a hydrophilic compound that is trapped within cells, which prevents washout. Cerebral uptake is complete within 2 minutes and less than 5% is redistributed later. The activity in the brain remains essentially constant for hours after injection and proportional to regional perfusion at the time of administration. Its distribution is not affected by subsequent changes in cerebral blood flow or pharmacologic intervention. Given the regional stability of fixation of these radiopharmaceuticals with minimal regional washout (Ichise et al., 1997), static SPECT scans can be acquired up to 240 minutes after their intravenous administration.

Dementia

Perfusion SPECT can be used for early diagnosis of Alzheimer's disease (AD), for differentiating AD from other types of dementia, and for prediction of progression from mild cognitive impairment (MCI) to AD. This is based on the specific regional pattern of hypoperfusion, which is correlated to glucose consumption and reflects neuronal activity (Torosyan and Silverman, 2012). AD patients show decreased cerebral blood flow in the temporal and parietal association cortex, as well as in the posterior cingulate/precuneus areas, and in more advanced cases also in the frontal cortex. There is a relative preservation of blood flow in the sensorimotor cortex, basal ganglia, primary visual cortex, brainstem, and cerebellum. The extent of perfusion abnormalities is well correlated with the severity of cognitive impairment and the clinical stage of dementia (Farid et al., 2011). Regional, and particularly posterior cingulate, hypoperfusion can be an indicator in evaluating which MCI patients are at risk for developing AD (Park et al., 2012). Overall, side-by-side studies of AD patients with mild symptoms reveal that positron emission tomography (PET) with ^{18}F-fluorodeoxyglucose (FDG) is 15–20% more accurate than perfusion SPECT in establishing the diagnosis of AD (Farid et al., 2011; O'Brien et al., 2014). Enhanced spatial resolution and the higher neurobiologic amplitude of hypometabolism compared to hypoperfusion make FDG-PET a more sensitive marker for early diagnosis of AD than SPECT measures of blood flow alterations (Van Heertum et al., 2009).

Because of overlapping phenotypes and imprecise clinical or neuropsychologic distinctions, the clinical differential diagnosis of dementia can be difficult, with values in the early stages of disease of about 60–70% in accuracy (Devous, 2002). Imaging can add significantly in improving accuracy in the differential diagnosis of AD versus frontotemporal dementia (FTD) versus dementia with Lewy bodies (DLB). In DLB, decreased activity is prominent in the visual cortex in a large number of cases. In FTD diminished activity in frontal and/or anterior temporal cortex is the main differentiating feature. In a meta-analysis, brain perfusion SPECT was shown to be useful in the differential diagnosis of AD versus FTD with a sensitivity of 71.5% and a specificity of 78.2% (Dougall et al., 2004). More recent studies found a sensitivity and specificity for differentiating FTD from AD of 80–91% and 75–81%, respectively (McNeill et al., 2007; Mendez et al., 2007). Accuracy of perfusion SPECT imaging in differentiating DLB from AD was 73–85% (Lobotesis et al., 2001; Shimizu et al., 2005).

Epilepsy

Despite multiple drug treatment, a group of patients with epilepsy will continue to have frequent seizures. These patients can benefit from surgical resection of the seizure onset zone. During the presurgical evaluation of such patients, imaging can aid in identifying whether there is a single and detectable epileptogenic zone. The epileptogenic zone is the cortical region that is indispensable for the generation of seizures, and which has to be removed in order to render a patient seizure-free. It is a theoretic construct, which is defined in terms of different cortical zones (Rosenow and Luders, 2001). The seizure onset zone is the region in which the seizures actually originate. Ictal perfusion SPECT is currently the only imaging modality that can define the ictal onset zone in a reliable and consistent manner. The epileptic lesion can sometimes be visualized on morphologic magnetic resonance imaging (MRI). On the other hand, the functional deficit zone, the part of the cortex with an abnormal function in between seizures due to morphologic or functional factors, or both, can be assessed by interictal FDG-PET and sometimes also using interictal perfusion SPECT, but with reduced accuracy. Epilepsy surgery has the best results when the different cortical zones are concordant, i.e., point towards the same cortical region, and provided that there is no overlap with eloquent cortex.

Several methods for a rapid and safe ictal injection have been described (Herrendorf et al., 1999; Smith et al., 1999; Vanbilloen et al., 1999). Whereas ^{99m}Tc-ECD is a stable ligand, also a stabilized form of ^{99m}Tc-HMPAO is commercially available, enabling early kit constitution and longer shelf-life for the logistics of ictal scanning. ^{99m}Tc-ECD is cleared more rapidly than ^{99m}Tc-HMPAO from the body, thus giving a higher brain/background ratio of activity and a better SPECT image quality. For both tracers, it is important to start tracer injection as early as possible after the seizure onset. For ictal SPECT interpretation, it is therefore also important to be aware of injected seizure type, timing of injection, ictal semiology and electroencephalography (EEG) data. Ictal SPECT has a poor time resolution and, therefore, the brain region of ictal hyperperfusion often includes not only the ictal onset zone, but also propagation pathways.

Interictal SPECT in partial epilepsy shows areas of low perfusion in a proportion of patients, mainly with temporal-lobe epilepsy. The usefulness of interictal SPECT as such for preoperative seizure focus localization is limited (Rowe et al., 1991; McNally et al., 2005). The interictal SPECT is more useful when compared to the ictal SPECT scan, to obtain subtraction ictal SPECT co-registered to MRI (SISCOM), i.e., an analysis technique comparing ictal and interictal studies and co-registering to MRI (Zubal et al., 1995; O'Brien et al., 1998a). The difference images are thresholded to highlight regions of hyperperfusion and SISCOM has improved localization and visualization of the region of hyperperfusion (O'Brien et al., 1998b). Especially in difficult cases with ictal propagation or in patients with semiologically plural expected ictal onset zones, composite ictal SPECT (Kaiboriboon et al., 2005) is particularly useful (Fig. 13.1 G, K). The technique requires two or more ictal SPECT scans in an individual patient. Regions of ictal hyperperfusion which are common in two or more ictal SPECT studies are more likely to represent the ictal onset zone, while other regions are more likely to represent propagated epileptic activity (Fig. 13.1).

In mesial temporal-lobe epilepsy with hippocampal sclerosis, ictal SPECT during a complex focal seizure usually shows early ipsilateral neocortical temporal-lobe hyperperfusion, frontal-lobe hypoperfusion, ipsilateral more than contralateral, contralateral cerebellar hypoperfusion, and later parietal-lobe hypoperfusion (Van Paesschen et al., 2003; Blumenfeld et al., 2004). Ictal SPECT during simple focal seizures in mesial temporal-lobe epilepsy with hippocampal sclerosis can show a small hyperperfusion cluster confined to the temporal lobe, or may reveal no hyperperfusion in around 40% of cases (Van Paesschen et al., 2000; Van Paesschen, 2004), probably because the hyperperfusion is below the spatial resolution of SPECT (around 7 mm full-width-at-half-maximum). Seizure propagation towards the ipsilateral basal ganglia together with hypoperfusion of associative brain regions correlates with contralateral dystonic posturing of the arm (Kim et al., 2007; Chassagnon et al., 2009). Seizures can propagate to the contralateral temporal lobe, and when the ictal SPECT injection is given after seizure propagation, SISCOM may show hyperperfusion in the contralateral temporal lobe (Cho et al., 2010). Early ictal SPECT injection can obviate this problem of seizure propagation (Van Paesschen et al., 2000). Different propagation patterns in mesial temporal-lobe epilepsy with hippocampal sclerosis are not of prognostic significance with respect to seizure outcome after epilepsy surgery (Kim et al., 2007).

Malformations of cortical development are intrinsic epileptogenic lesions, since the ictal onset zone is within the dysplastic cortex. Dysplastic cortex may not always be visible on MRI and, therefore, the ictal onset zone may be at the border of an MR-visible dysplastic lesion (Marusic et al., 2002; Blumcke et al., 2011). Ictal SPECT is particularly useful to delineate the ictal onset zone in focal dysplastic lesions, even when these are not visible on MRI (Dupont et al., 2006; Van Paesschen et al., 2007; Kim et al., 2011). Overlap between the SISCOM hyperperfusion cluster and an MRI-visible focal dysplastic lesion may suffice to proceed to epilepsy surgery aimed at removing the MRI-visible focal dysplastic lesion and the part of the hyperperfusion cluster within and immediately surrounding the focal dysplastic lesion (Dupont et al., 2006).

In MR-negative refractory focal epilepsy, re-evaluation of the MRI, guided by the ictal SPECT, reveals small focal dysplastic lesions in around 15% (Van Paesschen, 2004; Van Paesschen et al., 2007). SISCOM can be used to guide placement of intracranial electrodes (Ahnlide et al., 2007) and may alter and extend the strategy for electrode placement at invasive recording. Favorable surgical outcome has been observed when intracranial EEG was concordant with SISCOM hyperperfusion, but not when discordant. SISCOM localization, therefore, is an independent method with an impact in patients with refractory partial epilepsy scheduled for intracranial EEG studies. In comparison with MRI, FDG-PET, magnetoencephalography, and scalp EEG, ictal SPECT is probably the most sensitive technique to localize the ictal onset zone in extratemporal-lobe epilepsy and to predict a seizure-free outcome after epilepsy surgery (Knowlton et al., 2008; Kim et al., 2009b).

Vascular disorders

Cerebrovascular reactivity

Moyamoya disease is a rare chronic progressive cerebrovascular disease characterized by bilateral stenosis or occlusion of the arteries around the circle of Willis with prominent arterial collateral circulation. The clinical manifestations of moyamoya disease are variable and include transient ischemic attack (TIA), ischemic stroke, hemorrhagic stroke, and epilepsy. Cranial computed tomography (CT) and/or MRI are useful for the

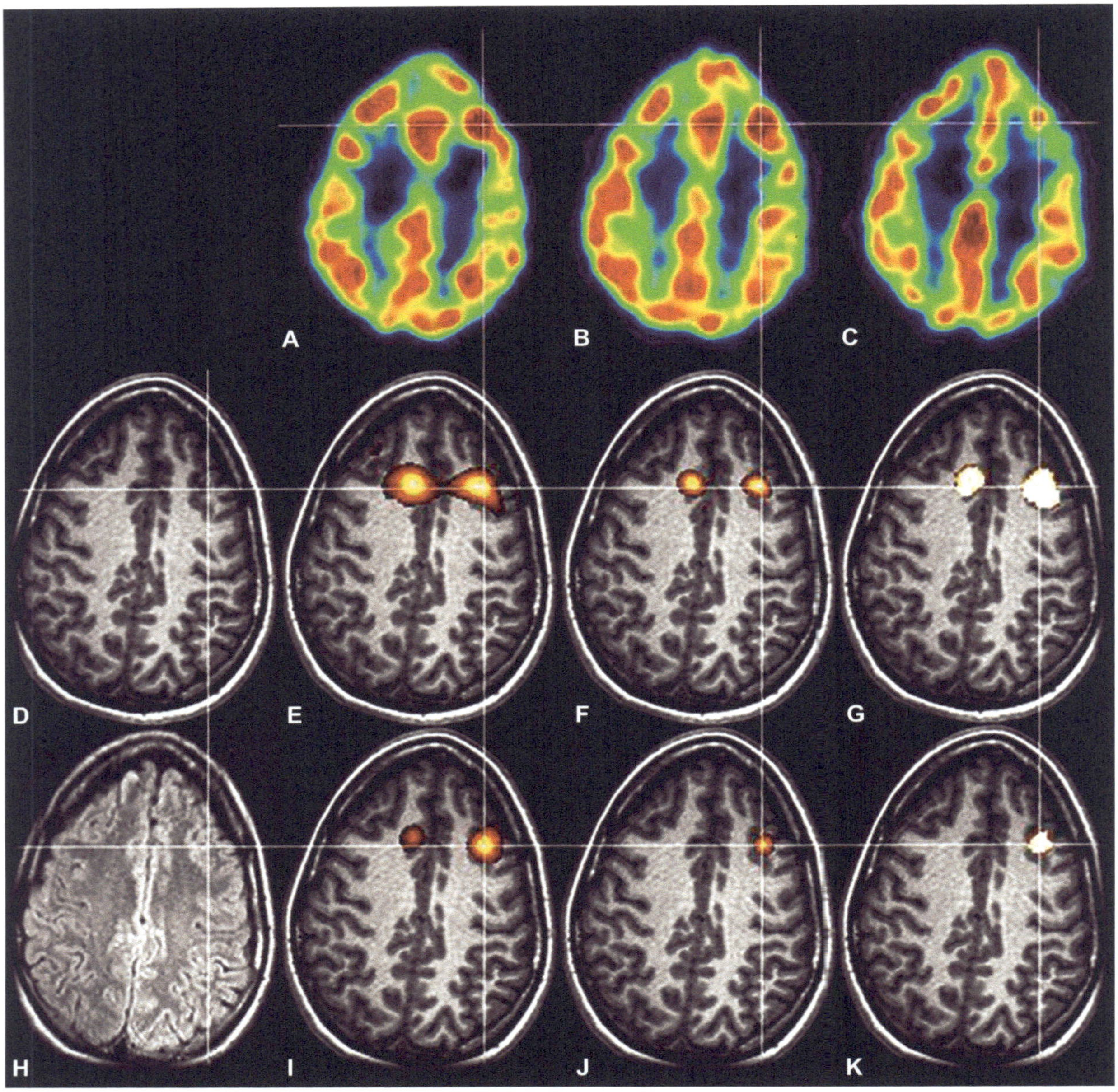

Fig. 13.1. (**A**) First ictal single-photon emission computed tomography (SPECT) scan. (**B**) Second ictal SPECT scan. (**C**) Interictal SPECT scan. Visual assessment showed areas of hyperfusion in the left frontal lobe and at the midline of the frontal lobes. (**E**) Subtraction ictal SPECT co-registered to magnetic resonance imaging (SISCOM) of ictal SPECT 1 thresholded at 2 standard deviations (SD) showed two hyperperfusion clusters of equal intensity connected with a small trail of hyperfusion. (**F**) SISCOM of ictal SPECT 2 thresholded at 2 SD showed two separate hyperfusion clusters. (**G**) The composite image of the two ictal SPECT images thresholded at 2 SD (**E** and **F**) confirmed that the frontal lobes had two regions in common displaying ictal hyperperfusion in two different seizures. (**I**) SISCOM of ictal SPECT 1 thresholded at 3 SD showed two separate hyperperfusion clusters. The hyperperfusion cluster in the left frontal lobe had a higher *z*-score than the one in the right frontal lobe. (**J**) SISCOM of ictal SPECT 2 thresholded at 3 SD showed one hyperfusion cluster in the left frontal lobe. (**K**) The composite ictal SPECT of the two ictal SPECT images thresholded at 3 SD (**I** and **J**) showed that the frontal lobes had one region in common displaying ictal hyperperfusion in two different seizures. Although this region did not reveal an epileptic lesion on a T1-weighted magnetic resonance image (**D**) and fluid-attenuated inversion recovery (FLAIR) (**H**), surgical resection of this region has rendered the patient seizure-free for more than 2 years. Pathology revealed a small area of dysplastic neurons (Van Paesschen and Goffin, 2011).

detection of brain infarction and hemorrhage in patients with moyamoya. Vascular imaging with MR angiography, CT angiography, or conventional catheter angiography is essential to demonstrate stenotic or occlusive lesions in the distal internal carotid arteries and the arteries around the circle of Willis (Yamada et al., 2001; Roach et al., 2008; Kim et al., 2009a). Cerebrovascular reactivity is a predictor of the autoregulatory reserve of the cerebral circulation in steno-occlusive diseases like moyamoya disease. Determining how much the cerebral arterioles can dilate to maintain a constant cerebral blood flow in a given arterial territory under stress may in turn influence treatment decisions regarding cerebral revascularization (Kohno et al., 1998). Several methods, including perfusion SPECT, have been shown to be able to measure the cerebral autoregulatory reserve when challenged with intravenous acetazolamide. SPECT cerebrovascular reserve can be determined by comparing brain perfusion SPECT in baseline and postacetazolamide (Mountz et al., 2003).

A similar approach can be taken in patients with a carotid artery stenosis. In patients with symptomatic carotid occlusive disease, decreased cerebrovascular reactivity is strongly predictive of subsequent stroke (Webster et al., 1995; Mountz et al., 2003). Similarly, it has been demonstrated that in patients with a critical carotid artery stenosis, preoperatively reduced cerebrovascular reactivity to acetazolamide was significantly associated with the development of new postoperative ischemic lesions on MRI (Aso et al., 2009), can predict the development of cerebral ischemia during carotid clamping (Kim et al., 2000) and can identify patients at risk for hyperperfusion after carotid endarterectomy (Ogasawara et al., 2003).

Acute stroke

Perfusion SPECT imaging can be used in acute stroke in patient selection for thrombolytic therapy and in therapy follow-up (Lewis et al., 2012). SPECT imaging has a sensitivity of 90% for detection of perfusion abnormalities within 8 hours of stroke (Lewis et al., 2012), which is less than diffusion/perfusion-weighted (DWI/PWI) MR imaging, with sensitivity close to 100% (Hakimelahi et al., 2012). Sensitivities of perfusion SPECT, perfusion CT, and DWI/PWI MRI become similar at 72 hours (Beauchamp et al., 1999; Abraham and Feng, 2011). A study of resting perfusion in 30 subjects who underwent successful intra-arterial thrombolysis of acute internal carotid artery occlusion showed that stroke-to-cerebellar ratios over 35% reliably predicted salvage of ischemic regions. Conversely, a stroke-to-cerebellar ratio below 35% was associated with increased risk of hemorrhage (Ueda et al., 1999). Similarly, the percentage improvement in perfusion derangements on resting perfusion SPECT from 24 to 48 hours after reperfusion therapy strongly correlated with stroke scores at 3 months (Baird et al., 1996).

Despite these encouraging data, perfusion SPECT imaging is not incorporated into stroke triage or follow-up algorithms, primarily because of the technical challenge of performing such a relatively lengthy study in a short time window (Lewis et al., 2012) and the higher accuracy of DWI/PWI MRI. In the setting of TIA, however, perfusion SPECT may play a role in the objectivation of delayed functional significance of a TIA. It has been shown that perfusion SPECT can distinguish TIA from stroke when performed within 6 hours of symptom onset in patients with presumed middle cerebral artery stroke ictus (Berrouschot et al., 1998). Sensitivity of perfusion SPECT decreases with time after TIA (Hartmann, 1985; De Roo et al., 1989).

Brain death

The diagnosis of brain death is a clinical diagnosis that is sometimes confirmed with technical investigations, including EEG and cerebral perfusion scintigraphy. Perfusion imaging can be useful when clinical assessment and EEG are less reliable because of conditions such as severe hypothermia, coma caused by barbiturates, electrolyte or acid–base imbalance, endocrine disturbances, drug intoxication, poisoning, and neuromuscular blockade (Donohoe et al., 2012). Brain death scintigraphy may also be helpful in patients who are being considered as possible organ donors or when family members require documentation of the lack of blood flow to the brain. In cases of brain death, brain perfusion is absent in the entire brain, including the cerebellum (Conrad and Sinha, 2003) and a typical "stop sign" is noted on early dynamic planar images, indicating absence of intracranial perfusion.

Traumatic brain injury

After patient stabilization upon traumatic brain injury, CT is the first imaging step to assess the need for immediate neurosurgical intervention, with high sensitivity and specificity for several conditions that are often suspected in traumatic head injuries such as skull fractures, brain herniation, and intracranial bleeding (Dubroff and Newberg, 2008). In the subacute setting, MRI can assist in optimal patient management with detection of brain swelling, bleeding, brain contusions, and axonal injury (Dubroff and Newberg, 2008).

In patients with mild traumatic brain injury, perfusion abnormalities can be detected using SPECT despite normal morphology, indicating areas of brain dysfunction (Gray et al., 1992; Dubroff and Newberg, 2008;

Kapucu et al., 2009). Furthermore, perfusion SPECT can detect areas of hyperemia in structurally normal tissue adjacent to intraparenchymal and extracerebral lesions, as determined by MRI or CT, indicating focal damage to the blood–brain barrier (Sakas et al., 1995).

It has also been shown that results of perfusion SPECT imaging have prognostic value for persistence of neuropsychologic sequelae after traumatic brain injury (Newberg and Alavi, 2003; Dubroff and Newberg, 2008).

MOVEMENT DISORDERS

Tracers

For imaging of the dopaminergic system in patients with movement disorders, two main types of SPECT tracers are utilized: (1) tracers of dopamine transporters (DAT) such as [^{123}I]-N-ω-fluoropropyl-2β-carbomethoxy-3β-(4-iodophenyl)-nortropane ([^{123}I]FP-CIT), [^{123}I]-2β – carbomethoxy-3β-(4-iodophenyl)-tropane ([^{123}I]β-CIT) (Neumeyer et al., 1991) or ^{99m}Tc-TRODAT (Kung et al., 1996) and (2) tracers of dopamine D2 receptors in the basal ganglia, such as [^{123}I] iodobenzamide (^{123}I-IBZM) (Kung et al., 1991). Currently β-CIT (DOPASCAN) and FP-CIT (DaTSCAN) are commercially available in Europe via MAP Medical Technologies Oy (Finland) and GE Healthcare (UK), respectively, and are widely used in the clinical evaluation of patients.

[^{123}I]-FP-CIT is stable 3–6 hours after intravenous administration and is best imaged 3–4 hours postinjection, when specific binding of the striatum, as compared to the rest of the brain, is highest (Darcourt et al., 2010). ^{123}I-IBZM, on the other hand, is stable in the striatum 1.5–3 hours after intravenous administration and is therefore best imaged at approximately 2 hours after injection (Darcourt et al., 2010).

Parkinson's disease

Parkinson's disease (PD) is a chronic and progressive degenerative neurologic disease characterized by the degeneration of dopaminergic neurons in the substantia nigra and formation of Lewy inclusion bodies (Lang and Lozano, 1998). The definitive diagnosis of PD can only be made postmortem by histologic demonstration of intraneuronal Lewy bodies in the pars compacta of the substantia nigra (SNpc) (Hughes et al., 1992, 2002). Loss of dopaminergic neurons begins several years before clinical onset of the parkinsonian syndrome. On average, the interval between onset of dopaminergic degeneration and appearance of symptoms is 5–6 years (Fearnley and Lees, 1991; Benamer et al., 2000a). At the onset of symptoms, putaminal dopamine is depleted ~80%, and ~60% of SNpc dopaminergic neurons have already been lost (Dauer and Przedborski, 2003).

Nuclear medicine techniques have been extensively used to investigate striatal dopaminergic function in PD. Using SPECT, the availability of presynaptic dopamine transporters can be visualized using several compounds, among which are [^{123}I]FP-CIT, [^{123}I]β-CIT or ^{99m}Tc-TRODAT. These ligands bind to dopamine, norepinephrine, and serotonin transporters, with a variable level of selectivity. Since the majority of transporters in the striatum are dopaminergic, reductions in striatal uptake of these tracers provide a useful marker of striatal DAT functional loss. Using PET, striatal aromatic amino acid decarboxylase activity can be imaged using ^{18}F-dopa and the density of vesicular monoamine transporters using ^{11}C- or ^{18}F-dihydrotetrabenazine (Brooks and Pavese, 2011), but also several compounds for DAT are available, among which are ^{11}C-PE2I and ^{18}F-FE-PE2I.

More than 90% of patients with clinically probable PD show reduced striatal DAT binding (Benamer et al., 2000b). DAT imaging has a reported sensitivity of 87–98% and specificity of 80–100% for differentiating PD from essential tremor (Lyons and Pahwa, 2011). Therefore, DAT imaging provides a valuable tool to support or reject a diagnosis of parkinsonism associated with striatal dopamine deficiency (Fig. 13.2). Procedure guidelines for brain neurotransmission SPECT using ^{123}I-labeled dopamine transporter ligands have been published by the European Association for Nuclear Medicine (Darcourt et al., 2010).

When using DAT imaging in diagnosing PD, one has to be aware of the fact that, also in healthy aging, there is a decline of DAT of 5.5% per decade (Varrone et al., 2013). Apart from visual interpretation of imaging data, a semiquantitative approach can be useful in unclear cases, comparing an individual DAT scan to scans of a group of age-matched controls. Such a database of control subjects has been described in 2013 in the ENC-DAT study (Nobili et al., 2013; Varrone et al., 2013). The database is however not yet available to the public.

It is likely that a significant proportion of the 4–15% of *de novo* patients recruited for recent clinical trials with antiparkinsonian drugs who have no evidence of nigrostriatal dopamine denervation on functional imaging (subjects without evidence of dopaminergic deficit (SWEDDs)) have tremulous syndromes other than PD (Bajaj et al., 2010). This is supported by long-term follow-up showing minimal clinical deterioration, no response to dopaminergic therapy, and in some cases no evidence on repeat functional imaging of dopamine denervation. Only 3% of SWEDDs showed clinical progression and were still felt to have PD 2 years later (Marek et al., 2005; Marshall et al., 2006; Stoessl, 2010).

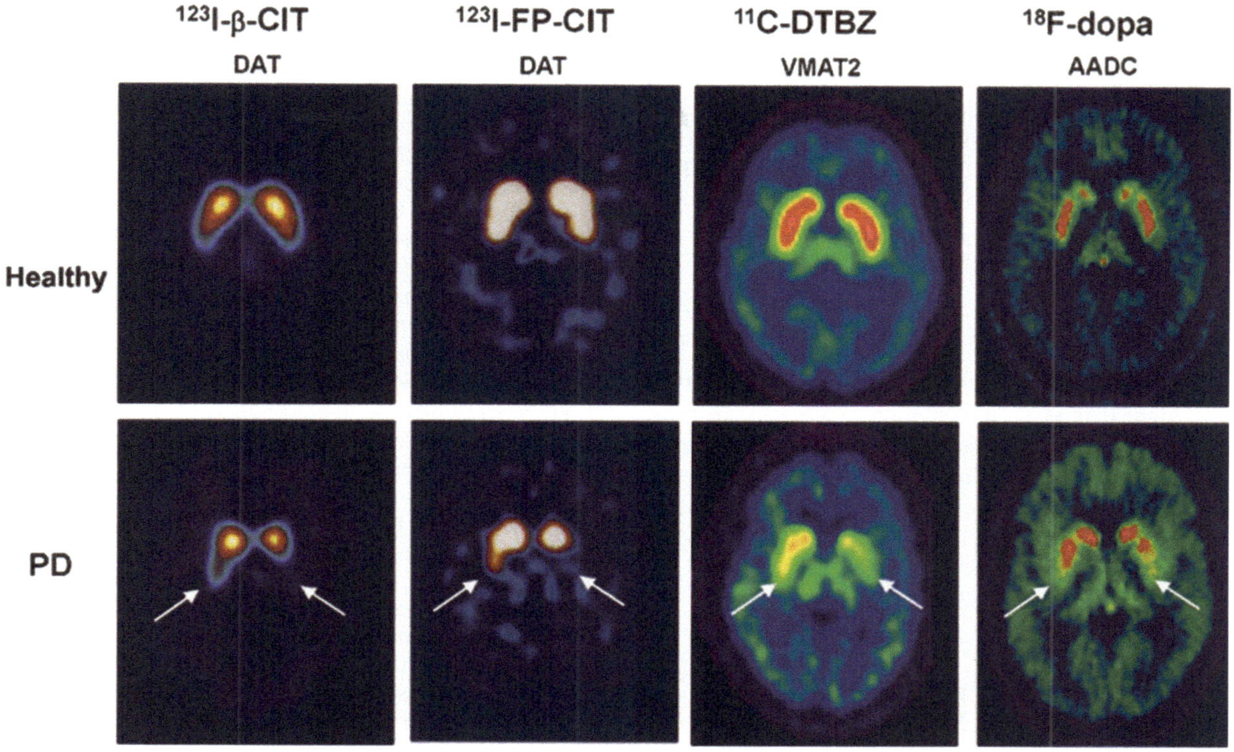

Fig. 13.2. Images of striatal beta-CIT single-photon emission computed tomography (SPECT) (DAT), FP-CIT SPECT (DAT), ^{11}C-DTBZ positron emission tomography (PET) (VMAT2), and ^{18}F-dopa PET (AADC) uptake in healthy volunteers and patients with early Parkinson's disease (PD). The four imaging modalities show asymmetrically reduced posterior putamen dopaminergic function in PD (Brooks and Pavese, 2011).

Parkinson-plus syndromes

Progressive supranuclear palsy (PSP) is a taupathy, characterized by midbrain atrophy, associated with deposition of aggregated tau-positive structures in neurons and glial cells in substantia nigra, periaqueductal gray matter, and variably in basal ganglia and frontal neocortex (Verny et al., 1996). Striatal DAT imaging shows generally more decreased binding in PSP compared to multiple system atrophy with predominant parkinsonism and PD with uniform involvement of dopamine terminals in the caudate and putamen (Antonini et al., 2003). Characteristic of PSP and useful for the differential diagnosis of PD in the early phase is the early, symmetric, and severe decrease of D2 receptors (van Royen et al., 1993). These D2 receptors can be imaged using ^{11}C-raclopride or ^{18}F-fallypride (or ^{18}F-desmethoxyfallipride) PET or [^{123}I]-labeled S(–)IBZM SPECT (Darcourt et al., 2010).

Decreased DAT binding and D2 receptor availability are present in patients with MSA as well as in PSP. To discriminate between Parkinson-plus disorders, a combination of perfusion SPECT (or metabolism FDG-PET) and DAT allows differentiation between PD, MSA, PSP, DLB, and essential tremor. Using a template-based discriminant analysis, MSA, PSP, and PD could be discriminated in 82% of cases at an early stage (Van Laere et al., 2006). Using FDG-PET in this differential diagnosis, sensitivity/specificity of in identifying subgroups of atypical parkinsonian syndromes is 77%/97% for MSA, 74%/95% for PSP, and 75%/92% for corticobasal degeneration. Also the discrimination between atypical parkinsonian syndromes and DLB was significantly larger for FDG-PET than for [(^{123})I]IBZM SPECT (Hellwig et al., 2012).

DLB is the second most common form of neurodegenerative dementia following AD, accounting for approximately 15% of cases at autopsy (McKeith et al., 2004). DLB is a type of dementia that shares clinical and pathologic features with other dementia subtypes, such as AD, vascular dementia, and PD, making it difficult to distinguish in clinical practice. Using perfusion SPECT imaging, presence of occipital hypoperfusion had a sensitivity and specificity of 75% in differentiating DLB from AD (Shimizu et al., 2005). A similar decrease in the occipital lobes can also be detected using FDG-PET, with sensitivity and specificity values that are higher (99% and 74%, respectively: Mosconi et al., 2008).

Apart from changes in occipital (and parietal) perfusion and metabolism, nigrostriatal degeneration, accompanied by profound reductions in the striatal dopamine transporter, has been demonstrated in subjects with DLB. It therefore is possible to use DAT imaging in differentiating DLB from AD (Walker et al., 2002; O'Brien et al., 2004; McKeith et al., 2007). In a meta-analysis of four studies, sensitivity and specificity were 86% and 94%, respectively (Papathanasiou et al., 2012).

CONCLUSIONS

Brain SPECT imaging is a technology that can provide important diagnostic information in a broad spectrum of neurologic and psychiatric disorders. In the differential diagnosis of dementia and in stroke, however, perfusion SPECT can no longer be considered state of the art and has been replaced by FDG-PET and DWI/PWI MRI, respectively.

REFERENCES

Abraham T, Feng J (2011). Evolution of brain imaging instrumentation. Semin Nucl Med 41: 202–219.

Ahnlide JA, Rosen I, Linden-Mickelsson Tech P et al. (2007). Does SISCOM contribute to favorable seizure outcome after epilepsy surgery? Epilepsia 48: 579–588.

Antonini A, Benti R, De Notaris R et al. (2003). ^{123}I-Ioflupane/SPECT binding to striatal dopamine transporter (DAT) uptake in patients with Parkinson's disease, multiple system atrophy, and progressive supranuclear palsy. Neurol Sci 24: 149–150.

Aso K, Ogasawara K, Sasaki M et al. (2009). Preoperative cerebrovascular reactivity to acetazolamide measured by brain perfusion SPECT predicts development of cerebral ischemic lesions caused by microemboli during carotid endarterectomy. Eur J Nucl Med Mol Imaging 36: 294–301.

Baird AE, Austin MC, McKay WJ et al. (1996). Changes in cerebral tissue perfusion during the first 48 hours of ischaemic stroke: relation to clinical outcome. J Neurol Neurosurg Psychiatry 61: 26–29.

Bajaj NP, Gontu V, Birchall J et al. (2010). Accuracy of clinical diagnosis in tremulous parkinsonian patients: a blinded video study. J Neurol Neurosurg Psychiatry 81: 1223–1228.

Beauchamp Jr NJ, Barker PB, Wang PY et al. (1999). Imaging of acute cerebral ischemia. Radiology 212: 307–324.

Benamer HT, Patterson J, Wyper DJ et al. (2000a). Correlation of Parkinson's disease severity and duration with ^{123}I-FP-CIT SPECT striatal uptake. Mov Disord 15: 692–698.

Benamer TS, Patterson J, Grosset DG et al. (2000b). Accurate differentiation of parkinsonism and essential tremor using visual assessment of [^{123}I]-FP-CIT SPECT imaging: the [^{123}I]-FP-CIT study group. Mov Disord 15: 503–510.

Berrouschot J, Barthel H, von Kummer R et al. (1998). 99 m technetium-ethyl-cysteinate-dimer single-photon emission CT can predict fatal ischemic brain edem. Stroke 29: 2556–2562.

Blumcke I, Thom M, Aronica E et al. (2011). The clinicopathologic spectrum of focal cortical dysplasias: a consensus classification proposed by an ad hoc Task Force of the ILAE Diagnostic Methods Commission. Epilepsia 52: 158–174.

Blumenfeld H, McNally KA, Vanderhill SD et al. (2004). Positive and negative network correlations in temporal lobe epilepsy. Cereb Cortex 14: 892–902.

Brooks DJ, Pavese N (2011). Imaging biomarkers in Parkinson's disease. Prog Neurobiol 95: 614–628.

Chassagnon S, Namer IJ, Armspach JP et al. (2009). SPM analysis of ictal-interictal SPECT in mesial temporal lobe epilepsy: relationships between ictal semiology and perfusion changes. Epilepsy Res 85: 252–260.

Cho JW, Hong SB, Lee JH et al. (2010). Contralateral hyperperfusion and ipsilateral hypoperfusion by ictal SPECT in patients with mesial temporal lobe epilepsy. Epilepsy Res 88: 247–254.

Conrad GR, Sinha P (2003). Scintigraphy as a confirmatory test of brain death. Semin Nucl Med 33: 312–323.

Darcourt J, Booij J, Tatsch K et al. (2010). EANM procedure guidelines for brain neurotransmission SPECT using (123) I-labelled dopamine transporter ligands, version 2. Eur J Nucl Med Mol Imaging 37: 443–450.

Dauer W, Przedborski S (2003). Parkinson's disease: mechanisms and models. Neuron 39: 889–909.

De Roo M, Mortelmans L, Devos P et al. (1989). Clinical experience with Tc-99 m HM-PAO high resolution SPECT of the brain in patients with cerebrovascular accidents. Eur J Nucl Med 15: 9–15.

Devous Sr MD (2002). Functional brain imaging in the dementias: role in early detection, differential diagnosis, and longitudinal studies. Eur J Nucl Med Mol Imag 29: 1685–1696.

Donohoe KJ, Agrawal G, Frey KA et al. (2012). SNM practice guideline for brain death scintigraphy 2.0. J Nucl Med Technol 40: 198–203.

Dougall NJ, Bruggink S Ebmeier KP (2004). Systematic review of the diagnostic accuracy of ^{99m}Tc-HMPAO-SPECT in dementia. Am J Geriatr Psychiatry 12: 554–570.

Dubroff JG, Newberg A (2008). Neuroimaging of traumatic brain injury. Semin Neurol 28: 548–557.

Dupont P, Van Paesschen W, Palmini A et al. (2006). Ictal perfusion patterns associated with single MRI-visible focal dysplastic lesions: implications for the noninvasive delineation of the epileptogenic zone. Epilepsia 47: 1550–1557.

Farid K, Caillat-Vigneron N, Sibon I (2011). Is brain SPECT useful in degenerative dementia diagnosis? J Comput Assist Tomogr 35: 1–3.

Fearnley JM, Lees AJ (1991). Ageing and Parkinson's disease: substantia nigra regional selectivity. Brain 114: 2283–2301.

Gray BG, Ichise M, Chung DG et al. (1992). Technetium-99 m-HMPAO SPECT in the evaluation of patients with a remote history of traumatic brain injury: a comparison with x-ray computed tomography. J Nucl Med 33: 52–58.

Hakimelahi R, Yoo AJ, He J et al. (2012). Rapid identification of a major diffusion/perfusion mismatch in distal internal carotid artery or middle cerebral artery ischemic stroke. BMC Neurol 12: 132.

Hartmann A (1985). Prolonged disturbances of regional cerebral blood flow in transient ischemic attacks. Stroke 16: 932–939.

Hellwig S, Amtage F, Kreft A et al. (2012). [18 F]FDG-PET is superior to [123I]IBZM-SPECT for the differential diagnosis of parkinsonism. Neurology 79: 1314–1322.

Herrendorf G, Steinhoff BJ, Bittermann HJ et al. (1999). An easy method to accelerate ictal SPECT. J Neuroimaging 9: 129–130.

Hughes AJ, Daniel SE, Kilford L et al. (1992). Accuracy of clinical diagnosis of idiopathic Parkinson's disease: a clinico-pathological study of 100 cases. J Neurol Neurosurg Psychiatry 55: 181–184.

Hughes AJ, Daniel SE, Ben-Shlomo Y et al. (2002). The accuracy of diagnosis of parkinsonian syndromes in a specialist movement disorder service. Brain 125: 861–870.

Ichise M, Golan H, Ballinger JR et al. (1997). Regional differences in technetium-99 m-ECD clearance on brain SPECT in healthy subjects. J Nucl Med 38: 1253–1260.

Kaiboriboon K, Bertrand ME, Osman MM et al. (2005). Quantitative analysis of cerebral blood flow patterns in mesial temporal lobe epilepsy using composite SISCOM. J Nucl Med 46: 38–43.

Kapucu OL, Nobili F, Varrone A et al. (2009). EANM procedure guideline for brain perfusion SPECT using ^{99m}Tc-labelled radiopharmaceuticals, version 2. Eur J Nucl Med Mol Imaging 36: 2093–2102.

Kim JS, Moon DH, Kim GE et al. (2000). Acetazolamide stress brain-perfusion SPECT predicts the need for carotid shunting during carotid endarterectomy. J Nucl Med 41: 1836–1841.

Kim JH, Im KC, Kim JS et al. (2007). Ictal hyperperfusion patterns in relation to ictal scalp EEG patterns in patients with unilateral hippocampal sclerosis: a SPECT study. Epilepsia 48: 270–277.

Kim JM, Lee SH, Roh JK (2009a). Changing ischaemic lesion patterns in adult moyamoya disease. J Neurol Neurosurg Psychiatry 80: 36–40.

Kim JT, Bai SJ, Choi KO et al. (2009b). Comparison of various imaging modalities in localization of epileptogenic lesion using epilepsy surgery outcome in pediatric patients. Seizure 18: 504–510.

Kim YH, Kang HC, Kim DS et al. (2011). Neuroimaging in identifying focal cortical dysplasia and prognostic factors in pediatric and adolescent epilepsy surgery. Epilepsia 52: 722–727.

Knowlton RC, Elgavish RA, Bartolucci A et al. (2008). Functional imaging: II. Prediction of epilepsy surgery outcome. Ann Neurol 64: 35–41.

Kohno K, Oka Y, Kohno S et al. (1998). Cerebral blood flow measurement as an indicator for an indirect revascularization procedure for adult patients with moyamoya disease. Neurosurgery 42: 752–757. discussion 757–8.

Kung MP, Liu BL, Yang YY et al. (1991). A kit formulation for preparation of iodine-123-IBZM: a new CNS D-2 dopamine receptor imaging agent. J Nucl Med 32: 339–342.

Kung HF, Kim HJ, Kung MP et al. (1996). Imaging of dopamine transporters in humans with technetium-99 m TRODAT-1. Eur J Nucl Med 23: 1527–1530.

Lang AE, Lozano AM (1998). Parkinson's disease. First of two parts. N Engl J Med 339: 1044–1053.

Lewis DH, Toney LK, Baron JC (2012). Nuclear medicine in cerebrovascular disease. Semin Nucl Med 42: 387–405.

Lobotesis K, Fenwick JD, Phipps A et al. (2001). Occipital hypoperfusion on SPECT in dementia with Lewy bodies but not AD. Neurol 56: 643–649.

Lyons KE, Pahwa R (2011). Diagnosis and initiation of treatment in Parkinson's disease. Int J Neurosci 121: 27–36.

Marek K, Jennings D, Seibyl J (2005). Long-term follow-up of patients with scans without evidence of dopaminergic deficit (SWEDD) in the ELLDOPA study. Neurology 64: A274.

Marshall VL, Patterson J, Hadley DM et al. (2006). Two-year follow-up in 150 consecutive cases with normal dopamine transporter imaging. Nucl Med Commun 27: 933–937.

Marusic P, Najm IM, Ying Z et al. (2002). Focal cortical dysplasias in eloquent cortex: functional characteristics and correlation with MRI and histopathologic changes. Epilepsia 43: 27–32.

McKeith I, Mintzer J, Aarsland D et al. (2004). Dementia with Lewy bodies. Lancet Neurol 3: 19–28.

McKeith I, O'Brien J, Walker Z et al. (2007). Sensitivity and specificity of dopamine transporter imaging with ^{123}I-FP-CIT SPECT in dementia with Lewy bodies: a phase III, multicentre study. Lancet Neurol 6: 305–313.

McNally KA, Paige AL, Varghese G et al. (2005). Localizing value of ictal-interictal SPECT analyzed by SPM (ISAS). Epilepsia 46: 1450–1464.

McNeill R, Sare GM, Manoharan M et al. (2007). Accuracy of single-photon emission computed tomography in differentiating frontotemporal dementia from Alzheimer's disease. J Neurol Neurosurg Psychiatry 78: 350–355.

Mendez MF, Shapira JS, McMurtray A et al. (2007). Accuracy of the clinical evaluation for frontotemporal dementia. Arch Neurol 64: 830–835.

Mosconi L, Tsui WH, Herholz K et al. (2008). Multicenter standardized ^{18}F-FDG PET diagnosis of mild cognitive impairment, Alzheimer's disease, and other dementias. J Nucl Med 49: 390–398.

Mountz JM, Liu HG, Deutsch G (2003). Neuroimaging in cerebrovascular disorders: measurement of cerebral physiology after stroke and assessment of stroke recovery. Semin Nucl Med 33: 56–76.

Neirinckx RD, Canning LR, Piper IM et al. (1987). Technetium-99 m d, l-HM-PAO: a new radiopharmaceutical for SPECT imaging of regional cerebral blood perfusion. J Nucl Med 28: 191–202.

Neumeyer JL, Wang SY, Milius RA et al. (1991). [^{123}I]-2 beta-carbomethoxy-3 beta-(4-iodophenyl)tropane: high-affinity SPECT radiotracer of monoamine reuptake sites in brain. J Med Chem 34: 3144–3146.

Newberg AB, Alavi A (2003). Neuroimaging in patients with head injury. Semin Nucl Med 33: 136–147.

Nobili F, Naseri M, De Carli F et al. (2013). Automatic semi-quantification of [(123)I]FP-CIT SPECT scans in healthy volunteers using BasGan version 2: results from the ENC-DAT database. Eur J Nucl Med Mol Imaging 40: 565–573.

O'Brien TJ, O'Connor MK, Mullan BP et al. (1998a). Subtraction ictal SPET co-registered to MRI in partial epilepsy: description and technical validation of the method with phantom and patient studies. Nucl Med Commun 19: 31–45.

O'Brien TJ, So EL, Mullan BP et al. (1998b). Subtraction ictal SPECT co-registered to MRI improves clinical usefulness of SPECT in localizing the surgical seizure focus. Neurology 50: 445–454.

O'Brien JT, Colloby S, Fenwick J et al. (2004). Dopamine transporter loss visualized with FP-CIT SPECT in the differential diagnosis of dementia with Lewy bodies. Arch Neurol 61: 919–925.

O'Brien TJ, Firbank TJ, Davison C et al. (2014). ^{18}F-FDG PET and perfusion SPECT in the diagnosis of Alzheimer and Lewy body dementias. J Nucl Med 55: 1959–1965.

Ogasawara K, Yukawa H, Kobayashi M et al. (2003). Prediction and monitoring of cerebral hyperperfusion after carotid endarterectomy by using single-photon emission computerized tomography scanning. J Neurosurg 99: 504–510.

Oku N, Matsumoto M, Hashikawa K et al. (1997). Intra-individual differences between technetium-99 m-HMPAO and technetium-99 m-ECD in the normal medial temporal lobe. J Nucl Med 38: 1109–1111.

Papathanasiou ND, Boutsiadis A, Dickson J et al. (2012). Diagnostic accuracy of ^{123}I-FP-CIT (DaTSCAN) in dementia with Lewy bodies: a meta-analysis of published studies. Parkinsonism Relat Disord 18: 225–229.

Park KW, Yoon HJ, Kang DY et al. (2012). Regional cerebral blood flow differences in patients with mild cognitive impairment between those who did and did not develop Alzheimer's disease. Psychiatry Res 203: 201–206.

Roach ES, Golomb MR, Adams R et al. (2008). Management of stroke in infants and children: a scientific statement from a Special Writing Group of the American Heart Association Stroke Council and the Council on Cardiovascular Disease in the Young. Stroke 39: 2644–2691.

Rosenow F, Luders H (2001). Presurgical evaluation of epilepsy. Brain 124: 1683–1700.

Rowe CC, Berkovic SF, Austin MC et al. (1991). Visual and quantitative analysis of interictal SPECT with technetium-99 m-HMPAO in temporal lobe epilepsy. J Nucl Med 32: 1688–1694.

Sakas DE, Bullock MR, Patterson J et al. (1995). Focal cerebral hyperemia after focal head injury in humans: a benign phenomenon? J Neurosurg 83: 277–284.

Shimizu S, Hanyu H, Kanetaka H et al. (2005). Differentiation of dementia with Lewy bodies from Alzheimer's disease using brain SPECT. Dement Geriatr Cogn Disord 20: 25–30.

Smith BJ, Karvelis KC, Cronan S et al. (1999). Developing an effective program to complete ictal SPECT in the epilepsy monitoring unit. Epilepsy Res 33: 189–197.

Stoessl AJ (2010). Scans without evidence of dopamine deficiency: the triumph of careful clinical assessment. Mov Disord 25: 529–530.

Torosyan N, Silverman DH (2012). Neuronuclear imaging in the evaluation of dementia and mild decline in cognition. Semin Nucl Med 42: 415–422.

Ueda T, Sakaki S, Yuh WT et al. (1999). Outcome in acute stroke with successful intra-arterial thrombolysis and predictive value of initial single-photon emission-computed tomography. J Cereb Blood Flow Metab 19: 99–108.

Vanbilloen H, Dupont P, Mesotten L et al. (1999). Simple design for rapid self-injection ictal SPET during aura. Eur J Nucl Med 26: 1380–1381.

Van Heertum RL, Tikofsky R, Ichise M (2009). Functional Cerebral SPECT and PET Imaging, 4th edn. Lippincott Williams and Wilkins, New York.

Van Laere K, Casteels C, De Ceuninck L et al. (2006). Dual-tracer dopamine transporter and perfusion SPECT in differential diagnosis of parkinsonism using template-based discriminant analysis. J Nucl Med 47: 384–392.

Van Paesschen W (2004). Ictal SPECT. Epilepsia 45: 35–40.

Van Paesschen W, Goffin K (2011). Ictal SPECT in extratemporal lobe epilepsy. In: MZ Koubeisi, R Maciunas (Eds.), Extratemporal Lobe Epilepsy Surgery. Progress in Epileptic Disorders, Editions John Libbey Eurotext, Cleveland, pp. 167–173.

Van Paesschen W, Dupont P, Van Heerden B et al. (2000). Self-injection ictal SPECT during partial seizures. Neurology 54: 1994–1997.

Van Paesschen W, Dupont P, Van Driel G et al. (2003). SPECT perfusion changes during complex partial seizures in patients with hippocampal sclerosis. Brain 126: 1103–1111.

Van Paesschen W, Dupont P, Sunaert S et al. (2007). The use of SPECT and PET in routine clinical practice in epilepsy. Curr Opin Neurol 20: 194–202.

van Royen E, Verhoeff NF, Speelman JD et al. (1993). Multiple system atrophy and progressive supranuclear palsy. Diminished striatal D2 dopamine receptor activity demonstrated by ^{123}I-IBZM single photon emission computed tomography. Arch Neurol 50: 513–516.

Varrone A, Dickson JC, Tossici-Bolt L et al. (2013). European multicentre database of healthy controls for [(123)I]FP-CIT SPECT (ENC-DAT): age-related effects, gender differences and evaluation of different methods of analysis. Eur J Nucl Med Mol Imaging 40: 213–227.

Verny M, Duyckaerts C, Agid Y et al. (1996). The significance of cortical pathology in progressive supranuclear palsy. Clinico-pathological data in 10 cases. Brain 119: 1123–1136.

Walker Z, Costa DC, Walker RW et al. (2002). Differentiation of dementia with Lewy bodies from Alzheimer's disease using a dopaminergic presynaptic ligand. J Neurol Neurosurg Psychiatry 73: 134–140.

Webster MW, Makaroun MS, Steed DL et al. (1995). Compromised cerebral blood flow reactivity is a predictor of stroke in patients with symptomatic carotid artery occlusive disease. J Vasc Surg 21: 338–344. discussion 344–5.

Yamada I, Nakagawa T, Matsushima Y et al. (2001). High-resolution turbo magnetic resonance angiography for diagnosis of Moyamoya disease. Stroke 32: 1825–1831.

Zubal IG, Spencer SS, Imam K et al. (1995). Difference images calculated from ictal and interictal technetium-99 m-HMPAO SPECT scans of epilepsy. J Nucl Med 36: 684–689.

Section 2

Brain diseases

Handbook of Clinical Neurology, Vol. 135 (3rd series)
Neuroimaging, Part I
J.C. Masdeu and R.G. González, Editors

Chapter 14

Intra-axial brain tumors

OTTO RAPALINO[1]*, TRACY BATCHELOR[2], AND R. GILBERTO GONZÁLEZ[1]

[1]*Division of Neuroradiology, Department of Radiology, Massachusetts General Hospital, Boston, MA, USA*

[2]*Departments of Neurology and Radiation Oncology, Division of Hematology/Oncology, Massachusetts General Hospital, Boston, MA, USA*

Abstract

There is a wide variety of intra-axial primary and secondary brain neoplasms. Many of them have characteristic imaging features while other tumors can present in a similar fashion. There are peculiar posttreatment imaging phenomena that can present as intra-axial mass-like lesions (such as pseudoprogression or radiation necrosis), further complicating the diagnosis and clinical follow-up of patients with intracerebral tumors. The purpose of this chapter is to present a general overview of the most common intra-axial brain tumors and peculiar posttreatment changes that are very important in the diagnosis and clinical follow-up of patients with brain tumors.

INTRODUCTION

Intra-axial brain tumors are responsible for significant morbidity and mortality and include a wide variety of pathologic subtypes with variable biologic aggressiveness. These tumors range from pseudotumoral lesions such as the dysplastic gangliocytoma of cerebellum (Lhermitte–Duclos disease: LDD) to highly malignant and aggressive tumors such as glioblastoma. Despite advances in diagnostic techniques, some of these primary tumors carry a dismal prognosis and limited response to current treatment protocols. The aim of this chapter is to present a general overview of the most relevant intra-axial brain tumors, currently available advanced imaging techniques, and frequently encountered diagnostic imaging problems after treatment of these neoplasms.

EPIDEMIOLOGY

Based on the 2005–2009 Central Brain Tumor Registry in the United States statistical report, glial tumors constitute approximately 29% of all intracranial tumors and 80% of malignant brain tumors (Dolecek et al., 2012). The most common intra-axial glial tumor is glioblastoma (54% of all gliomas; Dolecek et al., 2012). Astrocytomas and ependymal tumors constitute approximately 6.3% and 2.0% respectively of all intracranial tumors. Oligodendrogliomas represent about 1.8% of all intracranial tumors (Dolecek et al., 2012). Lymphoma is responsible for 2.2% of all primary brain tumors. Embryonal tumors constitute the most common histologic type (followed by pilocytic astrocytoma) during early childhood (0–4 years), while pilocytic astrocytoma becomes the most common type in later childhood and early adolescence (5–14 years) (Dolecek et al., 2012). Glioblastoma is the second most common intracranial tumor (after meningioma) in the 55–84-year age groups.

SUBTYPES

Astrocytic tumors

GLIOBLASTOMA (WORLD HEALTH ORGANIZATION (WHO) GRADE IV)

Clinical aspects

This is the most common and lethal primary cerebral neoplasm, responsible for 82% of malignant gliomas (Dolecek et al., 2012; Omuro and DeAngelis, 2013),

*Correspondence to: Otto Rapalino, MD, Department of Radiology, Massachusetts General Hospital, 55 Fruit Street, GRB 273A, Boston MA 02114-2696, USA. Tel: +1-617-726-8323, E-mail: orapalino@mgh.harvard.edu

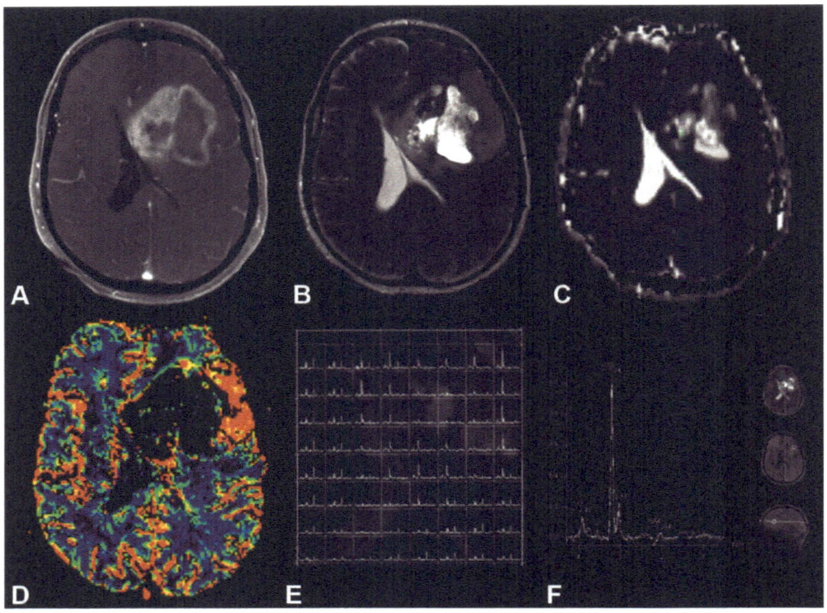

Fig. 14.1. Glioblastoma. (**A**) Postcontrast axial T1-weighted, (**B**) axial T2-weighted, (**C**) apparent diffusion coefficient map, (**D**) corrected relative cerebral blood volume (rCBV), and (**E, F**) multivoxel magnetic resonance spectroscopy (MRS) images. Centrally necrotic and heterogeneously enhancing mass in the left frontal lobe extending into the genu of the corpus callosum and producing prominent local mass effect with partial effacement of the left lateral ventricle and marked rightward midline shift. There are areas of abnormal restricted diffusion colocalized with some of the enhancing regions. rCBV values are markedly increased towards the superficial portion of the mass. MRS (intermediate echo time) shows pronounced decrease of *N*-acetyl aspartate/creatine and increase of choline/creatine ratios.

typically affecting young and middle-aged adult patients. Glioblastomas can develop from pre-existing gliomas and are called secondary glioblastomas. Tumors developing *de novo* without pre-existing lesions are referred to as primary glioblastomas. There are four subtypes of glioblastomas based on gene expression analysis, including the classic, mesenchymal, proneural, and neural subtypes. Isocitrate dehydrogenase 1 (*IDH1*) mutations are more prevalent in secondary glioblastomas, with a reported prevalence of approximately 73%, and carry a better prognosis (SongTao et al., 2012). *IDH1* mutated glioblastomas are typically located in the frontal lobes (Carrillo et al., 2012; Yan et al., 2012).

Glioblastomas are aggressive tumors, with high mitotic activity, variable but commonly rapid tumoral growth and frequent leptomeningeal metastases. Hematogenous or distant metastases have also been reported. These tumors demonstrate very prominent intratumoral neoangiogenesis, central areas of necrosis, and frequent intratumoral hemorrhage (Fig. 14.1).

There are special pathologic variants of glioblastoma, including gliosarcoma and giant cell glioblastoma. Gliosarcomas constitute up to 2% of glioblastomas and show prominent mesenchymal (sarcomatous) differentiation. These tumors are very aggressive, often infiltrating the adjacent dura, skull, and pericranial soft tissues, as well as producing distant metastases (including nodal metastases). Giant cell glioblastomas exhibit multinucleated giant cells pathologically and a prominent stromal reticulin network (Louis et al., 2007). These pathologic features are reflected in their macroscopic appearance in imaging studies as well-defined subcortical masses often mimicking a metastatic lesion. Microvascular proliferation is rare.

Imaging features

The most common presentation on imaging studies is as a heterogeneously enhancing mass with central areas of necrosis and extensive surrounding T2 hyperintense areas (likely a mix of edema and infiltrating tumoral cells) (Fig. 14.1). Areas of abnormal restricted diffusion within the tumor often correlate with tumoral components with high cell density. Magnetic resonance (MR) perfusion shows very high relative cerebral blood volume (rCBV) values reflecting intratumoral neoangiogenesis and vascular proliferation. MR spectroscopy shows marked decrease of *N*-acetyl aspartate (NAA)/creatine (Cr) and increased choline (Cho)/Cr ratios as well as prominent lipid peaks and lactate near/within the necrotic regions (Fig. 14.1). Nonenhancing lesions are also rarely seen.

Treatment

The standard treatment of patients with glioblastoma consists of maximal cytoreductive surgery (if possible), followed by radiation (60 Gy divided in 30 fractions) in combination with temozolomide, an oral methylating agent, with an additional 6–12 months of postradiation temozolomide (Stupp et al., 2005). Patients with tumors that have promoter methylation of the (O^6-methylguanine-DNA methyltransferase (MGMT) enzyme are particularly responsive to chemoradiation and demonstrate increased survival. After initial chemoradiation, most of the patients exhibit progression after an average of 7–10 months (Omuro and DeAngelis, 2013). Therapeutic options for recurrent disease include surgical resection, bevacizumab, or other cytotoxic agents. Bevacizumab is a monoclonal antibody that binds circulating vascular endothelial growth factor, resulting in radiographic response and improved progression-free survival (Friedman et al., 2009). Tumor progression during treatment with bevacizumab may develop as worsening enhancement at the initial tumoral site (46% of cases), new sites of enhancing disease (16%), or progression of nonenhancing tumoral elements (35% of cases) (Iwamoto et al., 2009).

Posttreatment imaging

Early postoperative period. Early postoperative imaging should be performed within 72 hours after the initial resection to avoid potential areas of nodular enhancement related to devitalized tissue or small subacute infarcts along the margins of the surgical cavity (Cairncross et al., 1985a, b; Forsting et al., 1993; Meyding-Lamade et al., 1993; Albert et al., 1994) (Fig. 14.2).

Pseudoprogression. This is a phenomenon initially described after radiation treatment of high-grade gliomas but it may have become more prevalent with the combined use of temozolomide and radiation. The reported prevalence of pseudoprogression after chemoradiation for high-grade gliomas is approximately 30%, but reports of up to 45% have been published. It is described as a transient worsening of the abnormal enhancement, T2 hyperintensity, or mass effect within 6–8 weeks after completion of chemoradiation (Figs 14.2 and 14.3). The conventional MR features of pseudoprogression are similar to true tumoral progression (Young et al., 2011). There is emerging evidence that MR perfusion can be very helpful to differentiate these two processes (Hu et al., 2012; Choi et al., 2013b; Gahramanov et al., 2013; Martinez-Martinez and Martinez-Bosch, 2013; Young et al., 2013) (Fig. 14.3). Based on the current Response Assessment

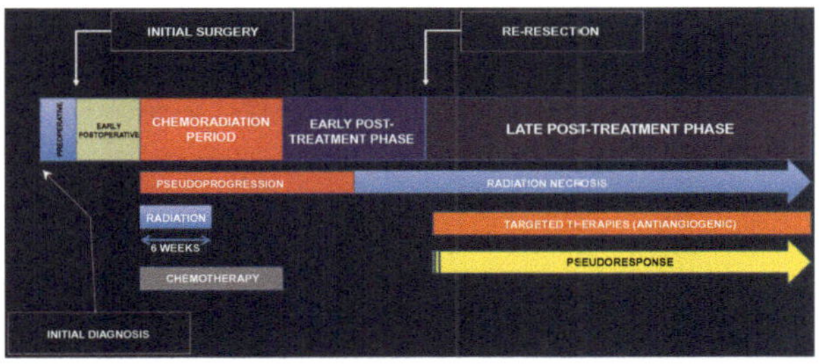

Fig. 14.2. Overview of the typical diagnostic and treatment stages of a patient with glioblastoma.

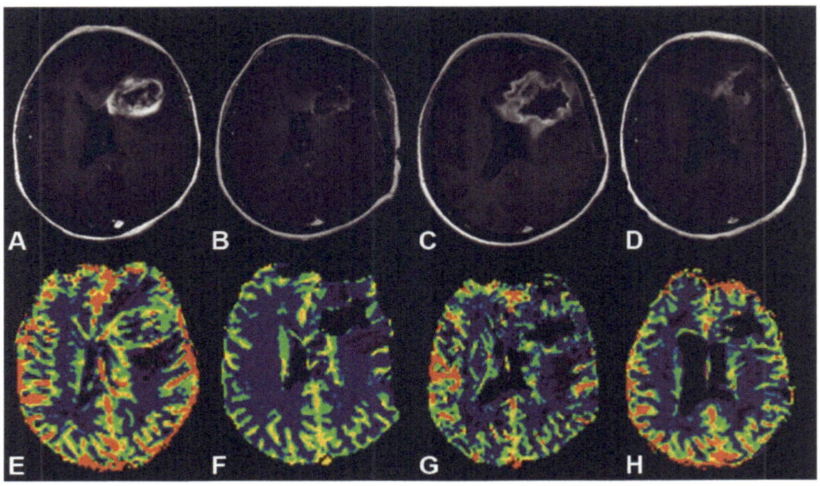

Fig. 14.3. Pseudoprogression in a patient with left frontal glioblastoma. Gadolinium-enhanced T1-weighted images (upper row) and leakage-corrected relative cerebral blood volume (rCBV) maps before surgery (**A, E**), immediately after resection (**B, F**), 70 days after chemoradiation (**C, G**), and 146 days after chemoradiation (**D, H**). There is transient increase of abnormal enhancement and mass effect on the first scan after chemoradiation (**C**) that decreased on the next scan compatible with pseudoprogression. Corrected rCBV maps (lower row) show a predominance of low rCBV values at the time of pseudoprogression (**G**).

in Neuro-oncology (RANO) criteria, tumoral progression can only be prospectively defined during the first 12 weeks after radiation treatment if there is a new enhancing focus outside of the radiation-treated areas or if there is pathologic proof of tumoral involvement (Wen et al., 2010).

Radiation necrosis versus tumoral recurrence. This is a clinical problem commonly encountered in irradiated brain tumor patients, typically appearing >6 months after radiotherapy and within the first 5 years (although longer latencies have been reported). The conventional MR features are similar between radiation necrosis and high-grade tumoral recurrence, although callosal and bilateral parenchymal involvement is typically seen with tumoral recurrence (Mullins et al., 2005). Advanced MR techniques, particularly MR spectroscopy (MRS) and MR perfusion, have been used in the discrimination of radiation necrosis from tumoral recurrence (Fig. 14.4). MRS often demonstrates low NAA, Cho, and Cr levels (particularly when corrected to contralateral levels) and prominent lipid or lactate peaks (see Fig. 14.21, below). rCBV values (using dynamic susceptibility contrast (DSC) MR perfusion) or cerebral blood flow values (using Arterial Spin Labeling (ASL)) are decreased or not significantly elevated within the areas of radiation necrosis (Ozsunar et al., 2010) (Fig. 14.4).

Imaging during antiangiogenic treatment and pseudoresponse. Antiangiogenic therapies such as bevacizumab have improved progression-free survival in newly diagnosed and recurrent glioblastoma patients. These drugs rapidly normalize the hyperpermeable intratumoral capillaries, resulting in decreased vasogenic brain edema, decreased contrast enhancement, and reduction of mass effect. However, whether antiangiogenic agents have a direct antitumoral effect remains a matter of debate. Due to their direct effect on the intratumoral vascular permeability, the degree of enhancement, T2/fluid-attenuated inversion recovery (FLAIR) hyperintensity and even rCBV values are affected by this type of therapy, making more challenging the imaging follow-up of these patients. Progressive nonenhancing tumoral infiltration is one of the imaging patterns that can develop after failure of treatment with bevacizumab (Fig. 14.5). MRS is an attractive imaging modality for the differentiation of progressive nonenhancing tumor versus posttreatment changes in this particular population of patients.

Assessment of treatment response. Previous criteria for treatment response in brain tumor patients relied on 2D measurements obtained from the enhancing components of the tumors (MacDonald criteria). However, due to the increasing recognition of the described

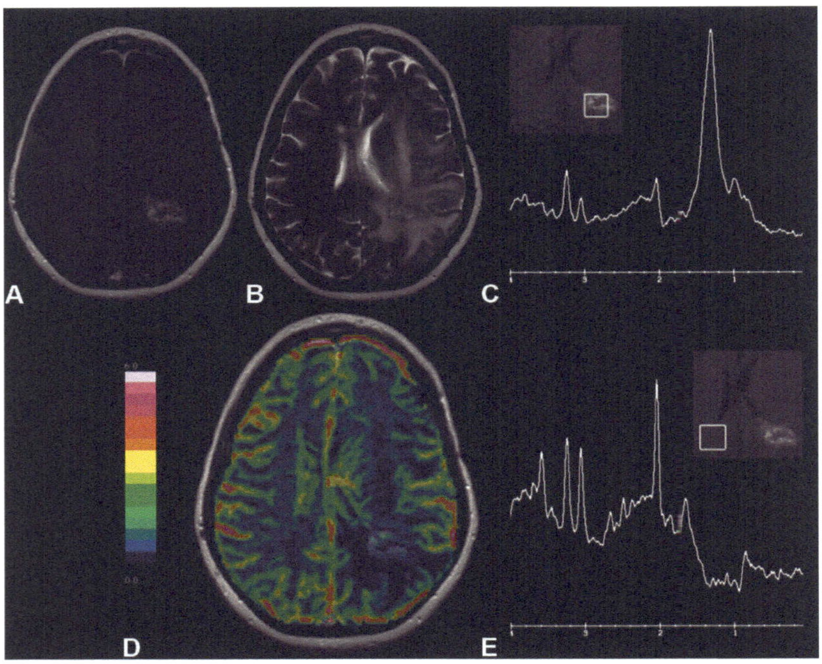

Fig. 14.4. Radiation necrosis in a patient with left temporal glioma. (**A**) Axial postcontrast T1-weighted, (**B**) axial T2-weighted, (**C**) axial corrected relative cerebral blood volume (rCBV), (**D**) intralesional magnetic resonance spectroscopy (MRS), and (**E**) contralateral MRS images. Heterogeneously enhancing lesion in the left periatrial white matter showing a predominance of relatively low rCBV values. MRS demonstrates prominent lipid peaks with generalized decrease of the remaining metabolites (compared to the contralateral spectrum).

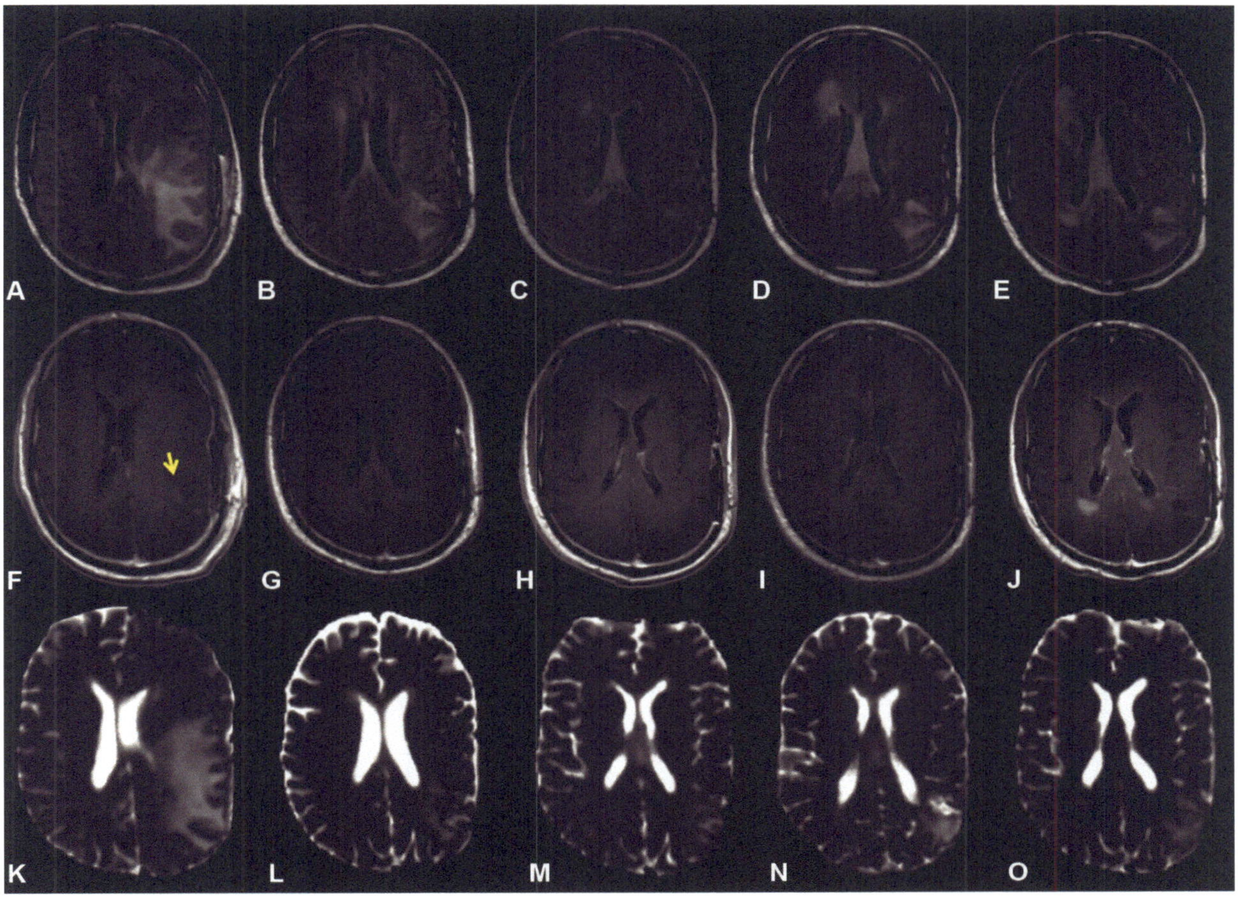

Fig. 14.5. Pseudoresponse and progressive nonenhancing tumoral infiltration during treatment with bevacizumab. Axial fluid-attenuated inversion recovery (FLAIR: upper row), postcontrast T1 (middle row), and apparent diffusion coefficient (bottom row) images at different time points before and during bevacizumab treatment: immediately after surgery (**A, F, K**) and before treatment showing residual enhancement in the left posterior temporal lobe (small yellow arrow), week #7 (**B, G, L**), week # 14 (**C, H, M**), week # 18 (**D, I, N**), and week # 21 (**E, J, O**) during treatment with bevacizumab. Abnormal enhancement and T2 hyperintensity rapidly improved after starting treatment with bevacizumab. However, there was slow progression of mildly expansile areas of abnormal T2 hyperintensity and restricted diffusion in the corpus callosum and periventricular white matter compatible with nonenhancing tumor. Abnormal nodular enhancement eventually recurred during the last time point.

pseudophenomena, patterns of tumoral recurrence of glioblastoma during antiangiogenic treatment and potential radiologic effects of some therapeutic agents (e.g., steroids), the RANO working group developed new imaging criteria for assessment of treatment response in glial tumors (Wen et al., 2010). These new criteria are are summarized in Table 14.1.

Diffuse astrocytoma (WHO grade II)

These are slowly growing infiltrating neoplasms that commonly present in young adult patients more often in a supratentorial location (but infratentorial cases also occur) (Louis et al., 2007). These tumors are slowly growing and can transform into anaplastic astrocytomas and glioblastomas. There are three pathologic subtypes: fibrillary, gemistocytic, and protoplasmic (Louis et al., 2007). The most common presentation in imaging studies is as a nonenhancing mass with ill-defined borders with variable mass effect (depending on the size), with increased diffusivity and relatively normal rCBV values (Fig. 14.6). MRS demonstrates variable decrease of NAA/Cr and increased Cho/Cr ratios (Fig. 14.6). Prominent lipid peaks, lactate, and changes in myo-inositol have also been described. Current imaging techniques cannot differentiate the different subtypes of diffuse astrocytomas.

There is growing evidence of the favorable prognostic impact of *IDH1* gene mutations in low- and high-grade astrocytic tumors (Houillier et al., 2010). The *IDH1* mutation is identified in approximately 73% of diffuse astrocytomas (Hartmann et al., 2009) and most

Table 14.1

Summarized Response Assessment in Neuro-oncology (RANO) criteria

Criterion	Complete response (CR)	Partial response (PR)	Stable disease (SD)	Progressive disease (PD)
Enhancement	No residual enhancement	≥50% reduction	<50% reduction to <25% increase	≥25% increase*
T2/FLAIR hyperintensity	Stable or decreased	Stable or decreased	Stable or decreased	Increased*
New lesion	No	No	No	Yes*
Corticosteroids	None	Stable or decreased	Stable or decreased	Not applicable
Clinical status	Stable or improved	Stable or improved	Stable or improved	Clinical worsening*
Required criteria	All	All	All	Any

*Response is considered PD if present.

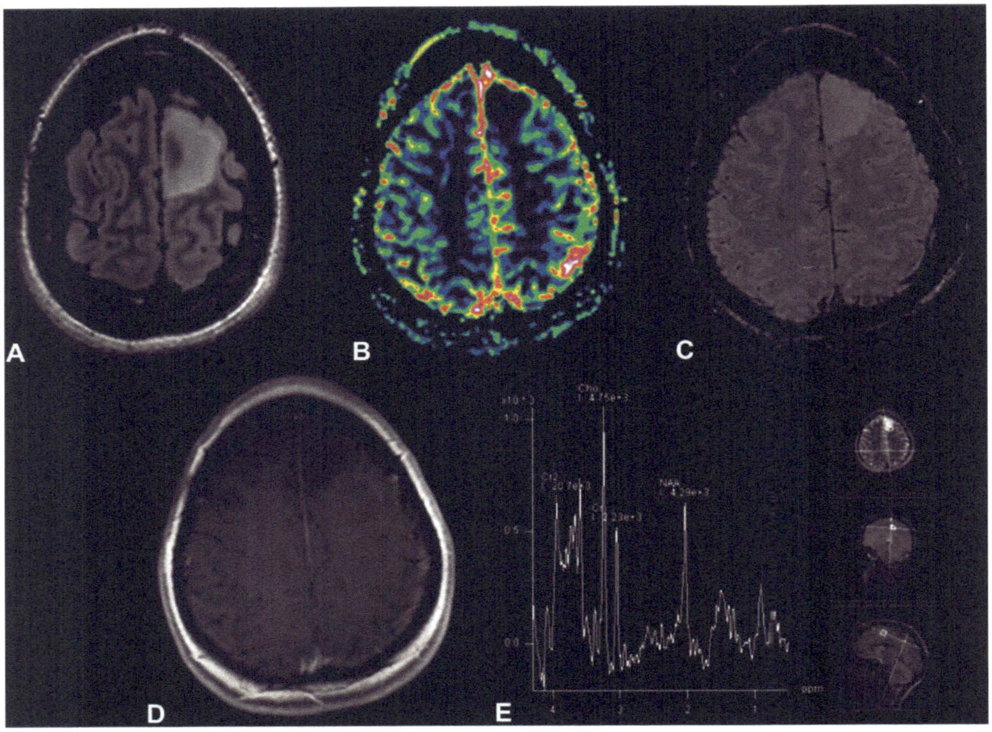

Fig. 14.6. Diffuse astrocytoma (World Health Organization grade II). Axial fluid-attenuated inversion recovery (FLAIR: **A**), axial corrected relative cerebral blood volume map (**B**), axial susceptibility-weighted imaging (**C**), axial postcontrast T1-weighted (**D**), and multivoxel magnetic resonance spectroscopy (MRS) (**E**) images. Expansile FLAIR hyperintense lesion in the left frontal lobe without internal hemorrhage, significant increase of rCBV values or nodular enhancement. MRS (echo time 30 ms) demonstrates mild decrease of *N*-acetyl aspartate/creatine and moderate increase of choline/creatine. Myo-inositol may also be mildly elevated.

of the *IDH1* mutated diffuse astrocytomas appear to have a frontal predominance (Stockhammer et al., 2012). 2-Hydroxyglutarate (2HG) is a potential imaging biomarker of the *IDH1* mutation that can be detected by MRS (Fig. 14.7) (Andronesi et al., 2012, 2013; Choi et al., 2012, 2013a; Elkhaled et al., 2012; Kalinina et al., 2012; Pope et al., 2012; Esmaeili et al., 2013).

Anaplastic astrocytoma (WHO grade III)

These are astrocytomas with atypical nuclear features and increased mitotic activity (with proliferation indexes in the 5–10% range) (Louis et al., 2007). Anaplastic astrocytomas commonly affect patients in their fourth or fifth decades and have similar anatomic distribution as

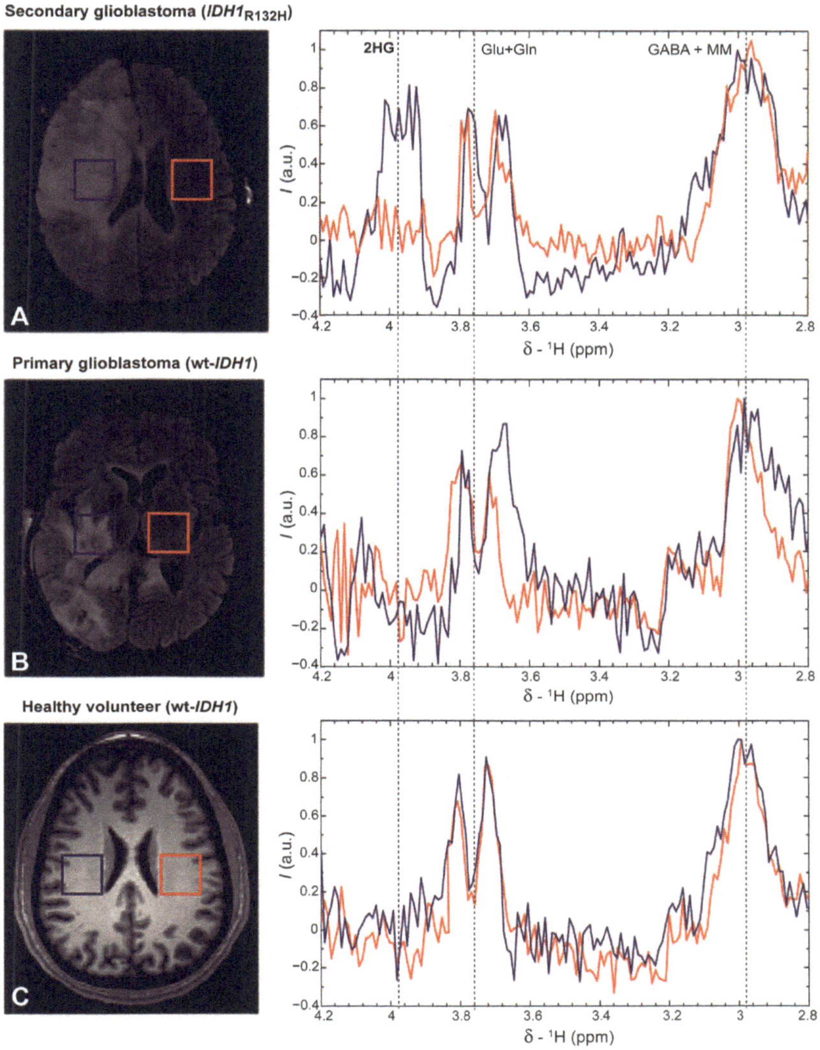

Fig. 14.7. Single-voxel mega-laser spectra *in vivo* at 3 T. (**A**) Secondary glioblastoma patient with IDH1R132H mutation. (**B**) Spectra from a patient with a primary glioblastoma and wild-type (WT) *IDH1*. (**C**) Healthy volunteer. There is a four-peak metabolite present in patients with the *IDH* mutation, compatible with 2HG. (Reproduced from Andronesi et al., 2012, with permission from AAAS.)

the diffuse astrocytomas (most commonly, supratentorial). *IDH1* mutations are observed in up to 64% of anaplastic astrocytomas (Hartmann et al., 2009). *IDH1* mutated anaplastic astrocytomas also exhibit a frontal predominance and better prognosis versus *IDH1* wild-type tumors (Zhang et al., 2014).

Anaplastic astrocytomas are typically expansile and show variable enhancement (often mild and ill defined) (Fig. 14.8). Previous MR perfusion literature suggested rCBV values intermediate between diffuse astrocytomas and glioblastomas, but the lack of vascular proliferation used in more recent pathologic classifications has redefined the perfusion features of these neoplasms. Based on the current pathologic criteria, these neoplasms more often will not show increased rCBV values (Fig. 14.3). Apparent diffusion coefficient (ADC) values are variable depending on the tumoral cell density (higher density producing lower ADC values). MRS shows even more pronounced changes when compared to lower-grade astrocytomas, with marked decrease of NAA/Cr and increased Cho/Cr ratios.

Gliomatosis cerebri (WHO grade I–III)

This term refers to a glial neoplasm diffusely infiltrating large areas of brain parenchyma (at least three cerebral lobes) (Louis et al., 2007; Chen et al., 2013). This tumor is most commonly fibrillary astrocytic and is considered WHO III in most cases (although grades II and IV have been described) (Chen et al., 2013). The MR imaging

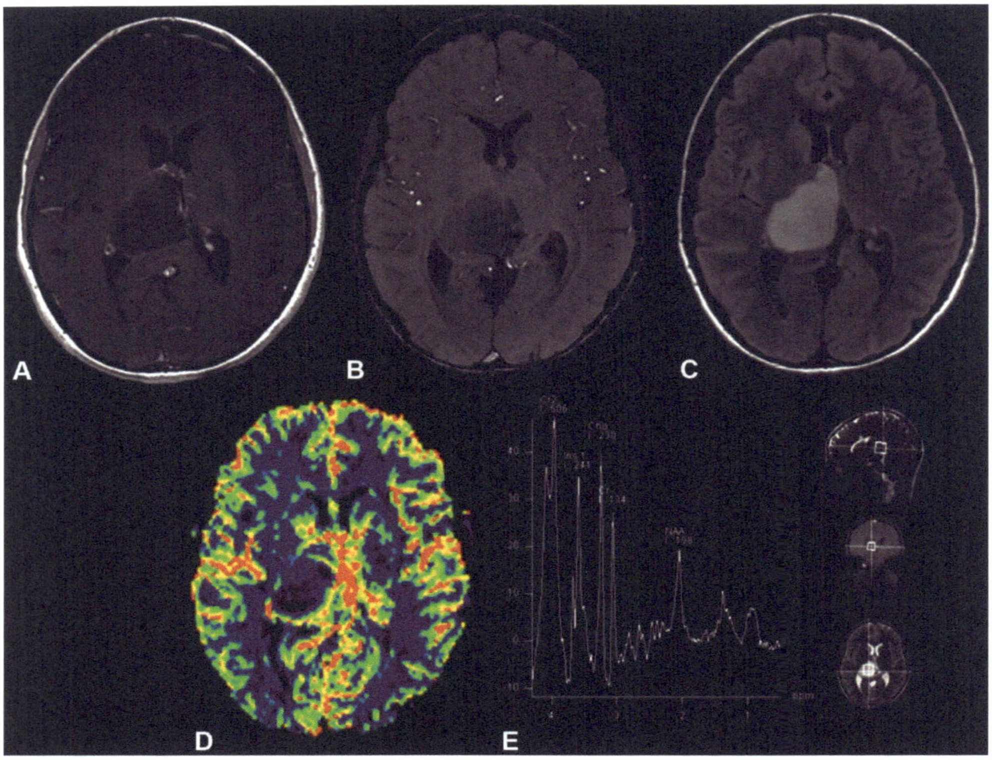

Fig. 14.8. Anaplastic astrocytoma. (**A**) Axial T1 postcontrast, (**B**) axial susceptibility-weighted imaging, (**C**) axial fluid-attenuated inversion recovery (FLAIR), (**D**) leakage-corrected relative cerebral blood volume (rCBV) map, and (**E**) multivoxel magnetic resonance spectroscopy (MRS) images. Expansile FLAIR hyperintense mass with minimal internal enhancement and without internal foci of susceptibility effect or significant increase of rCBV values. MRS shows significant decrease of *N*-acetyl aspartate/creatine and increased choline/creatine ratios.

(MRI) features include extensive, mildly expansile areas of increased T2 signal, increased diffusivity with variable degrees of enhancement, or increased rCBV values (Fig. 14.8). Abnormal enhancement is observed in some of these areas in up to 58% of cases (Chen et al., 2013). MRS is particularly helpful and demonstrates the classic findings seen with diffuse and anaplastic astrocytomas (Fig. 14.9).

Pilocytic and pilomyxoid astrocytoma (WHO grade I and II respectively)

Pilocytic astrocytomas are slowly growing neoplasms, most commonly affecting pediatric and young adult patients. They represent up to 6% of all gliomas and are often located in the cerebellum, optic pathways, or deep gray matter (Louis et al., 2007). These tumors most commonly appear as well-defined enhancing masses with intra- or peritumoral cystic components (Louis et al., 2007) (Fig. 14.10). Intratumoral hemorrhage is occasionally reported. MR perfusion shows marked increase of rCBV values within these masses likely related to glomeruloid vascular proliferation (Sie et al., 2010) (Fig. 14.10). Pilocytic astrocytomas may also involve adjacent leptomeningeal surfaces or, rarely, have distant seeding or anaplastic features (Louis et al., 2007).

Pilomyxoid astrocytomas are considered WHO grade II tumors, typically affecting the pediatric population, and represent a small fraction of pilocytic-like neoplasms (Louis et al., 2007). They are most commonly located in the suprasellar region, deep gray matter, and posterior fossa (Louis et al., 2007). These tumors behave in a more aggressive fashion with frequent local recurrences after resection or cerebrospinal seeding.

Subependymal giant cell astrocytoma (WHO grade I)

Subependymal giant cell astrocytoma (SEGA) is a slowly growing tumor most commonly located within the foramen of Monro region and originating from the adjacent ventricular wall (Fig. 14.11). Most of the cases are associated with tuberous sclerosis complex (TSC) and up to 14% of TSC patients have SEGAs (Louis et al., 2007). Calcifications and intratumoral hemorrhage are frequent. Radiographic regression and reduction in seizure

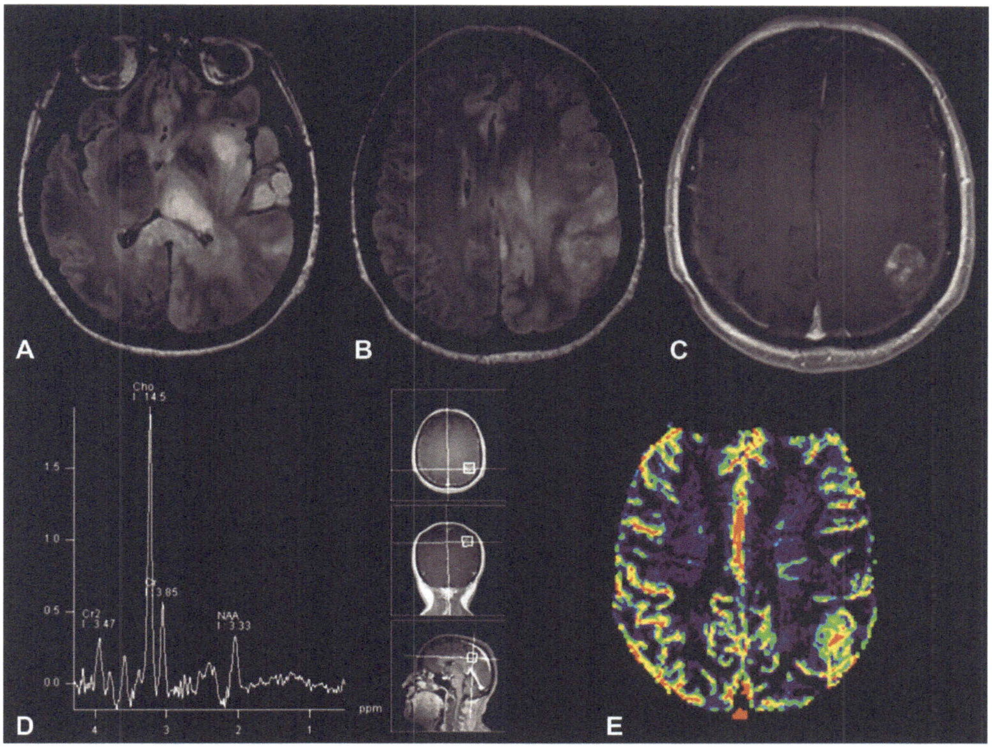

Fig. 14.9. Gliomatosis cerebri. Axial fluid-attenuated inversion recovery (FLAIR) images (**A**, **B**), postcontrast axial T1-weighted (**C**), multivoxel magnetic resonance spectroscopy (MRS) images (**D**), and corrected relative cerebral blood volume (rCBV) (**E**). There is an ill-defined, heterogeneously enhancing, left parietal mass with increased rCBV values (pathologically proven to be a higher-grade glioma, at least anaplastic) associated with more extensive FLAIR hyperintense areas involving the left frontoparietal white matter, corpus callosum, left thalamus, and left subinsular region compatible with gliomatosis cerebri (without increase of rCBV). MRS shows marked decrease of *N*-acetyl aspartate/creatine and increase of choline/creatine ratios within the left parietal enhancing lesion.

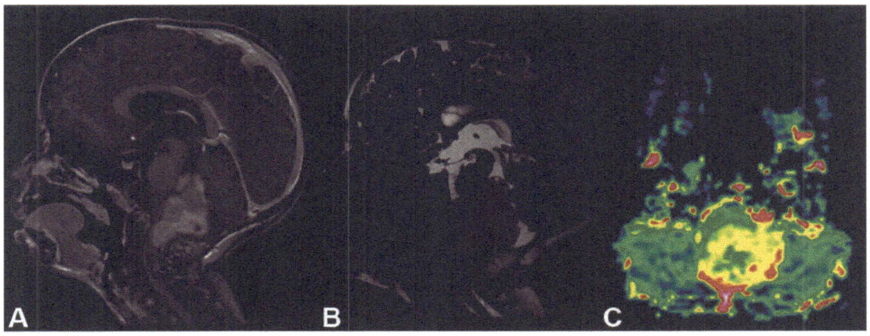

Fig. 14.10. Pilocytic astrocytoma. (**A**) Sagittal gadolinium-enhanced T1-weighted, (**B**) sagittal Fast Imaging Employing Steady-state Acquisition (FIESTA: GE Healthcare), and (**C**) axial relative cerebral blood volume (rCBV) map images. Exophytic enhancing mass occupying the inferior-two thirds of the fourth ventricle, foramen of Magendie, and adjacent dorsal cervical subarachnoid space, compressing the cervicomedullary junction. The mass demonstrates marked increase of rCBV values.

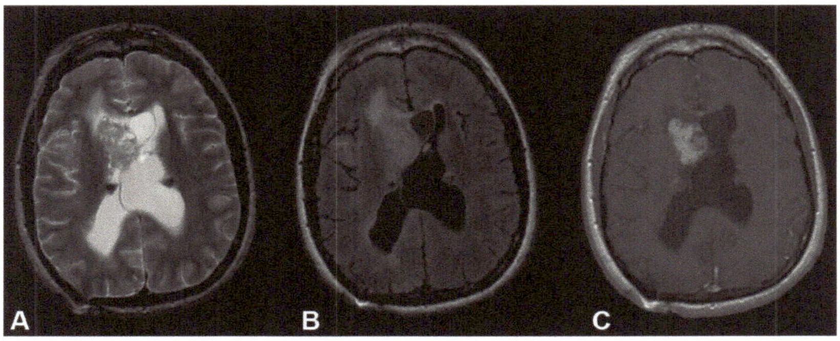

Fig. 14.11. Subependymal giant cell astrocytoma (SEGA). (**A**) Axial T2-weighted, (**B**) fluid-attenuated inversion recovery (FLAIR), and (**C**) postcontrast T1-weighted images. Ill-defined exophytic mass centered on the right anterior lateral ventricle and right foramen of Monro, with heterogeneous internal signal and enhancement.

frequency have been reported in some TSC patients treated with the mammalian target of rapamycin (mTOR) inhibitor, everolimus, which was recently approved by the US Food and Drug Administration for TSC-related SEGA (Krueger et al., 2010, 2013).

Pleomorphic xanthoastrocytoma (WHO grade II)

Pleomorphic xanthoastrocytoma (PXA) most commonly affects pediatric or young adult patients and represents less than 1% of all astrocytomas (Louis et al., 2007). The tumor typically presents superficially in a supratentorial location (more often in the temporal lobe), although other anatomic sites have been reported. They usually demonstrate prominent cystic/necrotic components mixed with solid enhancing portions with mild surrounding edema (Yu et al., 2011; Tien et al., 1992; Petropoulou et al., 1995) (Fig. 14.12). Vascular proliferation (Hirose et al., 2008) may be present in anaplastic PXA. Anaplastic tumors often demonstrate significant increase of rCBV values with MR perfusion (Fig. 14.12).

Oligodendroglial and oligoastrocytic tumors (WHO grade II–III)

Oligodendrogliomas are infiltrating glial neoplasms that are considered WHO II and represent up to 6% of all gliomas (Louis et al., 2007). They most commonly affect adult patients (peak in the fourth or fifth decade of life) and typically occur in a superficial (cortical/subcortical level) supratentorial location (Fig. 14.13). Oligoastrocytomas are histologic variants, demonstrating a combination of astrocytic and oligodendroglial features. Oligoastrocytomas do not have specific imaging features to differentiate them from oligodendrogliomas or pure astrocytomas (Koeller and Rushing, 2005). The WHO II oligodendroglial tumors (oligodendrogliomas and oligoastrocytomas) appear as relatively well-defined intraparenchymal masses with variable enhancement, internal calcifications, and/or hemorrhage and cystic changes (Koeller and Rushing, 2005) (Fig. 14.12). Computed tomography (CT) images show them as predominantly hypoattenuating masses with variable coarse calcifications (20–91% of cases) (Koeller and Rushing, 2005) (Fig. 14.13). Specific imaging features have been

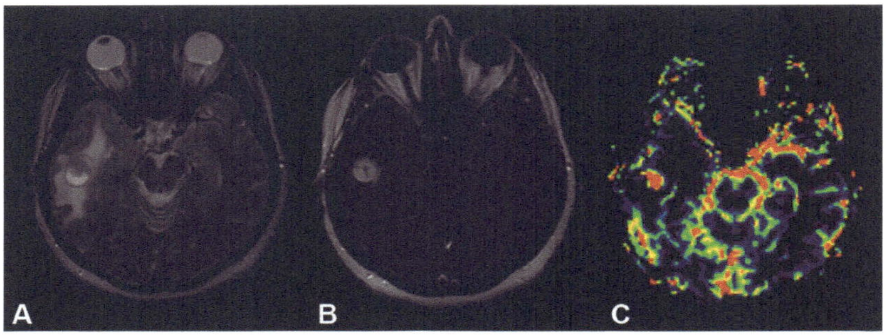

Fig. 14.12. Pleomorphic xanthoastrocytoma. (**A**) Axial T2-weighted, (**B**) postcontrast axial T1-weighted, and (**C**) axial corrected relative cerebral blood volume (rCBV) map images. Heterogeneously enhancing and partially cystic mass in the right temporal lobe showing significant focal increase of rCBV values and surrounded by moderate amount of T2 hyperintense areas.

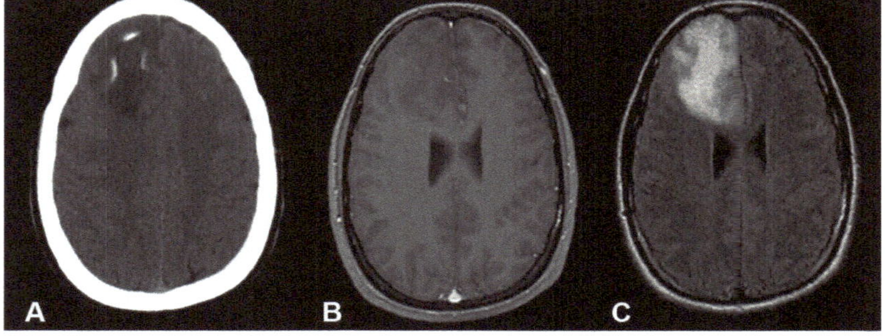

Fig. 14.13. Low-grade oligodendroglioma. (**A**) Axial unenhanced computed tomography, (**B**) axial postcontrast T1-weighted, (**C**) axial fluid-attenuated inversion recovery (FLAIR) images. Partially calcified mass in the right anterior frontal lobe producing mild local mass effect with minimal internal enhancement.

associated with the presence of chromosome 1p and 19q co-deletions, including ill-defined margins, heterogeneous signal, intratumoral calcifications, maximal intratumoral rCBV values, frontal location, and lower intratumoral normalized ADC values (Megyesi et al., 2004; Koeller and Rushing, 2005; Khayal et al., 2011; Kim et al., 2011; Chawla et al., 2013). MR perfusion predominantly demonstrates no significant elevation of rCBV values within these low grade oligodendroglial tumors. Areas of necrosis, lower ADC values, abnormal enhancement, increased rCBV and K_{trans} values are more often seen with anaplastic oligodendrogliomas (Fellah et al., 2012; Khalid et al., 2012; Jia et al., 2013).

Lymphomas and hematopoietic neoplasms

Lymphoma

Primary central nervous system lymphoma (PCNSL) is a rare extranodal variant of non-Hodgkin lymphoma. Greater than 90% of PCNSL cases consist of the diffuse large B-cell subtype. These tumors typically present as a single homogeneously enhancing mass in immunocompetent subjects, often preferentially involving the periventricular regions and corpus callosum. Intrinsic hyperdensity on CT images or abnormal restricted diffusion on diffusion-weighted imaging (DWI) is seen in many cases related to their high tumoral cellular density (Fig. 14.14). Peritumoral edema is typically less pronounced in comparison with metastatic lesions or high-grade gliomas. PCNSL in immunocompromised individuals (e.g., human immunodeficiency virus (HIV) infection) demonstrates different imaging features, often presenting as a ring-enhancing lesion (due to central necrosis) and more frequently involving the basal ganglia (Zacharia et al., 2008). PCNSL commonly shows mild to moderate increase of rCBV values in DSC MR perfusion (Abul-Kasim et al., 2008; Lee et al., 2010; Blasel et al., 2013).

Less common hematopoietic neoplasms

Plasmacytoma, granulocytic sarcoma, and leukemia rarely present as intraparenchymal masses, often with nonspecific features such as variable enhancement and abnormal restricted diffusion.

Ependymal tumors

Subependymoma (WHO grade I)

This type of tumor is considered a benign (WHO I) neoplasm exhibiting very slow growth, classically arising

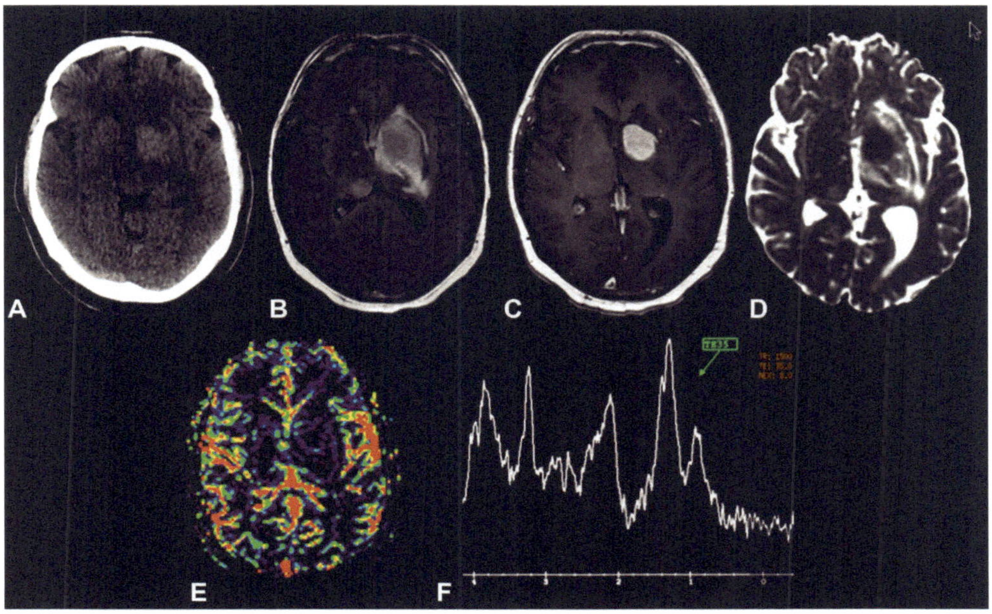

Fig. 14.14. Primary central nervous system lymphoma (PCNSL). (**A**) Axial noncontrast computed tomography, (**B**) axial fluid-attenuated inversion recovery (FLAIR), (**C**) postcontrast axial T1-weighted, (**D**) axial apparent diffusion coefficient, (**E**) axial leakage-corrected relative cerebral blood volume (rCBV) map, and (**F**) single-voxel short echo time magnetic resonance spectroscopy images. Intrinsically hyperdense (**A**) mass in the left basal ganglia region showing moderate surrounding T2 hyperintensity (**B**) and mass effect, homogeneous enhancement (**C**), and abnormal restricted diffusion (**D**). There is no significant increase of rCBV values on dynamic susceptibility contrast perfusion (**E**). Magnetic resonance spectroscopy demonstrates decreased *N*-acetyl aspartate/creatine ratio and prominent lipid peaks (**F**).

from the surface of one of the ventricles (Fig. 14.15). Subependymomas represent up to 8% of ependymal tumors, most commonly discovered in older patients and most frequently located in the fourth and lateral ventricles (Louis et al., 2007; Smith et al., 2013). These neoplasms present as well-circumscribed masses, most commonly without enhancement (but avid enhancement has also been described), with occasional calcifications or intratumoral hemorrhage (Chiechi et al., 1995a) (Fig. 14.15). There is no surrounding edema or T2 hyperintensity in the adjacent brain parenchyma and there have been no reports of metastases or subarachnoid seeding.

Ependymoma (WHO grade II-III)

Ependymomas account for up to 9% of intracranial tumors (higher proportion in the pediatric population) and are usually located near the ventricular system or spinal canal (Louis et al., 2007; Smith et al., 2013). There are several pathologic subtypes of ependymomas, including the cellular, papillary, clear cell, and tanycytic subtypes. These tumors appear as heterogeneous masses on CT and MR images, often with variable enhancement, areas of cystic/necrotic changes, intratumoral hemorrhage, and coarse calcifications (Yuh et al., 2009) (Fig. 14.15). Most of the supratentorial ependymomas present as intraparenchymal masses, difficult to distinguish radiographically from other glial neoplasms (Smith et al., 2013), possibly originating from remnants of ependymal tissue from embryonal development (Smith et al., 2013). Increased levels of glycine, myo-inositol, and glycerophosphocholine using MRS may be helpful in the differentiation of ependymomas from other neoplasms (Davies et al., 2008) (Fig. 14.16).

Choroid plexus tumors (papilloma – WHO grade I; atypical papilloma – WHO grade II; carcinoma – WHO grade III)

These tumors constitute less than 1% of all brain tumors and are more prevalent during childhood, particularly during the first year of life (up to 20% of intracranial tumors in this age group; Louis et al., 2007; Smith et al., 2013). Papillomas are the most common choroid plexus neoplasms (Fig. 14.17), at least five times more frequent than carcinomas (Louis et al., 2007). These lesions typically originate from epithelial cells in the choroid plexus and the most common locations are the lateral ventricular atrium, third and fourth ventricles (Smith et al., 2013). Current diagnostic imaging techniques cannot reliably differentiate choroid plexus papilloma from carcinoma (Naeini et al., 2009; Smith et al., 2013) and, in some cases, from other intraventricular neoplasms (Kim et al., 2012) due to significant overlap of most of their imaging features. Choroid plexus papillomas and carcinomas demonstrate absence of Cr and NAA as well as high levels of Cho and myo-inositol on MRS, and these features can be very helpful for their differentiation from other intraventricular neoplasms (Horska et al., 2001; Krieger et al., 2005; Shibata et al., 2008). Both papilloma (particularly atypical cases) and carcinoma can develop leptomeningeal seeding as well as parenchymal invasion (Naeini et al., 2009). The presence of extensive invasion and vasogenic edema of the adjacent brain parenchyma may favor atypical papilloma or carcinoma (Naeini et al., 2009).

Neuronal and mixed tumors

Dysplastic gangliocytoma of cerebellum (Lhermitte–Duclos disease)

This benign entity is considered a hamartomatous lesion (based on histopathology, lack of or minimal mitotic

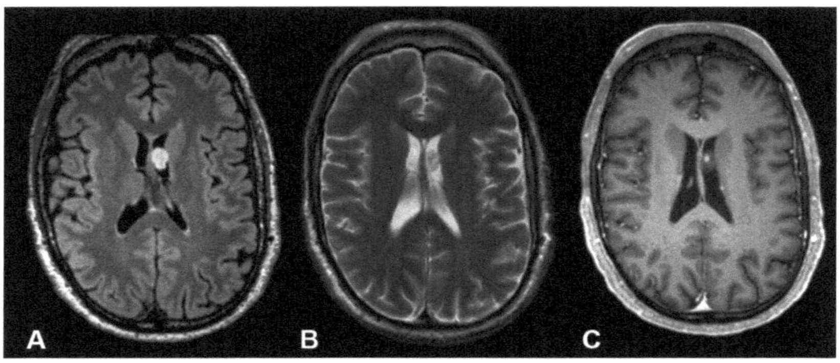

Fig. 14.15. Subependymoma. Axial fluid-attenuated inversion recovery (FLAIR: **A**), axial T2-weighted (**B**) and postcontrast axial T1-weighted (**C**) images. Well-defined T2 hyperintense mass in the anterior left lateral ventricle arising from the ependymal wall and showing mild focal internal enhancement.

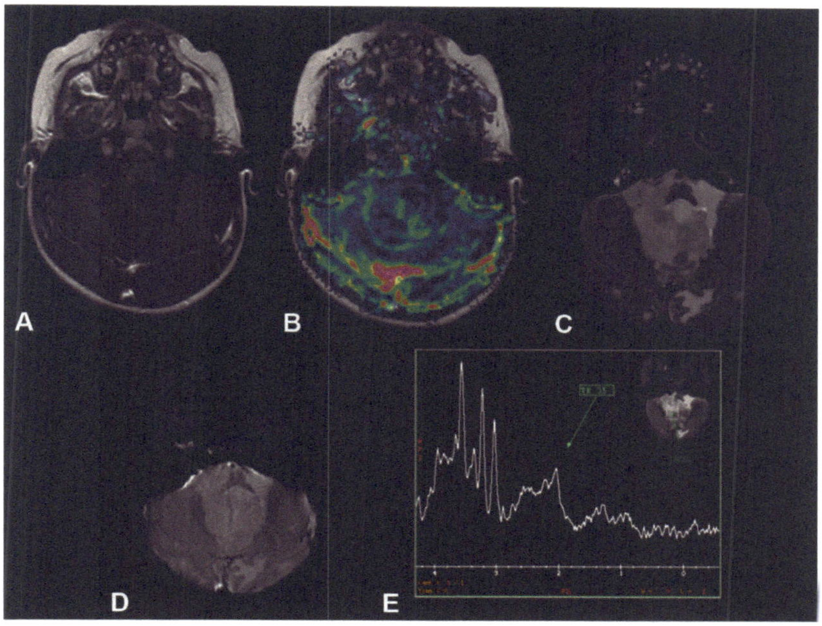

Fig. 14.16. Ependymoma (World Health Organization III). (**A**) Axial postcontrast T1-weighted, (**B**) corrected relative cerebral blood volume (rCBV) map, (**C**) T2-weighted, (**D**) gradient recalled echo, and (**E**) magnetic resonance spectroscopy (**E**) images. Irregular, minimally enhancing mass with internal cystic components and variable rCBV values involving the fourth ventricle and right foramen of Luschka. The mass demonstrates mild to moderate decrease of *N*-acetyl aspartate/creatine, mild increase of choline/creatine, and increase of myo-inositol. Mild elevation of glycine may also be present.

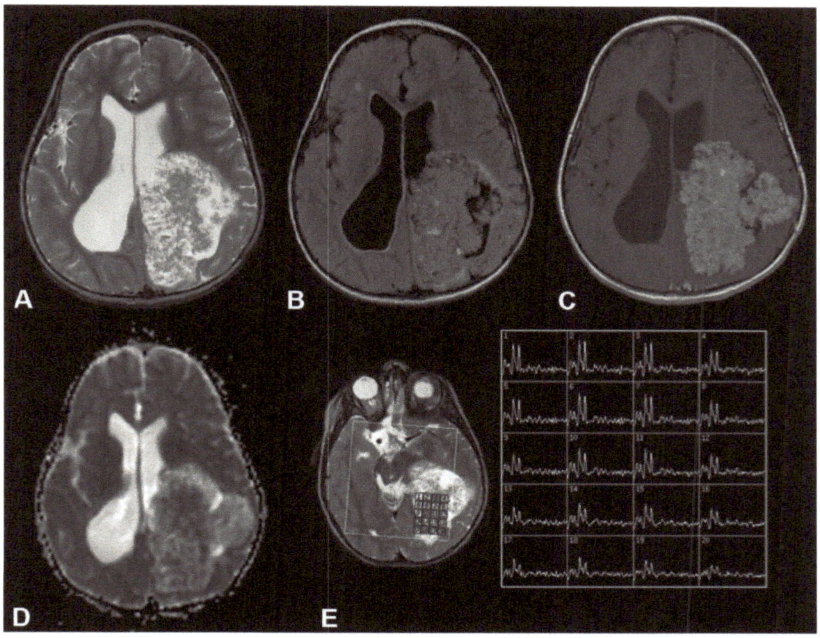

Fig. 14.17. Choroid plexus papilloma. (**A**) Axial T2-weighted, (**B**) axial fluid-attenuated inversion recovery (FLAIR), (**C**) axial T1-weighted postcontrast, (**D**) axial apparent diffusion coefficient map, and (**E**) multivoxel magnetic resonance spectroscopy (MRS) images. Large frond-like T2 hyperintense and homogeneously enhancing mass expanding the left ventricular atrium, producing local mass effect and mild hydrocephalus. MRS shows lack of *N*-acetyl aspartate peaks (suggesting a nonneuronal histology) and prominent choline/creatine ratios.

activity) containing ganglionic cells producing diffuse enlargement of the molecular and internal granular cerebellar layers (Louis et al., 2007). Most patients with LDD have mutations in PTEN (phosphatase and tensin homologue deleted on chromosome 10). LDD is also considered a major component of Cowden disease (multiple hamartoma syndrome, commonly associated with PTEN mutations) (Louis et al., 2007). MRI demonstrates mild expansion of the cerebellar folia, producing a "tiger-striped" appearance on T2-weighted images, without abnormal enhancement (Meltzer et al., 1995; Klisch et al., 2001; Thomas et al., 2007; Cianfoni et al., 2008; Moenninghoff et al., 2010) (Fig. 14.18).

Dysembryoplastic neuroepithelial tumor (WHO grade I)

This entity is considered a benign neoplasm typically involving the cortex and typically producing seizures. It can be identified in up to 13.5% of children having epilepsy surgery (Louis et al., 2007). Focal cortical dysplasia is often (up to 80% of cases) associated with these lesions (Louis et al., 2007). Dysembryoplastic neuroepithelial tumors are usually supratentorial, often involving the temporal lobes, and present as superficial (intracortical) expansile "bubbly" multicystic lesions with variable enhancement, and occasional intratumoral calcifications (<20%) without significant surrounding T2 hyperintensity or local mass effect (Shin et al., 2002) (Fig. 14.19).

Gangliocytoma and ganglioglioma (WHO grade I or III)

These tumors are neuroepithelial neoplasms that contain ganglion cells (gangliocytoma) or a combination of ganglion and glial cells (ganglioglioma) (Louis et al., 2007). Most gangliogliomas and gangliocytomas are considered WHO grade I lesions but some gangliogliomas can be anaplastic (WHO grade III) (Louis et al., 2007). These tumors can involve any anatomic location in the CNS but most gangliogliomas are located in the temporal lobes and often present clinically with seizures (Louis et al., 2007). Gangliogliomas are the most common mixed neuronal-glial CNS neoplasms (Shin et al., 2002), often presenting as a partially cystic mass associated with a mural nodule, variable enhancement of the solid component, and occasionally with intratumoral calcifications (30% of cases) (Shin et al., 2002) (Fig. 14.20). Local mass effect and surrounding T2 hyperintensity in the adjacent brain parenchyma are often mild (Fig. 14.20).

Central and extraventricular neurocytoma (WHO grade II)

This is an infrequent neuronal tumor that typically presents as a supratentorial, intraventricular, partially cystic, and heterogeneously enhancing mass. This tumor involves the anterior third ventricle in up to 50% of

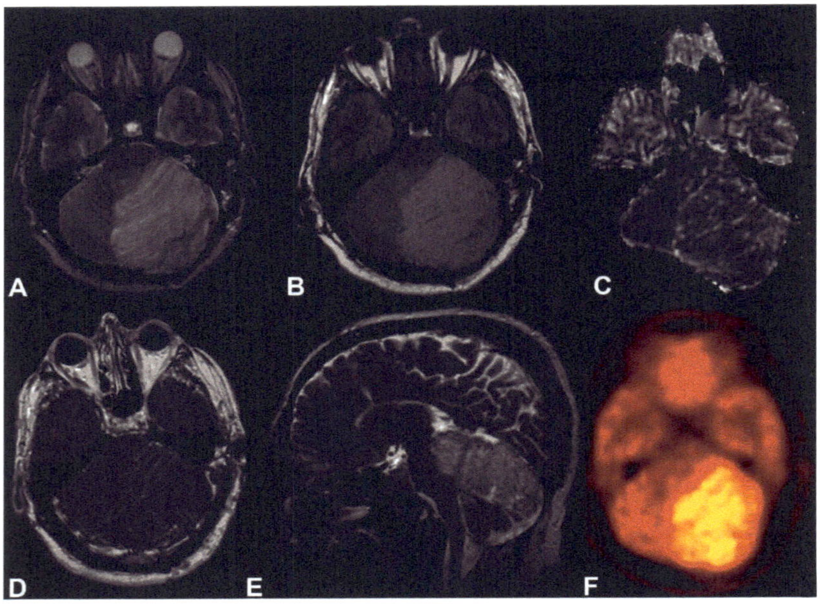

Fig. 14.18. Dysplastic gangliocytoma of cerebellum (Lhermitte–Duclos disease). (**A**) Axial T2-weighted, (**B**) axial fluid-attenuated inversion recovery (FLAIR), (**C**) axial apparent diffusion coefficient, (**D**) axial T1-weighted postcontrast, (**E**) sagittal T2-weighted, and (**F**) fluorodeoxyglucose (FDG) positron emission tomography (PET) images. Extensive areas of expansion of cerebellar folia and increased T2/FLAIR signal in the left cerebellar hemisphere with minimal overlying vascular enhancement and without abnormal restricted diffusion. FDG PET demonstrates increased FDG uptake in this abnormality.

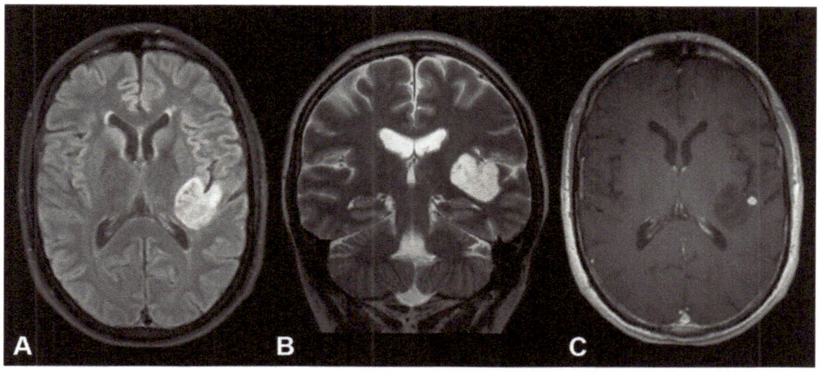

Fig. 14.19. Dysembryoplastic neuroepithelial tumor (DNET). (**A**) Axial fluid-attenuated inversion recovery (FLAIR), (**B**) coronal T2-weighted, and (**C**) axial T1-weighted postcontrast images. Expansile "bubbly" multicystic mass in the left posterior subinsular region with a focus of abnormal nodular enhancement in the left temporal opercular region.

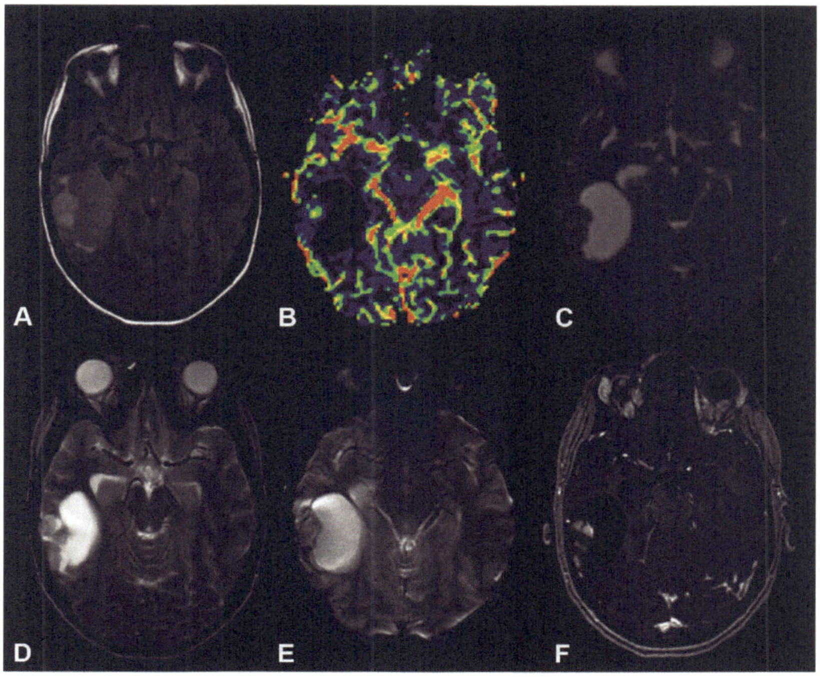

Fig. 14.20. Ganglioglioma (World Health Organization grade I). (**A**) Axial fluid-attenuated inversion recovery (FLAIR), (**B**) axial corrected relative cerebral blood volume (rCBV) map, (**C**) axial apparent diffusion coefficient, (**D**) T2-weighted, (**E**) gradient recalled echo, and (**F**) postcontrast axial T1-weighted images. Partially cystic mass in the right temporal lobe producing mild local mass effect. Laterally located enhancing nodular component shows significant increase of rCBV values.

cases, commonly adjacent to or attached to the septum pellucidum (Fig. 14.21) (Demetriades et al., 2013).

Pineal tumors

Pineocytoma (WHO grade I)

This is a rare, benign neoplasm typically developing in adults and presenting as a well-defined, small rounded homogeneously enhancing mass with occasional peripheral calcification (Chiechi et al., 1995b; Nakamura et al., 2000; Louis et al., 2007). Most pineocytomas are solid and, less frequently, partially cystic/solid neoplasms (Fakhran and Escott, 2008).

Pineoblastoma (WHO grade IV)

This is a highly malignant pineal parenchymal neoplasm containing immature pineal cells (Smirniotopoulos et al., 1992) and predominantly affecting the pediatric

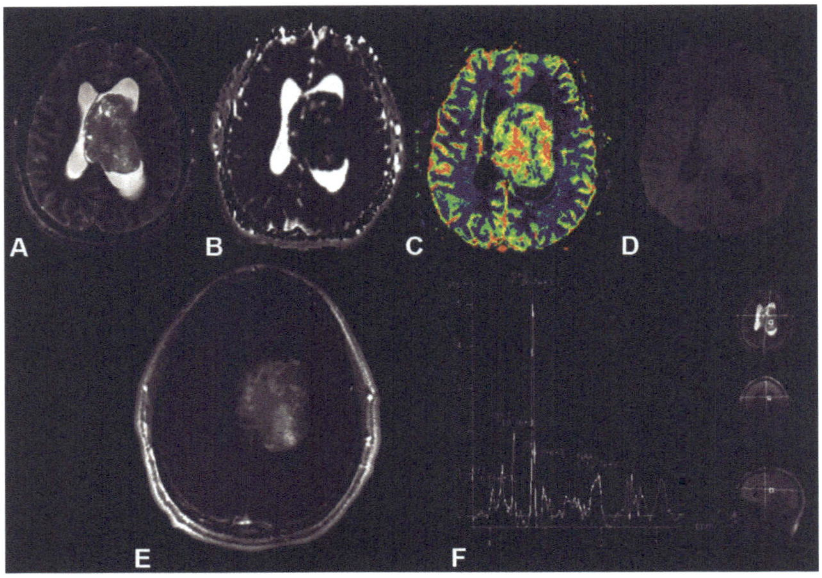

Fig. 14.21. Central neurocytoma. (**A**) Axial T2-weighted, (**B**) apparent diffusion coefficient, (**C**) corrected relative cerebral blood volume (rCBV), (**D**) susceptibility-weighted, (**E**) postcontrast T1-weighted, and (**F**) magnetic resonance spectroscopy (MRS) images. Multicystic mass centered on the left lateral ventricle and attached to the septum pellucidum. The mass has extensive areas of abnormal restricted diffusion, heterogeneous enhancement, and increased rCBV values. MRS shows marked decrease of *N*-acetyl aspartate/creatine and increase of choline/creatine ratios.

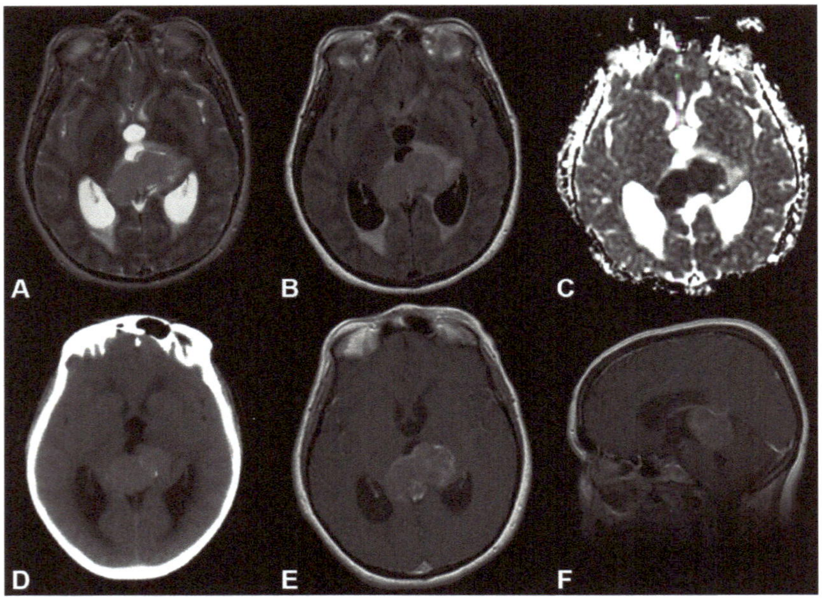

Fig. 14.22. Pineoblastoma. (**A**) Axial T2-weighted, (**B**) fluid-attenuated inversion recovery (FLAIR), (**C**) apparent diffusion coefficient map, (**D**) unenhanced computed tomography, (**E**) postcontrast T1-weighted axial, and (**F**) sagittal images. Homogeneously enhancing mass involving the thalami and pineal gland, producing local mass effect on the adjacent tectal place and effacement of the posterior third ventricle. Small calcifications are seen peripherally displaced by the mass on the computed tomography.

population. Pineoblastomas present as larger multilobulated or ill-defined, more infiltrating, and, rarely, calcified tumors with variable enhancement (Smirniotopoulos et al., 1992; Chiechi et al., 1995b; Nakamura et al., 2000) (Fig. 14.22). Prominent cystic changes are unusual in this type of tumor (Louis et al., 2007). Leptomeningeal and cerebrospinal fluid dissemination is frequently observed.

Pineal parenchymal tumor of intermediate differentiation (WHO grades II–III)

The pineal parenchymal tumor of intermediate differentiation is a WHO grade II or III pineal neoplasm, responsible for > 20% of pineal tumors, often with combined features of pineocytoma and pineoblastoma (Louis et al., 2007) and without a specific age preference. Metastases are rare and local relapse is observed in 22% of patients (Louis et al., 2007).

Embryonal tumors

Medulloblastoma (WHO grade IV)

Medulloblastoma is a malignant embryonal cerebellar neoplasm, predominantly affecting the pediatric population and often associated with leptomeningeal metastases. However, 30% of medulloblastomas present in patients older than 16 (Louis et al., 2007). There are four subtypes of medulloblastomas: desmoplastic/nodular, medulloblastoma with extensive nodularity, anaplastic medulloblastoma, and large cell medulloblastoma. Based on their transcriptional profiles, medulloblastomas can also be subdivided into four different subgroups: Wnt, Shh, group 3, and group 4 (Taylor et al., 2012). The majority of medulloblastomas originate from the vermis (>75% of cases) and the tumors that arise from the cerebellar hemispheres are typically encountered in older patients and are of the desmoplastic/nodular variety. The classic radiologic features of these tumors include solid masses with variable enhancement (from avidly enhancing to nonenhancing), abnormal restricted diffusion, and relative absence of intratumoral hemorrhage or calcifications (Fig. 14.23).

CNS primitive neuroectodermal tumors (WHO grade IV)

This is a group of neoplasms containing poorly differentiated neuroepithelial cells with variable neuronal, glial,

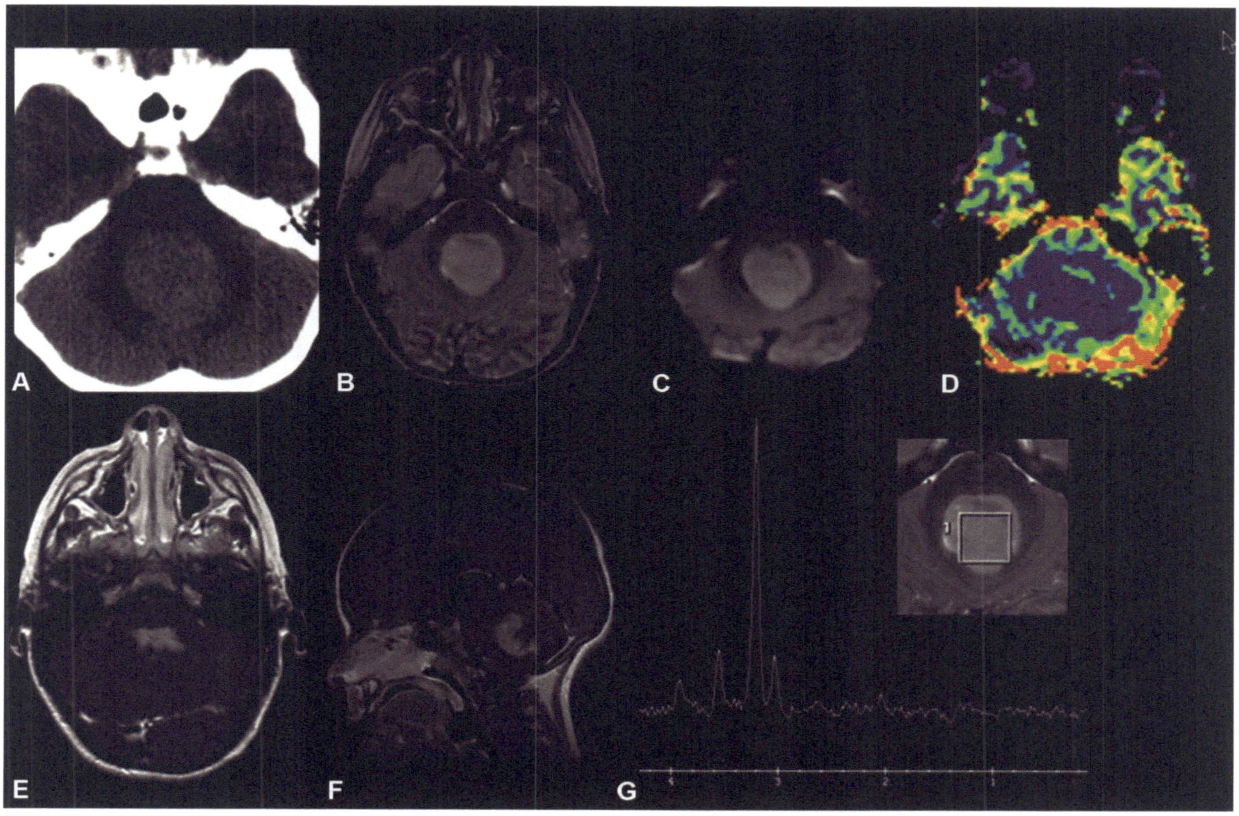

Fig. 14.23. Medulloblastoma. (**A**) Axial unenhanced computed tomography (CT), (**B**) axial T2-weighted, (**C**) axial diffusion-weighted imaging; (**D**) axial corrected relative cerebral blood volume (rCBV) map, (**E**) axial and (**F**) sagittal postcontrast T1-weighted images as well as (**G**) single-voxel magnetic resonance (MR) spectroscopy. CT hyperdense, T2 hyperintense mass centered on the anterior vermis and fourth ventricle. The mass shows homogeneous internal restricted diffusion and heterogeneous enhancement without significant increase of rCBV values. MR spectroscopy demonstrates marked decrease of *N*-acetyl aspartate/creatine and marked increase of choline/creatine ratios. A small taurine peak may also be present.

or ependymal differentiation, predominantly affecting pediatric patients. There are several subtypes, including CNS PNET NOS (not otherwise specified: also known as supratentorial PNET), CNS neuroblastoma, CNS ganglioneuroblastoma, medulloepithelioma, and ependymoblastoma. These tumors appear hyperdense on CT and demonstrate abnormal restricted diffusion on MRI, likely secondary to their high cellular density. They often contain cystic areas, calcifications (up to 70%), and mild surrounding T2 hyperintensity.

Atypical teratoid/rhabdoid tumor (WHO grade IV)

This is an intracranial tumor typically encountered in the pediatric population (first decade) and containing a combination of rhabdoid and primitive neuroectodermal cells (Louis et al., 2007). These tumors can be supra- or infratentorial, rarely involving the spinal cord. Leptomeningeal seeding and drop metastases are observed in up to 20–25% of cases (Louis et al., 2007). The MR features are very similar to medulloblastoma, with variable contrast enhancement, intrinsically hyperdense on CT, and with abnormal restricted diffusion on DWI sequences.

Germ cell tumors

These neoplasms can be extra- or intra-axial and have been described in detail in the extra-axial tumors chapter. Germ cell tumors can produce local parenchymal involvement in the pineal and hypothalamic regions.

Metastatic brain tumors

The most common neoplasms metastasizing to the brain in adults are lung cancer (50% of brain metastases), breast cancer (particularly small cell and adenocarcinoma) (15%) (Fig. 14.24), melanoma (11%), renal cell, and colon cancer. In 11% of all brain metastases, the primary cancer is unknown (Louis et al., 2007). CNS metastases are identified in up to 25% of patients dying of cancer at the time of autopsy (Louis et al., 2007). The most common neoplasms with metastatic involvement of the brain in children are leukemia, lymphoma, osteosarcoma, rhabdomyosarcoma, and Ewing sarcoma (Louis et al., 2007). Metastatic lesions often develop in the arterial "border zones" and at sites of gray–white-matter junction. Some neoplasms often present with hemorrhagic metastases, particularly melanoma, renal cell carcinoma, thyroid carcinoma, and choriocarcinoma. Metastases typically present as heterogeneously enhancing masses, often

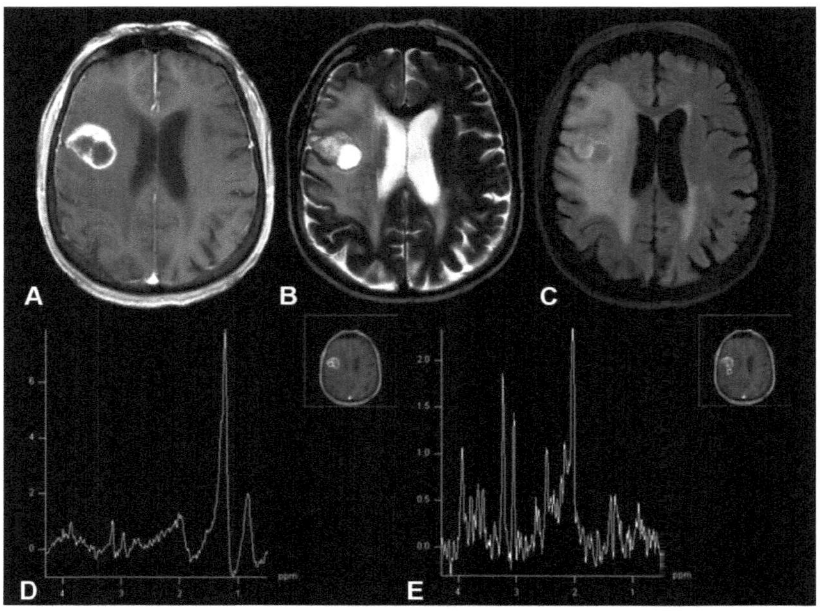

Fig. 14.24. Breast adenocarcinoma metastatic to the brain. (**A**) Axial postcontrast T1-weighted, (**B**) axial T2-weighted, (**C**) axial fluid-attenuated inversion recovery (FLAIR), (**D**) intralesional magnetic resonance spectroscopy (MRS), and (**E**) juxtalesional MRS images. Heterogeneously enhancing centrally necrotic mass in the right frontal white matter surrounded by extensive areas of vasogenic edema and producing local mass effect with effacement of overlying sulci. The MR spectrum from within the lesion shows prominent lipid peaks and marked decrease of the remaining metabolites. The MR spectrum from the white matter immediately surrounding the enhancing lesion demonstrates relatively preserved metabolic ratios compatible with areas of vasogenic edema.

necrotic or partially cystic, and with variable surrounding edema (Fig. 14.19). MRS and MR perfusion can be used for the differentiation of metastatic tumor from a high-grade glioma in cases with a solitary brain mass (Fig. 14.24).

ROLE OF ADVANCED IMAGING TECHNIQUES

Certain advanced MR techniques are very useful for the characterization of newly diagnosed intra-axial brain tumors or during follow-up for identification of tumoral recurrences (Al-Okaili et al., 2006). Some tumors, such as lymphoma, PNET, and medulloblastoma, often demonstrate abnormal restricted diffusion. DSC MR perfusion has shown a strong correlation with intratumoral vascularity and is very helpful in the diagnosis of high-grade gliomas and pilocytic astrocytomas (Hartmann et al., 2003; Cotton, 2006; Barajas et al., 2009; Liao et al., 2009; Valles et al., 2013) (Figs 14.1, 14.3, and 14.4). MRS offers the possibility of *in vivo* metabolic profiling of intra-axial tumors and characteristic MRS profiles have been described in meningiomas (elevated alanine), medulloblastomas (increased taurine and choline peaks) (Wilke et al., 2001), and astrocytomas (myo-inositol, Cho, and 2HG) (Andronesi et al., 2012; Kalinina et al., 2012) (Fig. 14.7).

Nuclear medicine techniques are also commonly used, particularly fluorodeoxyglucose (^{18}F-FDG) and methionine (^{11}C-MET) PET imaging, particularly for the differentiation of radiation necrosis and recurrent high-grade tumor (Kim et al., 2010; Okamoto et al., 2011; Glaudemans et al., 2013; Kickingereder et al., 2013).

CONCLUSION

There is a broad spectrum of intra-axial brain neoplasms, many of them with overlapping imaging features and with variable prognosis. Advanced MR techniques can be helpful to narrow the differential diagnosis and to identify higher-grade tumoral components. Peculiar posttreatment phenomena such as pseudoprogression, radiation necrosis, and pseudoresponse make the imaging diagnosis and follow-up of these patients even more complex and challenging. Awareness of these posttreatment changes, detailed clinical information, and appropriate use of advanced MRI techniques are key factors to improve patient management.

References

Abul-Kasim K, Maly P, Strombeck A et al. (2008). Perfusion weighted MR imaging may differentiate primary CNS lymphoma from other homogeneously enhancing brain tumors. Neuroradiol J 21: 637–644.

Albert FK, Forsting M, Sartor K et al. (1994). Early postoperative magnetic resonance imaging after resection of malignant glioma: objective evaluation of residual tumor and its influence on regrowth and prognosis. Neurosurgery 34: 45–60. discussion 60–1.

Al-Okaili RN, Krejza J, Wang S et al. (2006). Advanced MR imaging techniques in the diagnosis of intraaxial brain tumors in adults. Radiographics 26 (Suppl 1): S173–S189.

Andronesi OC, Kim GS, Gerstner E et al. (2012). Detection of 2-hydroxyglutarate in IDH-mutated glioma patients by in vivo spectral-editing and 2D correlation magnetic resonance spectroscopy. Sci Transl Med 4: 116ra4.

Andronesi OC, Rapalino O, Gerstner E et al. (2013). Detection of oncogenic IDH1 mutations using magnetic resonance spectroscopy of 2-hydroxyglutarate. J Clin Invest 123: 3659–3663.

Barajas RF, Chang JS, Sneed PK et al. (2009). Distinguishing recurrent intra-axial metastatic tumor from radiation necrosis following gamma knife radiosurgery using dynamic susceptibility-weighted contrast-enhanced perfusion MR imaging. AJNR Am J Neuroradiol 30: 367–372.

Blasel S, Jurcoane A, Bahr O et al. (2013). MR perfusion in and around the contrast-enhancement of primary CNS lymphomas. J Neurooncol 114: 127–134.

Cairncross JG, Pexman JH, Rathbone MP (1985a). Post-surgical contrast enhancement mimicking residual brain tumour. Can J Neurol Sci 12: 75.

Cairncross JG, Pexman JH, Rathbone MP et al. (1985b). Postoperative contrast enhancement in patients with brain tumor. Ann Neurol 17: 570–572.

Carrillo JA, Lai A, Nghiemphu PL et al. (2012). Relationship between tumor enhancement, edema, IDH1 mutational status, MGMT promoter methylation, and survival in glioblastoma. AJNR Am J Neuroradiol 33: 1349–1355.

Chawla S, Krejza J, Vossough A et al. (2013). Differentiation between oligodendroglioma genotypes using dynamic susceptibility contrast perfusion-weighted imaging and proton MR spectroscopy. AJNR Am J Neuroradiol 34: 1542–1549.

Chen S, Tanaka S, Giannini C et al. (2013). Gliomatosis cerebri: clinical characteristics, management, and outcomes. J Neurooncol 112: 267–275.

Chiechi MV, Smirniotopoulos JG, Jones RV (1995a). Intracranial subependymomas: CT and MR imaging features in 24 cases. AJR Am J Roentgenol 165: 1245–1250.

Chiechi MV, Smirniotopoulos JG, Mena H (1995b). Pineal parenchymal tumors: CT and MR features. J Comput Assist Tomogr 19: 509–517.

Choi C, Ganji SK, DeBerardinis RJ et al. (2012). 2-hydroxyglutarate detection by magnetic resonance spectroscopy in IDH-mutated patients with gliomas. Nat Med 18: 624–629.

Choi C, Ganji S, Hulsey K et al. (2013a). A comparative study of short- and long-TE (1)H MRS at 3 T for in vivo detection of 2-hydroxyglutarate in brain tumors. NMR Biomed 26: 1242–1250.

Choi YJ, Kim HS, Jahng GH et al. (2013b). Pseudoprogression in patients with glioblastoma: added value of arterial spin labeling to dynamic susceptibility contrast perfusion MR imaging. Acta Radiol 54: 448–454.

Cianfoni A, Wintermark M, Piludu F et al. (2008). Morphological and functional MR imaging of Lhermitte-Duclos disease with pathology correlate. J Neuroradiol 35: 297–300.

Cotton F (2006). Diffusion-perfusion in intra-axial brain tumors with high relaxivity contrast agents. Neuroradiology 48 (Suppl 1): 34–40.

Davies NP, Wilson M, Harris LM et al. (2008). Identification and characterisation of childhood cerebellar tumours by in vivo proton MRS. NMR Biomed 21: 908–918.

Demetriades AK, Al Hyassat S, Al-Sarraj S et al. (2013). Papillary glioneuronal tumour: a review of the literature with two illustrative cases. Br J Neurosurg 27: 401–404.

Dolecek TA, Propp JM, Stroup NE et al. (2012). CBTRUS statistical report: primary brain and central nervous system tumors diagnosed in the United States in 2005-2009. Neuro Oncol 14 (Suppl 5): v1–v49.

Elkhaled A, Jalbert LE, Phillips JJ et al. (2012). Magnetic resonance of 2-hydroxyglutarate in IDH1-mutated low-grade gliomas. Sci Transl Med 4: 116ra5.

Esmaeili M, Vettukattil R, Bathen TF (2013). 2-hydroxyglutarate as a magnetic resonance biomarker for glioma subtyping. Transl oncol 6: 92–98.

Fakhran S, Escott EJ (2008). Pineocytoma mimicking a pineal cyst on imaging: true diagnostic dilemma or a case of incomplete imaging? AJNR Am J Neuroradiol 29: 159–163.

Fellah S, Caudal D, De Paula AM et al. (2012). Multimodal MR imaging (diffusion, perfusion, and spectroscopy): is it possible to distinguish oligodendroglial tumor grade and 1p/19q codeletion in the pretherapeutic diagnosis? AJNR Am J Neuroradiol 34: 1326–1333.

Forsting M, Albert FK, Kunze S et al. (1993). Extirpation of glioblastomas: MR and CT follow-up of residual tumor and regrowth patterns. AJNR Am J Neuroradiol 14: 77–87.

Friedman HS, Prados MD, Wen PY et al. (2009). Bevacizumab alone and in combination with irinotecan in recurrent glioblastoma. J Clin Oncol 27: 4733–4740.

Gahramanov S, Muldoon LL, Varallyay CG et al. (2013). Pseudoprogression of glioblastoma after chemo- and radiation therapy: diagnosis by using dynamic susceptibility-weighted contrast-enhanced perfusion MR imaging with ferumoxytol versus gadoteridol and correlation with survival. Radiology 266: 842–852.

Glaudemans AW, Enting RH, Heesters MA et al. (2013). Value of 11C-methionine PET in imaging brain tumours and metastases. Eur J Nucl Med Mol Imaging 40: 615–635.

Hartmann M, Heiland S, Harting I et al. (2003). Distinguishing of primary cerebral lymphoma from high-grade glioma with perfusion-weighted magnetic resonance imaging. Neurosci Lett 338: 119–122.

Hartmann C, Meyer J, Balss J et al. (2009). Type and frequency of IDH1 and IDH2 mutations are related to astrocytic and oligodendroglial differentiation and age: a study of 1,010 diffuse gliomas. Acta Neuropathol 118: 469–474.

Hirose T, Ishizawa K, Sugiyama K et al. (2008). Pleomorphic xanthoastrocytoma: a comparative pathological study between conventional and anaplastic types. Histopathology 52: 183–193.

Horska A, Ulug AM, Melhem ER et al. (2001). Proton magnetic resonance spectroscopy of choroid plexus tumors in children. J Magn Reson Imaging 14: 78–82.

Houillier C, Wang X, Kaloshi G et al. (2010). IDH1 or IDH2 mutations predict longer survival and response to temozolomide in low-grade gliomas. Neurology 75: 1560–1566.

Hu LS, Eschbacher JM, Heiserman JE et al. (2012). Reevaluating the imaging definition of tumor progression: perfusion MRI quantifies recurrent glioblastoma tumor fraction, pseudoprogression, and radiation necrosis to predict survival. Neuro Oncol 14: 919–930.

Iwamoto FM, Abrey LE, Beal K et al. (2009). Patterns of relapse and prognosis after bevacizumab failure in recurrent glioblastoma. Neurology 73: 1200–1206.

Jia Z, Geng D, Liu Y et al. (2013). Low-grade and anaplastic oligodendrogliomas: differences in tumour microvascular permeability evaluated with dynamic contrast-enhanced magnetic resonance imaging. J Clin Neurosci 20: 1110–1113.

Kalinina J, Carroll A, Wang L et al. (2012). Detection of "oncometabolite" 2-hydroxyglutarate by magnetic resonance analysis as a biomarker of IDH1/2 mutations in glioma. J Mol Med 90: 1161–1171.

Khalid L, Carone M, Dumrongpisutikul N et al. (2012). Imaging characteristics of oligodendrogliomas that predict grade. AJNR Am J Neuroradiol 33: 852–857.

Khayal IS, Vandenberg SR, Smith KJ et al. (2011). MRI apparent diffusion coefficient reflects histopathologic subtype, axonal disruption, and tumor fraction in diffuse-type grade II gliomas. Neuro Oncol 13: 1192–1201.

Kickingereder P, Dorn F, Blau T et al. (2013). Differentiation of local tumor recurrence from radiation-induced changes after stereotactic radiosurgery for treatment of brain metastasis: case report and review of the literature. Radiat Oncol 8: 52.

Kim YH, Oh SW, Lim YJ et al. (2010). Differentiating radiation necrosis from tumor recurrence in high-grade gliomas: assessing the efficacy of 18 F-FDG PET, 11C-methionine PET and perfusion MRI. Clin Neurol Neurosurg 112: 758–765.

Kim JW, Park CK, Park SH et al. (2011). Relationship between radiological characteristics and combined 1p and 19q deletion in World Health Organization grade III oligodendroglial tumours. J Neurol Neurosurg Psychiatry 82: 224–227.

Kim TW, Jung TY, Jung S et al. (2012). Unusual radiologic findings and pathologic growth patterns on choroid plexus papillomas. J Korean Neurosurg Soc 51: 272–275.

Klisch J, Juengling F, Spreer J et al. (2001). Lhermitte-Duclos disease: assessment with MR imaging, positron emission tomography, single-photon emission CT, and MR spectroscopy. AJNR Am J Neuroradiol 22: 824–830.

Koeller KK, Rushing EJ (2005). From the archives of the AFIP: Oligodendroglioma and its variants: radiologic-pathologic correlation. Radiographics 25: 1669–1688.

Krieger MD, Panigrahy A, McComb JG et al. (2005). Differentiation of choroid plexus tumors by advanced magnetic resonance spectroscopy. Neurosurg Focus 18.

Krueger DA, Care MM, Holland K et al. (2010). Everolimus for subependymal giant-cell astrocytomas in tuberous sclerosis. N Engl J Med 363: 1801–1811.

Krueger DA, Care MM, Agricola K et al. (2013). Everolimus long-term safety and efficacy in subependymal giant cell astrocytoma. Neurology 80: 574–580.

Lee IH, Kim ST, Kim HJ et al. (2010). Analysis of perfusion weighted image of CNS lymphoma. Eur J Radiol 76: 48–51.

Liao W, Liu Y, Wang X et al. (2009). Differentiation of primary central nervous system lymphoma and high-grade glioma with dynamic susceptibility contrast-enhanced perfusion magnetic resonance imaging. Acta Radiol 50: 217–225.

Louis DN, International Agency for Research on Cancer, World Health Organization (2007). WHO classification of tumours of the central nervous system. Lyon, International Agency for Research on Cancer.

Martinez-Martinez A, Martinez-Bosch J (2013). Perfusion magnetic resonance imaging for high grade astrocytomas: can cerebral blood volume, peak height, and percentage of signal intensity recovery distinguish between progression and pseudoprogression? Radiologia 56: 35–43.

Megyesi JF, Kachur E, Lee DH et al. (2004). Imaging correlates of molecular signatures in oligodendrogliomas. Clin Cancer Res 10: 4303–4306.

Meltzer CC, Smirniotopoulos JG, Jones RV (1995). The striated cerebellum: an MR imaging sign in Lhermitte-Duclos disease (dysplastic gangliocytoma). Radiology 194: 699–703.

Meyding-Lamade U, Forsting M, Albert F et al. (1993). Accelerated methaemoglobin formation: potential pitfall in early postoperative MRI. Neuroradiology 35: 178–180.

Moenninghoff C, Kraff O, Schlamann M et al. (2010). Assessing a dysplastic cerebellar gangliocytoma (Lhermitte-Duclos disease) with 7 T MR imaging. Korean J Radiol 11: 244–248.

Mullins ME, Barest GD, Schaefer PW et al. (2005). Radiation necrosis versus glioma recurrence: conventional MR imaging clues to diagnosis. AJNR Am J Neuroradiol 26: 1967–1972.

Naeini RM, Yoo JH, Hunter JV (2009). Spectrum of choroid plexus lesions in children. AJR Am J Roentgenol 192: 32–40.

Nakamura M, Saeki N, Iwadate Y et al. (2000). Neuroradiological characteristics of pineocytoma and pineoblastoma. Neuroradiology 42: 509–514.

Okamoto S, Shiga T, Hattori N et al. (2011). Semiquantitative analysis of C-11 methionine PET may distinguish brain tumor recurrence from radiation necrosis even in small lesions. Ann Nucl Med 25: 213–220.

Omuro A, DeAngelis LM (2013). Glioblastoma and other malignant gliomas: a clinical review. JAMA 310: 1842–1850.

Ozsunar Y, Mullins ME, Kwong K et al. (2010). Glioma recurrence versus radiation necrosis? A pilot comparison of arterial spin-labeled, dynamic susceptibility contrast enhanced MRI, and FDG-PET imaging. Acad Radiol 17: 282–290.

Petropoulou K, Whiteman ML, Altman NR et al. (1995). CT and MRI of pleomorphic xanthoastrocytoma: unusual biologic behavior. J Comput Assist Tomogr 19: 860–865.

Pope WB, Prins RM, Albert Thomas M et al. (2012). Non-invasive detection of 2-hydroxyglutarate and other metabolites in IDH1 mutant glioma patients using magnetic resonance spectroscopy. J Neurooncol 107: 197–205.

Shibata Y, Katayama W, Kawamura H et al. (2008). Proton magnetic resonance spectroscopy and 201Thallium-, 99mTechnetium methoxyisobutylisonitrile single photon emission computed tomography findings of a patient with choroid plexus papilloma. Neuroradiology 50: 741–742.

Shin JH, Lee HK, Khang SK et al. (2002). Neuronal tumors of the central nervous system: radiologic findings and pathologic correlation. Radiographics 22: 1177–1189.

Sie M, de Bont ES, Scherpen FJ et al. (2010). Tumour vasculature and angiogenic profile of paediatric pilocytic astrocytoma; is it much different from glioblastoma? Neuropathol Appl Neurobiol 36: 636–647.

Smirniotopoulos JG, Rushing EJ, Mena H (1992). Pineal region masses: differential diagnosis. Radiographics 12: 577–596.

Smith AB, Smirniotopoulos JG, Horkanyne-Szakaly I (2013). From the radiologic pathology archives: intraventricular neoplasms: radiologic-pathologic correlation. Radiographics 33: 21–43.

SongTao Q, Lei Y, Si G et al. (2012). IDH mutations predict longer survival and response to temozolomide in secondary glioblastoma. Cancer Sci 103: 269–273.

Stockhammer F, Misch M, Helms HJ et al. (2012). IDH1/2 mutations in WHO grade II astrocytomas associated with localization and seizure as the initial symptom. Seizure 21: 194–197.

Stupp R, Mason WP, van den Bent MJ et al. (2005). Radiotherapy plus concomitant and adjuvant temozolomide for glioblastoma. N Engl J Med 352: 987–996.

Taylor MD, Northcott PA, Korshunov A et al. (2012). Molecular subgroups of medulloblastoma: the current consensus. Acta Neuropathol 123: 465–472.

Thomas B, Krishnamoorthy T, Radhakrishnan VV et al. (2007). Advanced MR imaging in Lhermitte-Duclos disease: moving closer to pathology and pathophysiology. Neuroradiology 49: 733–738.

Tien RD, Cardenas CA, Rajagopalan S (1992). Pleomorphic xanthoastrocytoma of the brain: MR findings in six patients. AJR Am J Roentgenol 159: 1287–1290.

Valles FE, Perez-Valles CL, Regalado S et al. (2013). Combined diffusion and perfusion MR imaging as biomarkers of prognosis in immunocompetent patients with primary central nervous system lymphoma. AJNR Am J Neuroradiol 34: 35–40.

Wen PY, Macdonald DR, Reardon DA et al. (2010). Updated response assessment criteria for high-grade gliomas: response assessment in neuro-oncology working group. J Clin Oncol 28: 1963–1972.

Wilke M, Eidenschink A, Muller-Weihrich S et al. (2001). MR diffusion imaging and 1H spectroscopy in a child with medulloblastoma. A case report. Acta Radiol 42: 39–42.

Yan W, Zhang W, You G et al. (2012). Correlation of IDH1 mutation with clinicopathologic factors and prognosis in primary glioblastoma: a report of 118 patients from China. PLoS One 7, e30339.

Young RJ, Gupta A, Shah AD et al. (2011). Potential utility of conventional MRI signs in diagnosing pseudoprogression in glioblastoma. Neurology 76: 1918–1924.

Young RJ, Gupta A, Shah AD et al. (2013). MRI perfusion in determining pseudoprogression in patients with glioblastoma. Clin Imaging 37: 41–49.

Yu S, He L, Zhuang X et al. (2011). Pleomorphic xanthoastrocytoma: MR imaging findings in 19 patients. Acta Radiol 52: 223–228.

Yuh EL, Barkovich AJ, Gupta N (2009). Imaging of ependymomas: MRI and CT. Childs Nerv Syst 25: 1203–1213.

Zacharia TT, Law M, Naidich TP et al. (2008). Central nervous system lymphoma characterization by diffusion-weighted imaging and MR spectroscopy. J Neuroimaging 18: 411–417.

Zhang CB, Bao ZS, Wang HJ et al. (2014). Correlation of IDH1/2 mutation with clinicopathologic factors and prognosis in anaplastic gliomas: a report of 203 patients from China. J Cancer Res Clin Oncol 140: 45–51.

Handbook of Clinical Neurology, Vol. 135 (3rd series)
Neuroimaging, Part I
J.C. Masdeu and R.G. González, Editors

Chapter 15

Extra-axial brain tumors

OTTO RAPALINO[1]* AND JAMES G. SMIRNIOTOPOULOS[2]

[1]*Division of Neuroradiology, Department of Radiology, Massachusetts General Hospital, Boston, MA, USA*

[2]*Department of Radiology and Radiological Sciences, Uniformed Services University of the Health Sciences, Bethesda, MD, USA*

Abstract

Extra-axial brain tumors are the most common adult intracranial neoplasms and encompass a broad spectrum of pathologic subtypes. Meningiomas are the most common extra-axial brain tumor (approximately one-third of all intracranial neoplasms) and typically present as slowly growing dural-based masses. Benign meningiomas are very common, and may occasionally be difficult to differentiate from more aggressive subtypes (i.e., atypical or malignant varieties) or other dural-based masses with more aggressive biologic behavior (e.g., hemangiopericytoma or dural-based metastases). Many neoplasms that typically affect the brain parenchyma (intra-axial), such as gliomas, may also present with primary or secondary extra-axial involvement. This chapter provides a general and concise overview of the common types of extra-axial tumors and their typical imaging features.

INTRODUCTION

The category of extra-axial brain tumors includes a large number of varied pathologic tumors grouped by their primarily extraparenchymal involvement, typically involving the meningeal layers of the brain. Extra-axial tumors are responsible for approximately half of all intracranial neoplasms in the USA (Dolecek et al., 2012). Many of these extra-axial tumors may involve anatomic sites outside the central nervous system (CNS) with similar imaging characteristics. Some of these neoplasms may also secondarily invade the brain parenchyma (e.g., meningioma, craniopharyngioma, metastatic disease).

EPIDEMIOLOGY

Based on the most recent data from the Central Brain Tumor Registry of the United States (2005–2009) (Dolecek et al., 2012), approximately 35% of all intracranial neoplasms (with more than 7.49 cases per 100 000/year) are meningeal-based neoplasms (Table 15.1). Among these tumors, benign meningiomas represent approximately 35.5% of all intracranial neoplasms, followed next by glioblastomas (15.8%). Meningiomas also become more common with advancing age and they constitute the most common intracranial tumor in age groups older than 35 years (Dolecek et al., 2012). Tumors of the pituitary gland constitute 14.1% of all intracranial tumors (Dolecek et al., 2012). See Table 15.1 for further description of the current prevalence of different extra-axial tumors. Nerve sheath tumors are the most common extra-axial tumors during childhood (<14 years of age), constituting approximately 4.9% of all intracranial neoplasms (Dolecek et al., 2012). Craniopharyngiomas have a slightly lower prevalence in this age group (4.1%) (Dolecek et al., 2012). Overall, vestibular schwannomas constitute the most common nerve sheath tumors (65% of these tumors), with an incidence of 1.1 per 100 000/year, and are responsible for 5% of all intracranial neoplasms (Dolecek et al., 2012).

DIFFERENTIAL DIAGNOSIS OF EXTRA-AXIAL MASSES

The differential diagnosis of extra-axial intracranial masses varies depending on their location. The main neoplasms affecting the most common anatomic locations

*Correspondence to: Otto Rapalino, M.D., Department of Radiology, Massachusetts General Hospital, 55 Fruit Street, GRB 273A, Boston MA 02114-2696, USA. Tel: +1-617-726-8323, E-mail: orapalino@partners.org

Table 15.1

Epidemiology of extra-axial intracranial tumors

Pathology	Number of cases (2005–2009)	Proportion of all intracranial neoplasms	Annual age-adjusted incidence*
Meningioma	110 359	35.5%	7.22
Pituitary tumors	43 882	14.1%	2.94
Nerve sheath tumors	25 926	8.3%	1.70
Lymphoma†	6774	2.2%	0.45
Other meningeal neoplasms	2706	0.9	0.18
Craniopharyngioma	2680	0.9%	0.18
Extra-axial mesenchymal tumors	1192	0.4%	0.08
Other extra-axial hematopoietic neoplasms	182	0.1%	0.01

*Per 100 000 individuals/year.

†The Central Brain Tumor Registry of the United States report does not separate the prevalence of intra- and extra-axial involvement for these tumors (Dolecek et al., 2012).

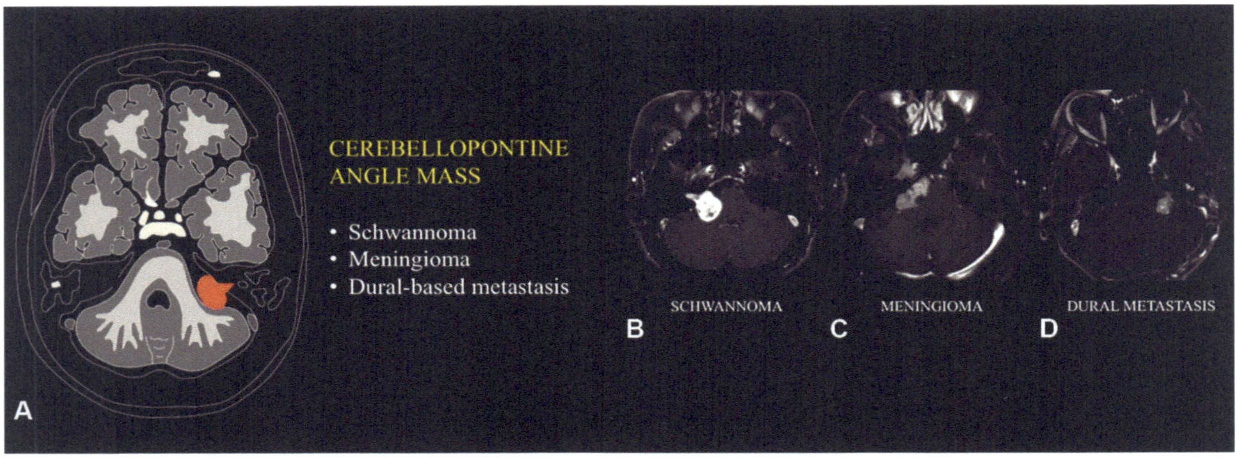

Fig. 15.1. (**A**) Differential diagnosis of cerebellopontine angle (CPA) masses. Gadolinium-enhanced axial T1-weighted images of a vestibular schwannoma (right CPA lesion extending into the right internal auditory canal (IAC) in **B**), (**C**) meningioma (also right CPA lesion but without IAC involvement), and (**D**) metastasis (relatively rare).

are summarized in Figures 15.1–15.5. The most frequent tumors involving the cerebellopontine angle cistern are schwannomas (typically arising from the vestibular nerves and extending into the internal auditory canals), followed by meningiomas or metastases (Fig. 15.1). Meningiomas, metastases, hemangiopericytomas, or dural-based lymphomas are responsible for most of the supratentorial extra-axial masses along the lateral cerebral convexities (Fig. 15.2). The differential diagnosis of pineal masses is broad, with pineal parenchymal tumors, germ cell tumors, and metastases being the most common neoplasms (Fig. 15.3). Intraventricular masses more often include ependymal and choroid plexus tumors, intraventricular meningiomas, central neurocytomas, or giant cell astrocytomas (Fig. 15.4). Some of these tumors have a neuroglial or neuronal histologic origin, commonly involve the brain parenchyma and are described in detail in the chapter dealing with intra-axial neoplasms. The most frequent sellar and suprasellar neoplasms are pituitary macroadenomas, meningiomas, and craniopharyngiomas (Fig. 15.5).

MENINGEAL TUMORS

Meningiomas

Meningiomas are the most common intracranial and dural-based neoplasms. They are twice as frequent in women (Rees and Wen, 2010; Dolecek et al., 2012) and show progressive increase in frequency with age. Radiation exposure is a well-characterized risk factor for development of meningiomas, and hormonal receptors (estrogen and progesterone) in these tumors likely contribute to their growth. Syndromes associated with an increased risk and prevalence of meningiomas, typically

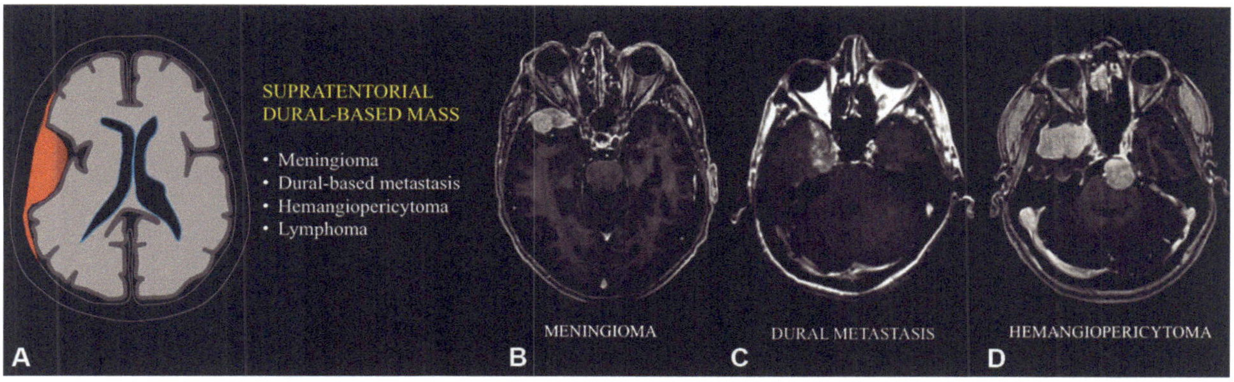

Fig. 15.2. (**A**) Differential diagnosis of supratentorial dural-based masses. (**B**) Gadolinium-enhanced axial T1-weighted images of a right middle cranial fossa meningioma, (**C**) dural metastasis, and (**D**) hemangiopericytoma (with multifocal involvement of the right middle cranial fossa and left prepontine cistern).

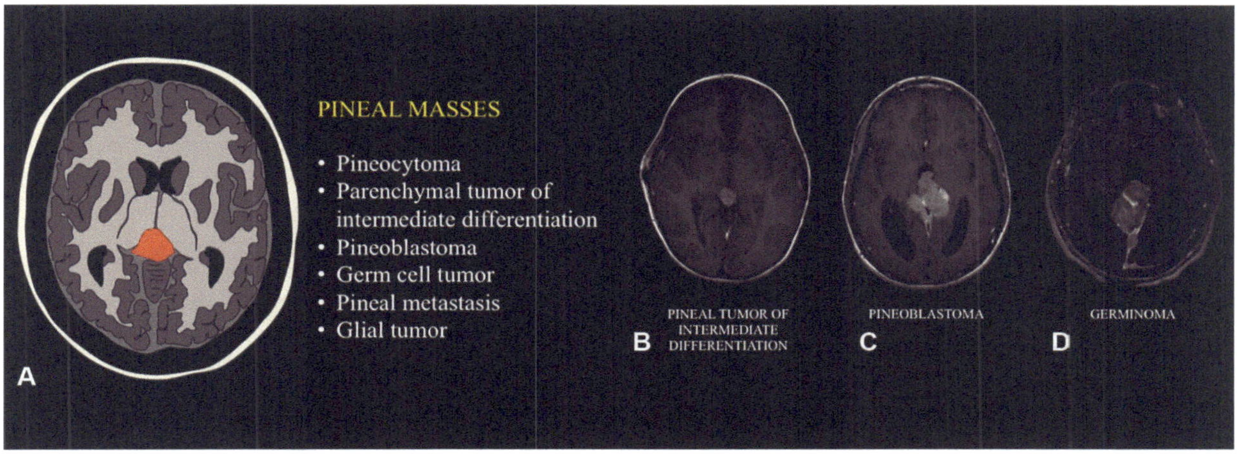

Fig. 15.3. (**A**) Differential diagnosis of pineal masses. (**B**) Gadolinium-enhanced axial T1-weighted images of a pineal tumor of intermediate differentiation, (**C**) pineoblastoma, and (**D**) germinoma. Pineoblastomas are often quite large at the time of diagnosis.

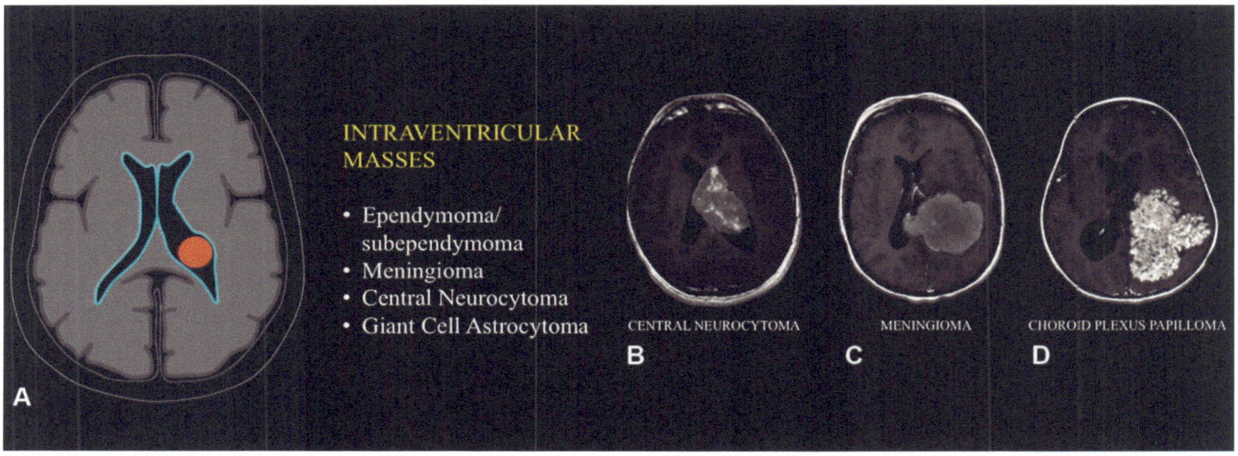

Fig. 15.4. (**A**) Differential diagnosis of intraventricular masses. (**B**) Gadolinium-enhanced axial T1-weighted images of a central neurocytoma, (**C**) meningioma, and (**D**) choroid plexus papilloma.

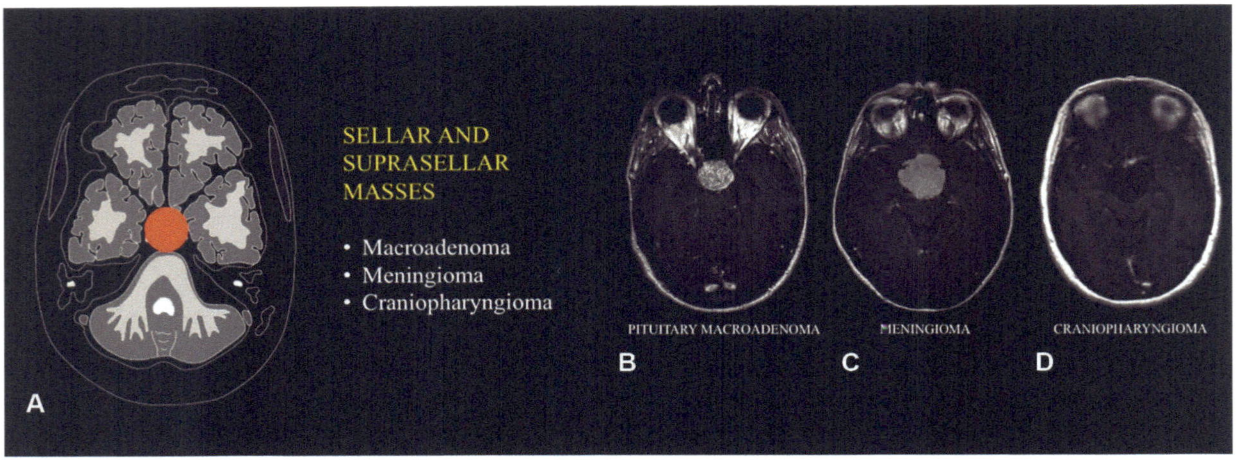

Fig. 15.5. (**A**) Differential diagnosis of sellar/suprasellar masses. (**B**) Gadolinium-enhanced axial T1-weighted images of a pituitary macroadenoma (sellar/suprasellar heterogeneously enhancing mass), (**C**) meningioma (homogeneously enhancing suprasellar mass), and (**D**) craniopharyngioma (large predominantly cystic suprasellar lesion).

presenting with multiple lesions, include neurofibromatosis type II, Gorlin syndrome, Cowden syndrome, and multiple endocrine neoplasia type 1 (MEN1), among other genetic conditions (Mawrin and Perry, 2010; Plotkin et al., 2013).

PATHOLOGIC SUBTYPES

Meningiomas originate from the arachnoidal cap cells in the arachnoid layer and they are currently subdivided into at least 16 neuropathologic subtypes (Louis et al., 2007; Mawrin and Perry, 2010) (Table 15.2). The vast majority, roughly 90%, are World Health Organization (WHO) grade I neoplasms. Based on their biologic behavior, these subtypes can be clustered into three different WHO grades (Table 15.2).

Table 15.2

Neuropathologic subtypes of meningiomas and World Health Organization (WHO) grading (based on WHO 2007 classification) (Louis et al., 2007; Alahmadi and Croul, 2011)

	WHO grading		
Neuropathologic subtype	I	II	III
Meningothelial	x		
Fibrous (fibroblastic)	x		
Transitional (mixed)	x		
Psammomatous	x		
Angiomatous	x		
Microcystic	x		
Secretory	x		
Lymphoplasmacyte-rich	x		
Metaplastic	x		
Chordoid		x	
Clear-cell		x	
Atypical		x	
Papillary			x
Rhabdoid			x
Anaplastic (malignant)			x

IMAGING FEATURES

Meningiomas typically present as homogeneously enhancing dural-based masses, often exhibiting smooth tapering extensions along the adjacent dura mater ("dural tails") (Figs 15.6 and 15.7). The most common locations for meningiomas include the cerebral convexity (up to 34% of cases), parafalcine region, sphenoid wings, parasellar compartment, posterior fossa (including the tentorium), and the olfactory groove (Drevelegas, 2005; Rockhill et al., 2007; Kaizer, 2010). On plain radiographs and computed tomography (CT) studies, meningiomas often demonstrate hyperostosis of the underlying adjacent bone (18–50% of benign cases) and intratumoral calcifications (up to 25–27% of meningiomas) (Drevelegas, 2005; Rockhill et al., 2007) (Fig. 15.6). Focal osteolysis is unusual and only seen in less than 3% of meningiomas (Drevelegas, 2005). Most meningiomas appear as well-defined hemispheric or lobulated masses with increased attenuation on plain CT images. On magnetic resonance imaging (MRI), meningiomas show avid homogeneous gadolinium enhancement, and are T1 iso- to mildy hypointense and T2 iso- to mildly hyperintense (in relation to gray matter) (Drevelegas, 2005). The presence of cerebrospinal fluid (CSF) clefts (crescentic between tumor and brain), white-matter buckling, or a signal void pseudocapsule (between tumor and brain) is very helpful in confirming an extra-axial location (Drevelegas, 2005). Gradient echo (T2*) sequences demonstrate the presence of

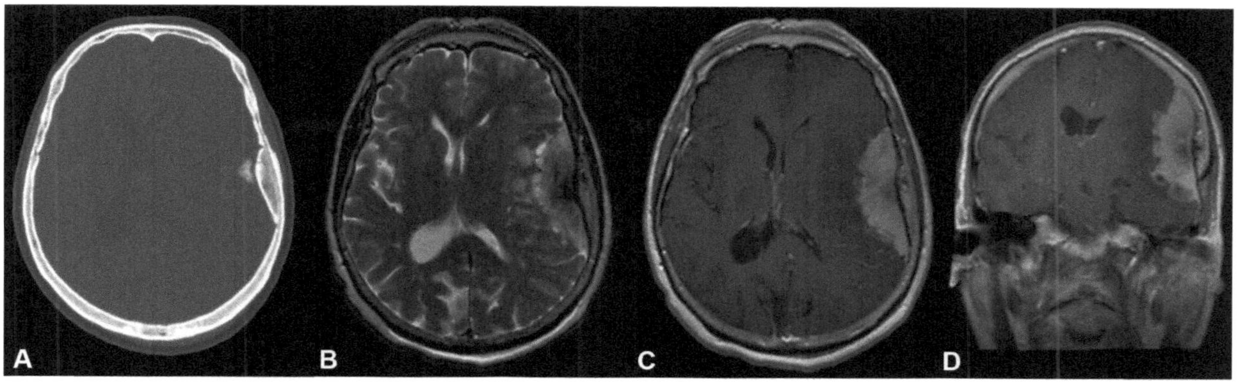

Fig. 15.6. Meningioma (World Health Organization grade I): angiomatous variant. (**A**) Axial computed tomography – bone window, (**B**) axial T2-weighted, (**C**) gadolinium-enhanced T1-weighted axial, and (**D**) coronal images. There is a dural-based mass in the left frontotemporal region with adjacent prominent hyperostosis, compatible with a meningioma (subclassified as an angiomatous meningioma after histopathologic analysis). Small dural tails are best seen along the inferior margin of the lesion on coronal images.

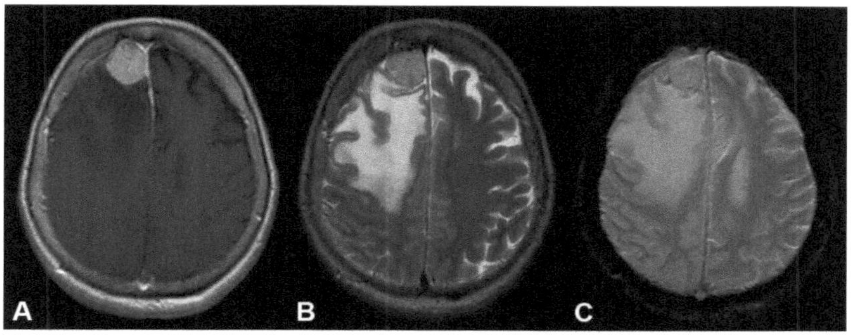

Fig. 15.7. Meningioma (World Health Organization grade I): secretory variant. (**A**) Gadolinium-enhanced axial T1-weighted; (**B**) axial T2-weighted and (**C**) axial gradient echo images. Dural-based mass in the right anterior frontal/parafalcine region without significant mineralization but associated with prominent vasogenic edema in the right cerebral hemisphere.

intratumoral foci of susceptibility artifact compatible with mineralization and/or intratumoral vascularity. Dural tails are seen in approximately 60% of meningiomas (Drevelegas, 2005; Rockhill et al., 2007). The correlation between direct dural invasion around the meningioma and the presence of dural tails is controversial and some authors have attributed the presence of dural tails to reactive dural thickening, dural hyperemia, and/or tumoral invasion (Drevelegas, 2005; Rokni-Yazdi et al., 2009; Sotoudeh and Yazdi, 2010). The extent of parenchymal vasogenic edema, irregular contour, and local osteolysis may be helpful for the differentiation between benign and atypical/malignant meningiomas (Chernov et al., 2010) (Fig. 15.8). The role of diffusion-weighted imaging in the identification of atypical and malignant subtypes is very controversial, with some reports showing no significant difference, while other reports suggest lower apparent diffusion coefficient values in these subtypes (Toh et al., 2008; Santelli et al., 2010; Sanverdi et al., 2012; Yin et al., 2012; Watanabe et al., 2013) (Fig. 15.8).

Meningiomas are highly vascular tumors with intense intratumoral blushes on conventional cerebral angiography and markedly elevated relative cerebral blood volume (rCBV)/cerebral blood flow values in dynamic susceptibility contrast and arterial spin labeling MR perfusion (Kimura et al., 2006) (Fig. 15.8). Intratumoral rCBV values within angiomatous meningiomas and in the surrounding brain parenchyma around anaplastic meningiomas appear to be statistically higher than with other subtypes (Zhang et al., 2008a, b) (Fig. 15.8). MR spectroscopy can be helpful in the distinction of meningiomas from other extra-axial or dural-based masses due to the presence of alanine peaks in well-differentiated tumors (Demir et al., 2006). MR spectroscopy has no role in the differentiation between benign and aggressive meningiomas (Demir et al., 2006; Zhang et al., 2008a; Chernov et al., 2010).

Meningiomas are considered "en plaque" when they appear as broad elongated flattened lesions infiltrating the dura and inner table of the skull, often associated with local hyperostosis (Kim et al., 1987; Drevelegas, 2005).

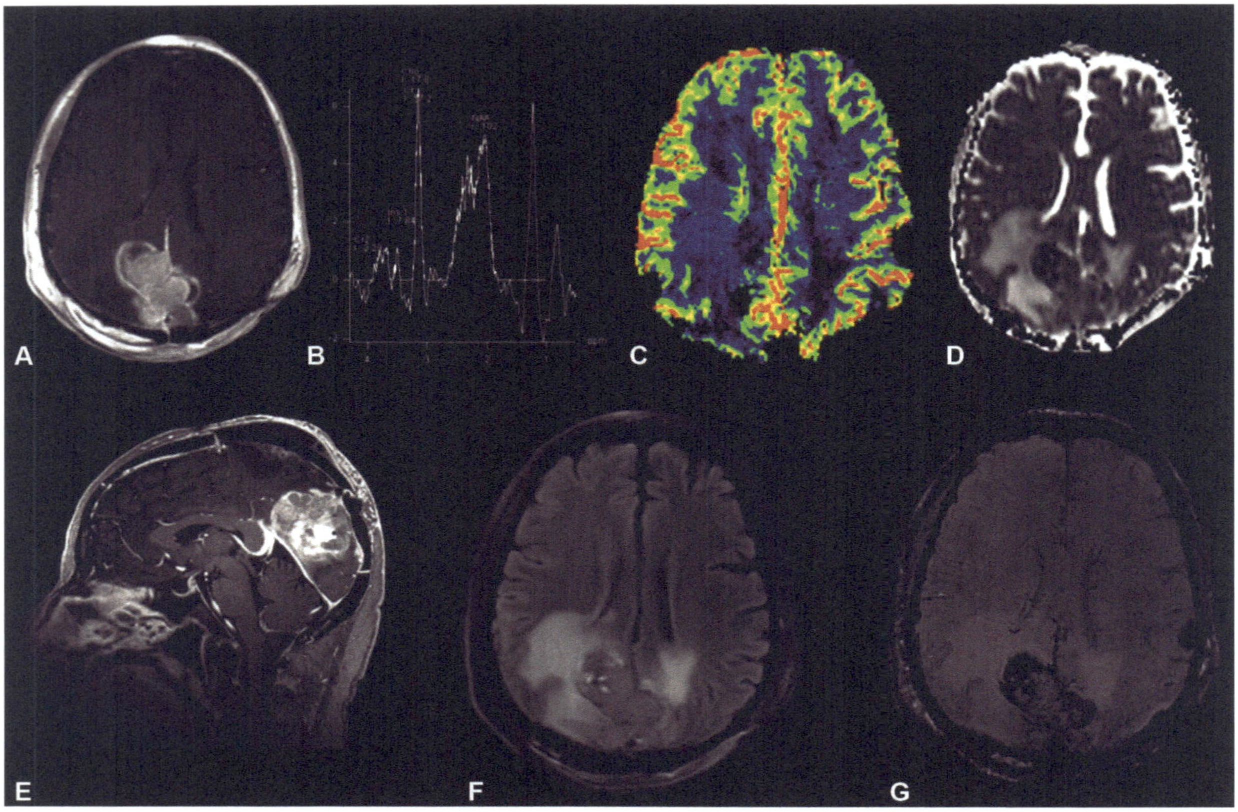

Fig. 15.8. Malignant meningioma (World Health Organization grade III). (**A**) Gadolinium-enhanced axial and (**E**) sagittal T1-weighted images; (**B**) magnetic resonance (MR) spectroscopy, (**C**) relative cerebral blood volume (rCBV) map, (**D**) apparent diffusion coefficient (ADC) map, (**F**) axial fluid-attenuated inversion recovery, and (**G**) axial susceptibility-weighted imaging sequences. These images demonstrate a large heterogeneously enhancing and rapidly growing recurrent meningioma centered on the posterior falx cerebri with foci of central necrosis, invading the adjacent superior sagittal sinus and producing significant vasogenic edema in the adjacent brain parenchyma. The mass also demonstrated internal foci of increased rCBV and low ADC values. MR spectroscopy shows significant decrease of *N*-acetyl aspartate/creatine ratio and prominent lipid peaks (although no definite alanine peak was identified). Pathology was consistent with a malignant meningioma.

Intradiploic or intraosseous meningiomas are rare meningiomas that develop within the diploic space of the skull, often expanding the diploic space and infiltrating the pericranial spaces (Arana et al., 1996; Changhong et al., 1997). Secondary osseous involvement is also seen commonly with meningiomas (up to 26% of cases) (Gasparetto et al., 2007). Involved bone should be resected to prevent recurrence. Hyperostosis may occur with or without bone involvement. Meningiomas often exhibit prominent intra-axial vasogenic edema in the surrounding brain parenchyma (up to 90% of cases) (Gasparetto et al., 2007), that appears to correlate with intratumoral vasculature (Pistolesi et al., 2003; Schmid et al., 2010) and also with a close apposition of the tumor to brain parenchyma. More extensive areas of peritumoral vasogenic edema have been described with meningothelial (Ide et al., 1994; Tamiya et al., 2001) and other uncommon subtypes (including angiomatous, microcystic, lymphoplasmacyte-rich, and secretory meningiomas (Tamiya et al., 2001; Paek et al., 2005; Osawa et al., 2013), as well as with tumors with higher proliferation indexes (Osawa et al., 2013) (Fig. 15.7).

Additional features described with meningiomas include the presence of cystic changes within (intratumoral) and around these tumors ("acquired arachnoid cyst") (Demir et al., 2007; Zhang et al., 2009), metaplasia with intratumoral fat (Sacher et al., 1985; Okamoto et al., 1996), and intracranial hemorrhage (Latchaw et al., 1981).

Mesenchymal nonmeningothelial tumors

This category includes a broad spectrum of mesenchymal pathologies, ranging from fat-containing tumors, chondroid or osseous-matrix tumors, to highly vascularized dural-based mesenchymal tumors with variable biologic behavior and aggressiveness. Hemangiopericytoma is the most common mesenchymal nonmeningothelial tumor. Sarcomas represent less than 0.1–0.2% of intracranial neoplasms (Louis et al., 2007) and can occur intracranially as a delayed sequela of craniofacial irradiation (particularly fibrosarcoma, malignant fibrous histiocytoma, chondrosarcoma, and osteosarcoma) (Louis et al., 2007). Primary sarcomas are rare and most of the intracranial sarcomas are secondary to metastatic CNS involvement (Al-Gahtany et al., 2003).

FAT-CONTAINING TUMORS

These tumors represent approximately 0.4% of intracranial neoplasms and include lipomas (Fig. 15.9), osteolipomas, angiolipomas, hibernomas, complex lipomatous lesions, epidural lipomatosis, and intracranial liposarcoma. Fat-containing tumors are, in general, benign (except for the rare intracranial liposarcoma) (Jabot et al., 2009). Osteolipomas are characteristically seen in the tuber cinereum region (Bognar et al., 2002; Moschopulos et al., 2006; Louis et al., 2007).

HEMANGIOPERICYTOMA

Hemangiopericytoma is classically described as a highly cellular and vascularized neoplasm, almost always dural-based, with a high recurrence/metastatic rate and variable pathologic grading (WHO II or III) (Uttley et al., 1995; Louis et al., 2007; Sibtain et al., 2007) (Fig. 15.10). There is recent debate regarding the origin of these tumors, and many soft-tissue pathologists call them "solitary fibrous tumors," while neuropathologists retain the nosology of hemangiopericytoma (Penel et al., 2012). These tumors are uncommon (when compared to meningiomas) and represent approximately 0.4% of all primary intracranial tumors (Chiechi et al., 1996; Louis et al., 2007). Primary hemangiopericytomas commonly present as a solitary dural-based mass, more frequently in the occipital region near the sinus confluence (Louis et al., 2007) and typically without calcifications (Osborne et al., 1981; Akiyama et al., 2004) (Fig. 15.10). On CT studies, the presence of focal osteolysis of the adjacent bone (instead of hyperostosis) may be suggestive of hemangiopericytoma (Ruscalleda et al., 1994;

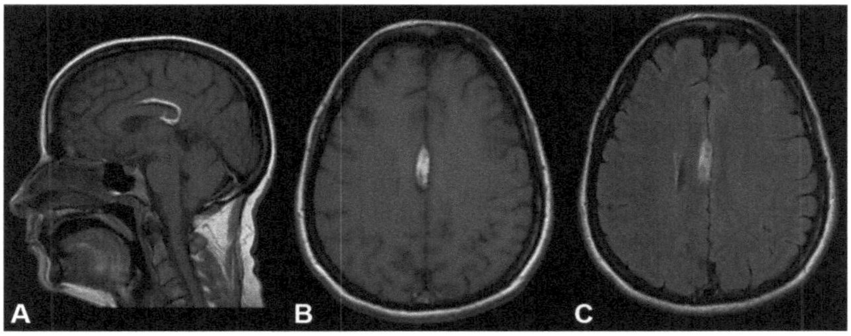

Fig. 15.9. Intracranial lipoma. (**A**) Sagittal T1-weighted, (**B**) axial T1-weighted, and (**C**) axial fluid-attenuated inversion recovery images without intravenous contrast. There is an intrinsically T1/T2 hyperintense abnormality partially surrounding the posterior corpus callosum, compatible with a lipoma.

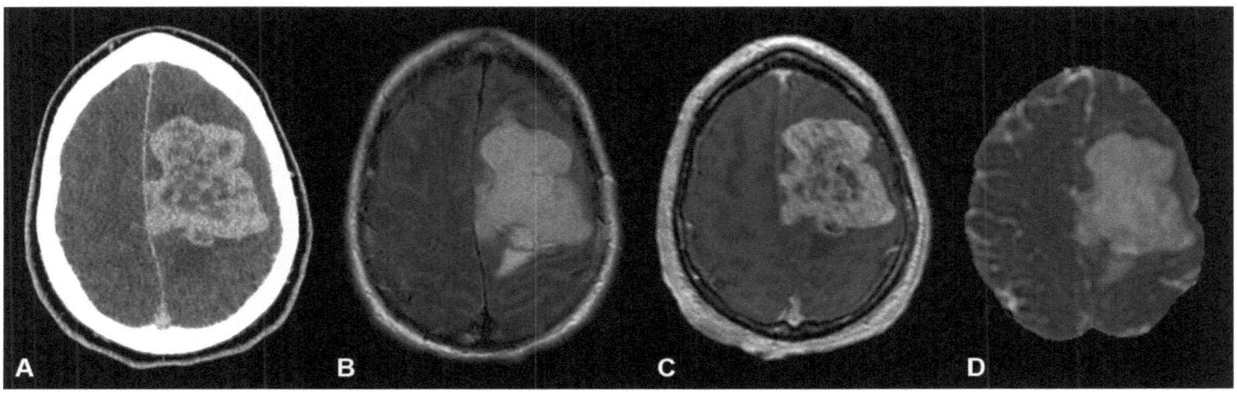

Fig. 15.10. Hemangiopericytoma. (**A**) Axial contrast-enhanced computed tomography, (**B**) axial fluid-attenuated inversion recovery , (**C**) axial gadolinium-enhanced T1-weighted and (**D**) axial apparent diffusion coefficient images. Heterogeneously enhancing noncalcified dural-based mass in the left posterior frontal region was pathologically confirmed as a hemangiopericytoma.

Chiechi et al., 1996; Tayoro et al., 2002). Angiographic studies depict the marked vascularity of these tumors, occasionally with intratumoral "corkscrew-like" vessels (Akiyama et al., 2004).

OSTEOCARTILAGINOUS TUMORS

Most commonly, these tumors arise from the skull base osseous structures – especially the synchondroses – and extend intracranially, often involving the adjacent dura. They include chondrosarcoma and osteosarcoma.

VASCULAR TUMORS

The most common intracranial vascular tumors include benign hemangiomas (subdivided into capillary and cavernous, involving the skull and/or dura) (Perry et al., 1993; Ito et al., 2009; Joshi et al., 2009; Patnaik et al., 2012), hemangioendothelioma (intermediate grade) (Parajon and Vaquero, 2008), and more malignant subtypes, particularly angiosarcoma (Choi et al., 2008) and Kaposi sarcoma (Louis et al., 2007; Pantanowitz and Dezube, 2008). Intracranial involvement by these tumors is, in general, very rare.

OTHER MESENCHYMAL TUMORS

Meningeal sarcomatosis and Ewing sarcoma-peripheral primitive neuroectodermal tumor (EWS-pPNET) are included in this group. Both pathologies are very rare and present as diffuse leptomeningeal involvement (in the case of leptomeningeal sarcomatosis) (Grier and Yachnis, 2004; Uluc et al., 2004) and as a focal dural-based mass (for EWS-pPNET) (Antunes et al., 2001).

CHORDOMA

Chordoma appears to originate from notochordal remnants and is considered to have low-to-intermediate biologic aggressiveness (Gangadhar and Santhosh, 2012), although systemic hematogenous metastases may occur in more aggressive lesions. This tumor most commonly presents as an extra-axial and extradural lobulated, locally infiltrating and destructive mass in the sacrococcygeal (up to 60% of cases) and skull base (up to 40%) regions (Gangadhar and Santhosh, 2012) (Fig. 15.11). Rarely, chordoma can also present as a primarily intradural extra-axial mass (Roberti et al., 2007). CT may be the study of choice to demonstrate the osteolytic changes and presence of internal calcifications (Erdem et al., 2003). However, MRI is more sensitive for detection of tumoral invasion and extension into the adjacent soft tissues and intracranial spaces. The tumor is composed of physaliferous (having bubbles or vacuoles) cells with intracytoplasmic fluid, making them typically T2 hyperintense/T1 hypointense with variable enhancement (Erdem et al., 2003) (Fig. 15.11). Some chordomas can exhibit internal foci of T1 hyperintensity from the physaliferous cells that are characteristic of this neoplasm (Bonneville et al., 2006). Steady-state sequences such as CISS/FIESTA sequences are very helpful for better evaluation of intracranial extension. Previous studies have suggested that clival chordomas often originate more centrally while chondrosarcomas involving the skull base are more lateral, and most commonly develop near the petroclival fissure and foramen lacerum (Weber et al., 1994; Chapman et al., 2011). However, other studies have concluded that there are no specific imaging features that could help with their accurate diagnosis and there is significant anatomic overlap between these two skull base tumors (Pamir and Ozduman, 2006).

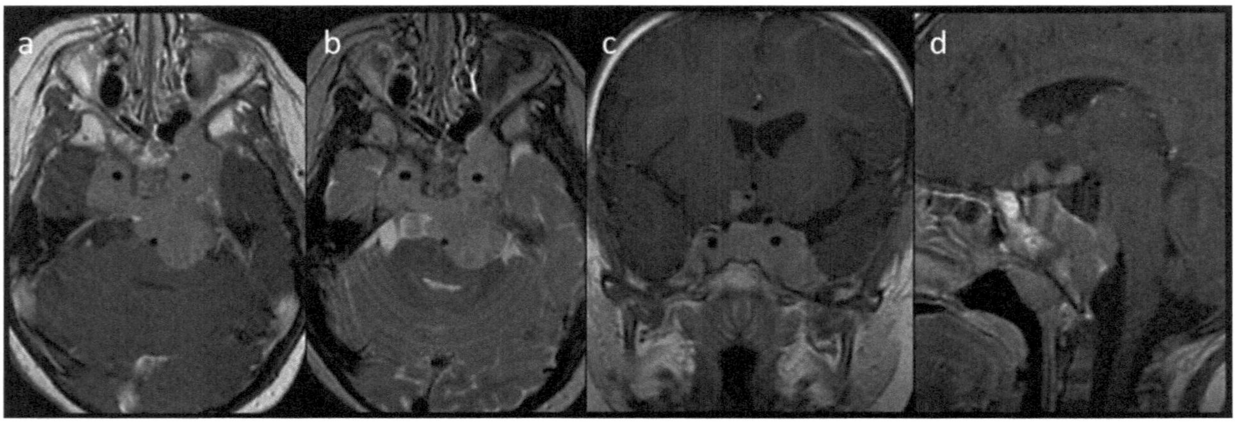

Fig. 15.11. Chordoma. (**A**) Gadolinium-enhanced axial, (**C**) coronal, and (**D**) sagittal T1-weighted images, as well as (**B**) axial T2-weighted image. Large irregular and infiltrative central skull base mass extending to the cavernous sinuses, medial aspects of the middle cranial fossa, and prepontine cistern. Biopsy confirmed the clinical diagnosis of chordoma.

TUMORS OF THE CRANIAL NERVES

Schwannomas

These are benign encapsulated neoplasms arising from Schwann cells that surround the peripheral portions of the cranial and spinal nerves. Schwannomas are the second most common extra-axial intracranial tumor and constitute approximately 8% of intracranial neoplasms (Drevelegas, 2005; Louis et al., 2007). These tumors are well-defined, typically encapsulated, tumors (Drevelegas, 2005) (Fig. 15.12) that may often be dissected free from the parent nerve. There are two histologic components: Dense Antoni A and looser Antoni B tissue patterns. Schwannomas most commonly affect the inferior vestibular division of the eighth nerve and, less often, the fifth cranial nerve (Fig. 15.12). Because they grow slowly, secondary arachnoid cysts are often seen around large tumors. In addition, intratumoral benign cystic degeneration may occur in larger tumors. Signal intensity varies depending on the relative proportions of tissue, with the predominantly Antoni type A lesions appearing more homogeneous and hypointense of T2-weighted images, while those with more Antoni B tissue are T2 hyperintense and are more heterogeneous, often with internal foci of cystic change or hemorrhage (Drevelegas, 2005). Schwannomas, particularly in the cerebellopontine-angle cistern region, often have associated arachnoid cysts. Dural tails are also occasionally seen with schwannomas, and they are the second most common tumor to show this feature, after meningiomas. The presence of calcifications within the tumor is rare and statistically argues against the diagnosis of schwannoma (Drevelegas, 2005).

Neurofibromas

These WHO grade I neoplasms typically involve the spine and, sporadically, skull base in patients with neurofibromatosis type 1, but they only rarely arise intracranially from cranial nerves (Rodriguez and Berthrong, 1966; Drevelegas, 2005).

LYMPHOMAS AND HEMATOPOIETIC NEOPLASMS

Lymphoma

Primary CNS lymphomas (PCNSLs) are defined as extranodal lymphomas involving CNS structures without evidence of extension outside the CNS (different from the secondary CNS involvement seen in cases of peripheral lymphoma). Most of the PCNSLs are classified as diffuse large B-cell lymphomas. PCNSLs involving immunocompetent individuals are more frequent in older male patients but are seen in younger immunocompromised individuals (e.g., posttransplant, acquired immunodeficiency syndrome (AIDS), inherited immunodeficiencies) (Louis et al., 2007). PCNSL presents more commonly with intraparenchymal involvement, often as an ill-defined hyperdense mass on CT (due to high cell density and high nuclear-to-cytoplasm ratio) involving the subependymal and periventricular regions or corpus callosum. Meningeal involvement by primary CNS lymphoma is occasionally seen (up to 30–40% of cases) (Louis et al., 2007). Primary dural involvement is very unusual and pathologically is usually classified as low-grade marginal-zone B-cell type (Mneimneh et al., 2013). Dural-based lymphoma typically presents as a homogeneously enhancing dural-based mass with abnormal restricted diffusion, somewhat similar to a meningioma (Iwamoto and Abrey, 2006; Kulkarni et al., 2012; Tandon et al., 2012) (Fig. 15.13). There have been also reports of dural lymphoma confused with epidural hematomas (Iaccarino et al., 2013). Steroid treatment has a dramatic effect in these cases and lesions can disappear very rapidly after treatment (Louis et al., 2007). For this reason, they are often called "ghost tumors."

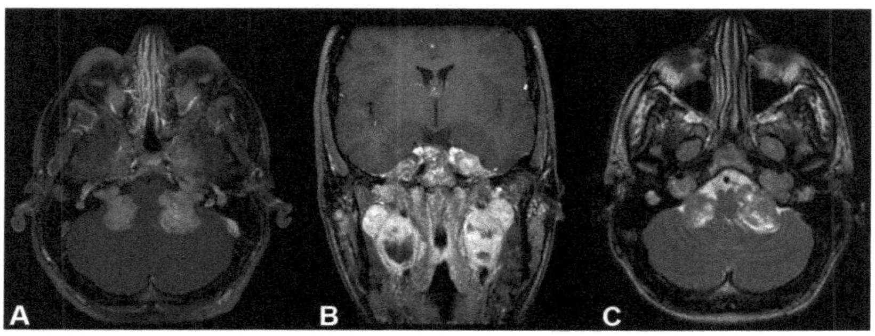

Fig. 15.12. Bilateral schwannomas. (**A**) Gadolinium-enhanced axial and (**B**) coronal T1-weighted images; (**C**) axial T2-weighted image. Multiple large bilateral enhancement masses along the trajectories of multiple cranial nerves in a patient with neurofibromatosis type II, compatible with schwannomas.

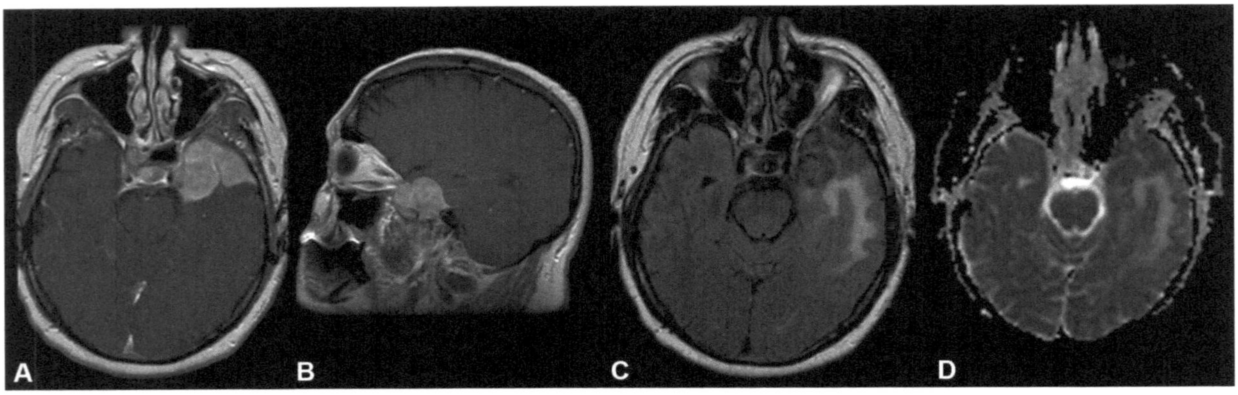

Fig. 15.13. Dural lymphoma. (**A**) Gadolinium-enhanced axial and (**B**) sagittal T1-weighted; (**C**) axial fluid-attenuated inversion recovery (FLAIR) and (**D**) axial apparent diffusion coefficient (ADC) images. There is a large dural-based mass in the left middle cranial fossa with abnormal restricted diffusion and adjacent parenchymal T2 hyperintensities. The mass demonstrates low ADC values, potentially helpful in their differentiation from other extra-axial masses.

Plasmacytomas

These tumors can develop in patients with multiple myeloma as intra- or extraosseous lesions and rarely involve the CNS (Cerase et al., 2008). Plasmacytomas can present as an intraosseous masses involving the central skull base with secondary intracranial involvement or as a dural-based mass in cases of solitary intracranial plasmacytomas (Cerase et al., 2008; Cao et al., 2010). Most of the solitary intracranial plasmacytomas occur in older patients (fifth and sixth decades) and are iso- to hyperdense on CT (Cerase et al., 2008; Cao et al., 2010). They show nonspecific MRI findings, variable T1/T2 signal, variable enhancement, and abnormal restricted diffusion (Cerase et al., 2008; Cao et al., 2010). Their imaging features can very similar to other intracranial pathologies, such as meningiomas, lymphomas, metastases, and nonneoplastic processes (Cerase et al., 2008).

Myeloid sarcoma

Previously called chloroma or granulocytic sarcoma, this is a rare tumor composed of immature granulocytic cells and seen in patients with acute myeloid leukemia (or other myeloproliferative disorders) that can involve intracranial structures in 2–3% of cases (Hakyemez et al., 2007; Grier et al., 2008). The intracranial cases more often present as dural-based masses and are considered to originate from the bone marrow in the skull, extending intracranially (Hakyemez et al., 2007). Differentiation from lymphoma can be difficult, even in histologic analysis (Hakyemez et al., 2007; Grier et al., 2008). Myeloid sarcomas are typically iso- to hypointense in T1- and T2-weighted images, with homogeneous enhancement and often with abnormal restricted diffusivity (Hakyemez et al., 2007).

GERM CELL TUMORS

Germinomas (formerly called "atypical teratoma," and identical to testicular seminoma and ovarian dysgerminoma) are rare tumors, probably arising from totipotential germ cells. These tumors constitute less than 3% of all primary intracranial neoplasms and usually present in or the near the midline, in children or young adults (Takeshima et al., 2012; Wang et al., 2010). These neoplasms can be extra- or intra-axial and often involve the suprasellar and pineal regions (Wang et al., 2010). Germinomas often demonstrate secondary leptomeningeal dissemination following the CSF pathways (up to 10% of cases) but rarely can also disseminate as primarily dural-based lesions (Takeshima et al., 2012). Teratomas, which also arise from pluripotent cells, more often present as midline lesions, often located in the pineal and suprasellar regions (Fig. 15.14). Teratomas may show heterogeneous components, including sebaceous lipid, watery fluid, and solid enhancing tissues.

Germ cell tumors are subdivided in several histopathologic subtypes, including germinoma, teratoma, mature teratoma, yolk sac tumor, embryonal carcinoma, and choriocarcinoma (Louis et al., 2007).

The CT and MR features of germ cell tumors are predominantly nonspecific, particularly with extra-axial involvement. Nonteratomatous germ cell tumors often are T1/T2 iso- to hypointense and show homogeneous enhancement (Wang et al., 2010). Because germinomas are typically hypercellular and often contain a lymphocytic component (probably reactive), they may be homogeneously hyperattenuating on plain CT and have restricted diffusivity on MRI (Ogiwara et al., 2015). These can be very useful differentiating imaging features. Calcification and necrosis can be seen occasionally (Wang et al., 2010). Teratomas classically

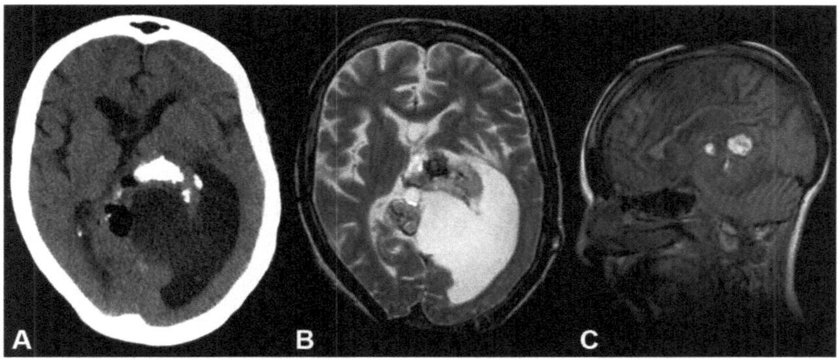

Fig. 15.14. Teratoma. (**A**) Axial computed tomography, (**B**) axial T2-weighted, and (**C**) sagittal noncontrast T1-weighted images demonstrate a large partially calcified and cystic mass centered on the left posterior aspect of the third ventricle and pineal region. The mass also shows internal foci of fat attenuation, compatible with a teratoma (confirmed by pathology).

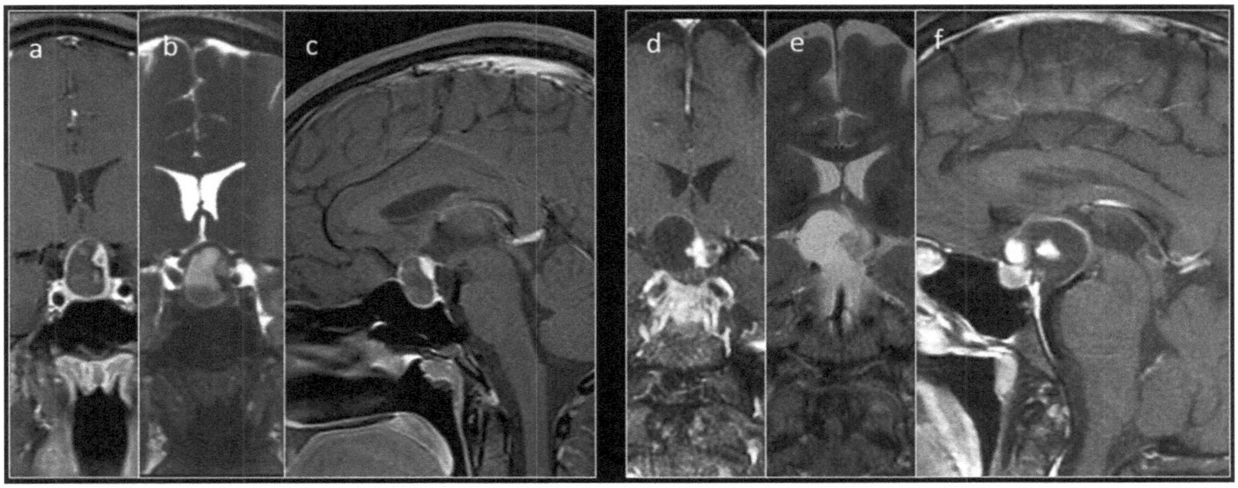

Fig. 15.15. Craniopharyngioma: (**A–C**) adamantinomatous and papillary (**D–F**) variants. Gadolinium-enhanced coronal (**A, D**) and sagittal (**C, F**) T1-weighted images, coronal T2-weighted images (**B, E**). Partially cystic and heterogeneously enhancing masses in the sellar and suprasellar regions, with internal nodularity within the cystic components, compatible with craniopharyngiomas. Papillary type (**D–F**) shows slightly more prominent solid components and T1 hypointense cystic components.

present as mixed lesions with cystic, calcified, and fatty components (Fig. 15.14). Neoplasms with chorocarcinomatous or syncitiotrophoblastic components often show intratumoral hemorrhage (Louis et al., 2007) that will cause T1 shortening. Leptomeningeal and dural metastases of germ cell tumors are difficult to differentiate from other neoplastic conditions.

TUMORS OF THE SELLAR REGION

Craniopharyngioma

These are intracranial cystic tumors that are considered benign (WHO grade I), typically suprasellar in location, and may be derived from Rathke's pouch remnants. They represent up to 4.6% of all intracranial tumors (5–10% in children) (Louis et al., 2007). Craniopharyngiomas demonstrate a bimodal distribution with two age peaks: one during the first and second decades and a second during the fourth and fifth decades. Despite their benign pathologic designation, craniopharyngiomas often recur locally because of adherence to surrounding brain and depending on the extent of surgical resection. There are two histopathologic subtypes: adamantinomatous (mostly younger patients) and papillary craniopharyngiomas (mostly older patients).

Adamantinomatous craniopharyngiomas are typically mixed cystic and solid masses with internal or ring calcifications and occasional hemorrhagic foci (Fig. 15.15A–C). Papillary craniopharyngiomas are more solid and intratumoral calcifications are seen less frequently but may be present in this subtype (Fig. 15.15D–F). Most of the papillary subtype cases have been reported in adults. Vascular encasement, lobulated contour, and

T1 hyperintense cysts are more often seen with the adamantinomatous subtype, while hypointense cysts and a predominantly solid appearance are more commonly seen with the papillary tumors (Sartoretti-Schefer et al., 1997) (Fig. 15.15).

Pituitary adenomas

Pituitary adenomas represent the most frequent intrasellar masses and are typically classified based on their size into micro- and macroadenomas (< or > 10 mm respectively). The vast majority of pituitary adenomas are considered functional (up to 75%) (Kumar et al., 2007), and, the most common functional subtype are the prolactin-secreting adenomas. Adenomas can manifest clinically due to endocrinologic disturbances (which vary by hormone production) or due to local mass effect (usually with visual disturbance due to chiasmatic compression or other cranial nerve palsies). Microadenomas may appear as areas of relatively decreased enhancement within the pituitary gland during early postcontrast images (dynamic scanning), often hypointense on precontrast T1-weighted images (Kumar et al., 2007). Macroadenomas, by definition, will expand the sella and/or extend into the suprasellar cistern. They often appear as T1 isointense, T2 hyperintense, with heterogeneous enhancement, and often exhibit intralesional necrotic/cystic changes (in up to 18% of macroadenomas) (Kumar et al., 2007) (Fig. 15.16). Macroadenomas frequently show intratumoral hemorrhage (up to 30% of cases) with fluid levels. Absence of vascular narrowing of the adjacent cavernous internal carotid arteries is a frequently described sign favoring a macroadenoma (Fig. 15.16).

Rathke's cleft cysts

These cystic lesions are also originated from remnants of the Rathke's pouch and are more commonly intrasellar, located at the level of the pars intermedia (but can also be occasionally present along the infundibular stalk and suprasellar region). Their T1 and T2-weighted MR appearance is variable and depends on the amount of intracystic debris/proteinaceous content. Mild peripheral enhancement can be present and intracystic nodules have been reported in the literature as a useful imaging finding to differentiate them from other cystic pathologies (Binning et al., 2005).

METASTATIC EXTRA-AXIAL TUMORS

Dural metastases develop by direct/contiguous extension or via hematogenous seeding. Pelvic malignancies may disseminate via the Batson retrovertebral plexus, which communicates intracranially with the retroclival veins. The most prevalent primary neoplasms presenting as dural-based masses in adults include breast cancer, prostate cancer (Fig. 15.17), lung adenocarcinoma, renal cell carcinoma, and multiple myeloma (Maroldi et al., 2005). For children, neuroblastoma and sarcoma represent the most common tumors presenting as dural-based metastases. Leptomeningeal metastases can also have a hematogenous mechanism (arterial seeding or venous hematogenous access) (Maroldi et al., 2005).

OTHER NONNEOPLASTIC CYSTIC LESIONS

Dermoid and epidermoid cysts

These are considered to be slowly growing developmental pathologies, representing up to 1% of all intracranial tumors (Gelabert-Gonzalez, 1998). Dermoid and epidermoid cysts are thought to be the result of abnormal inclusion of ectodermal tissue intracranially during development (Orakcioglu et al., 2008), probably from incomplete separation of the surface ectoderm from

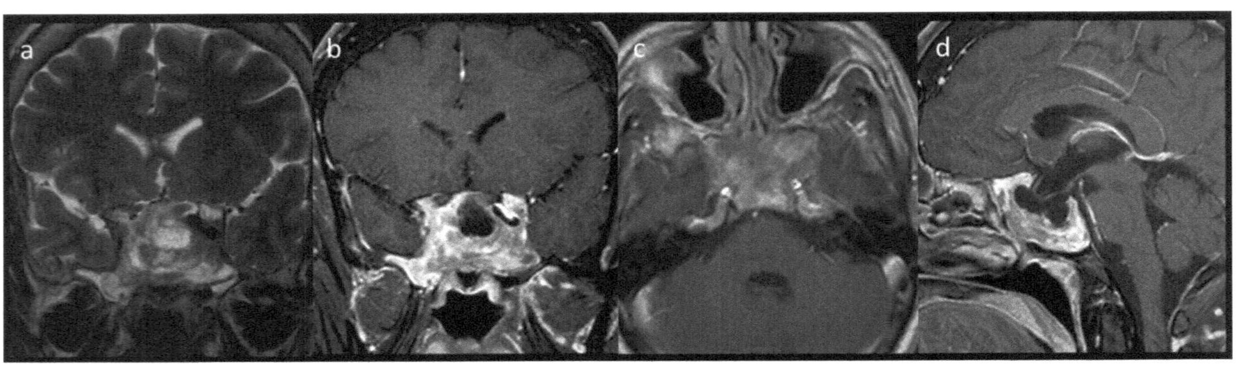

Fig. 15.16. Pituitary macroadenoma. (**A**) Coronal T2-weighted, (**B**) gadolinium-enhanced coronal, (**C**) axial, and (**D**) sagittal T1-weighted images. Large infiltrative mass involving the sellar and suprasellar component, extending into the sphenoid sinus and cavernous sinuses bilaterally. Pathology was consistent with a pituitary macroadenoma.

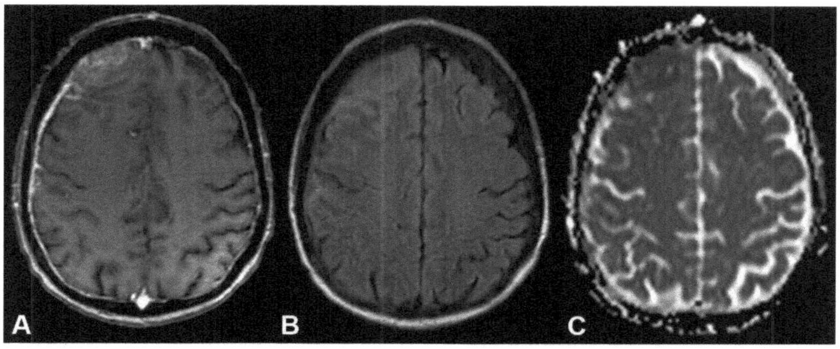

Fig. 15.17. Dural metastasis from prostate carcinoma. (**A**) Gadolinium-enhanced axial T1-weighted, (**B**) axial fluid-attenuated inversion recovery (FLAIR), and (**C**) axial apparent diffusion coefficient (ADC) images. Large, heterogeneously enhancing intracranial extradural mass in the right frontal region without significant T2 hyperintensities in the adjacent brain parenchyma. ADC maps show slight decrease of ADC values within this mass.

the neural tube or related to the invaginations of the otic capsule or during development of the eye and orbit. Dermoid cysts are generally benign sebaceous lipid-containing lesions, often located near the midline, that can occasionally rupture, producing chemical meningitis, vasospasm, and hydrocephalus (Orakcioglu et al., 2008). They are often T1 hyperintense, T2 hypointense but occasionally can show CSF-like signal similar to epidermoid cysts (Orakcioglu et al., 2008). Dermoid and epidermoid cysts increase in size due to desquamation and secretions related to the epithelial components lining the cysts. Epidermoid cysts often present as heterogeneously fluid-attenuated inversion recovery (FLAIR) and diffusion-weighted imaging (DWI) hyperintense extra-axial lesions involving the basilar cisterns (Hakyemez et al., 2005) and in the cerebellopontine angle (Fig. 15.18). Atypical appearances have been reported in up to 5.6% of epidermoid cysts (Ren et al., 2012) due to intralesional hemorrhage.

Arachnoid cysts

Arachnoid cysts are considered nonneoplastic intra-arachnoid cysts constituting approximately 1% of all intracranial mass-like lesions (Cincu et al., 2007), often involving the middle cranial fossa. These cysts are likely developmental in etiology and related to focal splitting/duplication of the arachnoid membrane (Cincu et al., 2007). Arachnoid cysts follow the appearance of the cerebrospinal fluid in CT and MR images, with variable local mass effect on the adjacent structures (Fig. 15.19).

Neurenteric cysts and ecchordosis physaliphora

Neurenteric cysts are rare cystic endodermal-derived developmental lesions typically located in the spinal canal and posterior fossa (most commonly within the cerebellopontine angle and prepontine cisterns (Preece et al., 2006). These cysts are typically CSF isointense on T1- and T2-weighted images, without internal enhancement, and often show increased FLAIR signal and variable appearance of DW images (Preece et al., 2006) (Fig. 15.20). Ecchordosis physaliphora are also rare cystic endodermal-derived developmental pathologies, typically located in the prepontine cistern and often associated with an osseous spicule or small stalk in the adjacent clivus (Mehnert et al., 2004) (Fig. 15.21).

CONCLUSION

There are many different types of intracranial neoplasms and nonneoplastic conditions that can present as extra-axial intracranial masses. The differential diagnosis can often be narrowed if specific imaging findings (such as focal hyperostosis for meningiomas or presence of abnormal DWI hyperintensity in cases of epidermoid cysts) are present. The ultimate diagnosis often requires pathologic sampling or long-term follow-up to confirm stability. The challenge of the radiologic assessment of these lesions is to develop new, more accurate noninvasive imaging techniques, decreasing the need for pathologic sampling and accelerating their treatment.

DISCLAIMER

The views and opinions expressed herein are those of the authors and should not be construed as being official, nor as representing the Uniformed Services University of the Health Sciences, the Department of Defense, nor the federal government.

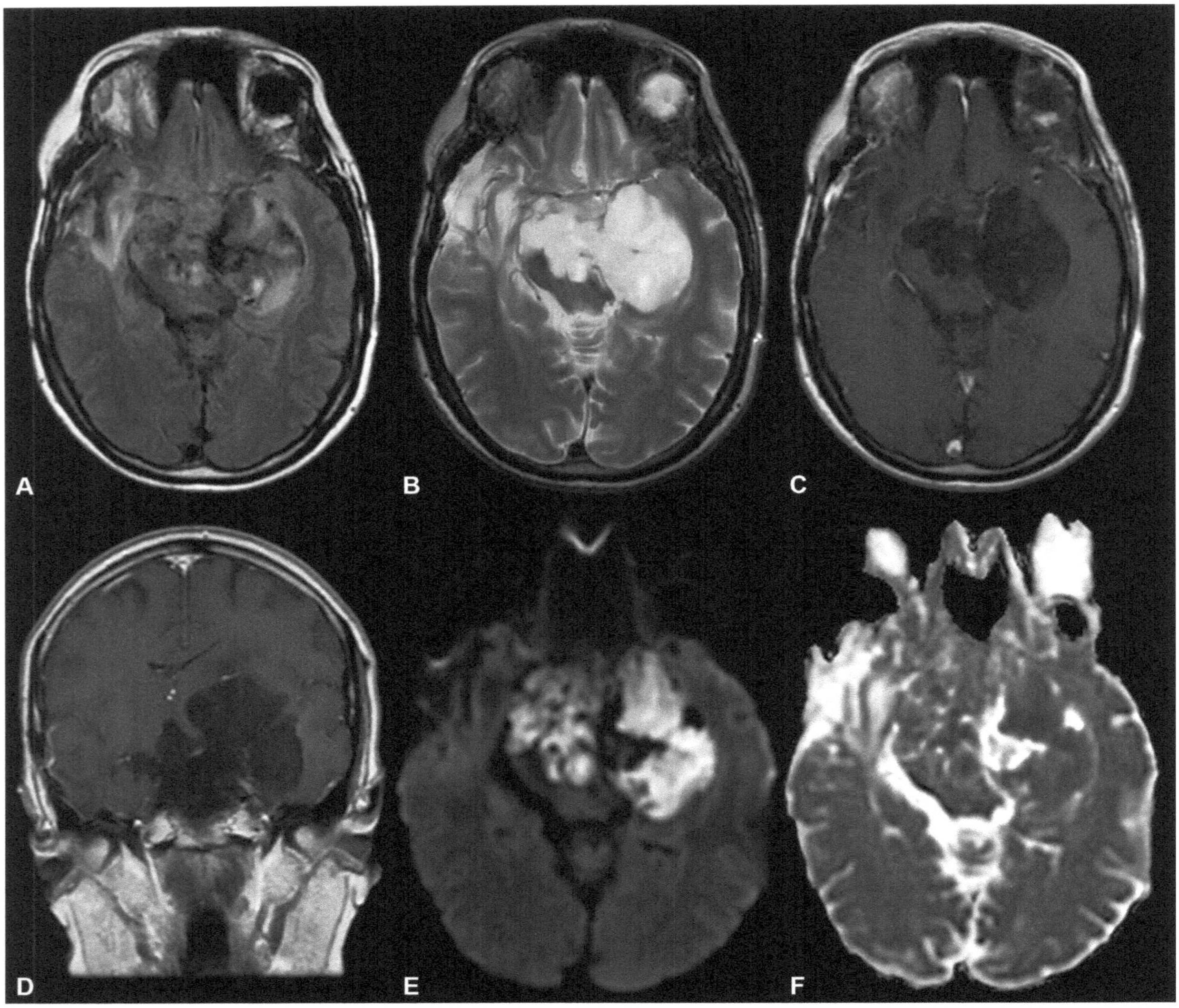

Fig. 15.18. Epidermoid cyst. (**A**) Axial fluid-attenuated inversion recovery (FLAIR), (**B**) axial T2-weighted, (**C**) axial, and (**D**) coronal postcontrast T1-weighted images, as well as axial diffusion-weighted (B = 1000) (**E**) and axial apparent diffusion coefficient (ADC) (**F**) images. There is a large T2 hyperintense mass-like lesion in the basilar cisterns and medial aspect of the left temporal lobe, producing local mass effect, without abnormal nodular enhancement but with increased diffusion-weighted imaging signal (**E**) (isointense on the ADC map), compatible with a large epidermoid cyst.

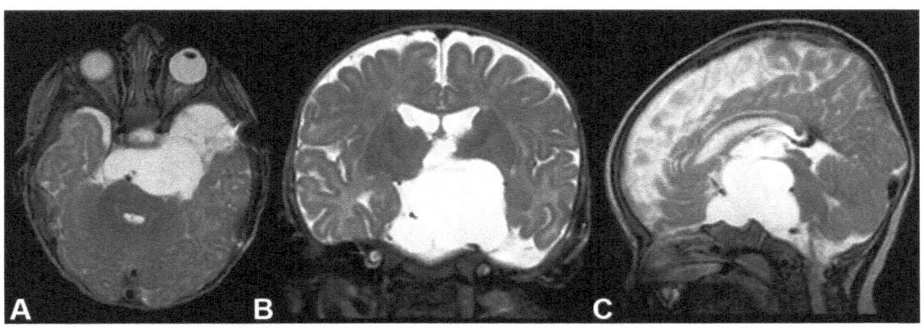

Fig. 15.19. Arachnoid cyst. Axial, coronal, and sagittal T2-weighted images. There is a large arachnoid cyst (isointense to cerebrospinal fluid on all sequences) centered on the basilar and left middle cerebral artery cisterns.

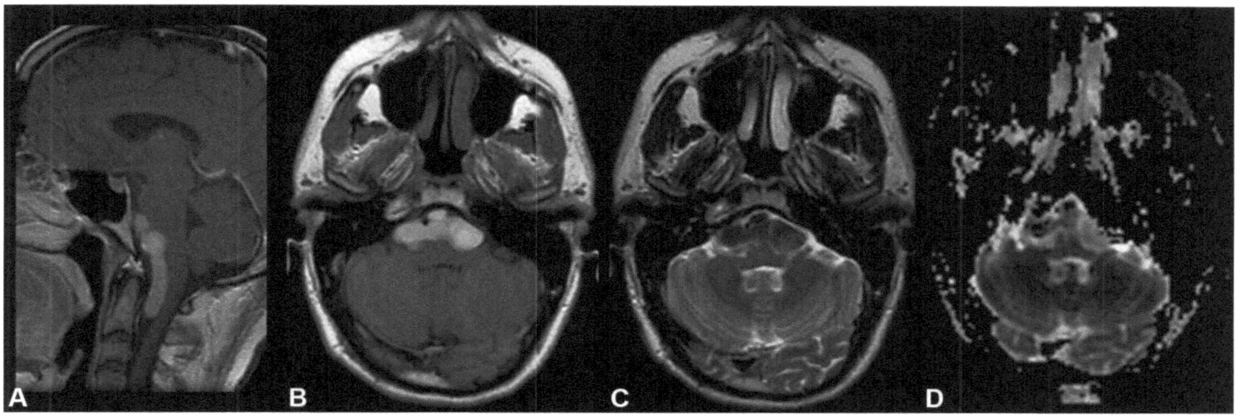

Fig. 15.20. Neurenteric cyst. (**A**) Sagittal and (**B**) axial postcontrast T1-weighted; (**C**) axial T2-weighted and (**D**) axial apparent diffusion coefficient images. There is an intrinsically T1 hyperintense tubular structure in the prepontine and premedullary cisterns, compatible with a neurenteric cyst (confirmed by pathology).

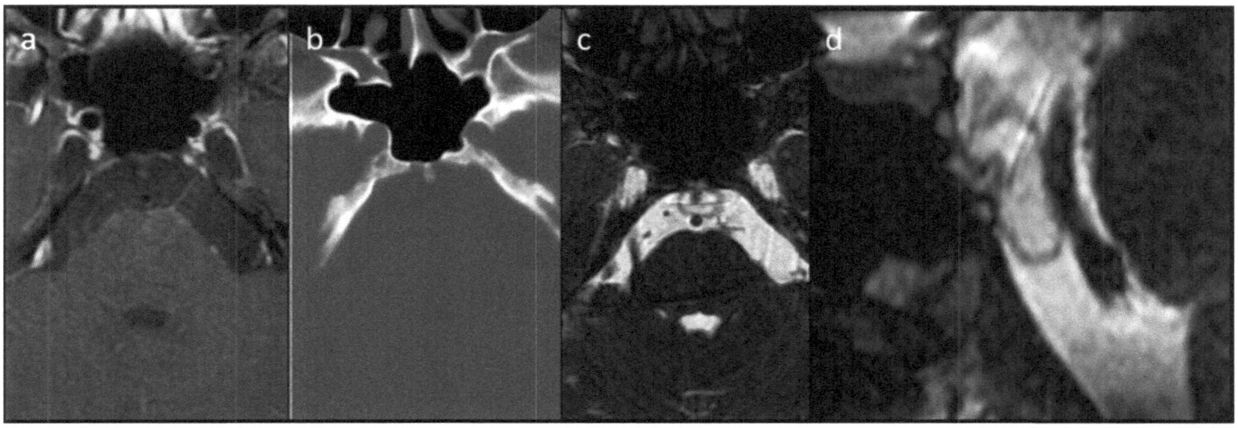

Fig. 15.21. Ecchordosis physaliphora. (**A**) Axial T1 – post, (**B**) axial computed tomography – bone window, (**C**) axial CISS, and (**D**) sagittal reformatted CISS images. A nonenhancing cystic structure in the prepontine cistern associated with a small midline spicule along the clivus is compatible with ecchordosis physaliphora.

References

Akiyama M, Sakai H, Onoue H et al. (2004). Imaging intracranial haemangiopericytomas: study of seven cases. Neuroradiology 46: 194–197.

Alahmadi H, Croul SE (2011). Pathology and genetics of meningiomas. Semin Diagn Pathol 28: 314–324.

Al-Gahtany M, Shroff M, Bouffet E et al. (2003). Primary central nervous system sarcomas in children: clinical, radiological, and pathological features. Childs Nerv Syst 19: 808–817.

Antunes NL, Lellouch-Tubiana A, Kalifa C et al. (2001). Intracranial Ewing sarcoma/'peripheral' primitive neuroectodermal tumor of dural origin with molecular genetic confirmation. J Neurooncol 51: 51–56.

Arana E, Diaz C, Latorre FF et al. (1996). Primary intraosseous meningiomas. Acta Radiol 37: 937–942.

Binning MJ, Gottfried ON, Osborn AG et al. (2005). Rathke cleft cyst intracystic nodule: a characteristic magnetic resonance imaging finding. J Neurosurg 103: 837–840.

Bognar L, Balint K, Bardoczy Z (2002). Symptomatic osteolipoma of the tuber cinereum. Case report. J Neurosurg 96: 361–363.

Bonneville F, Cattin F, Marsot-Dupuch K et al. (2006). T1 signal hyperintensity in the sellar region: spectrum of findings. Radiographics 26: 93–113.

Cao X, Luan S, Sun L et al. (2010). Impaired vision associated with a solitary intracranial plasmacytoma. J Clin Neurosci 17: 1215–1217.

Cerase A, Tarantino A, Gozzetti A et al. (2008). Intracranial involvement in plasmacytomas and multiple myeloma: a pictorial essay. Neuroradiology 50: 665–674.

Changhong L, Naiyin C, Yuehuan G et al. (1997). Primary intraosseous meningiomas of the skull. Clin Radiol 52: 546–549.

Chapman PR, Shah R, Cure JK et al. (2011). Petrous apex lesions: pictorial review. AJR Am J Roentgenol 196. WS26-37 Quiz S40-3.

Chernov MF, Kasuya H, Nakaya K et al. (2010). (1)H-MRS of intracranial meningiomas: what it can add to known

clinical and MRI predictors of the histopathological and biological characteristics of the tumor? Clin Neurol Neurosurg 113: 202–212.
Chiechi MV, Smirniotopoulos JG, Mena H (1996). Intracranial hemangiopericytomas: MR and CT features. AJNR Am J Neuroradiol 17: 1365–1371.
Choi KS, Chun HJ, Yi HJ et al. (2008). Intracranial invasion from recurrent angiosarcoma of the scalp. J Korean Neurosurg Soc 43: 201–204.
Cincu R, Agrawal A, Eiras J (2007). Intracranial arachnoid cysts: current concepts and treatment alternatives. Clin Neurol Neurosurg 109: 837–843.
Demir MK, Iplikcioglu AC, Dincer A et al. (2006). Single voxel proton MR spectroscopy findings of typical and atypical intracranial meningiomas. Eur J Radiol 60: 48–55.
Demir MK, Musluman M, Kilicoglu G et al. (2007). Imaging features of unusual intracranial cystic meningiomas. Can Assoc Radiol J 58: 109–115.
Dolecek TA, Propp JM, Stroup NE et al. (2012). CBTRUS statistical report: primary brain and central nervous system tumors diagnosed in the United States in 2005–2009. Neuro Oncol 14 (Suppl 5): v1–v49.
Drevelegas A (2005). Extra-axial brain tumors. Eur Radiol 15: 453–467.
Erdem E, Angtuaco EC, Van Hemert R et al. (2003). Comprehensive review of intracranial chordoma. Radiographics 23: 995–1009.
Gangadhar K, Santhosh D (2012). Radiopathological evaluation of primary malignant skull tumors: a review. Clin Neurol Neurosurg 114: 833–839.
Gasparetto EL, Leite Cda C, Lucato LT et al. (2007). Intracranial meningiomas: magnetic resonance imaging findings in 78 cases. Arq Neuropsiquiatr 65: 610–614.
Gelabert-Gonzalez M (1998). [Intracranial epidermoid and dermoid cysts]. Rev Neurol 27: 777–782.
Grier DD, Yachnis AT (2004). Secondary leptomeningeal sarcomatosis. Arch Pathol Lab Med 128: 1303–1304.
Grier DD, Al-Quran SZ, Gray B et al. (2008). Intracranial myeloid sarcoma. Br J Haematol 142: 681.
Hakyemez B, Aksoy U, Yildiz H et al. (2005). Intracranial epidermoid cysts: diffusion-weighted, FLAIR and conventional MR findings. Eur J Radiol 54: 214–220.
Hakyemez B, Yildirim N, Taskapilioglu O et al. (2007). Intracranial myeloid sarcoma: conventional and advanced MRI findings. Br J Radiol 80: e109–e112.
Iaccarino C, Schiavi P, Crafa P et al. (2013). Primary dural lymphoma mimicking a chronic epidural hematoma. Differential diagnosis of two rare conditions. Clin Neurol Neurosurg 115: 1276–1280.
Ide M, Jimbo M, Kubo O et al. (1994). Peritumoral brain edema and cortical damage by meningioma. Acta Neurochir Suppl (Wien) 60: 369–372.
Ito M, Kamiyama H, Nakamura T et al. (2009). Dural cavernous hemangioma of the cerebellar falx. Neurol Med Chir (Tokyo) 49: 410–412.
Iwamoto FM, Abrey LE (2006). Primary dural lymphomas: a review. Neurosurg Focus 21, E5.
Jabot G, Stoquart-Elsankari S, Saliou G et al. (2009). Intracranial lipomas: clinical appearances on neuroimaging and clinical significance. J Neurol 256: 851–855.
Joshi V, Muzumdar D, Dange N et al. (2009). Supratentorial convexity dural-based cavernous hemangioma mimicking a meningioma in a child. Pediatr Neurosurg 45: 141–145.
Kim KS, Rogers LF, Goldblatt D (1987). CT features of hyperostosing meningioma en plaque. AJR Am J Roentgenol 149: 1017–1023.
Kimura H, Takeuchi H, Koshimoto Y et al. (2006). Perfusion imaging of meningioma by using continuous arterial spin-labeling: comparison with dynamic susceptibility-weighted contrast-enhanced MR images and histopathologic features. AJNR Am J Neuroradiol 27: 85–93.
Kulkarni KM, Sternau L, Dubovy SR et al. (2012). Primary dural lymphoma masquerading as a meningioma. J Neuroophthalmol 32: 240–242.
Kumar J, Kumar A, Sharma R et al. (2007). Magnetic resonance imaging of sellar and suprasellar pathology: a pictorial review. Curr Probl Diagn Radiol 36: 227–236.
Latchaw Jr JP, Dohn DF, Hahn JF et al. (1981). Subarachnoid hemorrhage from an intracranial meningioma. Neurosurgery 9: 433–435.
Louis DN, International Agency for Research on Cancer, World Health Organization (2007). WHO classification of tumours of the central nervous system. International Agency for Research on Cancer, Lyon.
Maroldi R, Ambrosi C, Farina D (2005). Metastatic disease of the brain: extra-axial metastases (skull, dura, leptomeningeal) and tumour spread. Eur Radiol 15: 617–626.
Mawrin C, Perry A (2010). Pathological classification and molecular genetics of meningiomas. J Neurooncol 99: 379–391.
Mehnert F, Beschorner R, Kuker W et al. (2004). Retroclival ecchordosis physaliphora: MR imaging and review of the literature. AJNR Am J Neuroradiol 25: 1851–1855.
Mneimneh WS, Ashraf MA, Li L et al. (2013). Primary dural lymphoma: A novel concept of heterogeneous disease. Pathol Int 63: 68–72.
Moschopulos M, Becheanu G, Stamm B (2006). Hypothalamic osteolipoma of the tuber cinereum. J Cell Mol Med 10: 240–242.
Ogiwara H, Tsutsumi Y, Matsuoka K et al. (2015). Apparent diffusion coefficient of intracranial germ cell tumors. J Neurooncol 121 (3): 565–571.
Okamoto K, Ito J, Tokiguchi S et al. (1996). Development of fat within a meningioma. Neuroradiology 38: 214–216.
Orakcioglu B, Halatsch ME, Fortunati M et al. (2008). Intracranial dermoid cysts: variations of radiological and clinical features. Acta Neurochir (Wien) 150: 1227–1234. discussion 1234.
Osawa T, Tosaka M, Nagaishi M et al. (2013). Factors affecting peritumoral brain edema in meningioma: special histological subtypes with prominently extensive edema. J Neurooncol 111: 49–57.
Osborne DR, Dubois P, Drayer B et al. (1981). Primary intracranial meningeal and spinal hemangiopericytoma: radiologic manifestations. AJNR Am J Neuroradiol 2: 69–74.
Paek SH, Kim SH, Chang KH et al. (2005). Microcystic meningiomas: radiological characteristics of 16 cases. Acta Neurochir (Wien) 147: 965–972. discussion 972.

Pamir MN, Ozduman K (2006). Analysis of radiological features relative to histopathology in 42 skull-base chordomas and chondrosarcomas. Eur J Radiol 58: 461–470.

Pantanowitz L, Dezube BJ (2008). Kaposi sarcoma in unusual locations. BMC Cancer 8: 190.

Parajon A, Vaquero J (2008). Meningeal intracranial epithelioid hemangioendothelioma: case report and literature review. J Neurooncol 88: 169–173.

Patnaik A, Mishra SS, Mishra S et al. (2012). Intradiploic ossified giant cavernous hemangioma of skull with a dural tail sign mimicking primary calvarial meningioma. Neurol India 60: 250–252.

Penel N, Amela EY, Decanter G et al. (2012). Solitary fibrous tumors and so-called hemangiopericytoma. Sarcoma 2012: 690251.

Perry JR, Tucker WS, Chui M et al. (1993). Dural cavernous hemangioma: an under-recognized lesion mimicking meningioma. Can J Neurol Sci 20: 230–233.

Pistolesi S, Fontanini G, Boldrini L et al. (2003). The role of somatostatin in vasogenic meningioma associated brain edema. Tumori 89: 136–140.

Plotkin SR, Blakeley JO, Evans DG et al. (2013). Update from the 2011 International Schwannomatosis Workshop: from genetics to diagnostic criteria. Am J Med Genet A 161: 405–416.

Preece MT, Osborn AG, Chin SS et al. (2006). Intracranial neurenteric cysts: imaging and pathology spectrum. AJNR Am J Neuroradiol 27: 1211–1216.

Raizer J (2010). Meningiomas. Curr Treat Options Neurol 12: 360–368.

Rees JH, Wen PY (2010). Neuro-oncology. Saunders/Elsevier, Philadelphia.

Ren X, Lin S, Wang Z et al. (2012). Clinical, radiological, and pathological features of 24 atypical intracranial epidermoid cysts. J Neurosurg 116: 611–621.

Roberti F, Sekhar LN, Jones RV et al. (2007). Intradural cranial chordoma: a rare presentation of an uncommon tumor. Surgical experience and review of the literature. J Neurosurg 106: 270–274.

Rockhill J, Mrugala M, Chamberlain MC (2007). Intracranial meningiomas: an overview of diagnosis and treatment. Neurosurg Focus 23, E1.

Rodriguez HA, Berthrong M (1966). Multiple primary intracranial tumors in von Recklinghausen's neurofibromatosis. Arch Neurol 14: 467–475.

Rokni-Yazdi H, Azmoudeh Ardalan F, Asadzandi Z et al. (2009). Pathologic significance of the "dural tail sign". Eur J Radiol 70: 10–16.

Ruscalleda J, Feliciani M, Avila A et al. (1994). Neuroradiological features of intracranial and intraorbital meningeal haemangiopericytomas. Neuroradiology 36: 440–445.

Sacher M, Lanzieri CF, Huang YP et al. (1985). Meningioma with intratumoral fat. J Comput Tomogr 9: 83–85.

Santelli L, Ramondo G, Della Puppa A et al. (2010). Diffusion-weighted imaging does not predict histological grading in meningiomas. Acta Neurochir (Wien) 152: 1315–1319. discussion 1319.

Sanverdi SE, Ozgen B, Oguz KK et al. (2012). Is diffusion-weighted imaging useful in grading and differentiating histopathological subtypes of meningiomas? Eur J Radiol 81: 2389–2395.

Sartoretti-Schefer S, Wichmann W, Aguzzi A et al. (1997). MR differentiation of adamantinous and squamous-papillary craniopharyngiomas. AJNR Am J Neuroradiol 18: 77–87.

Schmid S, Aboul-Enein F, Pfisterer W et al. (2010). Vascular endothelial growth factor: the major factor for tumor neovascularization and edema formation in meningioma patients. Neurosurgery 67: 1703–1708. discussion 1708.

Sibtain NA, Butt S, Connor SE (2007). Imaging features of central nervous system haemangiopericytomas. Eur Radiol 17: 1685–1693.

Sotoudeh H, Yazdi HR (2010). A review on dural tail sign. World J Radiol 2: 188–192.

Takeshima Y, Yamada S, Motoyama Y et al. (2012). An unusual case of primary central nervous system germinoma with meningeal dissemination. Childs Nerv Syst 28: 2173–2176.

Tamiya T, Ono Y, Matsumoto K et al. (2001). Peritumoral brain edema in intracranial meningiomas: effects of radiological and histological factors. Neurosurgery 49: 1046–1051. discussion 1051–2.

Tandon R, Mukherjee U, Abrari A et al. (2012). Primary dural follicular lymphoma masquerading a meningioma: a case report. Br J Neurosurg 26: 905–906.

Tayoro K, Cottier J, Jan M et al. (2002). [Imaging of meningeal hemangiopericytomas]. J Radiol 83: 459–465.

Toh CH, Castillo M, Wong AM et al. (2008). Differentiation between classic and atypical meningiomas with use of diffusion tensor imaging. AJNR Am J Neuroradiol 29: 1630–1635.

Uluc K, Arsava EM, Ozkan B et al. (2004). Primary leptomeningeal sarcomatosis; a pathology proven case with challenging MRI and clinical findings. J Neurooncol 66: 307–312.

Uttley D, Clifton AC, Wilkins PR (1995). Haemangiopericytoma: a clinical and radiological comparison with atypical meningiomas. Br J Neurosurg 9: 127–134.

Wang Y, Zou L, Gao B (2010). Intracranial germinoma: clinical and MRI findings in 56 patients. Childs Nerv Syst 26: 1773–1777.

Watanabe Y, Yamasaki F, Kajiwara Y et al. (2013). Preoperative histological grading of meningiomas using apparent diffusion coefficient at 3 T MRI. Eur J Radiol 82: 658–663.

Weber AL, Liebsch NJ, Sanchez R et al. (1994). Chordomas of the skull base. Radiologic and clinical evaluation. Neuroimaging Clin N Am 4: 515–527.

Yin B, Liu L, Zhang BY et al. (2012). Correlating apparent diffusion coefficients with histopathologic findings on meningiomas. Eur J Radiol 81: 4050–4056.

Zhang H, Rodiger LA, Shen T et al. (2008a). Perfusion MR imaging for differentiation of benign and malignant meningiomas. Neuroradiology 50: 525–530.

Zhang H, Rodiger LA, Shen T et al. (2008b). Preoperative subtyping of meningiomas by perfusion MR imaging. Neuroradiology 50: 835–840.

Zhang D, Hu LB, Zhen JW et al. (2009). MRI findings of intracranial cystic meningiomas. Clin Radiol 64: 792–800.

Handbook of Clinical Neurology, Vol. 135 (3rd series)
Neuroimaging, Part I
J.C. Masdeu and R.G. González, Editors

Chapter 16

Imaging acute ischemic stroke

R. GILBERTO GONZÁLEZ[1]* AND LEE H. SCHWAMM[2]

[1]*Neuroradiology Division, Massachusetts General Hospital and Harvard Medical School, Boston, MA, USA*

[2]*Department of Neurology, Massachusetts General Hospital and Harvard Medical School, Boston, MA, USA*

Abstract

Acute ischemic stroke is common and often treatable, but treatment requires reliable information on the state of the brain that may be provided by modern neuroimaging. Critical information includes: the presence of hemorrhage; the site of arterial occlusion; the size of the early infarct "core"; and the size of underperfused, potentially threatened brain parenchyma, commonly referred to as the "penumbra." In this chapter we review the major determinants of outcomes in ischemic stroke patients, and the clinical value of various advanced computed tomography and magnetic resonance imaging methods that may provide key physiologic information in these patients. The focus is on major strokes due to occlusions of large arteries of the anterior circulation, the most common cause of a severe stroke syndrome. The current evidence-based approach to imaging the acute stroke patient at the Massachusetts General Hospital is presented, which is applicable for all stroke types. We conclude with new information on time and stroke evolution that imaging has revealed, and how it may open the possibilities of treating many more patients.

IMAGING ACUTE ISCHEMIC STROKE

Acute ischemic stroke is common and often treatable. But successful treatment of the stroke patient often requires reliable information on the state of the brain. Modern neuroimaging provides information on the physiologic basis for the patient's neurologic deficits including: the presence of hemorrhage; the site of arterial occlusion; the size of the early infarct "core"; and the size of underperfused, potentially threatened brain parenchyma, commonly referred to as the "penumbra." However, not all the information provided by computed tomography (CT) and magnetic resonance imaging (MRI) is equally reliable or clinically relevant in an individual patient. Indeed, these technologies reveal complementary information, and both may be required for the proper evaluation of a specific patient. Here we describe the major determinants of stroke patient outcomes and how neuroimaging may reveal them. We then review the clinical value of various CT and MRI methods. This is followed by the current evidence-based approach to imaging the acute stroke patient at the Massachusetts General Hospital. A primary focus is on major strokes due to occlusions of large arteries of the anterior circulation, the most common cause of a severe stroke syndrome, but the algorithm is applicable for all stroke types. We conclude with new information on time and stroke evolution that imaging has revealed, and how it may open the possibilities of treating many more patients.

CLINICAL AND NEUROIMAGING DETERMINANTS OF STROKE OUTCOMES

Neurologic status

The single most important factor that predicts outcome and guides management of patients that present with an acute ischemic stroke syndrome is the severity of the neurologic deficit, which may be reliably assessed using the National Institutes of Health Stroke Scale

*Correspondence to: R. Gilberto González, Neuroradiology Division, Massachusetts General Hospital, Harvard Medical School, Boston MA 02114, USA. Tel: +1-617-726-8628, Fax: +1-617-724-3338, E-mail: rggonzalez@mgh.harvard.edu

Table 16.1

National Institutes of Health Stroke Scale (NIHSS)

1a. Level of consciousness:
- 0 Alert
- 1 Not alert, but rousable with minimal stimulation
- 2 Not alert, requires repeated stimulation to attend
- 3 Coma

1b. Ask patient the month and the patient's age:
- 0 Answers both correctly
- 1 Answers one correctly
- 2 Both incorrect

1c. Ask patient to open and close eyes:
- 0 Obeys both correctly
- 1 Obeys one correctly
- 2 Both incorrect

2. Best gaze (only horizontal eye movement):
- 0 Normal
- 1 Partial gaze palsy
- 2 Forced deviation

3. Visual field testing:
- 0 No visual field loss
- 1 Partial hemianopia
- 2 Complete hemianopia
- 3 Bilateral hemianopia (blind, including cortical blindness)

4. Facial paresis (ask patient to show teeth or raise eyebrows and close eyes tightly):
- 0 Normal symmetric movement
- 1 Minor paralysis (flattened nasolabial fold, asymmetry on smiling)
- 2 Partial paralysis (total or near-total paralysis of lower face)
- 3 Complete paralysis of one or both sides (absence of facial movement in the upper and lower face)

5. Motor function – arm (right and left):
- 0 Normal (extends arms 90° (or 45°) for 10 seconds without drift)
- 1 Drift
- 2 Some effort against gravity
- 3 No effort against gravity
- 4 No movement
- 9 Untestable (joint fused or limb amputated)

6. Motor function – leg (right and left):
- 0 Normal (holds leg 30° position for 5 seconds)
- 1 Drift
- 2 Some effort against gravity
- 3 No effort against gravity
- 4 No movement
- 9 Untestable (joint fused or limb amputated)

7. Limb ataxia
- 0 No ataxia
- 1 Present in one limb
- 2 Present in two limbs

8. Sensory (use pinprick to test arms, legs, trunk and face – compare side to side)
- 0 Normal
- 1 Mild to moderate decrease in sensation
- 2 Severe to total sensory loss

9. Best language (describe picture, name items, read sentences)
- 0 No aphasia
- 1 Mild to moderate aphasia
- 2 Severe aphasia
- 3 Mute

10. Dysarthria (read several words)
- 0 Normal articulation
- 1 Mild to moderate slurring of words
- 2 Near unintelligible or unable to speak
- 9 Intubated or other physical barrier

11. Extinction and inattention
- 0 Normal
- 1 Inattention or extinction to bilateral simultaneous stimulation in one of the sensory modalities
- 2 Severe hemi-inattention or hemi-inattention to more than one modality

Total score:

(NIHSS: Table 16.1). The neurologic exam provides critical diagnostic and prognostic information in stroke, and provides pretest probabilities on whether imaging will reveal a major artery occlusion and the size of territory at risk. Simply put, patients with mild neurologic deficits are likely to have minor imaging abnormalities and to have good outcomes, while those that present with severe symptoms have a high probability of having significant findings on imaging and a poor outcome. The most widely used clinical measurement instrument is the NIHSS, and it has proven value in predicting stroke outcomes and assessing new treatments (Adams et al., 1999). The NIHSS has been shown to predict length of stay, hospital cost, clinical outcomes, and hospital discharge disposition (Rundek et al., 2000; Chang et al., 2002; Johnston et al., 2003). The major drawback of the NIHSS is that it cannot distinguish between the neurologic dysfunction due to: irreversible brain injury (infarction); ongoing ischemia of still viable tissue; "stunned" but normally perfused tissue; or a combination of these conditions. The NIHSS is an excellent indicator of functional significance of an ischemic insult, but it alone is limited in assessing the amount of irreversible brain injury and the likelihood of recovery for tissue at risk.

Based on data from the Screening Technology and Outcome Project in Stroke (STOPStroke) Study, a large prospective study performed at the Massachusetts General Hospital (MGH) and University of California, San Francisco, nearly two-thirds of acute ischemic stroke patients will present with mild to moderate symptoms (NIHSS 0–10). Most of these patients will have favorable outcomes, as shown in Figure 16.1 (Gonzalez et al., 2012). Over half of all stroke patients present with mild symptoms (NIHSS 0–5). The majority of these patients will have good outcomes, and thrombolytic therapy is not indicated. While the majority of patients with moderate symptoms (NIHSS 6–10) will have good outcomes, the evidence supports the use of thrombolytic therapy with intravenous (IV) tissue plasminogen activator (t-PA) in these patients. The majority of patients who present with severe symptoms (NIHSS > 10) are likely to have poor outcomes (modified Rankin scale greater than 2), but many may be helped with treatment.

Arterial occlusion location

The identification of an occlusion of a major cerebral artery by vascular imaging in addition to the neurologic examination significantly improves outcome prediction (Fig. 16.2) (Gonzalez et al., 2012). The presence of a major artery occlusion in patients with severe neurologic symptoms result in a probability of a poor outcome of close to 90%, which is significantly higher than the presence of only one of these factors. Conversely, patients with mild to moderate symptoms and an absence of a major artery occlusion have a high probability of good outcomes even in the absence of therapy. In addition to prognostic information, vascular imaging may identify a potential target for therapy – the site of the embolus that has produced the stroke syndrome. These data support obtaining vascular imaging as soon as practicable. Since most patients in these circumstances will initially undergo noncontrast CT scanning, the acquisition of a CT angiography (CTA) immediately afterwards is highly efficient in obtaining this critical information.

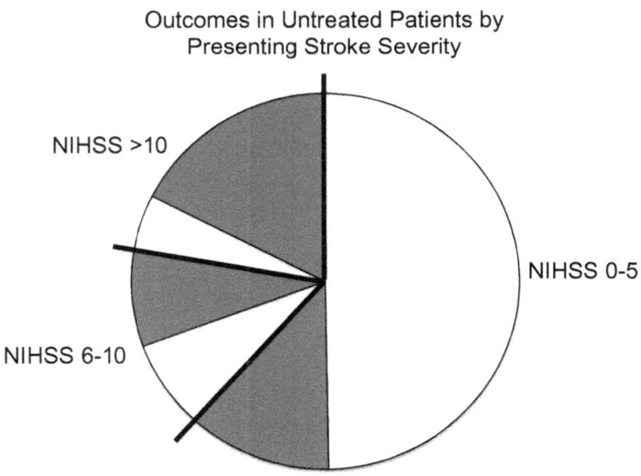

Fig. 16.1. Untreated acute stroke patient outcomes. Data are from the Screening Technology and Outcome Project in Stroke (STOPStroke) study. Prospectively, acute stroke patients had admission National Institutes of Health Stroke Scale (NIHSS) scores, noncontrast computed tomography (CT), CT angiography, and 6-month outcome assessed using modified Rankin scale (mRS), with good outcomes defined as mRS equal to 2 or less. Good outcomes are in white and poor outcomes are in gray. The outcomes data displayed here include 544 patients who did not receive intravenous tissue plasminogen activator treatment. The majority of patients presented with mild symptoms and ~80% (276/342) had good outcomes. Of the patients with NIHSS between 6 and 10, over half (43/82) had good outcomes. Of patients with NIHSS >10, ~78% (97/124) had poor outcomes. (Adapted from Gonzalez et al., 2012.)

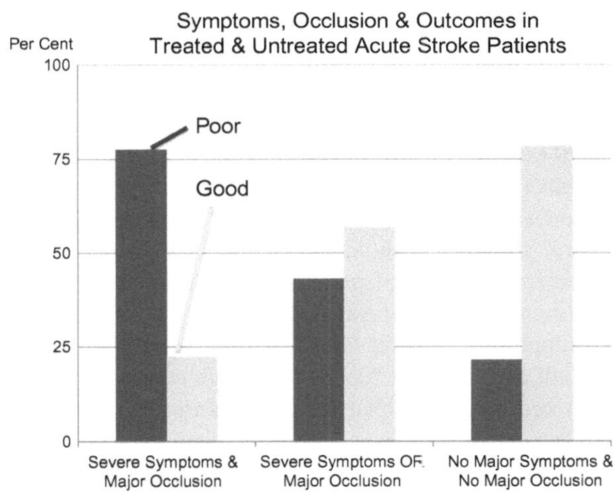

Fig. 16.2. Patient outcomes by vascular occlusion status and National Institutes of Health Stroke Scale (NIHSS) classification. Patient outcomes, regardless of treatment, are grouped into possible combinations of major artery occlusion and stroke severity. Severe symptom classifications are given to patients with NIHSS >10, and major occlusion classification is given to patients with occlusion of the basilar, distal internal carotid, and/or proximal middle cerebral arteries or infarction due to such occlusions. There are significant differences in outcomes amongst the categories (3 × 2 contingency table; $p < 0.0001$). Both the severe symptom/major occlusion and the no severe symptom/no major occlusion groups are significantly different from each other and from the other categories ($p < 0.0001$). (Adapted from Gonzalez et al., 2012.)

Infarct size

Another important factor in determining the outcome of a patient with an ischemic stroke is the presence and size of irreversibly injured brain, commonly referred to as the infarct core. Stroke physiology is dynamic; the infarction process begins with stroke onset and may continue during hospitalization. The cerebral infarct may grow substantially in the absence of treatment. However, the presence of a large completed infarct has been shown to make revascularization treatment futile or worse by raising the probability of hemorrhage. The exclusion of patients with a large infarction (i.e., >70–100 mL) is desirable because such patients have a low probability of a good outcome (Yoo et al., 2009; Lansberg et al., 2012). Additionally, the risk of reperfusion hemorrhage increases with pretreatment infarct size, especially when infarcts are larger than 100 mL (Lansberg et al., 2007; Singer et al., 2008). Several groups have demonstrated the importance of core infarct size in predicting outcomes in patients who undergo endovascular stroke treatment (Hill et al., 2003, 2006; Jovin et al., 2003; Yoo et al., 2009; Lansberg et al., 2012). Diffusion MRI is the most reliable method to estimate the size of an early infarct, and studies have shown that a diffusion-weighted imaging (DWI) abnormality volume of greater than 70 mL is highly specific for a poor outcome (Sanak et al., 2006; Yoo et al., 2010). This threshold volume is useful in selecting patients for endovascular intervention (Yoo et al., 2009). A DWI threshold volume of 70 mL was also employed in the DEFUSE II trial (Lansberg et al., 2012) to identify patients most likely to benefit by undergoing endovascular treatment. This infarct volume threshold was adopted by the Cleveland Clinic for inclusion of patients for endovascular stroke treatment; they demonstrated superior outcomes after its adoption (Wisco et al., 2014). The identification of a small early infarct "core" for triage decisions is also bolstered by reports that the final infarct volume is the single best predictor of good outcome at 90 days in patients with anterior circulation occlusion who were treated endovascularly (Yoo et al., 2012; Zaidi et al., 2012).

Treatment

The administration of IV t-PA improves outcomes in patients with moderate to severe symptoms and is recommended if the drug can be administered within 3 hours, or in some cases 4.5 hours, after stroke onset (Jauch et al., 2013). The drug is particularly effective in patients with moderate symptoms (Fig. 16.3A). In these patients good outcomes occur in approximately 55% without therapy. The administration of IV t-PA increases good outcomes to approximately 75%, whether or not there is an identifiable arterial occlusion. In patients with occlusion of the distal internal carotid artery (ICA) and/or proximal middle cerebral artery (MCA), the administration of IV t-PA improves outcomes from approximately 17% to 35% (Fig. 16.3B) (Gonzalez et al., 2013b). There are two intravenous fibrinolytic drugs under investigation, desmoteplase (Hacke et al., 2005, 2009; Furlan et al., 2006) and tenectoplase (Parsons et al., 2012), but phase III trials have not been completed.

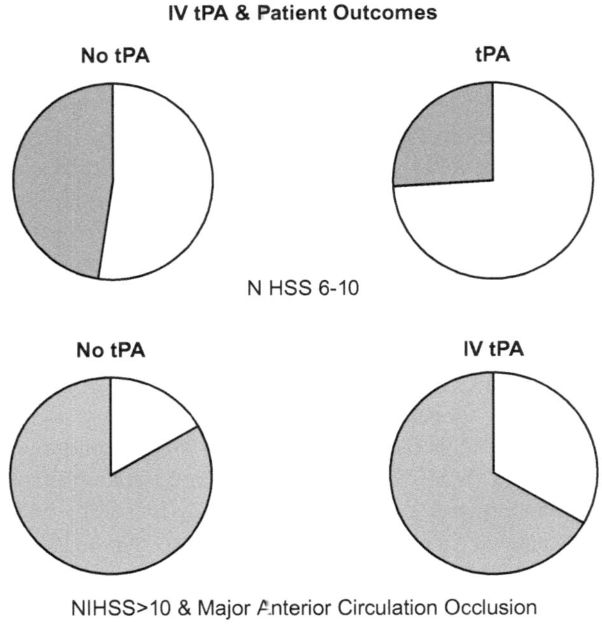

Fig. 16.3. Efficacy of intravenous (IV) tissue plasminogen activator (tPA) in patients with moderate and severe symptoms. (Top) Patients from the Screening Technology and Outcome Project in Stroke (STOPStroke) cohort with National Institutes of Health Stroke Scale (NIHSS) 6–10 irrespective of intracranial occlusions were stratified into those who did not receive IV-tPA, and those received IV-tPA. Good outcomes (modified Rankin scale (mRS)$\leq$2) are in white and poor outcomes (mRS >2) are in gray. Approximately 75% (20/27) of these moderately symptomatic patients who were treated with IV-tPA had good outcomes, compared to approximately 50% (43/82) of those not treated with IV-tPA. (Bottom) Patients from the STOPStroke cohort with NIHSS >10 and major intracranial occlusions were stratified into two groups: those who did not receive IV-tPA, and those who did receive IV-tPA. Good outcomes (mRS <2) are in white and poor outcomes (mRS >2) are in gray. Patients with severe symptoms and major occlusions who were treated with IV-tPA had significantly more good outcomes (approximately 35%) compared to those who were not treated with IV-tPA (approximately 17%). (Adapted from Gonzalez et al., 2013b.)

Endovascular recanalization of major artery occlusions may be employed in patients with severe symptoms

(Jauch et al., 2013). Successful treatment of patients using the intra-arterial route was demonstrated in 1999 (Furlan et al., 1999). In subsequent years fibrinolytic therapy has been replaced with endovascular mechanical recanalization, most recently with devices known as stentrievers (Nogueira et al., 2012; Saver et al., 2012; Jauch et al., 2013). Recent trial results, including IMS 3 (Broderick et al., 2013) and MR Rescue (Kidwell et al., 2013), had disappointing results. One possible reason is suboptimal patient selection. As shown in Figure 16.4 (Yoo et al., 2012), good outcomes in patients treated endovascularly were observed in nearly 70% of such patients when the final infarct volume was 30 mL or less. The rate of good outcomes rapidly declines with infarcts that are larger. To insure the probability of a good outcome it is best to determine the size of the core infarct before treatment is initiated.

A major advance has occurred in the treatment of severe strokes caused by occlusions of large anterior circulation arteries that is documented in the publication in the *New England Journal of Medicine* or three prospective randomized trials: MR CLEAN (Berkhemer et al., 2015), ESCAPE (Goyal et al., 2015), and EXTEND IA (Campbell et al., 2015). There is also a fourth positive trial with similar results, SWIFT PRIME, reported at a major conference. There are two major differences between the latest successful trial and prior failures. First, the new trials employed modern thrombectomy devices that are highly effective; second, advanced imaging was employed to identify a target occlusion (all trials) and favorable physiology (all trials except MR CLEAN).

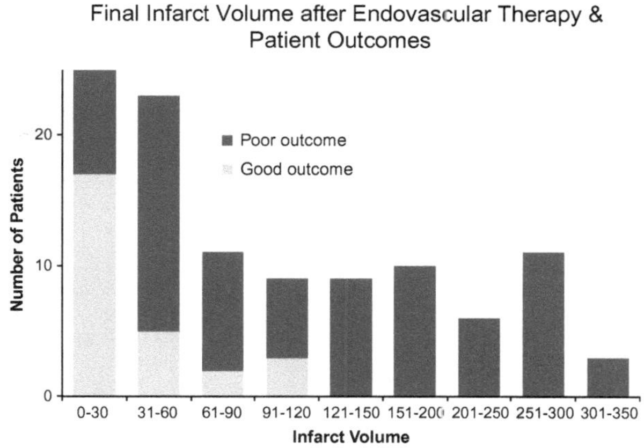

Fig. 16.4. Final infarct volume and outcomes in patients treated endovascularly. Depicted is the relationship between final infarct volume and long-term functional outcome in a prospective cohort of 107 endovascularly treated patients. The bar graphs show the proportion of 3-month good (modified Rankin Scale (mRS) 0–2) or poor outcomes in groups of patients stratified by final infarct volume. Reperfusion was achieved in 78 (72.9%) patients. Twenty-seven (25.2%) patients achieved a 3-month good outcome (mRS 0–2), and 30 (28.0%) died. Final infarct volume independently correlated with functional outcome across the entire mRS. In receiver operating characteristic analysis, it was the best discriminator of both good outcome and mortality. A final infarct of approximately 50 cm^3 demonstrated the greatest accuracy for distinguishing good versus poor outcome, and a final infarct volume of approximately 90 cm^3 was highly specific for a poor outcome. The interaction term between final infarct volume and age was the only independent predictor of good outcome ($p < 0.0001$). (Adapted from Yoo et al., 2012.)

IMAGING STROKE PHYSIOLOGY BY CT AND MRI

Modern CT and MRI are powerful tools for interrogating the physiologic state of the brain during and after an ischemic insult. The choice of CT and/or MRI when the stroke patients first presents depends on the clinical state of the patient and the therapeutic options. Table 16.2 lists the relationships between neurologic status, treatment options, key physiologic parameters, and imaging options. The key parameters in ischemic stroke and the CT and MRI methods available to measure them are shown in Figure 16.5. The figure represents a patient with an acute MCA occlusion, the most common type of severe stroke. An MCA occlusion produces two distinct brain regions distal to it: a volume of irreversibly injured brain tissue, commonly referred to as the "core," and a region of abnormally perfused (and possibly

Table 16.2

Clinical status, treatment, and imaging

NIHSS	% Stroke patient population	Treatment	Key factors for treatment	Imaging for treatment
<5	55%	None	–	–
5–10	10%	IV t-PA	Time, hemorrhage	CT
>10	35%	IV t-PA	Time, hemorrhage	CT
		IA	Time, hemorrhage, core, penumbra	CT+MR or MR alone

NIHSS, National Institutes of Health Stroke Scale; IV t-PA, intravenous tissue plasminogen activator; IA, intra-arterial; CT, computed tomography; MR, magnetic resonance.

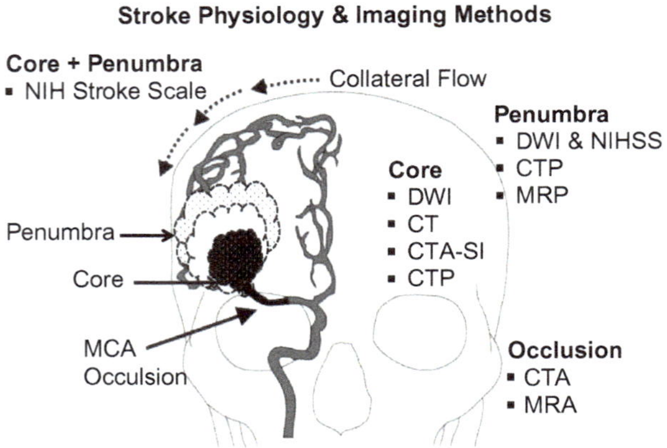

Fig. 16.5. Middle cerebral artery (MCA) stroke physiology and imaging methods. The figure represents a patient who has embolic occlusion of the proximal right MCA. The occlusion produces two abnormal brain regions: a region of irreversible brain injury (core) and abnormally perfused region (penumbra). The sizes of these two regions are linked by the quality of the collateral circulation. The relative sizes of the ischemic core and penumbra will change with time. Typically with the passage of time there is shrinkage of the ischemic penumbra and a corresponding growth of the infarct core. With good collaterals, the shrinkage of the penumbra and growth of the core are slow, while with poor collaterals very rapid growth of the core and shrinkage of the penumbra are observed. The physiology of the MCA depicted here may be evaluated using several neuroimaging methods, including computed tomography (CT), CT angiography (CTA), CTA source images (CTA-SI), CT perfusion (CTP), diffusion-weighted images (DWI), magnetic resonance (MR) angiography (MRA), and MR perfusion (MRP). The neurologic exam including the National Institutes of Health (NIH) Stroke Scale provides physiologic information on the functional penumbra, but cannot distinguish it from the infarct core. The clinical use and value of each method are listed in Tables 16.2 and 16.3.

symptomatic) parenchyma, also known as the "penumbra." The relative sizes of the core and the penumbra are determined by the vigor of the collateral circulation. An important concept is that the core and penumbra are not independent parameters, but rather are dependent variables that are linked by the collateral circulation. Hence, in the case of an MCA occlusion, measurement of the core is sufficient to deduce the size of the penumbra: if the core is small, the penumbra must be large, and vice versa. CT (including CT perfusion (CTP)) and MRI are not equivalent in reliably identifying the core. Indeed, CT and MRI have complementary strengths in revealing stroke physiology and sometimes it is best if both are used.

Identifying hemorrhage

The presence of intracranial hemorrhage is a critical bifurcation point in the evaluation of the stroke patient. The presence of hemorrhage has diagnostic value on the cause of the neurologic deficit, which may be due to a vascular malformation, aneurysm, mass lesion, coagulopathy, hypertension, hemorrhagic transformation of an ischemic stroke, as well as other causes. Also, the presence of hemorrhage in ischemic stroke patients has therapeutic implications by precluding the use of IV t-PA or endovascular therapy in most cases. Noncontrast CT can definitively identify parenchymal hemorrhage (Jauch et al., 2013). It has also been shown that MRI is highly reliable in identifying parenchymal hemorrhages, especially when magnetic susceptibility-weighted imaging sequences are employed. The one area where MRI is weaker than CT is in the identification of early subarachnoid hemorrhage because the high oxygen tension of the cerebrospinal fluid maintains a high oxyhemoglobin content in blood cells.

Vascular imaging

After the finding of a significant neurologic deficit in a patient with ischemic stroke, identifying the vascular occlusion responsible for the stroke syndrome is the next most valuable piece of information needed for formulating a treatment plan. This may be accomplished with CT or MR angiography (MRA) (Almandoz et al., 2011; Kim et al., 2011). Since such a patient usually undergoes noncontrast computed tomography (NCCT imaging), it is convenient and efficient to proceed with a CTA immediately after review of the noncontrast images. With modern multidetector CT technology, the arterial system can be visualized from the aortic arch to the vertex in less than a minute. The reliability of CTA is very high (Torres-Mozqueda et al., 2008; Cipriano et al., 2009; Deipolyi et al., 2012; Jauch et al., 2013). CTA has been shown to have >95% sensitivity and specificity compared to digital subtraction angiography (Lev et al., 2001; Bash et al., 2005). An important aspect in the use of CTA is the rapid reconstruction and presentation of images for review. Thick-slab (30 mm), overlapping (5 mm slice interval) maximal-intensity projection (MIP) images in the three cardinal planes may be created at the CT console immediately after data acquisition, and may be performed in less than 5 minutes (Pomerantz et al., 2006; Almandoz et al., 2011). An example of overlapping, thick-slab MIPs is shown in Figure 16.6.

Modern multidetector CT scanners facilitate the direct visualization of the embolus that is the cause of occlusions of major cerebral arteries. Such scanners obtain imaging data at very high resolution and can reconstruct thin cross-sectional images with a thickness of 1.25 or 2.5 mm. Most emboli are red blood cell-rich and around 90% appear hyperdense on thin-section CT scans. The thinner slice thickness produces higher

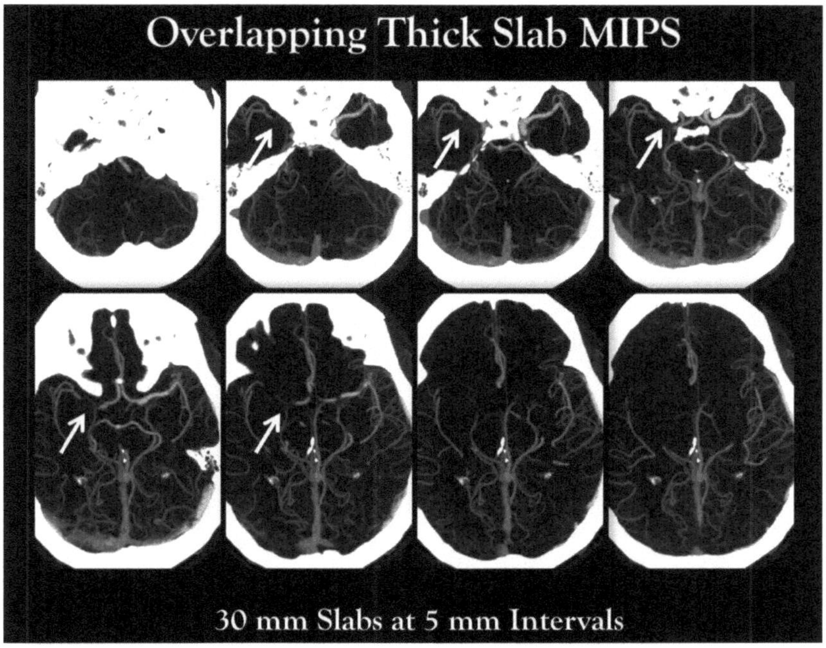

Fig. 16.6. Axial overlapping thick-slab maximal-intensity projections (MIPs). A sequential set of eight images from a series of 30-mm thick-slab, MIP reconstructions that overlap at 5-mm intervals. In these eight images the distal internal carotids, anterior cerebral, middle cerebral, posterior cerebral, and basilar arteries as well as many of their branches are well visualized. The M1 segment of the right middle cerebral artery is occluded (arrows). The thick slab helps identify occlusions that can be neglected on the thin, nonoverlapping sections. The overlapping aspect of this method also helps to identify occlusions that may occur at the border of nonoverlapping consecutive thick-slab MIPs.

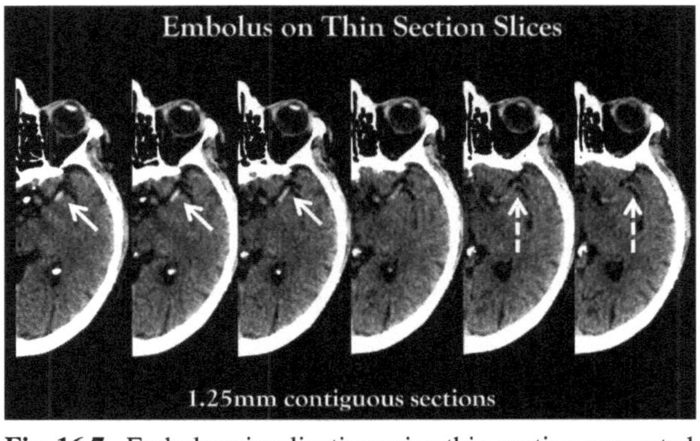

Fig. 16.7. Embolus visualization using thin-section computed tomography. Image slices have a thickness 1.25 mm. An embolus within the proximal left middle cerebral artery is well seen (solid arrows). No embolus is identified more distally within this artery (dashed arrows).

embolus contrast because of less volume averaging with adjacent brain tissue and cerebrospinal fluid (Fig. 16.7). Additionally, the length of the embolus may be measured and the length may provide prognostic information on the efficacy of thrombolytic therapy (Marder et al., 2006; Riedel et al., 2010, 2011; Liebeskind et al., 2011; Yuki et al., 2012; Yoo et al., 2013).

Vascular imaging using MRI is also reliable, although less so than CTA. Three-dimensional time-of-flight MRA of the intracranial circulation has been shown to identify proximal occlusions of major arteries with sensitivity of 84–87% and specificity of 85–98% (Bash et al., 2005; Tomanek et al., 2006). However, MRA requires substantially more time to acquire, making the likelihood of patient motion artifact higher, especially in a confused patient with a major stroke syndrome. Flow artifacts and the inability to distinguish slow flow from occlusion are additional problems (Bash et al., 2005).

Imaging the infarct core

Imaging of the early infarct core is amongst the most important factors for assessing prognosis and guiding treatment. With the presence of an MCA or/and a distal ICA embolic occlusion, the core size not only provides information on what is most likely the minimal final infarct size, but is also an indirect measure of the collateral circulation: a small core (<70 mL) is a reliable marker of an excellent collateral circulation. Because of the critical nature of this information, it is important that its measurement be reliable at early times after ictus and precise to within 10 mL.

Diffusion MRI

Diffusion MRI is highly reliable and the best available method for the early detection of infarct core. It is nearly 100% sensitive and specific in diagnosing acute stroke, and is clearly superior to NCCT (Fig. 16.8) (Lovblad et al., 1998; Singer et al., 1998; van Everdingen et al., 1998; Gonzalez et al., 1999; Urbach et al., 2000; Perkins et al., 2001; Fiebach et al., 2002; Mullins et al., 2002; Schellinger et al., 2010; Jauch et al., 2013). Acute infarction produces a high-contrast abnormality on DWI, the volume of which is relatively simple to quantify (Sims et al., 2009). It is not perfect in identifying the infarct core, and it has been shown using positron emission tomography (PET) that some infarcted tissue may not demonstrate restricted diffusion (Guadagno et al., 2005; Shimosegawa et al., 2005). DWI abnormalities sometimes reverse (Kidwell et al., 2000, 2002; Neumann-Haefelin et al., 2000; Fiehler et al., 2002; Oppenheim et al., 2006; Campbell et al., 2012), but this is unusual (Grant et al., 2001), and when it occurs, it usually involves only a small part of the lesion (Campbell et al., 2012). Additionally, a DWI reversal is often a pseudo-reversal, in that such tissue proceeds to infarction despite apparent temporary normalization of the DWI signal abnormality (Kidwell et al., 2002; Campbell et al., 2012).

Noncontrast CT

The widespread availability of CT scanners and their reliability for detection of intracranial blood makes CT nearly always the front-line imaging method in acute stroke. Also advantageous is that CTA may be acquired during the same imaging session. However, the ability of NCCT to reliably detect and estimate the size of the early infarct core is limited, and it is substantially inferior to diffusion MRI. NCCT is highly specific for infarction when a hypodensity is clearly visible, but such changes occur later and NCCT has low sensitivity early in the course of ischemic infarction (Fiehler et al., 2002).

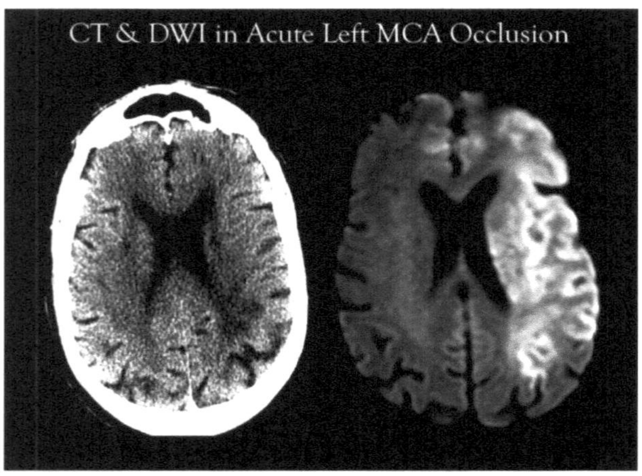

Fig. 16.8. Computed tomography (CT) and diffusion-weighted imaging (DWI) in a patient with acute-onset right hemiparesis. The head CT (left) was obtained ~15 minutes before the magnetic resonance imaging (right) diffusion study and reveals chronic changes, but not the large acute infarction revealed by the DWI study. MCA, middle cerebral artery.

Ischemic infarction reduces the normal attenuation of radiation as it passes through brain tissue and appears hypodense compared to normal tissue (Almandoz et al., 2011). This finding of early parenchymal hypodensity in stroke is due to increased water content of the tissue. Early there is cytotoxic edema, caused by lactic acidosis and failure of cell membrane ion pumps due to reduced adenosine triphosphate (Bell et al., 1985). This will result in redistribution of water from the extracellular to the intracellular space. However, there is little net change in tissue water, and consequently only minimal reduction in gray- and white-matter brain parenchymal attenuation. Subsequently, vasogenic edema that is a result of endothelial cell tight junction dysfunction produces CT-detectable changes. The attenuation of ischemic brain parenchyma is directly proportional to the degree of edema: X-ray attenuation decreases by 3–5% for every 1% increase in tissue water content, resulting in a drop of approximately 2.5 HU on CT images (Torack et al., 1976; Unger et al., 1988; Marks, 1998). The clinical observations have been confirmed in a rat model of acute MCA occlusion (Dzialowski et al., 2004). Such small changes are difficult to detect and require optimal "window width" and "center level" when the images are reviewed on the workstation (Lev et al., 1999; Almandoz et al., 2011). Also apparent early in ischemic stroke is loss of distinction of gray and white matter. This effect is due in part to edema, but it is also likely due to reduced blood content within gray-matter capillaries.

CT perfusion

The widespread availability of CT scanners makes it an attractive option for applying it for infarct core size estimation, if sufficiently reliable and precise. As stated above, NCCT is usually inadequate early after stroke onset. The source images from CTA have also been shown to be problematic (Pulli et al., 2012). A large amount of research effort has been devoted to developing CTP techniques for identification and quantification of the early infarct core (Konstas et al., 2011). High expectations for CTP are likely due in part by clinical observations that sometimes it appears very accurate (Fig. 16.9). This occurs in the special case when there is little or no collateral circulation. However, the more

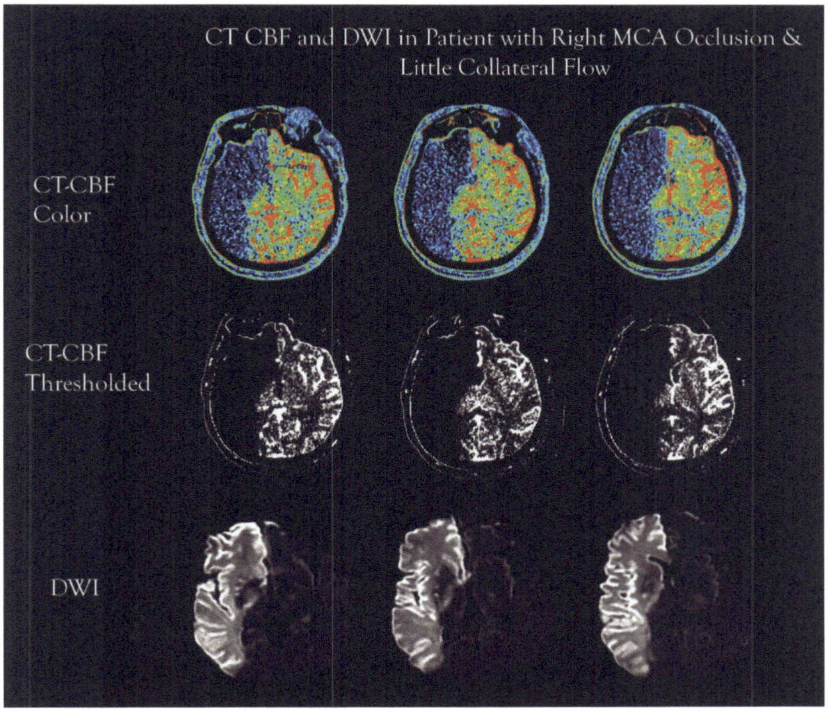

Fig. 16.9. Matching computed tomography (CT) perfusion and magnetic resonance diffusion lesions. Images are from a 61-year-old man with atrial fibrillation who stopped taking coumadin. He had a witnessed sudden onset of a left hemiparesis and was found to have a National Institutes of Health Stroke Scale of 23. A right middle cerebral artery occlusion was documented on CT angiography. Color-rendered, wide-window (top row) and 15% threshold narrow-window CT cerebral blood flow (CBF) images (middle row) are strikingly similar to the diffusion-weighted imaging abnormalities (lower row). The correspondence between the imaging methods is explained by an isolated right anterior circulation system due to an incomplete circle of Willis, resulting in little collateral flow.

common situation of significant collateral blood flow makes images from CTP much less likely to clearly delineate the infarct core (Fig. 16.10). Another reason for the adoption of CTP for core infarct estimation is its "validation" through the use of correlation and regression to compare CTP-derived images to DWI or another reference standard. Despite these efforts, a recent evidence-based analysis of diffusion and perfusion imaging in stroke by the Therapeutics and Technology Assessment Subcommittee of the American Academy of Neurology found that, while diffusion MR was a level A/class I method, there was insufficient evidence to even classify perfusion imaging (Schellinger et al., 2010).

There is no consensus on how to best apply CTP in acute stroke. Many different perfusion data acquisition parameters have been used, as well as many different data-processing methods. Additionally, different parameters (e.g., cerebral blood volume (CBV) or flow (CBF) thresholds) have been proposed for defining infarcted tissue (Dani et al., 2011). The variability in data processing has been shown to produce different results for the same patient (Konstas et al., 2009; Christensen et al., 2009). There are significant differences in opinion whether CBV or CBF is the best parameter to define the infarct core (Wintermark et al., 2006; Schaefer et al., 2008; Bivard et al., 2011; Kamalian et al., 2011), but the evidence suggests that CBF may be better. Moreover, it has been shown that different commercial software packages result in large differences in estimates of infarct size using the same patient data (Fahmi et al., 2012). Because of these difficulties there is general agreement that standardization and validation are needed for CTP (Hacke et al., 2009; Latchaw et al., 2009).

However, while CTP standardization is possible, validation of CTP as a reliable method to measure the infarct core is unlikely (Deipolyi et al., 2012; Gonzalez et al., 2013a). Copen et al. (2009) summarized the expected changes in the major CTP parameters that result from the reduced cerebral perfusion pressure that result in occlusive stroke (Fig. 16.11). This understanding informs us that CBV is unlikely to be able to reliably measure the infarct core size because the CBV may be elevated or depressed in core tissue. This prediction has been empirically confirmed, as shown in Figure 16.12 (Deipolyi et al., 2012). CBF is the only

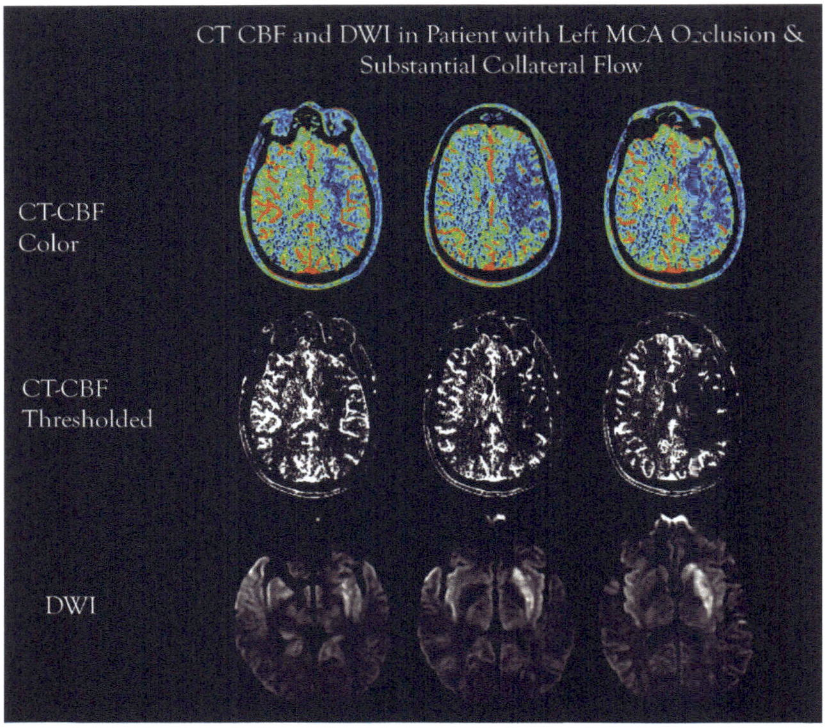

Fig. 16.10. Computed tomography (CT) perfusion and magnetic resonance diffusion lesions that do not match. Images are from a 53-year-old man who presented with aphasia and right-sided face, arm, and leg weakness the day after he had suffered whiplash in his car and sustained neck pain. CT angiography demonstrated occlusion of the left internal carotid artery from its origin to the cavernous segment, as well as in the mid to distal M1 segment of the left middle cerebral artery (MCA). Color-coded, wide-windowed (top row), and 15% thresholded, narrow-windowed (middle row) CT cerebral blood flow (CT-CBF) abnormalities appear significantly larger than the diffusion-weighted imaging (DWI) abnormalities (lower row). The lack of correspondence between the imaging methods is explained by a robust collateral flow that maintained tissue viability in the majority of the MCA territory but hemodynamically was sufficiently abnormal to produce larger apparent abnormalities on the cerebral blood flow images.

Cerebral Perfusion Pressure and Hemodynamic Parameters

	CBV	CBF	MTT	Tmax
Alternate pathway, CPP preserved	—	—	—	↑
Compensated low CPP	↑	—	↑	↑
Underperfused	↑↓	↓	↑↓	↑
Overperfused (post-ischemic hyperperfusion)	↑	↑	↑↓	↑↓

William A. Copen, MD

Fig. 16.11. Cerebral perfusion pressure (CPP) changes and resultant hemodynamic parameter changes that may occur in major anterior circulation occlusions. The change in CPP that follows a major artery occlusion may or may not be fully compensated by the collateral circulation. In each of the four scenarios, arrows indicate possible increase or decrease in cerebral blood volume (CBV), cerebral blood flow (CBF), mean transit time (MTT) and T_{max}. This is a derivation of the more detailed graph shown in the appendix (from Gonzalez et al., 2013a.)

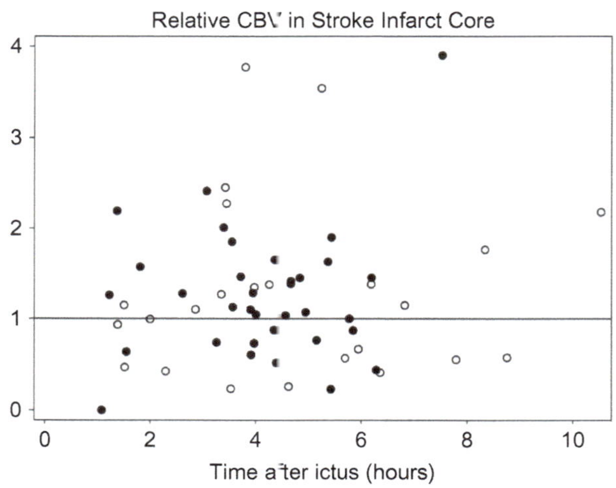

Fig. 16.12. Increased and decreased relative cerebral blood volume (CBV) at center of infarct core identified by diffusion-weighted imaging (DWI). Scatter plot of 58 patients who underwenDWI and magnetic resonance perfusion imaging within 12 hours of stroke onset. CBV in each DWI lesion's center was divided by CBV in the normal-appearing contralateral hemisphere to yield relative regional CBV. The plot demonstrates that relative CBV is not reliably decreased in the infarct core as defined by reduced diffusion. The majority of lesions demonstrated relative CBV >1, whether the patient had (filled circles) or had not (open circles) received intravenous tissue plasminogen activator. (Adapted from (Deipolyi et al., 2012.)

CTP-derived parameter that might be able to provide reliable information on infarct core size. The reasoning here is that, below a certain CBF threshold, brain tissue is very unlikely to be viable after a short period of time, such as an hour. A consideration of imaging physics related to the signal-to-noise ratio (SNR) of CTP measurements casts doubt on the reliability of this approach.

Images derived from CTP data, including CBF and CBV, are "noisy." How noise affects the appearance of a feature in an image (such as an infarct) is well understood. The processing of CTP source images into derivative images such as CBF requires certain assumptions and multiple steps. Each assumption and each processing step adds uncertainty that is reflected as noise in the final image. Added noise will reduce the contrast-to-noise ratio (CNR). It is well established that a CNR of 4 or greater allows a feature to be identified 100% of the time. A feature with any CNR of less than 4 may still be identified, but with less confidence. The CNRs of infarct cores on DWI images are substantially superior to CTP images. This is illustrated in Figure 16.13. The figure shows the DWI and CTP-derived CBF images from a patient with a documented left MCA stem occlusion. While the outline of the core is easily identified on the DWI because of a high CNR, the boundaries are unclear on the low CNR CBF images.

The inherently poor SNR of CTP-derived images is a fundamental weakness of the technique. Researchers may derive meaningful information from low SNR measurements by repeating a measurement multiple times and calculating a mean. This cannot be done with CTP scans in individual patients. Despite the poor SNR, high correlations have repeatedly been reported between CTP-derived images and a reference standard such as DWI. An example of this effect is shown in Figure 16.14 (Souza et al., 2011). Some investigators extrapolate a high correlation in a population of measurements to high accuracy of the measurement in an individual. As Bland and Altman (1986) pointed out more than 25 years ago, correlation and regression analyses are not appropriate to judge the validity of a quantitative clinical test. More appropriate are difference

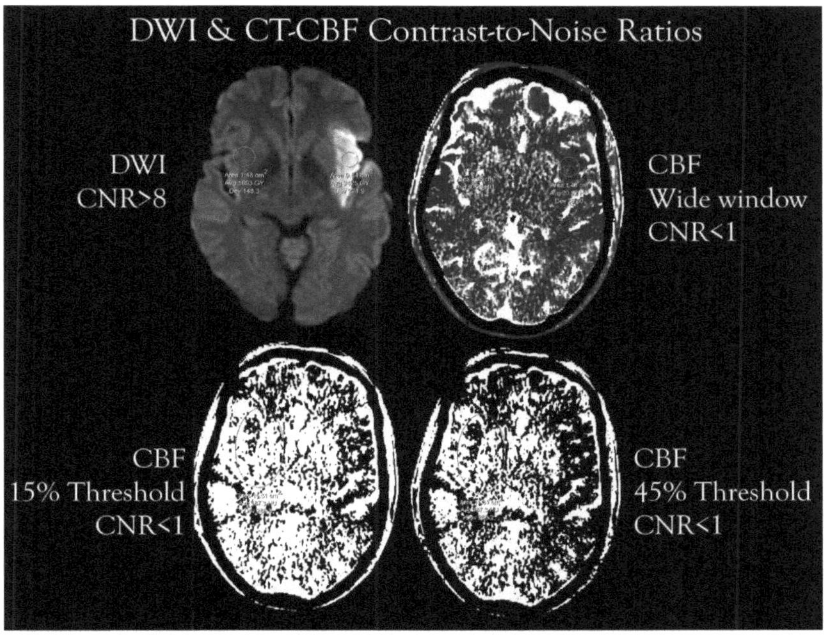

Fig. 16.13. Contrast-to-noise ratios and distinctness of infarct volume borders on diffusion-weighted imaging (DWI) and computed tomography perfusion (CTP)-derived cerebral blood flow (CBF) images. Images are from a patient with an acute stroke syndrome and documented left middle cerebral artery stem occlusion. DWI is at top left, while the others are the same CTP-derived CBF image at different window settings. The top right image is the CBF image at a wide window. The bottom left CBF image is displayed with a very narrow window, with the center set at a level of 15% of the mean signal within a normal-appearing region. The bottom right CBF image is displayed with a very narrow window with the center set at a level of 45% of the mean signal within a normal-appearing region. A region of interest (roi) was drawn within the DWI hyperintense area and the mean signal intensity and signal standard deviation from within that roi was obtained. The mean signal intensity and signal standard deviation from a roi in the contralateral hemisphere were also obtained. These values were used to calculate the signal-to-noise and contrast-to-noise ratios (CNR). A similar procedure was done on the CBF image. CNR was above 8 at the center of the DWI lesion, while it was <1 in the same region on the CBF image. The much higher clarity of the infarct border on the DWI compared to the CBF images is easily appreciated and is attributable to differences in the CNR for the respective images.

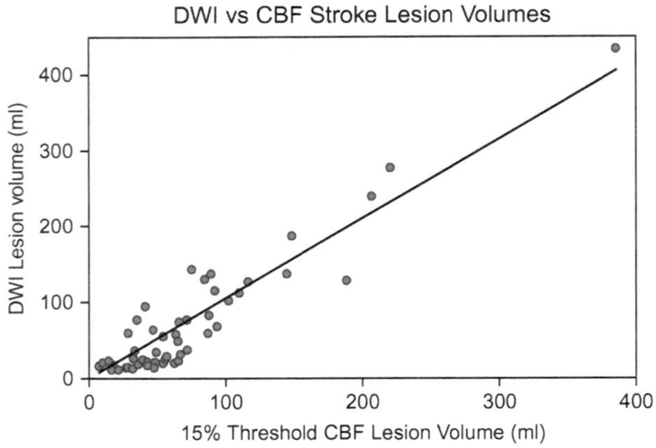

Fig. 16.14. Correlation between diffusion-weighted imaging (DWI) and computed tomography perfusion (CTP) estimates of infarct core volumes. Linear regression of admission CTP and DWI scans of 55 patients with major anterior circulation artery occlusion documented with computed tomography angiography. The core infarct was estimated by DWI by visual inspection and on CTP by applying 15% threshold (relative to normal thalamus) to the CT-cerebral blood flow (CBF) maps. A high correlation was found between the admission DWI (*y*-axis), and the 15% thresholded CT-CBF map volumes (slope = 1.1, $r^2 = 0.87$, $p < 0.001$). (Adapted from Souza et al., 2011.)

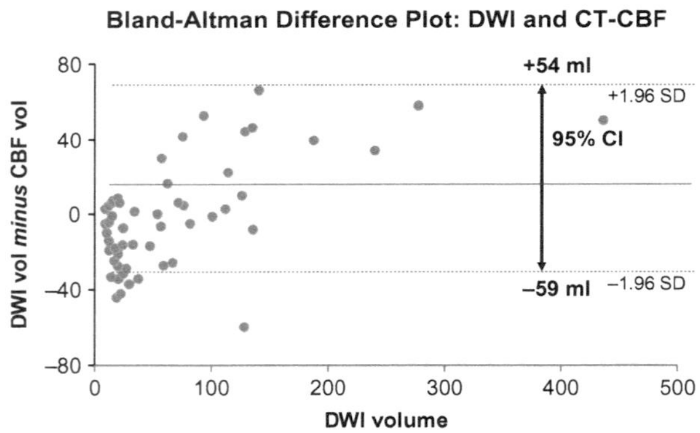

Fig. 16.15. Bland–Altman difference plot between diffusion-weighted imaging (DWI) and computed tomography perfusion (CTP) estimates of core infarct volumes. Analysis of the same data shown in Figure 16.14, assuming that the DWI lesion volume is the reference standard. The difference plot reveals that the 95% confidence interval for a cerebral blood flow (CBF)-determined volume is −59 mL to +54 mL of the same infarct core volume determined by DWI. Such a large confidence interval precludes confidence in the volume estimates given by CT-CBF measurements.

tests, as exemplified in Figure 16.15 (Souza et al., 2011), which is an analysis of the same data shown in Figure 16.14. It demonstrates that the 95% confidence limits of a core volume measurement by CBF of 70 mL would be between 11 mL and 124 mL. Such a wide confidence interval severely limits the number of patients for whom a decision could be justified on whether to proceed with endovascular therapy based on core infarct size.

Despite the high error inherent in CTP-CBF images, there are two special conditions in which such imaging may be applied successfully. One is the situation of very poor or absent collaterals, as noted above. The other circumstance is to use it to select patients with small core infarcts. When the core infarct is small, even a large error in its measurement will not result in adverse selection. This may explain the EXTENTD IA key result of small core lesions of less than 20 mL on average (Campbell et al., 2015). There is a cost to this strategy, and it is the screening out of many patients who may benefit from thrombectomy.

ESTIMATING THE PENUMBRA

The ischemic penumbra is generally defined as severely hypoperfused brain tissue that may eventually be recruited into the infarct core, in the absence of timely reperfusion (Baron, 1999). The diffusion/perfusion mismatch (as an operational penumbra) has been used to identify those patients with occlusion of the terminal ICA and/or proximal MCA who are most likely to benefit from therapy. Diffusion MRI is used to estimate the core infarct, and perfusion-weighted imaging (PWI) is used to delineate hypoperfused tissue. This approach has been successfully used in treating patients with IV t-PA outside the 3-hour limit (Ribo et al., 2005). In the DEFUSE trial (Furlan et al., 2006), it was shown that the use of t-PA after 3 hours was effective if there was a significant diffusion/perfusion mismatch that included a DWI lesion of less than 100 mL. It has also been used as inclusion criteria in successful phase II trials of desmoteplase, Desmoteplase in Acute Ischemic Stroke (DIAS) and Dose Escalation of Desmoteplase for Acute Ischemic Stroke (DEDAS) (Hacke et al., 2005; Furlan et al., 2006), in which patients were given the drug outside the 3-hour limit. Most recently, it was used in the DEFUSE II trial (Lansberg et al., 2012), in which endovascular therapy was used.

However, trial failures as well as a meta-analysis of the mismatch trials have raised questions regarding the effectiveness of the mismatch approach (Hacke et al., 2009; Mishra et al., 2010). For the reasons described above, there is concern over the reliability of perfusion imaging data (Wintermark et al., 2008), and there may be simpler alternatives. Hakimelahi et al. (2012) reported that a proximal anterior circulation artery occlusion with a DWI lesion of 70 mL or less predicts a diffusion/perfusion mismatch of at least 100%, and is a simple alternative to perfusion methods for identifying major stroke

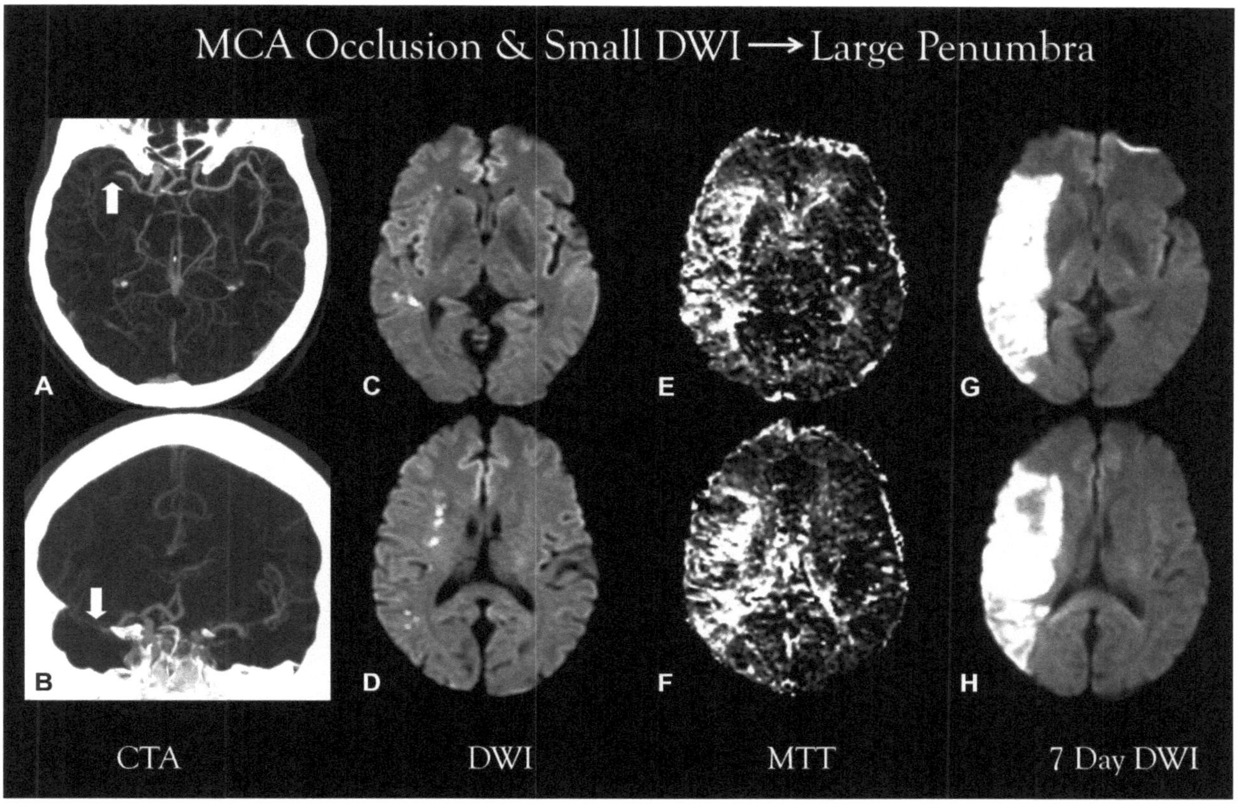

Fig. 16.16. Middle cerebral artery (MCA) occlusion and small diffusion-weighted imaging (DWI) lesion volume predicts a large penumbra. A 61-year-old male presented with left facial droop and dysarthria. (**A**, **B**) Computed tomography angiography (CTA) demonstrated a proximal right MCA occlusion (white arrows). (**C**, **D**) Initial DWI performed 12.7 hours after stroke onset showed multiple small foci of diffusion abnormality in the right centrum semiovale and corona radiata consistent with small acute infarcts. (**E**, **F**) Mean transit time (MTT) magnetic resonance perfusion map demonstrated a large volume of hypoperfusion involving the majority of the right MCA territory confirming a large penumbra. The patient did not undergo thrombolytic therapy because of the long time between stroke onset and diagnosis. (**G**, **H**) Follow-up magnetic resonance imaging showed a large increase in the infarcted tissue that now involves the majority of the right MCA territory.

patients most likely to benefit from treatment. This method takes advantage of our understanding of the relevant physiology. Occlusion of the distal ICA and/or the proximal MCA puts at risk a large brain region that typically measures well over 200 mL (van der Zwan et al., 1993). In this situation, the state of the brain depends on the vigor of the collateral flow, which determines the volumes of the infarct core and penumbra that produce the diffusion/perfusion mismatch. The collateral flow that arises after ICA/MCA occlusion makes the core and penumbra interdependent parameters (Christoforidis et al., 2005; Yoo et al., 2009). Figures 16.16 and 16.17 illustrate this principle. In both cases, the patients underwent imaging that included CTA followed by diffusion/perfusion MRI. Both patients were found to have proximal anterior circulation artery occlusion. However, one had a small DWI lesion volume (Fig. 16.16) at presentation, while the other (Fig. 16.17) had a very large DWI lesion volume.

The proposed method predicts that the patient with the small DWI lesion will have a large diffusion/perfusion mismatch, but not the patient with the large DWI abnormality. Excellent collateral flow accompanying a major occlusion will result in a small diffusion abnormality and a large mismatch (Fig. 16.16), with the opposite result in the setting of poor collateral flow (Fig. 16.17). Hakimelahi et al. (2012) reported that this simple approach predicts a diffusion/perfusion mismatch of at least 100% when the DWI is less than 70 mL (Fig. 16.18), and it is a simple alternative to perfusion methods for identifying major stroke patients most likely to benefit from treatment.

Complementary to the simple method described by Hakimelahi et al. is the clinical/DWI mismatch, which uses the fact that the neurologic examination is a sensitive indicator of reduced perfusion, and that the DWI lesion is a reliable indicator of irreversible injury. Davalos and colleagues (2004) used the NIHSS score

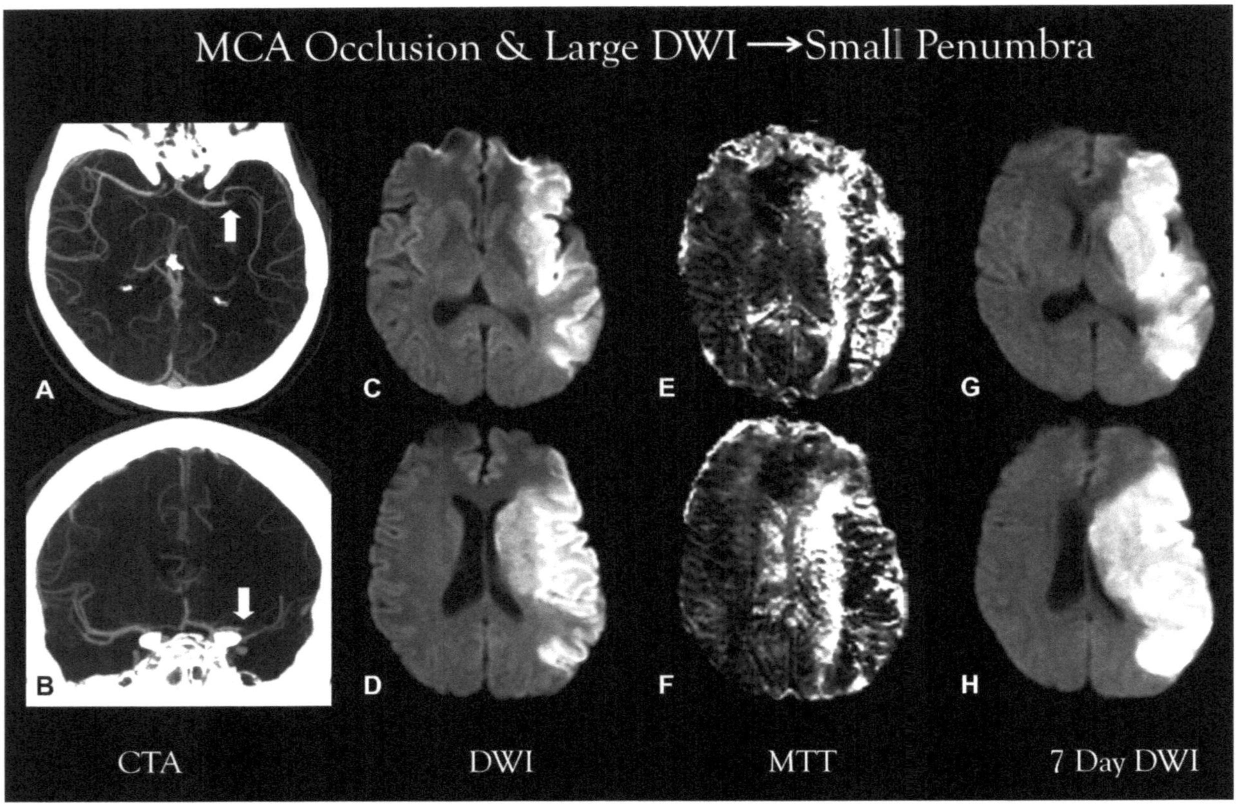

Fig. 16.17. Middle cerebral artery (MCA) occlusion and large diffusion-weighted imaging lesion volume predicts a large penumbra. A 51-year-old male presented with a right hemiparesis and aphasia. (**A**, **B**) Computed tomography angiography (CTA) demonstrated occlusion of the proximal left MCA (white arrows). (**C**, **D**) Initial DWI performed 4.8 hours after stroke onset showed large infarction involving the left MCA territory. (**E**, **F**) Magnetic resonance perfusion mean transit time (MTT) maps demonstrated abnormal transit times in almost the same area as the diffusion abnormality, confirming a small penumbra. (**G**, **H**) Follow-up magnetic resonance imaging showed no significant enlargement of the initial lesion.

and the volume of DWI lesion for this purpose. There is considerable experimental and clinical evidence supporting the use of the neurologic exam to identify in functional terms the areas of eloquent brain that have reduced perfusion. This functional penumbra is likely to be superior for outcome predictions to a volume derived from perfusion imaging because the outcomes themselves are clinical functional measurements.

MGH ACUTE STROKE IMAGING ALGORITHM

The MGH Neuroradiology Division and the Stroke Service undertook a critical evaluation of stroke imaging methods in order to develop a neuroimaging algorithm that optimizes outcomes in patients with severe ischemic strokes caused by anterior circulation occlusions (Gonzalez, 2013; Gonzalez et al., 2013a). Each method was assessed for its capability to provide reliable information on the presence of hemorrhage, the site of arterial occlusion, the extent of irreversibly injured tissue ("infarct core"), the size of the ischemic penumbra, and possible stroke treatment (Table 16.3). Based on the review of the evidence, a new imaging algorithm was adopted (Fig. 16.19). All patients presenting with a stroke syndrome undergo a neurologic evaluation, including the NIHSS, followed by an NCCT and a CTA. If the patient is eligible, t-PA is prepared while the CTA is performed, and infusion begins once it is prepared. If the CTA reveals a treatable occlusion, diffusion MRI is performed. If the DWI lesion is small (<70 mL), the patient is considered likely to benefit and proceeds to endovascular therapy, if the patient meets all other criteria for such treatment. If the DWI lesion is 70–100 mL in size, the patient is considered uncertain to benefit and will also undergo thrombectomy if there are no other negative factors that make a favorable outcome after intervention unlikely. Perfusion imaging with CT or MRI may be performed if the patient is not eligible for MRI or for intra-arterial therapy.

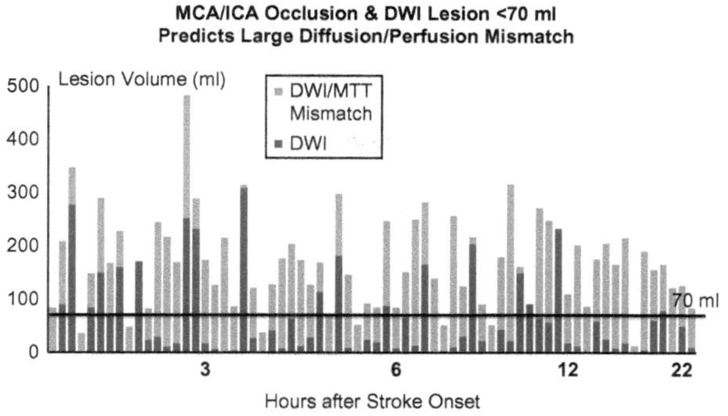

Fig. 16.18. Middle cerebral artery (MCA)/internal carotid artery (ICA) occlusion and diffusion-weighted imaging (DWI) lesion <70 mL predicts a large diffusion/perfusion mismatch. Diffusion/perfusion mismatch in 68 consecutive patients with distal ICA and/or proximal MCA occlusions that presented to the emergency department. Abnormal DWI volume of each patient is depicted as a black bar. Gray bars represent DWI/mean transit time (MTT) mismatch. The horizontal line demarcates 70 mL. There were 49 (72%) patients with volumes ≤70 mL and 19 (28%) patients with volumes >70 mL. A mismatch of 100% or greater was found in all 49 patients with DWI lesion volume ≤70 mL, but in only 4 of 19 (21%) patients with a larger DWI abnormality ($p<0.0001$). No patient with an abnormal DWI volume >100 mL had a mismatch of 100% or greater ($p<0.0001$). (Adapted from Copen et al., 2009, and Hakimelahi et al., 2012.)

An example of how the algorithm is commonly employed is shown in Figure 16.20. The management of this patient illustrates how advanced imaging can be incorporated into sophisticated stroke management without significant time delays. While this algorithm is optimized for patients who may undergo endovascular treatment, it is employed for the majority of patients with acute stroke or transient ischemic attack because it efficiently provides the maximum amount of information. The Cleveland Clinic has adopted a similar approach and demonstrated significantly better outcomes despite a sharp reduction in the number of interventions performed (Wisco et al., 2014).

TIME, IMAGING, AND OPPORTUNITIES FOR EXPANDING STROKE THERAPY

The parameter that determines treatment decisions in most acute ischemic stroke patients is the time since stroke onset. The effect of time after ictus on the odds ratio of a good outcome was demonstrated in an analysis of the original National Institute of Neurological Disorders and Stroke t-PA trial (Marler et al., 2000) and has been validated (Jauch et al., 2013). Less well validated are guidelines for endovascular therapy, although a widely used guideline is that intervention should be performed less than 8 hours after ictus. The main problem with using time as the principal parameter is that the majority of patients arrive too late to be treated. But data are emerging that show that infarct growth is highly variable, and this variability offers the opportunity to treat some – perhaps many more – patients outside the traditional time windows.

Prevalence of a significant clinical ischemic penumbra at late time points

Similar to studies based on PET, clinical investigations employing diffusion and perfusion MRI have found that a substantial proportion of patients have a small core/large penumbra many hours after the onset of stroke symptoms. Early studies involving small numbers of patients found significant diffusion/perfusion mismatches after 10 hours (Sorensen et al., 1999) and up to 24 hours (Darby et al., 1999; Neumann-Haefelin et al., 1999) after stroke onset. In a study by Ribo et al. (2005), 43 of 56 stroke patients (77%) presenting 3–6 hours after stroke onset had a large DWI/PWI mismatch of ≥50% of DWI lesion volume. Amongst the largest studies to date was a report that included 109 patients with anterior circulation strokes (Copen et al., 2009). All patients had diffusion and perfusion MRI performed within 24 hours of stroke onset, and more than 50% had DWI/mean transit time mismatch volume of 160% or greater. This mismatch was most common

Table 16.3

Identification of key factors in stroke

	Hemorrhage	Major artery occlusion	Late infarct	Early infarct core	Penumbra
CT/CTA	+	+	+	–	–
CT perfusion	–	–	–	–	+
MRI/MRA	+	+	+	+	–
MR perfusion	–	–	–	–	+
NIHSS	–	–	–	–	+

CT, computed tomography; CTA, computed tomography angiography; MRI, magnetic resonance imaging; MRA, magnetic resonance angiography; NIHSS, National Institutes of Health Stroke Scale.

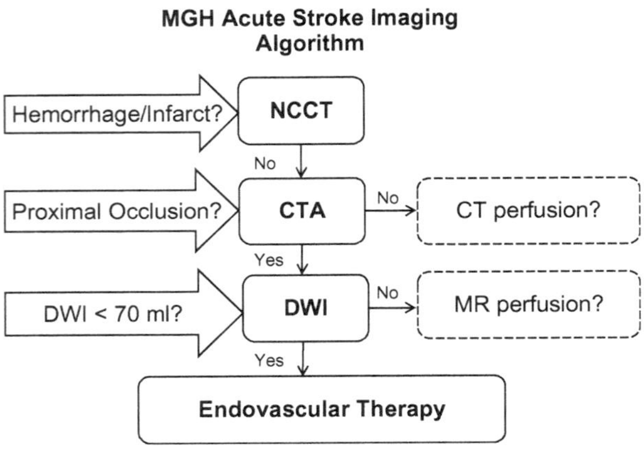

Fig. 16.19. Massachusetts General Hospital (MGH) acute ischemic stroke imaging algorithm. All patients who present with a new onset of a significant neurologic deficit undergo noncontrast computed tomography (NCCT) scan that is followed immediately by CT angiography (CTA). If hemorrhage is excluded then a head and neck CTA is performed. While the patient is undergoing CT examination, it is determined whether the patient is able to undergo magnetic resonance imaging (MRI), including that there are no contraindications to MRI. If the patient is able and the scanner is available, a diffusion MRI scan (DWI) is acquired. The next step is dependent on the findings on vessel imaging and DWI. If there is an occlusion of a major artery (internal carotid artery, proximal middle cerebral artery), and there is a small diffusion abnormality (defined as less than 70 mL in an anterior circulation stroke), then the patient is considered likely to benefit and proceeds to interventional radiology suite for endovascular therapy, if the patient meets all other criteria for such treatment. If the DWI lesion is 70–100 mL in size, the patient is considered uncertain to benefit and will also undergo thrombectomy if there are no other negative factors, such as age >80 years, National Institutes of Health Stroke Scale >20, baseline modified Rankin Scale >1 or untenable vascular anatomy that makes a favorable outcome after intervention very unlikely. If endovascular therapy is not indicated; if the DWI abnormality is large (>100 mL); or if there is no large artery occlusion, then the patient will typically proceed to MRI perfusion. CT perfusion (CTP) is provided to patients who are not able to undergo MRI. Perfusion imaging information obtained by CT or MRI may help to fully delineate the patient's physiology for consideration of other potential treatment. Patients who are eligible and are within the 4.5-hour time limit for intravenous tissue plasminogen activator will receive the treatment in the CT scanner suite before proceeding to MRI, if that is the next step.

among patients with proximal artery occlusions involving the distal ICA and/or the proximal MCA identified by CTA or MRA. Of particular interest was the observation of the presence of large mismatches many hours after ictus: 69% of patients who were scanned within 9 hours had at least a 160% mismatch, which was very similar to the 68% of patients who were scanned after 9 hours. This study suggests that persistence of mismatch after 9 hours is common and occurs most often in patients with proximal occlusions of the anterior circulation.

High variability of infarct core rate of growth

The finding that a large proportion of patients who present many hours after the onset of stroke symptoms have large diffusion/perfusion mismatches suggests that there are substantial differences in the infarct growth rates amongst patients. It is commonly assumed that infarct growth is similar amongst patients, and a widely cited rate of tissue loss is that ~1.9 million neurons are lost every minute (5.4 mL brain tissue loss per hour) (Saver, 2006). However, this estimate is an average value. Two clinical examples that illustrate the variability of the ischemic core growth rates are shown in Figures 16.21 and 16.22. The patient whose images are shown in Figure 16.21 had an apparent core infarct growth rate that is over 50 times greater than the average estimate by Saver. The opposite is illustrated in Figure 16.22. This individual, with a documented proximal right MCA occlusion, had a small DWI lesion and no detectable infarct growth over a 4-hour period. The very large difference in core infarct growth in these two patients' proximal anterior circulation occlusions is most likely due to differences in the collateral circulation which appears absent in the first patient, and well endowed in the second.

To investigate the variability in the rate of infarct growth amongst patients with severe strokes, we studied 188 consecutive patients who had occlusions of major arteries of the anterior circulation and had presented within 24 hours of stroke onset. The results are shown in Figure 16.23. While these data are from single measurements in each individual, the only explanation for these findings is that there is a very wide variability in infarct growth rates, most likely governed by wide variations in collateral circulation competency.

Stability of the clinical ischemic penumbra

Imaging studies are showing that, for many patients, core infarct growth changes at a very slow rate and may be stable for long periods. These stroke patients are sometimes referred to as "slow progressors" and must have an excellent collateral circulation that keeps the core infarct small for many hours after stroke onset (Figs 16.17 and 16.22). A few longitudinal studies have been performed that have documented the rate of change of the infarct over the first few hours and days, but they do exist. For example, the stability of ischemic core volume during the initial hours of acute large-vessel

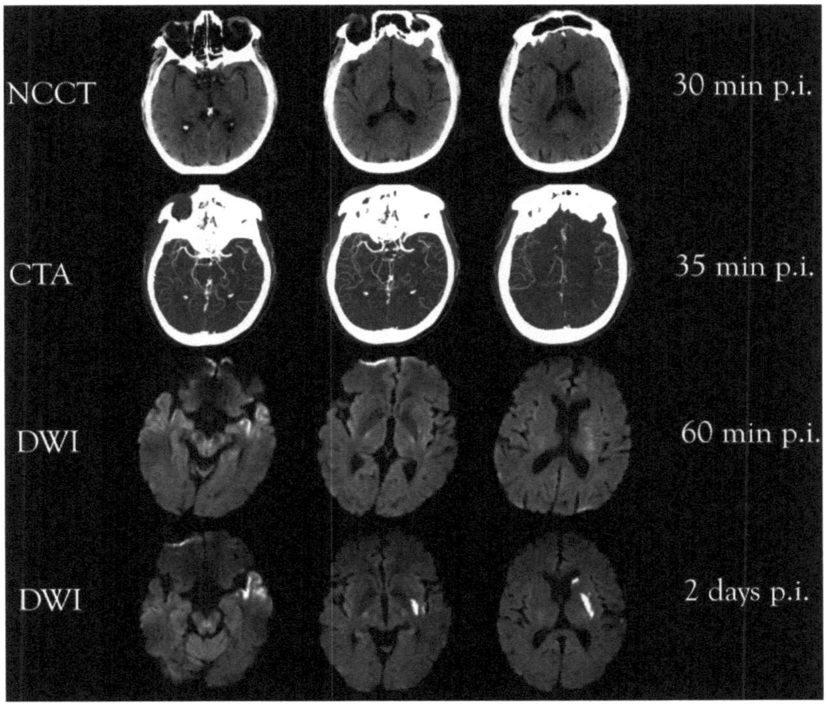

Fig. 16.20. Patient managed using Massachusetts General Hospital (MGH) acute stroke imaging algorithm. Selected images are from a 62-year-old man with a history of atrial fibrillation who had a sudden onset of right face/arm/leg weakness and aphasia who had a witnessed stroke and was immediately taken to MGH Emergency Department. The computed tomography (CT) scan was started within 15 minutes of arrival. It did not demonstrate hemorrhage or evidence of a completed infarction, but did reveal a hyperdense left middle cerebral artery. While the tissue plasminogen activator (t-PA) was being prepared, CT angiography (CTA) was performed. Intravenous administration of t-PA was begun, and review of the CTA maximum-intensity projection (MIP) images on the CT scanner console demonstrated occlusion of the M1 segment of the left middle cerebral artery. The patient was rapidly transferred to the magnetic resonance imaging (MRI) scanner and only a diffusion MR scan was performed; it revealed a small diffusion abnormality involving the left temporal lobe, and a very subtle abnormality of the left corona radiata. The patient met all the criteria for endovascular treatment and was transferred to the angiography suite, where successful recanalization of the left middle cerebral artery was achieved approximately 3 hours after stroke onset. The patient made a complete recovery at the time of the follow-up MRI 2 days later, which showed small infarctions of the left temporal lobe, basal ganglia, and corona radiata. NCCT, noncontrast computed tomography; DWI, diffusion-weighted imaging.

ischemic stroke in a subgroup of mechanically revascularized patients has been reported (Finitsis et al., 2014).

A remarkable degree of core infarct stability was observed in a prospective study designed to study the effect of normobaric oxygen (Gonzalez et al., 2010). Patients underwent a diffusion-perfusion imaging at study entry, at 4 hours, and at 24 hours after the initial study; a final scan was performed 1 week later. There were 14 patients with ICA and/or proximal MCA occlusion. In these patients there was no significant interval change in the mean abnormal DWI volume (29.4 vs 28.1 mL) or abnormal mean transit time volumes (137 vs 130.9 mL). By 24 hours, only two patients did not maintain a mismatch of 20% or greater. Figure 16.23 displays DWI data from the first three time points. The stability of the penumbra in these patients was most likely due to excellent collateral circulation. To be eligible for the study, patients had to be outside the therapeutic window for thrombolysis, have an MCA occlusion, and have a large diffusion–perfusion mismatch. These criteria resulted in selection for patients with a stable clinical ischemic penumbra. These results were replicated and extended in another study of normobaric oxygen (Singhal, 2006). Inclusion criteria for these patients were that they were not eligible for IV t-PA, but a specific occlusion or diffusion/perfusion mismatch was not required. Patients underwent DWI/PWI at presentation and at multiple times for up to 48 hours. Approximately one-third of the total, 38 patients, presented with occlusions of a distal ICA and/or proximal MCA. Remarkably, over 80% had stable or slow growth of the DWI lesion volume over 24 hours. DWI lesion growth data from a subset of these patients are shown in Figure 16.24 (Singhal, 2006).

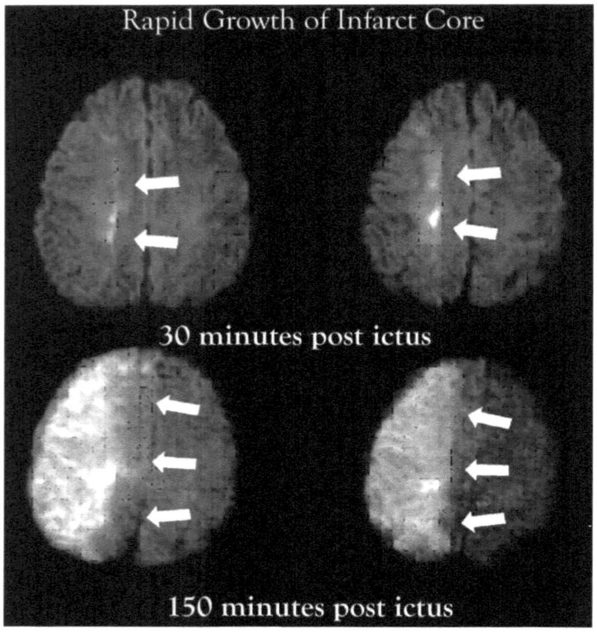

Fig. 16.21. High rate of infarct growth. Diffusion-weighted imaging (DWI) is from a young woman who presented with a right cervical internal carotid artery dissection. She had a sudden onset of a left hemiplegia while being examined by a neurologist. DWI performed 30 minutes after hemiplegia onset demonstrated DWI lesions in a watershed distribution. Repeat DWI at 150 minutes after ictus demonstrated severe reduction in the diffusion of water throughout the right cerebral hemisphere. The very high rate of infarct growth in this individual is nearly 50 times higher than the average infarct growth estimated by Saver (2006).

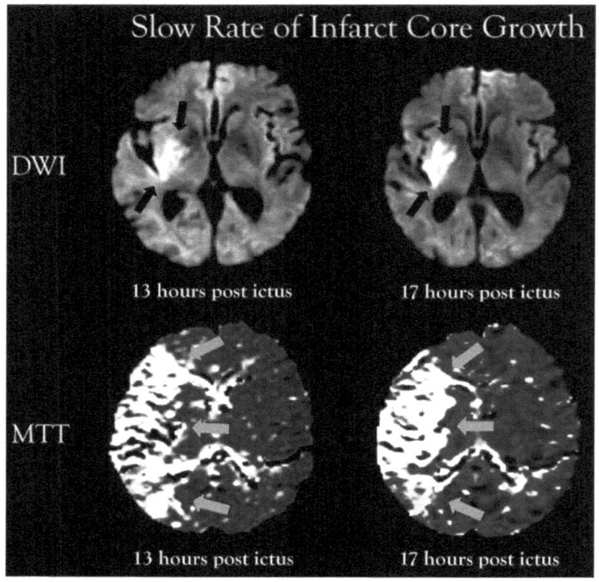

Fig. 16.22. Slow infarct growth rate. A 72-year-old woman presented 13 hours after stroke onset with left-sided weakness and neglect (National Institutes of Health Stroke Scale of 11). Computed tomography angiography revealed occlusion of the right middle cerebral artery. Diffusion and perfusion studies revealed a small diffusion abnormality (top left) and a very large perfusion abnormality (bottom left). Repeat study performed 4 hours after the initial imaging study showed very little growth in the size of the diffusion abnormality (top right), despite the persistence of a very large perfusion abnormality (bottom right). The stability of the small infarct core is most likely due to a good collateral circulation. MTT, mean transit time.

These data indicate that a robust collateral circulation capable of keeping the infarct core stable for many hours exists for many patients, possibly the majority of them. Consideration of these with studies published by several groups (Ribo et al., 2005; Copen et al., 2009; Finitsis et al., 2014) suggests that there may be opportunities to successfully treat many more patients than are permitted by current time restrictions. It reinforces the arguments put forth by Baron et al. (1995) that strict reliance on time alone in the management of patients with ischemic stroke is perhaps ill considered, and may lead to circumstances in which institutions are not properly prepared to help a significant number of patients who could benefit by treatment of a major artery occlusion, even many hours after the onset of symptoms.

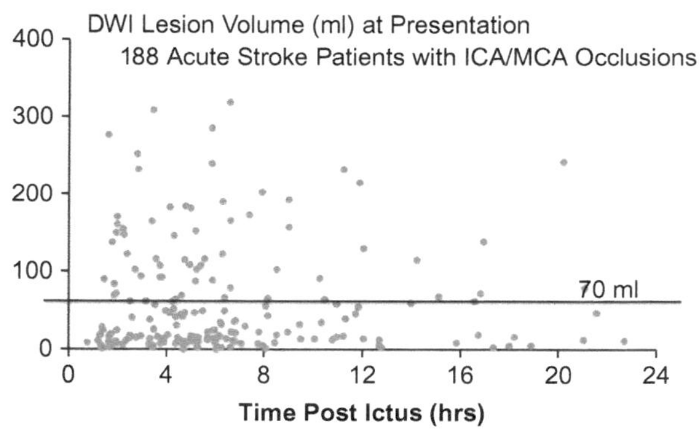

Fig. 16.23. No correlation between infarct core volume and time since stroke onset in patients with major anterior circulation occlusions. Scatter plot of diffusion-weighted imaging (DWI) lesion volumes of 188 patients with acute stroke syndromes who presented to the emergency department. All had M1-segment middle cerebral artery (MCA) and/or distal internal carotid artery (ICA) occlusion documented by computed tomography angiography or magnetic resonance angiography. The data are from consecutive patients in two separate time periods of 18 and 22 months. There was no correlation between core infarct size and time since stroke onset ($r^2 < 0.001; p > 0.5$).

Using imaging to "witness" time of stroke onset

An important new application of imaging to inform stroke treatment decisions is using MRI to estimate the time of stroke onset in patients with an unknown time

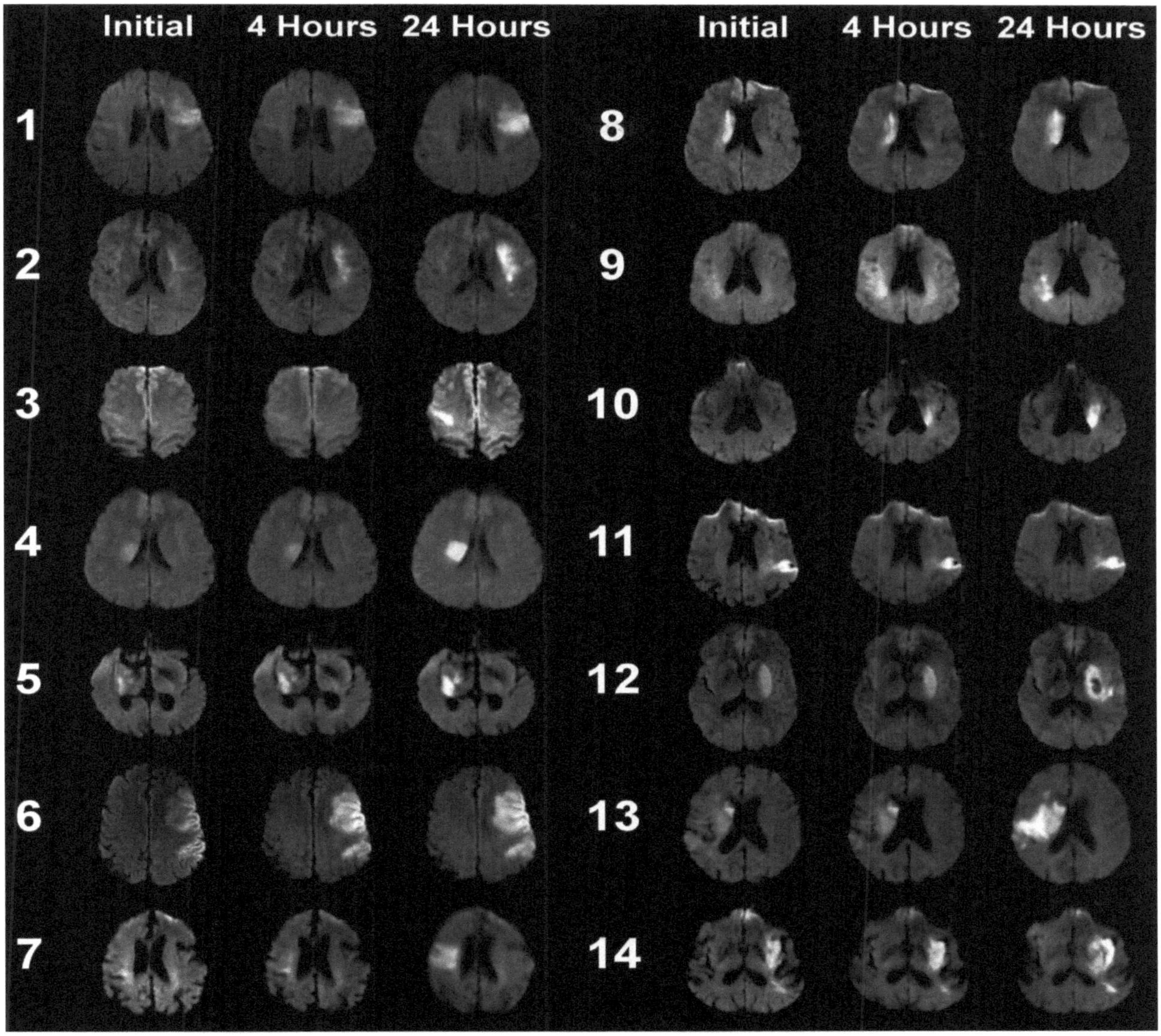

Fig. 16.24. Stability of diffusion abnormalities for 4 or more hours in patients with proximal middle cerebral artery (MCA) occlusions. Serial magnetic resonance imaging scans that included diffusion and perfusion were acquired in 14 patients. Patients presented an average of 7.1 hours after stroke onset. All 14 patients had proximal MCA occlusion and were not eligible for thrombolytic therapy. All 14 patients had large perfusion abnormalities. Imaging performed ~4 hours after the initial study demonstrates striking stability in nearly all the patients. At 24 hours there is significant growth of the diffusion abnormality in several of the patients. This study is fully described in Gonzalez et al. (2010).

of ictus. This approach exploits the observation that fluid-attenuated inversion recovery (FLAIR) signal abnormalities become apparent several hours after the diffusion signal changes. In a large retrospective study, Thomalla et al. (2011) reported that a DWI-FLAIR mismatch identified patients within 4.5 hours of symptom onset with 62% sensitivity, 78% specificity, 83% positive predictive value, and 54% negative predictive value. These observations have led to clinical trials to see if it is safe and effective to give IV recombinant t-PA to people with unwitnessed stroke but with MRI evidence of early ischemic stroke. One of these trials is MR Witness, which is a multicenter, open-label, phase IIa safety study in adult acute ischemic stroke patients to determine if it is safe to extend IV thrombolytic treatment to subjects who are evaluated within 24 hours from when last known well, and eligible to receive thrombolytic treatment within 4.5 hours from symptom discovery with the assistance of an MRI-based "witness" when no human witness of stroke onset is available (Schwamm, 2011). The study is designed to investigate the safety in using standard diagnostic MRI in selecting patients for thrombolytic therapy when the last-known-well time places the patient beyond the current IV thrombolytic time window.

CONCLUSIONS

Imaging the acute ischemic stroke patient with CT and MRI provides valuable diagnostic and prognostic information. These technologies can inform on the presence of hemorrhage, vessel occlusion, irreversible injury, and tissue at risk, which are of great importance for making the most appropriate management decisions. CT and MRI provide complementary information, and the most comprehensive understanding of the state of the brain in the patient with a stroke syndrome is attained using both. It may not be possible to employ both, so a clear understanding of the limits of only using one is essential in making clinical decisions. Much progress has been made in treating stroke, and new insights on stoke physiology, especially on the presence of robust collateral circulations, in individual patients provided by imaging suggest that there are major opportunities to effectively treat many more patients.

ACKNOWLEDGMENT

The authors wish to thank Dr. Julian He for his many efforts in the preparation of this manuscript.

References

Adams Jr HP, Davis PH, Leira EC et al. (1999). Baseline NIH Stroke Scale score strongly predicts outcome after stroke: a report of the Trial of Org 10172 in Acute Stroke Treatment (TOAST). Neurology 53: 126–131.

Almandoz DJE, Kamalian S, Lev MH et al. (2011). Acute Ischemic Stroke Imaging and Intervention, Springer, Berlin.

Baron JC (1999). Mapping the ischaemic penumbra with PET: implications for acute stroke treatment. Cerebrovasc Dis 9: 193–201.

Baron JC, von Kummer R, del Zoppo GJ (1995). Treatment of acute ischemic stroke. Challenging the concept of a rigid and universal time window. Stroke 26: 2219–2221.

Bash S, Villablanca JP, Jahan R et al. (2005). Intracranial vascular stenosis and occlusive disease: evaluation with CT angiography, MR angiography, and digital subtraction angiography. AJNR Am J Neuroradiol 26: 1012–1021.

Bell BA, Symon L, Branston NM (1985). CBF and time thresholds for the formation of ischemic cerebral edema, and effect of reperfusion in baboons. J Neurosurg 62: 31–41.

Berkhemer OA, Fransen PS, Beumer D et al. (2015). A randomized trial of intraarterial treatment for acute ischemic stroke. N Engl J Med 372: 11–20.

Bivard A, McElduff P, Spratt N et al. (2011). Defining the extent of irreversible brain ischemia using perfusion computed tomography. Cerebrovasc Dis 31: 238–245.

Bland JM, Altman DG (1986). Statistical methods for assessing agreement between two methods of clinical measurement. Lancet 1: 307–310.

Broderick JP, Palesch YY, Demchuk AM et al. (2013). Endovascular therapy after intravenous t-PA versus t-PA alone for stroke. N Engl J Med 368: 893–903.

Campbell BC, Purushotham A, Christensen S et al. (2012). The infarct core is well represented by the acute diffusion lesion: sustained reversal is infrequent. J Cereb Blood Flow Metab 32: 50–56.

Campbell BC, Mitchell PJ, Kleinig TJ et al. (2015). Endovascular therapy for ischemic stroke with perfusion-imaging selection. N Engl J Med 372: 1009–1018.

Chang KC, Tseng MC, Weng HH et al. (2002). Prediction of length of stay of first-ever ischemic stroke. Stroke 33: 2670–2674.

Christensen S, Mouridsen K, Wu O et al. (2009). Comparison of 10 perfusion MRI parameters in 97 sub-6-hour stroke patients using voxel-based receiver operating characteristics analysis. Stroke 40: 2055–2061.

Christoforidis GA, Mohammad Y, Kehagias D et al. (2005). Angiographic assessment of pial collaterals as a prognostic indicator following intra-arterial thrombolysis for acute ischemic stroke. AJNR Am J Neuroradiol 26: 1789–1797.

Cipriano LE, Steinberg ML, Gazelle GS et al. (2009). Comparing and predicting the costs and outcomes of patients with major and minor stroke using the Boston Acute Stroke Imaging Scale neuroimaging classification system. AJNR Am J Neuroradiol 30: 703–709.

Copen WA, Rezai Gharai L, Barak ER et al. (2009). Existence of the diffusion-perfusion mismatch within 24 hours after onset of acute stroke: dependence on proximal arterial occlusion. Radiology 250: 878–886.

Dani KA, Thomas RG, Chappell FM et al. (2011). Computed tomography and magnetic resonance perfusion imaging in ischemic stroke: definitions and thresholds. Ann Neurol 70: 384–401.

Darby DG, Barber PA, Gerraty RP et al. (1999). Pathophysiological topography of acute ischemia by combined diffusion-weighted and perfusion MRI. Stroke 30: 2043–2052.

Davalos A, Blanco M, Pedraza S et al. (2004). The clinical-DWI mismatch: a new diagnostic approach to the brain tissue at risk of infarction. Neurology 62: 2187–2192.

Deipolyi AR, Wu O, Macklin EA et al. (2012). Reliability of cerebral blood volume maps as a substitute for diffusion-weighted imaging in acute ischemic stroke. J Magn Reson Imaging 36: 1083–1087.

Dzialowski I, Weber J, Doerfler A et al. (2004). Brain tissue water uptake after middle cerebral artery occlusion assessed with CT. J Neuroimaging 14: 42–48.

Fahmi F, Marquering HA, Streekstra GJ et al. (2012). Differences in CT perfusion summary maps for patients with acute ischemic stroke generated by 2 software packages. AJNR Am J Neuroradiol 33: 2074–2080.

Fiebach JB, Schellinger PD, Jansen O et al. (2002). CT and diffusion-weighted MR imaging in randomized order: diffusion-weighted imaging results in higher accuracy and lower interrater variability in the diagnosis of hyperacute ischemic stroke. Stroke 33: 2206–2210.

Fiehler J, Foth M, Kucinski T et al. (2002). Severe ADC decreases do not predict irreversible tissue damage in humans. Stroke 33: 79–86.

Finitsis S, Kemmling A, Havemeister S et al. (2014). Stability of ischemic core volume during the initial hours of acute large vessel ischemic stroke in a subgroup of mechanically revascularized patients. Neuroradiology 56 (4): 325–332.

Furlan A, Higashida R, Wechsler L et al. (1999). Intra-arterial prourokinase for acute ischemic stroke. The PROACT II study: a randomized controlled trial. Prolyse in Acute Cerebral Thromboembolism. JAMA 282: 2003–2011.

Furlan AJ, Eyding D, Albers GW et al. (2006). Dose Escalation of Desmoteplase for Acute Ischemic Stroke (DEDAS): evidence of safety and efficacy 3 to 9 hours after stroke onset. Stroke 37: 1227–1231.

Gonzalez RG (2013). Current state of acute stroke imaging. Stroke 44: 3260–3264.

Gonzalez RG, Schaefer PW, Buonanno FS et al. (1999). Diffusion-weighted MR imaging: diagnostic accuracy in patients imaged within 6 hours of stroke symptom onset. Radiology 210: 155–162.

Gonzalez RG, Hakimelahi R, Schaefer PW et al. (2010). Stability of large diffusion/perfusion mismatch in anterior circulation strokes for 4 or more hours. BMC Neurol 10: 13.

Gonzalez RG, Lev MH, Goldmacher GV et al. (2012). Improved outcome prediction using CT angiography in addition to standard ischemic stroke assessment: results from the STOPStroke study. PLoS One 7: e30352.

Gonzalez RG, Copen WA, Schaefer PW et al. (2013a). The Massachusetts General Hospital acute stroke imaging algorithm: an experience and evidence based approach. J Neurointerv Surg 5 (Suppl 1): i7–i12.

Gonzalez RG, Furie KL, Goldmacher GV et al. (2013b). Good outcome rate of 35% in IV-tPA-treated patients with computed tomography angiography confirmed severe anterior circulation occlusive stroke. Stroke 44: 3109–3113.

Goyal M, Demchuk AM, Menon BK et al. (2015). Randomized assessment of rapid endovascular treatment of ischemic stroke. N Engl J Med 372: 1019–1030.

Grant PE, He J, Halpern EF et al. (2001). Frequency and clinical context of decreased apparent diffusion coefficient reversal in the human brain. Radiology 221: 43–50.

Guadagno JV, Warburton EA, Jones PS et al. (2005). The diffusion-weighted lesion in acute stroke: heterogeneous patterns of flow/metabolism uncoupling as assessed by quantitative positron emission tomography. Cerebrovasc Dis 19: 239–246.

Hacke W, Albers G, Al-Rawi Y et al. (2005). The Desmoteplase in Acute Ischemic Stroke Trial (DIAS): a phase II MRI-based 9-hour window acute stroke thrombolysis trial with intravenous desmoteplase. Stroke 36: 66–73.

Hacke W, Furlan AJ, Al-Rawi Y et al. (2009). Intravenous desmoteplase in patients with acute ischaemic stroke selected by MRI perfusion-diffusion weighted imaging or perfusion CT (DIAS-2): a prospective, randomised, double-blind, placebo-controlled study. Lancet Neurol 8: 141–150.

Hakimelahi R, Yoo AJ, He J et al. (2012). Rapid identification of a major diffusion/perfusion mismatch in distal internal carotid artery or middle cerebral artery ischemic stroke. BMC Neurol 12: 132.

Hill MD, Rowley HA, Adler F et al. (2003). Selection of acute ischemic stroke patients for intra-arterial thrombolysis with pro-urokinase by using ASPECTS. Stroke 34: 1925–1931.

Hill MD, Demchuk AM, Tomsick TA et al. (2006). Using the baseline CT scan to select acute stroke patients for IV-IA therapy. AJNR Am J Neuroradiol 27: 1612–1616.

Jauch EC, Saver JL, Adams Jr HP et al. (2013). Guidelines for the early management of patients with acute ischemic stroke: a guideline for healthcare professionals from the American Heart Association/American Stroke Association. Stroke 44: 870–947.

Johnston KC, Connors Jr AF, Wagner DP et al. (2003). Predicting outcome in ischemic stroke: external validation of predictive risk models. Stroke 34: 200–202.

Jovin TG, Yonas H, Gebel JM et al. (2003). The cortical ischemic core and not the consistently present penumbra is a determinant of clinical outcome in acute middle cerebral artery occlusion. Stroke 34: 2426–2433.

Kamalian S, Maas MB, Goldmacher GV et al. (2011). CT cerebral blood flow maps optimally correlate with admission diffusion-weighted imaging in acute stroke but thresholds vary by postprocessing platform. Stroke 42: 1923–1928.

Kidwell CS, Saver JL, Mattiello J et al. (2000). Thrombolytic reversal of acute human cerebral ischemic injury shown by diffusion/perfusion magnetic resonance imaging. Ann Neurol 47: 462–469.

Kidwell CS, Saver JL, Starkman S et al. (2002). Late secondary ischemic injury in patients receiving intraarterial thrombolysis. Ann Neurol 52: 698–703.

Kidwell CS, Jahan R, Gornbein J et al. (2013). A trial of imaging selection and endovascular treatment for ischemic stroke. N Engl J Med 368: 914–923.

Kim AC, Vu D, González RG et al. (2011). Acute Ischemic Stroke Imaging and Intervention, Springer, Berlin.

Konstas AA, Goldmakher GV, Lee TY et al. (2009). Theoretic basis and technical implementations of CT perfusion in acute ischemic stroke, part 2: technical implementations. AJNR Am J Neuroradiol 30: 885–892.

Konstas AA, González RG, Lev MH (2011). Acute Ischemic Stroke Imaging and Intervention, Springer, Berlin.

Lansberg MG, Thijs VN, Bammer R et al. (2007). Risk factors of symptomatic intracerebral hemorrhage after tPA therapy for acute stroke. Stroke 38: 2275–2278.

Lansberg MG, Straka M, Kemp S et al. (2012). MRI profile and response to endovascular reperfusion after stroke (DEFUSE 2): a prospective cohort study. Lancet Neurol 11: 860–867.

Latchaw RE, Alberts MJ, Lev MH et al. (2009). Recommendations for imaging of acute ischemic stroke: a scientific statement from the American Heart Association. Stroke 40: 3646–3678.

Lev MH, Farkas J, Gemmete JJ et al. (1999). Acute stroke: improved nonenhanced CT detection – benefits of soft-copy interpretation by using variable window width and center level settings. Radiology 213: 150–155.

Lev MH, Farkas J, Rodriguez VR et al. (2001). CT angiography in the rapid triage of patients with hyperacute stroke to intraarterial thrombolysis: accuracy in the detection of large vessel thrombus. J Comput Assist Tomogr 25: 520–528.

Liebeskind DS, Sanossian N, Yong WH et al. (2011). CT and MRI early vessel signs reflect clot composition in acute stroke. Stroke 42: 1237–1243.

Lovblad KO, Laubach HJ, Baird AE et al. (1998). Clinical experience with diffusion-weighted MR in patients with acute stroke. AJNR Am J Neuroradiol 19: 1061–1066.

Marder VJ, Chute DJ, Starkman S et al. (2006). Analysis of thrombi retrieved from cerebral arteries of patients with acute ischemic stroke. Stroke 37: 2086–2093.

Marks MP (1998). CT in ischemic stroke. Neuroimaging Clin N Am 8: 515–523.

Marler JR, Tilley BC, Lu M et al. (2000). Early stroke treatment associated with better outcome: the NINDS rt-PA stroke study. Neurology 55: 1649–1655.

Mishra NK, Albers GW, Davis SM et al. (2010). Mismatch-based delayed thrombolysis: a meta-analysis. Stroke 41: e25–e33.

Mullins ME, Schaefer PW, Sorensen AG et al. (2002). CT and conventional and diffusion-weighted MR imaging in acute stroke: study in 691 patients at presentation to the emergency department. Radiology 224: 353–360.

Neumann-Haefelin T, Wittsack HJ, Wenserski F et al. (1999). Diffusion- and perfusion-weighted MRI. The DWI/PWI mismatch region in acute stroke. Stroke 30: 1591–1597.

Neumann-Haefelin T, Wittsack HJ, Wenserski F et al. (2000). Diffusion- and perfusion-weighted MRI in a patient with a prolonged reversible ischaemic neurological deficit. Neuroradiology 42: 444–447.

Nogueira RG, Lutsep HL, Gupta R et al. (2012). Trevo versus Merci retrievers for thrombectomy revascularisation of large vessel occlusions in acute ischaemic stroke (TREVO 2): a randomised trial. Lancet 380: 1231–1240.

Oppenheim C, Lamy C, Touze E et al. (2006). Do transient ischemic attacks with diffusion-weighted imaging abnormalities correspond to brain infarctions? AJNR Am J Neuroradiol 27: 1782–1787.

Parsons M, Spratt N, Bivard A et al. (2012). A randomized trial of tenecteplase versus alteplase for acute ischemic stroke. N Engl J Med 366: 1099–1107.

Perkins CJ, Kahya E, Roque CT et al. (2001). Fluid-attenuated inversion recovery and diffusion- and perfusion-weighted MRI abnormalities in 117 consecutive patients with stroke symptoms. Stroke 32: 2774–2781.

Pomerantz SR, Harris GJ, Desai HJ et al. (2006). Computed tomography angiography and computed tomography perfusion in ischemic stroke: a step-by-step approach to image acquisition and three-dimensional postprocessing. Semin Ultrasound CT MR 27: 243–270.

Pulli B, Schaefer PW, Hakimelahi R et al. (2012). Acute ischemic stroke: infarct core estimation on CT angiography source images depends on CT angiography protocol. Radiology 262: 593–604.

Ribo M, Molina CA, Rovira A et al. (2005). Safety and efficacy of intravenous tissue plasminogen activator stroke treatment in the 3- to 6-hour window using multimodal transcranial Doppler/MRI selection protocol. Stroke 36: 602–606.

Riedel CH, Jensen U, Rohr A et al. (2010). Assessment of thrombus in acute middle cerebral artery occlusion using thin-slice nonenhanced computed tomography reconstructions. Stroke 41: 1659–1664.

Riedel CH, Zimmermann P, Jensen-Kondering U et al. (2011). The importance of size: successful recanalization by intravenous thrombolysis in acute anterior stroke depends on thrombus length. Stroke 42: 1775–1777.

Rundek T, Mast H, Hartmann A et al. (2000). Predictors of resource use after acute hospitalization: the Northern Manhattan Stroke Study. Neurology 55: 1180–1187.

Sanak D, Nosal V, Horak D et al. (2006). Impact of diffusion-weighted MRI-measured initial cerebral infarction volume on clinical outcome in acute stroke patients with middle cerebral artery occlusion treated by thrombolysis. Neuroradiology 48: 632–639.

Saver JL (2006). Time is brain – quantified. Stroke 37: 263–266.

Saver JL, Jahan R, Levy EI et al. (2012). Solitaire flow restoration device versus the Merci Retriever in patients with acute ischaemic stroke (SWIFT): a randomised, parallel-group, non-inferiority trial. Lancet 380: 1241–1249.

Schaefer PW, Barak ER, Kamalian S et al. (2008). Quantitative assessment of core/penumbra mismatch in acute stroke: CT and MR perfusion imaging are strongly correlated when sufficient brain volume is imaged. Stroke 39: 2986–2992.

Schellinger PD, Bryan RN, Caplan LR et al. (2010). Evidence-based guideline: The role of diffusion and perfusion MRI for the diagnosis of acute ischemic stroke: report of the Therapeutics and Technology Assessment Subcommittee of the American Academy of Neurology. Neurology 75: 177–185.

Schwamm L (2011). MR WITNESS: A Study of Intravenous Thrombolysis With Alteplase in MRI-Selected Patients (MR WITNESS) trial. Available online at http://www.clinicaltrials.gov/show/NCT01282242.

Shimosegawa E, Hatazawa J, Ibaraki M et al. (2005). Metabolic penumbra of acute brain infarction: a correlation with infarct growth. Ann Neurol 57: 495–504.

Sims JR, Gharai LR, Schaefer PW et al. (2009). ABC/2 for rapid clinical estimate of infarct, perfusion, and mismatch volumes. Neurology 72: 2104–2110.

Singer MB, Chong J, Lu D et al. (1998). Diffusion-weighted MRI in acute subcortical infarction. Stroke 29: 133–136.

Singer OC, Humpich MC, Fiehler J et al. (2008). Risk for symptomatic intracerebral hemorrhage after thrombolysis assessed by diffusion-weighted magnetic resonance imaging. Ann Neurol 63: 52–60.

Singhal AB (2006). Normobaric oxygen therapy in acute ischemic stroke trial [online]. In: ClinicalTrials.gov [Internet],

National Library of Medicine (US), Bethesda (MD). 2000- [cited 2013 April 6], http://clinicaltrials.gov/show/NCT0041 4726. NLM Identifier: NCT00414726..

Sorensen AG, Copen WA, Ostergaard L et al. (1999). Hyperacute stroke: simultaneous measurement of relative cerebral blood volume, relative cerebral blood flow, and mean tissue transit time. Radiology 210: 519–527.

Souza L, Lev M, Franceschi A et al. (Nov. 27-Dec. 2 2011). Thresholded CTP maps can accurately determine infarct core when dwi is unavailable, and have similar specificity in identifying patients unlikely to benefit from thrombolysis. In: 97th RSNA Scientific Assembly and Annual Meeting, RSNA, Chicago, IL, USA. 84.

Thomalla G, Cheng B, Ebinger M et al. (2011). DWI-FLAIR mismatch for the identification of patients with acute ischaemic stroke within 4.5 h of symptom onset (PRE-FLAIR): a multicentre observational study. Lancet Neurol 10: 978–986.

Tomanek AI, Coutts SB, Demchuk AM et al. (2006). MR angiography compared to conventional selective angiography in acute stroke. Can J Neurol Sci 33: 58–62.

Torack RM, Alcala H, Gado M et al. (1976). Correlative assay of computerized cranial tomography CCT, water content and specific gravity in normal and pathological postmortem brain. J Neuropathol Exp Neurol 35: 385–392.

Torres-Mozqueda F, He J, Yeh IB et al. (2008). An acute ischemic stroke classification instrument that includes CT or MR angiography: the Boston Acute Stroke Imaging Scale. AJNR Am J Neuroradiol 29: 1111–1117.

Unger E, Littlefield J, Gado M (1988). Water content and water structure in CT and MR signal changes: possible influence in detection of early stroke. AJNR Am J Neuroradiol 9: 687–691.

Urbach H, Flacke S, Keller E et al. (2000). Detectability and detection rate of acute cerebral hemisphere infarcts on CT and diffusion-weighted MRI. Neuroradiology 42: 722–727.

van der Zwan A, Hillen B, Tulleken CA et al. (1993). A quantitative investigation of the variability of the major cerebral arterial territories. Stroke 24: 1951–1959.

van Everdingen KJ, van der Grond J, Kappelle LJ et al. (1998). Diffusion-weighted magnetic resonance imaging in acute stroke. Stroke 29: 1783–1790.

Wintermark M, Flanders AE, Velthuis B et al. (2006). Perfusion-CT assessment of infarct core and penumbra: receiver operating characteristic curve analysis in 130 patients suspected of acute hemispheric stroke. Stroke 37: 979–985.

Wintermark M, Albers GW, Alexandrov AV et al. (2008). Acute stroke imaging research roadmap. AJNR Am J Neuroradiol 29: e23–e30.

Wisco D, Uchino K, Saqqur M et al. (2014). Addition of hyperacute MRI AIDS in patient selection, decreasing the use of endovascular stroke therapy. Stroke 45: 467–472.

Yoo AJ, Verduzco LA, Schaefer PW et al. (2009). MRI-based selection for intra-arterial stroke therapy: value of pretreatment diffusion-weighted imaging lesion volume in selecting patients with acute stroke who will benefit from early recanalization. Stroke 40: 2046–2054.

Yoo AJ, Barak ER, Copen WA et al. (2010). Combining acute diffusion-weighted imaging and mean transmit time lesion volumes with National Institutes of Health Stroke Scale Score improves the prediction of acute stroke outcome. Stroke 41: 1728–1735.

Yoo AJ, Chaudhry ZA, Nogueira RG et al. (2012). Infarct volume is a pivotal biomarker after intra-arterial stroke therapy. Stroke 43: 1323–1330.

Yoo AJ, Heck DV, Frei D et al. (2013). Preliminary clot length analysis of anterior circulation large vessel occlusions. Stroke 44: A193.

Yuki I, Kan I, Vinters HV et al. (2012). The impact of thromboemboli histology on the performance of a mechanical thrombectomy device. AJNR Am J Neuroradiol 33: 643–648.

Zaidi SF, Aghaebrahim A, Urra X et al. (2012). Final infarct volume is a stronger predictor of outcome than recanalization in patients with proximal middle cerebral artery occlusion treated with endovascular therapy. Stroke 43: 3238–3244.

Handbook of Clinical Neurology, Vol. 135 (3rd series)
Neuroimaging, Part I
J.C. Masdeu and R.G. González, Editors

Chapter 17

Other cerebrovascular occlusive disease

ERICA C.S. CAMARGO[1], PAMELA W. SCHAEFER[2], AND ANEESH B. SINGHAL[1*]

[1]*Department of Neurology, Massachusetts General Hospital, Boston, MA, USA*

[2]*Department of Radiology, Massachusetts General Hospital, Boston, MA, USA*

Abstract

In this chapter we review the optimal imaging modalities for subacute and chronic stroke. We discuss the utility of computed tomography (CT) and multimodal CT imaging. Further, we analyze the importance of specific magnetic resonance imaging sequences, such as diffusion-weighted imaging for acute ischemic stroke, T2/fluid-attenuated inversion recovery for subacute and chronic stroke, and susceptibility imaging for detection of intracranial hemorrhages. Different ischemic stroke mechanisms are reviewed, and how these imaging modalities may aid in the determination of such. Further, we analyze how topographic patterns in ischemic stroke may provide important clues to the diagnosis, in addition to the temporal evolution of the stroke. Lastly, specific cerebrovascular occlusive diseases are reviewed, with emphasis on the optimal imaging modalities and their findings in each condition.

INTRODUCTION

Patients with symptoms of acute stroke require urgent brain imaging to confirm the diagnosis of ischemic or hemorrhagic stroke, to understand mechanisms, and for acute management decisions. After the acute phase, brain imaging studies may still be required to determine the etiology of stroke, assess lesion evolution, exclude complications of stroke treatment, and to guide subsequent management, including secondary stroke prevention. Chapter 15 addresses acute stroke neuroimaging. In this chapter, we will discuss the utility of computed tomography (CT) and magnetic resonance imaging (MRI) in nonacute stroke, and present the typical imaging findings of several common conditions that cause stroke.

DIAGNOSTIC WORKUP

Several imaging modalities are available for stroke evaluation, as described in detail in Chapters 1, 2, 6, 7, 10, 16, and 18. Here we briefly summarize the modalities and their utility in ischemic stroke.

Computed tomography

Noncontrast head CT

As discussed in Chapter 1, noncontrast CT (NCCT) imaging is the first-line modality for the evaluation of a patient with suspected acute ischemic or hemorrhagic stroke. NCCT has high sensitivity and specificity for all types of brain hemorrhage. NCCT has low sensitivity for early ischemic stroke as compared to MRI; however, in patients with suspected acute ischemic stroke, its main utility is to exclude mimics such as brain hemorrhages and tumors. NCCT may show early ischemic changes, such as the loss of gray–white-matter differentiation in the insula or hemispheric convexities, attenuation of the lentiform nucleus, and the hyperdense vessel sign. After the first few hours, the sensitivity of NCCT for ischemic change becomes higher, so it is more useful for detecting subacute and chronic infarctions. It is useful for the evaluation of periventricular white-matter disease. In cerebrovenous disorders, NCCT can reveal thrombus within the cerebral venous sinus or

*Correspondence to: Aneesh B. Singhal, MD, Vice Chair of Neurology, Quality and Safety, Associate Professor of Neurology, Harvard Medical School, Department of Neurology, Stroke Service, Massachusetts General Hospital, 55 Fruit Street, WACC 729C, Boston MA 02114, USA. Tel: +1-617-726-8459 x 4, Fax: +1-617-726-5043, E-mail: asinghal@partners.org

cortical vein, and any associated vasogenic brain edema or hemorrhage.

CT angiography and CT venography

CT angiography and CT venography (CTA/CTV) are excellent imaging tools for the rapid and relatively noninvasive evaluation of the intracranial and extracranial arteries and veins. CTA/CTV is highly sensitive and specific, comparable to digital subtraction angiography (DSA) for most conditions, and has good interrater reliability. Further, images can be reconstructed or collapsed into maximum-intensity pixel (MIP) projections, which allow for improved detection of vascular abnormalities. Limitations of this technique include limited resolution for the evaluation of the distal vasculature, and risks associated with exposure to iodinated contrast dye and cranial radiation (Knauth et al., 1997; Lev et al., 2001).

Magnetic resonance imaging

Diffusion-weighted imaging (DWI)

DWI is an MRI technique that is extremely sensitive for the detection of cytotoxic edema. It is highly specific and sensitive (>95% for both) for the detection of acute ischemic infarcts and can differentiate acute from chronic infarctions. It has high signal-to-noise ratio and excellent interrater reliability. Acquisition of high-resolution coronal DWI images can help in the detection of small strokes such as those located in the brainstem. False-positive DWI lesions can be seen in prolonged seizures, hypoglycemia, cerebral abscesses, highly cellular solid tumors, and demyelination disorders (Grant et al., 2001; Mullins et al., 2002).

Fluid attenuation inversion recovery imaging (FLAIR)

FLAIR images are highly sensitive to T2 prolongation in brain tissue. Because the cerebrospinal fluid (CSF) has low signal, FLAIR allows for improved detection of parenchymal lesions adjacent to CSF in the ventricles and sulci, as well as subarachnoid lesions. Due to the differential evolution of ischemia-related signal intensity on DWI and FLAIR, a comparison of signal intensity on these two sequences allows estimation of the age of ischemic stroke. For example, in the first 6 hours, ischemic stroke typically has little to no signal abnormality on FLAIR images and is hyperintense on DWI; in the subacute stage, a stroke will be hyperintense on both FLAIR and DWI images; and in the chronic stage, a stroke remains hyperintense on FLAIR images but is no longer hyperintense on DWI images. FLAIR images further allow for optimal detection of white-matter lesions and vasogenic edema. FLAIR imaging is useful in acute stroke and cerebral arteriopathies as it can show indirect signs of embolism or of increased collateral circulation, visualized as linear or dot-shaped hyperintensities within the sulcal spaces (collateral vessels appear hyperintense on FLAIR images due to slow flow or thrombus). Finally FLAIR is sensitive to detect subarachnoid hemorrhage (SAH) (Stuckey et al., 2007; Lee et al., 2009a).

Perfusion-weighted imaging (PWI)

PWI provides information about hemodynamic parameters such as cerebral blood volume, cerebral blood flow and transit time (e.g., mean transit time, time to peak, time to peak of the residue function). In the acute setting, the combination of DWI and PWI is used to estimate potentially salvageable ischemic brain tissue by assessing the "mismatch" between the DWI and the hypoperfused lesion volume on PWI sequences. PWI determines if other vascular territories with no DWI abnormality are also at risk of infarction, allowing for expedited medical management (Sorensen et al., 1996; Rordorf et al., 1998; Albers, 1999). After arterial recanalization, regions of cerebral hyperperfusion may be seen. In the subacute and chronic phase, PWI can be useful in providing information about areas of reduced perfusion (oligemic or ischemic brain tissue) in conditions like severe carotid artery stenosis, moyamoya disease (MMD), or other arterial occlusive diseases.

Gradient echo imaging (GRE)

This MRI technique detects inhomogeneities of the brain magnetic field, such as those produced by certain products of hemorrhage such as deoxyhemoglobin, intracellular methemoglobin, and hemosiderin. It allows visualization of intraparenchymal hemorrhages with high sensitivity and accuracy. It also demonstrates intravascular clot in the acute stages of thrombo-embolism, and identifies postischemic hemorrhage as well as extra-axial hemorrhage (Hermier and Nighoghossian, 2004).

Magnetic resonance angiography and venography

Magnetic resonance angiography (MRA) and magnetic resonance venography (MRV) are excellent alternatives to CTA/CTV. Images are acquired with flow-dependent techniques such as time of flight (TOF) and phase contrast techniques, or contrast-enhanced flow-independent techniques. Contrast-enhanced flow-independent techniques are typically used for imaging of the carotid and vertebral arteries; the three-dimensional TOF technique is typically used for imaging the intracranial arteries, and the 3D phase contrast technique is typically used for imaging the intracranial venous structures. Similar to CTV, MIPs are typically reconstructed in order to improve lesion detection. MRA has been shown to have good correlation with DSA. As with CTA, MRA has limited resolution for the evaluation of distal arteries and leptomeningeal collaterals. 3D TOF MRA is used to evaluate the circle of Willis vessels because it has superior spatial resolution and to evaluate the neck vessels when contrast is contraindicated, but it may overestimate the degree of arterial stenoses. In general, CTA and CTV are probably more accurate than MRA and MRV, but since the latter are not associated with radiation risks, they are more useful for serial imaging during disease monitoring (Nederkoorn et al., 2003a, b).

Digital subtraction angiography

Given the widespread availability of relatively noninvasive modalities such as CTA and MRA and their excellent correlation with transfemoral cerebral angiography or DSA, the latter is now typically reserved for specific diagnostic questions that are not answered by CTA or MRA. This includes the assessment of distal arteries, for example in cerebral vasculitis, or to exclude mycotic aneurysms in bacterial endocarditis. DSA is useful for the assessment and embolization of arteriovenous vascular malformations and fistulas, for aneurysm coiling, and for preoperative surgical planning for bypass surgery such as encephaloduroarteriosynangiosi s for MMD. Complications of DSA include symptomatic stroke (0.5–1%) and groin hematomas (up to 8%) (U-King-Im et al., 2009).

LESION TOPOGRAPHY AND STROKE ETIOLOGY

Careful analysis of the size, nature, age, location, and distribution of lesions on NCCT or MRI can help uncover specific stroke etiologies, guide diagnostic testing, and optimize the management of stroke patients. Single ischemic lesions (see Figs 17.7 and 17.8, below) have different mechanistic implications than multiple ischemic lesions (see Figs 17.3, 17.5, 17.11, 17.13, and 17.14, below); for example, they may suggest a specific underlying stroke mechanism such as lipohyalinotic small-vessel disease (Roh et al., 2000). Further, the arterial territories involved can provide clues to the underlying mechanism: single arterial territory (e.g., lacunar infarction, artery-to-artery embolism) vs multiple arterial territorial involvement (e.g., cardiac embolism). If the stroke lesion does not respect an arterial distribution, then venous or metabolic diseases should be considered.

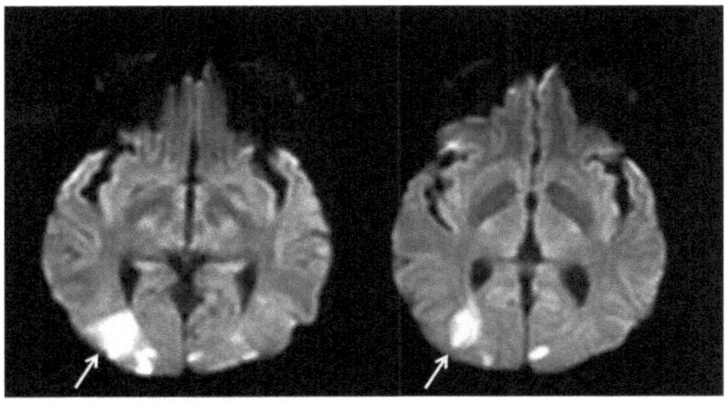

Fig. 17.1. External borderzone infarct. Diffusion-weighted images show restricted diffusion consistent with acute infarction in the external borderzone between the middle cerebral artery and posterior cerebral artery territories (arrows).

Watershed ischemic pattern

Watershed infarcts occur at the junction of the distal fields of two arterial systems. Classic neuropathologic studies have described two types of watershed infarction patterns: (1) cortical watershed, or "external borderzone" infarcts: these are supratentorial lesions located in the frontal, parietal, and occipital lobes, between the arterial territories of the anterior, middle, and posterior cerebral arteries in one or both hemispheres (Fig. 17.1); and (2) internal watershed or "internal borderzone" infarcts: these lesions are located in the white matter, along and slightly above the lateral ventricle, between the deep and the superficial arterial systems of the middle cerebral artery (MCA), or between the superficial systems of the MCA and anterior cerebral artery (ACA) (Fig. 17.2). Together, watershed infarcts account for approximately 10% of all ischemic lesions.

Unilateral watershed lesions develop in patients with hemodynamically significant arterial stenosis or occlusions typically involving the ipsilateral MCA or the ipsilateral internal carotid artery (ICA). The most common etiology of proximal arterial narrowing is atherosclerosis, resulting in a "string-of-pearls" appearance of lesions resulting either from small emboli that settle in watershed regions due to poor washout, or, less commonly, a low-flow state (Caplan and Hennerici, 1998). In young adults, watershed infarcts can develop in patients with cervical artery dissections (CAD), the reversible cerebral vasoconstriction syndromes (RCVS), sickle cell anemia, and other large- or medium-vessel cerebral arteriopathies. This pattern is not exclusively seen in large-vessel disease, and sometimes can be present in cardioembolic stroke (Mangla et al., 2011) (Fig. 17.3).

Subcortical white-matter infarcts

Predominantly subcortical white-matter infarcts are associated with a number of uncommon stroke

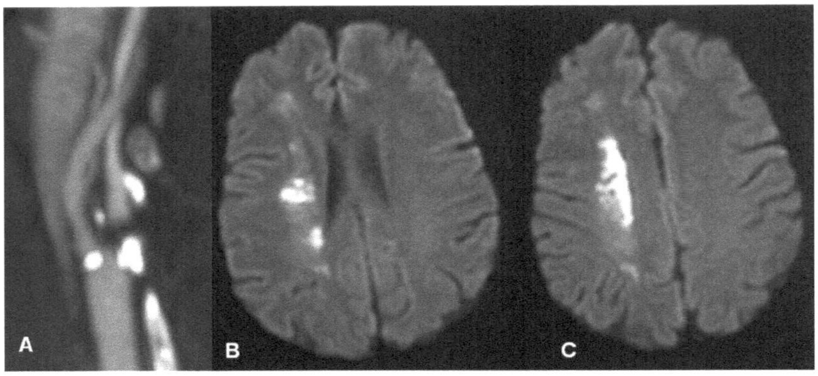

Fig. 17.2. Internal borderzone infarction due to severe internal carotid artery stenosis. A 60-year woman developed acute left hemiplegia and a right gaze preference after starting a new antihypertensive agent. Computed tomography-angiography (**A**) shows a critical stenosis at the origin of the right internal carotid artery. Diffusion-weighted images (**B, C**) show restricted diffusion consistent with acute infarction in the right corona radiata and centrum semiovale.

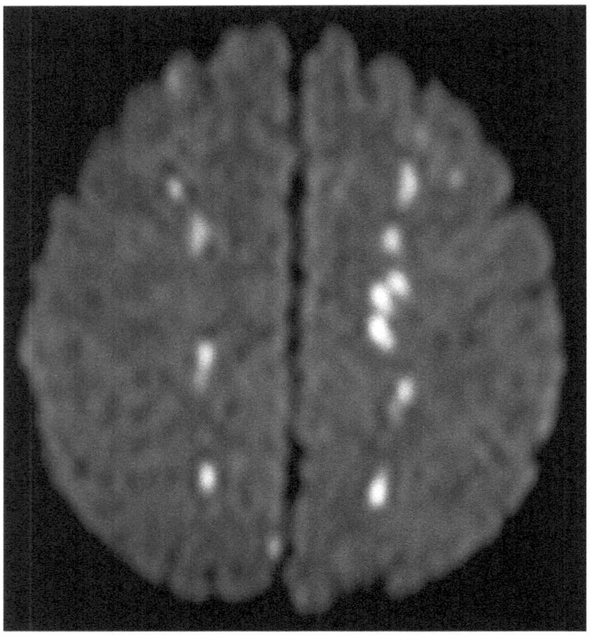

Fig. 17.3. Internal borderzone infarctions with string-of-pearls appearance.

disorders, including primary central nervous system (CNS) vasculitis and Behçet's disease. However, certain patterns suggest specific diagnoses. In cerebral autosomal-dominant arteriopathy with subcortical infarcts and leukoencephalopthy (CADASIL), the typical finding of symmetric periventricular white-matter lesions as well as lesions involving the external capsule and anterior temporal lobe is pathognomonic (Chabriat et al., 2009). In Susac's syndrome, white-matter lesions typically involve the central portion of the corpus callosum and have a "snowball" appearance (Susac et al., 2003).

It should be noted that subcortical white-matter infarctions are different from periventricular white-matter hyperintensities commonly attributed to microvascular disease from hypertension or other vascular risk factors. The Fazekas scale (Table 17.1) was established as a method to quantify white-matter lesions in patients with Alzheimer's disease and vascular dementia (Fazekas et al., 1987). It has since been used extensively as a rating scale for white-matter hyperintensities. In their original study, Fazekas and colleagues (1987) noted punctate or early confluent high-signal abnormalities in the deep white matter in 60% of Alzheimer's subjects and controls, in the absence of vascular risk factors. Additionally, an extensive smooth "halo" of periventricular hyperintensity was more commonly seen in Alzhimer's patients than controls. Conversely, vascular dementia was associated with deep white-matter hyperintensities and extensive, irregular, periventricular hyperintensities. Small isolated foci of deep white-matter hyperintensities were not characteristic of Alzheimer's disease or of vascular dementia (Fazekas et al., 1987). Stroke patients are found to have clinically silent white-matter lesions in 44%, which can be confluent in 19%. The degree of white-matter burden is directly associated with increasing age, diabetes mellitus, cardiac disease, carotid atherosclerosis, and hypertension (Schmidt et al., 1992) (Fig. 17.4).

Lesions in multiple arterial territories

Ischemic lesions in multiple arterial territories should elicit consideration of proximal sources of emboli such as intracardiac thrombus or nonbacterial thrombotic endocarditis (Fig. 17.5), cardiac valve diseases, atrial fibrillation, and aortic arch atheromatosis. In carotid diseases with a fetal posterior cerebral artery (PCA), strokes may involve the anterior circulation and the PCA territory simultaneously. Multifocal cerebral arteriopathies, such as human immunodeficiency virus

Table 17.1

Fazekas score variable definitions per grade

	Periventricular white-matter hyperintensity extent	Deep white-matter hyperintensity extent	Deep white-matter hyperintensity lesion count
0	Absent	Absent	Absent
1	Capping or pencil-thin lining	Punctate foci	1–4 lesions
2	Smooth halo	Initial confluence	5–9 lesions
3	Irregular periventricular signal extending into the deep white matter	Large confluent areas	>9 lesions

Reproduced from: Fazekas et al. (1987).

(HIV), varicella-zoster and primary angiitis of the CNS (PACNS) can cause infarcts in different vascular territories over time.

In a large study of consecutive ischemic stroke patients, multiple brain infarcts were seen in 29%. Of these, 65% were seen in the anterior circulation, 23% in the posterior circulation, and 12% in both anterior and posterior circulation. When involving the anterior circulation, multiple brain infarcts were more often unilateral (64%) than bilateral and predominantly due to large-artery atherosclerosis, though cardioembolism was also noted. The majority of these infarcts involved the cortical and deep territories simultaneously. When unilateral, these most commonly involved the territories of the perforating and leptomeningeal branches of the MCA. Multiple infarcts in the posterior circulation were

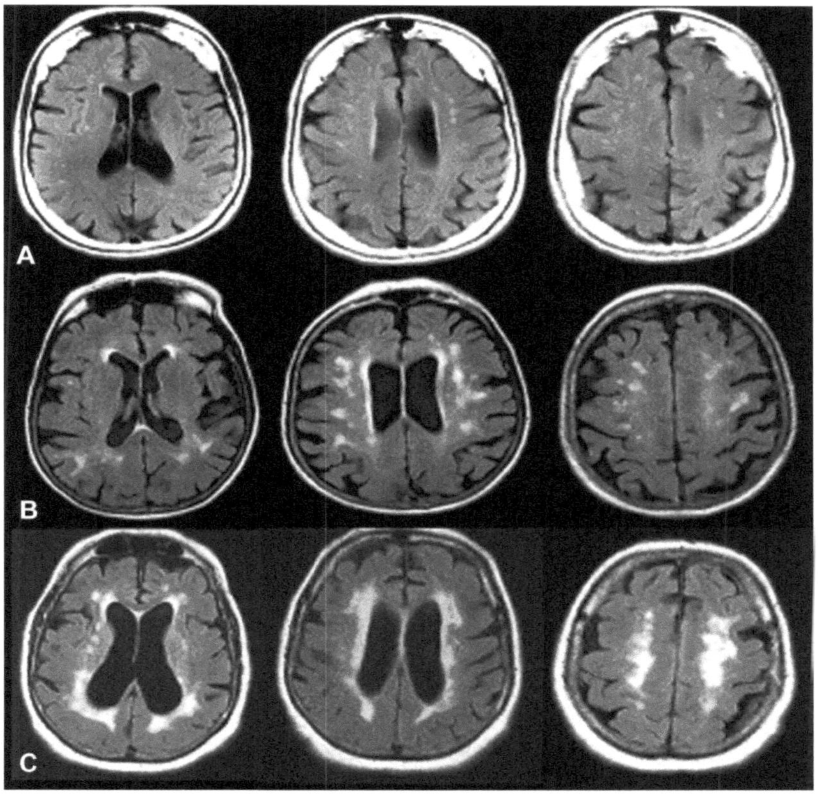

Fig. 17.4. White-matter hyperintensities: Fazekas grades. Examples for grade 0 for each variable are not included. (**A**) Three images from the same patient showing periventricular white-matter hyperintensity grade 1 and deep white-matter hyperintensity grade 1. (**B**) Three images from the same patient showing periventricular white-matter hyperintensity grade 2 and deep white-matter hyperintensity grade 2. (**C**) Three images from the same patient showing periventricular white-matter hyperintensity grade 3 and deep white-matter hyperintensity grade 3.

due to large-artery atherosclerosis in 68%. Infarcts were most frequently located in the territory of the PCA, followed by the posterior inferior cerebellar artery, superior cerebellar artery, anterior inferior cerebellar artery territories and the territory of the perforating branch of the basilar artery. The majority of patients with infarcts involving the anterior and posterior circulation had cardioembolism (55%). Small-artery occlusion was exclusively associated with bilateral anterior circulation infarcts. Of interest, in patients with strokes in both hemispheres or involving anterior and posterior circulations simultaneously, anatomic variations of the ACA or PCA or patent posterior communicating arteries were evident in some cases (Roh et al., 2000).

Lesions in nonarterial distributions

Suspicion for nonarterial vasculopathies such as venous infarctions and mitochondrial encephalomyopathy, lactic acidosis, and stroke-like episodes (MELAS) should be raised once it is clear that the infarct distribution does not conform to arterial territories of the anterior and posterior circulations (Bianchi et al., 1998; Yoneda et al., 1999; Kim et al., 2011; Saposnik et al., 2011).

Lesions with concomitant subarachnoid and/or intraparenchymal hemorrhage and ischemia

The combination of acute ischemia with subarachnoid or intraparenchymal hemorrhage should lead to the suspicion of a few specific cerebral vasculopathies. In RCVS ischemic strokes can coexist with convexal SAH (cSAH) or intraparenchymal hemorrhages (Ducros et al., 2010). MMD frequently presents with intraparenchymal hemorrhage in adult patients who may have already experienced ischemic stroke symptoms in childhood (Kuroda and Houkin, 2008). Small acute or subacute infarcts can be seen in subjects with brain hemorrhage from cerebral amyloid angiopathy. These are often present in the cortex and subcortical region, and their presence is associated with a higher burden of hemorrhages (Kimberly et al., 2009). Cerebral microbleeds are also seen in patients with other vasculopathies that have ischemic stroke as their hallmark. In CADASIL, microbleeds can be seen in up to 31% of symptomatic Notch-3 mutation carriers. These are most commonly found in the thalamus, and are associated with increasing age and the Notch-3 gene mutation (Lesnik Oberstein et al., 2001). Likewise, cerebral microhemorrhages may be seen in subacute bacterial endocarditis and may point to patients who are at high risk for mycotic aneurysm formation (Subramaniam et al., 2006).

SPECIFIC CONDITIONS

Arterial disorders

Arterial stroke can be classified according to the underlying mechanism leading to brain ischemia. Such a classification is important to determine optimal medical management. To that end, a classification scheme was devised called the "TOAST" classification which is used extensively for clinical and research purposes. The main stroke subtypes according to the TOAST classification are: (1) large-artery atherosclerosis; (2) cardioembolism; (3) small-vessel occlusion; (4) stroke of other determined etiology; and (5) stroke of undetermined etiology (Adams et al., 1993). More recently we developed an automated algorithm to classify ischemic strokes according to the original TOAST criteria. This web-based classification system, the Causative Classification of Stroke System (CCSS), further divides the undetermined category into cryptogenic embolism, other cryptogenic, incomplete evaluation, and unclassified categories. The CCSS has excellent intra- and interrater reliability (Ay et al., 2007). We will explore each of these major ischemic stroke categories below.

CARDIOEMBOLISM (FIG. 17.5)

Cardioembolism is responsible for 14–30% of ischemic strokes (Arboix and Alio, 2012). It can be due to multiple etiologies, including atrial fibrillation, cardiac valvular disease (mitral stenosis, mechanical prosthetic valve, endocarditis, calcific aortic valve disease, intraventricular thrombus (especially after anterior wall myocardial infarction and apical aneurysm), dilated cardiomyopathy, and other less common causes such as atrial myxoma. Additionally, patent foramen ovale (PFO) with or without atrial septal aneurysm, and aortic arch atheromatosis are recognized as causes of cardioembolic strokes. These strokes may lead to prominent disability and mortality given their association with large territorial infarcts and their high risk of recurrence (Ferro, 2003). Clinically, cardioembolism may affect the brain and other arterial territories simultaneously. Common manifestations include limb ischemia, mesenteric ischemia, and acute renal failure. Strokes may be seen simultaneously in the anterior and posterior circulation territories, bilaterally, and infarcts may be of varying ages. Cardiac emboli may be large and occlude the proximal cerebral vessels leading to large territorial infarcts. In a population-based study, cardioembolic strokes involved preferentially the posterior division of the MCA, ACA, cerebellum, and multiple territories (Bogousslavsky et al., 1991). Hemorrhagic transformation of an ischemic stroke is highly suggestive of cardioembolism and may be seen in 70% of cases (Ferro, 2003;

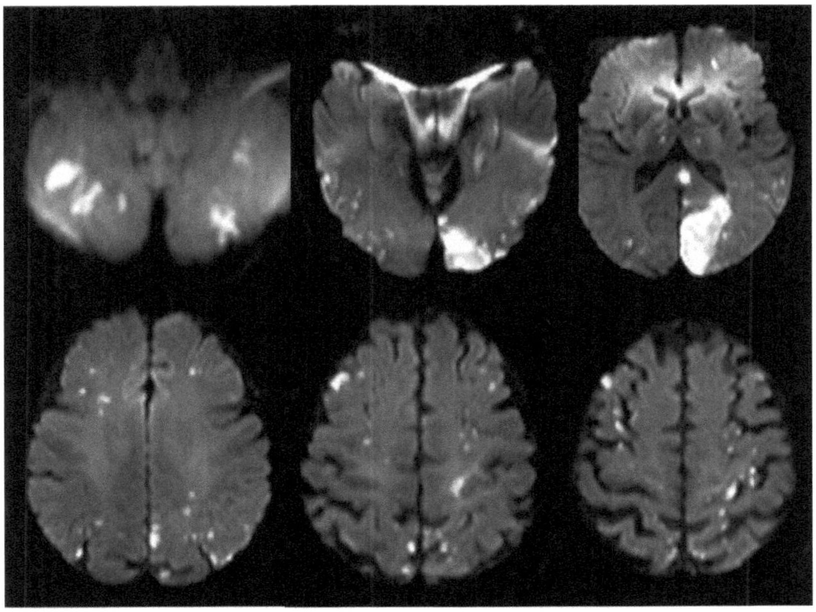

Fig. 17.5. Cardioembolic stroke. Diffusion-weighted images show numerous foci of restricted diffusion throughout the supratentorial and infratentorial brain, suggesting cardioembolic emboli.

Arboix and Alio, 2012). An additional pattern of involvement is that of multiple small infarcts in distal arterial branches, which may be in borderzone distribution (Fig. 17.3).

In nonbacterial thrombotic endocarditis strokes are nearly always numerous, widely distributed, and small (<10 mm), medium (10–30 mm), or large (>30 mm). In infective endocarditis, strokes may have different patterns, including disseminated punctate lesions often presenting as encephalopathy; multiple small to large strokes in multiple territories; single lesions; and territorial infarctions (Singhal et al., 2002). In PFO-related cardioembolism, strokes are usually single, moderate-sized, subcortical, and often without evidence of prior infarction (Thaler et al., 2013).

Treatment of cardioembolic stroke will depend on the etiology and extent of the lesion, but often involves the use of antithrombotic agents for secondary stroke prevention.

Large-vessel atherosclerosis (Figs. 17.2 and 17.6)

Large vessel atherosclerosis accounts for 20% of ischemic strokes. These strokes can be due to artery-to-artery embolism of atherosclerotic plaque and debris from unstable plaques, or from hemodynamic compromise within the dependent arterial territory. The incidence of strokes due to large-artery atherosclerosis is directly related to the degree of stenosis. Large-vessel disease may be seen in the extracranial and intracranial arteries. The clinical syndrome will depend on the arterial territory involved. One particular feature of large-vessel disease is the often stereotyped nature of the stroke syndrome. Carotid disease is more prevalent in Caucasians. It is most frequently seen at the bifurcation of the common carotid artery. ICA disease will often lead to ischemia in a borderzone between the MCA and ACA territories. Of interest, in a study of extracranial large-artery carotid disease, multiple infarcts were seen in 83%. Patterns of stroke distribution included territorial lesions, often wedge-shaped, without borderzone infarctions in about two-thirds of cases; borderzone infarcts in 28%; and, interestingly, bilateral hemispheric lesions in 11.5% (Kang et al., 2002). Common clinical syndromes in ICA stenosis include ipsilateral amaurosis fugax, contralateral limb-shaking transient ischemic attacks (TIA), and TIA with proximal weakness of the contralateral arm and leg. If a stroke occurs, it will usually affect the MCA territory and may include hemiparesis, cortical hemisensory loss, visual field defects, aphasia, dysarthria, and neglect. In addition to carotid disease, large-artery atherosclerosis can involve the extracranial vertebral artery, leading to hemodynamic or embolic TIAs involving the posterior circulation. Intracranial atherosclerosis is a disease more prevalent in Asians and African Americans. It can involve multiple arterial territories such as the MCA, ACA, basilar artery or PCA territories. The clinical presentation will again depend on the diseased vessel. An uncommon cause of artery-to-artery embolism from large-vessel disease is embolism from a thrombosed extracranial or intracranial aneurysm (Fig. 17.7). This is more likely to occur when

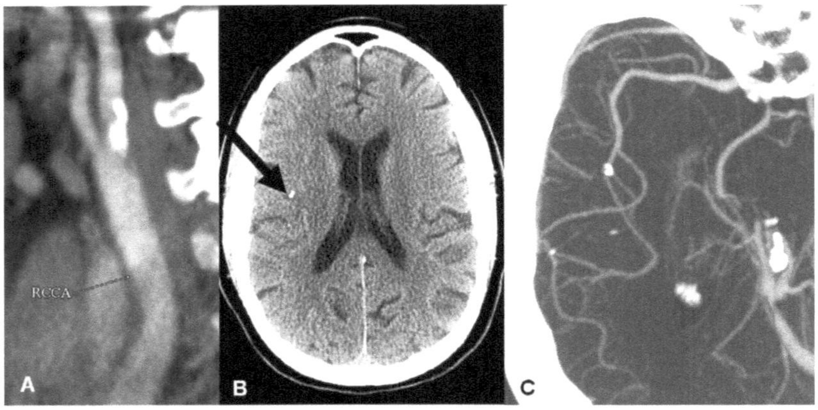

Fig. 17.6. Calcific microemboli. A 62-year-old man with hypertension and hyperlipidemia presented with acute dysarthria and left arm and face weakness. (**A**) Computed tomography-angiography (CTA) shows atherosclerotic plaque at the right common carotid artery (RCCA) bifurcation with severe stenosis at the origin of the right internal carotid artery. (**B**) Noncontrast head CT demonstrates a calcific focus in the upper right sylvian fissure (arrow). (**C**) CTA of the head shows that the calcific deposit is within a sylvian branch of the right middle cerebral artery.

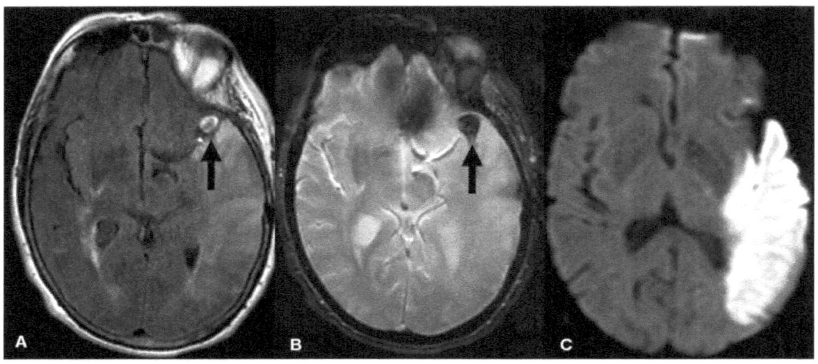

Fig. 17.7. Thrombosed aneurysm. Patient presenting with acute right hemiparesis. (**A**) Fluid-attenuated inversion recovery image shows an aneurysm (arrow) that is hyperintense, consistent with slow flow or occlusion. (**B**) Gradient echo image shows susceptibility in the aneurysm (arrow), consistent with occlusion. (**C**) Diffusion-weighted image shows a large left middle cerebral artery infarction.

aneurysms are large and thus prone to thrombus formation from turbulent blood flow (Ha et al., 2009).

DSA is still considered the gold-standard method for evaluation of the degree of vessel stenosis (Barnett et al., 1998; European Carotid Surgery Trialists' Collaborative Group, 1998). However, given its invasive nature, use of contrast, and radiation exposure, it is rarely used. Doppler ultrasound is an accurate noninvasive method for assessment of carotid stenosis, with reported sensitivities of 85–92% and specificities of 77–89% for severe carotid stenosis (Wardlaw et al., 2006). Its main limitations are related to operator dependence, susceptibility to artifacts from calcified plaques, and difficulty in distinguishing subtotal from complete arterial occlusion (Mikkonen et al., 1996; Grant et al., 2003). Contrast-enhanced MRA is an excellent alternative method for diagnosis of severe stenoses, with reported sensitivities and specificities of 88–97% and 89–96%, respectively, for detection of severe carotid stenosis (Cloft et al., 1996; Huston et al., 1999). Its main limitation is spatial resolution. CTA is also a very good diagnostic method, with 68–84% sensitivity and 91–97% specificity for severe carotid stenosis, with its main limitation related to beam-hardening artifacts from dense calcification (Wardlaw et al., 2006).

Small-vessel disease

Lacunar infarctions comprise 20–25% of all strokes (Chamorro et al., 1991). They are small strokes, characteristically ranging between 5 and 15 mm in diameter (up to 20 mm on DWI), located in the distribution of small penetrating arteries, including the lenticulostriate, anterior choroidal, thalamoperforator, and basilar artery branches. These arteries are 40–900 μm in diameter. Pathologically the diseased arteries have characteristic abnormalities, lipohyalinosis, and fibrinoid degeneration, which are mainly caused by hypertension. A small subset of lacunar strokes are suspected to be caused by microthrombi at the site of arterial occlusion (Fisher, 1968). Additional mechanisms of small strokes (often misinterpreted as lacunar infarcts, which imply a lacunar mechanism) include decreased perfusion of penetrating arteries from narrowing of proximal large vessels, and embolism (Gan et al., 1997). Lacunar strokes present with classic syndromes. The most common, seen in 50–66% of strokes, is pure motor hemiparesis involving the face, arm, and leg. In this syndrome, the stroke may be located in the corona radiata, posterior limb of the internal capsule, pons, or in the medullary pyramids. It may be preceded by a "capsular warning syndrome," in which stuttering motor deficits recur multiple times before the stroke is completed. Other lacunar syndromes include sensorimotor stroke (20%, posteroventral thalamus plus posterior limb of the internal capsule), homolateral ataxia and crural paresis (18%, corona radiata, internal capsule, or upper basis pontis), dysarthria clumsy-hand syndrome (2–16%, paramedian basis pontis, internal capsule, or between the internal capsule and corona radiata), and pure sensory stroke (6–7%, posteroventral thalamus) (Fisher, 1965a, b; Fisher and Cole, 1965; Fisher and Curry, 1965). Risk factors for lacunar stroke include hypertension, diabetes mellitus, hyperlipidemia, and race (more frequent in African Americans and Hispanics) (Gan et al., 1997). The diagnosis of lacunar stroke relies heavily on the clinical presentation, and neuroimaging may aid in the diagnosis. The lesions are small and lack edema or reperfusion hemorrhage. Thus, NCCT is not sensitive for the detection of acute lacunar infarctions. Additionally, lacunar strokes may be difficult to identify on FLAIR and T2-weighted sequences because most patients have concomitant white-matter disease. In fact, FLAIR and T2 imaging may fail to identify or misidentify a lacunar infarction in 25% of cases (Oliveira-Filho et al., 2000). Thus, DWI is key to diagnosis, with 94.6% accuracy, 95% sensitivity, and 94% specificity for small subcortical infarcts (Singer et al., 1998). Furthermore, DWI may help determine the stroke mechanism in small infarcts. Small subsidiary lesions in the leptomeningeal territory have been reported in 16% of patients with small strokes. This subset of patients is more likely to have an embolic etiology (Ay et al., 1999; Gerraty et al., 2002). Management in lacunar stroke includes antiplatelet therapy and control of vascular risk factors such as hypertension, hyperlipidemia, and diabetes.

Transient ischemic attack with and without infarct

TIA refers to a constellation of neurologic signs and symptoms that are attributable to vascular disease, resolve spontaneously within 24 hours, and are not associated with permanent cerebral infarction (Easton et al., 2009). Most TIAs last 5–10 minutes. When of longer duration, they usually resolve within 2–3 hours (Levy, 1988). NCCT imaging of TIA patients is usually normal. However, MRI may reveal DWI hyperintense/apparent diffusion coefficient (ADC) hypointense lesions in 21–70% of patients imaged after 17 hours of symptom onset. DWI positivity is usually directly correlated with TIA duration. Additionally, motor deficits and aphasia are independently associated with DWI abnormalities in TIA subjects. Lesions are invariably punctate or small, ranging from 5 to 40 mm in diameter, and may be both cortical and subcortical. The pattern of DWI lesion distribution may help determine the underlying etiology (Engelter et al., 1999; Kidwell et al., 1999; Ay et al., 2002; Rovira et al., 2002; Crisostomo et al., 2003). DWI positivity in TIAs has prognostic importance. In a large study evaluating TIA patients diagnosed by time-based criteria, DWI was positive in 70%. Seven-day recurrent stroke rates were 7.1% for DWI-positive TIAs and 0.4% for DWI-negative TIAs ($p < 0.0001$). Furthermore, DWI-positive TIAs with a low "ABCD2 score" and DWI-negative events with a high "ABCD2 score" had similar stroke risks, especially after 90 days (Giles et al., 2011).

Other specific causes

Carotid and vertebral artery dissection (Fig. 17.8)

CAD occurs when there is separation of different layers of the arterial wall, leading to luminal stenosis and/or pseudoaneurysm formation. CAD comprises approximately 2% of all ischemic strokes, and 25% of strokes in young adults, with peak incidence in the fifth decade (Arnold et al., 2006; Lee et al., 2006). Pathologically, an intimal tear with bleeding within the arterial wall due to ruptured vasa vasorum creates a false arterial lumen and a hematoma in the wall of the artery. The intramural hematoma expands, resulting in stenosis. The dissection plane can also lie between the tunica media and adventitia, resulting in aneurysmal dilatation of the artery (Schievink, 2001). CAD can occur spontaneously, after minor trauma or torsion of the neck from innocuous physical activities, or from more severe head and neck trauma. Other risk factors include aortic root diameter >34 mm, migraine, high homocysteine levels, and recent infection (Rubinstein et al., 2005). Fibromuscular dysplasia is seen in 15% of CAD cases (Debette and Leys,

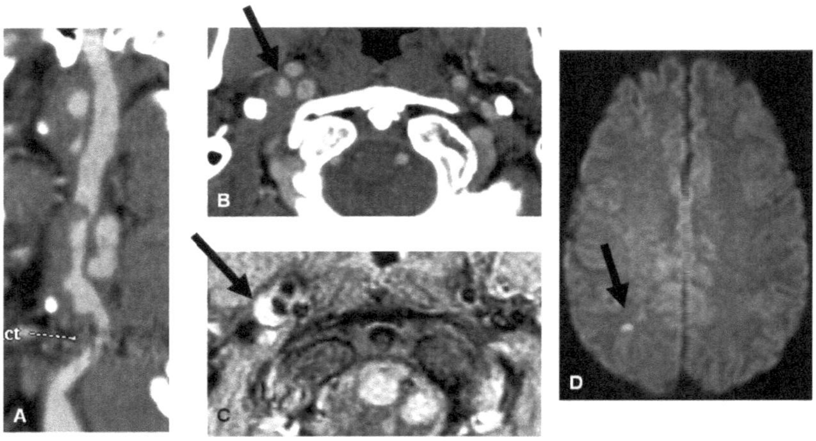

Fig. 17.8. Right internal carotid artery dissection. A 60-year woman presented with neck pain and transient weakness after chiropractic manipulation. (**A**) Computed tomography-angiography (CTA) maximum-intensity pixel images show irregularity with severe narrowing, consistent with dissection, in the distal cervical right internal carotid artery. (**B**) CTA axial source image shows right internal carotid artery luminal narrowing with a thickened lateral wall (arrow). (**C**) Fat-suppressed axial T1-weighted image shows hyperintensity, consistent with subacute blood in the false lumen (arrow). (**D**) Diffusion-weighted imaging shows a punctate acute infarction (arrow) in the right parietal lobe.

2009). Genetic causes, such as vascular Ehlers–Danlos syndrome polymorphisms in ICAM-1 and COL3A1, and an association with MTHFR677TT genotype, have also been reported (Debette and Markus, 2009). Ischemic and local signs and symptoms typically occur within the first few days after the inciting event (Biousse et al., 1995). Local signs and symptoms, such as ipsilateral headache or neck pain and partial Horner's syndrome, occur in 23–40% (Fisher, 1982). Ischemic stroke is seen in >50% of carotid dissections and 89% of vertebral artery dissections (Lee et al., 2006; Arnold et al., 2010). SAH can occur with intracranial extension of CAD (Debette and Leys, 2009).

The diagnosis of CAD is based on neuroimaging findings. The most specific feature is an enlarged artery with a mural hematoma, termed the "crescent sign" (Debette and Leys, 2009). Morphologically, frequent findings include pathognomonic intimal flaps, long tapered stenoses ("flame sign," 48%), tapered occlusions (35%), long stenosis ("string sign") and dissecting pseudoaneurysms (17%) (Lee et al., 2006). These are usually seen in the ICA at the level of the skull base or in the V3–V4 vertebral artery segment. CT/CTA and MR with T1 fat-suppressed images and MRA are now preferred over conventional angiography for the diagnosis of CAD, since conventional angiography is invasive and does not allow visualization of the mural hematoma (Debette and Leys, 2009). CT/CTA and MRI/MRA are comparable, though one study has found that CT/CTA detected more intimal flaps, pseudoaneurysms, and high-grade stenoses than MRI/MRA, especially for vertebral artery dissections (Vertinsky et al., 2008). On MRI, findings include an iso- or hyperintense crescentic signal in the dissection flap, due to acute or subacute blood products, on T1 fat-suppressed images; loss of flow void within the vessel on T2-weighted images; and multiple brain infarcts on DWI, usually in the vascular territory of the dissected cervical vessel or in a borderzone distribution.

Management of acute CAD includes either antiplatelet agents or anticoagulation in the first few days after symptom onset. Thereafter, and for secondary prevention, antiplatelet agents have been shown to be as affective as anticoagulants (CADISS Trial Investigators, 2015). Repeat CTA or MRA are often useful for management decisions. Resolution of dissection is seen in 46% for stenoses, 33% for occlusions, and 12% for dissecting aneurysms (Lee et al., 2006).

Inflammatory CNS vasculitis

Giant cell arteritis (GCA, Horton's disease). GCA is the most common primary systemic vasculitis. It involves large and medium-sized arteries such as the aorta and its branches, with a predilection for the extracranial branches of the carotid artery, including the superficial temporal, posterior ciliary, ophthalmic, internal maxillary, facial, and occipital arteries (Borchers and Gershwin, 2012). Pathologically, there is a granulomatous giant cell inflammatory infiltrate within the arterial wall leading to intimal hyperplasia and partial or complete lumen occlusion (Borchers and Gershwin, 2012). GCA affects persons above the age of 50 (peaking at 70–80 years), and women twice as commonly as men (Salvarani et al., 2004). There is significant overlap with polymyalgia rheumatica (Salvarani et al., 2002).

Symptoms are both ischemic (headache, in two-thirds of patients; jaw claudication, scalp tenderness) and inflammatory (malaise, anorexia, depression, fever). Constitutional symptoms are present in approximately 50% of cases (Salvarani et al., 2002). Elevated erythrocyte sedimentation rate (ESR), usually $\geq$50 mm/h, is present in most cases, though up to 22% of patients have normal ESR (Hunder et al., 1990; Salvarani and Hunder, 2001; Borchers and Gershwin, 2012). A c-reactive protein > 2.45 mg/dL may be more sensitive than ESR for GCA (Hayreh et al., 1997). Visual symptoms, due to arteritis of ophthalmic or posterior ciliary artery branches, occur early in 30% (Gonzalez-Gay et al., 1998). They can occur in one or both eyes and include amaurosis fugax, diplopia, and visual loss. Permanent visual loss may ensue in up to 20% (Salvarani and Hunder, 2001). Neurologic symptoms have been reported in 31% and strokes in 3–7%, most commonly involving the carotid and vertebral arteries (Caselli et al., 1988; Gonzalez-Gay et al., 1998).

Once clinically suspected, a 1–2-cm long biopsy of the temporal artery is considered the diagnostic gold standard for GCA. Sensitivity for biopsy is 70–90% and false negatives are seen in 13–15%. Predictors of a positive biopsy are headache, jaw claudication, and abnormal temporal artery on palpation (Gonzalez-Gay et al., 2001; Mari et al., 2009). Temporal artery biopsy should not delay treatment with steroids, including high-dose intravenous methylprednisolone in cases of acute or impending visual loss. A combination of color Doppler and ultrasonography of the temporal arteries is an excellent alternative to biopsy. This will show the characteristic "halo sign," a dark hypoechoic circumferential wall thickening around the arterial lumen. On color and Doppler ultrasound turbulent flow and stenosis of the affected vessel may be seen (Schmidt et al., 1997). A unilateral halo sign has a specificity of 83–91% and a sensitivity of 68–75% for GCA (Arida et al., 2010; Ball et al., 2010; Borchers and Gershwin, 2012). Ultrasound may also be used to assess response to therapy. The main limitation to the technique is operator dependence, though interrater agreement >95% has been reported (Schmidt et al., 1997). Contrast-enhanced high-resolution MRI of the temporal artery is also sensitive and specific, demonstrating mural thickening and enhancement of the vessel wall; however, this technique is still not widely accepted (Bley et al., 2008). For extracranial GCA, ^{14}F-fluorodeoxyglucose (FDG) positron emission tomography (PET) scanning is the method of choice. It will show smooth linear or long segmental FDG uptake in the aorta and its main branches, with sensitivity and specificity of 80% and 89% for GCA, respectively (Besson et al., 2011). Additionally, CTA and MRA are usually indicated for extracranial GCA, especially focusing on mural thickening and enhancement of the aorta and its main branches. Angiography will typically show bilateral stenosis or occlusion of the subclavian, axillary, and proximal brachial arteries, with a smooth, tapered appearance. The presence of aortic wall thickening is suggestive of active inflammatory disease. Aortic aneurysms can also be seen (Stanson, 2000).

Takayasu's arteritis (pulseless disease). Takayasu's arteritis is a rare, idiopathic, chronic inflammatory disease characterized by granulomatous panarteritis of the aorta and its major branches, most commonly the subclavian and carotid arteries (Mason, 2010). It peaks at ages 20–30 years and the female-to-male ratio is 4.5:1 to 11:1 (Hotchi, 1992; Mason, 2010). It is most commonly seen in Japan, China, India, and other Asian countries (Johnston et al., 2002). Histopathology reveals adventitial thickening, focal leukocytic infiltration of the tunica media, and intimal hyperplasia (Hotchi, 1992). This leads to stenotic lesions in >90% of patients, and aneurysms in 25% (Mason, 2010). Clinical presentation includes secondary hypertension in 77%, limb claudication, paresthesias, fever, headaches in up to 42%, carotidynia in 10–30%, and elevated ESR in 70% (Kerr, 1995). Stroke occurs in 20% of cases (Mwipatayi et al., 2005). The common carotid artery is affected in 50%, commonly on the left. Morbidity is substantial in Takayasu arteritis, with 74% of patients reporting considerable compromise of daily activities. Mortality is high. Cardiac complications are common and include aortic valve insufficiency, cardiac ischemia, and myocardial infarction complicated by cardiac failure and death (Mason, 2010). Given its clinical and pathologic similarities with GCA, it has been postulated that these two diseases may represent different phenotypes within the spectrum of a single disorder (Maksimowicz-McKinnon et al., 2009).

In the absence of serologic markers, the diagnosis of Takayasu arteritis is based on clinical suspicion and radiologic findings. Neuroimaging techniques may have a complementary role to one another. Conventional angiography is being replaced by CTA and MRA, as it is invasive and may fail to detect early disease with normal lumen diameter, while CTA and MRA may detect the presence of arterial wall enhancement, edema, or wall thickening in pre-stenotic disease. Nonetheless, conventional angiography is superior to CTA and MRA for the assessment of smaller aortic branches, allows blood pressure measurements, and is used for preoperative evaluation (Mason, 2010). Contrast-enhanced CTA and MRA allow noninvasive imaging of the entire aorta and branches, and stenoses and aneurysms are readily identified and monitored. (Yoshida et al., 2001; Steeds and Mohiaddin, 2006;

Mason, 2010). As in GCA, ^{18}F-FDG-PET and ^{18}F-FDG-PET CT have been increasingly used for assessment of pre-stenotic active Takayasu arteritis, with intense linear uptake seen in the aorta, common carotid, and pulmonary arteries (Walter, 2007). However, it has limited utility for assessment of treatment response (Arnaud et al., 2009). Thus, MRA may be more favorable for long-term disease monitoring (Mason, 2010).

Isolated primary or granulomatous angiitis of the central nervous system (Fig. 17.9). PACNS is an idiopathic vasculitis restricted to the small and medium-sized arteries and veins/venules of the brain, spinal cord, and leptomeninges (Calabrese and Mallek, 1988; Salvarani et al., 2007). It results from an immunologic nonspecific T-cell-mediated inflammatory reaction affecting the vessel wall, which expresses itself as three

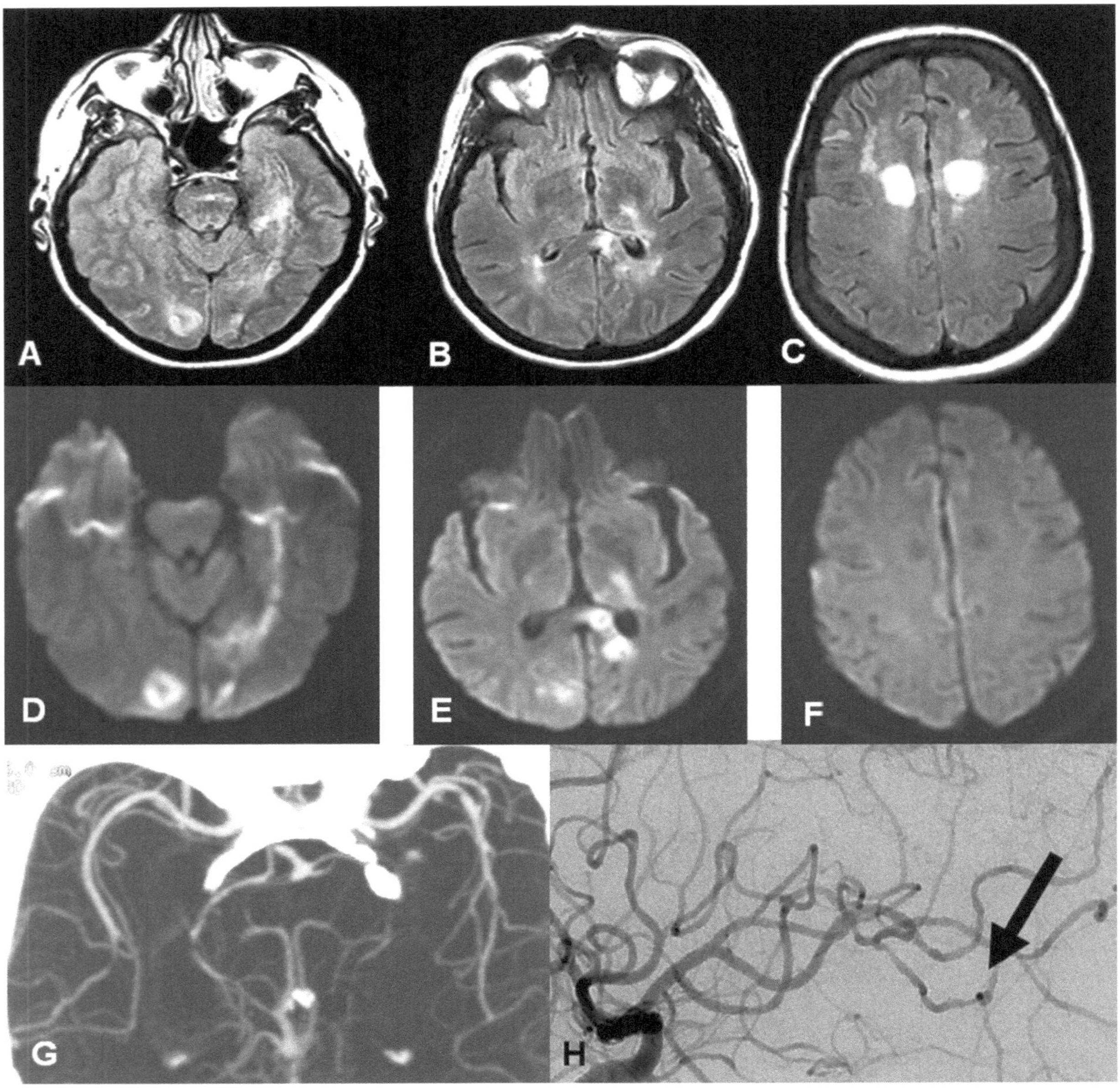

Fig. 17.9. Primary angiitis of the central nervous system. A 48 year-old woman presented with acute visual loss and hemiparesis. There are fluid-attenuated inversion recovery (FLAIR) hyperintense lesions (**A, B**) with restricted diffusion (**D, E**) in both occipital lobes, the left splenium of the corpus callosum, the left thalamus and the left posterior limb of the internal capsule, consistent with acute infarctions. There are FLAIR hyperintense lesions (**C**) with elevated diffusion (**F**) in both frontal lobes, consistent with chronic strokes. (**G**) Computed tomography-angiography demonstrates mulitfocal stenoses, most prominent in both posterior cerebral arteries and the inferior division of the left middle cerebral artery. (**H**) Digital subtraction angiography of the left middle cerebral artery shows multifocal middle cerebral artery stenoses, most prominent in the posterior inferior parietal branches (arrow).

pathologic subtypes: granulomatous, lymphocytic, and acute necrotizing vasculitis. Furthermore, congophilic amyloid angiopathy may be associated with angiocentric inflammatory infiltrates similar to those seen in PACNS (amyloid-β-related angiitis, or ABRA) (Miller et al., 2009). These changes are seen focally and/or segmentally, and lead to tissue infarction or hemorrhage, loss of myelin, and axonal degeneration. PACNS is rare, with an estimated incidence of 2.4 cases/1 000 000 person-years (Salvarani et al., 2007). The disease can occur at all ages but peaks between ages 40–60 years, and men are more commonly affected than women (Hajj-Ali et al., 2011). The onset is usually insidious. Symptoms routinely precede an angiographic diagnosis by 1.5–4.5 months and a pathologic diagnosis by 6 months (Siva, 2001). Three clinical patterns have been described: (1) acute or subacute encephalopathy; (2) multiple sclerosis-like presentation; and (3) rapidly progressive mass lesion, which is more common in patients with ABRA (Molloy et al., 2008). The most frequent symptom in PACNS is headache, which is usually mild to moderate, dull and aching, and almost never thunderclap-like. Encephalopathy and dementia are common. Strokes are seen in 30–50% of cases (Hajj-Ali et al., 2011). Other manifestations include cranial nerve involvement, myelopathy, seizures, and ataxia. Signs and symptoms of systemic vasculitis are very rare in PACNS, and likewise serologic markers of systemic inflammation are usually normal (Hajj-Ali et al., 2011). The clinical findings are accompanied by chronic inflammatory changes suggestive of aseptic meningitis in the CSF in 90% (Birnbaum and Hellmann, 2009).

Leptomeningeal and brain biopsy are considered the gold standard in the diagnosis of PACNS, though it carries a false-negative rate of 25–50% given the focal and segmental nature of the disease (Hajj-Ali et al., 2011). The most useful radiologic technique in PACNS is MRI, with sensitivity of 90–100% (Birnbaum and Hellmann, 2009; Hajj-Ali et al., 2011). The absence of infarcts and white-matter change on parenchymal imaging virtually rules out PACNS. Cerebral infarcts are often multiple, distributed nearly equally among cortical, subcortical, and deep gray-matter structures, and involve multiple arterial territories, both in large- and small-artery patterns (Pomper et al., 1999). They are usually of different ages and do not necessarily bear correlation with angiographic changes (Greenan et al., 1992). Nonspecific high-intensity T2WI/FLAIR lesions in white matter are seen in up to 41% (Appenzeller et al., 2008). Additional findings include: gadolinium-enhanced intracranial lesions in one-third; leptomeningeal enhancement in 8%; and mass lesions mimicking tumor or abscess in 5% (Salvarani et al., 2007, 2008; Molloy et al., 2008). Three-Tesla high-resolution MRI through the circle of Willis with pre- and postcontrast T1-weighted FLAIR images and T2-weighted images may demonstrate characteristic inflammatory changes in the anatomically detailed vessel wall (Kuker et al., 2008; Swartz et al., 2009). The sensitivity of cerebral angiography ranges from 40% to 90%, but the specificity is as low as 30% (Vollmer et al., 1993; Duna and Calabrese, 1995; Kadkhodayan et al., 2004; Calabrese et al., 2007; Hajj-Ali et al., 2011). When present, the most common angiographic findings are areas of ectasia and irregularity usually in multiple vascular distributions, but sometimes in a single artery. Single stenotic areas in multiple vessels are more frequent than multiple stenotic areas along one vessel segment. Additionally, vascular occlusions, collateral circulation, and prolonged circulation time may be present (Alhalabi and Moore, 1994). The most important disease in the differential diagnosis of PACNS with abnormal angiogram is RCVS, given its clinical similarity to PACNS. However, the angiographic changes in RCVS are more severe, with affected arteries showing smoothly tapering segments alternating with dilated segments ("sausaging") rather than an irregular notched appearance. Further, neuroimaging may show SAH or parenchymal hemorrhages, which are uncommon in PACNS (Chen et al., 2010). Treatment of PACNS includes prolonged immunosuppression with high-dose steroids or cyclophosphamide.

Susac's syndrome (retinocochleocerebral arteriopathy: Fig. 17.10). Susac's syndrome is a rare microangiopathy of the precapillary arteries of the brain, eye, and inner ear characterized by a triad of encephalopathy, branch retinal artery occlusions, and hearing loss. The pathologic findings include necrosis of the endothelial cells and C4d deposition in the endothelium, indicating an autoimmune mechanism. Disease onset occurs between ages 9 and 58 years and the female-to-male ratio is 3:1. Headache is usually the initial manifestation and is later followed by confusion, behavioral changes, and dementia. Ocular symptoms can be seen at onset and include photopsia, black spots, scintillating scotoma, and vision loss. Hearing loss may not be apparent in the encephalopathic patient; lower tones are usually affected. It is uncommon to see all three components of the triad present at onset (Susac et al., 2007). The disease usually presents with one to eight acute exacerbations and then stabilizes over a period of 2–4 years. Disease activity is not directly related to radiologic changes (Aubart-Cohen et al., 2007). Brain MRI is key for diagnosis. There is a predominance of supratentorial white-matter abnormalities with a predilection for the central portion of the corpus callosum. The microinfarcts in the central corpus callosum may become

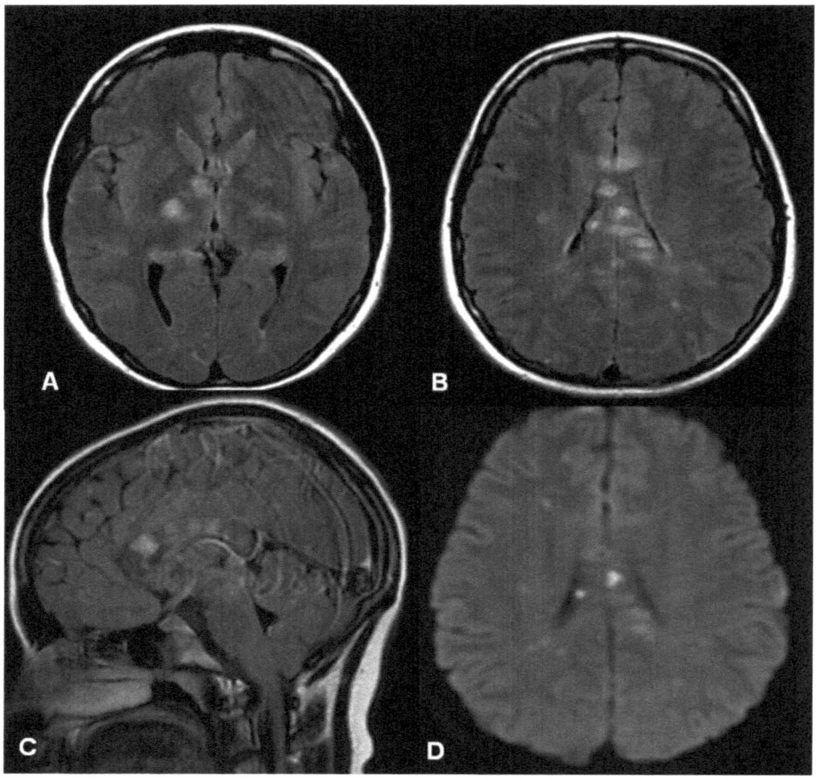

Fig. 17.10. Susac's syndrome. A 25-year man with right-eye visual loss and hearing loss. (**A, B**) Fluid-attenuated inversion recovery (FLAIR) images show numerous hyperintense ischemic lesions in the internal capsules, corpus callosum, periventricular white matter, and subcortical white matter. (**C**) Sagittal FLAIR shows that callosal lesions span the whole thickness of the corpus callosum. (**D**) Diffusion-weighted image shows restricted diffusion in some of the lesions, consistent with acute ischemia.

confluent and have a classic, snowball appearance. Additionally, other corpus callosum lesions may appear as linear defects extending from the callosal septal surface to the superior callosal margin. Callosal lesions may ultimately develop cavitation, considered pathognomonic of the disease. Furthermore, involvement of the deep gray nuclei and parenchymal enhancement can both occur in up to 70%, and leptomeningeal enhancement in up to 33% (Susac et al., 2003, 2007). CSF usually shows mild pleocytosis and elevated protein (Susac et al., 2007). Treatment includes steroids, immune globulin, and cyclophosphamide, often simultaneously (Susac et al., 2007).

Infectious CNS vasculitis

When faced with a patient with a CNS arteriopathy, infectious etiologies should be included in the differential diagnosis. Infections can lead to vasculopathies by direct invasion of the pathogen into the arterial wall, or more commonly, by immune-mediated mechanisms promoting vascular inflammation and thrombosis. The vasculopathy can involve both medium-sized and small vessels (Salvarani et al., 2012). In the case of HIV vasculopathy, patients may develop an infectious or inflammatory arteritis and/or aneurysmal dilatation, small-vessel arteriopathy, hypercoagulability, and premature atherosclerosis from metabolic disorders associated with highly active antiretroviral therapy (Ortiz et al., 2007; Monsuez et al., 2009). Clinical presentation of infectious vasculopathies may include fever, systemic infection, altered sensorium, and focal neurologic deficits. Inflammatory markers may be elevated and there may be leukocytosis. Small- and large-artery strokes may ensue. Potential infectious organisms in this setting include meningovascular syphilis, tuberculous meningitis, Lyme disease, cysticercosis, aspergillosis, mucormycosis, varicella-zoster virus, HIV, and other bacterial, parasitic, and fungal diseases. The diagnosis will usually be determined by CSF analysis and cultures. Prognosis is dependent on the pathogen, aggressiveness of the disease, and response to therapy.

Radiologic clues can help determine the diagnosis. Tuberculous meningitis (Fig. 17.11) typically involves the basilar cisterns with prominent enhancement of the basal meninges on postcontrast T1-weighted MRI.

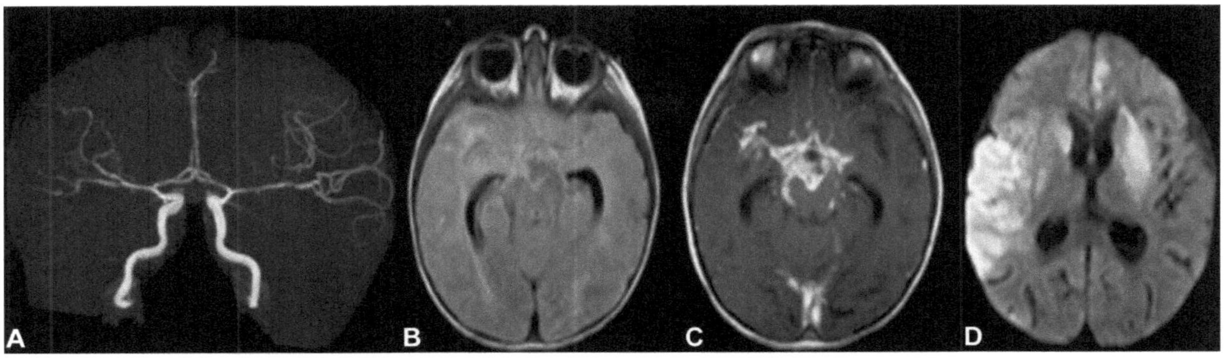

Fig. 17.11. Tuberculous meningitis. A 15-year-old child presented with acute right hemiparesis. (**A**) Three-dimensional train-of-flight magnetic resonance angiography shows multifocal narrowing of the proximal middle cerebral arteries. (**B**) There is hyperintense material in the subarachnoid space on fluid-attenuated inversion recovery images that enhances on postcontrast T1-weighted sequences (**C**), consistent with meningeal inflammation. (**D**) Diffusion-weighted imaging shows bilateral middle cerebral artery and left anterior cerebral artery acute infarctions.

Strokes can complicate meningovascular tuberculosis in more than a third of cases. The vasculopathy usually involves the lenticulostriate and thalamoperforator arteries, leading to small ischemic strokes in the basal ganglia and brainstem (Leiguarda et al., 1988). In meningovascular neurosyphilis, the presentation is commonly that of an ischemic stroke involving the MCA or basilar artery territory in a young patient (Gaa et al., 2004). Varicella-zoster virus vasculopathy can rarely affect a focal artery in association with zoster ophthalmicus. More often than not, varicella-zoster virus vasculopathy involves small and large vessels diffusely, usually in immunocompromised patients (Fig. 17.12) (Nagel et al., 2008). Mucormycosis may spread from the nasopharynx, oropharynx, or facial sinuses to the cavernous sinus and ICA, with ensuing thrombosis and ischemic or hemorrhagic stroke (Garg, 2011). Mycotic aneurysms develop in 2–5% of patient with infective endocarditis. They are most commonly found at arterial branch points, especially those involving the distal MCA (Bayer et al., 1998).

Moyamoya disease and syndrome (Fig. 17.13)

MMD is an idiopathic, nonatherosclerotic, noninflammatory condition characterized by chronic progressive and bilateral stenosis of the terminal ICA and the proximal portions of the ACA and MCA with formation of a fine network of collateral blood vessels at the base of the brain that angiographically resembles a puff of smoke, termed "moyamoya" in Japanese (Kuroda and Houkin, 2008; Scott and Smith, 2009). There is compensatory development of collateral vasculature by small vessels near the apex of the carotid artery, on the cortical surface, on the leptomeninges, and in the branches of the external carotid artery supplying the dura and skull base (Scott and Smith, 2009). "Moyamoya phenomenon" or "angiographic moyamoya" is used in the setting of secondary severe unilateral or bilateral ICA stenosis, such as is seen with sickle cell disease (SSD), atherosclerosis, cranial irradiation, Down syndrome, neurofibromatosis, exposure to vasoactive drugs, neonatal anoxia, and head trauma (Ullrich et al., 2007; Scott and Smith, 2009). Pathologic features include intimal thickening from smooth-muscle cell proliferation, reduplication of the elastic lamina, minimal to no lipid deposition, arterial thrombosis, and formation of collateral vessels and microaneurysms (Masuda et al., 1993; Scott and Smith, 2009). The disease is most prevalent in Asia (Yilmaz et al., 2001; Scott and Smith, 2009). The annual incidence and prevalence in Japan have been estimated at 3.16/100 000 and 0.35/100 000, respectively (Kuroda and Houkin, 2008). Disease peaks at ages 5–9 and 40–49 years, and the female-to-male ratio is 1.4 to 2:1 (Baba et al., 2008; Kuroda and Houkin, 2008; Scott and Smith, 2009). A positive family history of MMD is present in 7–12%, and inheritance can be autosomal dominant with incomplete penetrance or X-linked recessive (Mineharu et al., 2006; Herve et al., 2010). MMD is the most common vascular etiology of childhood stroke. However, nearly 18% of individuals with MMD may be asymptomatic. The disease may begin as an asymptomatic isolated stenosis of the MCA stem, progressing to symptomatic MMD over a few years. The annual stroke risk is 3%. Ischemic manifestations are more common in children than in adults and involve the MCA and ACA territories (Scott and Smith, 2009). Cerebral hemorrhage typically occurs in the deep gray nuclei and deep white matter, but may be intraventricular or subarachnoid, and is more common in adults. Migraine-like and intractable headaches are a frequent presenting symptom and may improve after pial revascularization (Scott and Smith,

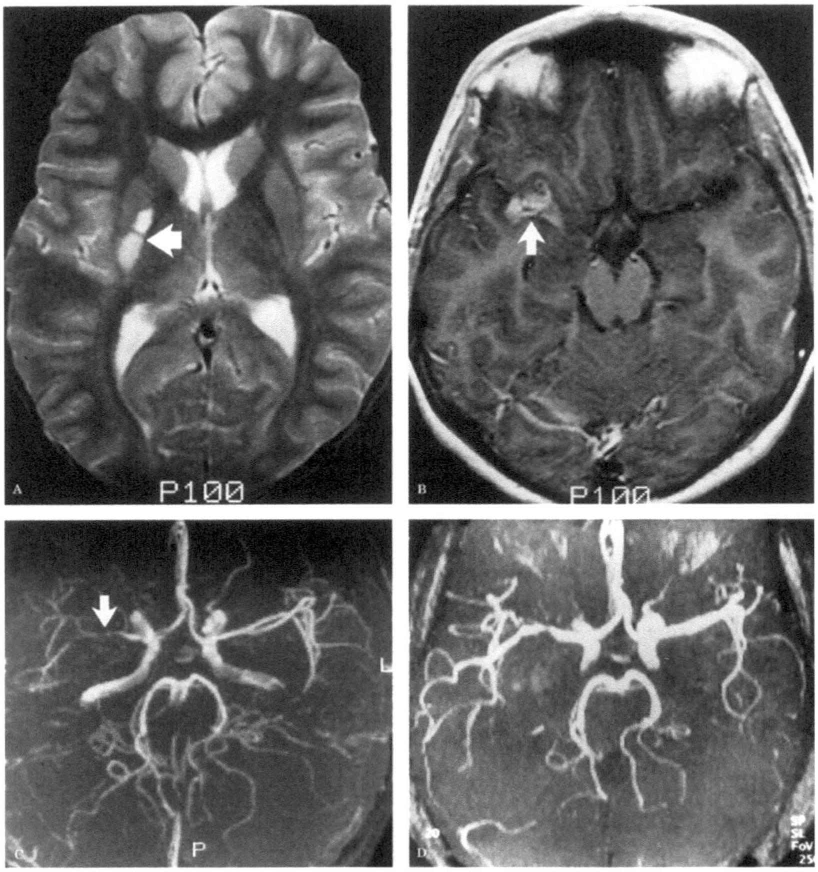

Fig. 17.12. Varicella-zoster virus vasculitis. Findings of brain magnetic resonance (MR) imaging. (**A**) Axial T2-weighted scan at presentation shows infarction (arrow) in the right putamen. (**B**) Axial gadolinium-enhanced T1-weighted scan at presentation shows contrast enhancement within and surrounding the right middle cerebral artery (arrow). (**C**) Initial MR angiogram shows focal stenosis in the right middle cerebral artery (arrow) with reduced distal flow signal. (**D**) Follow-up MR angiogram at 6 months shows partial resolution of middle cerebral artery stenosis and normal distal flow signal. Reproduced from Singhal et al. (2001), with permission.

2009). The disease has an inevitable progressive nature, more so in women than men and despite therapy (Kuroda et al., 2005).

The diagnosis of MMD relies on conventional angiography, considered the diagnostic gold standard. A definite diagnosis requires an angiographic finding of stenosis of the distal intracranial ICA extending to the proximal ACA and MCA. The degree of disease progression is angiographically classified into six stages by the Suzuki grading system. The characteristic "puff of smoke" is seen in the intermediate stages of disease (Suzuki and Takaku, 1969). MRI and MRA are helpful for the diagnosis and for monitoring of disease progression. On MRA, decreased flow-related enhancement in the distribution of the distal ICA, MCA, and ACA with associated prominence of flow-related enhancement in the basal ganglia and thalami due to collateral vessels are characteristic findings. Contrast-enhanced T1 may be superior to FLAIR imaging in showing the characteristic "ivy sign," a depiction of superficial pial vascular collateral networks (Yoon et al., 2002). Contrast imaging may also show vascular enhancement in the basal ganglia. MRI may also show nonspecific sulcal or ventricular dilatation. Ischemic strokes are seen commonly in the anterior borderzone and/or in the distribution of the deep penetrator arteries. Microbleeds can be seen in about 40% of MMD patients (Kikuta et al., 2008). Hemorrhages may be deep intraparenchymal, intraventricular, and, less commonly, subdural or subarachnoid. Assessment of cerebral blood flow and cerebrovascular reserve is crucial in MMD, and can be done with multiple modalities such as PET, single-photon emission CT (SPECT), transcranial Doppler (TCD), perfusion MRI, and perfusion CT (Lee et al., 2009b). For assessment of progression of arterial stenoses or postsurgical improvement, TCD can be useful and has excellent correlation with conventional angiography (Perren et al., 2005).

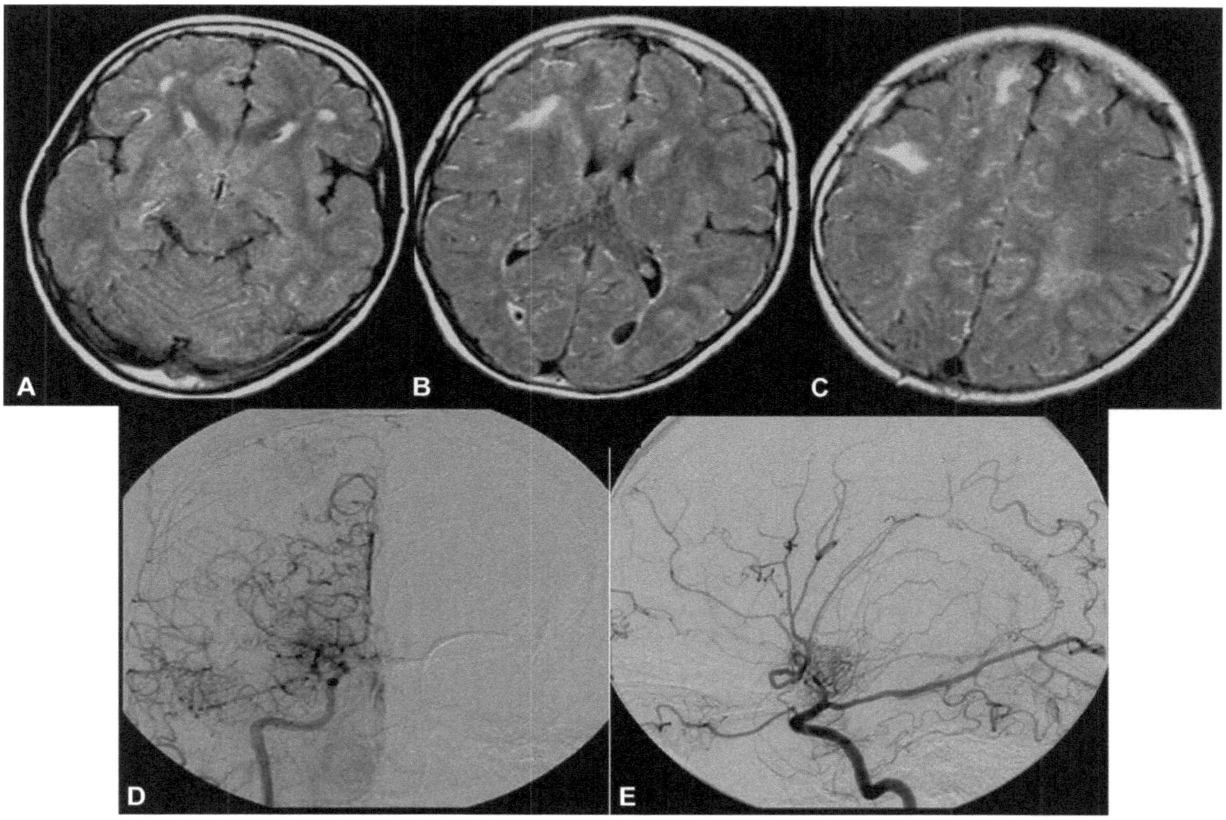

Fig. 17.13. Moyamoya syndrome. Axial fluid-attenuated inversion recovery (FLAIR) images (**A–C**) from a child with moyamoya disease demonstrate multiple hyperintense subcortical white-matter lesions consistent with chronic infarctions. FLAIR images also show hyperintense collateral vessels in the basal ganglia and subarachnoid spaces. The vessels are probably hyperintense due to slow flow. (**D**) Anteroposterior and (**E**) lateral digital subtraction angiographic images from another patient show severe stenosis of the distal right internal carotid artery and proximal anterior and middle cerebral arteries. There is poor direct filling of the anterior cerebral artery and middle cerebral artery branches. There are prominent pial–pial collateral vessels from the posterior to middle and anterior cerebral artery branches. There are also prominent collateral vessels in the region of the basal ganglia.

Reversible cerebral vasoconstriction syndrome (Fig. 17.14)**.** RCVS comprises a group of disorders characterized by prolonged but reversible segmental vasoconstriction and vasodilatation ("sausaging") of the circle of Willis arteries and their branches, usually associated with acute-onset, severe, recurrent headaches, with or without additional neurologic signs and symptoms. This group of disorders has also received many epynomic or syndromic labels, reflecting its varied etiology: Call–Fleming syndrome, benign angiopathy of the CNS, postpartum cerebral angiopathy, migraine angiitis, and cerebral vasoconstriction associated with vasoactive drugs, tumors, and recurrent thunderclap headaches (Calabrese et al., 2007). The etiology of RCVS is unknown, but it is believed to be triggered by a disturbance in the control of cerebral vascular tone, which may be spontaneous or induced by external or internal factors (Calabrese et al., 2007). The syndrome affects mainly women (4:1 ratio) of all races between ages 20 and 50 years. Children can also be affected (Calabrese et al., 2007; Singhal et al., 2011). Disease onset is usually dramatic, with 90% of patients presenting with worst-ever thunderclap headaches prompting urgent medical evaluation. Headaches are often occipital or diffuse, can recur over a period of weeks to months in 80% of cases and are worsened or precipitated by exertion or the Valsalva maneuver (Singhal et al., 2011). Additional symptoms include transient or permanent visual defects, hemiplegia, dysarthria, aphasia, numbness, ataxia, seizures, and transient hypertension (Calabrese et al., 2007). Such symptoms are commonly due to stroke, which usually presents itself at the onset of RCVS or within a few days. In rare cases infarction may progress and lead to death and is presumed to be secondary to severe vasoconstriction (Geraghty et al., 1991; Singhal et al., 2009). Resolution of the vasoconstriction may be complicated by reperfusion injury and disturbed autoregulation, leading to hemorrhages and reversible

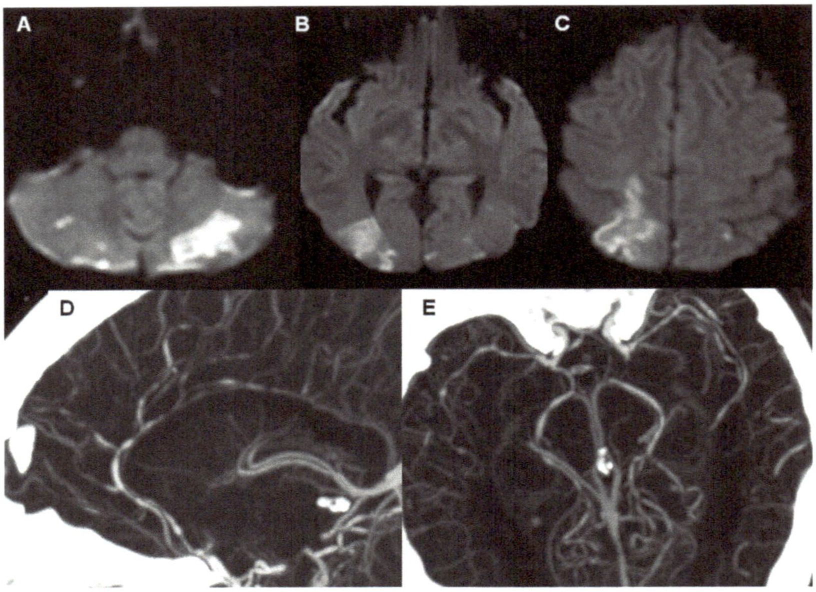

Fig. 17.14. Reversible cerebral vasoconstriction syndrome. A 55-year-old woman on serotonergic antidepressants, with recurrent thunderclap headaches followed by motor deficits. (**A–C**) Diffusion-weighted images show acute infarctions in both cerebellar hemispheres, both occipital lobes and both parietal lobes. There are also punctate infarctions in the right frontal lobe. (**D, E**) Sagittal and axial computed tomography-angiography images show multifocal stenoses ("sausaging") throughout the intracranial vasculature, more prominent in the middle cerebral artery and anterior cerebral artery territories than in the posterior cerebral artery territory.

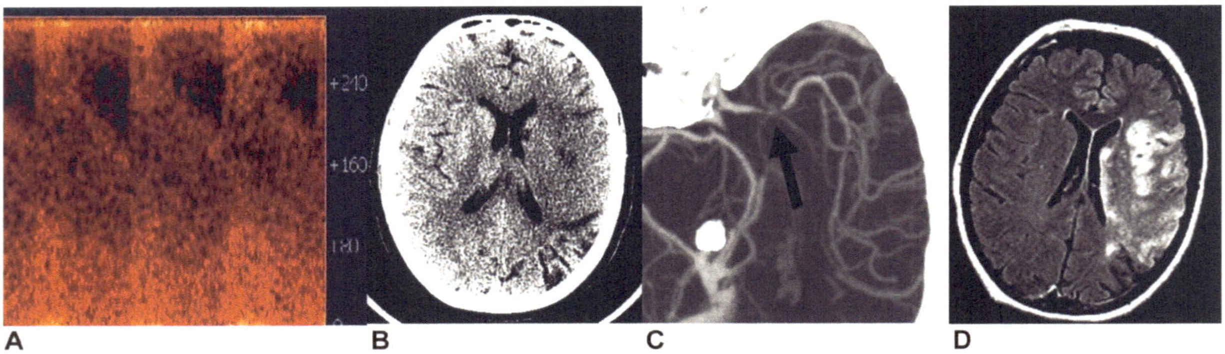

Fig. 17.15. Stroke from cocaine-induced vasospasm. (**A**) Transcranial Doppler of the left middle cerebral artery shows severely elevated velocities. (**B**) Noncontrast computed tomography (CT) shows loss of gray–white differentiation in the left basal ganglia and deep white matter as well as the perisylvian cortex, consistent with acute left middle cerebral artery infarction. More well-defined hypodense foci in the left insula, left caudate head, and left parietal lobe represent more chronic infarctions. (**C**) CT angiography shows severe stenosis in the M1 segment of the left middle cerebral artery (arrow). (**D**) Fluid-attenuated inversion recovery magnetic resonance imaging image obtained 5 days later confirms a subacute left middle cerebral artery infarction.

cerebral edema. Precipitating factors in RCVS are found in two-thirds of cases and include postpartum state (postpartum angiopathy), pre-eclampsia/eclampsia, migraine, use of vasoactive drugs (cocaine, pseudoephedrine, sumatriptan, selective serotonin reuptake inhibitors, ergot derivatives) and cannabis (Calabrese et al., 2007; Ducros et al., 2007) (Fig. 17.15). CSF analysis is entirely normal in 80% of cases and may show minor abnormalities related to the underlying infarct of hemorrhage in the rest (Calabrese et al., 2007).

The diagnosis of RCVS is usually made based on the clinical suspicion and after exclusion of other conditions that can also present with thunderclap headache, such as SAH due to aneurysmal rupture. Neuroimaging is key to establishing the diagnosis. Noncontrast head CT should be performed initially to exclude aneurysmal SAH and other mimics. Initial parenchymal neuroimaging by CT or MRI is normal in 55% of cases; however, serial imaging reveals infarcts, edema, or hemorrhage in approximately 80% of cases in inpatient studies (Singhal et al., 2011). Parenchymal imaging may show strokes in up to 54% of RCVS cases, which are usually in a watershed distribution (Calabrese et al., 2007; Singhal et al., 2011). Hemorrhages (lobar in 6%, cortical surface SAH in 22–33%, and subdural hematomas) have been seen in up to 34% (Ducros et al., 2010; Singhal et al., 2011). Furthermore, reversible cerebral edema in a posterior distribution similar to that seen in posterior reversible encephalopathy syndrome (PRES) is found in more than one-third of patients (Singhal, 2004; Ducros et al., 2007, 2010; Bartynski and Boardman, 2008; Singhal et al., 2011). Vascular imaging helps ascertain the diagnosis. Conventional cerebral angiography is still considered the gold standard, but there is utility for MRA and CTA (Chen et al., 2010). Vascular imaging will show alternating areas of arterial constriction and dilatation in multiple vascular beds involving large and medium-sized cerebral arteries of the anterior and posterior cerebral circulation. On MRI, dilated segments of cortical surface arteries can result in linear or dot-shaped hyperintensities (dot sign) within the deep sulcal spaces on FLAIR imaging (Iancu-Gontard et al., 2003). This has been reported in 70% of RCVS cases (Singhal et al., 2011). MRA and CTA are the preferred methods of choice for monitoring the resolution of the arterial abnormalities in RCVS. Additionally, TCD can be used to follow these dynamic vasoconstrictive arterial changes until resolution occurs.

Genetic, inherited, and developmental vascular anomalies

Fabry's disease. Fabry's disease is a multisystem, X-linked recessive lysosomal storage disorder caused by a mutation in the GLA gene on chromosome Xq22, resulting in alpha-galactosidase A enzyme deficiency. This leads to deposition of glycosphingolipids in the endothelium and smooth muscle with secondary vessel occlusion and ischemic organ dysfunction. The disease most commonly affects hemizygous males, but disease in heterozygous females can occur. Initial clinical findings present in childhood and include renal dysfunction with proteinuria, cardiac dysfunction, painful peripheral and autonomic neuropathy, and strokes. Mean age of onset of strokes is 33–46 years in men and 40–52 years in women. Recurrent stroke occurs in 77% with high mortality rates. Ischemic stroke is most commonly seen in the vertebrobasilar territory, in association with typical dolichoectatic vessels (Rolfs et al., 2005). Unrecognized Fabry's disease may be an important etiology of cryptogenic ischemic stroke in the young: one study found an incidence of 4.9% in men and 2.4% in women with cryptogenic stroke, and >24% in men with recurrent cryptogenic strokes (Rolfs et al., 2005). Intracerebral hemorrhages and SAH may also occur. In addition to the findings mentioned above, the pulvinar of the thalami may appear hyperintense on T1-weighted MRI images (Bersano et al., 2012).

Fibromuscular dysplasia (Fig. 17.16). FMD is a nonatherosclerotic, noninflammatory vascular disease that most commonly affects medium-sized arteries. There are three histologic subtypes: medial dysplasia, intimal fibroplasia, and adventitial fibroplasia. The most common pathologic finding is medial fibroplasia (75–80% of cases), with exclusive involvement of the media. This results in rings of fibrous tissue and smooth-muscle segments, characterized by a "string-of-beads" appearance in the middle to distal portion of the affected artery. The beads are usually larger than the arterial diameter. The second most common is perimedial fibroplasia, seen in 10% of cases. This is characterized histologically by a homogeneous collar of elastic tissue at the junction of the media and the adventitia with preservation of their elastic components. Radiologically this leads to focal stenoses and, occasionally, multiple constrictions with

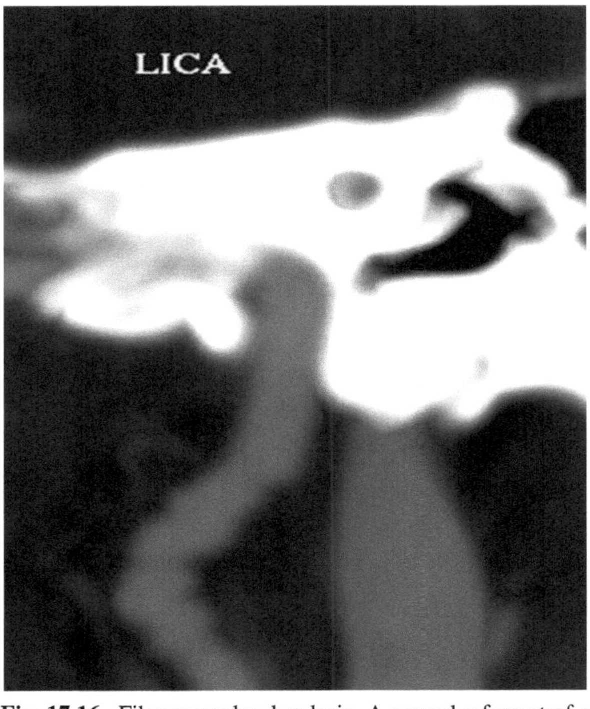

Fig. 17.16. Fibromuscular dysplasia. A curved reformat of a neck computed tomography-angiography shows diffuse irregularity with multiple dilated foci, consistent with fibromuscular dysplasia of the distal cervical left internal carotid artery (LICA) in a 50-year-old patient.

good collateral vascularization (Slovut and Olin, 2004). Macroaneurysms and dissections occur as well. The most commonly involved arteries are renal (60–75% of cases) and cerebrovascular (25–30%). When cerebral arteries are involved, the ICAs are affected in 95% and vertebral arteries in 12–40%. Cervical artery FMD is associated with intracranial aneurysms in 7–51% of cases (Olin, 2007). Additional affected arterial beds include the visceral (10%) and limb arteries (5%) (Olin, 2007). Risk factors for the disease include smoking, hypertension, and angiotensin-converting enzyme allele ACE-I (Slovut and Olin, 2004). An association with collagen and elastin mutations has not been confirmed and there is weak familial transmission. The disease is most commonly seen in Caucasian women 15–50 years old, and patients are usually asymptomatic at the time of diagnosis. Cervical FMD may be diagnosed during investigation of a high cervical bruit. Cervical artery FMD is more commonly diagnosed at age 50 years (Olin, 2007). Nonspecific symptoms such as headaches, dizziness, neck pain, and tinnitus may be present, as well as amaurosis fugax, other TIA syndromes, and cranial nerve palsies. Strokes are usually ischemic and due to arterial dissections or result from progressive arterial stenosis and occlusion. Spontaneous cervical dissections are seen in 15% of FMD patients, may be multiple, and are sometimes associated with pseudoaneurysms. SAH may also occur in the setting of intracranial aneurysm rupture. Duplex ultrasonography may show irregular patterns of stenosis and aneurysms, but its sensitivity is lower than angiography given the distal location of the cervical artery disease. Conventional angiography is still the gold-standard method for diagnosis, but CTA and MRA of the intra- and extracranial vasculature are good alternatives (Slovut and Olin, 2004).

Dolichoectasia (dilatative arteriopathy: Fig. 17.17**).** Dolichoectasia is a nonatherosclerotic vasculopathy that occurs due to disruption of the internal elastic lamina. It is characterized by elongated and tortuous arteries, sometimes with fusiform aneurysmal dilatation. It preferentially involves the intracranial vessels, especially the basilar and vertebral arteries. Dolichoectasia has been associated with hypertension, older age, male sex, cardiovascular risk factors, decreased matrix metalloproteinase (MMP)-3 levels, MMP-3 gene polymorphisms, Marfan's and Ehlers–Danlos syndromes, Fabry's disease, and SSD (Pico et al., 2010; Gutierrez et al., 2011). Associated vascular findings include extensive leukoaraiosis, severe "etat criblé" and multiple lacunar infarcts (Pico et al., 2005). The disease may be asymptomatic or present with ischemic strokes and TIAs secondary to distortion of the origins of penetrator arteries or atherosclerosis involving the penetrating arteries, especially those arising from the basilar artery (Kwon et al., 2009). Hemorrhagic strokes and SAH have been reported in 18% of patients with vertebrobasilar dolichoectasia, and their occurrence is associated with the degree of ectasia and elongation of the basilar artery (Passero et al., 2005). Often patients will have symptoms of compression of the brainstem, such as trigeminal neuralgia and hemifacial spasm. Diagnosis can be made with conventional angiography, MRA, or CTA. Smoker's criteria have been used to diagnose dolichoectasia. These criteria include the basilar artery diameter, laterality of the vessel, and the height of the vertebral-basilar junction (Smoker et al., 1986). There is no known treatment for this condition, though surgery to relieve compressive symptoms can be performed.

Cerebral autosomal-dominant arteriopathy with subcortical infarcts and leukoencephalopathy (Fig. 17.18). CADASIL is an inherited autosomal-dominant disease due to Notch-3 gene mutations on chromosome 19p13.2–13.1 (Joutel et al., 1996). This gene encodes a transmembrane receptor expressed in systemic arterial smooth-muscle cells. Pathologically the vasculopathy affects the small penetrating and leptomeningeal arteries. There is arterial wall thickening, luminal stenosis, deposits of nonamyloid granular

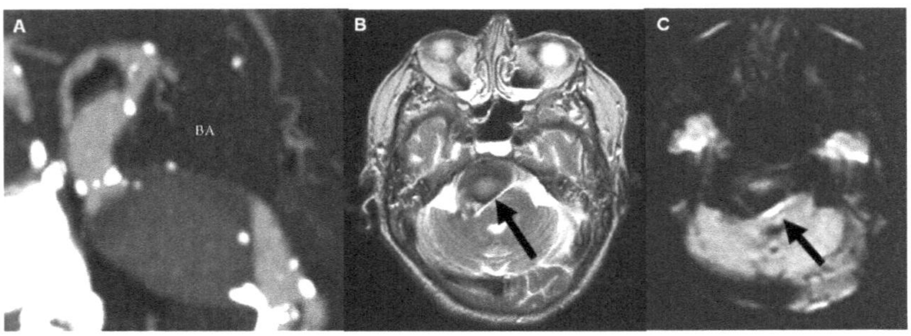

Fig. 17.17. Dolichoectasia. A 70-year-old woman presenting with somnolence and hemiparesis. (**A**) Computed tomography-angiography shows impressive fusiform dilatation of the basilar artery (BA) with nonopacification of the proximal portion, consistent with acute clot. Brain magnetic resonance imaging was obtained 6 hours later. There is an acute infarction in the left pons characterized by hyperintensity on the T2 image (**B**, arrow), and restricted diffusion on diffusion-weighted imaging (**C**, arrow).

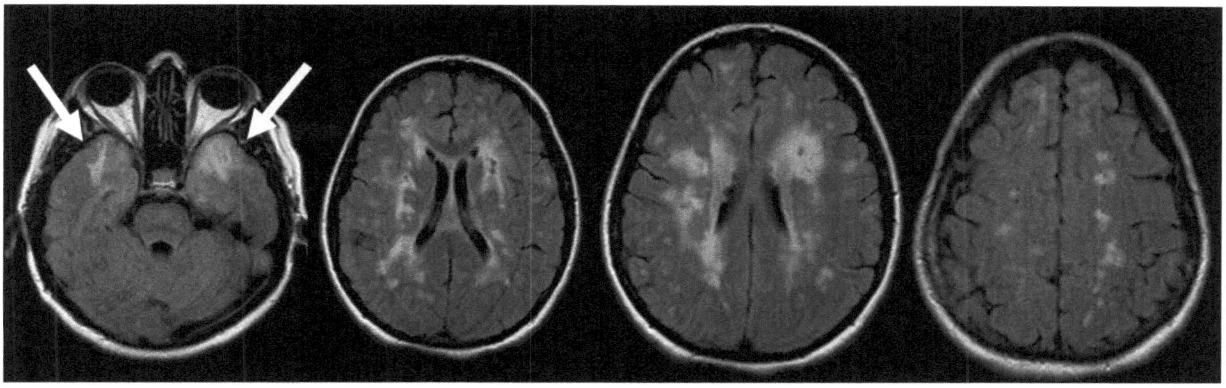

Fig. 17.18. Cerebral autosomal-dominant arteriopathy with subcortical infarcts and leukoencephalopathy (CADASIL). Axial fluid-attenuated inversion recovery images at multiple levels show patchy periventricular and subcortical hyperintense foci with some areas of cavitation. Lesions in the anterior temporal subcortical white matter (arrows) are characteristic of CADASIL.

osmophilic material in the media and adventitia, and morphologic changes to the smooth-muscle cells (Baudrimont et al., 1993; Okeda et al., 2002). The prevalence of CADASIL is unknown, but it has been reported in 11% of patients younger than age 50 who present with lacunar strokes and leukoaraiosis (Chabriat et al., 2009). Clinical manifestations include migraine with aura in 20–40%; subcortical TIAs or strokes in 60–80%, often in the absence of vascular risk factors and usually presenting with classic lacunar syndromes; mood disturbance and apathy in 20%; and cognitive impairment and dementia. Cognitive decline is the second most common manifestation and usually begins with executive dysfunction (Chabriat et al., 2009; Reyes et al., 2009). Progression to dementia is directly associated with an increasing lacunar burden (Viswanathan et al., 2007). Migraine with aura is the initial manifestation and starts approximately at age 30, followed by ischemic events and mood disturbances between ages 40 and 60 years, and later by dementia between 50 and 60 years (Chabriat et al., 2009). MRI findings are usually evident by age 30 and may precede clinical manifestations by 10–15 years. The most common findings are areas of increased signal on T2 or FLAIR images in the periventricular region and centrum semiovale, later progressing in a symmetric and confluent fashion to involve the external capsule and anterior temporal subcortical white matter, which is nearly pathognomonic of this disease. Multiple lacunar infarctions can be seen, usually of various ages (Markus et al., 2002). Cerebral microbleeds are seen in 25–69% of cases and may contribute further to cognitive impairment. Dilated perivascular spaces can also be noted, conforming to a condition called "état criblé" (Chabriat et al., 2009). Rapidly progressing brain atrophy is also present. There is no clear role for conventional angiography or CT imaging in CADASIL. Additional diagnostic techniques include skin biopsy and genetic mutation testing (Markus et al., 2002). Unfortunately there is no disease-specific treatment for CADASIL, although stroke risk factor modification is recommended to decrease cerebrovascular burden. Acetazolamide can be used to improve cerebral perfusion and decrease migrainous manifestations (Chabriat et al., 2000).

Of interest, a recessive disease similar to CADASIL has been described, entitled CARASIL (cerebral autosomal-recessive arteriopathy with subcortical infarcts and leukoencephalopathy). This disease is present in younger patients (ages 25–30 years) and is more frequent in women. Clinical manifestations include ischemic cerebral small-vessel disease without hypertension, alopecia, spondylosis, progressive cognitive impairment, pyramidal syndrome, and pseudobulbar palsy. MRI reveals diffuse white-matter changes (Fukutake and Hirayama, 1995).

Retinovasculopathy and cerebral leukodystrophy (RVCL). Cerebroretinal vasculopathy (CRV), hereditary endotheliopathy with retinopathy, neuropathy, and stroke (HERNS), hereditary vascular retinopathy (HVR) and hereditary systemic angiopathy (HSA) – subsequently combined as RVCL – are devastating autosomal-dominant genetic disorders linked to TREX-1 mutations that present in early to middle age with characteristic neurologic and ophthalmologic findings. Histologic examination shows characteristic multilaminated basement membranes in the brain, kidney, stomach, appendix, and skin. Linkage to chromosome 3p21 has been shown (Vahedi et al., 2003). HERNS first presents with neuropsychiatric symptoms in the second decade of life. This is followed by visual loss and renal dysfunction, including proteinuria and hematuria in the third to fourth decades. Neurologic manifestations such as migraine, and signs of multifocal cortical and subcortical dysfunction from recurrent strokes, culminating with dementia, begin 4–10 years later. In the presymptomatic phase, MRI shows multiple FLAIR and T2 hyperintense lesions in the deep white matter. Once neurologic signs and symptoms ensue, contrast-enhancing lesions with surrounding vasogenic edema appear, predominantly in the deep frontoparietal white matter. Ophthalmologic changes include macular edema, capillary dropout, and perifoveal microangiopathic telangectasias (Jen et al., 1997). Unfortunately, there is no known disease-specific treatment for HERNS.

Sickle cell disease

SSD is a hemoglobinopathy caused by an autosomal-recessive point mutation in the hemoglobin β chain. The disease occurs mainly in African Americans, with an estimated prevalence of 1/500 births in the USA. Under conditions of acidosis and hypoxemia, the abnormal hemoglobin polymerizes into a gel. This changes the red cell morphology and increases blood viscosity. There is sludging in the arterial microcirculation and adherence of hemoglobin to the arterial wall. A cascade of inflammation and clotting ensues, promoting intimal proliferation, increase in arterial fibroblasts and smooth-muscle cells, and progressive vascular occlusions (Switzer et al., 2006). This arterial pathology is frequently seen in the distal ICA, circle of Willis, and proximal branches of the major intracranial arteries (Switzer et al., 2006). Symptoms of SSD begin in early childhood, usually as painful vascular occlusive crises. There is an increased risk of recurrent vascular occlusive events, including ischemic stroke and infarctions of the kidney, lung, bone, skin, and eye. SSD is the most common cause of childhood stroke. The highest risk for stroke is between ages 2 and 5, and peaks again after age 29. Eleven percent of SSD patients will have strokes by age 10, and 24% by 45 years. Recurrent strokes are reported in two-thirds of patients, usually within 2–3 years of the initial event. Silent infarcts occur in 17–35% of patients. Risk factors for ischemic stroke include TIA, acute chest syndrome within 2 weeks, anemia with persistent hemoglobin levels <7 g/dL, elevated systolic blood pressure, moyamoya phenomenon, silent brain infarcts, and elevated velocities on TCD (Switzer et al., 2006). Stroke neuroimaging in SSD is usually performed with MRI and MRA. Ischemic strokes can be seen in the distribution of large anterior circulation vessels (27–41%), in cortical borderzones (31–88%), and in the basal ganglia (22%) (Adams et al., 1988; Pavlakis et al., 1988). Spinal cord ischemia and venous sinus thrombosis have also been reported. Hemorrhagic strokes occur in SSD patients aged 20–30 years. MRA will often show stenosis or occlusion of the large intracranial vessels, with a moyamoya-like pattern in 20–40% (Wiznitzer et al., 1990; Dobson et al., 2002). MRA and TCDs have good correlation with angiography. In children, TCD velocities >200 cm/s are associated with a 10% annual risk of stroke and may help guide prophylactic blood transfusion therapy (Switzer et al., 2006). PET and xenon-133 inhalation studies can be done to assess vascular reserve in SSD, and usually demonstrate increased cerebral blood flow and blood volume with normal oxygen extraction. CTA is not typically performed in SSD patients because high osmolar iodinated contrast media were thought to increase the risk of sickling of erythrocytes, although there is no evidence that the currently used osmolar CT contrast agents increase this risk.

Stroke prevention involves hydroxyurea and serial blood transfusions aiming at hemoglobin S levels $<30\%$. This treatment has been shown to promote a 92% risk reduction of first ever stroke over 2 years (Adams et al., 1998).

Venous disorders

CEREBRAL VEIN AND DURAL SINUS THROMBOSIS (CVST: FIG. 17.19)

CVST is an uncommon cerebrovascular disease that involves thrombosis of cerebral sinuses and cerebral veins, accounting for 0.5–1% of all strokes (Bousser and Ferro, 2007). It can affect all ages, from neonates to the elderly, but is most commonly seen in those younger than 50 years of age (Ferro et al., 2004; Bousser and Ferro, 2007). There is a female predominance, with 75% of cases occurring in women in the largest CVST series to date (Ferro et al., 2004). It has a favorable outcome in 80% of cases, with mortality rates of approximately 8% (Ferro et al., 2004). Symptoms may present acutely in 37%, subacutely in 56%, or chronically in 7% (Ferro et al., 2004). The most common symptoms and signs are headaches, seizures, focal neurologic deficits, altered consciousness, and papilledema. These may be seen in isolation or combined, with or without other signs and symptoms. The most common clinical syndromes include isolated intracranial hypertension (10–40%), focal syndrome (40–75%), and subacute encephalopathy (31%). Isolated headaches are being more commonly recognized, often with a thunderclap quality (Biousse et al., 1999; Ferro et al., 2001; Cumurciuc et al., 2005). Risk factors for CVST are multiple and include genetic and acquired thrombophilias in 34%, oral contraceptives in 54%, and other conditions, such as malignancy, hematologic disorders (thrombocytemia, polycythemia, anemia), pregnancy, puerperium (14%), and infections, among others. A combination of risk factors is seen in approximately 44% of cases (Ferro et al., 2004). The superior sagittal sinus is the most frequently involved sinus (62%), followed by the transverse sinus (41–45%), straight sinus (18%), deep venous system (11%), and cortical veins (17%) (Ferro et al., 2004).

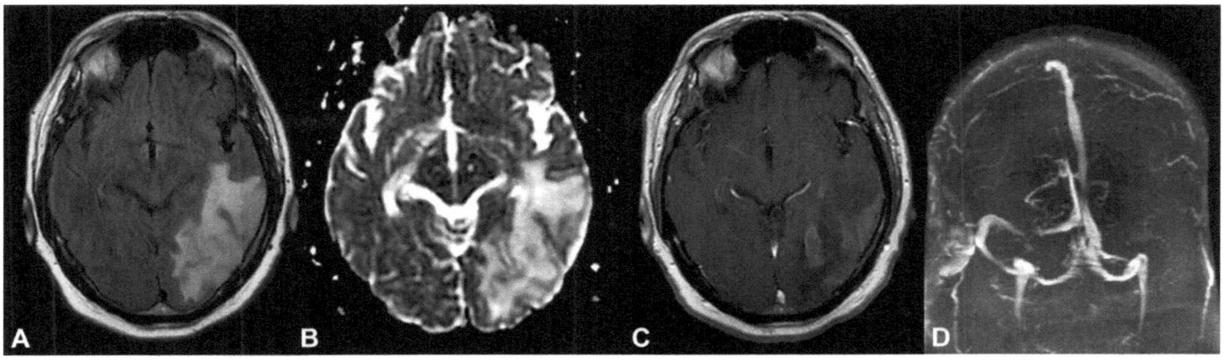

Fig. 17.19. Venous infarction. A 59-year-old man with worsening headaches for 2 weeks and word-finding difficulties. (**A**) A fluid-attenuated inversion recovery image demonstrates confluent hyperintensity, consistent with vasogenic edema, involving the gray and white matter of the left temporal and occipital lobes, with mild mass effect. The lesion is hyperintense on an apparent diffusion coefficient map (**B**), consistent with elevated diffusion typical of vasogenic edema. (**C**) On a gadolinium-enhanced T1-weighted image, there is gyriform enhancement due to breakdown of the blood–brain barrier. (**D**) Magnetic resonance venogram shows no flow-related enhancement, consistent with thrombosis, in the left transverse and sigmoid sinuses and proximal internal jugular vein.

Management involves anticoagulation with either unfractionated or low-molecular-weight heparin in the acute phase, followed by oral warfarin for 3–6 months or indefinitely, depending on the underlying etiology. Anticoagulation leads to an absolute risk reduction of 14% in mortality, and relative risk reduction of 56–70% in death or disability. Anticoagulation is deemed safe in the presence of intracerebral hemorrhage (Einhaupl et al., 1991, 2010; de Bruijn and Stam, 1999).

CVST may be difficult to recognize given its multiple clinical presentations and modes of onset, often leading to diagnostic delays (Ferro et al., 2004; Bousser and Ferro, 2007). Neuroimaging is required for confirmation of the diagnosis. NCCT imaging is insensitive for the diagnosis of CVST, with abnormalities only present in 30% of cases. Direct signs of CVST on NCCT include hyperdensities of the venous sinuses, often seen in the transverse sinus, torcula (dense triangle sign) and superior sagittal sinus, or of the cortical veins (cord sign) in the cerebral convexity. Indirect signs include parenchymal hemorrhages and edema in nonarterial distributions as well as cortical surface SAH (Ford and Sarwar, 1981). Contrast-enhanced CT imaging may show the classic empty delta sign. This is characterized by peripheral enhancement of the superior sagittal sinus at the torcula accompanied by central hypodensity due to clot (Buonanno et al., 1978). MRI is more sensitive than CT for detection of a venous thrombus within a sinus or vein. Brain MRI will show absence of flow voids in the venous structures and signal changes suggestive of thrombosis. Further, on contrast-enhanced MRI, a central nonenhancing lesion with peripheral enhancement may be seen, akin to the CT empty delta sign (Yuh et al., 1994). Thrombus has variable signal on brain MRI depending on the stage of thrombus. Acutely, the clot is isointense on T1 and hyperintense on T2-weighted images due to oxyhemoglobin. As deoxyhemoglobin forms, the clot becomes hypointense on T2-weighted images. As intracellular methemoglobin forms, the clot becomes hyperintense on T1-weighted images. With the formation of extracellular methemoglobin in the subacute stage, the clot becomes hyperintense on T1- and T2-weighted sequences. Chronic clot is isointense on T1 and isointense to hypointense on T2-weighted images (Bianchi et al., 1998). Adding susceptibility-weighted imaging for detection of thrombosis increases the sensitivity of MRI for CVST, especially for isolated cortical vein thrombosis (Idbaih et al., 2006). MRI is also more sensitive than NCCT for parenchymal changes. MRI may show normal parenchyma or edema and cerebral hemorrhages (Yuh et al., 1994). On DWI, edema may have elevated or decreased diffusion or a mixed pattern (Chu et al., 2001; Lovblad et al., 2001; Mullins et al., 2004). The distribution of parenchymal changes may provide clues as to the location of the venous thrombosis. In superior sagittal sinus thrombosis parenchymal changes may be seen bilaterally in frontal, parietal, and occipital lobes. Transverse sinus thrombosis will lead to parenchymal abnormalities of the ipsilateral temporal lobe. When deep parenchymal changes are seen bilaterally, such as in both thalami, thrombosis of the internal cerebral veins, vein of Galen, or straight sinus should be considered. Thrombosis of these structures can also lead to intraventricular hemorrhages (Saposnik et al., 2011). Both CTV and MRV can be used for anatomic visualization of CVST. For MRV, 2-D TOF has excellent sensitivity for slow flow (Saposnik et al., 2011), but newer, phase contrast techniques provide superior visualization of the sinuses in general. Multiplanar CT/CTV has 95% sensitivity and 91% specificity for CVST as compared to conventional cerebral angiogram (Wetzel et al., 1999). CTV and MRV have nearly replaced conventional angiography for the diagnosis of CVST.

Behçet's disease (Fig. 17.20)

Behçet's disease is a rare idiopathic systemic vasculitis, with a predilection for the venular system, most commonly seen in Turkey as well as in other Mediterranean countries, Japan, and Asia. The hallmark clinical manifestation is recurrent oral ulceration, which must occur at least three times over 1 year for a diagnosis of Behçet's disease. Other diagnostic clinical features include any two of: recurrent genital ulcerations; eye lesions such as uveitis or retinal vasculitis; skin lesions such as erythema nodosum-like lesions and papulopustular lesions; or a positive pathergy skin test (Ambrose and Haskard, 2013). Neurologic manifestations of Behçet's disease occur in 10–50% of cases and can be parenchymal (neuro-Behçet's disease, 80% of cases with CNS involvement) or vascular (vascular Behçet's disease, 20% of cases with CNS involvement). Cerebrovascular Behçet's disease usually presents with cerebral venous thrombosis or benign intracranial hypertension (Wechsler et al., 1992). Neuro-Behçet's disease can present with subacute meningoencephalitis, headache, and signs of brainstem, pyramidal, and cerebellar dysfunction. Brain MRI shows scattered or confluent T2-hyperintense lesions in the white matter (70% of cases), brainstem and cerebellum (60%), and basal ganglia or thalamus (40%), which can progress over time (Gerber et al., 1996). The CSF is invariably abnormal. Treatment of the disease usually involves immunosuppression in the acute phase and colchicine to prevent relapses (Hatemi et al., 2008). In cerebrovascular Behçet's disease, treatment usually consists of anticoagulation followed by lifelong antiplatelet therapy (Ambrose and Haskard, 2013).

Miscellaneous cerebrovascular disorders

Air and fat embolism (Figs 17.21 and 17.22)

Air embolism is an uncommon condition that can affect both the venous and arterial circulation. Venous air embolism is more frequent than arterial, and is most commonly seen during placement, manipulation, or removal of venous lines in the subclavian or jugular veins; during venous power injection for radiologic procedures; during neurosurgery with patients in the sitting position; or in neck, craniofacial, orthopedic, and cardiac surgery (Muth and Shank, 2000). Arterial air embolism is less common and may be seen during transthoracic needle aspiration and biopsy, or secondary to barotrauma from positive-pressure ventilation or chronic lung disease. Air

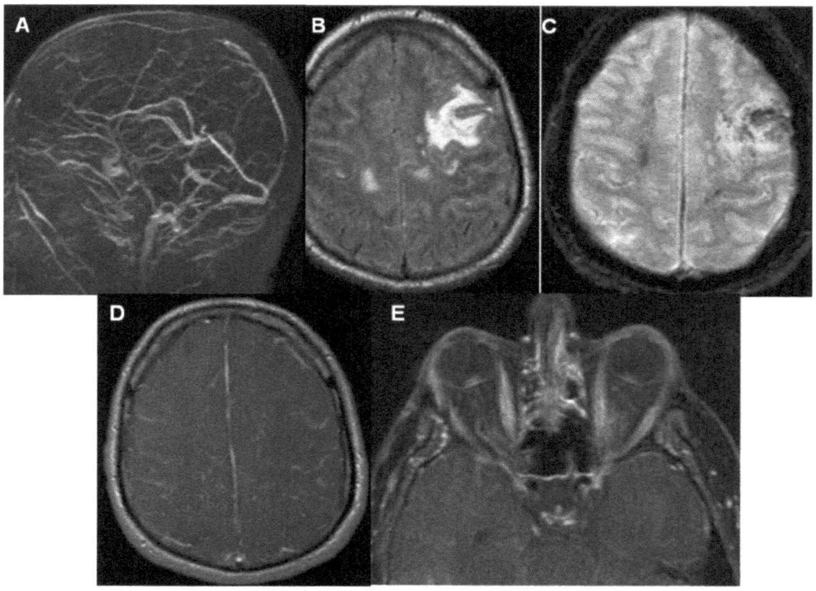

Fig. 17.20. Behçet's disease. Sagittal magnetic resonance venogram (**A**) shows no flow-related enhancement due to thrombosis of the anterior half of the superior sagittal sinus. (**B**) Fluid-attenuated inversion recovery image shows hyperintense lesions, consistent with edema, in frontal white matter bilaterally. (**C**) Gradient echo image shows foci of susceptibility, consistent with hemorrhage, in frontal white matter bilaterally. (**D**) A gadolinium-enhanced T1-weighted image shows leptomeningeal enhancement due to meningeal inflammation and/or collateral veins. (**E**) A gadolinium-enhanced fat-suppressed T1-weighted image through the orbits shows focal enhancement along the posterior portion of the eye globes, consistent with uveitis.

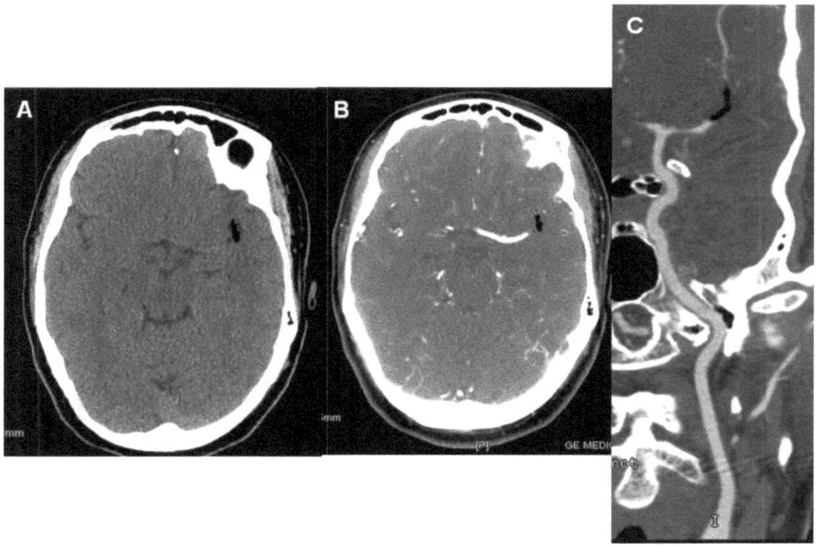

Fig. 17.21. Air embolism. A 38-year-old woman with a patent foramen ovale was undergoing sclerotherapy of varicose veins when she developed sudden onset of right-sided arm and leg weakness. (**A**) Nonconstrast computed tomography (CT) shows air in the expected location of the left middle cerebral artery bifurcation. (**B**) CT angiography source image shows contrast in the left middle cerebral artery contiguous with the air. (**C**) Curved reformatted images of the left internal carotid artery and middle cerebral artery show that the air is located within the middle cerebral artery in the region of the bifurcation.

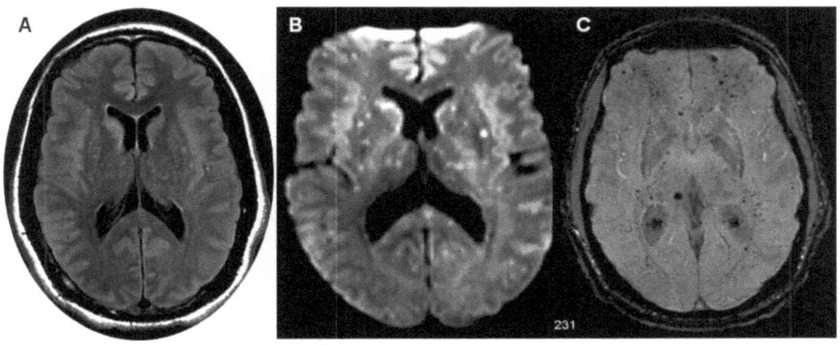

Fig. 17.22. Fat embolism. A 25-year-old with humerus fracture status posttrauma. There are numerous fluid-attenuated inversion recovery (**A**) and diffusion-weighted imaging (**B**) hyperintense punctate lesions scattered throughout the brain, consistent with acute infarctions secondary to fat emboli. (**C**) A susceptibility-weighted image shows numerous punctate foci of susceptibility, consistent with microhemorrhages due to blood vessel injury from free fatty acids.

embolism is enabled due to a pressure gradient favoring embolism towards a negative intravascular pressure. In the presence of a PFO, venous emboli can reach the arterial circulation as well. Air embolism can affect the lungs, heart, large vessels, and the brain. Clinical presentation includes dyspnea, chest pain, tachypnea, tachycardia, hemodynamic instability, agitation, confusion, seizures, coma and, rarely, cardiogenic shock and arrest. CT imaging is more sensitive than plain radiographs for detection of air embolism and will show nondependent air bubbles in the intrathoracic veins, heart, and arteries. On CT imaging air is very hypodense. In venous air embolism air is seen in the right heart, systemic veins, and cavernous sinus, whereas in arterial air embolism it is seen in the left heart, aorta, and cerebral arteries. Echocardiographic imaging may also show air in the right or left side of the heart and in the pulmonary arteries or veins. In venous embolism, the mainstay of treatment is prevention of additional entry of gas, volume expansion with fluids, 100% inhaled oxygen, and measures to maintain cardiorespiratory stability. In arterial gas embolism, treatment is hyperbaric oxygen therapy (Muth and Shank, 2000).

Fat embolization is a similar condition that occurs mainly after long bony or pelvic fractures, hip or knee replacement surgery, or after cardiac surgery. It is rare, seen in 0.7–2% of fractures. The small fat emboli can bypass the pulmonary vasculature and reach the arterial circulation, leading to embolization to the brain and other organs. Clinical manifestations are similar to those seen in air embolization. In addition there may be petechiae, anemia, thrombocytopenia, and fever. Neurologic manifestations include stroke-like syndromes, confusion, encephalopathy, seizures, and coma. Death can ensue in up to 7% of cases (Bulger et al., 1997). On neuroimaging, NCCT may be normal, though a "hypodense MCA sign" may be seen, representing a fat embolus in the MCA (Lee et al., 2005). MRI is the method of choice for diagnosis. T1-weighted images may be normal. On T2 and FLAIR there may be multiple, small and nonconfluent hyperintensities involving both the gray and white matter as well as deep nuclei, sometimes also in a borderzone distribution. These lesions typically demonstrate restricted diffusion on DWI and ADC. Acute ischemia involving large-artery brain territories may also be seen (Parizel et al., 2001). The release of fatty acids from the fat globules causes local toxic injury to endothelium and susceptibility-weighted images typically show numerous microhemorrhages.

Mitochondrial myopathy, encephalopathy, lactic acidosis, and stroke-like episodes (Fig. 17.23)

MELAS is an uncommon mitochondrial disorder involving multiple organ systems. It is most commonly seen in children and young adults and is inexorably progressive, leading to severe neurologic disability and death (Pavlakis et al., 1984). There have been several genetic mutations identified in this disease, but the most common one is the mitochondrial m.3243A > G mutation, which is seen in greater than 80% of cases (Ciafaloni et al., 1992; Goto et al., 1992). This genetic mutation is related to the respiratory transport chain, and its dysfunction leads to oxidative stress in highly metabolic

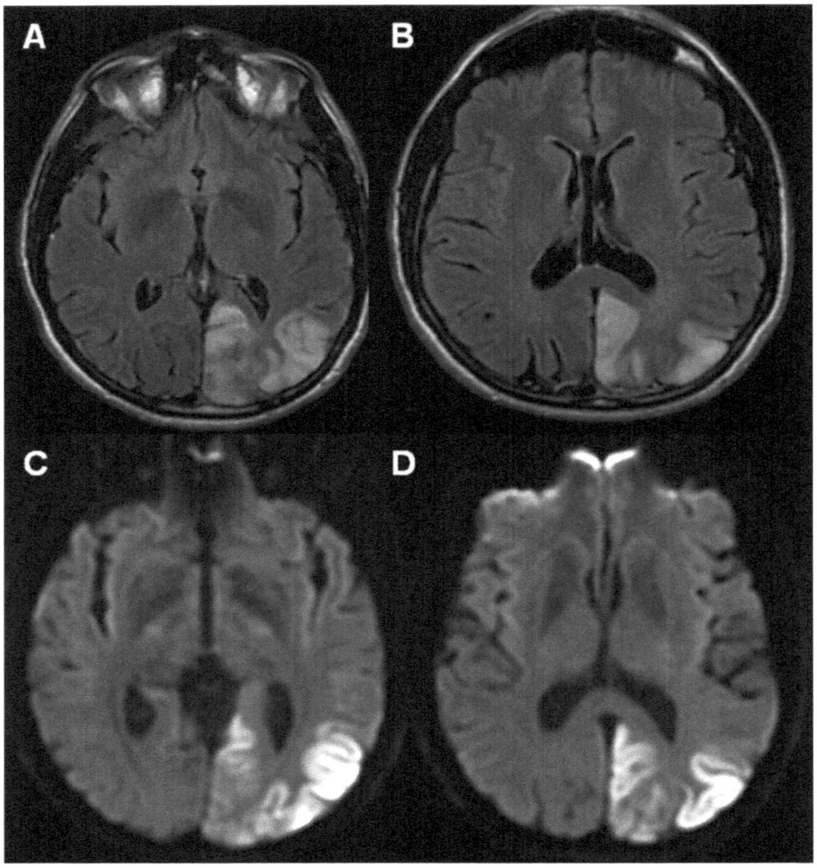

Fig. 17.23. Mitochondrial encephalomyopathy, lactic acidosis, and stroke-like episodes (MELAS). A 48-year-old man with homonymous hemianopsia and neurobehavioral deficits. There is a fluid-attenuated inversion recovery (**A, B**) hyperintense lesion involving cortex and subcortical white matter in the left parietal and occipital lobes. The lesion is hyperintense on diffusion-weighted imaging (**C, D**) due to restricted diffusion. The lesion involves both the posterior cerebral artery and middle cerebral artery territories.

organs such as muscle and brain. MELAS has a maternal pattern of inheritance with heteroplasmy and a threshold effect (Ciafaloni et al., 1992; Goto et al., 1992). Clinical findings include short stature, seizures, hearing loss, migraine-like headaches, fluctuating stroke-like episodes often seen as cortical blindness, hemianopsia and hemiparesis, developmental delay, cognitive impairment, and diabetes mellitus (Goto et al., 1992; Kaufmann et al., 2011; Yatsuga et al., 2012).

The diagnosis of MELAS relies on clinical suspicion, and is corroborated by neuroimaging findings. NCCT is usually unremarkable, although it may sometimes show lesions suggestive of ischemic infarcts, bilateral calcifications of the basal ganglia, and cerebral atrophy in the late stages of the disease (Hirano and Pavlakis, 1994; Kim et al., 1996). MRI shows cortical and subcortical cerebral lesions that do not respect arterial boundaries and that may migrate to other cerebral regions over time (Abe et al., 1990). These are most commonly seen in the occipital and parietal lobes. They usually affect the cortical ribbon, with relatively little involvement of the white-matter fibers. Similar lesions may also be seen in the thalami (Kim et al., 1996; Sue et al., 1998). The lesions are FLAIR and T2 hyperintense and most commonly have restricted diffusion during the acute phase, although they can have elevated diffusion (Yoneda et al., 1999; Wang et al., 2003; Sheerin et al., 2008; Kim et al., 2011). Over time there may be focal or diffuse cerebral atrophy, most often involving the cerebellum or occipital lobes (Kim et al., 1996). Magnetic resonance spectroscopy may reveal elevated levels of lactate and decreased *N*-acetyl aspartate/*N*-acetyl aspartatyl glutamate (Bianchi et al., 2003). Direct arterial and venous imaging is normal in MELAS (Abe et al., 1990). Additional diagnostic findings include elevated serum or CSF lactate in 97–100% of cases (Goto et al., 1992). Muscle biopsy will show characteristic ragged-red fibers on Gomori

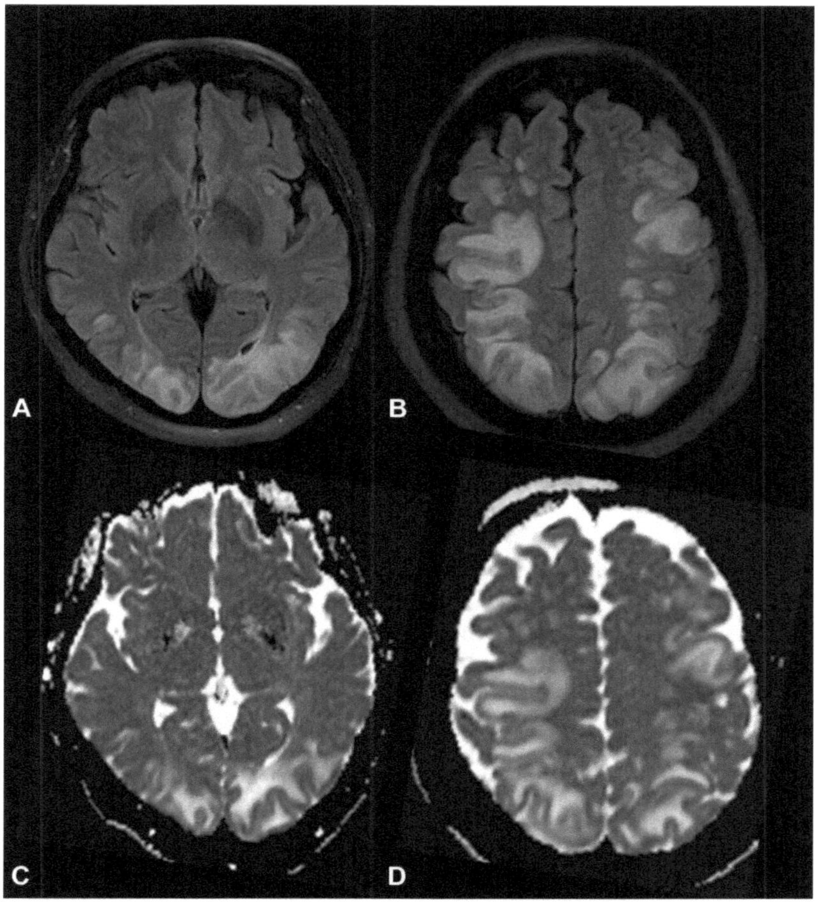

Fig. 17.24. Posterior reversible encephalopathy syndrome (PRES). A 64-year-old woman with hypertension and seizures. Fluid-attenuated inversion recovery images (**A, B**) show hyperintense lesions involving the posterior temporal and occipital cortex and subcortical white matter (**A**), as well as the frontal and parietal cortex and subcortical white matter in a borderzone distribution (**B**). The lesions are hyperintense on apparent diffusion coefficient images (**C, D**), because they represent vasogenic edema.

stains, and genetic testing may show the characteristic mutation in 80% of cases (Sato et al., 1992; Sarnat and Marin-Garcia, 2005). There is unfortunately no specific treatment for MELAS. Therapies that have been used include coenzyme Q10, ketogenic diet, idebenone, L-arginine, and dichloroacetate, but all with inconclusive results (Goodfellow et al., 2012).

Posterior reversible encephalopthy syndrome (Fig. 17.24)

PRES is a condition characterized by neurologic dysfunction due to reversible vasogenic cerebral edema. Edema develops due to transmembrane flow of intravascular fluid and protein in the setting of abnormal capillary filtration pressure and disruption of the blood–brain barrier (Hansson et al., 1975). Histopathology reveals vasogenic edema, arteriolar and capillary thrombosis with microinfarcts, and petechial hemorrhages (Chester et al., 1978). The classic clinical presentation includes a combination of headaches, cortical visual symptoms, seizures, and altered level of consciousness in the background of elevated blood pressure (Feske, 2011). The degree of blood pressure elevation is variable, and the rapid rise of blood pressure rather than the absolute blood pressure value is the most important determinant of PRES (Schwartz et al., 2000). PRES may be precipitated by medical conditions and drugs that can cause endothelial dysfunction and/or secondary hypertension. These include malignant hypertension, eclampsia/pre-eclampsia, critical medical illness, medications that promote hypertension, and imunosuppressants such as cyclosporine and tacrolimus (Feske, 2011).

The diagnosis of PRES should be based mainly on clinical suspicion as rarely neuroimaging may be normal. However, neuroimaging findings are usually present and may strongly support the diagnosis. MRI typically demonstrates T2/FLAIR hyperintensites with elevated diffusion in the occipital and parietal regions bilaterally, involving both white and gray matter. The frontal lobes, bilateral occipital-temporal regions, cerebellum, brainstem, basal ganglia, and thalami may also be involved. Hemorrhage may be seen in 15% of cases, typically as a cortical hematoma or cortical surface SAH. Rarely, reversible restricted diffusion may be seen on DWI and ADC images (McKinney et al., 2007; Stevens and Heran, 2012). Cerebral angiography often shows segmental arterial narrowing, suggesting a shared pathophysiology with RCVS. The mainstay of medical management involves aggressive blood pressure control and treatment of associated complications such as seizures (Feske, 2011).

References

Abe K, Inui T, Hirono N et al. (1990). Fluctuating MR images with mitochondrial encephalopathy, lactic acidosis, stroke-like syndrome (MELAS). Neuroradiology 32: 77.

Adams RJ, Nichols FT, McKie V et al. (1988). Cerebral infarction in sickle cell anemia: mechanism based on CT and MRI. Neurology 38: 1012–1017.

Adams Jr HP, Bendixen BH, Kappelle LJ et al. (1993). Classification of subtype of acute ischemic stroke. Definitions for use in a multicenter clinical trial. TOAST. Trial of Org 10172 in Acute Stroke Treatment. Stroke 24: 35–41.

Adams RJ, McKie VC, Hsu L et al. (1998). Prevention of a first stroke by transfusions in children with sickle cell anemia and abnormal results on transcranial Doppler ultrasonography. N Engl J Med 339: 5–11.

Albers GW (1999). Expanding the window for thrombolytic therapy in acute stroke. The potential role of acute MRI for patient selection. Stroke 30: 2230–2237.

Alhalabi M, Moore PM (1994). Serial angiography in isolated angiitis of the central nervous system. Neurology 44: 1221–1226.

Ambrose NL, Haskard DO (2013). Differential diagnosis and management of Behcet syndrome. Nat Rev Rheumatol 9: 79–89.

Appenzeller S, Faria AV, Zanardi VA et al. (2008). Vascular involvement of the central nervous system and systemic diseases: etiologies and MRI findings. Rheumatol Int 28: 1229–1237.

Arboix A, Alio J (2012). Acute cardioembolic cerebral infarction: answers to clinical questions. Curr Cardiol Rev 8: 54–67.

Arida A, Kyprianou M, Kanakis M et al. (2010). The diagnostic value of ultrasonography-derived edema of the temporal artery wall in giant cell arteritis: a second meta-analysis. BMC Musculoskelet Disord 11: 44.

Arnaud L, Haroche J, Malek Z et al. (2009). Is (18)F-fluorodeoxyglucose positron emission tomography scanning a reliable way to assess disease activity in Takayasu arteritis? Arthritis Rheum 60: 1193–1200.

Arnold M, Kappeler L, Georgiadis D et al. (2006). Gender differences in spontaneous cervical artery dissection. Neurology 67: 1050–1052.

Arnold M, Kurmann R, Galimanis A et al. (2010). Differences in demographic characteristics and risk factors in patients with spontaneous vertebral artery dissections with and without ischemic events. Stroke 41: 802–804.

Aubart-Cohen F, Klein I, Alexandra JF et al. (2007). Long-term outcome in Susac syndrome. Medicine (Baltimore) 86: 93–102.

Ay H, Oliveira-Filho J, Buonanno FS et al. (1999). Diffusion-weighted imaging identifies a subset of lacunar infarction associated with embolic source. Stroke 30: 2644–2650.

Ay H, Oliveira-Filho J, Buonanno FS et al. (2002). 'Footprints' of transient ischemic attacks: a diffusion-weighted MRI study. Cerebrovasc Dis 14: 177–186.

Ay H, Benner T, Arsava EM et al. (2007). A computerized algorithm for etiologic classification of ischemic stroke: the Causative Classification of Stroke System. Stroke 38: 2979–2984.

Baba T, Houkin K, Kuroda S (2008). Novel epidemiological features of moyamoya disease. J Neurol Neurosurg Psychiatry 79: 900–904.

Ball EL, Walsh SR, Tang TY et al. (2010). Role of ultrasonography in the diagnosis of temporal arteritis. Br J Surg 97: 1765–1771.

Barnett HJ, Taylor DW, Eliasziw M et al. (1998). Benefit of carotid endarterectomy in patients with symptomatic moderate or severe stenosis. North American Symptomatic Carotid Endarterectomy Trial Collaborators. N Engl J Med 339: 1415–1425.

Bartynski WS, Boardman JF (2008). Catheter angiography, MR angiography, and MR perfusion in posterior reversible encephalopathy syndrome. AJNR Am J Neuroradiol 29: 447–455.

Baudrimont M, Dubas F, Joutel A et al. (1993). Autosomal dominant leukoencephalopathy and subcortical ischemic stroke. A clinicopathological study. Stroke 24: 122–125.

Bayer AS, Bolger AF, Taubert KA et al. (1998). Diagnosis and management of infective endocarditis and its complications. Circulation 98: 2936–2948.

Bersano A, Lanfranconi S, Valcarenghi C et al. (2012). Neurological features of Fabry disease: clinical, pathophysiological aspects and therapy. Acta Neurol Scand 126: 77–97.

Besson FL, Parienti JJ, Bienvenu B et al. (2011). Diagnostic performance of (1)(8)F-fluorodeoxyglucose positron emission tomography in giant cell arteritis: a systematic review and meta-analysis. Eur J Nucl Med Mol Imaging 38: 1764–1772.

Bianchi D, Maeder P, Bogousslavsky J et al. (1998). Diagnosis of cerebral venous thrombosis with routine magnetic resonance: an update. Eur Neurol 40: 179–190.

Bianchi MC, Tosetti M, Battini R et al. (2003). Proton MR spectroscopy of mitochondrial diseases: analysis of brain metabolic abnormalities and their possible diagnostic relevance. AJNR Am J Neuroradiol 24: 1958–1966.

Biousse V, D'Anglejan-Chatillon J, Touboul PJ et al. (1995). Time course of symptoms in extracranial carotid artery dissections. A series of 80 patients. Stroke 26: 235–239.

Biousse V, Ameri A, Bousser MG (1999). Isolated intracranial hypertension as the only sign of cerebral venous thrombosis. Neurology 53: 1537–1542.

Birnbaum J, Hellmann DB (2009). Primary angiitis of the central nervous system. Arch Neurol 66: 704–709.

Bley TA, Reinhard M, Hauenstein C et al. (2008). Comparison of duplex sonography and high-resolution magnetic resonance imaging in the diagnosis of giant cell (temporal) arteritis. Arthritis Rheum 58: 2574–2578.

Bogousslavsky J, Cachin C, Regli F et al. (1991). Cardiac sources of embolism and cerebral infarction – clinical consequences and vascular concomitants: the Lausanne Stroke Registry. Neurology 41: 855–859.

Borchers AT, Gershwin ME (2012). Giant cell arteritis: a review of classification, pathophysiology, geoepidemiology and treatment. Autoimmun Rev 11: A544–A554.

Bousser MG, Ferro JM (2007). Cerebral venous thrombosis: an update. Lancet Neurol 6: 162–170.

Bulger EM, Smith DG, Maier RV et al. (1997). Fat embolism syndrome. A 10-year review. Arch Surg 132: 435–439.

Buonanno FS, Moody DM, Ball MR et al. (1978). Computed cranial tomographic findings in cerebral sinovenous occlusion. J Comput Assist Tomogr 2: 281–290.

CADISS trial investigators, Markus HS, Hayter E et al. (2015). Antiplatelet treatment compared with anticoagulation treatment for cervical artery dissection (CADISS): a randomised trial. Lancet Neurol 14 (4): 361–367.

Calabrese LH, Mallek JA (1988). Primary angiitis of the central nervous system. Report of 8 new cases, review of the literature, and proposal for diagnostic criteria. Medicine (Baltimore) 67: 20–39.

Calabrese LH, Dodick DW, Schwedt TJ et al. (2007). Narrative review: reversible cerebral vasoconstriction syndromes. Ann Intern Med 146: 34–44.

Caplan LR, Hennerici M (1998). Impaired clearance of emboli (washout) is an important link between hypoperfusion, embolism, and ischemic stroke. Arch Neurol 55: 1475–1482.

Caselli RJ, Hunder GG, Whisnant JP (1988). Neurologic disease in biopsy-proven giant cell (temporal) arteritis. Neurology 38: 352–359.

Chabriat H, Pappata S, Ostergaard L et al. (2000). Cerebral hemodynamics in CADASIL before and after acetazolamide challenge assessed with MRI bolus tracking. Stroke 31: 1904–1912.

Chabriat H, Joutel A, Dichgans M et al. (2009). Cadasil. Lancet Neurol 8: 643–653.

Chamorro A, Sacco RL, Mohr JP et al. (1991). Clinical-computed tomographic correlations of lacunar infarction in the Stroke Data Bank. Stroke 22: 175–181.

Chen SP, Fuh JL, Wang SJ et al. (2010). Magnetic resonance angiography in reversible cerebral vasoconstriction syndromes. Ann Neurol 67: 648–656.

Chester EM, Agamanolis DP, Banker BQ et al. (1978). Hypertensive encephalopathy: a clinicopathologic study of 20 cases. Neurology 28: 928–939.

Chu K, Kang DW, Yoon BW et al. (2001). Diffusion-weighted magnetic resonance in cerebral venous thrombosis. Arch Neurol 58: 1569–1576.

Ciafaloni E, Ricci E, Shanske S et al. (1992). MELAS: clinical features, biochemistry, and molecular genetics. Ann Neurol 31: 391–398.

Cloft HJ, Murphy KJ, Prince MR et al. (1996). 3D gadolinium-enhanced MR angiography of the carotid arteries. Magn Reson Imaging 14: 593–600.

Crisostomo RA, Garcia MM, Tong DC (2003). Detection of diffusion-weighted MRI abnormalities in patients with transient ischemic attack: correlation with clinical characteristics. Stroke 34: 932–937.

Cumurciuc R, Crassard I, Sarov M et al. (2005). Headache as the only neurological sign of cerebral venous thrombosis: a series of 17 cases. J Neurol Neurosurg Psychiatry 76: 1084–1087.

Debette S, Leys D (2009). Cervical-artery dissections: predisposing factors, diagnosis, and outcome. Lancet Neurol 8: 668–678.

Debette S, Markus HS (2009). The genetics of cervical artery dissection: a systematic review. Stroke 40: e459–e466.

de Bruijn SF, Stam J (1999). Randomized, placebo-controlled trial of anticoagulant treatment with low-molecular-weight heparin for cerebral sinus thrombosis. Stroke 30: 484–488.

Dobson SR, Holden KR, Nietert PJ et al. (2002). Moyamoya syndrome in childhood sickle cell disease: a predictive factor for recurrent cerebrovascular events. Blood 99: 3144–3150.

Ducros A, Boukobza M, Porcher R et al. (2007). The clinical and radiological spectrum of reversible cerebral vasoconstriction syndrome. A prospective series of 67 patients. Brain 130: 3091–3101.

Ducros A, Fiedler U, Porcher R et al. (2010). Hemorrhagic manifestations of reversible cerebral vasoconstriction syndrome: frequency, features, and risk factors. Stroke 41: 2505–2511.

Duna GF, Calabrese LH (1995). Limitations of invasive modalities in the diagnosis of primary angiitis of the central nervous system. J Rheumatol 22: 662–667.

Easton JD, Saver JL, Albers GW et al. (2009). Definition and evaluation of transient ischemic attack. Stroke 40: 2276–2293.

Einhaupl KM, Villringer A, Meister W et al. (1991). Heparin treatment in sinus venous thrombosis. Lancet 338: 597–600.

Einhaupl K, Stam J, Bousser MG et al. (2010). EFNS guideline on the treatment of cerebral venous and sinus thrombosis in adult patients. Eur J Neurol 17: 1229–1235.

Engelter ST, Provenzale JM, Petrella JR et al. (1999). Diffusion MR imaging and transient ischemic attacks. Stroke 30: 2762–2763.

European Carotid Surgery Trialists' Collaborative Group (1998). Randomised trial of endarterectomy for recently symptomatic carotid stenosis: final results of the MRC European Carotid Surgery Trial (ECST). Lancet 351: 1379–1387.

Fazekas F, Chawluk JB, Alavi A et al. (1987). MR signal abnormalities at 1.5 T in Alzheimer's dementia and normal aging. AJR Am J Roentgenol 149: 351–356.

Ferro JM (2003). Cardioembolic stroke: an update. Lancet Neurol 2: 177–188.

Ferro JM, Correia M, Pontes C et al. (2001). Cerebral vein and dural sinus thrombosis in Portugal: 1980–1998. Cerebrovasc Dis 11: 177–182.

Ferro JM, Canhao P, Stam J et al. (2004). Prognosis of cerebral vein and dural sinus thrombosis: results of the International Study on Cerebral Vein and Dural Sinus Thrombosis (ISCVT). Stroke 35: 664–670.

Feske SK (2011). Posterior reversible encephalopathy syndrome: a review. Semin Neurol 31: 202–215.

Fisher CM (1965a). Lacunes: small, deep cerebral infarcts. Neurology 15: 774–784.

Fisher CM (1965b). Pure sensory stroke involving face, arm, and leg. Neurology 15: 76–80.

Fisher CM (1968). The arterial lesions underlying lacunes. Acta Neuropathol 12: 1–15.

Fisher CM (1982). The headache and pain of spontaneous carotid dissection. Headache 22: 60–65.

Fisher CM, Cole M (1965). Homolateral ataxia and crural paresis: a vascular syndrome. J Neurol Neurosurg Psychiatry 28: 48–55.

Fisher CM, Curry HB (1965). Pure motor hemiplegia of vascular origin. Arch Neurol 13: 30–44.

Ford K, Sarwar M (1981). Computed tomography of dural sinus thrombosis. AJNR Am J Neuroradiol 2: 539–543.

Fukutake T, Hirayama K (1995). Familial young-adult-onset arteriosclerotic leukoencephalopathy with alopecia and lumbago without arterial hypertension. Eur Neurol 35: 69–79.

Gaa J, Weidauer S, Sitzer M et al. (2004). Cerebral vasculitis due to *Treponema pallidum* infection: MRI and MRA findings. Eur Radiol 14: 746–747.

Gan R, Sacco RL, Kargman DE et al. (1997). Testing the validity of the lacunar hypothesis: the Northern Manhattan Stroke Study experience. Neurology 48: 1204–1211.

Garg A (2011). Vascular brain pathologies. Neuroimaging Clin N Am 21: 897–926. ix.

Geraghty JJ, Hoch DB, Robert ME et al. (1991). Fatal puerperal cerebral vasospasm and stroke in a young woman. Neurology 41: 1145–1147.

Gerber S, Biondi A, Dormont D et al. (1996). Long-term MR follow-up of cerebral lesions in neuro-Behcet's disease. Neuroradiology 38: 761–768.

Gerraty RP, Parsons MW, Barber PA et al. (2002). Examining the lacunar hypothesis with diffusion and perfusion magnetic resonance imaging. Stroke 33: 2019–2024.

Giles MF, Albers GW, Amarenco P et al. (2011). Early stroke risk and ABCD2 score performance in tissue- vs time-defined TIA: a multicenter study. Neurology 77: 1222–1228.

Gonzalez-Gay MA, Blanco R, Rodriguez-Valverde V et al. (1998). Permanent visual loss and cerebrovascular accidents in giant cell arteritis: predictors and response to treatment. Arthritis Rheum 41: 1497–1504.

Gonzalez-Gay MA, Garcia-Porrua C, Llorca J et al. (2001). Biopsy-negative giant cell arteritis: clinical spectrum and predictive factors for positive temporal artery biopsy. Semin Arthritis Rheum 30: 249–256.

Goodfellow JA, Dani K, Stewart W et al. (2012). Mitochondrial myopathy, encephalopathy, lactic acidosis and stroke-like episodes: an important cause of stroke in young people. Postgrad Med J 88: 326–334.

Goto Y, Horai S, Matsuoka T et al. (1992). Mitochondrial myopathy, encephalopathy, lactic acidosis, and stroke-like episodes (MELAS): a correlative study of the clinical features and mitochondrial DNA mutation. Neurology 42: 545–550.

Grant PE, He J, Halpern EF et al. (2001). Frequency and clinical context of decreased apparent diffusion coefficient reversal in the human brain. Radiology 221: 43–50.

Grant EG, Benson CB, Moneta GL et al. (2003). Carotid artery stenosis: gray-scale and Doppler US diagnosis –Society of Radiologists in Ultrasound Consensus Conference. Radiology 229: 340–346.

Greenan TJ, Grossman RI, Goldberg HI (1992). Cerebral vasculitis: MR imaging and angiographic correlation. Radiology 182: 65–72.

Gutierrez J, Sacco RL, Wright CB (2011). Dolichoectasia – an evolving arterial disease. Nat Rev Neurol 7: 41–50.

Ha SY, Park KY, Youn YC et al. (2009). Teaching NeuroImages: artery-to-artery embolism from a thrombosed cerebral aneurysm. Neurology 73: e63.

Hajj-Ali RA, Singhal AB, Benseler S et al. (2011). Primary angiitis of the CNS. Lancet Neurol 10: 561–572.

Hansson HA, Johansson B, Blomstrand C (1975). Ultrastructural studies on cerebrovascular permeability in acute hypertension. Acta Neuropathol 32: 187–198.

Hatemi G, Silman A, Bang D et al. (2008). EULAR recommendations for the management of Behcet disease. Ann Rheum Dis 67: 1656–1662.

Hayreh SS, Podhajsky PA, Raman R et al. (1997). Giant cell arteritis: validity and reliability of various diagnostic criteria. Am J Ophthalmol 123: 285–296.

Hermier M, Nighoghossian N (2004). Contribution of susceptibility-weighted imaging to acute stroke assessment. Stroke 35: 1989–1994.

Herve D, Touraine P, Verloes A et al. (2010). A hereditary moyamoya syndrome with multisystemic manifestations. Neurology 75: 259–264.

Hirano M, Pavlakis SG (1994). Mitochondrial myopathy, encephalopathy, lactic acidosis, and strokelike episodes (MELAS): current concepts. J Child Neurol 9: 4–13.

Hotchi M (1992). Pathological studies on Takayasu arteritis. Heart Vessels Suppl 7: 11–17.

Hunder GG, Bloch DA, Michel BA et al. (1990). The American College of Rheumatology 1990 criteria for the classification of giant cell arteritis. Arthritis Rheum 33: 1122–1128.

Huston 3rd J, Fain SB, Riederer SJ et al. (1999). Carotid arteries: maximizing arterial to venous contrast in fluoroscopically triggered contrast-enhanced MR angiography with elliptic centric view ordering. Radiology 211: 265–273.

Iancu-Gontard D, Oppenheim C, Touze E et al. (2003). Evaluation of hyperintense vessels on FLAIR MRI for the diagnosis of multiple intracerebral arterial stenoses. Stroke 34: 1886–1891.

Idbaih A, Boukobza M, Crassard I et al. (2006). MRI of clot in cerebral venous thrombosis: high diagnostic value of susceptibility-weighted images. Stroke 37: 991–995.

Jen J, Cohen AH, Yue Q et al. (1997). Hereditary endotheliopathy with retinopathy, nephropathy, and stroke (HERNS). Neurology 49: 1322–1330.

Johnston SL, Lock RJ, Gompels MM (2002). Takayasu arteritis: a review. J Clin Pathol 55: 481–486.

Joutel A, Corpechot C, Ducros A et al. (1996). Notch3 mutations in CADASIL, a hereditary adult-onset condition causing stroke and dementia. Nature 383: 707–710.

Kadkhodayan Y, Alreshaid A, Moran CJ et al. (2004). Primary angiitis of the central nervous system at conventional angiography. Radiology 233: 878–882.

Kang DW, Chu K, Ko SB et al. (2002). Lesion patterns and mechanism of ischemia in internal carotid artery disease: a diffusion-weighted imaging study. Arch Neurol 59: 1577–1582.

Kaufmann P, Engelstad K, Wei Y et al. (2011). Natural history of MELAS associated with mitochondrial DNA m.3243A > G genotype. Neurology 77: 1965–1971.

Kerr GS (1995). Takayasu's arteritis. Rheum Dis Clin North Am 21: 1041–1058.

Kidwell CS, Alger JR, Di Salle F et al. (1999). Diffusion MRI in patients with transient ischemic attacks. Stroke 30: 1174–1180.

Kikuta K, Takagi Y, Nozaki K et al. (2008). The presence of multiple microbleeds as a predictor of subsequent cerebral hemorrhage in patients with moyamoya disease. Neurosurgery 62: 104–111. discussion 111–102.

Kim IO, Kim JH, Kim WS et al. (1996). Mitochondrial myopathy-encephalopathy-lactic acidosis-and strokelike episodes (MELAS) syndrome: CT and MR findings in seven children. AJR Am J Roentgenol 166: 641–645.

Kim JH, Lim MK, Jeon TY et al. (2011). Diffusion and perfusion characteristics of MELAS (mitochondrial myopathy, encephalopathy, lactic acidosis, and stroke-like episode) in thirteen patients. Korean J Radiol 12: 15–24.

Kimberly WT, Gilson A, Rost NS et al. (2009). Silent ischemic infarcts are associated with hemorrhage burden in cerebral amyloid angiopathy. Neurology 72: 1230–1235.

Knauth M, von Kummer R, Jansen O et al. (1997). Potential of CT angiography in acute ischemic stroke. AJNR Am J Neuroradiol 18: 1001–1010.

Kuker W, Gaertner S, Nagele T et al. (2008). Vessel wall contrast enhancement: a diagnostic sign of cerebral vasculitis. Cerebrovasc Dis 26: 23–29.

Kuroda S, Houkin K (2008). Moyamoya disease: current concepts and future perspectives. Lancet Neurol 7: 1056–1066.

Kuroda S, Ishikawa T, Houkin K et al. (2005). Incidence and clinical features of disease progression in adult moyamoya disease. Stroke 36: 2148–2153.

Kwon HM, Kim JH, Lim JS et al. (2009). Basilar artery dolichoectasia is associated with paramedian pontine infarction. Cerebrovasc Dis 27: 114–118.

Lee TC, Bartlett ES, Fox AJ et al. (2005). The hypodense artery sign. AJNR Am J Neuroradiol 26: 2027–2029.

Lee VH, Brown RD, Mandrekar JN et al. (2006). Incidence and outcome of cervical artery dissection: a population-based study. Neurology 67: 1809–1812.

Lee KY, Latour LL, Luby M et al. (2009a). Distal hyperintense vessels on FLAIR: an MRI marker for collateral circulation in acute stroke? Neurology 72: 1134–1139.

Lee M, Zaharchuk G, Guzman R et al. (2009b). Quantitative hemodynamic studies in moyamoya disease: a review. Neurosurg Focus 26: E5.

Leiguarda R, Berthier M, Starkstein S et al. (1988). Ischemic infarction in 25 children with tuberculous meningitis. Stroke 19: 200–204.

Lesnik Oberstein SA, van den Boom R, van Buchem MA et al. (2001). Cerebral microbleeds in CADASIL. Neurology 57: 1066–1070.

Lev MH, Farkas J, Rodriguez VR et al. (2001). CT angiography in the rapid triage of patients with hyperacute stroke to intraarterial thrombolysis: accuracy in the detection of large vessel thrombus. J Comput Assist Tomogr 25: 520–528.

Levy DE (1988). How transient are transient ischemic attacks? Neurology 38: 674–677.

Lovblad KO, Bassetti C, Schneider J et al. (2001). Diffusion-weighted mr in cerebral venous thrombosis. Cerebrovasc Dis 11: 169–176.

Maksimowicz-McKinnon K, Clark TM, Hoffman GS (2009). Takayasu arteritis and giant cell arteritis: a spectrum within the same disease? Medicine (Baltimore) 88: 221–226.

Mangla R, Kolar B, Almast J et al. (2011). Border zone infarcts: pathophysiologic and imaging characteristics. Radiographics 31: 1201–1214.

Mari B, Monteagudo M, Bustamante E et al. (2009). Analysis of temporal artery biopsies in an 18-year period at a community hospital. Eur J Intern Med 20: 533–536.

Markus HS, Martin RJ, Simpson MA et al. (2002). Diagnostic strategies in CADASIL. Neurology 59: 1134–1138.

Mason JC (2010). Takayasu arteritis – advances in diagnosis and management. Nat Rev Rheumatol 6: 406–415.

Masuda J, Ogata J, Yutani C (1993). Smooth muscle cell proliferation and localization of macrophages and T cells in the occlusive intracranial major arteries in moyamoya disease. Stroke 24: 1960–1967.

McKinney AM, Short J, Truwit CL et al. (2007). Posterior reversible encephalopathy syndrome: incidence of atypical regions of involvement and imaging findings. AJR Am J Roentgenol 189: 904–912.

Mikkonen RH, Kreula JM, Virkkunen PJ (1996). Reproducibility of Doppler ultrasound measurements. Acta Radiol 37: 545–550.

Miller DV, Salvarani C, Hunder GG et al. (2009). Biopsy findings in primary angiitis of the central nervous system. Am J Surg Pathol 33: 35–43.

Mineharu Y, Takenaka K, Yamakawa H et al. (2006). Inheritance pattern of familial moyamoya disease: autosomal dominant mode and genomic imprinting. J Neurol Neurosurg Psychiatry 77: 1025–1029.

Molloy ES, Singhal AB, Calabrese LH (2008). Tumour-like mass lesion: an under-recognised presentation of primary angiitis of the central nervous system. Ann Rheum Dis 67: 1732–1735.

Monsuez JJ, Goujon C, Wyplosz B et al. (2009). Cerebrovascular diseases in HIV-infected patients. Curr HIV Res 7: 475–480.

Mullins ME, Schaefer PW, Sorensen AG et al. (2002). CT and conventional and diffusion-weighted MR imaging in acute stroke: study in 691 patients at presentation to the emergency department. Radiology 224: 353–360.

Mullins ME, Grant PE, Wang B et al. (2004). Parenchymal abnormalities associated with cerebral venous sinus thrombosis: assessment with diffusion-weighted MR imaging. AJNR Am J Neuroradiol 25: 1666–1675.

Muth CM, Shank ES (2000). Gas embolism. N Engl J Med 342: 476–482.

Mwipatayi BP, Jeffery PC, Beningfield SJ et al. (2005). Takayasu arteritis: clinical features and management: report of 272 cases. ANZ J Surg 75: 110–117.

Nagel MA, Cohrs RJ, Mahalingam R et al. (2008). The varicella zoster virus vasculopathies: clinical, CSF, imaging, and virologic features. Neurology 70: 853–860.

Nederkoorn PJ, Elgersma OE, van der Graaf Y et al. (2003a). Carotid artery stenosis: accuracy of contrast-enhanced MR angiography for diagnosis. Radiology 228: 677–682.

Nederkoorn PJ, van der Graaf Y, Hunink MG (2003b). Duplex ultrasound and magnetic resonance angiography compared with digital subtraction angiography in carotid artery stenosis: a systematic review. Stroke 34: 1324–1332.

Okeda R, Arima K, Kawai M (2002). Arterial changes in cerebral autosomal dominant arteriopathy with subcortical infarcts and leukoencephalopathy (CADASIL) in relation to pathogenesis of diffuse myelin loss of cerebral white matter: examination of cerebral medullary arteries by reconstruction of serial sections of an autopsy case. Stroke 33: 2565–2569.

Olin JW (2007). Recognizing and managing fibromuscular dysplasia. Cleve Clin J Med 74: 273–274. 277–282.

Oliveira-Filho J, Ay H, Schaefer PW et al. (2000). Diffusion-weighted magnetic resonance imaging identifies the "clinically relevant" small-penetrator infarcts. Arch Neurol 57: 1009–1014.

Ortiz G, Koch S, Romano JG et al. (2007). Mechanisms of ischemic stroke in HIV-infected patients. Neurology 68: 1257–1261.

Parizel PM, Demey HE, Veeckmans G et al. (2001). Early diagnosis of cerebral fat embolism syndrome by diffusion-weighted MRI (starfield pattern). Stroke 32: 2942–2944.

Passero SG, Calchetti B, Bartalini S (2005). Intracranial bleeding in patients with vertebrobasilar dolichoectasia. Stroke 36: 1421–1425.

Pavlakis SG, Phillips PC, DiMauro S et al. (1984). Mitochondrial myopathy, encephalopathy, lactic acidosis, and strokelike episodes: a distinctive clinical syndrome. Ann Neurol 16: 481–488.

Pavlakis SG, Bello J, Prohovnik I et al. (1988). Brain infarction in sickle cell anemia: magnetic resonance imaging correlates. Ann Neurol 23: 125–130.

Perren F, Horn P, Vajkoczy P et al. (2005). Power Doppler imaging in detection of surgically induced indirect neoangiogenesis in adult moyamoya disease. J Neurosurg 103: 869–872.

Pico F, Labreuche J, Touboul PJ et al. (2005). Intracranial arterial dolichoectasia and small-vessel disease in stroke patients. Ann Neurol 57: 472–479.

Pico F, Jacob MP, Labreuche J et al. (2010). Matrix metalloproteinase-3 and intracranial arterial dolichoectasia. Ann Neurol 67: 508–515.

Pomper MG, Miller TJ, Stone JH et al. (1999). CNS vasculitis in autoimmune disease: MR imaging findings and correlation with angiography. AJNR Am J Neuroradiol 20: 75–85.

Reyes S, Viswanathan A, Godin O et al. (2009). Apathy: a major symptom in CADASIL. Neurology 72: 905–910.

Roh JK, Kang DW, Lee SH et al. (2000). Significance of acute multiple brain infarction on diffusion-weighted imaging. Stroke 31: 688–694.

Rolfs A, Bottcher T, Zschiesche M et al. (2005). Prevalence of Fabry disease in patients with cryptogenic stroke: a prospective study. Lancet 366: 1794–1796.

Rordorf G, Koroshetz WJ, Copen WA et al. (1998). Regional ischemia and ischemic injury in patients with acute middle cerebral artery stroke as defined by early diffusion-weighted and perfusion-weighted MRI. Stroke 29: 939–943.

Rovira A, Rovira-Gols A, Pedraza S et al. (2002). Diffusion-weighted MR imaging in the acute phase of transient ischemic attacks. AJNR Am J Neuroradiol 23: 77–83.

Rubinstein SM, Peerdeman SM, van Tulder MW et al. (2005). A Systematic Review of the Risk Factors for Cervical Artery Dissection. Stroke 36: 1575–1580.

Salvarani C, Hunder GG (2001). Giant cell arteritis with low erythrocyte sedimentation rate: frequency of occurrence in a population-based study. Arthritis Rheum 45: 140–145.

Salvarani C, Cantini F, Boiardi L et al. (2002). Polymyalgia rheumatica and giant-cell arteritis. N Engl J Med 347: 261–271.

Salvarani C, Crowson CS, O'Fallon WM et al. (2004). Reappraisal of the epidemiology of giant cell arteritis in Olmsted County, Minnesota, over a fifty-year period. Arthritis Rheum 51: 264–268.

Salvarani C, Brown Jr RD, Calamia KT et al. (2007). Primary central nervous system vasculitis: analysis of 101 patients. Ann Neurol 62: 442–451.

Salvarani C, Brown Jr RD, Calamia KT et al. (2008). Primary central nervous system vasculitis with prominent leptomeningeal enhancement: a subset with a benign outcome. Arthritis Rheum 58: 595–603.

Salvarani C, Brown Jr RD, Hunder GG (2012). Adult primary central nervous system vasculitis. Lancet 380: 767–777.

Saposnik G, Barinagarrementeria F, Brown Jr RD et al. (2011). Diagnosis and management of cerebral venous thrombosis: a statement for healthcare professionals from the American Heart Association/American Stroke Association. Stroke 42: 1158–1192.

Sarnat HB, Marin-Garcia J (2005). Pathology of mitochondrial encephalomyopathies. Can J Neurol Sci 32: 152–166.

Sato W, Hayasaka K, Komatsu K et al. (1992). Genetic analysis of three pedigrees of mitochondrial myopathy, encephalopathy, lactic acidosis, and strokelike episodes (MELAS). Am J Hum Genet 50: 655–657.

Schievink WI (2001). Spontaneous dissection of the carotid and vertebral arteries. N Engl J Med 344: 898–906.

Schmidt R, Fazekas F, Kleinert G et al. (1992). Magnetic resonance imaging signal hyperintensities in the deep and subcortical white matter. A comparative study between stroke patients and normal volunteers. Arch Neurol 49: 825–827.

Schmidt WA, Kraft HE, Vorpahl K et al. (1997). Color duplex ultrasonography in the diagnosis of temporal arteritis. N Engl J Med 337: 1336–1342.

Schwartz RB, Feske SK, Polak JF et al. (2000). Preeclampsia-eclampsia: clinical and neuroradiographic correlates and insights into the pathogenesis of hypertensive encephalopathy. Radiology 217: 371–376.

Scott RM, Smith ER (2009). Moyamoya disease and moyamoya syndrome. N Engl J Med 360: 1226–1237.

Sheerin F, Pretorius PM, Briley D et al. (2008). Differential diagnosis of restricted diffusion confined to the cerebral cortex. Clin Radiol 63: 1245–1253.

Singer MB, Chong J, Lu D et al. (1998). Diffusion-weighted MRI in acute subcortical infarction. Stroke 29: 133–136.

Singhal AB (2004). Postpartum angiopathy with reversible posterior leukoencephalopathy. Arch Neurol 61: 411–416.

Singhal AB, Singhal BS, Ursekar MA et al. (2001). Serial MR angiography and contrast-enhanced MRI in chickenpox-associated stroke. Neurology 56: 815–817.

Singhal AB, Topcuoglu MA, Buonanno FS (2002). Acute ischemic stroke patterns in infective and nonbacterial thrombotic endocarditis: a diffusion-weighted magnetic resonance imaging study. Stroke 33: 1267–1273.

Singhal AB, Kimberly WT, Schaefer PW et al. (2009). Case records of the Massachusetts General Hospital. Case 8-2009. A 36-year-old woman with headache, hypertension, and seizure 2 weeks post partum. N Engl J Med 360: 1126–1137.

Singhal AB, Hajj-Ali RA, Topcuoglu MA et al. (2011). Reversible cerebral vasoconstriction syndromes: analysis of 139 cases. Arch Neurol 68: 1005–1012.

Siva A (2001). Vasculitis of the nervous system. J Neurol 248: 451–468.

Slovut DP, Olin JW (2004). Fibromuscular dysplasia. N Engl J Med 350: 1862–1871.

Smoker WR, Corbett JJ, Gentry LR et al. (1986). High-resolution computed tomography of the basilar artery: 2. Vertebrobasilar dolichoectasia: clinical-pathologic correlation and review. AJNR Am J Neuroradiol 7: 61–72.

Sorensen AG, Buonanno FS, Gonzalez RG et al. (1996). Hyperacute stroke: evaluation with combined multisection diffusion-weighted and hemodynamically weighted echo-planar MR imaging. Radiology 199 (2): 391–401.

Stanson AW (2000). Imaging findings in extracranial (giant cell) temporal arteritis. Clin Exp Rheumatol 18: S43–S48.

Steeds RP, Mohiaddin R (2006). Takayasu arteritis: role of cardiovascular magnetic imaging. Int J Cardiol 109: 1–6.

Stevens CJ, Heran MK (2012). The many faces of posterior reversible encephalopathy syndrome. Br J Radiol 85: 1566–1575.

Stuckey SL, Goh TD, Heffernan T et al. (2007). Hyperintensity in the subarachnoid space on FLAIR MRI. AJR Am J Roentgenol 189: 913–921.

Subramaniam S, Puetz V, Dzialowski I et al. (2006). Cerebral microhemorrhages in a patient with mycotic aneurysm: relevance of T2-GRE imaging in SBE. Neurology 67: 1697.

Sue CM, Crimmins DS, Soo YS et al. (1998). Neuroradiological features of six kindreds with MELAS tRNA(Leu) A2343G point mutation: implications for pathogenesis. J Neurol Neurosurg Psychiatry 65: 233–240.

Susac JO, Murtagh FR, Egan RA et al. (2003). MRI findings in Susac's syndrome. Neurology 61: 1783–1787.

Susac JO, Egan RA, Rennebohm RM et al. (2007). Susac's syndrome: 1975–2005 microangiopathy/autoimmune endotheliopathy. J Neurol Sci 257: 270–272.

Suzuki J, Takaku A (1969). Cerebrovascular "moyamoya" disease. Disease showing abnormal net-like vessels in base of brain. Arch Neurol 20: 288–299.

Swartz RH, Bhuta SS, Farb RI et al. (2009). Intracranial arterial wall imaging using high-resolution 3-tesla contrast-enhanced MRI. Neurology 72: 627–634.

Switzer JA, Hess DC, Nichols FT et al. (2006). Pathophysiology and treatment of stroke in sickle-cell disease: present and future. Lancet Neurol 5: 501–512.

Thaler DE, Ruthazer R, Di Angelantonio E et al. (2013). Neuroimaging findings in cryptogenic stroke patients with and without patent foramen ovale. Stroke 44: 675–680.

U-King-Im JM, Young V, Gillard JH (2009). Carotid-artery imaging in the diagnosis and management of patients at risk of stroke. Lancet Neurol 8: 569–580.

Ullrich NJ, Robertson R, Kinnamon DD et al. (2007). Moyamoya following cranial irradiation for primary brain tumors in children. Neurology 68: 932–938.

Vahedi K, Massin P, Guichard JP et al. (2003). Hereditary infantile hemiparesis, retinal arteriolar tortuosity, and leukoencephalopathy. Neurology 60: 57–63.

Vertinsky AT, Schwartz NE, Fischbein NJ et al. (2008). Comparison of multidetector CT angiography and MR imaging of cervical artery dissection. AJNR Am J Neuroradiol 29: 1753–1760.

Viswanathan A, Gschwendtner A, Guichard JP et al. (2007). Lacunar lesions are independently associated with disability and cognitive impairment in CADASIL. Neurology 69: 172–179.

Vollmer TL, Guarnaccia J, Harrington W et al. (1993). Idiopathic granulomatous angiitis of the central nervous system. Diagnostic challenges. Arch Neurol 50: 925–930.

Walter MA (2007). [(18)F]fluorodeoxyglucose PET in large vessel vasculitis. Radiol Clin North Am 45: 735–744. viii.

Wang XY, Noguchi K, Takashima S et al. (2003). Serial diffusion-weighted imaging in a patient with MELAS and presumed cytotoxic oedema. Neuroradiology 45: 640–643.

Wardlaw JM, Chappell FM, Best JJ et al. (2006). Non-invasive imaging compared with intra-arterial angiography in the diagnosis of symptomatic carotid stenosis: a meta-analysis. Lancet 367: 1503–1512.

Wechsler B, Vidailhet M, Piette JC et al. (1992). Cerebral venous thrombosis in Behcet's disease: clinical study and long-term follow-up of 25 cases. Neurology 42: 614–618.

Wetzel SG, Kirsch E, Stock KW et al. (1999). Cerebral veins: comparative study of CT venography with intraarterial digital subtraction angiography. AJNR Am J Neuroradiol 20: 249–255.

Wiznitzer M, Ruggieri PM, Masaryk TJ et al. (1990). Diagnosis of cerebrovascular disease in sickle cell anemia by magnetic resonance angiography. J Pediatr 117: 551–555.

Yatsuga S, Povalko N, Nishioka J et al. (2012). MELAS: a nationwide prospective cohort study of 96 patients in Japan. Biochim Biophys Acta 1820: 619–624.

Yilmaz EY, Pritz MB, Bruno A et al. (2001). Moyamoya: Indiana University Medical Center experience. Arch Neurol 58: 1274–1278.

Yoneda M, Maeda M, Kimura H et al. (1999). Vasogenic edema on MELAS: a serial study with diffusion-weighted MR imaging. Neurology 53: 2182–2184.

Yoon HK, Shin HJ, Chang YW (2002). "Ivy sign" in childhood moyamoya disease: depiction on FLAIR and contrast-enhanced T1-weighted MR images. Radiology 223: 384–389.

Yoshida S, Akiba H, Tamakawa M et al. (2001). The spectrum of findings in supra-aortic Takayasu's arteritis as seen on spiral CT angiography and digital subtraction angiography. Cardiovasc Intervent Radiol 24: 117–121.

Yuh WT, Simonson TM, Wang AM et al. (1994). Venous sinus occlusive disease: MR findings. AJNR Am J Neuroradiol 15: 309–316.

Handbook of Clinical Neurology, Vol. 135 (3rd series)
Neuroimaging, Part I
J.C. Masdeu and R.G. González, Editors

Chapter 18

Hemorrhagic cerebrovascular disease

JAVIER M. ROMERO[1]* AND JONATHAN ROSAND[2]

[1]*Department of Neuroradiology, Massachusetts General Hospital, Harvard Medical School, Boston, MA, USA*

[2]*Neuroscience Intensive Care Unit, Department of Neurology, Massachusetts General Hospital, Boston, MA, USA*

Abstract

Primary or nontraumatic spontaneous intracerebral hemorrhage (ICH) accounts for 10–15% of all strokes, and has a poor prognosis. ICH has a mortality rate of almost 50% when associated with intraventricular hemorrhage within the first month, and 80% rate of dependency at 6 months from onset. Neuroimaging is critical in identifying the underlying etiology and thus assisting in the important therapeutic decisions. There are several imaging modalities available in the workup of patients who present with ICH, including computed tomography (CT), magnetic resonance imaging (MRI), and digital subtraction angiography (DSA). A review of the current imaging approach, as well as a differential diagnosis of etiologies and imaging manifestations of primary versus secondary intraparenchymal hemorrhage, is presented. Active bleeding occurs in the first hours after symptom onset, with early neurologic deterioration. Identifying those patients who are more likely to have hematoma expansion is an active area of research, and there are many ongoing therapeutic trials targeting this specific patient population at risk.

PRIMARY INTRACEREBRAL HEMORRHAGE (ICH)

Primary or non-traumatic spontaneous ICH accounts for 10–15% of all strokes (Sudlow and Warlow, 1997) and has a poor prognosis. ICH has a mortality rate of almost 50% when associated with intraventricular hemorrhage within the first month, and 80% rate of dependency at 6 months from onset (Flaherty et al., 2006). Active bleeding occurs in the first hours after symptom onset, often accompanied by early neurologic deterioration. Identifying patients who are more likely to have hematoma expansion is an active area of research. The "spot sign," a radiologic sign of active extravasation, has a strong positive predictive value for hematoma expansion and has been adopted by multiple trials. There are ongoing therapeutic trials targeting this specific patient population at risk, including Antihypertensive Treatment of Acute Cerebral Hemorrhage (ATACH-II), the Spot Sign for Predicting and Treating ICH Growth Study (STOP-IT), and "Spot Sign" Selection of Intracerebral Hemorrhage to Guide Hemostatic Therapy (SPOTLIGHT).

IMAGING OF INTRACEREBRAL HEMORRHAGE

Neuroimaging is critical in identifying the underlying etiology and thus assisting in making important therapeutic decisions. There are several imaging modalities available in the workup of patients who present with ICH, including computed tomography (CT), magnetic resonance imaging (MRI), and digital subtraction angiography (DSA).

Computed tomography

Noncontrast CT (NCCT) is the cornerstone imaging modality to evaluate a patient with stroke-like symptoms. NCCT has near-perfect accuracy in detecting not only ICH, but also subarachnoid, intraventricular, and extradural hemorrhage. In the initial minutes, intracranial blood has 30–60 Hounsfield units (HU). The Hounsfield unit is a scale that measures material radiodensity. After 3 days the density may increase to 80 HU. This high density is the reason for the high detection rate of hemorrhage within the brain (Bergstrom et al., 1977).

*Correspondence to: Javier M. Romero, Neuroradiology, Gray Building Floor 2, Room 267B, Massachusetts General Hospital, 55 Fruit Street, Boston MA 02114, USA. Tel: +1-617-724-7095, Fax: +1-617-726-8395, E-mail: jmromero@partners.org

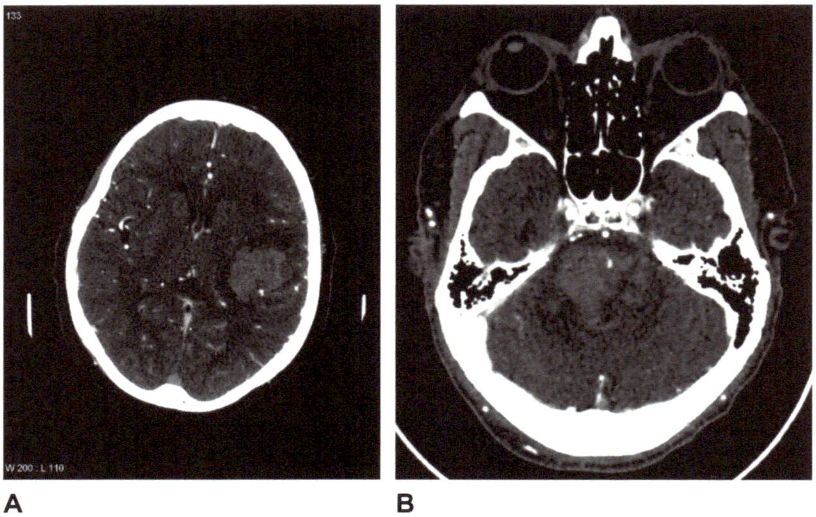

Fig. 18.1. (**A**) Axial computed tomography angiography of the brain demonstrates a spot sign in the posterior aspect of the left frontal intracerebral hemorrhage (ICH) (arrow). (**B**) Spot sign (arrow) in the pons ICH.

Multidetector CT angiography (MDCTA) is highly sensitive for detecting the vascular etiologies of ICH, and is a useful tool for identifying the spot sign in both primary and secondary ICH. The spot sign is an indicator of active bleeding that has been shown to be a predictor of hematoma expansion and poor outcome in multiple studies Wada et al., 2007; Demchuk et al., 2012). Examples of the spot sign are shown in Figure 18.1.

Spot sign

First described in 1999 (Wada et al., 2007), the MDCTA spot sign is based on the concept of active leakage of high-density contrast material within the hematoma, on MDCTA source images. The spot sign score was developed based on radiologic characteristics of the spot sign. This score incorporated the number, maximum attenuation (in Hounsfield units), and maximum dimension of spot signs (Romero et al., 2013) (Table 18.1). Most commonly, the term contrast extravasation refers to the presence of contrast within the hematoma on postcontrast CT; however, we believe that the spot sign is a continuum of the same phenomenon and not a different entity (Ederies et al., 2009; Hallevi et al., 2010).

Three prospective trials have evaluated the value of the spot sign in the prediction of ICH expansion and poor clinical outcome (Li et al., 2011; Demchuk et al., 2012; Romero et al., 2013). These studies have validated in heterogeneous and distinct populations that the spot sign is a predictor of ICH expansion, mortality, and poor clinical outcome after primary ICH. Our data suggest that the stop sign score categorizes expansion and mortality risk in a stepwise fashion for those patients with a positive spot sign (Romero et al., 2013) (Fig. 18.2).

Table 18.1

Spot sign scoring

Spot sign characteristics	
Number of spot signs	
1–2	1
≥3	2
Maximum axial attenuation	
1–4 mm	0
≥5 mm	1
Maximum attenuation	
120–179 HU	0
180 HU	1

HU, Hounsfield units.

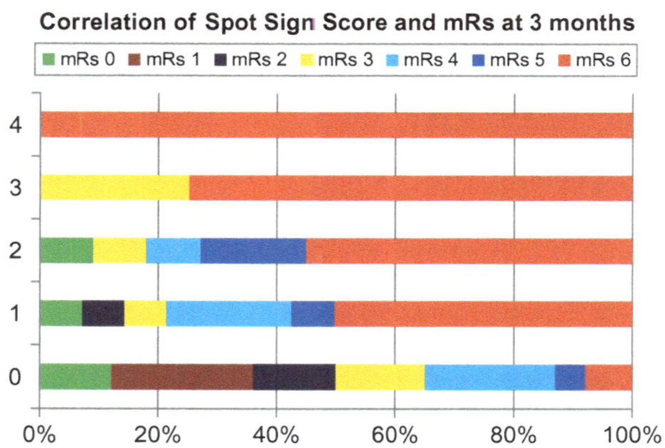

Fig. 18.2. Correlation of spot sign score and modified Rankin score (mRs) at 3 months after discharge. From Romero et al. (2013).

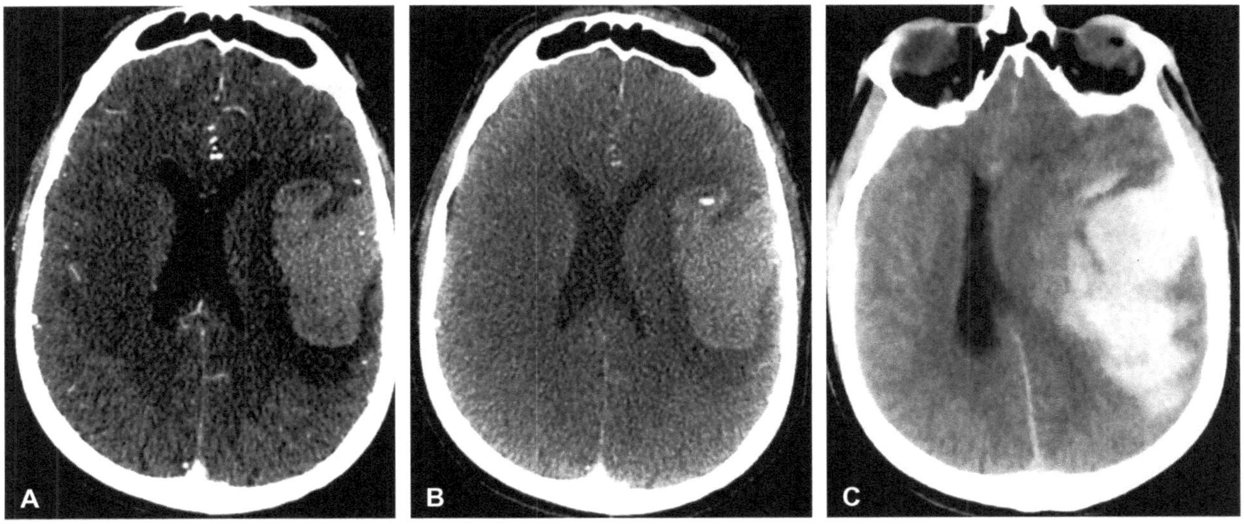

Fig. 18.3. (**A**) Computed tomography (CT) angiography first-pass shows a left frontal intracerebral hemorrhage (ICH); no spot sign is detected. (**B**) 90-second delay image shows a spot sign in the most anterior aspect of the ICH. (**C**) A 4-hour follow-up noncontrast CT of the head shows significant enlargement of the ICH.

Delayed MDCTA imaging has been proposed as a method to increase the sensitivity in the detection of the spot sign. Our group has prospectively changed the imaging protocol of acute patients with ICH to include a 90-second delayed imaging of the brain after contrast injection. This approach has a double purpose: it improves the venous phase imaging of the cerebral veins and venous sinuses, and it will also demonstrate the dynamic changes of the spot sign during this interval. We observed a sensitivity of 55% for predicting hematoma expansion if the spot sign was present on first-pass MDCTA, which increased to 64% if the spot sign was present on either MDCTA acquisition (Fig. 18.3).

SECONDARY HEMORRHAGE

Computed tomography and multidetector CT angiography

The incidence of underlying vascular etiologies as the cause of ICH depends on the patient's clinical characteristics. The patient's age and presence of hypertension are the most important variables. The frequency of secondary ICH ranges from 13% to 28% in patients older than 18 years (Delgado Almandoz et al., 2009a, b; Yoon et al., 2009), to 65% in patients 40 years or younger in MDCTA studies (Romero et al., 2009). Table 18.2 shows the different types and relative frequencies of causative vascular lesions in a cohort of 845 ICH patients evaluated with MDCTA at the authors' institution over a 10-year period (Delgado Almandoz et al., 2009a).

MDCTA can accurately identify patients with ICH that have an underlying vascular etiology (secondary ICH). Several recent studies comparing MDCTA to

Table 18.2

Relative frequency of different vascular etiologies in a cohort of 845 hemorrhagic stroke patients evaluated with multidetector computed tomography angiography

Vascular etiology	*n*	%
Arteriovenous malformations	55	45.8
Aneurysms with purely intracerebral hemorrhage	26*	21.7
Dural venous sinus/cortical vein thrombosis	20†	16.7
Arteriovenous fistula	11	9.2
Vasculopathy	4‡	3.3
Moyamoya	4‡	3.3

*Includes three pseudoaneurysms.
†Includes two cases of isolated cortical vein thrombosis.
‡Includes a patient in whom vasculitis led to pseudoaneurysm formation and rupture.

conventional angiography and autopsy findings demonstrated sensitivities ranging from 89% to 96% and overall accuracy rates of 91–99% for MDCTA (Delgado Almandoz et al., 2009a; Romero et al., 2009; Yeung et al., 2009; Yoon et al., 2009) (Fig. 18.4). Rapid identification of patients with secondary ICH is important because these patients may benefit from prompt surgical or endovascular treatment once an underlying vascular abnormality has been identified. This approach will decrease the high rate of re-hemorrhage, morbidity, and mortality (Jane et al., 1985; Ondra et al., 1990; Qureshi et al., 2001, 2009; Badjatia and Rosand, 2005). Although conventional catheter angiography

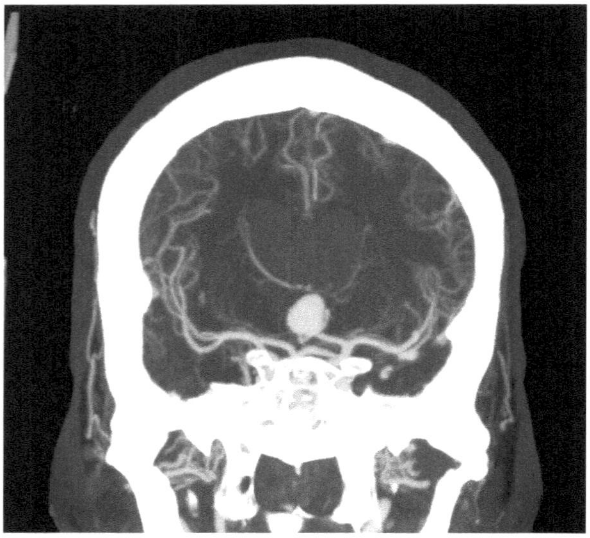

Fig. 18.4. Computed tomography angiogram maximum-intensity projection; coronal view of a tip of the basilar aneurysm.

remains the gold standard for the detection of underlying vascular etiologies in patients with hemorrhagic stroke, thanks to its widespread availability, rapidity of acquisition, lower cost, and favorable risk profile, MDCTA is rapidly becoming the favored diagnostic tool in the initial evaluation of this patient population.

Radiation dose from CT is a concern; however, the risks and benefits of the procedure and the drawbacks of not making a timely diagnosis need to be considered. It is important that CT protocols be optimized to deliver the lowest radiation dose possible while still obtaining diagnostic-quality images.

Magnetic resonance imaging

MRI is as accurate as, or more accurate than, CT in identifying acute ICH, and more accurate than CT in identifying chronic hemorrhage, particularly chronic microbleeds associated with cerebral amyloid angiopathy (CAA) or hypertension (Patel et al., 1996).

The MRI signal characteristics of ICH are variable depending on the oxidation state of hemoglobin and time. These differences are useful in estimating an approximate age of the hematoma. The hyperacute phase (hours) of the hematoma appears isointense on T1-weighted images and isointense to slightly hyperintense on T2-weighted images. The red cell membrane is intact in this phase, and the hemoglobin molecule is saturated with oxygen (oxyhemoglobin).

In the acute phase, which occurs in the first 48 hours, the ICH demonstrates iso- or slight hypointensity on T1-weighted images. Occasionally, a thin rim of T1 hyperintensity can be seen in the margins of the hematoma, resulting from early oxidation of intracellular deoxyhemoglobin to intracellular methemoglobin. On T2-weighted images the hematoma becomes hypointense. The late subacute phase occurs after several days to weeks. There is increased signal intensity on T1- and T2-weighted images. There is slight loss of the susceptibility effect, secondary to the absence of intracellular met-hemoglobin (Gomori et al., 1985). Ultimately the chronic phase occurs after the first month. There is a significant decrease of the degree of signal intensity on T1- and T2-weighted images. Residual iron deposition in the margins of the hematoma cavity demonstrates significant susceptibility effect without significant dipole–dipole interactions, leading to marked hypointensity on T2-weighted images (Table 18.3) (Patel et al., 1996; Linfante et al., 1999; Wiesmann et al., 2001; Wintermark et al., 2002). The magnetic susceptibility effect of paramagnetic blood products (deoxyhemoglobin, methemoglobin, and hemosiderin) is exploited on gradient recalled echo (GRE) pulse sequences. In this sequence, blood products appear as areas of loss of signal (Wiesmann et al., 2001; Wintermark et al., 2002; Allkemper et al., 2004) (Fig. 18.5).

Susceptibility-weighted imaging (SWI), a type of GRE sequence that utilizes both magnitude and phase images, has demonstrated higher sensitivity than conventional T2*-weighted gradient echo sequences for

Table 18.3

Phases of intracerebral hemorrhage and imaging patterns

	Predominant hemoglobin state	T1-weighted signal intensity	T2-weighted signal intensity	Gradient echo and susceptibility-weighted artifact
Hyperacute phase	Oxyhemoglobin	Isointense	Isointense to slight high	Thin artifact in the periphery
Acute phase	Deoxyhemoglobin	Isointense to slight low	Low	Progression towards center
Subacute phase	Methemoglobin	High	High	Significant portions
Chronic phase	Methemoglobin and hemosiderin	Low	Low	Artifact in cavity

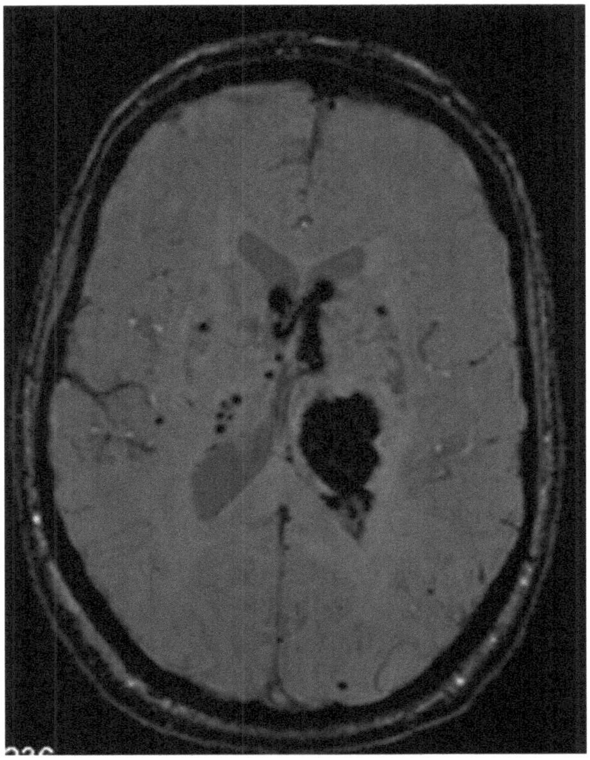

Fig. 18.5. Magnetic resonance imaging, axial susceptibility-weighted image, demonstrates multiple punctate blooming lesions secondary to microhemorrhage in the basal ganglia. A larger intracerebral hemorrhage is noted in the left thalamus secondary to chronic hypertension.

the detection of small intracranial hemorrhage (Wycliffe et al., 2004; Akter et al., 2007). Vascular etiologies are better seen in other MRI sequences, including post-contrast imaging and time-of-flight MR angiography (TOF-MRA). TOF-MRA as well as GRE/SWI sequences have high sensitivity for assessment of blood flow without intravenous contrast agents, and are capable of identifying arteriovenous shunting (Chen et al., 1992; Jagadeesan et al., 2012) (Fig. 18.6). MRI is the exam of choice when a hemorrhagic intracranial neoplasm is suspected, given the high sensitivity of MRI detecting the enhancing portions of the neoplasm and changes in the expected evolution of blood products.

There are a few limitations to the use of MRI, particularly in the emergent setting, which include MRI availability, time, cost, proximity to the Emergency Department, patient tolerance and clinical status, and contraindicated medical implants, including pacemakers (Chen et al., 1992).

Digital subtraction angiography

DSA, or conventional angiography, is a technique with higher resolution, which is usually reserved for those cases where a cause for hemorrhage is not identified with less invasive imaging modalities. It should be considered in all patients who have subarachnoid blood associated with ICH, and young patients < 45 years, with negative MDCTA or MR workup (Qureshi et al., 2009). A study of patients with spontaneous ICH found that, in patients younger than 45 without pre-existing hypertension, the angiographic yield was 48% in those with putaminal, thalamic, or posterior fossa ICH and 65% in those with lobar ICH, compared to 0% and 10% respectively in patients older than 65 with pre-existing hypertension (Zhu et al., 1997). This finding justifies the use of angiography in patients below 45 when the noninvasive imaging results are negative (Fig. 18.7).

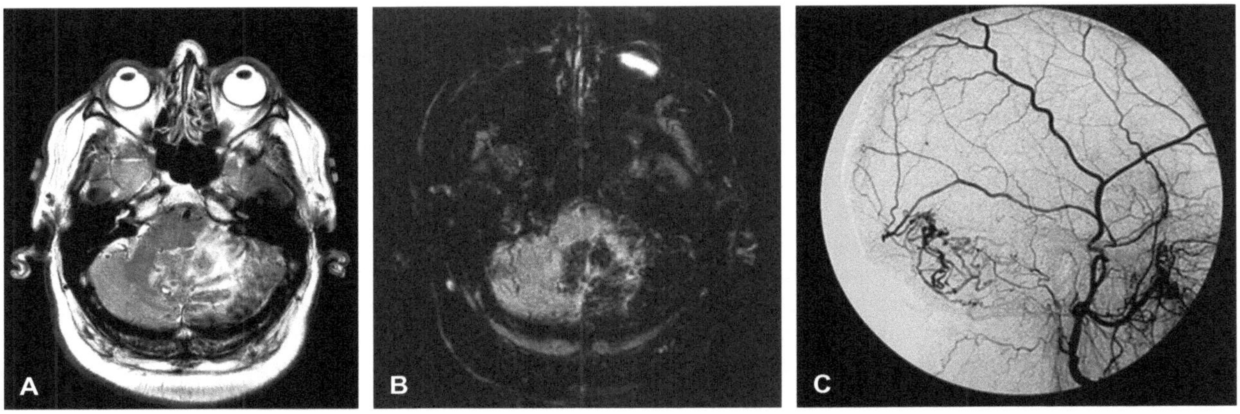

Fig. 18.6. (**A, B**) Axial magnetic resonance imaging T2-weighted image and gradient recalled echo images demonstrate a large left cerebellar intracerebral hemorrhage. (**C**) Digital subtraction angiography of the external carotid artery demonstrates arterial to venous shunting, representing an arteriovenous fistula.

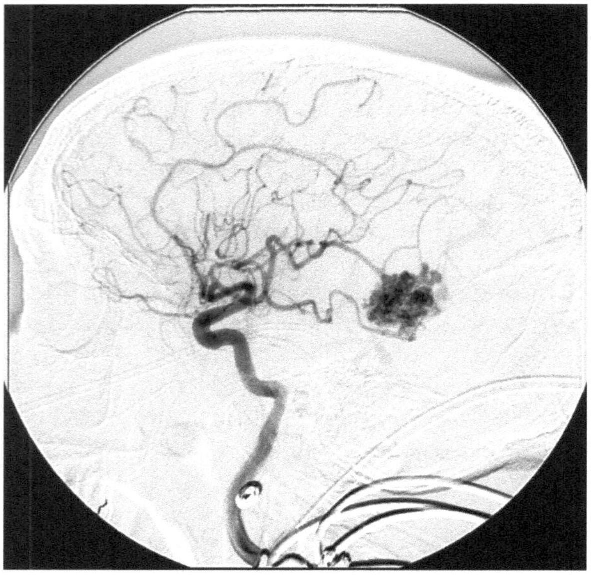

Fig. 18.7. Digital subtraction angiography of brain demonstrates an arteriovenous malformation of the left posterior cerebral artery.

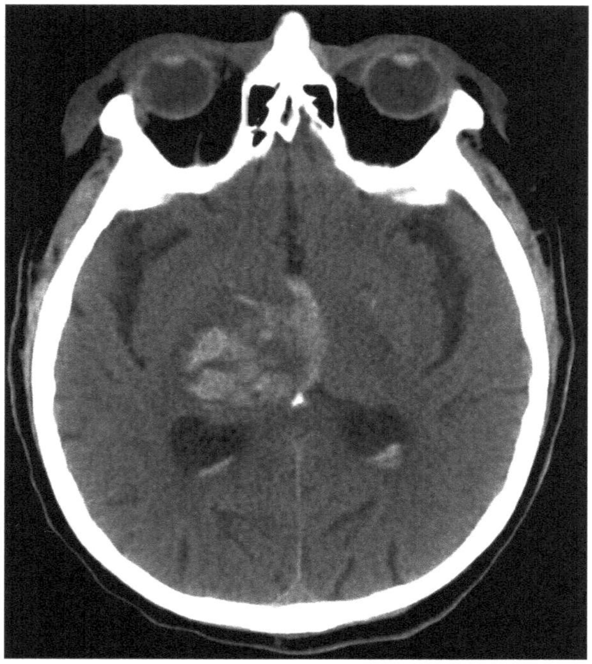

Fig. 18.8. Noncontrast computed tomography axial images demonstrate a right thalamic intracerebral hemorrhage (ICH), with intraventricular extension. Secondary to the patient's chronic hypertensive history and ICH location, this lesion likely represents a hypertensive hemorrhage.

CAUSES OF INTRACEREBRAL HEMORRHAGE

ICH may be either primary or secondary, depending on the underlying cause of bleeding. Primary ICH is due to an abrupt rupture of small damaged vessels, usually as a result of chronic hypertension or amyloid angiopathy. The incidence of primary hemorrhage is 78–88% of all cases of ICH (Foulkes et al., 1988). Secondary ICH occurs in about 15% of all ICHs. Secondary ICH occurs in patients with impaired coagulation, underlying neoplasms or vascular anomalies, venous infarction, hemorrhagic transformation of an arterial infarct, underlying vasculopathies, and certain infectious conditions.

Primary intracerebral hemorrhage

Hypertension

Hypertension is the leading risk factor for spontaneous intracranial hemorrhage (Brott et al., 1986). Chronic hypertension leads to hypertensive cerebral angiopathy, characterized by intimal hyperplasia and hyalinosis in deep penetrating brain arterioles, which become prone to rupture. A landmark trial demonstrated that the 5-year incidence of all strokes (including ICH) in patients greater than 60 years of age who had a systolic blood pressure of at least 160 mmHg was 5.2 per 100 in patients with antihypertensive treatment, compared to 8.2 per 100 with placebo treatment (SHEP, 1991). Hypertensive ICH occurs in characteristic locations – the striatocapsular region (60–65%), the thalamus (15–20%), the cerebellum and pons (10%) and, least commonly, in a lobar location (5–10%) (Fig. 18.8).

Cerebral amyloid angiopathy

CAA results from the progressive deposition of amyloid protein within small- to medium-sized blood vessels of the cerebral cortex and leptomeninges. This accumulation theoretically leads to fibrinoid necrosis and vascular rupture, and is another risk factor for ICH, particularly in the elderly. Studies have shown that the apolipoprotein E genotype (and specifically the $\epsilon 2$ and $\epsilon 4$ alleles, whose expression is thought to augment the vasculopathic effect of amyloid deposition) is associated with increased risk of CAA-related hemorrhage and triples the risk of recurrent hemorrhage in these patients (McCarron and Nicoll, 2000; O'Donnell et al., 2000). CAA is also characterized by the presence of microhemorrhages seen on MRI, typically distributed at the corticomedullary junction. Symptomatic parenchymal hemorrhage in CAA most commonly occurs in a cortical-subcortical (lobar) location, although less commonly patients may present with focal nontraumatic subarachnoid or intraventricular hemorrhage (Chao et al., 2006; Alexander et al., 2013). CAA should be suspected in patients with two or more lobar hemorrhages of any age, areas of high T2 signal intensity in the cerebral white matter, and corticomedullary cerebral microhemorrhages represented by small foci of susceptibility blooming on T2-weighted, GRE, and SWI (Blitstein and Tung, 2007) (Fig. 18.9).

Secondary intracerebral hemorrhage

Vascular malformations

Vascular malformations comprise many different types of vascular anomalies, including arteriovenous malformations (Fig. 18.10), dural arteriovenous fistulas, cavernous malformations, developmental venous anomalies, and capillary telangiectasias. With the exception of capillary telangiectasias, and, rarely, developmental venous anomalies (Ku et al., 2009), these can all be causes of secondary ICH. Cavernous malformation is the most frequent vascular malformation in humans. They consist of single lesions or may be multiple, particularly in the hereditary form of the disorder, and may have a coexistent developmental venous anomaly in approximately 23% of cases (Abe et al., 1998). Cavernous malformations have a 4.5% rate of re-hemorrhage. On CT scanning cavernous malformation appear as a hyperdense lesion, which is also present in diseases such as low-grade tumors and neurocysticersosis, among other entities, reducing the specificity of NCCT in detecting cavernous malformation. Fortunately, cavernous malformations have a specific and classic imaging pattern on MRI: they demonstrate an irregular central cluster of high signal on T1-weighted images with peripheral low signal on T2-weighted images, greatly increasing the specificity of MRI compared with CT images.

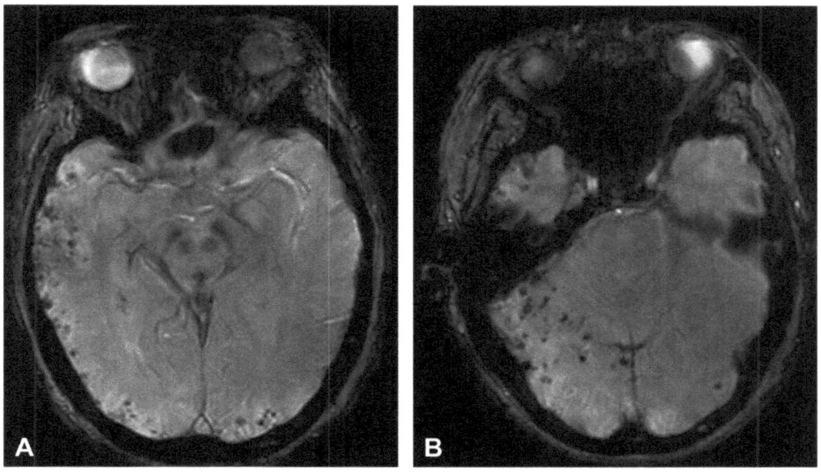

Fig. 18.9. (**A, B**) Axial magnetic resonance imaging gradient recalled echo demonstrates multiple foci of susceptibility blooming involving the right temporal and bilateral occipital lobes, representing cerebral amyloid angiopathy.

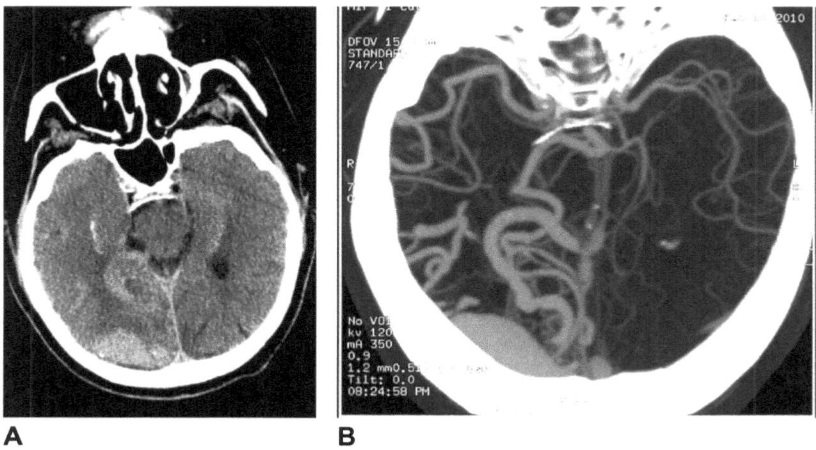

Fig. 18.10. (**A, B**) Noncontrast computed tomography axial images show a hyperdense lesion in the right occipital lobe. Computed tomography angiography of the head demonstrates enlarged tubular structures of the right posterior cerebral artery and an aneurysmal dilatation in the venous drainage.

Additionally, GRE and SWI, with its high sensitivity to susceptibility blooming, is useful in detecting smaller lesions, which may not be detected with a traditional MRI imaging protocol (Pinker et al., 2007).

In young patients (less than 45 years old) presenting with ICH, there should be careful assessment for an underlying vascular malformation. Many vascular anomalies can be detected with noninvasive CT angiography, with overall accuracy rates of 91–99% (Delgado Almandoz et al., 2009a; Romero et al., 2009; Yeung et al., 2009; Yoon et al., 2009). Arteriovenous malformations demonstrate multiple serpentine or round flow voids adjacent to the ICH on T2-weighted images. Minimal parenchymal high signal intensity, representing gliosis, may be seen adjacent to the abnormal vasculature. MRA has excellent resolution, depicting feeding arteries and draining veins. There are a few morphologic characteristics of arteriovenous malformations that have been related to increased risk of rupture and ICH: intranidal or venous aneurysm, stenosis of the draining vein, smaller size and previous rupture are risk factors for ICH (Spetzler et al., 1992). It is highly recommended to perform a conventional angiogram in these young patients with unknown cause for ICH given the high incidence of vascular malformations (Romero et al., 2009).

Aneurysms

Although aneurysms are better known to result in subarachnoid hemorrhage (SAH), recent studies have demonstrated incidences as high as 18% in patients with large ICH and small focal SAH (Romero et al., 2009). Commonly, these aneurysms are located in the M1 segment or middle cerebral artery bifurcation or in the anterior cerebral artery. The proximity of this aneurysm to the brain parenchyma results in smaller foci of SAH and large ICH (Fig. 18.11).

SAH is blood leakage into the space between the brain parenchyma and the arachnoid, called the subarachnoid space. Radiologic detection of SAH is currently performed with NCCT and MRI of the brain. The sensitivity of NCCT is of approximately 90% in the first 24 hours and later declines with changes in clot density (van Gijn and van Dongen, 1982). Despite the high sensitivity of fluid-attenuated inversion recovery (FLAIR) MRI for the detection of SAH (Noguchi et al., 1994; Woodcock et al., 2001), small acute SAH is poorly detected by FLAIR MRI, and NCCT shows superior sensitivity in these cases (Mohamed et al., 2004). Benign perimesencephalic hemorrhage is defined as blood isolated to the perimesencephalic cisterns anterior to the brainstem and ambient cisterns. In contrast to extensive SAH, perimesencephalic hemorrhage is not secondary to aneurysmal rupture and invasive diagnostic procedures may be withheld (van Gijn et al., 1985).

Hemorrhagic venous infarction

Cerebral venous thrombosis (CVT) is a difficult disease to diagnose, and requires a high degree of suspicion for ordering the appropriate radiologic test. CVT is more common in young females. Risk factors include hypercoagulable states, including underlying prothrombotic conditions, pregnancy and the peripartum period, oral contraceptive pills, and cancer.

Approximately 30–40% of patients with CVT present with ICH, most commonly parenchymal and rarely subarachnoid (Girot et al., 2007; Poon et al., 2007). Other imaging findings of CVT on noncontrast CT include

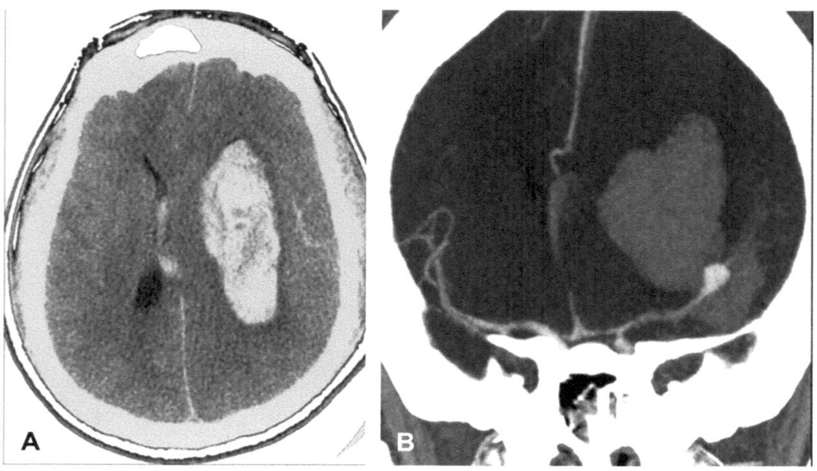

Fig. 18.11. (**A**) Noncontrast computed tomography axial images demonstrate an intracerebral hemorrhage in the left basal ganglia, with a small trace of subarachnoid hemorrhage in the left Sylvian fissure. (**B**) Computed tomography angiography; coronal view demonstrates a left middle cerebral artery aneurysm rupturing into the frontal lobe.

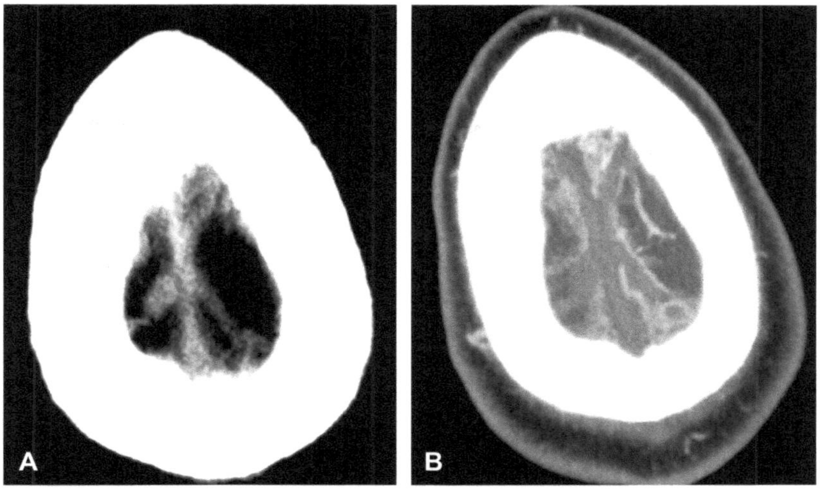

Fig. 18.12. (**A**) Noncontrast computed tomography of the head demonstrates tubular hyperdensity at the vertex. (**B**) There is thrombosis within a superior sagittal sinus, and the "cord sign" of a thrombosed cortical vein.

the "empty delta sign" of thrombosis within a dural sinus, the "cord sign" of a thrombosed cortical vein (as demonstrated in Fig. 18.12), infarction not conforming to a major arterial vascular territory and extending over more than one arterial distribution (Poon et al., 2007). The location of the ICH is a good indicator of the occluded or stenotic venous structure; for example, bilateral thalamic venous infarctions likely represent a flow-limiting lesion at the vein of Galen or the more distal venous stuctures. On the other hand, bilateral parasagittal ICH in the high frontal convexity should raise concern for a superior sagittal sinus thrombosis. Cerebral venous sinus thrombosis can be confirmed with CT venography or time-of-flight MR venography. In our institution we prefer CT venography given the flow-related artifact MR venography can present. However, recent research with MR venography in conjunction with SWI has demonstrated higher sensitivity for the detection of venous sinus thrombus. Direct imaging of a venous thrombus by MRI depends on the age of the thrombus. A T1 hyperintensity filling a venous structure can be diagnostic (Idbaih et al., 2006; Khandelwal et al., 2006).

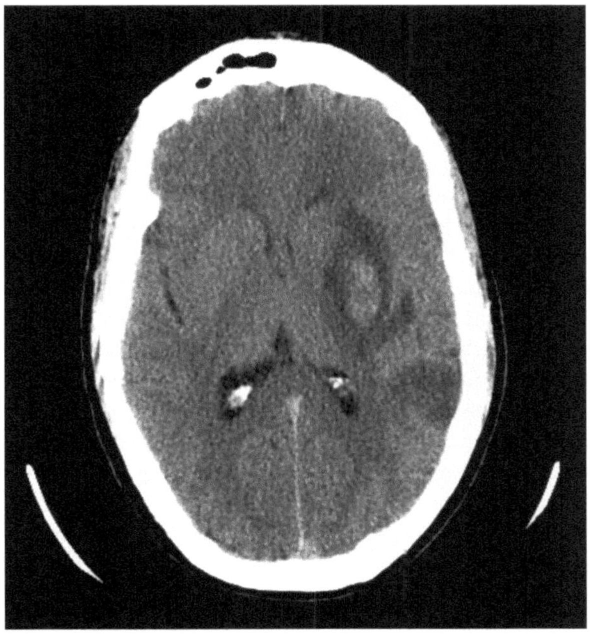

Fig. 18.13. Hemorrhagic transformation cf a left middle cerebral artery territory infarct. Noncontrast computed tomography shows a hyperdense lesion in the left putamen.

Hemorrhagic transformation of ischemic arterial infarction

Secondary hemorrhagic conversion of a cerebral infarct can occur after administration of thrombolytic therapy. Spontaneous ICH may also occur in the evolution of the infarct, typically within the first 3 days to a week after the infarct (Bozzao et al., 1991; Moulin et al., 1994; Toni et al., 1996). Although the appearance of an intrainfarct hematoma can mimic other causes of primary and secondary ICH on CT, careful observation of the surrounding areas of low density compromising a specific arterial territory may help in reaching the correct diagnosis (Fig. 18.13). Evidence of hemorrhage in the first few days after ischemic injury is very common on MRI, and is usually due to small petechial hemorrhage (Xavier et al., 2003).

Vasculitis

Vasculitis is characterized by inflammation and necrosis of the blood vessel wall. There are multiple subtypes of

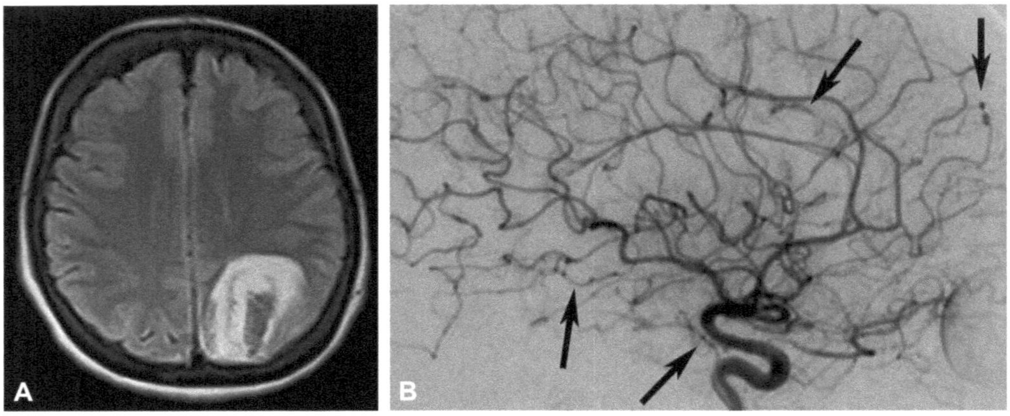

Fig. 18.14. (**A**) Axial magnetic resonance imaging, fluid-attenuated inversion recovery, demonstrates a left parietal intracerebral hemorrhage. (**B**) Conventional angiography demonstrates multiple segments of stenosis and beading appearance of the left anterior choroidal artery and branches of the left middle and anterior cerebral arteries (arrows).

vasculitis, either isolated to the central nervous system, such as primary central nervous system vasculitis (Fig. 18.14), or associated with systemic disease such as systemic lupus erythematosus, Wegener's granulomatosis, rheumatoid vasculitis, Behçet's disease, or relapsing polychondritis (Toni et al., 1996; Pomper et al., 1999). Laboratory findings include elevated erythrocyte sedimentation rate and C-reactive protein. Patients may present with ischemic or hemorrhagic lesions of different ages, findings of focal or diffuse inflammation (Pomper et al., 1999), and typical angiographic findings of segmental and often multifocal narrowing of the cerebral arteries with areas of localized dilatation or beading. Conventional catheter angiography is the gold standard for diagnosing vasculitis of the central nervous system; MDCTA and MRA are useful modalities for screening for vascular anomalies. Intracranial hemorrhage occurs in approximately 11% of patients with central nervous system vasculitis, most commonly parenchymal hemorrhage, followed by SAH (Pomper et al., 1999).

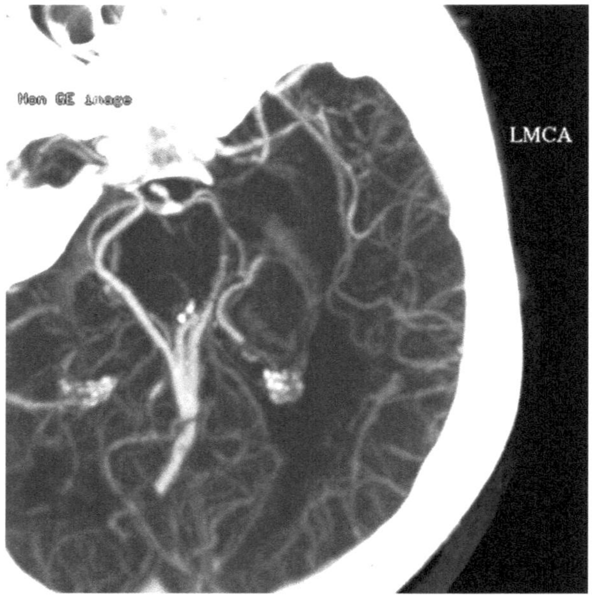

Fig. 18.15. Reversible cerebral vasoconstriction syndrome, with multiple segments of beading appearance. LMCA, left middle cerebral artery.

Miscellaneous vasculopathies

There are other rarer causes of ICH caused by abnormalities of the underlying cerebral arteries, including, but not limited, to vasculitis and moyamoya disease. Posterior reversible encephalopathy syndrome (PRES), and its overlap with reversible cerebral vasoconstriction syndrome (RCVS), are also important uncommon causes of ICH (Fig. 18.15).

Moyamoya disease is an idiopathic vaso-occlusive disease involving the terminal internal carotid artery and circle of Willis. Prominent collateral vessels develop, giving a "puff of smoke" appearance on cerebral angiography. Its appearance on MRA is demonstrated in Figure 18.16. Certain entities, such as sickle cell disease and neurofibromatosis type I, are associated with moyamoya phenomenon (in these cases it is referred to as moyamoya syndrome). Adults with the disease typically present with intracranial hemorrhage from abnormal vessels; this is classically in the later phases of the disease (Scott and Smith, 2009). The rate of hemorrhage in adults with moyamoya phenomenon is up to 20% (Hallemeier et al., 2006). Moyamoya-related ICH often presents with intraventricular hemorrhage (Nah et al., 2012). Ischemic infarction is more common than hemorrhage in children.

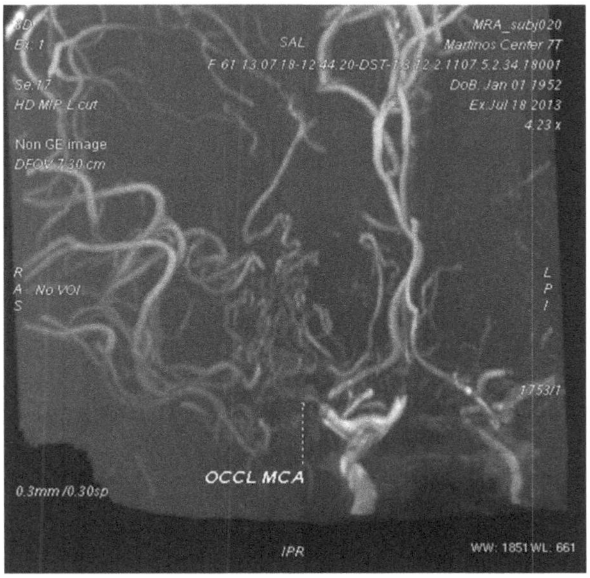

Fig. 18.16. Magnetic resonance angiography, coronal maximum-intensity projection, demonstrates prominent collateral vessels developing, giving a "puff of smoke" appearance. There is an occlusion of the right middle cerebral artery (MCA).

PRES is a vasoneurotoxic state which appears to be related to a number of conditions, including hypertension, pre-eclampsia/eclampsia, bone marrow and organ transplantation, and high-dose chemotherapy, with characteristic imaging findings of cerebral vasogenic edema typically affecting white matter and, to a lesser extent, the cortex of the occipital and parietal lobes (Bartynski, 2008). Patients typically present with altered level of consciousness, visual disturbances, and seizure. Approximately 15% of patients with PRES present with either parenchymal hemorrhage or SAH (Bartynski and Boardman, 2007; McKinney et al., 2007) (Fig. 18.17). RCVS has many underlying features that overlap with PRES; however, patients classically present with a thunderclap headache, with evidence of vasoconstriction on angiography. Imaging findings include cerebral infarction, typically in a watershed distribution; however, parenchymal hemorrhage and/or cortical subarachnoid hemorrhage can also be seen. The pathophysiology of PRES and RCVS in some patients suggests that a disturbance in cerebral arterial tone and autoregulation is the underlying cause of both syndromes, although there is some evidence of a neurotoxic effect as well (Calabrese et al., 2007).

Hemorrhagic intracranial masses

Hemorrhage occurs in 3–14% of all brain metastases and in 1–3% of primary cerebral gliomas (Davis et al., 1982). The most common metastases to hemorrhage are renal cell carcinoma, melanoma, choriocarcinoma, thyroid carcinoma, lung, and breast carcinoma (Lieu et al., 1999). Detection of neoplastic tissue in hemorrhagic lesions is challenging given the amount of mass effect over adjacent tissue. However, gadolinium-enhanced MRI of the brain is superior in the detection of enhancing neoplastic tissue compared to contrast-enhanced CT and is the technique of choice for this purpose (Russell et al., 1987; Van Dijk et al., 1997). Other imaging clues to an underlying neoplastic mass are the heterogeneous phases of blood product evolution and persistent peripheral edema, even in the late stages (Atlas et al., 1987). Patients with a clinical history suggesting metastatic disease and negative initial MRI evaluation should be re-evaluated in 1–3 months, once the hematoma has at least partially resolved.

CONCLUSION AND FUTURE DIRECTION

Imaging of patients with ICH is pivotal in the management, prognosis, and diagnosis. A practical imaging algorithm should be applied in order to reach a diagnosis and also provide prognostic detail of the patient's clinical outcome. MDCTA spot sign represents a substantial

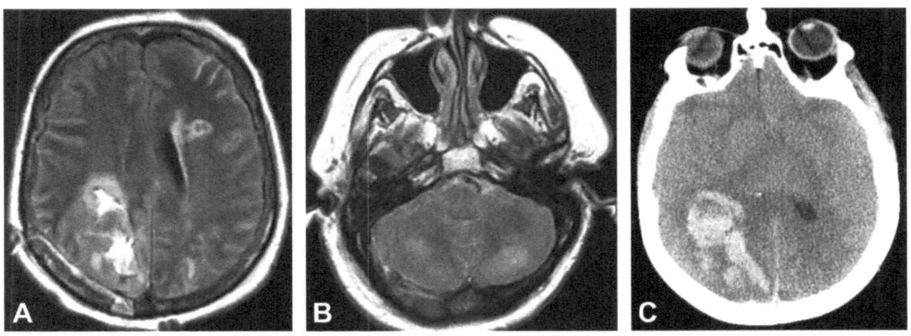

Fig. 18.17. (**A, B**) Axial magnetic resonance imaging fluid-attenuated inversion recovery (FLAIR) images demonstrating cortical and subcortical hyperintensity in the occipital and parietal lobes. There is increased FLAIR signal in the subarachnoid space, likely representing subarachnoid hemorrhage (**C**) Axial noncontrast computed tomography of the head demonstrates an intracerebral hemorrhage in the right parietal lobe secondary to posterior reversible encephalopathy syndrome.

advance for the prediction of hematoma expansion in ICH. Multiple challenges are ahead of this field of research, including the relatively low sensitivity of the current definition of the spot sign. In PREDICT, only 37 (51%) of 73 patients with hematoma expansion demonstrated a spot sign, highlighting that in a substantial number of patients hematomas will expand despite the absence of a spot sign (Brouwers et al., 2012). This is also the case for other prospective trials that demonstrate low sensitivity of 63–76% (Li et al., 2011; Romero et al., 2013). Technical refinement of the MDCTA spot sign may increase the sensitivity of the spot sign to capture more patients destined to expand and thus reduce the number of potentially treatable patients excluded from any trial. Future directions include phase II and phase III clinical trials to evaluate the spot sign as a selection tool for aggressive medical or surgical management.

References

Abe T, Singer RJ, Marks MP et al. (1998). Coexistence of occult vascular malformations and developmental venous anomalies in the central nervous system: MR evaluation. AJNR Am J Neuroradiol 19: 51–57.

Akter M, Hirai T, Hiai Y et al. (2007). Detection of hemorrhagic hypointense foci in the brain on susceptibility-weighted imaging clinical and phantom studies. Acad Radiol 14: 1011–1019.

Alexander M, Patil AK, Mathew V et al. (2013). Recurrent craniospinal subarachnoid hemorrhage in cerebral amyloid angiopathy. Ann Indian Acad Neurol 16: 97–99.

Allkemper T, Tombach B, Schwindt W et al. (2004). Acute and subacute intracerebral hemorrhages: comparison of MR imaging at 1.5 and 3.0 T – initial experience. Radiology 232: 874–881.

Atlas SW, Grossman RI, Gomori JM et al. (1987). Hemorrhagic intracranial malignant neoplasms: spin-echo MR imaging. Radiology 164: 71–77.

Badjatia N, Rosand J (2005). Intracerebral hemorrhage. Neurologist 11: 311–324.

Bartynski WS (2008). Posterior reversible encephalopathy syndrome, part 1: fundamental imaging and clinical features. AJNR Am J Neuroradiol 29: 1036–1042.

Bartynski WS, Boardman JF (2007). Distinct imaging patterns and lesion distribution in posterior reversible encephalopathy syndrome. AJNR Am J Neuroradiol 28: 1320–1327.

Bergstrom M, Ericson K, Levander B et al. (1977). Variation with time of the attenuation values of intracranial hematomas. J Comput Assist Tomogr 1: 57–63.

Blitstein MK, Tung GA (2007). MRI of cerebral microhemorrhages. AJR Am J Roentgenol 189: 720–725.

Bozzao L, Angeloni U, Bastianello S et al. (1991). Early angiographic and CT findings in patients with hemorrhagic infarction in the distribution of the middle cerebral artery. AJNR Am J Neuroradiol 12: 1115–1121.

Brott T, Thalinger K, Hertzberg V (1986). Hypertension as a risk factor for spontaneous intracerebral hemorrhage. Stroke 17: 1078–1083.

Brouwers HB, Goldstein JN, Romero JM et al. (2012). Clinical applications of the computed tomography angiography spot sign in acute intracerebral hemorrhage: a review. Stroke 43: 3427–3432.

Calabrese LH, Dodick DW, Schwedt TJ et al. (2007). Narrative review: reversible cerebral vasoconstriction syndromes. Ann Intern Med 146: 34–44.

Chao CP, Kotsenas AL, Broderick DF (2006). Cerebral amyloid angiopathy: CT and MR imaging findings. Radiographics 26: 1517–1531.

Chen JC, Tsuruda JS, Halbach VV (1992). Suspected dural arteriovenous fistula: results with screening MR angiography in seven patients. Radiology 183: 265–271.

Davis JM, Zimmerman RA, Bilaniuk LT (1982). Metastases to the central nervous system. Radiol Clin North Am 20: 417–435.

Delgado Almandoz JE, Schaefer PW, Forero NP et al. (2009a). Diagnostic accuracy and yield of multidetector CT angiography in the evaluation of spontaneous intraparenchymal cerebral hemorrhage. AJNR Am J Neuroradiol 30: 1213–1221.

Delgado Almandoz JE, Yoo AJ, Stone MJ et al. (2009b). Systematic characterization of the computed tomography angiography spot sign in primary intracerebral hemorrhage identifies patients at highest risk for hematoma expansion: the spot sign score. Stroke 40: 2994–3000.

Demchuk AM, Dowlatshahi D, Rodriguez-Luna D et al. (2012). Prediction of haematoma growth and outcome in patients with intracerebral haemorrhage using the CT-angiography spot sign (PREDICT): a prospective observational study. Lancet Neurol 11: 307–314.

Ederies A, Demchuk A, Chia T et al. (2009). Postcontrast CT extravasation is associated with hematoma expansion in CTA spot negative patients. Stroke 40: 1672–1676.

Flaherty ML, Haverbusch M, Sekar P et al. (2006). Long-term mortality after intracerebral hemorrhage. Neurology 66: 1182–1186.

Foulkes MA, Wolf PA, Price TR et al. (1988). The Stroke Data Bank: design, methods, and baseline characteristics. Stroke 19: 547–554.

Girot M, Ferro JM, Canhao P et al. (2007). Predictors of outcome in patients with cerebral venous thrombosis and intracerebral hemorrhage. Stroke 38: 337–342.

Gomori JM, Grossman RI, Bilaniuk LT et al. (1985). High-field MR imaging of superficial siderosis of the central nervous system. J Comput Assist Tomogr 9: 972–975.

Hallemeier CL, Rich KM, Grubb Jr RL et al. (2006). Clinical features and outcome in North American adults with moyamoya phenomenon. Stroke 37: 1490–1496.

Hallevi H, Abraham AT, Barreto AD et al. (2010). The spot sign in intracerebral hemorrhage: the importance of looking for contrast extravasation. Cerebrovasc Dis 29: 217–220.

Idbaih A, Boukobza M, Crassard I et al. (2006). MRI of clot in cerebral venous thrombosis: high diagnostic value of susceptibility-weighted images. Stroke 37: 991–995.

Jagadeesan BD, Delgado Almandoz JE, Moran CJ et al. (2012). Accuracy of susceptibility-weighted imaging for the detection of arteriovenous shunting in vascular malformations of the brain. Stroke 42: 87–92.

Jane JA, Kassell NF, Torner JC et al. (1985). The natural history of aneurysms and arteriovenous malformations. J Neurosurg 62: 321–323.

Khandelwal N, Agarwal A, Kochhar R et al. (2006). Comparison of CT venography with MR venography in cerebral sinovenous thrombosis. AJR Am J Roentgenol 187: 1637–1643.

Ku MG, Rhee DY, Park HS et al. (2009). Repeated intracerebral hemorrhage from developmental venous anomaly alone. J Korean Neurosurg Soc 45: 46–49.

Li N, Wang Y, Wang W et al. (2011). Contrast extravasation on computed tomography angiography predicts clinical outcome in primary intracerebral hemorrhage: a prospective study of 139 cases. Stroke 42: 3441–3446.

Lieu AS, Hwang SL, Howng SL et al. (1999). Brain tumors with hemorrhage. J Formos Med Assoc 98: 365–367.

Linfante I, Llinas RH, Caplan LR et al. (1999). MRI features of intracerebral hemorrhage within 2 hours from symptom onset. Stroke 30: 2263–2267.

McCarron MO, Nicoll JA (2000). Apolipoprotein E genotype and cerebral amyloid angiopathy-related hemorrhage. Ann N Y Acad Sci 903: 176–179.

McKinney AM, Short J, Truwit CL et al. (2007). Posterior reversible encephalopathy syndrome: incidence of atypical regions of involvement and imaging findings. AJR Am J Roentgenol 189: 904–912.

Mohamed M, Heasly DC, Yagmurlu B et al. (2004). Fluid-attenuated inversion recovery MR imaging and subarachnoid hemorrhage: not a panacea. AJNR Am J Neuroradiol 25: 545–550.

Moulin T, Crepin-Leblond T, Chopard JL et al. (1994). Hemorrhagic infarcts. Eur Neurol 34: 64–77.

Nah HW, Kwon SU, Kang DW et al. (2012). Moyamoya disease-related versus primary intracerebral hemorrhage: [corrected] location and outcomes are different. Stroke 43: 1947–1950.

Noguchi K, Ogawa T, Inugami A et al. (1994). MR of acute subarachnoid hemorrhage: a preliminary report of fluid-attenuated inversion-recovery pulse sequences. AJNR Am J Neuroradiol 15: 1940–1943.

O'Donnell HC, Rosand J, Knudsen KA et al. (2000). Apolipoprotein E genotype and the risk of recurrent lobar intracerebral hemorrhage. N Engl J Med 342: 240–245.

Ondra SL, Troupp H, George ED et al. (1990). The natural history of symptomatic arteriovenous malformations of the brain: a 24-year follow-up assessment. J Neurosurg 73: 387–391.

Patel MR, Edelman RR, Warach S (1996). Detection of hyperacute primary intraparenchymal hemorrhage by magnetic resonance imaging. Stroke 27: 2321–2324.

Pinker K, Stavrou I, Szomolanyi P et al. (2007). Improved preoperative evaluation of cerebral cavernomas by high-field, high-resolution susceptibility-weighted magnetic resonance imaging at 3 Tesla: comparison with standard (1.5 T) magnetic resonance imaging and correlation with histopathological findings – preliminary results. Invest Radiol 42: 346–351.

Pomper MG, Miller TJ, Stone JH et al. (1999). CNS vasculitis in autoimmune disease: MR imaging findings and correlation with angiography. AJNR Am J Neuroradiol 20: 75–85.

Poon CS, Chang JK, Swarnkar A et al. (2007). Radiologic diagnosis of cerebral venous thrombosis: pictorial review. AJR Am J Roentgenol 189: S64–S75.

Qureshi AI, Tuhrim S, Broderick JP et al. (2001). Spontaneous intracerebral hemorrhage. N Engl J Med 344: 1450–1460.

Qureshi AI, Mendelow AD, Hanley DF (2009). Intracerebral haemorrhage. Lancet 373: 1632–1644.

Romero JM, Artunduaga M, Forero NP et al. (2009). Accuracy of CT angiography for the diagnosis of vascular abnormalities causing intraparenchymal hemorrhage in young patients. Emerg Radiol 16: 195–201.

Romero JM, Brouwers HB, Lu J et al. (2013). Prospective validation of the computed tomographic angiography spot sign score for intracerebral hemorrhage. Stroke 44: 3097–3102.

Russell EJ, Geremia GK, Johnson CE et al. (1987). Multiple cerebral metastases: detectability with Gd-DTPA-enhanced MR imaging. Radiology 165: 609–617.

Scott RM, Smith ER (2009). Moyamoya disease and moyamoya syndrome. N Engl J Med 360: 1226–1237.

SHEP (1991). Prevention of stroke by antihypertensive drug treatment in older persons with isolated systolic hypertension. Final results of the Systolic Hypertension in the Elderly Program (SHEP). SHEP Cooperative Research Group. JAMA 265: 3255–3264.

Spetzler RF, Hargraves RW, McCormick FW et al. (1992). Relationship of perfusion pressure and size to risk of hemorrhage from arteriovenous malformations. J Neurosurg 76: 918–923.

Sudlow CL, Warlow CP (1997). Comparable studies of the incidence of stroke and its pathological types: results from an international collaboration. International Stroke Incidence Collaboration. Stroke 28: 491–499.

Toni D, Fiorelli M, Bastianello S et al. (1995). Hemorrhagic transformation of brain infarct: predictability in the first 5 hours from stroke onset and influence on clinical outcome. Neurology 46: 341–345.

Van Dijk P, Sijens PE, Schmitz PI et al. (1997). Gd-enhanced MR imaging of brain metastases: contrast as a function of dose and lesion size. Magn Reson Imaging 15: 535–541.

van Gijn J, van Dongen KJ (1982). The time course of aneurysmal haemorrhage on computed tomograms. Neuroradiology 23: 153–156.

van Gijn J, van Dongen KJ, Vermeulen M et al. (1985). Perimesencephalic hemorrhage: a nonaneurysmal and benign form of subarachnoid hemorrhage. Neurology 35: 493–497.

Wada R, Aviv RI, Fox AJ et al. (2007). CT angiography "spot sign" predicts hematoma expansion in acute intracerebral hemorrhage. Stroke 38: 1257–1262.

Wiesmann M, Mayer TE, Yousry I et al. (2001). Detection of hyperacute parenchymal hemorrhage of the brain using echo-planar T2*-weighted and diffusion-weighted MRI. Eur Radiol 11: 849–853.

Wintermark M, Maeder P, Reichhart M et al. (2002). MR pattern of hyperacute cerebral hemorrhage. J Magn Reson Imaging 15: 705–709.

Woodcock Jr RJ, Short J, Do HM et al. (2001). Imaging of acute subarachnoid hemorrhage with a fluid-attenuated inversion recovery sequence in an animal model: comparison with non-contrast-enhanced CT. AJNR Am J Neuroradiol 22: 1698–1703.

Wycliffe ND, Choe J, Holshouser B et al. (2004). Reliability in detection of hemorrhage in acute stroke by a new three-dimensional gradient recalled echo susceptibility-weighted imaging technique compared to computed tomography: a retrospective study. J Magn Reson Imaging 20: 372–377.

Xavier AR, Qureshi AI, Kirmani JF et al. (2003). Neuroimaging of stroke: a review. South Med J 96: 367–379.

Yeung R, Ahmad T, Aviv RI et al. (2009). Comparison of CTA to DSA in determining the etiology of spontaneous ICH. Can J Neurol Sci 36: 176–180.

Yoon DY, Chang SK, Choi CS et al. (2009). Multidetector row CT angiography in spontaneous lobar intracerebral hemorrhage: a prospective comparison with conventional angiography. AJNR Am J Neuroradiol 30: 962–967.

Zhu XL, Chan MS, Poon WS (1997). Spontaneous intracranial hemorrhage: which patients need diagnostic cerebral angiography? A prospective study of 206 cases and review of the literature. Stroke 28: 1406–1409.

Handbook of Clinical Neurology, Vol. 135 (3rd series)
Neuroimaging, Part I
J.C. Masdeu and R.G. González, Editors

Chapter 19

Infection

GAURAV SAIGAL*, NATALYA NAGORNAYA, AND M. JUDITH D. POST
Department of Radiology, University of Miami Miller School of Medicine, Miami, FL, USA

Abstract

Imaging is useful in the diagnosis and management of infections of the central nervous system. Typically, imaging findings at the outset of the disease are subtle and nonspecific, but they often evolve to more definite imaging patterns in a few days, with less rapidity than for stroke but faster than for neoplastic lesions. This timing is similar to that of noninfectious inflammatory brain disease, such as multiple sclerosis. Fortunately, imaging patterns help to distinguish the two kinds of processes. Other than for sarcoidosis, the meninges are seldom involved in noninfectious inflammation; in contrast, many infectious processes involve the meninges, which then enhance with contrast on computed tomography (CT) or magnetic resonance imaging (MRI). However, brain infection causes a vast array of imaging patterns. Although CT is useful when hemorrhage or calcification is suspected or bony detail needs to be determined, MRI is the imaging modality of choice in the investigation of intracranial infections. Imaging sequences such as diffusion-weighted imaging help in accurately depicting the location and characterizing pyogenic infections and are particularly useful in differentiating bacterial infections from other etiologies. Susceptibility-weighted imaging is extremely useful for the detection of hemorrhage. Although MR spectroscopy findings can frequently be nonspecific, certain conditions such as bacterial abscesses show a relatively specific spectral pattern and are useful in diagnosing and constituting immediate therapy. In this chapter we review first the imaging patterns associated with involvement of various brain structures, such as the epidural and subdural spaces, the meninges, the brain parenchyma, and the ventricles. Involvement of these regions is illustrated with bacterial infections. Next we illustrate the patterns associated with viral and prion diseases, followed by mycobacterial and fungal infections, to conclude with a review of imaging findings in parasitic infections.

INTRODUCTION

Central nervous system (CNS) infections can be life-threatening and rapid diagnosis of a specific microorganism is essential for effective treatment. Neuroimaging not only plays a critical role in the diagnosis and therapeutic strategies involving intracranial infections, but is also essential in the monitoring of treatment response. Intracranial infections can be categorized according to their preferential location in the neuraxis (meningitis, ventriculitis, cerebritis) or whether they are caused by: (1) bacterial; (2) mycobacterial; (3) viral; (4) fungal; or (5) parasitic microorganisms. Discussing infections caused by each and every specific microorganism is beyond the scope of this chapter. Particular emphasis is given to certain organisms which have associated specific imaging characteristics, helpful in the diagnosis and treatment of those infections. Infections in both immunocompetent and immunocompromised hosts are described.

REGIONAL PATTERNS OF INVOLVEMENT

Meningitis

Meningitis is an infectious/inflammatory infiltration of the leptomeninges (pia and arachnoid mater) which can be acute (bacterial or viral) or chronic (tuberculosis or

*Correspondence to: Gaurav Saigal, MBBS, MD, Department of Radiology, University of Miami Miller School of Medicine, 1611 NW 12th Avenue WW279, Miami FL 33136, USA. Tel: +1-305-585-7500, E-mail: GSaigal@med.miami.edu

fungal) (Wong and Quint, 1999). The spread of infection can be hematogenous, directly via implantation or due to a local infection such as sinusitis, mastoiditis, or orbital cellulitis (Kanamalla et al., 2000). Patients typically present with headache, fever, neck stiffness, photophobia, and altered mental status (van de Beek et al., 2004).

Meningitis is associated with leptomeningeal enhancement. While dural enhancement can be seen normally, leptomeningeal enhancement is considered abnormal (Sze and Zimmerman, 1988; Smirniotopoulos et al., 2007). Normal enhancement of the dura is thin, markedly discontinuous, and most prominent in the parasagittal regions (Smirniotopoulos et al., 2007). It appears symmetric and does not usually extend into the sulci. Meningeal enhancement due to meningitis is seen extending to the base of the sulci and is asymmetric (Mohan et al., 2012). Leptomeningeal enhancement can occur due to many causes, but is mainly seen associated with infectious meningitis, which may be bacterial, viral, or fungal, tubercular or parasitic. Bacterial and viral meningitis typically exhibit thin and linear enhancement, whereas fungal meningitis usually produces thicker, lumpy, or nodular enhancement (Sage et al., 1998). In acute meningitis the pathologic enhancement is preferentially located over the cerebral convexity, whereas in chronic meningitis, as seen with tuberculous or fungal organisms, the enhancement is most prominent in the basal cisterns (Kanamalla et al., 2000).

Typically, the diagnosis of meningitis is made clinically and by cerebrospinal fluid (CSF) cultures. The role of computed tomography (CT) and magnetic resonance imaging (MRI) is not for the diagnosis of meningitis *per se*, as only 50% of patients show imaging features consistent with meningitis. Imaging studies are performed mainly to exclude increased intracranial pressure prior to lumbar puncture, to rule out meningitis mimics, and to evaluate for any complications of meningitis (Kastrup et al., 2008).

Early in the disease process, the initial CT or MRI study may be normal. Later, an unenhanced CT might show mild hydrocephalus and loss of the gray–white-matter differentiation suggesting cerebral edema. Obliteration of the CSF spaces and basal cisterns with exudate may be seen in the more advanced cases. MRI is more sensitive for the detection of enhancement in the subarachnoid spaces (Osborne, 1994; Wong and Quint, 1999). The exudate is isointense on T1 and hyperintense on T2/fluid-attenuated in version recovery (FLAIR) images and demonstrates restricted diffusion (Karagulle-Kendi and Truwit, 2010).

Leptomeningeal involvement is best seen on postcontrast MRI (Figs 19.1–19.3) (Parmar et al., 2006; Karagulle-Kendi and Truwit, 2010). Postcontrast FLAIR imaging has been shown to be more sensitive than regular postcontrast T1-weighted imaging in the detection of early abnormal meningeal enhancement (Parmar et al., 2006). On the other hand, T1 postcontrast images are more sensitive in the detection of parenchymal enhancement (Karagulle-Kendi and Truwit, 2010). Meningeal enhancement by itself is a nonspecific finding and can be due to infectious and noninfectious causes such as neoplastic, inflammatory, chemical, drug-induced, and collagen vascular disorders (Dietemann et al., 2005). A common noninfectious cause is carcinomatous meningitis. Carcinomatous meningitis more commonly involves both the dura and the leptomeninges, rather than the leptomeninges in isolation, whereas infectious meningitis more frequently involves the leptomeninges (Kioumehr et al., 1995). Similarly, other entities which can result in both dural and leptomenininngeal enhancement, and should be kept in mind while evaluating meningeal enhancement, include lymphoma, and granulomatous diseases such as sarcoidosis (Dietemann et al., 2005). In chronic meningitis, abnormal enhancement may be seen several years after the initial infection, and calcification may be seen in some cases in the basilar cisterns (Jinkins, 1991).

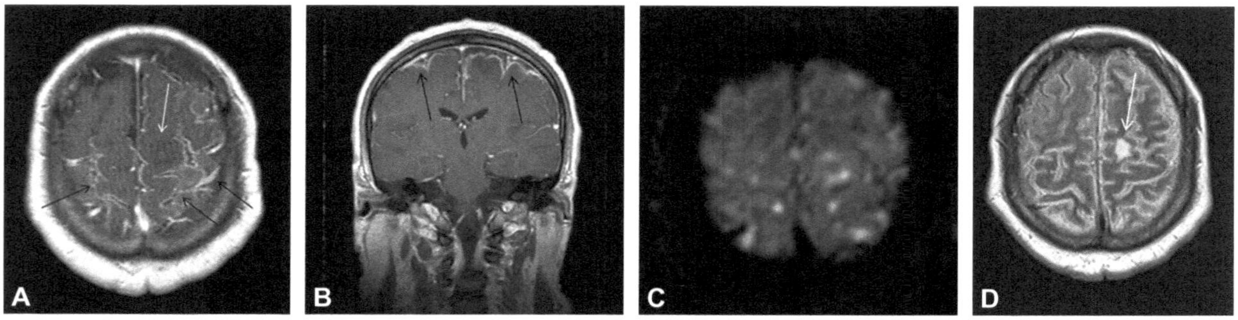

Fig. 19.1. A 47-year-old-male with *Escherichia coli* bacterial meningitis. (**A**) Axial and (**B**) coronal postcontrast T1, (**C**) axial diffusion and (**D**) fluid-attenuated inversion recovery (FLAIR) magnetic resonance images demonstrating abnormal leptomeningeal enhancement (black arrows). Enhancement can be clearly seen to extend into the sulci. There is corresponding restricted diffusion (apparent diffusion coefficient maps not shown) and abnormal FLAIR hyperintensity. Small focus of parenchymal FLAIR hyperintensity and T1 hypointensity (white arrows) was felt to represent a focus of cerebritis which later developed into an abscess.

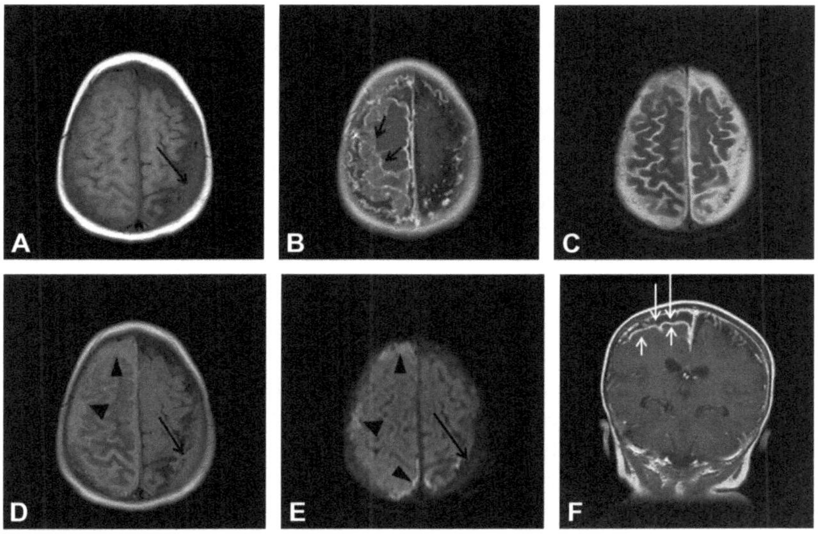

Fig. 19.2. A 12-month-old female with diagnosis of *Haemophilus* influenza (obtained from a blood culture), presenting with altered mental status. (**A**) Axial T1, (**B**) postcontrast T1, (**C**) T2, (**D**) fluid-attenuated inversion recovery (FLAIR), (**E**) diffusion, and (**F**) coronal postcontrast T1-weighted magnetic resonance images demonstrate prominence of the subarachnoid spaces, best identified on the coronal postcontrast images (long white arrows). There are multiple linear areas of enhancement within the subarachnoid spaces bilaterally, which likely represent a combination of vessels and septations. Pial enhancement of the right frontal lobe is also appreciated (short white arrows). Leptomeningeal and adjacent cortical enhancement is noted on the axial postcontrast images (short black arrows). The right-sided subarachnoid space demonstrates FLAIR hyperintensity as well as restricted diffusion (triangular black arrows). There is a left frontal extra-axial collection (long black arrows), without any evidence of restricted diffusion, demonstrating T1 and FLAIR isointensity, consistent with a subdural effusion. Overall, findings were consistent with pyogenic meningitis with underlying cerebritis and an associated subdural effusion.

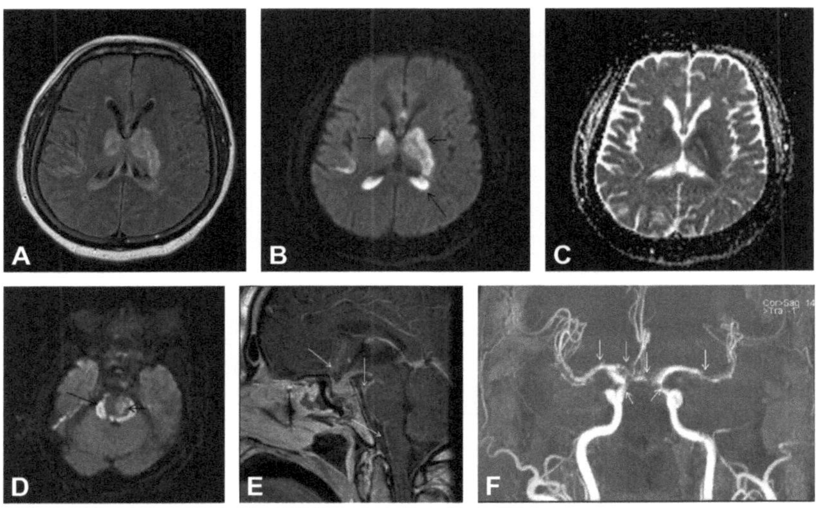

Fig. 19.3. A 63-year-old man with known *Pseudomonas* meningitis. (**A**) Axial fluid-attenuated inversion recovery, diffusion and apparent diffusion coefficient (ADC)at the level of the basal ganglia (**B, C**), and diffusion at the level of the brainstem (**D**), demonstrating multiple acute infarcts in the basal ganglia bilaterally and the left thalamus as well as the left pons (short black arrows). Corresponding low signal on the ADC map is noted. Diffusion signal noted within the ventricles and surrounding the brainstem (long black arrows), which is consistent with purulent material within the ventricles and the subarachnoid spaces. (**E**) Sagittal postcontrast image demonstrates the enhancing exudates in the basal cisterns and along the brainstem (short white arrows), consistent with meningitis. (**F**) Three-dimensional time-of-flight magnetic resonance angiography coronal maximum-intensity projection image demonstrates marked irregularity and narrowing of the A1, M1 segments of both middle cerebral arteries, as well the supraclinoid segments of both internal cerebral arteries (short white arrows), findings consistent with vasculitis.

Besides evaluating for meningeal enhancement, MRI is also extremely useful in the evaluation of complications of meningitis such as hydrocephalus, cerebritis and brain abscess, ventriculitis and choroid plexitis, and vascular complications such as vasculopathy and infarction (Fig. 19.3) and involvement of the cranial nerves. Extra-axial collections such as sterile subdural effusions and empyema (subdural/epidural) can also be well depicted (Hughes et al., 2010).

Effusions/empyema

Extra-axial fluid collections may be sterile (effusions/hygromas) or purulent (empyemas or abscesses). Subdural and epidural empyemas account for approximately 20–33% of all intracranial infections (Danziger et al., 1980; Weingarten et al., 1989). These infections need to be recognized early since they are associated with a high mortality rate, nearing 10%.

Effusions are sterile collections which occur due to irritation of the dura from adjacent parenchymal infection or secondary to inflammation of the subdural veins (Fig. 19.2) (Ferreira et al., 2005). These can be seen in up to a third of patients with meningitis. On imaging, effusions are seen as extra-axial crescenteric collections which are low in density on CT and similar to CSF intensity on MRI (Tsuchiya et al., 2003; Ferreira et al., 2005). Some may be slightly hyperintense on T1-weighted images due to the presence of serosanguineous fluid and high concentrations of protein and may show underlying septations which may enhance, making it difficult to differentiate from empyemas (Hughes et al., 2010).

Approximately 15% of subdural effusions become empyemas (Castillo, 2004). An epidural abscess or empyema refers to an infection between the inner table of the skull and the dura. Subdural abscesses or empyemas, on the other hand, occur beneath the dura in the subdural space. Subdural empyemas, which usually are secondary to sinus or ear infections or meningitis, have a more fulminant clinical course than epidural empyemas, because they can occlude cortical veins and cause adjacent parenchymal edema and even infarction. They therefore require urgent surgical intervention.

Subdural and epidural empyemas appear as crescenteric or lentiform extracerebral collections with an intensely enhancing membrane surrounding the empyema (Figs 19.2 and 19.4) (Weingarten et al., 1989). The T1

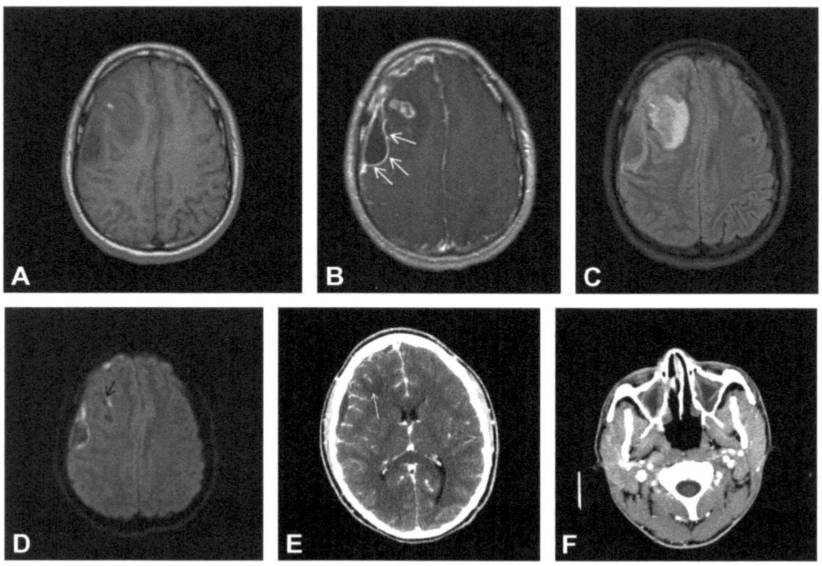

Fig. 19.4. An 18-year-old with sickle cell disease presents with headache and fever. (**A**) Axial T1, (**B**) axial postcontrast T1, (**C**) axial fluid-attenuated inversion recovery (FLAIR), and (**D**) diffusion magnetic resonance imaging (MRI) images of the brain demonstrate a small, irregular, peripherally enhancing collection in the right frontal lobe at the gray–white-matter junction, demonstrating underlying restricted diffusion (short black arrow) consistent with a brain abscess Significant surrounding FLAIR signal abnormality, consistent with edema and mass effect on the adjacent brain parenchyma and midline shift, is noted. An adjacent large subdural collection is noted (short white arrows), also demonstrating some degree of restricted diffusion. (**E**) Axial postcontrast computed tomography scan of the brain (done 7 days prior to the MRI study) at the level of the lateral ventricles demonstrates an ill-defined hypodensity in the right frontal lobe with a small focus of underlying enhancement, likely cerebritis (long white arrow). There is an associated adjacent extra-axial crescenteric hypodensity. These findings correlate well with the frontal-lobe abscess and the subdural empyema seen on the follow-up MRI study. (**F**) Postcontrast axial image at the level of the maxillary sinuses demonstrates complete opacification of both the maxillary sinuses. An air fluid level was noted in the right frontal sinus (not shown), suggesting acute sinusitis.

hyperintensity as well as the FLAIR hyperintensity seen in empyemas is much higher than that seen in most effusions (Tsuchiya et al., 2003). Also, bacterial empyemas show restricted diffusion (as they contain pus), whereas effusions do not (Wong et al., 2004).

The dura serves as a barrier to brain inflammation in cases of epidural empyemas and therefore these have a less fulminant course. Differentiation between these two collections requires correct identification of the dura, which can be seen as low signal on the T1- and T2-weighted images (Weingarten et al., 1989). Epidural empyemas may extend across the midline in the frontal region, which may help differentiate them from subdural empyemas, which do not cross the midline.

Ventriculitis

Ventriculitis may be the cause of persistent infection and failure of therapy in cases of meningitis (Rahal et al., 1974; Kaiser and McGee, 1975). Early recognition and treatment of ventriculitis are essential because, if untreated, ventriculitis could lead to fatal complications (Mangi et al., 1977). Neuroimaging plays an important role in the diagnosis of this potentially lethal condition. Cranial sonography is useful in diagnosing this condition in infants and young children (Yikilmaz and Taylor, 2008). Findings include increased echogenicity of the ventricular wall, increased thickness of the ventricular walls, and presence of septations and debris in the ventricles (Han et al., 1985). On CT and MRI, ependymal enhancement and thickening with surrounding FLAIR signal hyperintensity, suggestive of parenchymal edema, may be seen (Figs 19.3 and 19.5) (Fukui et al., 2001). Dilated ventricles, increased T2 hyperintensity in the ventricular wall, and debris in the dependent portion of the ventricle are other imaging findings. In ventriculitis secondary to a pyogenic organism, restricted diffusion may be seen in the dependent purulent intraventricular fluid (Pezzullo et al., 2003). Purulent material in the ventricle may be strongly hyperintense on diffusion-weighted images (DWI). However, apparent diffusion coefficient (ADC) maps may demonstrate variable intensity secondary to dilution of pus with CSF and regional variation of the concentration of protein in the purulent material (Fig. 19.6) (Rana et al., 2002). Ventricular debris, seen as an irregular level on CT or MRI, is considered to be the most reliable sign of ventriculitis (Fukui et al., 2001).

Cerebritis and brain abscess

Parenchymal infection most commonly occurs due to direct spread from penetrating head injury or skull fractures or indirect spread of infection from the paranasal sinuses, middle ear, or teeth (Wong and Quint, 1999). Meningitis may be the cause or may result from brain abscesses (Hughes et al., 2010). Most cerebral abscesses are caused by pyogenic bacteria. Other less common

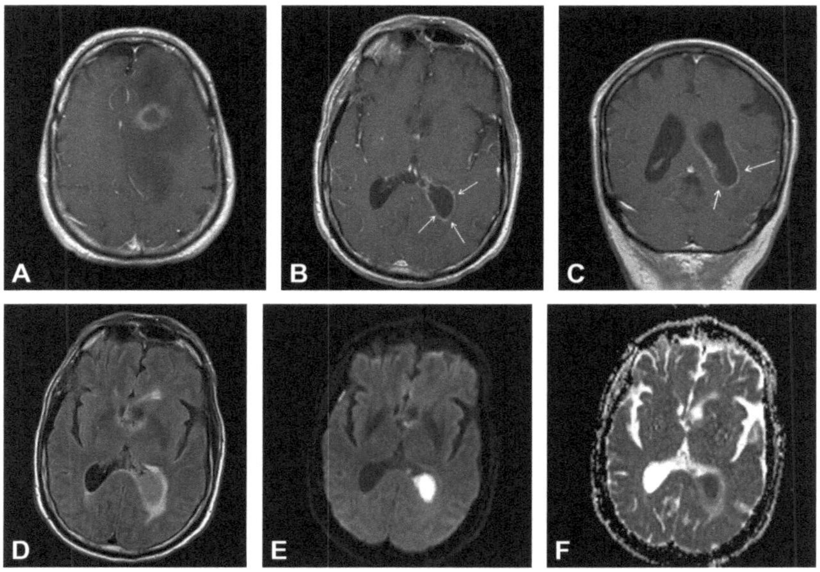

Fig. 19.5. A 70-year old man with known intracranial abscess with rupture into the left ventricle. (**A**) Axial T1-weighted postcontrast magnetic resonance (MR) image demonstrates a mass with thick and irregular ring enhancement in the medial left frontal lobe, just above the body of the left lateral ventricle, consistent with a brain abscess. T1-weighted postcontrast axial (**B**) and coronal (**C**), axial fluid-attenuated inversion recovery (FLAIR) (**D**) and axial diffusion (**E**) and apparent diffusion coefficient (**F**) MR images at the level of the atrium of the lateral ventricle demonstrate restricted diffusion within the dependent portion of the occipital horn of the left lateral ventricle with associated ependymal enhancement (arrows), consistent with ventriculitis. The adjacent brain parenchyma demonstrates significant FLAIR signal hyperintensity, consistent with vasogenic edema.

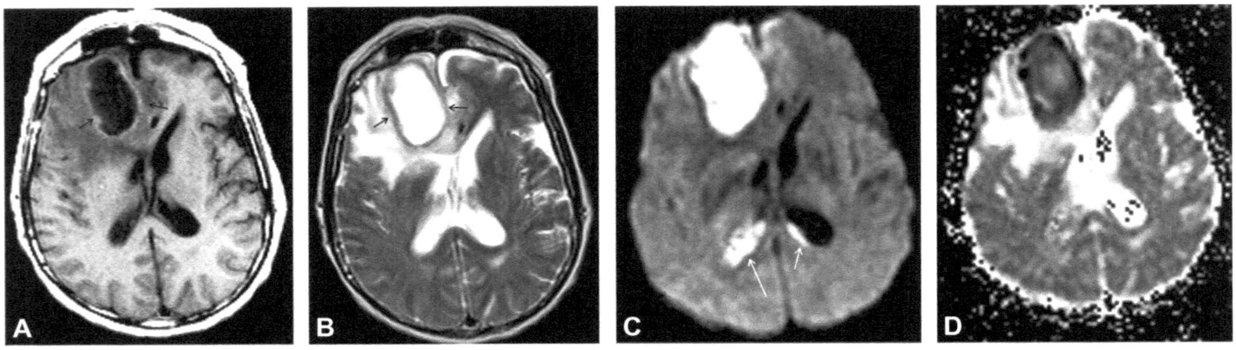

Fig. 19.6. A 71-year-old who presents with altered mental status and lethargy. (**A**) Axial T1- and (**B**) T2-weighted magnetic resonance images demonstrate a large cystic mass in the right frontal lobe with significant surrounding edema and mass effect. The rim of the mass is iso/hyperintense on the T1- and hypointense on the T2-weighted sequence (short black arrows). Restricted diffusion is noted within the center of the mass, based on the diffusion (**C**) and the apparent diffusion coefficient (**D**) maps, findings which are consistent with a pyogenic abscess, rather than tumor, which was also being considered in the differential at presentation. *Streptococcus mitis* was cultured from the pus. Note the restricted diffusion within the posterior aspect of the right lateral ventricle (long white arrow). The diffusion signal appears slightly less hyperintense than that within the abscess, which is likely due to mixing with the ventricular cerebrospinal fluid. Restricted diffusion is also noted along the ventricular margin (short white arrow), consistent with ventriculitis.

causes include *Mycobacterium tuberculosis*, fungi, and parasitic organisms. Abscesses are rare in children but, when they do occur, evaluation for congenital heart disease should be performed since it can be a predisposing factor (Saez-Llorens et al., 1989).

The initial parenchymal infection starts as a cerebritis and then progresses through multiple stages to form an abscess (Wong and Quint, 1999). On imaging studies, cerebritis is seen as a nonspecific focus of edema with or without enhancement (Fig. 19.1). It is seen as an ill-defined hypodensity on CT and hypointense T1/hyperintense T2 and FLAIR signal abnormality on MRI. The cerebritis phase lasts for 10–14 days, during which time there is progressive development into an abscess with the formation of a thin, peripheral capsule and central necrosis. Abscesses are typically seen in the frontal, temporal, or parietal lobes at the gray–white-matter interface or in the white matter. Because of the increased amounts of water present in pyogenic infections, bacterial abscesses can be readily detected on plain MR (Sze and Zimmerman, 1988; Haimes et al., 1989; Bowen and Post, 1990). This increased water content is seen as an area of low-intensity signal on T1-weighted imaging (T1WI) and high-intensity signal on T2WI. The cavity fluid may approximate the signal intensity of CSF but, if the fluid is proteinaceous, the protein and other macromolecular components can shorten the T1 relaxation value and result in T1 hyperintensity. Mature abscesses have a well-defined, smooth, complete capsular ring that enhances on postcontrast imaging and demonstrates significant surrounding vasogenic edema (Figs 19.5–19.7). On plain (noncontrast) MR, the peripheral rim is isointense to hyperintense on T1WI and hypointense on T2WI. These signal properties of the abscess rim may be due to collagen, hemorrhage, or to paramagnetic free radicals present within the heterogeneously distributed phagocytosing macrophages in the abscess periphery (Sze and Zimmerman, 1988; Bowen and Post, 1990). The hypointense rim seen on the T2WI, which does not exactly correspond to the usually thin enhancing rim of the abscess seen on contrast-enhanced MR, will resolve with successful medical or surgical therapy, and has been reported to be a better indicator of therapeutic response than the residual contrast-enhancing rim or nodule which may persist for months following completion of medical therapy (Sze and Zimmerman, 1988; Bowen and Post, 1990). The peripheral enhancement seen is thicker along the lateral margin compared to the medial (ependymal) margin due to better blood supply laterally. This finding can help differentiate from cystic neoplasms which often have the opposite pattern, with a thicker medial margin (Karampekios and Hesselink, 2005), or, demyelinating lesions (tumefactive plaques) where the ring of enhancement may be incomplete in the boundary with the cortex (open-ring sign) (Masdeu et al., 2000).

While evaluating a pyogenic abscess, the main differential to be considered is a cystic necrotic neoplasm (Rumboldt et al., 2007). DWI and MR spectroscopy (MRS) can be helpful in distinguishing pyogenic abscesses from cystic primary or secondary neoplasms. Pyogenic abscesses demonstrate significant restricted diffusion (hyperintense signal on DWI and reduced signal on ADC maps) due to the presence of pus which restricts water motion. Necrotic or cystic tumors show low to intermediate DWI signal and increased ADC values. Diffusion

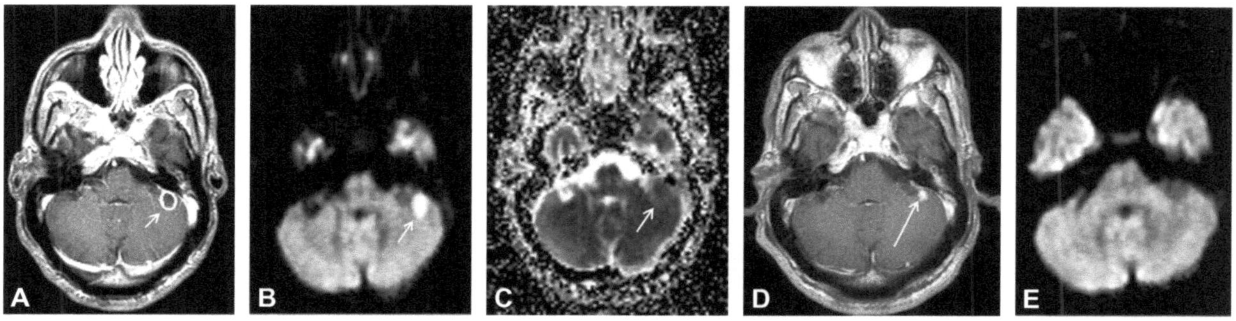

Fig. 19.7. Immunocompromised man who presents with earache and fever. (**A**) Axial postcontrast T1-weighted images of the brain demonstrate a small ring enhancing mass in the left cerebellopontine region demonstrating restricted diffusion, as noted on the diffusion (**B**) and apparent diffusion coefficient (**C**) maps (short white arrows). Previously performed computed tomography scan of the brain (not shown) demonstrated left mastoid sinus opacification. Imaging findings are consistent with mastoiditis with an associated left cerebellar brain abscess. Blood and cerebrospinal fluid cultures were positive for *Streptococcus viridans*. Patient was started on appropriate antibiotic treatment and the magnetic resonance imaging (MRI) was repeated in 14 days. Repeat MRI demonstrated resolution of the ring enhancement on the axial postcontrast T1-weighted image (**D**), with some residual nodular enhancement (long white arrow). (**E**) Diffusion imaging done at the same time showed complete resolution of the previously seen restricted diffusion, suggesting abscess resolution.

imaging is helpful also in monitoring the therapeutic response, because on follow-up it may show progressive decreases in the amount of restricted diffusion with treatment response (Fig. 19.7) (Cartes-Zumelzu et al., 2004). Similar findings of restricted diffusion in cases of cerebritis, and resolution on serial DWI/ADC, have also been reported (Tung and Rogg, 2003).

MRS is useful in the evaluation and diagnosis of abscesses, particularly differentiating pyogenic abscesses from necrotic tumors (Lai et al., 2002). The centers of mature abscesses have shown peaks of acetate (1.92 ppm), succinate (2.4 ppm), and other amino acids such as valine, leucine, and isoleucine (0.9 ppm) as well as lactate(1.3 ppm), whereas cystic necrotic tumors only show the presence of lactate with or without lipids (Fig. 19.8) (Lai et al., 2002). Amino acids and lactate are noted in abscesses with aerobic organisms, whereas additional acetate and succinate peaks are seen in anaerobic infections (Garg et al., 2004). The main brain metabolites (*N*-acetyl aspartate, choline, and creatine) are not seen in abscesses. Similarly, the spectral signature of a tumor (elevated choline creatine ratio above 2.5) can be seen in the peripheral enhancing solid component of a necrotic tumor, which would not be seen in an abscess, either peripherally or centrally. Recently diffusion tensor imaging has been found to be useful in differentiating brain abscesses from necrotic cystic tumors in the brain (Gupta et al., 2005a). Pyogenic abscesses show increased fractional anisotropy (FA) within the abscess cavity as opposed to necrotic brain tumors and other cystic lesions in the brain which show decreased FA. Increased FA values in pyogenic brain abscesses are felt to be due to the clumping of inflammatory cells (leukocytes) and to the restricting matrix in which they reside as well as the upregulation of various cellular adhesive molecules on the surfaces of endothelial cells.

Brain abscesses can be caused not only by bacteria but by other organisms as well, such as fungi and parasites. Table 19.1 summarizes some imaging characteristics of these lesions. Since the findings are not pathognomonic, it is meant only as a guide to the differential diagnosis of intracranial infection – a tool to aid in the differential diagnosis. Obviously close clinical and laboratory correlation is essential and monitoring of the efficacy of treatment with serial neuroimaging remains important.

VIRAL INFECTIONS

Viral infections of the CNS are uncommon, but when they do occur, can involve the brain, meninges, or the spinal cord, in isolation or in combination (Handique, 2011). Viral meningitis is characterized by headache, fever, photophobia, and neck stiffness (Studahl et al., 2013). Viral encephalitis is an infection of the brain parenchyma and can be focal or diffuse (Roos, 1999; Solbrig et al., 2008). When focal, patients usually present with aphasia, visual disturbances, hemiparesis, or ataxia. Diffuse involvement can manifest as altered mental status or seizures. Most viral infections present as a combination of meningitis and encephalitis, hence the term meningoencephalitis.

Herpes simplex

Herpes simplex virus (HSV) encephalitis is the most common cause of fatal encephalitis in the USA (Kennedy, 2004). The majority of cases (90%) are caused by herpes simplex 1 and the remainder (10%) are caused

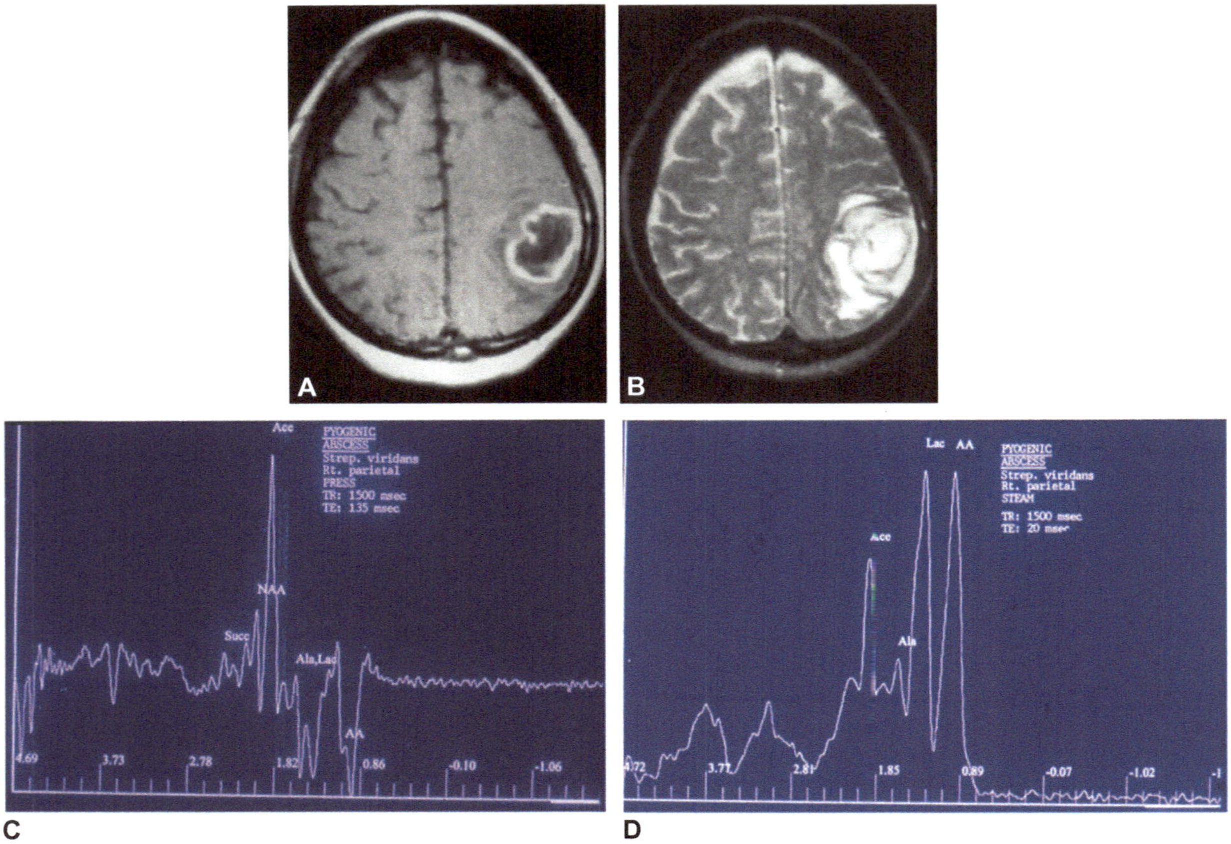

Fig. 19.8. A healthy middle-aged man with no pertinent past medical history and no fever. Axial postcontrast (**A**) T1- and (**B**) T2-weighted magnetic resonance (MR) images of the brain demonstrated a thick-walled ring enhancing lesion in the left parietal lobe. The wall of the lesion demonstrates low T2 signal. Surrounding T2 hyperintensity is noted, consistent with surrounding edema. Primary differentials considered were a brain abscess and a metastasis. MR spectroscopy using a long echo time (TE) of 135 ms (**C**) and short TE of 20 ms (**D**) over the lesion was performed. Elevated peaks at 1.92 ppm (consistent with acetate) were noted on the short-TE sequence. Elevated peaks were also noted at 1.3 ppm and 0.9 ppm (short TE), which demonstrated reversal below the baseline (long TE) consistent with increased lactate and amino acids. Based on the spectroscopy findings, a diagnosis of a pyogenic abscess was made. The final path came back as a bacterial abscess secondary to *Streptococcus viridans*.

by herpes simplex 2, which more frequently affects neonates (Kennedy, 2004).

The gold standard for making the diagnosis is either polymerase chain reaction or viral culture (Cinque et al., 1996; Foerster et al., 2007). Red blood cells may be seen in the CSF, which helps in distinguishing HSV from other infections. Since mortality with this infection is so high, treatment with antiviral therapy (acyclovir) is started as soon as there is a clinical suspicion. Untreated, HSV has a 70% mortality, reduced to 20–30% by treatment with acyclovir (Steiner et al., 2010).

HSV infection has a predilection for the limbic system, with predominant involvement of the medial temporal and inferior frontal lobes and less frequent involvement of the cingulate gyri and insula (Fig. 19.9) (Falcone and Post, 2000). The characteristic involvement of the temporal and frontal lobes is thought to be due to the probable mechanism of spread of infection intracranially along the small meningeal branches of the trigeminal nerve from the trigeminal ganglion (Tien et al., 1993).

CT findings are usually subtle, with low-attenuation areas noted in the involved lobes, causing mass effect. Petechial hemorrhage may occur; this is more easily detected on MRI than CT (Tien et al., 1993). MRI is clearly superior to CT in the early detection of signs of this necrotizing encephalitis, which can demonstrate increased T2/FLAIR signal abnormality in the involved brain within the first 48 hours (Tien et al., 1993; Falcone and Post, 2000). The involved cortex and the underlying subcortical white matter appear swollen and edematous. Gyriform enhancement may be seen in later stages (Noguchi et al., 2010). DWI appears to be more sensitive than T2 and FLAIR sequences in the detection of cytotoxic edema, which is seen as restricted diffusion (Kuker

Table 19.1

Characteristics of brain abscesses caused by various organisms

Lesion type	Conventional MR	DWI/ADC	DTI and FA	MR spectroscopy
Bacterial abscess	T2WI: hypointense rim; high signal centrally; thin ring enhancement	↓↓ diffusibility Restricted diffusion	↑↑ FA	Amino acids; acetate+succinate; lactate
Parasitic				
Toxoplasmosis	Variable T2WI signal and enhancement	Majority: ↑ diffusibility	Likely ↓ FA	Lactate; depletion of all normal metabolites
Cysticercosis	CSF equivalent on T1- and T2-weighted images Thin peripheral enhancement Calcifications on CT	↑↑ diffusibility Patchy restricted diffusion restriction may be in intracavitary projections	Likely ↑ FA	Amino acids; lactate; lipids; trehalose
Fungal abscess	Variable signal and enhancement pattern	↓ Diffusibility Patchy restricted diffusion Restriction may be in intracavitary projections as well as the periphery	Likely ↑ FA	Amino acids; lactate; lipids; trehalose
Cystic tumor				
Primary or metastaic	Heterogeneous signal on T1 and T2WI Thick irregular nodular ring enhancement	↑ diffusibility in cystic central portion Restricted diffusion in eccentric peripheral solid portion of tumor	↓ FA	↑↑ Choline/creatine ratio in solid portion of tumor and lactate; depletion centrally of all normal metabolites

Clinical and laboratory correlation with all the imaging findings is essential.
MR, magnetic resonance; DWI, diffusion-weighted imaging; ADC, apparent diffusion coefficient; DTI, diffusion tensor imaging; FA, fractional anisotropy; T2WI, T2-weighted imaging; CSF, cerebrospinal fluid; CT, computed tomography.

et al., 2004). Restricted diffusion usually disappears within 14 days after symptom onset, while T2/FLAIR hyperintensities may persist longer (Noguchi et al., 2010).

Neonatal HSV-2 encephalitis can involve the temporal lobes, brainstem, or cerebellum (Gilden et al., 2007; Vossough et al., 2008). Unlike HSV-1, the basal ganglia as well as the white matter can be involved and hemorrhage can be seen in more than half the patients. Meningeal enhancement may also be seen. DWI may be useful in the early stage of the disease and may be better than T2/FLAIR imaging to delineate the areas of involvement (Dhawan et al., 2006).

Varicella-zoster virus

Varicella-zoster virus, a member of the Herpesviridae family, causes varicella or chickenpox when it first infects an individual, usually early in childhood (Arvin, 1996). The virus becomes latent in the dorsal root ganglia after the primary infection (Gilden et al., 2009). It can become reactivated during episodes of immunosuppression or in the elderly and causes shingles or herpes zoster, which presents as a painful vesicular rash involving one or adjacent dermatomes. CNS manifestations include cerebellar ataxia, meningoencephalitis, vasculopathy, and cranial neuropathy (Tien et al., 1993). The fifth and the seventh cranial nerves are most frequently affected. If the trigeminal ganglion is affected, patients present with trigeminal neuralgia, headaches, and orbital blisters. The ophthalmic division of the fifth nerve is most frequently affected and its involvement can be seen as enhancement of the intraorbital portion of the ophthalmic division of the trigeminal nerve. If the seventh nerve is involved, facial nerve palsy can be the presenting symptom. Due to inflammation of the seventh nerve, involvement of the adjacent eighth nerve can occur and patients can present with ipsilateral hearing loss and/or vertigo with painful herpetic lesions

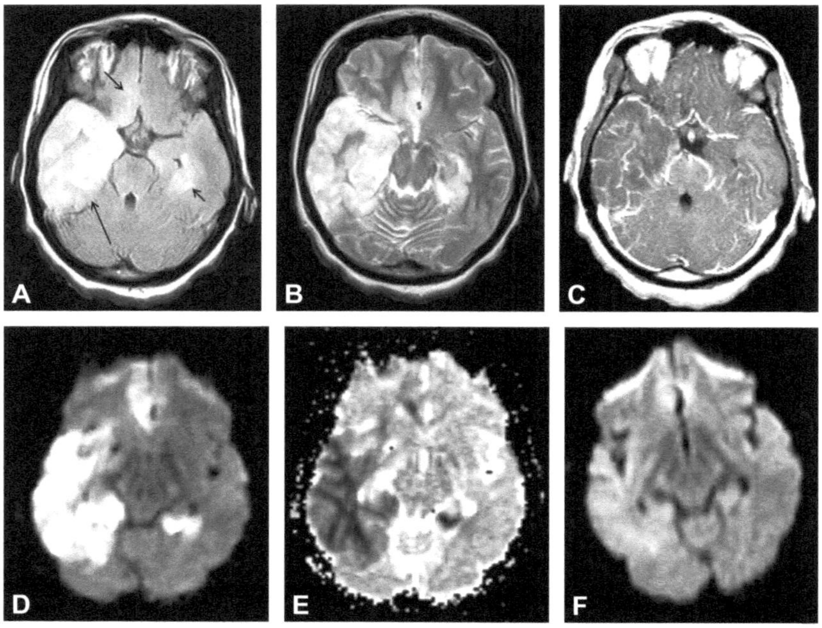

Fig. 19.9. A 16-year-old female who presented with headaches, fever, and seizures. (**A**) Axial fluid-attenuated inversion recovery and (**B**) T2 images demonstrate extensive hyperintense signal abnormality involving nearly the entire right temporal lobe (long arrow). Smaller areas of involvement are also noted in the right frontal and the left posterior temporal lobes (short arrows). (**C**) Axial postcontrast T1-weighted image demonstrates an overall hypointense right temporal lobe with no appreciable postcontrast enhancement. Significant restricted diffusion is noted on the diffusion (**D**) and corresponding apparent diffusion coefficient maps (**E**). Presumptive diagnosis of herpes simplex encephalitis was made and the patient was immediately started on acyclovir therapy. Polymerase chain reaction in the cerebrospinal fluid was positive for herpes simplex. Diffusion image from a follow-up MRI scan (**F**) at the level of the temporal lobes demonstrates resolution of the diffusion signal seen on the prior MRI study.

in and around the external auditory canal and seventh-nerve palsy (Ramsay Hunt syndrome). Ipsilateral asymmetric enhancement of the seventh and eighth nerves can occur, best seen on postcontrast fat-saturated MR images (Fig. 19.10) (Anderson and Laskoff, 1990; Tien et al., 1990; Iwasaki et al., 2013).

CNS vasculopathy can involve both the small and the large vessels either in combination or alone (Gilden et al., 2009). Patients can present with symptoms of an acute stroke or transient ischemic attacks. On imaging,

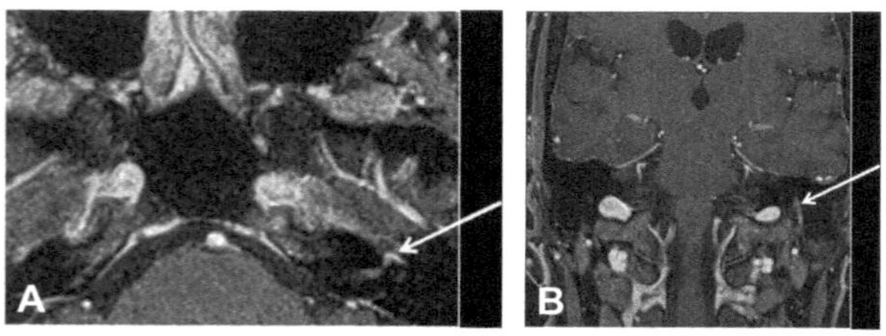

Fig. 19.10. Young man with clinical suspicion of herpes zoster, presenting with a painful rash around the left ear and facial nerve palsy. (**A**) Axial and (**B**) coronal postcontrast T1-weighted fat-saturated images demonstrating ipsilateral thickening and enhancement of the entire left facial nerve. Arrows indicate enhancement of the geniculate ganglion and the vertical portion of the facial nerve.

superficial or deep infarcts seen as multiple areas of increased T2/FLAIR signal abnormality involving the gray–white-matter junction, some with associated hemorrhage and restricted diffusion, may be seen. Less frequently, varicella-zoster virus vasculopathy results in aneurysm formation, subarachnoid or parenchymal hemorrhage, vascular ectasia, or dissection (Gilden et al., 2009).

West Nile virus

West Nile virus is a flavivirus transmitted to humans by mosquitoes from various species of birds that possibly act as both carriers and amplifiers of the disease (Handique, 2011). West Nile virus appeared in the western hemisphere with an outbreak of encephalitis in the greater New York area and, since then, has become an emerging infection with increasing incidence (Centers for Disease Control and Prevention, 2002). The majority of the patients infected with West Nile virus are asymptomatic. Less than 1% of infected individuals develop CNS disease, with the elderly, immunocompromised, and young children being most frequently affected (Petersen and Marfin, 2002; Samuel and Diamond, 2006). Findings are nonspecific on MRI. Increased

T2/FLAIR signal abnormality and restricted diffusion have been reported in the lobar gray and white matter, deep gray matter, brainstem, mesial temporal lobes, and cerebellum (Fig. 19.11) (Agid et al., 2003; Ali et al., 2005; Petropoulou et al., 2005). Postcontrast enhancement of the leptomeninges is rare but has been reported (Olsan et al., 2003). Concomitant flaccid paralysis and anterior myelitis due to involvement of the anterior horn cells are not uncommon. MR findings in the spine include signal abnormality involving the anterior horn cells and enhancement of the cauda equina (Fig. 19.11) (Ali et al., 2005; Petropoulou et al., 2005).

Creutzfeldt–Jakob disease

Creutzfeldt–Jakob disease (CJD) is a transmissible, rapidly progressive, invariably fatal spongiform encephalopathy caused by a protein known as prion (Masters et al., 1979; Prusiner, 1986). There are three known subtypes, with the sporadic form (sCJD) being the commonest (approximately 85%), followed by the familial form (approximately 15%). In 1996, a new and clinicopathologically different form of bovine spongiform encephalopathy was found in the UK and named variant CJD (vCJD); after the initial outbreak it has become rare (Will et al., 1996).

Diagnostic criteria for sCJD include a combination of rapidly progressive dementia, characteristic EEG findings of periodic synchronous discharges, and the demonstration of the 14-3-3 protein in the CSF (World Health Organization, 1998). Definite CJD requires pathologic confirmation on brain biopsy or autopsy.

MRI is highly sensitive and specific in making a diagnosis of both the sporadic and variant forms of CJD (Collie et al., 2003; Young et al., 2005). Both DWI and FLAIR have demonstrated high sensitivity and specificity in aiding in the diagnosis of CJD; however, DWI has been shown to be more useful in the early diagnosis of

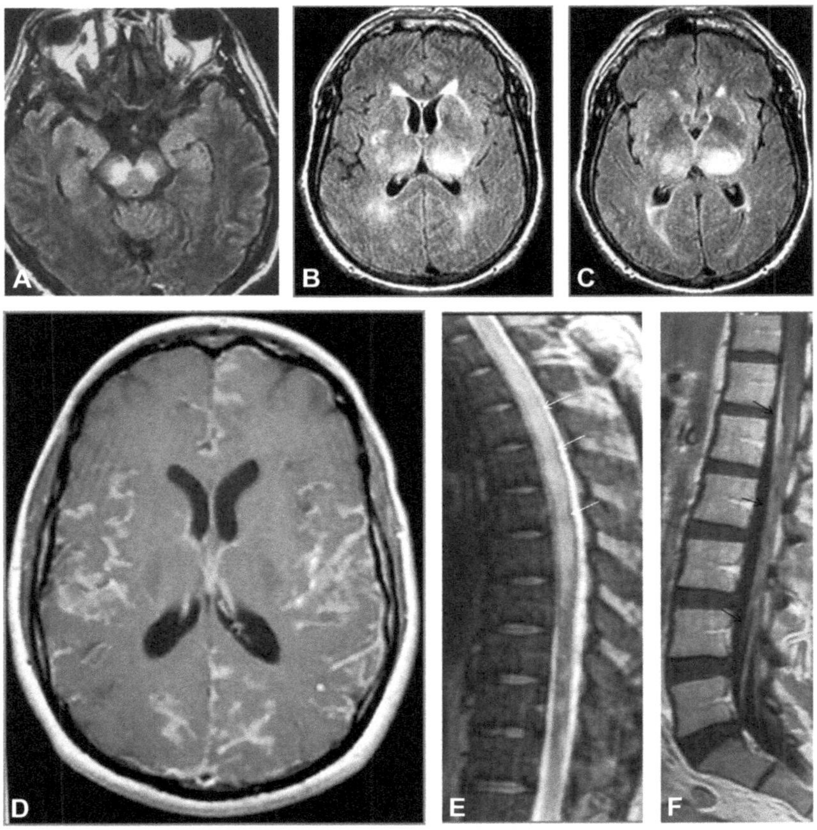

Fig. 19.11. Patient with proven West Nile virus infection who presented with the clinical picture of meningoencephalitis and Guillain–Barré-like syndrome. (**A–C**) Multiple axial fluid-attenuated inversion recovery (FLAIR) images demonstrate areas of FLAIR signal abnormality in the periventricular white-matter regions bilaterally, both basal ganglia/thalami, and the midbrain. (**D**) Axial postcontrast T1-weighted image demonstrating diffuse leptomeningeal enhancement consistent with meningitis. (**E**) Sagittal short T1 inversion recovery of the thoracic spine and sagittal postcontrast T1-weighted image (**F**) of the lumbar spine demonstrating diffuse intramedullary cord signal abnormality (short white arrows) and enhancement of the cauda equina nerve roots (short black arrows) (Courtesy of Dr. Enrique Palacios).

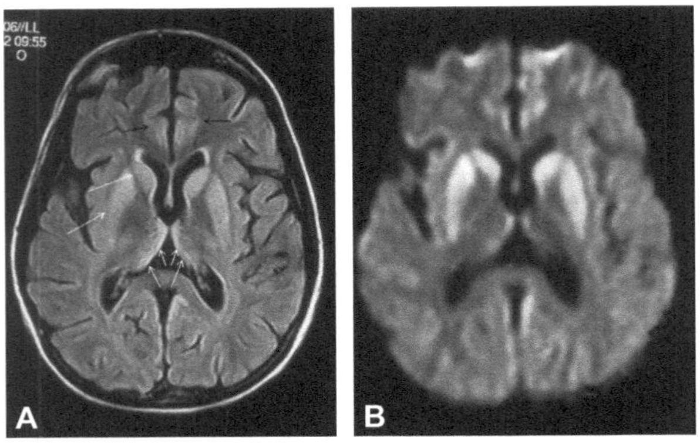

Fig. 19.12. Patient with Creutzfeldt–Jakob disease (proven by pathology). Axial fluid-attenuated inversion recovery (FLAIR) (**A**) and diffusion (**B**) images showing symmetric increased FLAIR and diffusion signal abnormality involving the caudate and the putamen nuclei bilaterally(long arrows). Subtle signal abnormality in the medial thalami and pulvinar (short white arrows) and the frontal-lobe cortex (short black arrows) is also seen. The involvement of the dorsomedial nuclei and the pulvinar nuclei in the thalamus is known as the "hockey stick sign."

CJD and monitoring disease progression (Matoba et al., 2001; Murata et al., 2002; Ukisu et al., 2005).

Typical MR findings in sCJD include extensive abnormal T2/FLAIR hyperintensity in the cortical gray matter and the corpus striatum with or without thalamic involvement and corresponding restricted diffusion (Young et al., 2005). Characteristic MR findings in vCJD includeT2/FLAIR hyperintensity involving the pulvinar nuclei and the dorsomedial nuclei, a combination of which is called the "hockey stick" sign (Fig. 19.12) (Collie et al., 2003). The pulvinar sign on MR images is the most accurate noninvasive diagnostic test of vCJD and has been included in the current World Health Organization diagnostic criteria and categories for vCJD (Collie et al., 2003).

Human immunodeficiency virus (HIV)

Infection by HIV-1 can result in meningitis (both acute and chronic), subacute encephalitis, myelopathy, and peripheral neuropathy (Britton and Miller, 1984; Navia et al., 1986; Berger et al., 1987). In the early stage of the infection, termed minor cognitive motor disorder, the bedside mini-mental status examination is normal, as are conventional MRI and CT studies. However, proton MRS has been reported to show biochemical alterations, such as elevations in choline/creatine and myoinositol-to-creatine ratios (Laubenberger et al., 1996; Navia and Gonzalez, 1997). These spectroscopic changes can be used to stage the infection and potentially to monitor the effectiveness of medical therapy. As the infection progresses into ADC stages I, II, and III, further abnormalities in metabolites can be discerned, including progressive decreases in *N*-acetyl-aspartate and further increases in choline and myo-inositol (Navia and Gonzalez, 1997). Imaging abnormalities that can be seen in these later stages of acquired immunodeficiency syndrome (AIDS)–dementia complex are cortical and deep atrophy (usually moderate to severe), and white-matter lesions (WML) (Olsen et al., 1988; Post, 1990; Post et al., 1993). While CT scans show atrophy and the low-density WML caused by HIV, MR can detect a greater number of WML and show their extent to better advantage (Post et al., 1988). Fast FLAIR has provided an excellent means of detecting these WML. The WML are most common in the periventricular white matter and centrum semiovale and are usually symmetric. They have no mass effect and no enhancement. They usually are bilateral and progress slowly over time to become more confluent and diffuse. The brainstem and cerebellar white matter can be involved, but this involvement is usually late and typically seen in conjunction with WML. Highly active antiretroviral therapy (HAART) therapy has been reported to induce a regression of WML on MR (Thurnher et al., 2000).

JC virus (progressive multifocal leukoencephalopathy: PML)

PML, occurring in 3–16% of poorly treated AIDS patients, is an opportunistic infection caused by the JC virus (Blum et al., 1985; Whiteman et al., 1993). This papovavirus, which causes subclinical infection in childhood in up to 80% of the human population, remains latent until reactivated by an immunodeficient state. When reactivated, progressive neurologic dysfunction occurs: thiscan include altered mental status, personality changes, motor and sensory deficits, visual deterioration, cognitive and speech difficulties, and memory loss. This neurologic deterioration is caused by the JC virus infecting oligodendrocytes, which then fail to maintain myelination. The resultant demyelination causes a PML and neurologic decline that usually culminate in death (Berger and Concha, 1995). Imaging findings in PML include low-density lesions on CT and high signal intensity lesions on T2-weighted MRI (Krupp et al., 1985) The lesions typically are located in the white matter, usually do not enhance, and usually do not have any mass effect (Fig. 19.13). Involvement of the supratentorial white matter predominates. A favorite site of involvement is the parietal-occipital white matter, although frontal or temporal white matter can also be affected When the subcortical white matter is involved, a common occurrence in PML, a typical

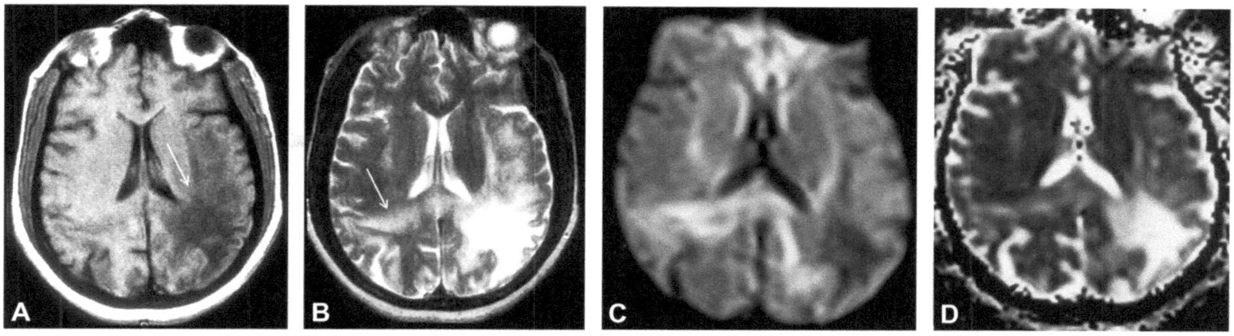

Fig. 19.13. Patient with acquired immunodeficiency syndrome (AIDS) who presents with altered mental status. Axial T1- (**A**) and T2- (**B**) weighted images demonstrate ill-defined, confluent T1 hypointense and T2 hyperintense areas in the left temporoparietal region and the right parieto-occipital region without mass effect (arrows). There is no restricted diffusion (**C, D**) or abnormal enhancement (not shown) noted. Polymerase chain reaction analysis showed JC virus infection, consistent with progressive multifocal leukoencephalopathy.

scalloped appearance will be seen because of U-fiber involvement. Internal and external capsules may also appear demyelinated. While the WML may be single and focal, it is more common to see multiple abnormal areas of white matter. Both cerebral hemispheres may be affected, but often one side is more severely affected than the other. The brainstem and cerebellar white matter may also be involved. Occasionally the posterior fossa can be the only site of disease (Whiteman et al., 1993). While occasionally in PML the deep gray matter may appear abnormal, such as the basal ganglia and thalamus, the involvement is usually a minor part of the disease and, when affected, it is felt likely due to involvement of the white-matter tracts which course through the deep gray matter (Whiteman et al., 1993). Serial MR or CT scans in PML show a progressive increase in the size and number of the WML becoming diffuse and confluent. On T1-weighted MRI, the WML show a progressive decrease in intensity. With HAART therapy, initial MR scans may demonstrate an apparent worsening with contrast leakage out of a disrupted blood–brain barrier and the development of more mass effect and edema (Thurnher et al., 2001).

On MRS, even early PML lesions have decreased *N*-acetyl-aspartate, elevated choline, presence of lactate and increased lipids; this technique can be used to monitor the effectiveness of therapeutic trials. Differentiation of PML from HIV encephalitis can be difficult, but some imaging features might help differentiate the two (Whiteman et al., 1993).

On MRI or CT, the finding of WML in a parietal-occipital location strongly favors PML, as does subcortical white-matter disease. The finding of asymmetric white-matter involvement of the cerebral or cerebellar hemispheres is another clue to the diagnosis of PML. While HIV encephalitis usually affects the deep white matter in a symmetric fashion, PML typically causes more severe demyelination in one hemisphere compared to the other. Furthermore, cortical and deep atrophy is usually absent or mild earlier on in the course of PML while moderate to severe cortical deep atrophy typifies HIV encephalitis. In addition, the lesions caused by this papovavirus more often appear hypointense on T1-weighted MRI than do those caused by HIV. Magnetization transfer ratios have also been shown to be decreased in PML lesions, which are thought to be due to demyelination (Ernst et al., 1999). From a clinical standpoint PML usually presents with a focal neurologic deficit and with visual disturbances and not with dementia, while dementia predominates in the presentation of patients with HIV encephalitis.

It should be noted that a different imaging appearance may be seen in a small number of HIV-positive patients with PML, namely in those in whom HAART therapy is initiated. Because of an intense inflammatory reaction that may occur from a dysregulated immune response, known as CNS immune reconstitution inflammatory syndrome (IRIS), patients with PML may paradoxically develop increasing FLAIR signal abnormalities due to interstitial edema, restricted diffusion, mass effect, and contrast enhancement related to their PML lesions (Fig. 19.14) (Post et al., 2012). These imaging findings, atypical for PML, are not seen in the untreated HIV-positive patients with PML and may occur while the patient is experiencing new symptoms. This imaging appearance is due to an exuberant inflammatory response from CD8 T-cell infiltration into the leptomeningeal and perivascular spaces and into the blood vessels and parenchyma (Post et al., 2012). These atypical imaging findings of PML IRIS are important to recognize because steroid therapy may help to alleviate this intense inflammatory response, leading to improved patient outcome.

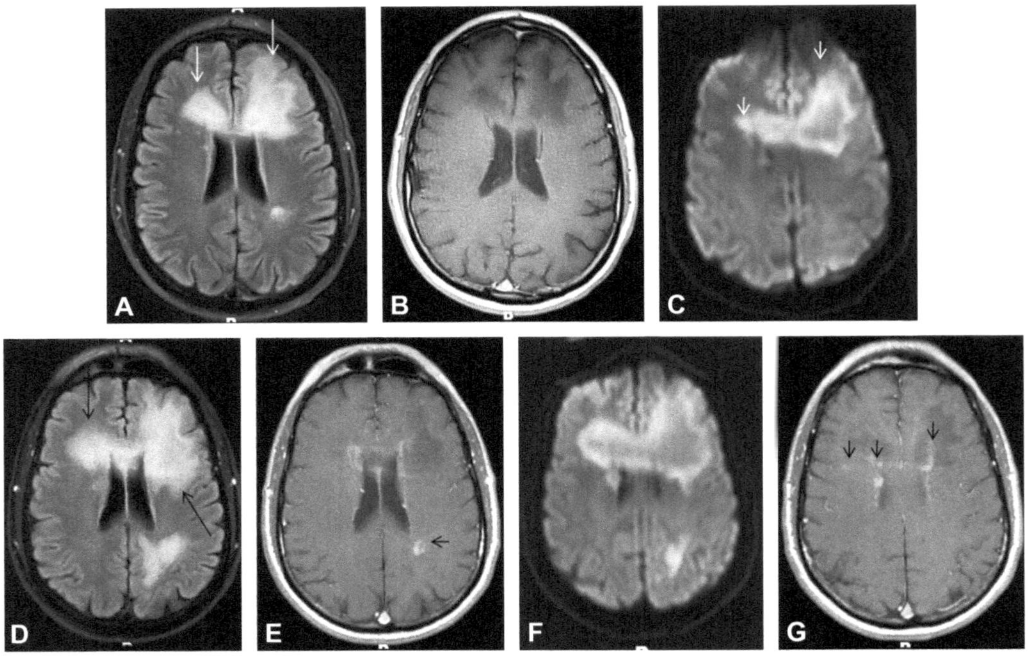

Fig. 19.14. Human immunodeficiency virus (HIV)-infected patient with personality changes and dysphasia on antiretroviral therapy but noncompliant. (**A**) Axial fluid-attenuated inversion recovery (FLAIR) shows predominantly bifrontal hyperintense white-matter lesions (long white arrows) with matching low signal on axial postcontrast T1-weighted images (**B**) without enhancement but with some peripheral restricted diffusion(short white arrows) on axial diffusion-weighted imaging (DWI) images (**C**), findings suggestive of progressive multifocal leukoencephalopathy. Five weeks later, following initiation of maraviroc, magnetic resonance (MR) demonstrates progression of the white-matter lesions (long black arrows) on axial FLAIR (**D**), the development of some mild patchy enhancement at multiple sites (short black arrows) evident on axial gadolinium MR (**E, G**) and increasing and new areas of peripheral restricted diffusion on axial DWI, (**F**) compatible with immune reconstitution inflammatory syndrome. The patient was placed on steroid therapy to decrease the inflammatory response. Reproduced with permission from Post et al. (2013).

TUBERCULOSIS

CNS infection caused by *Mycobacterium tuberculosis* is a devastating disease carrying exceptionally high mortality and morbidity rates. Disease disproportionately affects infants and young children less than 5 years of age and individuals who are infected with HIV or immunocompromised due to other conditions (Klein et al., 1985; Bidstrup et al., 2002; Cherian and Thomas, 2011).

Multiple forms of CNS tuberculosis exist. Those include tuberculous meningitis, vasculitis, tuberculoma, tuberculous abscess, cerebritis, spinal cord tuberculoma, and spinal arachnoiditis (Patkar et al., 2012). These forms refer more to the predominant involvement observed than to strictly different pathologies; most common is the involvement of both meninges and brain, with what could be called a meningoencephalitis.

Tuberculous meningitis

In the early stages, imaging studies may show little or no meningeal abnormality, as the radiographic manifestation of the disease can be subtle. CT and MRI scans can demonstrate hydrocephalus, basal exudates, and pathologic enhancement of the meninges in the basal cisterns, infarcts, and intraparenchymal or subarachnoid tuberculomas.

On CT, many imaging findings are not specific, as there is significant overlap with the findings of meningitides caused by other pathogens. Demonstrations of any of the imaging features of tuberculosis, such as basal enhancement, hydrocephalus, and infarction, are highly suggestive, but not diagnostic, of tuberculous meningitis (Andronikou et al., 2004; Botha et al., 2012). Presence of high-density exudates in the basal cisterns on noncontrast CT scan, however, was found to be very specific for tuberculous meningitis, with a reported specificity of 100% (Fig. 19.15) (Andronikou et al., 2004). MRI with DWI and administration of intravenous gadolinium contrast proved to detect more cases of meningeal enhancement and identified more cerebral infarcts in the strategic locations such as basal ganglia and brainstem (Pienaar et al., 2009). As the disease progresses,

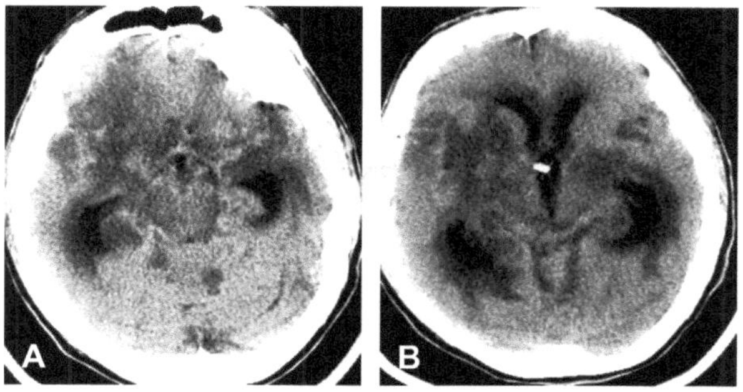

Fig. 19.15. Computed tomography (CT) findings of tuberculous meningitis with hyperdense exudate and hydrocephalus. (**A, B**) Noncontrast CT images obtained on a 38-year-old human immunodeficiency virus (HIV) patient with altered mental status for 2 weeks demonstrate severe communicating hydrocephalus with extensive confluent periventricular white-matter hypodensities representing transependymal cerebrospinal fluid edema. Note copious amount of high-density exudate in the skull base cisterns and bilateral basal ganglia hypodensities representing evolving infarcts.

a large amount of the exudates collected at the skull base cisterns will shorten T1 relaxation time, causing modest increase in T1 signal in the affected subarachnoid space. Suprasellar cisterns, prepontine cisterns, interpeduncular fossa, and perimesencephalic cisterns are commonly involved. Postcontrast T1-weighted images will demonstrate abnormal meningeal enhancement in the basal cisterns, Sylvian fissures, or, less frequently, over the cerebral convexities. Abnormal enhancement along the ependymal lining of the ventricles can occur (Trivedi et al., 2009).

On MR or CT angiography, arterial abnormalities manifested by multiple segmental areas of narrowing, irregular beaded appearance of the arteries, paucity of terminal branches, and vascular occlusion are observed in the majority of patients (50.7–70.2%) (Fig. 19.16) (Shukla et al., 2008; Kalita et al., 2012; Singh et al., 2012). Arterial narrowing and occlusion are more often seen in the anterior cerebral circulation. The most frequently involved arteries are supraclinoid internal carotid arteries, proximal middle and anterior cerebral arteries (Singh et al., 2012). An extremely rare vascular complication of tuberculous meningitis is development of mycotic aneurysms.

Cerebral infarctions are seen in 15–57% of patients with tuberculous meningitis and when present are commonly multiple and bilateral (Misra et al., 2011). Both ischemic and hemorrhagic strokes can occur. The most commonly reported sites of cerebral infarcts are basal ganglia, internal capsule, and thalamus.

Hydrocephalus is another common feature of tuberculous meningitis, reported in 75–100% of cases (Andronikou et al., 2004). Both communicating and noncommunicating types, or a combination of both, can occur in the same patient. Communicating hydrocephalus usually develops secondary to obstruction of the skull base cisterns and arachnoid villi by inflammatory exudate. Obstructive hydrocephalus is caused by the extrinsic compression of the ventricular system by parenchymal tuberculomas or tuberculous abscesses or due to the obstruction of part of the ventricular system as a result of development of inflammatory adhesions with the ventricular system secondary to granulomatous ventriculitis (Fig. 19.17) (Trivedi et al., 2009). Various degrees of transependymal CSF edema manifested by periventricular hyperintensities on T2 and FLAIR images or areas of low attenuation on CT scans can develop in patients with acute hydrocephalus. Abnormal signal along the ependymal lining of the ventricles and pathologic enhancement can be due to accompanying ventriculitis.

Cranial nerve involvement is seen in 17–45% of patients with tuberculous meningitis. Cranial

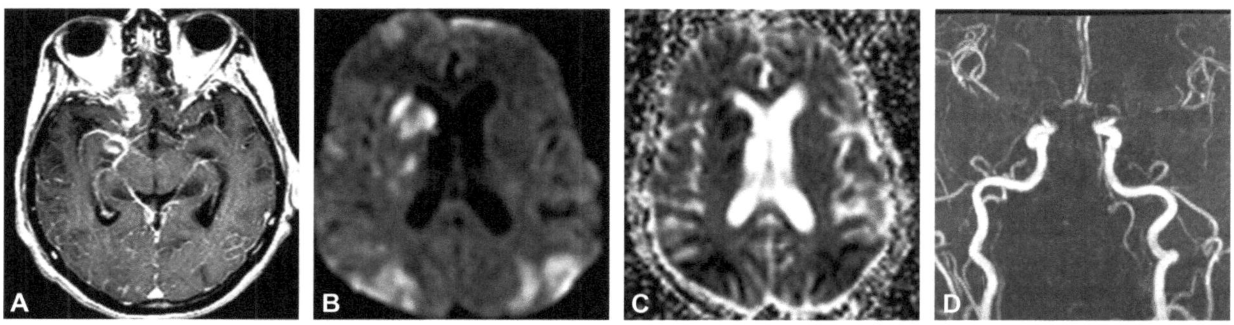

Fig. 19.16. Tuberculous meningitis with vasculitis and infarcts. (**A**) Postcontrast axial T1-weighted image demonstrates abnormal leptomeningeal enhancement along the basal cisterns representing tuberculous meningitis. (**B**) Diffusion-weighted and (**C**) apparent diffusion coefficient map images show multiple bilateral areas of restricted diffusion consistent with acute infarcts in the right basal ganglia and in the watershed territories of the bilateral cerebral hemispheres. (**D**) Maximum-intensity projection image from magnetic resonance angiogram of the circle of Willis reveals marked irregularity and high-grade stenosis of the bilateral supraclinoid internal cerebral arteries, M1, A1, and P1 segments and severe irregularity and paucity of the distal flow in the bilateral posterior cerebral arteries consistent with vasculitis.

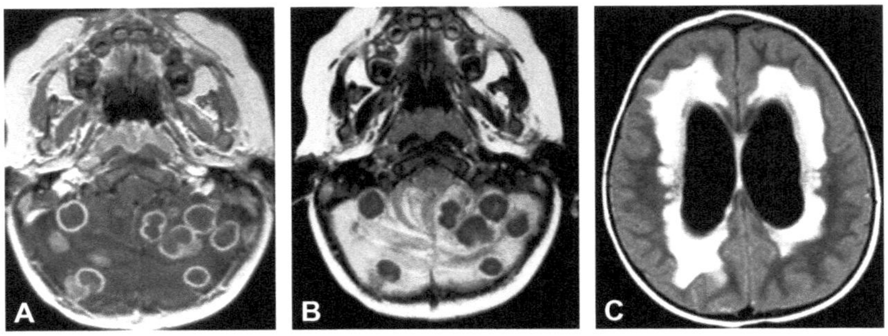

Fig. 19.17. Solid caseating tuberculomas with hypointense T2 signal resulting in obstructive hydrocephalus. (**A**) Postcontrast axial T1-weighted and (**B**) axial T2-weighted images demonstrate multiple peripherally enhancing lesions in both cerebellar hemispheres with markedly hypointense T2 signal representing caseating tuberculomas with solid caseation. No restricted diffusion was seen on diffusion-weighted images in these tuberculomas. (**C**) Axial fluid-attenuated inversion recovery (FLAIR) image obtained through the level of the lateral ventricles reveals moderate obstructive hydrocephalus with prominent confluent FLAIR hyperintensities within the periventricular regions representing transependymal cerebrospinal fluid edema. (Courtesy of Dr. Majda Thurnher.)

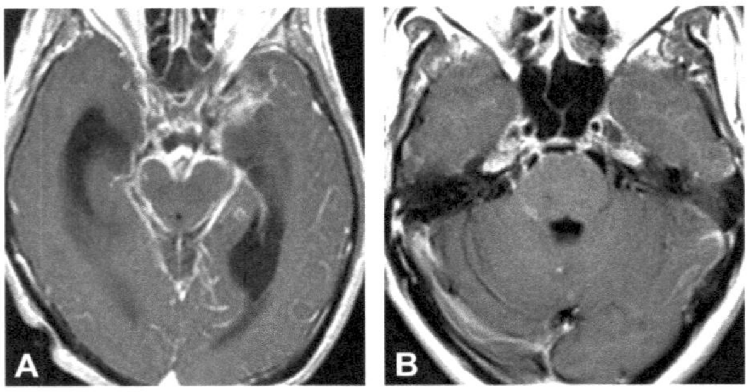

Fig. 19.18. Tuberculous meningitis with cranial nerve involvement in two different patients with multiple cranial neuropathies. (**A**) Axial postcontrast T1-weighted image obtained on a patient with tuberculous meningitis demonstrates abnormal leptomeningeal enhancement in the skull base cisterns extending along the optic chiasm and the cisternal segments of the bilateral cranial nerve 3. (**B**) Axial postcontrast T1-weighted image obtained on another patient with tuberculous meningitis and multiple cranial nerve palsies demonstrates abnormal leptomeningeal enhancement of the cisternal segments of the bilateral trigeminal nerves.

nerves 2, 3, 4, and 7 are most commonly affected (Leiguarda et al., 1988; Pienaar et al., 2009). High-resolution contrast-enhanced skull base MRI with fat saturation is the most sensitive imaging technique in demonstrating cranial nerve involvement. Abnormal increased signal on T2-weighted images, with or without enlargement of the involved nerve, and pathologic contrast enhancement can be observed (Fig. 19.18) (Gupta et al., 1994).

Sequelae of intracranial tuberculosis include cerebral atrophy and focal areas of encephalomalacia secondary to infarcts and hydrocephalus, parenchymal, meningeal, or ependymal calcifications (Harisinghani et al., 2000; Patkar et al., 2012). CT can confirm the presence of calcifications in patients with chronic tuberculosis, differentiating these old lesions from active caseating tuberculomas with hypointense T2 signal (Fig. 19.19).

Parenchymal tuberculosis

Tuberculous granuloma, tuberculous abscess, and tuberculous cerebritis are forms of parenchymal tuberculosis.

Tuberculous granuloma (tuberculoma)

Tuberculous granuloma (tuberculoma) is the most common form of parenchymal tuberculosis, which may develop with or without concomitant tuberculous meningitis or miliary tuberculosis. Tuberculomas arise from tuberculous foci, which did not rupture into the subarachnoid space. Initially, these begin as noncaseating granulomas characterized by central multinucleated giant cells surrounded by epithelioid cells without central necrosis, but ultimately progressing to caseating granulomas with or without liquefied necrosis.

Tuberculomas are commonly solitary lesions, typically seen at the gray–white junction or in the periventricular regions. In adults, tuberculomas are usually supratentorial, commonly involving frontal and parietal lobes and basal ganglia. On postcontrast CT images, tuberculomas can demonstrate either solid nodular or peripheral ring enhancement with perilesional edema and variable degree of mass effect. Many tuberculomas demonstrate a central nidus of calcification or central focus of enhancement surrounded by a rim of enhancement, also known as "target" sign. These central areas of enhancement or calcification can vary in appearance from small and regular to large and irregular (Bargallo et al., 1996). It is important to mention that the "target" sign demonstrating central enhancement

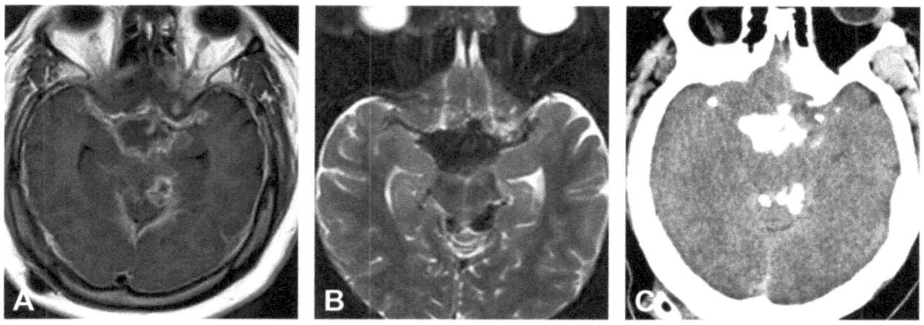

Fig. 19.19. Sequelae of tuberculous meningitis. (**A**) Postcontrast axial T1-weighted image obtained on a 34-year-old patient with prior history of multiple episodes of tuberculous meningitis treated medically demonstrates diffuse leptomeningeal and pachymeningeal enhancement. (**B**) Axial T2-weighted image shows markedly hypointense T2 signal of the large peripherally enhancing skull base tuberculomas. (**C**) Corresponding noncontrast computed tomography reveals heavy calcifications representing findings of chronic tuberculous meningitis.

Table 19.2

MRI characteristics of tuberculomas

Type of tuberculoma	Conventional MRI	DWI/ADC	MT/MTR	MRS	Histology
Noncaseating tuberculoma	Hyperintense T2 signal, isointense or hypointense T1 signal, hyperintense FLAIR signal Nodular or ring contrast enhancement	±Restricted diffusion (high DWI, low ADC)	Hyperintense rim on MT T1WI Low MTR	Lipid signal, depletion of NAA and creatine	Central giant cells surrounded by epitheliod cells Central necrosis is absent
Caseating tuberculoma with solid caseation	Hypointense T2 signal, isointense or hypointense T1 signal in the center Hyperintense T1 and T2 signal in the wall of the lesion Peripheral rim of enhancement No blooming on SWI	Absence of restricted diffusion (low DWI, high ADC)	Hyperintense rim on MT T1 images with solid hypointense center Low MTR: MTR in the rim of the lesion lower than MTR in the core of the lesion	Lipid signal, Depletion of NAA and creatine	Histiocytes, giant cells, epithelioid cells, lymphocytes surrounding a central area of solid caseation
Caseating tuberculoma with central liquefaction	Hyperintense T2 signal, hypointense T1 signal in the center Hypointense T2 signal in the wall of the lesion Peripheral rim of enhancement	Restricted diffusion (high DWI, low ADC)	Hyperintense rim on MT T1WI Low MTR	Lipid signal, depletion of NAA and creatine	Histiocytes, giant cells, epithelioid cells, lymphocytes surrounding a central area of liquid caseation

MRI, magnetic resonance imaging; DWI, diffusion-weighted imaging; ADC, apparent diffusion coefficient; MT, magnetization transfer; MTR, magnetization transfer ratio; MRS, magnetic resonance spectroscopy; FLAIR, fluid-attenuated inversion recovery; T1WI, T1-weighted imaging; NAA, *N*-acetyl aspartate; SWI, susceptibility-weighted images.

is nonspecific for tuberculous granuloma and can be seen in other space-occupying CNS lesions, such as CNS toxoplasmosis and primary CNS lymphoma. By contrast, central calcification with peripheral enhancement is characteristic of tuberculous granuloma (Bargallo et al., 1996; Patkar et al., 2012).

MRI characteristics of tuberculous granulomas vary depending on the type of the lesion (noncaseating vs caseating granuloma) and the presence or absence of liquefaction in the necrotic center of the caseating granulomas (Table 19.2 and Fig. 19.17A and B) (Karagulle-Kendi and Truwit, 2010; Gupta and Kumar, 2011).

The paradoxic development of tuberculomas has been described in patients undergoing therapy for tuberculosis and as a part of IRIS syndrome in HIV-infected patients after initiation of HAART therapy (Starke, 2010).

Tuberculous abscess

Tuberculous abscess is a rare form of parenchymal tuberculosis, constituting approximately 4–7% of total cases of CNS tuberculosis (Gupta and Kumar, 2011). Pathologically, tuberculous abscess represents an encapsulated collection of semiliquid pus with viable tuberculous bacili. The wall of the abscess is formed by a vascularized granulation tissue with mycobacteria without typical giant cell and epithelioid cell granulomatous reaction (Karagulle-Kendi and Truwit, 2010).

Tuberculous abscesses typically are large solitary lesions with a well-defined rim of enhancement, commonly multiloculated, with central hypointense T1, hyperintense T2 signal, perilesional edema, and mass effect. DWI demonstrates restricted diffusion within the cavity of the abscess (Gupta et al., 2005b; Luthra et al., 2007; Gupta and Kumar, 2011). Imaging features of tuberculous abscesses are nonspecific, mimicking bacterial abscess or caseating tuberculous granuloma with liquid caseation on conventional MRI and CT images. Tuberculous abscesses are larger, more often multiloculated, and have thicker walls than bacterial abscesses. Similarly, larger size (>4 cm), solitary and multiloculated nature of these lesions can help in differentiation of tuberculous abscesses from tuberculomas (Karagulle-Kendi and Truwit, 2010).

FUNGAL INFECTION

Fungal pathogens of the CNS can be classified as primary pathogens that affect immunocompetent hosts and opportunistic pathogens that primarily cause CNS infection in the clinical setting of immunosuppression (Lyons and Andriole, 1986). Most common opportunistic pathogens are *Candida* species, *Aspergillus* species, and *Mucoraceae* species. The most common pathogens seen in patients with normal immune systems are *Cryptococcus neoformans*, *Coccidioides immitis, Histoplasma capsulatum,* and *Blastomyces dermatitidis* (Gottfredsson and Perfect, 2000). *Cryptococcus neoformans* and *Coccidioides immitis* can cause infection in both patient populations, with increased incidence among immunosuppressed individuals (Lyons and Andriole, 1986; Mathur et al., 2012).

Aspergillosis

The most common human pathogen accounting for most of the cases of invasive aspergillosis is *Aspergillus fumigatus* (Nadkarni and Goel, 2005). Invasive aspergillosis can affect both immunocompetent and immunocompromised individuals. In patients with disseminated aspergillosis, CNS involvement is extremely common, reported as high as 81–94%, with mortality approaching 100% (Kleinschmidt-DeMasters, 2002; Tempkin et al., 2006).

Invasive cerebral aspergillosis is characterized by a marked tendency for angioinvasion, producing necrotizing vasculitis, thrombosis, and secondary hemorrhages (Nadkarni and Goel, 2005). *In situ* thrombosis and distal embolization of fungal organisms are responsible for the development of bland or hemorrhagic cerebral infarcts. Cerebral infarcts can be multiple and hemorrhagic, usually affecting a large vascular territory secondary to occlusion of the proximal vessels. Most commonly reported sites are distributions of the middle and anterior cerebral artery, including involvement of small perforators (DeLone et al., 1999; Hurst et al., 2001). Imaging reveals typical findings of multiple focal lesions with hyperintense signal on T2-weighted and FLAIR images, with corresponding restricted diffusion on DWI sequences with low ADC values (Fig. 19.20). Presence of hemorrhage is common and can be identified on both CT and susceptibility-weighted MR images (Mathur et al., 2012). Subtle peripheral enhancement can be detected on postcontrast MRI scans (DeLone et al., 1999).

Cerebral abscesses caused by *Aspergillus* are nonspecific, typically demonstrating multiple ring-enhancing lesions, predominantly located at the gray–white junction, suggesting hematogenous spread, with thick irregular enhancing walls (Ashdown et al., 1994). Restricted diffusion is usually present within the wall of the abscess and not in the central necrotic core (Luthra et al., 2007) (Fig. 19.21). They typically demonstrate a hypointense rim on T2 and gradient echo (GRE) images, attributed to the presence of hemorrhage and high concentration of *Aspergillus* hyphal elements in the abscess wall (Cox et al., 1992). Hemorrhages can be present within the central core of the abscesses, with similar findings of hypointense T2 signal and susceptibility artifact on GRE and susceptibility-weighted images (Tempkin et al., 2006).

Weakening of the vessel wall due to direct invasion with *Aspergillus* hyphae and necrosis can result in the formation of mycotic aneurysms. Septic aneurysms caused by aspergillosis are typically large, with average size 5–15 mm, arising from the major cerebral arteries at the skull base. The intradural segment of the internal cerebral artery is the most commonly reported site. Involvement of a long segment of the vessel wall is not uncommon, and this can result in the formation of fusiform aneurysms (Hurst et al., 2001). This is in

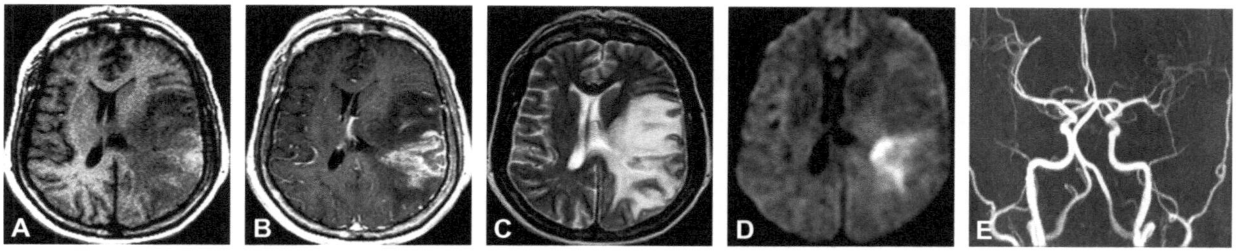

Fig. 19.20. Parenchymal aspergillosis. (**A, B**) Axial pre- and postcontrast T1-weighted images obtained on a patient with systemic lupus erythematosus and acute lymphoblastic leukemia on chemotherapy with new onset of mental status change demonstrate a large hemorrhagic lesion with adjacent edema in the left cerebral hemisphere. Note areas of irregular linear enhancement postcontrast and patchy T1 hyperintensity on precontrast T1-weighted image representing subacute hemorrhage. (**C**) Axial T2-weighted image reveals predominantly hyperintense signal with regions of T2 hypointensity within the lesion, which may represent hemorrhages or fungal elements. (**D**) Diffusion-weighted image demonstrates a smaller area of restricted diffusion consistent with ischemia. (**E**) Maximum-intensity projection image from a time-of-flight angiogram of the brain demonstrates paucity of distal left middle cerebral artery branches. The patient was treated empirically for presumed intracranial aspergillosis.

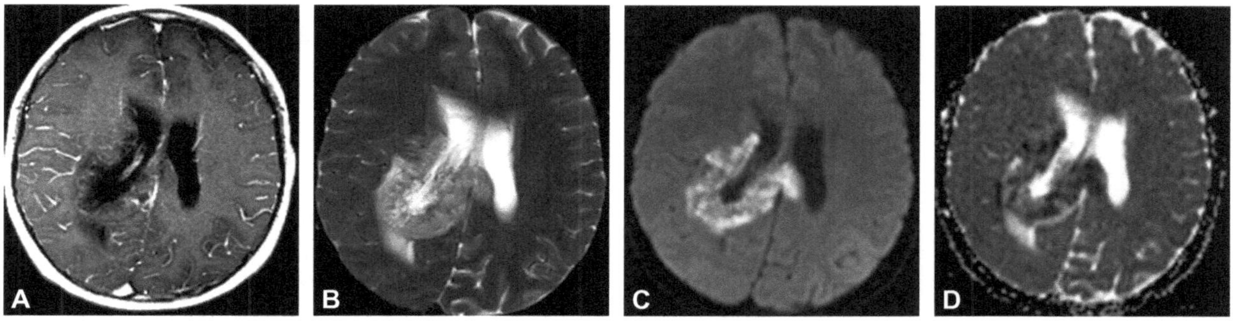

Fig. 19.21. Fungal abscess. (**A**) Axial postcontrast T1- and (**B**) T2-weighted images obtained on a 14-year-old patient with a history of intestinal transplant and recent fever and headaches show a large right parietal-lobe mass with irregular borders and only faint peripheral contrast enhancement representing fungal abscess due to *Aspergillus* spp. in this immunocompromised patient. The central portion of the abscess cavity reveals hyperintense T2 hypointense T1 signal and surrounded by isointense to slightly hypointense T2 signal intensity rim. Note nonenhancing intracavitary projections extending from the wall of the lesion representing fungal hyphae which are hypointense on T2 and isointense to hypointense on T1-weighted images. (**C**) Diffusion-weighted and (**D**) apparent diffusion coefficient map images demonstrate diffusion restriction in the wall and intracavitary projections of the lesion but not in the central portion of the abscess cavity.

contrast to the typical appearance of the bacterial mycotic aneurysms, which are usually multiple, small (2–5 mm in size), spherical, and peripheral. Aneurysmal rupture can occur, resulting in massive cerebral hemorrhage, with fatal outcome in most cases (Horten et al., 1976; Komatsu et al., 1991; Hurst et al., 2001).

In addition to the hematogenous spread from the lungs, *Aspergillus* can gain access to the brain from adjacent sinus infection or via direct inoculation of the organism during sinus surgery (Hurst et al., 2001; Riddell and Shuman, 2012). From the infected sinuses, fungal hyphae can extend intracranially through the sinus mucosa and walls, gaining access to the critical structures at the skull base. Skull base osteomyelitis, orbital involvement, cavernous sinus thrombosis, invasion of the carotid arteries with subsequent infarcts and development of mycotic aneurysms, meningitis, meningoencephalitis, and brain abscesses are potential fatal complications (Hurst et al., 2001) (Fig. 19.22).

CT of the paranasal sinuses is very useful for assessment of bony changes and can detect evidence of bony remodeling or erosion. Sinus opacification and high-density material within the sinuses can be observed on noncontrast CT (Chang et al., 1992; Hurst et al., 2001). MRII is superior to CT in evaluating intracranial complications and orbital extension of invasive sinus aspergillosis. If skull base osteomyelitis develops, characteristic loss of hyperintense T1 signal of the skull base marrow on noncontrast T1-weighted images is observed. Postcontrast T1 fat-suppressed images reveal intense enhancement of the skull base and meninges, with involvement of the cavernous sinuses and internal carotid arteries (Fig. 19.23). Extension of the disease process into the orbit can occur, manifesting as

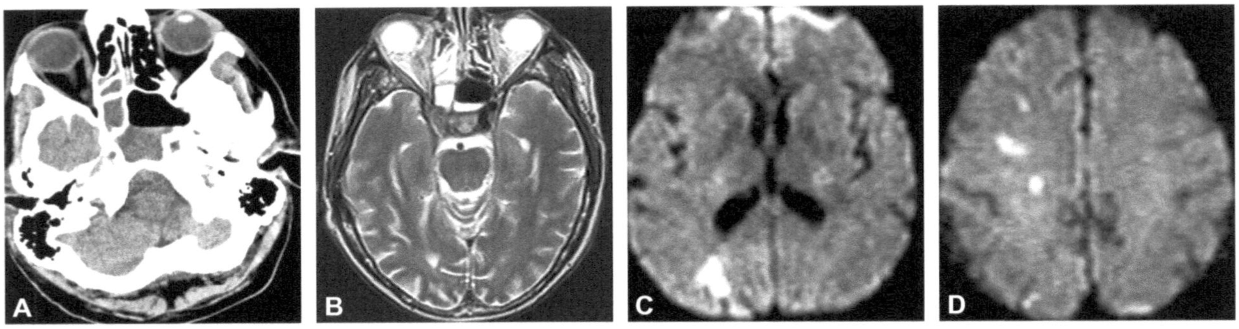

Fig. 19.22. Vascular complications of fungal sinusitis. (**A**) Noncontrast axial computed tomography obtained in a leukemic patient with altered mental status reveals air fluid levels in the sphenoid and ethmoid sinuses consistent with acute sinusitis. (**B**) Axial T2-weighted image demonstrates lack of vascular flow void in the right cavernous carotid artery. (**C, D**) Diffusion-weighted reveal multiple foci of restricted diffusion in right internal cerebral artery distribution compatible with acute infarcts. Corresponding low signal was seen on apparent diffusion coefficient map images.

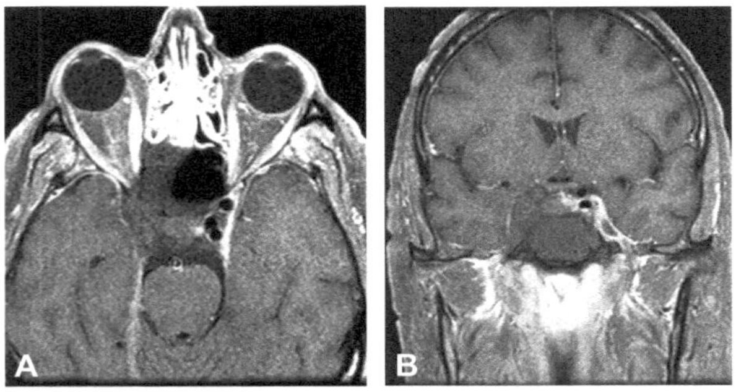

Fig. 19.23. Skull base involvement with arterial occlusion in a patient with fungal infection. (**A, B**) Axial and coronal post-contrast fat-suppressed T1-weighted images obtained on a leukemic patient with altered mental status (same patient as illustrated in Fig. 19.22) demonstrate sphenoid and ethmoid sinusitis with orbital inflammation and cavernous sinus involvement with absent flow in the right internal carotid artery.

abnormal enhancing soft tissue within the orbit, commonly involving the orbital apex, optic nerve–sheath complex, and orbital fat (Ashdown et al., 1994; DeLone et al., 1999).

Mucormycosis

Rhinocerebral mucormycosis is an acute, life-threatening opportunistic infection caused by fungi of the mucoraceal family, almost uniformly affecting immunocompromised individuals. Infection commonly presents as acute sinusitis or periorbital cellulitis with eye and facial pain, which can rapidly progress to blurry vision, facial swelling, with unilateral orbital apex syndrome and symptoms of cavernous sinus involvement (Chan et al., 2000; Spellberg et al., 2005).

Both CT and MRI are useful in the evaluation of patients with invasive fungal sinusitis. Initial imaging findings can be subtle. CT of the paranasal sinuses may only demonstrate mild nonspecific mucosal thickening without air fluid levels (Spellberg et al., 2005). Soft-tissue opacification of paranasal sinuses with high-density material can be seen. MR signal characteristics within the infected paranasal sinuses are variable. Heterogeneous hyperintense T2 or, more typically, strikingly hypointense T2 signal is observed, reflecting increased concentration of iron, manganese, and calcium in fungal elements (Zinreich et al., 1988). CT is extremely sensitive in the detection of bone erosion and presence of bone destruction is highly suspicious for mucormycosis when encountered in the appropriate clinical settings. However, it should be emphasized that erosive bone changes are not uncommonly absent, despite clinical evidence of progressive disease (Talmi et al., 2002), and intracranial and orbital extension of the infection can occur along the emissary vessels despite seemingly intact bony walls of the paranasal sinuses (Aribandi et al., 2007).

In advanced stages, high-resolution MRI of the skull base plays an important role in defining the extent of involvement and presence of intracranial and orbital disease. Heterogeneous contrast enhancement on postcontrast T1 fat-suppressed images and obliteration of the normal fat planes of the retorantral fat, infratemporal fossa, pterygopalatine fossa, pterygomaxillary fissure, and deep soft-tissue infiltration are often observed on noncontrast T1-weighted images without fat suppression (Fig. 19.24). Palate involvement is common, in some series affecting as many as 26–39% of patients (Talmi et al., 2002). When orbital invasion is present, images demonstrate characteristic findings of proptosis, periorbital inflammatory changes, inflammation in the orbital fat, thickening and lateral displacement of the medial rectus muscle, destruction of the lamina papyracea, and development of subperiosteal abscesses. Ischemic necrosis of

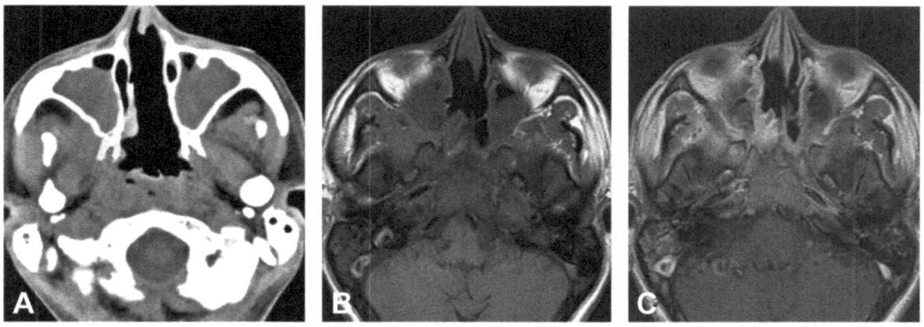

Fig. 19.24. Skull base involvement in a patient with fungal sinusitis. Skull base osteomyelitis in a patient with fungal sinusitis. (**A**) Axial computed tomography of the paranasal sinusitis obtained on a 31-year-old patient with a history of acute myeloid leukemia demonstrates bilateral maxillary sinusitis with extension of soft tissue into the right retromaxillary fat. Note intact bony walls of the maxillary sinuses and absence of nasal septum due to invasive septal aspergillosis. (**B**) Axial precontrast and (**C**) postcontrast fat-suppressed T1-weighted images demonstrate obliteration of normal fat planes in the retromaxillary fat, bilateral pterygopalatine fossa, infratemporal fossa, and extensive involvement of the skull base with loss of characteristic hyperintense marrow signal on precontrast images and diffuse heterogeneous contrast enhancement of the skull base on postcontrast study.

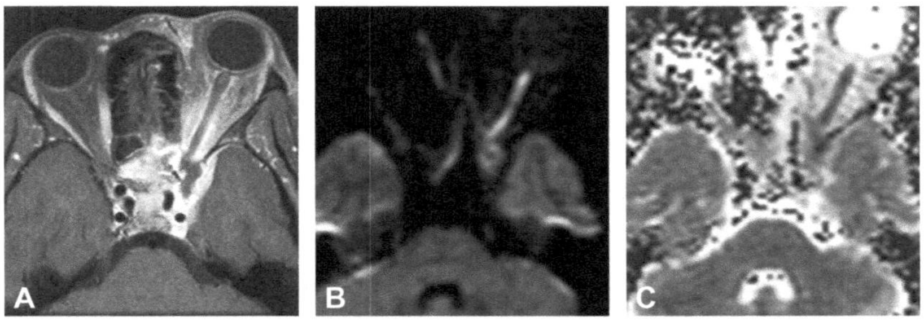

Fig. 19.25. Orbital and intracranial complications of mucormycosis. (**A**) Axial postcontrast fat-suppressed T1-weighted image obtained on an immunocompromised patient with altered mental status, orbital pain, and decreased vision in the left eye demonstrates mild proptosis and extensive orbital inflammation and cavernous sinus involvement. Hypointense T2 signal was present on T2-weighted images. Nonenhancing tissue along the anterior aspect of the cavernous sinus represents a focal abscess. (**B**) Diffusion-weighted and (**C**) apparent diffusion coefficient map images demonstrate restricted diffusion of the left optic nerve representing ischemia.

the optic nerve has been described (McLean et al., 1996). In such cases, DWI can demonstrate optic nerve infarction with restricted diffusion and low ADC values (Fig. 19.25) without signal abnormality on T2 or postcontrast T1-weighted sequences (Mathur et al., 2007). Meningeal enhancement, lack of enhancement of the superior orbital veins, distention with lack of enhancement of the cavernous sinus and carotid artery are indicative of intracranial spread with vascular thrombosis (Chan et al., 2000; Aribandi et al., 2007). MR angiography can be of particular value to document vascular involvement. Late intracranial complications related to vascular thrombosis include cerebral infarcts, mycotic embolization, and abscess formation.

Cryptococcosis

Cryptococcus neoformans is a ubiquitous organism found in mammal and bird feces, particularly in pigeon droppings (Mitchell and Perfect, 1995). Cryptococcosis is an opportunistic fungal infection that affects the CNS in HIV and other immunocompromised patients. It can rarely be seen in immunocompetent patients as well (Awasthi et al., 2001; Saigal et al., 2005). Headache is the most common symptom, but patients may also present with meningeal signs, confusion, seizures, blurred vision, and, rarely, focal deficits. Fever and nuchal rigidity may be mild or absent. The India ink test in CSF helps in demonstrating the fungus. The level of antigen titer corresponds to the severity of disease (Everett et al., 1978).

CNS involvement can be either meningeal or parenchymal. Infection usually starts as a meningitis. Parenchymal involvement is seen as cryptococcomas (also known as toruloma), with dilated Virchow–Robin spaces, or enhancing cortical nodules (Tien et al., 1991). It is believed that the meningeal infection along the base of the skull may involve the adjacent brain parenchyma, giving rise to cryptococcomas, or may extend along the Virchow–Robin spaces (Cornell and Jacoby, 1982). Virchow–Robin spaces are perivascular

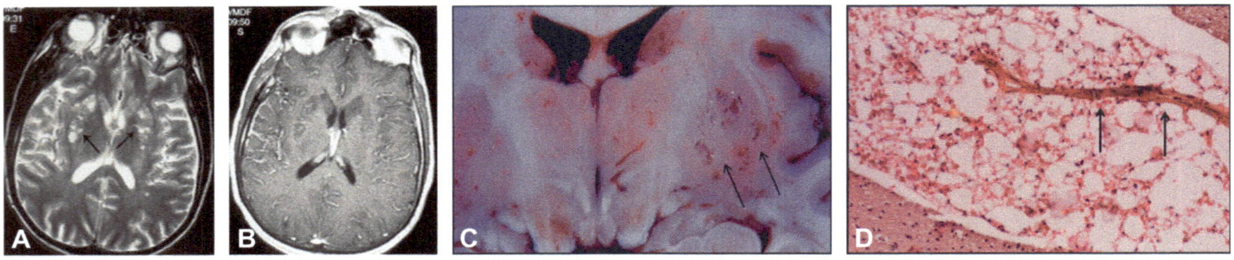

Fig. 19.26. Crytocococcosis: 30-year-old immunocompromised man presenting with altered mental status. (**A**) Axial T2 and (**B**) postcontrast T1-weighted images demonstrate multiple small rounded T2 hyperintense and T1 hypointense lesions in the basal ganglia bilaterally (short thick arrows), suggestive of dilated perivascular spaces. *Cryptococcus neoformans* was confirmed on Indian ink stain. (**C**) Gross specimen and (**D**) pathology slide from a different patient with cryptococcal meningitis showing multiple dilated perivascular spaces particularly on the left (thin arrows). Similar thin-walled cysts surrounding a lenticulostriate vessel can be seen on the pathology slide (long thick arrows).

spaces seen accompanying the lenticulostriate, perforating branches of the middle cerebral arteries in the basal ganglia. Perivascular spaces are also seen in the thalamus, periventricular white matter, midbrain, and the cerebellum (Ruiz et al., 1997b). As the infection spreads along the Virchow–Robin spaces, the perivascular spaces may dilate, with mucoid gelatinous material produced by the capsule of the organism (Everett et al., 1978; Wehn et al., 1989; Tien et al., 1991). These cysts have, therefore, also been called "gelatinous pseudocysts" (Tien et al., 1991). Imaging tests may provide useful diagnostic information (although the findings are not pathognomonic and other infectious processes may simulate cryptococcal infection in the brain). A communicating hydrocephalus may occur because of the acute meningeal exudate and also may occur late in the course of the infection because of meningeal adhesions. Gelatinous pseudocysts are seen as multiple CSF-equivalent round or oval cysts in the basal ganglia, thalami, midbrain, cerebellum, and the periventricular regions. On MRI, these are seen as multiple hypointense T1 and hyperintense T2 lesions (Fig. 19.26). Demonstration of clusters of these cysts in the basal ganglia and thalami is fairly specific and strongly suggestive of this infection (Wehn et al., 1989; Tien et al., 1991). In most cases, enhancement of these lesions does not occur. This is because, firstly, the lesions are perivascular and do not cross the blood–brain barrier, and secondly, the infection most often occurs in immunocompromised patients who are unable to mount an immune response (Saigal et al., 2005). Postcontrast enhancement may occur in rare instances when the infection occurs in immunocompetent patients who are able to mount an immune response to the infection, resulting in an inflammatory reaction (Saigal et al., 2005). Rarely, restricted diffusion may occur in these cysts (Saigal et al., 2005).

PARASITIC DISEASES

Parasitic diseases, such as neurocysticercosis (NCC), toxoplasmosis, echinococcosis, malariasis, amebiasis, toxocariasis, and African and American trypanosomiases, may affect the CNS and have a worldwide distribution, with increased prevalence in developing countries.

Neurocysticercosis

NCC is caused by the larval form of the pork tapeworm *Taenia solium*. Infection develops when humans ingest tapeworm eggs, resulting in subsequent hematogenous spread into the CNS with development of larvae (cysticerci) in the brain parenchyma, ventricular system, or subarachnoid space. During their life cycle, cysticerci pass a number of stages, with a complex host–parasite interaction (vesicular stage, colloidal stage, granular nodular stage, and calcified stage). First, viable cysticerci (vesicular stage) inhibit host immune response and have only minimal associated inflammation. Subsequently (colloidal stage), the parasites die and release their antigens into surrounding tissue, triggering an intense inflammatory reaction and losing their ability to control a host immune response. During this stage, there is progressive development of cyst wall fibrosis and eventual collapse of the cyst cavity (granular-nodular stage). In the terminal stage, the parasites are eventually replaced by fibrosis and calcify (nodular calcified stage) (Restrepo et al., 1998; White, 2000). The location of the parasitic cysts in the brain can influence the magnitude of the host inflammatory response. Parenchymal lesions appear to produce the least amount of inflammatory reaction and therefore are commonly asymptomatic. By contrast, ventricular and meningeal cysts typically elicit intense inflammation and can cause severe mass effect, hydrocephalus, and death (Restrepo et al., 1998). Diagnosis is usually made by a combination of compatible clinical history, positive serum and CSF serology, and typical imaging findings on CT and MRI scans (Rodriguez et al., 2009). Seizure is the most frequent symptom at presentation, reported in 60% of affected patients, followed by hydrocephalus and headaches, seen in 16% and 15% of cases respectively (Wallin and Kurtzke, 2004).

Parenchymal neurocysticercosis

Parenchymal NCC is the most common form, affecting about 70% of patients (Lucato et al., 2007). Lesions are typically multiple, located at the corticomedullary junction of the cerebral hemispheres. Typical imaging features of NCC are highly variable, depending on the stage of evolution and location of the cysts, reflecting underlying changes in the disease process and host response.

Vesicular stage

At this stage, a parasite larva appears on imaging as a cyst with an invaginated scolex or a cluster of multiple cysts of variable sizes with little or no edema or mass effect (Fig. 19.27). A mature cyst typically reaches 5–20 mm in size, with clear cyst fluid, demonstrating signal intensity similar to that of CSF (Kimura-Hayama et al., 2010). The cyst wall is commonly very thin and smooth with absent or only minimal contrast enhancement. Scolex can be seen in up to 50% of cases and appears as a small mural nodule, slightly hyperintense on T1 and FLAIR images and hypointense on T2-weighted images (Noujaim et al., 1999; Sinha and Sharma, 2009; Kimura-Hayama et al., 2010). It also may be detectable on ADC map and DWI as a restricting nodule within the hypointense signal of the vesicle fluid (do Amaral et al., 2005). During this stage, the classic imaging findings of a cystic lesion with a scolex are considered to be pathognomonic of NCC (Del Brutto et al., 2001; Lucato et al., 2007).

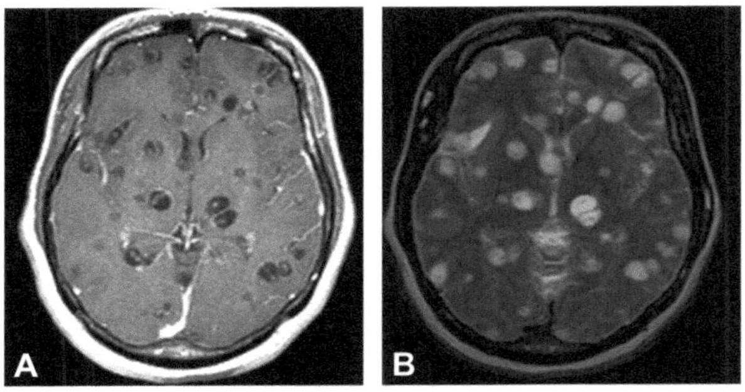

Fig. 19.27. Vesicular stage of neurocysticercosis. (**A**) Axial postcontrast T1-weighted and (**B**) T2-weighted images obtained on a 41-year-old women with headaches and seizures reveal innumerable well-defined cystic lesions in both cerebral hemispheres. Note the lack of adjacent edema and only minimal peripheral enhancement of the wall of a few lesions on postcontrast images, characteristic of the vesicular stage of neurocysticercosis. The fluid content follows the cerebrospinal fluid signal intensity. Scolices can be seen as hyperintense eccentrically located nodular structures within the cysts on T1-weighted images and as hypointense foci on T2-weighted images.

Colloidal vesicular stage

During the colloidal vesicular stage, death of the organism occurs, resulting in degeneration of larva with disintegration of scolex (Fig. 19.28). This triggers an intense host inflammatory reaction with pericystic edema and inflammation. Cyst fluid becomes more proteinaceous, which manifests on MR images as mildly hyperintense signal on T1 and FLAIR images. A scolex is typically not seen. Postcontrast images demonstrate thickening and enhancement of the cyst wall (Abdel Razek et al., 2011; Lerner et al., 2012). At this stage, NCC can mimic other lesions, including cystic neoplasms, pyogenic abscesses, and tuberculomas.

Granular nodular stage

During this stage, the cyst continues to degenerate, retracts, and begins to mineralize, eventually forming a small nodule. Imaging features can appear similar to the colloidal vesicular stage, demonstrating peripheral enhancement of the lesion (Fig. 19.29). The cyst wall

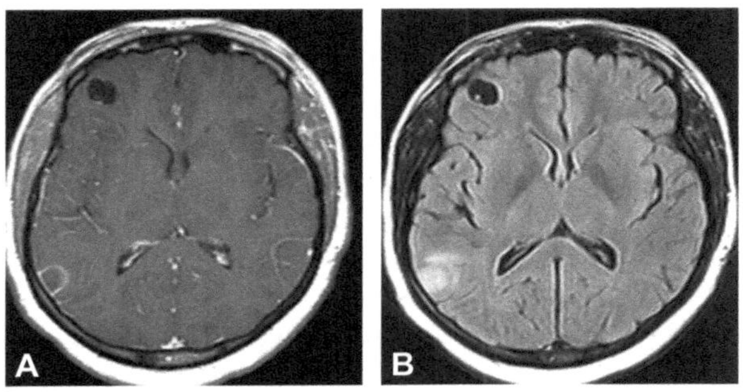

Fig. 19.28. Coexisting vesicular and colloidal vesicular stage of neurocysticercosis. (**A**) Axial postcontrast T1-weighted image reveals two focal lesions in the right frontal and the right parietal lobe. The right frontal-lobe lesion is cystic, well defined, with no discernible wall, adjacent edema or contrast enhancement, representing the vesicular stage of neurocysticercosis. The scolex is seen as a hyperintense eccentric nodule. The cyst content is similar to cerebrospinal fluid on all sequences. The second lesion in the right parietal lobe demonstrates peripheral contrast enhancement and moderate amount of adjacent vasogenic edema with no identifiable scolex. The cyst content is hyperintense on a fluid-attenuated inversion recovery image (**B**). The findings are characteristic of the colloidal vesicular stage of neurocysticercosis.

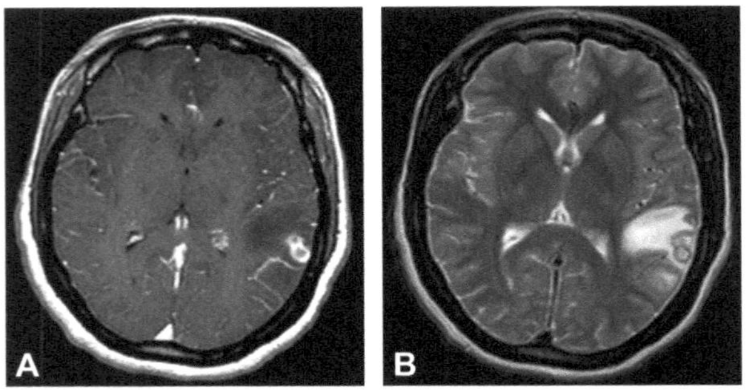

Fig. 19.29. Granular nodular stage of neurocysticercosis. Axial postcontrast T1-weighted (**A**) and T2-weighted (**B**) images obtained on a 36-year-old patient who presented with a recent seizure reveal a cystic lesion with marked surrounding edema, thick intense contrast enhancement, and hypointense T2 signal of the cyst wall. The cyst content is hyperintense to cerebrospinal fluid on T1-weighted images.

usually is thicker with more intense postcontrast enhancement (Abdel Razek et al., 2011). Some lesions may demonstrate nodular enhancement and hypointense T2 signal (Noujaim et al., 1999; Lerner et al., 2012). Various degrees of associated brain edema can be present, ranging from mild to severe. At this stage, differentiation of NCC from other infectious lesions or intracranial metastases is difficult.

Calcified stage

The calcified nodular stage represents a final stage of the disease, during which the parasite completely involutes, degenerating into a small, calcified granulomatous lesion. Clinically, it is considered to be an inactive stage. However, some patients continue to have associated seizure activity. Typical imaging features during this stage are multiple small calcified lesions, ranging in size from 2 to 8 mm, without edema or contrast enhancement (Fig. 19.30) (Abdel Razek et al., 2011). Noncontrast CT is highly sensitive in identifying parenchymal calcifications associated with calcified NCC lesions. On MR, lesions are typically hypointense on T1- and T2-weighted images. Thin perilesional FLAIR hyperintensity can be seen in some cases, potentially indicating the presence of gliosis in surrounding tissue. Calcified lesions typically appear markedly hypointense (demonstrating "blooming artifact") on T2* GRE and SWI. Occasionally, persistent contrast enhancement and intermittent perilesional edema can be observed in association with calcified NCC lesions; this has been postulated to be a result of either sporadic release of pathogen antigen or sporadic recognition of pathogen antigen by the host (Sheth et al., 1998; Nash et al., 2001, 2008; Nash and Garcia, 2011).

Intraventricular neurocysticercosis

Intraventricular NCC is the second most common type of NCC, encountered in 7–33% of cases (Govindappa et al., 2000; Kimura-Hayama et al., 2010). This form more commonly occurs in isolation but may coexist with parenchymal lesions. The fourth ventricle is the most common site of involvement, followed by the third ventricle and lateral ventricles (Sinha and Sharma, 2009). Intraventricular cysts can migrate and potentially cause ventricular outlet obstruction (Araujo et al., 2008; Chowdhary et al., 2010). Obstructive hydrocephalus is the most serious complication of intraventricular cysticercosis, which can develop due to obstruction of the ventricular system by a cyst (usually at the level of the fourth ventricle) or secondary to accompanying ependymitis, resulting in the development of inflammatory adhesions within the ventricular system (Fig. 19.30). In some cases, chronic hydrocephalus can persist after shunting (Kimura-Hayama et al., 2010).

Diagnosis of intraventricular cysticercosis on imaging can be challenging because the cyst content and

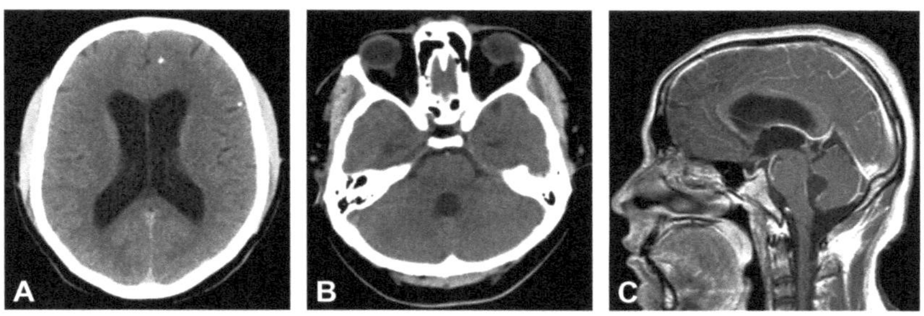

Fig. 19.30. Coexisting intraventricular and parenchymal neurocysticercosis. (**A, B**) Axial noncontrast computed tomography obtained on a 29-year-old patient with a history of headaches demonstrates moderate hydrocephalus of the lateral and fourth ventricles and two small parenchymal calcifications in the left frontal lobe. (**C**) Postcontrast sagittal T1-weighted image reveals a thin-walled cystic lesion within the fourth ventricle with only minimal wall enhancement on postcontrast images. Note that the cyst content is slightly hyperintense to cerebrospinal fluid. Calcified parenchymal lesions represent cysticerci in the calcified nodular stage in this patient with coexisting parenchymal and intraventricular form of neurocysticercosis.

surrounding CSF have similar intensity. Intraventricular cysts can be suspected when disproportionate enlargement, distortion, abnormal contour of the ventricles, or hydrocephalus are observed. Transependymal CSF edema is typically present in cases of acute hydrocephalus (Kimura-Hayama et al., 2010). Occasionally, the cysts appear slightly higher in signal than CSF on FLAIR images and, rarely, the cyst content can demonstrate hyperintense T1 and hypointense T2 signal (Govindappa et al., 2000; Abdel Razek et al., 2011). The wall of the cyst may appear as a thin curvilinear structure, hypointense on T2 and slightly hyperintense on T1 and FLAIR images. Contrast enhancement is usually absent. Similar to parenchymal cysts, detection of scolex within the ventricular cyst can greatly aid in diagnosis of intraventricular NCC (Fig. 19.31). Diffusion is usually unrestricted in the cyst fluid, demonstrating low DWI signal and high ADC values (do Amaral et al., 2005; Lucato et al., 2007). When routine MR sequences are unable to identify a cause of the ventricular abnormality or delineate all features of intraventricular NCC, alternative MR techniques such as three-dimensional constructive interference in steady state (3D-CISS) can be used (Kimura-Hayama et al., 2010). 3D-CISS sequences are found to be more sensitive and specific than routine spin-echo MR images in detecting and characterizing intraventricular cysts of NCC due to their higher resolution, faster acquisition time leading to less motion, and capability to accentuate the T2 value differences between the cystic fluid and surrounding CSF (Govindappa et al., 2000; Verma et al., 2011). The T2 signal intensity of the cyst fluid typically appears slightly lower than the adjacent CSF and both the cyst wall and the scolex can be seen as hypointense structures (do Amaral et al., 2005).

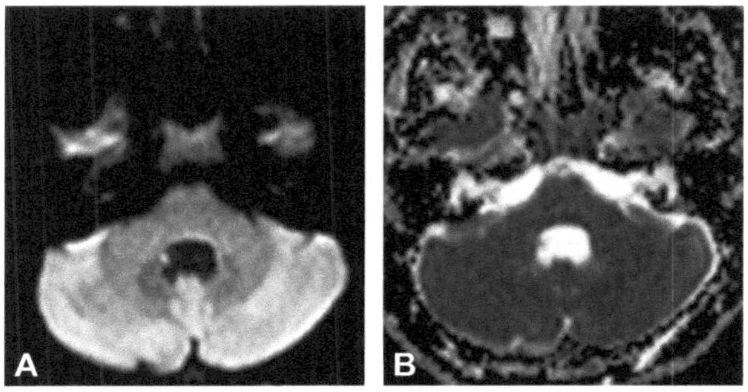

Fig. 19.31. Detection of scolex within the intraventricular cyst. (**A**) Axial diffusion-weighted imaging (DWI) and (**B**) apparent diffusion coefficient (ADC) map images obtained on a patient with a fourth ventricular cyst (same patient as illustrated in Fig. 19.30) identify a scolex as an eccentric small nodule within a cyst. Scolex is mildly hyperintense on DWI and isointense to hypointense on ADC map images.

Subarachnoid neurocysticercosis

The subarachnoid location is the least common site of involvement, accounting only for 3.5% of cases of NCC, with increased predilection for the basal cisterns (Arriada-Mendicoa et al., 2003; Hauptman et al., 2005; Kimura-Hayama et al., 2010). Due to lack of resistance within the subarachnoid space, cystic lesions in this location tend to be large, not uncommonly reaching up to 10 cm in size or even larger. In contrast to parenchymal cysts, the scolex is only rarely seen. Typically, multiple complex cystic structures develop within the subarachnoid space, forming so-called "cluster of grapes." This form is also known as "racemose" type of NCC (Fig. 19.32A, B). Similar to the intraventricular form

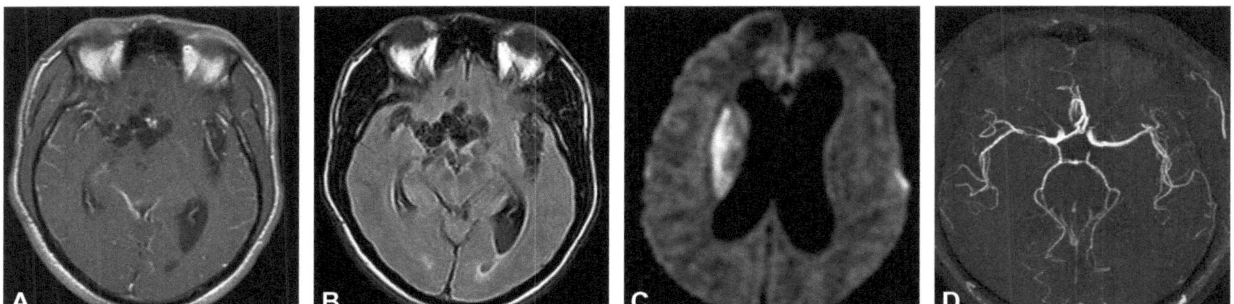

Fig. 19.32. Arachnoiditis and vascular complications of racemose neurocysticercosis. (**A**) Axial postcontrast T1-weighted and (**B**) fluid-attenuated inversion recovery images demonstrate distortion and marked expansion of the skull base cisterns containing multiple fluid-filled cysts lacking scolices representing subarachnoid neurocysticercosis. Note the multiloculated appearance of those cysts, resembling "cluster of grapes," characteristic of a "racemose" form of neurocysticercosis. Postcontrast images demonstrate irregular enhancement in the subarachnoid space at the skull base representing arachnoiditis. (**C**) Diffusion-weighted images show a large area of restricted diffusion with dark signal on apparent diffusion coefficient map images (not shown) in the right middle cerebral artery territory consistent with acute infarct. (**D**) Time-of-flight maximum-intensity projection magnetic resonance angiogram reveals a focal area of high-grade stenosis in the right M1 segment and loss of flow-related enhancement at the origin of the left posterior communicating artery.

of NCC, fluid within the cysts can be obscured by the adjacent CSF due to its similar signal intensity. Usually, there is no or only minimal enhancement within the wall of the cysts. However, the degree of enhancement can significantly vary, and some lesions can demonstrate significant enhancement in the cyst walls (Abdel Razek et al., 2011). On imaging, the lesions can be detected by the presence of mass effect, unusual distortion, or asymmetric enlargement of the affected cisterns. 3D-CISS MR acquisition has been shown to improve visualization of lesions, accentuating subtle differences in T2 signal between the cyst content and surrounding subarachnoid space (Govindappa et al., 2000; Kimura-Hayama et al., 2010; Verma et al., 2011).

Initially, enhancement in the subarachnoid space is usually absent, but as the disease progresses, the inflammatory process can affect the adjacent meninges, resulting in focal or diffuse arachnoiditis. Arachnoiditis is one of the most severe complications of NCC, associated with hydrocephalus, multiple cranial nerve dysfunction, and vasculitis (Arriada-Mendicoa et al., 2003). Meningeal thickening and enhancement are observed on postcontrast T1-weighted images and communicating hydrocephalus can develop as a result of obstruction of normal CSF flow at the level of the skull base cisterns. Eventually, leptomeningeal adhesions, scarring, and calcifications can develop. During this stage, the differential diagnosis of arachnoiditis due to NCC includes other causes of chronic meningitis, such as tuberculosis, sarcoidosis, cryptococcosis, and leptomeningeal carcinomatosis.

Vasculitis is present in approximately 53% of patients with the subarachnoid form of NCC, frequently affecting small perforating arteries at the skull base (Fig. 19.32C, D) (Kimura-Hayama et al., 2010; Abdel Razek et al., 2011). Common angiographic findings include focal segmental arterial narrowing, beaded appearance of vessels, luminal irregularity, and vascular occlusion.

Toxoplasmosis

Toxoplasma gondii is an obligate intracellular protozoan with worldwide distribution. In the immunologically intact individual it causes a subclinical and benign infection but in the immunocompromised patient it may cause a necrotizing encephalitis (Snider et al., 1983; Luft et al., 1984; Levy et al., 1985; Post et al., 1986; Grant et al., 1987).

Toxoplasma encephalitis appears on conventional imaging studies as focal lesions with mass effect and edema. The lesions are most commonly located in the cerebral hemispheres at the corticomedullary junction, with the basal ganglia being the second most common site of predilection (Post et al., 1986; Porter and Sande, 1992). Hemorrhage is rarely evident (Casado-Naranjo et al., 1989; Chaudhari et al., 1989; Wijdicks et al., 1991). Lesions due to *Toxoplasma* encephalitis typically range in size from 0.5 to 3.0 cm (Krick and Remington, 1978; Post et al., 1983, 1986). Lesions under 2 cm in size, especially those small lesions located in the cortical and subcortical regions, may be better appreciated on fast FLAIR images than on fast-spin echo T2WI scans (Thurnher et al., 1997). The parenchymal lesions in *Toxoplasma* encephalitis typically enhance, either homogeneously and/or inhomogeneously (Fig. 19.33A). Both nodular and ring enhancement, therefore, can be seen on either contrast CT or contrast MR scans.

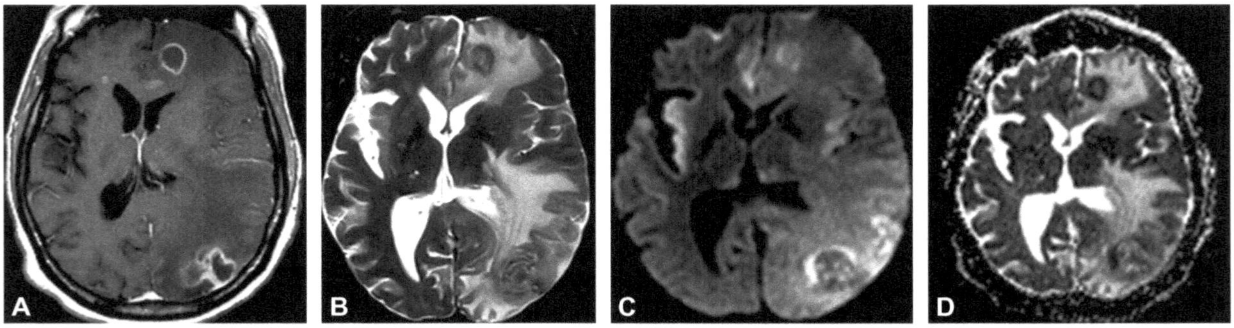

Fig. 19.33. Multiple enhancing lesions due to toxoplasmosis. (**A**) Axial postcontrast T1-weighted and (**B**) T2-weighted images obtained on a 43-year-old patient with end-stage acquired immunodeficiency syndrome (AIDS) who presented with altered mental status reveal multiple bilateral frontal and left occipital-lobe enhancing lesions with mass effect and edema. Note smooth peripheral rim enhancement of the left frontal lesion and irregular inhomogeneous contrast enhancement of the left occipital lobe lesion on postcontrast T1-weighted images. On T2-weighted images, left occipital lesion demonstrates a concentric T2 "target" sign with characteristic central hypointensity surrounded by concentric zones of alternating hyperintense and hypointense T2 signal. Similar alternating rings of hypointense and iso- to hyperintense T2 signal are seen in the left frontal lesion. Both lesions show peripheral restricted diffusion on diffusion-weighted (**C**) and apparent diffusion coefficient (ADC) map (**D**) images with increased diffusion-weighted imaging signal and low ADC values.

Toxoplasmosis lesions characterized by necrotizing encephalitis at neuropathology are mainly seen on T2-weighted images as hyperintense lesions because of the poorly demarcated necrosis and increased water concentration (Brightbill et al., 1996). In contrast, toxoplasmosis lesions found neuropathologically to be organizing abscesses are mainly isointense to gray matter on T2-weighted images because of the presence of a well-defined coagulative necrosis and decreased water concentration (Falangola et al., 1994; Brightbill et al., 1996). The "concentric target sign" was recently described in the literature as a new MRI sign in imaging of intracranial toxoplasmosis (Fig. 19.33B) (Mahadevan et al., 2013). The central hypointense core is surrounded by alternating concentric-zone hyper-, iso-, and hypointensities on T2-weighted images. The sign is more often seen in deep parenchymal lesions and was found to be present in 29% of cases in some series (Mahadevan et al., 2013). Histologically, it correlates to the presence of hemorrhage (hypointense core) and the alternating bands of fibrin-rich necrosis with edema and histiocytes (hyperintense zone) and coagulative necrosis (isointense zone) (Mahadevan et al., 2013).

Multiple enhancing lesions are more commonly seen than single lesions in AIDS patients with *Toxoplasma* encephalitis (Krick and Remington, 1978; Post et al., 1985, 1986; Ciricillo and Rosenblum, 1991; Thurnher et al., 1997). However, a single intracranial lesion due to *Toxoplasma gondii* in AIDS patients is not a rare occurrence and has been reported in between 14% and 27% of toxoplasmosis patients (Ciricillo and Rosenblum, 1991; Porter and Sande, 1992).

Typically, imaging studies show improvement in 2–4 weeks after treatment, with a decrease in the size and number of enhancing lesions and a progressive decrease in edema and mass effect. In the chronic stages, AIDS patients on treatment can show calcifications, encephalomalacia, atrophy, or even reversion of the scan to normal (Post et al., 1983, 1985, 1986).

Despite the fact that MR or CT can provide imaging clues to the diagnosis of toxoplasmosis and other AIDS-related pathology, it is crucial to remember that these findings are not pathognomonic and that a definitive diagnosis cannot be made on these imaging studies. To overcome the limitations of conventional MR and CT, numerous investigators have turned their attention to additional diagnostic methods, such as thallium-201 single-photon emission computed tomography (SPECT), positron emission tomography (PET) scans and also diffusion and perfusion imaging (Ernst et al., 1998).

Thallium-201 SPECT has been found to be useful in differentiating focal intracranial mass lesions in AIDS patients and especially in distinguishing *Toxoplasma* encephalitis from lymphoma (Ruiz et al., 1994, 1997a, b). The focal intense uptake of thallium-201 correlates with the focal area of contrast enhancement seen on the CT or MR in lymphoma patients (Fig. 19.34) (Ruiz et al., 1994). Conversely, negative thallium scans were seen in patients with intracranial toxoplasmosis. Alternatively, PET scanning could be considered.

Diffusion and perfusion imaging may be employed to help in the differentiation of CNS infection from neoplasm (Chang and Ernst, 1997; Ernst et al., 1998). Lymphomas demonstrate increased perfusion, while toxoplasmosis lesions do not (Ernst et al., 1998; Cha et al., 2002; Al-Okaili et al., 2006). These differences are postulated to be due to the presence of hypervascularity in the actively growing neoplasms (and hence the increase in regional cerebral blood volume) and lack of vascularity in toxoplasmosis lesion (and hence the decreased regional cerebral blood volume).

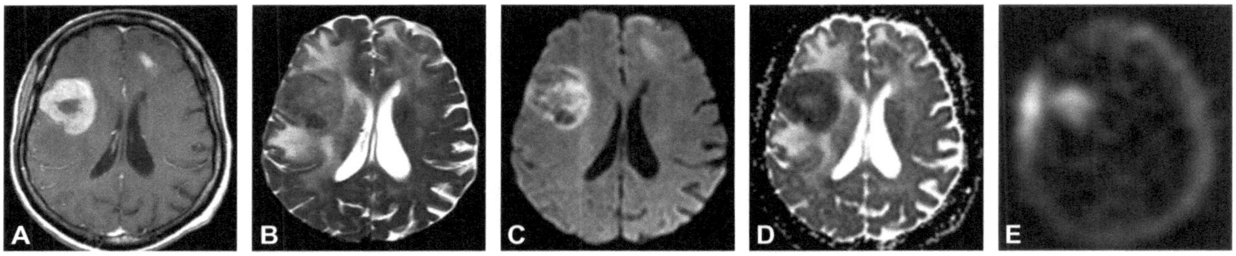

Fig. 19.34. Lymphoma mimicking toxoplasma encephalitis in a patient with human immunodeficiency virus (HIV). Axial post-contrast T1- (**A**) and T2-weighted (**B**) images obtained on a 49-year-old patient with acquired immunodeficiency syndrome (AIDS) demonstrate a large right frontal mass with thick peripheral enhancement and heterogeneous hypointense T2 signal. (**C**) Diffusion-weighted imaging (DWI) and (**D**) apparent diffusion coefficient (ADC) map images show low ADC signal mainly along the periphery of the lesion and inhomogeneous peripheral high DWI signal. Note overlapping imaging features with toxoplasmosis, illustrated in Figure 19.33. Blood *Toxoplasma* titers were negative. (**E**) 201-Thallium single-photon emission computed tomography demonstrates intense activity in the right frontal lesion suggestive of a lymphoma. At surgery, the lesion was proved to be central nervous system lymphoma.

With respect to diffusion imaging, the results have been more variable. ADC values were found to be helpful in the differentiation of some, but not all, cases of lymphoma and toxoplasmosis (Camacho et al., 2003; Schroeder et al., 2006). Increased diffusibility was more characteristic of toxoplasmosis lesions and restricted diffusion was more characteristic of lymphoma (Camacho et al., 2003; Al-Okaili et al., 2006). However, in patients who had lesions with ADC ratios between 1.0 and 1.6, there was overlap and the distinction could not be made (Figs 19.33C, D and Fig. 19.34C, D) (Camacho et al., 2003; Schroeder et al., 2006).

References

Abdel Razek AA, Watcharakorn A, Castillo M (2011). Parasitic diseases of the central nervous system. Neuroimaging Clin N Am 21: 815–841. viii.

Agid R, Ducreux D, Halliday WC et al. (2003). MR diffusion-weighted imaging in a case of West Nile virus encephalitis. Neurology 61: 1821–1823.

Ali M, Safriel Y, Sohi J et al. (2005). West Nile virus infection: MR imaging findings in the nervous system. AJNR. Am J neuroradiology 26: 289–297.

Al-Okaili RN, Krejza J, Wang S et al. (2006). Advanced MR imaging techniques in the diagnosis of intraaxial brain tumors in adults. Radiographics: a Review Publication of the Radiological Society of North America, Inc 26: S173–S189.

Anderson RE, Laskoff JM (1990). Ramsay Hunt syndrome mimicking intracanalicular acoustic neuroma on contrast-enhanced MR. AJNR. Am J Neuroradiology 11: 409.

Andronikou S, Smith B, Hatherhill M et al. (2004). Definitive neuroradiological diagnostic features of tuberculous meningitis in children. Pediatr Radiol 34: 876–885.

Araujo AL, Rodrigues RS, Marchiori E et al. (2008). Migrating intraventricular cysticercosis: magnetic resonance imaging findings. Arq Neuropsiquiatr 66: 111–113.

Aribandi M, McCoy VA, Bazan 3rd C (2007). Imaging features of invasive and noninvasive fungal sinusitis: a review. Radiographics: a review publication of the Radiological Society of North America, Inc 27: 1283–1296.

Arriada-Mendicoa N, Celis-Lopez MA, Higuera-Calleja J et al. (2003). Imaging features of sellar cysticercosis. AJNR. Am J Neuroradiology 24: 1386–1389.

Arvin AM (1996). Varicella-zoster virus. Clin Microbiol Rev 9: 361–381.

Ashdown BC, Tien RD, Felsberg GJ (1994). Aspergillosis of the brain and paranasal sinuses in immunocompromised patients: CT and MR imaging findings. AJR. Am J Roentgenology 162: 155–159.

Awasthi M, Patankar T, Shah P et al. (2001). Cerebral cryptococcosis: atypical appearances on CT. Br J Radiol 74: 83–85.

Bargallo J, Berenguer J, Garcia-Barrionuevo J et al. (1996). The "target sign": is it a specific sign of CNS tuberculoma? Neuroradiology 38: 547–550.

Berger JR, Concha M (1995). Progressive multifocal leukoencephalopathy: the evolution of a disease once considered rare. J Neurovirol 1: 5–18.

Berger JR, Moskowitz L, Fischl M et al. (1987). Neurologic disease as the presenting manifestation of acquired immunodeficiency syndrome. South Med J 80: 683–686.

Bidstrup C, Andersen PH, Skinhoj P et al. (2002). Tuberculous meningitis in a country with a low incidence of tuberculosis: still a serious disease and a diagnostic challenge. Scand J Infect Dis 34: 811–814.

Blum LW, Chambers RA, Schwartzman RJ et al. (1985). Progressive multifocal leukoencephalopathy in acquired immune deficiency syndrome. Arch Neurol 42: 137–139.

Botha H, Ackerman C, Candy S et al. (2012). Reliability and diagnostic performance of CT imaging criteria in the diagnosis of tuberculous meningitis. PLoS One 7: e38982.

Bowen BC, Post MJD (1990). Intracranial Infections, Raven Press, New York.

Brightbill TC, Post MJ, Hensley GT et al. (1996). MR of Toxoplasma encephalitis: signal characteristics on T2-weighted images and pathologic correlation. J Comput Assist Tomogr 20: 417–422.

Britton CB, Miller JR (1984). Neurologic complications in acquired immunodeficiency syndrome (AIDS). Neurol Clin 2: 315–339.

Camacho DL, Smith JK, Castillo M (2003). Differentiation of toxoplasmosis and lymphoma in AIDS patients by using apparent diffusion coefficients. AJNR. Am J Neuroradiology 24: 633–637.

Cartes-Zumelzu FW, Stavrou I, Castillo M et al. (2004). Diffusion-weighted imaging in the assessment of brain abscesses therapy. AJNR. Am J Neuroradiology 25: 1310–1317.

Casado-Naranjo I, Lopez-Trigo J, Ferrandiz A et al. (1989). Hemorrhagic abscess in a patient with the acquired immunodeficiency syndrome. Neuroradiology 31: 289.

Castillo M (2004). Imaging of meningitis. Semin Roentgenol 39: 458–464.

Centers for Disease Control and Prevention (2002). Acute flaccid paralysis syndrome associated with West Nile virus infection – Mississippi and Louisiana, July–August 2002. MMWR. Morbidity and mortality weekly report 51: 825–828.

Cha S, Knopp EA, Johnson G et al. (2002). Intracranial mass lesions: dynamic contrast-enhanced susceptibility-weighted echo-planar perfusion MR imaging. Radiology 223: 11–29.

Chan LL, Singh S, Jones D et al. (2000). Imaging of mucormycosis skull base osteomyelitis. AJNR. Am J Neuroradiology 21: 828–831.

Chang L, Ernst T (1997). MR spectroscopy and diffusion-weighted MR imaging in focal brain lesions in AIDS. Neuroimaging Clin N Am 7: 409–426.

Chang T, Teng MM, Wang SF et al. (1992). Aspergillosis of the paranasal sinuses. Neuroradiology 34: 520–523.

Chaudhari AB, Singh A, Jindal S et al. (1989). Haemorrhage in cerebral toxoplasmosis. A report on a patient with the acquired immunodeficiency syndrome. South African

medical journal = Suid-Afrikaanse tydskrif vir genees-kunde 76: 272–274.
Cherian A, Thomas SV (2011). Central nervous system tuberculosis. Afr Health Sci 11: 116–127.
Chowdhary A, Abel TJ, Gabikian P et al. (2010). Resolution of acute hydrocephalus and migration of neurocysticercosis cyst with external ventricular drainage. Case reports in medicine 2010: 245–259.
Cinque P, Cleator GM, Weber T et al. (1996). The role of laboratory investigation in the diagnosis and management of patients with suspected herpes simplex encephalitis: a consensus report. The EU Concerted Action on Virus Meningitis and Encephalitis. J Neurol Neurosurg psychiatr 61: 339–345.
Ciricillo SF, Rosenblum ML (1991). Imaging of solitary lesions in AIDS. J Neurosurg 74: 1029.
Collie DA, Summers DM, Sellar RJ et al. (2003). Diagnosing variant Creutzfeldt–Jakob disease with the pulvinar sign: MR imaging findings in 86 neuropathologically confirmed cases. AJNR. Am J Neuroradiology 24: 1560–1569.
Cornell SH, Jacoby CG (1982). The varied computed tomographic appearance of intracranial cryptococcosis. Radiology 143: 703–707.
Cox J, Murtagh FR, Wilfong A et al. (1992). Cerebral aspergillosis: MR imaging and histopathologic correlation. AJNR. Am J Neuroradiology 13: 1489–1492.
Danziger A, Price H, Schechter MM (1980). An analysis of 113 intracranial infections. Neuroradiology 19: 31–34.
Del Brutto OH, Rajshekhar V, White Jr AC et al. (2001). Proposed diagnostic criteria for neurocysticercosis. Neurology 57: 177–183.
DeLone DR, Goldstein RA, Petermann G et al. (1999). Disseminated aspergillosis involving the brain: distribution and imaging characteristics. AJNR. Am J Neuroradiology 20: 1597–1604.
Dhawan A, Kecskes Z, Jyoti R et al. (2006). Early diffusion-weighted magnetic resonance imaging findings in neonatal herpes encephalitis. J Paediatr Child Health 42: 824–826.
Dietemann JL, Correia Bernardo R, Bogorin A et al. (2005). Normal and abnormal meningeal enhancement: MRI features. J Radiol 86: 1659–1683.
do Amaral LL, Ferreira RM, da Rocha AJ et al. (2005). Neurocysticercosis: evaluation with advanced magnetic resonance techniques and atypical forms. Topics in magnetic resonance imaging: TMRI 16: 127–144.
Ernst TM, Chang L, Witt MD et al. (1998). Cerebral toxoplasmosis and lymphoma in AIDS: perfusion MR imaging experience in 13 patients. Radiology 208: 663–669.
Ernst T, Chang L, Witt M et al. (1999). Progressive multifocal leukoencephalopathy and human immunodeficiency virus-associated white matter lesions in AIDS: magnetization transfer MR imaging. Radiology 210: 539–543.
Everett BA, Kusske JA, Rush JL et al. (1978). Cryptococcal infection of the central nervous system. Surg Neurol 9: 157–163.
Falangola MF, Reichler BS, Petito CK (1994). Histopathology of cerebral toxoplasmosis in human immunodeficiency virus infection: a comparison between patients with early-onset and late-onset acquired immunodeficiency syndrome. Hum Pathol 25: 1091–1097.
Falcone S, Post MJ (2000). Encephalitis, cerebritis, and brain abscess: pathophysiology and imaging findings. Neuroimaging Clin N Am 10: 333–353.
Ferreira NP, Otta GM, do Amaral LL et al. (2005). Imaging aspects of pyogenic infections of the central nervous system. Topics in magnetic resonance imaging: TMRI 16: 145–154.
Foerster BR, Thurnher MM, Malani PN et al. (2007). Intracranial infections: clinical and imaging characteristics. Acta Radiol (Stockholm, Sweden: 1987) 48: 875–893.
Fukui MB, Williams RL, Mudigonda S (2001). CT and MR imaging features of pyogenic ventriculitis. AJNR. Am J Neuroradiology 22: 1510–1516.
Garg M, Gupta RK, Husain M et al. (2004). Brain abscesses: etiologic categorization with in vivo proton MR spectroscopy. Radiology 230: 519–527.
Gilden DH, Mahalingam R, Cohrs RJ et al. (2007). Herpesvirus infections of the nervous system. Nat Clin Pract Neurol 3: 82–94.
Gilden D, Cohrs RJ, Mahalingam R et al. (2009). Varicella zoster virus vasculopathies: diverse clinical manifestations, laboratory features, pathogenesis, and treatment. Lancet Neurol 8: 731–740.
Gottfredsson M, Perfect JR (2000). Fungal meningitis. Semin Neurol 20: 307–322.
Govindappa SS, Narayanan JP, Krishnamoorthy VM et al. (2000). Improved detection of intraventricular cysticercal cysts with the use of three-dimensional constructive interference in steady state MR sequences. AJNR. Am J Neuroradiology 21: 679–684.
Grant I, Atkinson JH, Hesselink JR et al. (1987). Evidence for early central nervous system involvement in the acquired immunodeficiency syndrome (AIDS) and other human immunodeficiency virus (HIV) infections. Studies with neuropsychologic testing and magnetic resonance imaging. Ann Intern Med 107: 828–836.
Gupta RK, Kumar S (2011). Central nervous system tuberculosis. Neuroimaging Clin N Am 21: 795–814. vii–viii.
Gupta RK, Gupta S, Singh D et al. (1994). MR imaging and angiography in tuberculous meningitis. Neuroradiology 36: 87–92.
Gupta RK, Hasan KM, Mishra AM et al. (2005a). High fractional anisotropy in brain abscesses versus other cystic intracranial lesions. AJNR Am J Neuroradiology 26: 1107–1114.
Gupta RK, Prakash M, Mishra AM et al. (2005b). Role of diffusion weighted imaging in differentiation of intracranial tuberculoma and tuberculous abscess from cysticercus granulomas – a report of more than 100 lesions. Eur J Radiol 55: 384–392.
Haimes AB, Zimmerman RD, Morgello S et al. (1989). MR imaging of brain abscesses. AJR Am J Roentgenology 152: 1073–1085.
Han BK, Babcock DS, McAdams L (1985). Bacterial meningitis in infants: sonographic findings. Radiology 154: 645–650.

Handique SK (2011). Viral infections of the central nervous system. Neuroimaging Clin N Am 21: 777–794. vii.

Harisinghani MG, McLoud TC, Shepard JA et al. (2000). Tuberculosis from head to toe. Radiographics: a Review Publication of the Radiological Society of North America, Inc 20: 449–470. quiz 528-9, 532.

Hauptman JS, Hinrichs C, Mele C et al. (2005). Radiologic manifestations of intraventricular and subarachnoid racemose neurocysticercosis. Emerg Radiol 11: 153–157.

Horten BC, Abbott GF, Porro RS (1976). Fungal aneurysms of intracranial vessels. Arch Neurol 33: 577–579.

Hughes DC, Raghavan A, Mordekar SR et al. (2010). Role of imaging in the diagnosis of acute bacterial meningitis and its complications. Postgrad Med J 86: 478–485.

Hurst RW, Judkins A, Bolger W et al. (2001). Mycotic aneurysm and cerebral infarction resulting from fungal sinusitis: imaging and pathologic correlation. AJNR. Am J Neuroradiology 22: 858–863.

Iwasaki H, Toda N, Takahashi M et al. (2013). Vestibular and cochlear neuritis in patients with Ramsay Hunt syndrome: a Gd-enhanced MRI study. Acta Otolaryngol 133: 373–377.

Jinkins JR (1991). Computed tomography of intracranial tuberculosis. Neuroradiology 33: 126–135.

Kaiser AB, McGee ZA (1975). Aminoglycoside therapy of gram-negative bacillary meningitis. N Engl J Med 293: 1215–1220.

Kalita J, Prasad S, Maurya PK et al. (2012). MR angiography in tuberculous meningitis. Acta Radiol (Stockholm, Sweden: 1987) 53: 324–329.

Kanamalla US, Ibarra RA, Jinkins JR (2000). Imaging of cranial meningitis and ventriculitis. Neuroimaging Clin N Am 10: 309–331.

Karagulle-Kendi AT, Truwit C (2010). Neuroimaging of central nervous system infections. In: PJ Vinken, GW Bruyn (Eds.), Handbook of Clinical Neurology, vol. 96. Elsevier, Amsterdam, pp. 239–255.

Karampekios S, Hesselink J (2005). Cerebral infections. Eur Radiol 15: 485–493.

Kastrup O, Wanke I, Maschke M (2008). Neuroimaging of infections of the central nervous system. Semin Neurol 28: 511–522.

Kennedy PG (2004). Viral encephalitis: causes, differential diagnosis, and management. J Neurol Neurosurg Psychiatry 75: i10–i15.

Kimura-Hayama ET, Higuera JA, Corona-Cedillo R et al. (2010). Neurocysticercosis: radiologic-pathologic correlation. Radiographics: a Review Publication of the Radiological Society of North America, Inc 30: 1705–1719.

Kioumehr F, Dadsetan MR, Feldman N et al. (1995). Postcontrast MRI of cranial meninges: leptomeningitis versus pachymeningitis. J Comput Assist Tomogr 19: 713–720.

Klein NC, Damsker B, Hirschman SZ (1985). Mycobacterial meningitis. Retrospective analysis from 1970 to 1983. Am J Med 79: 29–34.

Kleinschmidt-DeMasters BK (2002). Central nervous system aspergillosis: a 20-year retrospective series. Hum Pathol 33: 116–124.

Komatsu Y, Narushima K, Kobayashi E et al. (1991). Aspergillus mycotic aneurysm – case report. Neurol Med Chir 31: 346–350.

Krick JA, Remington JS (1978). Toxoplasmosis in the adult – an overview. N Engl J Med 298: 550–553.

Krupp LB, Lipton RB, Swerdlow ML et al. (1985). Progressive multifocal leukoencephalopathy: clinical and radiographic features. Ann Neurol 17: 344–349.

Kuker W, Nagele T, Schmidt F et al. (2004). Diffusion-weighted MRI in herpes simplex encephalitis: a report of three cases. Neuroradiology 46: 122–125.

Lai PH, Ho JT, Chen WL et al. (2002). Brain abscess and necrotic brain tumor: discrimination with proton MR spectroscopy and diffusion-weighted imaging. AJNR Am J Neuroradiology 23: 1369–1377.

Laubenberger J, Haussinger D, Bayer S et al. (1996). HIV-related metabolic abnormalities in the brain: depiction with proton MR spectroscopy with short echo times. Radiology 199: 805–810.

Leiguarda R, Berthier M, Starkstein S et al. (1988). Ischemic infarction in 25 children with tuberculous meningitis. Stroke; a Journal of Cerebral Circulation 19: 200–204.

Lerner A, Shiroishi MS, Zee CS et al. (2012). Imaging of neurocysticercosis. Neuroimaging Clin N Am 22: 659–676.

Levy RM, Bredesen DE, Rosenblum ML (1985). Neurological manifestations of the acquired immunodeficiency syndrome (AIDS): experience at UCSF and review of the literature. J Neurosurg 62: 475–495.

Lucato LT, Guedes MS, Sato JR et al. (2007). The role of conventional MR imaging sequences in the evaluation of neurocysticercosis: impact on characterization of the scolex and lesion burden. AJNR Am J Neuroradiology 28: 1501–1504.

Luft BJ, Brooks RG, Conley FK et al. (1984). Toxoplasmic encephalitis in patients with acquired immune deficiency syndrome. JAMA 252: 913–917.

Luthra G, Parihar A, Nath K et al. (2007). Comparative evaluation of fungal, tubercular, and pyogenic brain abscesses with conventional and diffusion MR imaging and proton MR spectroscopy. AJNR. Am J Neuroradiology 28: 1332–1338.

Lyons RW, Andriole VT (1986). Fungal infections of the CNS. Neurol Clin 4: 159–170.

Mahadevan A, Ramalingaiah AH, Parthasarathy S et al. (2013). Neuropathological correlate of the “concentric target sign” in MRI of HIV-associated cerebral toxoplasmosis. Journal of Magnetic Resonance Imaging: JMRI 38: 488–495.

Mangi RJ, Holstein LL, Andriole VT (1977). Treatment of Gram-negative bacillary meningitis with intrathecal gentamicin. Yale J Biol Med 50: 31–41.

Masdeu JC, Quinto C, Olivera C et al. (2000). Open-ring imaging sign: highly specific for atypical brain demyelination. Neurology 54: 1427–1433.

Masters CL, Harris JO, Gajdusek DC et al. (1979). Creutzfeldt-Jakob disease: patterns of worldwide occurrence and the significance of familial and sporadic clustering. Ann Neurol 5: 177–188.

Mathur S, Karimi A, Mafee MF (2007). Acute optic nerve infarction demonstrated by diffusion-weighted imaging in a case of rhinocerebral mucormycosis. AJNR Am J Neuroradiology 28: 489–490.

Mathur M, Johnson CE, Sze G (2012). Fungal infections of the central nervous system. Neuroimaging Clin N Am 22: 609–632.

Matoba M, Tonami H, Miyaji H et al. (2001). Creutzfeldt–Jakob disease: serial changes on diffusion-weighted MRI. J Comput Assist Tomogr 25: 274–277.

McLean FM, Ginsberg LE, Stanton CA (1996). Perineural spread of rhinocerebral mucormycosis. AJNR Am J Neuroradiology 17: 114–116.

Misra UK, Kalita J, Maurya PK (2011). Stroke in tuberculous meningitis. J Neurol Sci 303: 22–30.

Mitchell TG, Perfect JR (1995). Cryptococcosis in the era of AIDS – 100 years after the discovery of Cryptococcus neoformans. Clin Microbiol Rev 8: 515–548.

Mohan S, Jain KK, Arabi M et al. (2012). Imaging of meningitis and ventriculitis. Neuroimaging Clin N Am 22: 557–583.

Murata T, Shiga Y, Higano S et al. (2002). Conspicuity and evolution of lesions in Creutzfeldt–Jakob disease at diffusion-weighted imaging. AJNR. Am J Neuroradiology 23: 1164–1172.

Nadkarni T, Goel A (2005). Aspergilloma of the brain: an overview. J Postgrad Med 51: S37–S41.

Nash TE, Garcia HH (2011). Diagnosis and treatment of neurocysticercosis. Nat Rev Neurol 7: 584–594.

Nash TE, Pretell J, Garcia HH (2001). Calcified cysticerci provoke perilesional edema and seizures. Clinical Infectious Diseases: an Official Publication of the Infectious Diseases Society of America 33: 1649–1653.

Nash TE, Pretell EJ, Lescano AG et al. (2008). Perilesional brain oedema and seizure activity in patients with calcified neurocysticercosis: a prospective cohort and nested case-control study. Lancet Neurol 7: 1099–1105.

Navia BA, Gonzalez RG (1997). Functional imaging of the AIDS dementia complex and the metabolic pathology of the HIV-1-infected brain. Neuroimaging Clin N Am 7: 431–445.

Navia BA, Jordan BD, Price RW (1986). The AIDS dementia complex: I. Clinical features. Ann Neurol 19: 517–524.

Noguchi T, Yoshiura T, Hiwatashi A et al. (2010). CT and MRI findings of human herpesvirus 6-associated encephalopathy: comparison with findings of herpes simplex virus encephalitis. AJR Am J Roentgenology 194: 754–760.

Noujaim SE, Rossi MD, Rao SK et al. (1999). CT and MR imaging of neurocysticercosis. AJR Am J Roentgenology 173: 1485–1490.

Olsan AD, Milburn JM, Baumgarten KL et al. (2003). Leptomeningeal enhancement in a patient with proven West Nile virus infection. AJR Am J Roentgenology 181: 591–592.

Olsen WL, Longo FM, Mills CM et al. (1988). White matter disease in AIDS: findings at MR imaging. Radiology 169: 445–448.

Osborne AG (1994). Infections of the brain and its linings. Diagnostic Neuroradiology, St Louis, Mosby, pp. 673–715.

Parmar H, Sitoh YY, Anand P et al. (2006). Contrast-enhanced flair imaging in the evaluation of infectious leptomeningeal diseases. Eur J Radiol 58: 89–95.

Patkar D, Narang J, Yanamandala R et al. (2012). Central nervous system tuberculosis: pathophysiology and imaging findings. Neuroimaging Clin N Am 22: 677–705.

Petersen LR, Marfin AA (2002). West Nile virus: a primer for the clinician. Ann Intern Med 137: 173–179.

Petropoulou KA, Gordon SM, Prayson RA et al. (2005). West Nile virus meningoencephalitis: MR imaging findings. AJNR. Am J Neuroradiology 26: 1986–1995.

Pezzullo JA, Tung GA, Mudigonda S et al. (2003). Diffusion-weighted MR imaging of pyogenic ventriculitis. AJR Am J Roentgenology 180: 71–75.

Pienaar M, Andronikou S, van Toorn R (2009). MRI to demonstrate diagnostic features and complications of TBM not seen with CT. Child's Nervous System: ChNS: Official Journal of the International Society for Pediatric Neurosurgery 25: 941–947.

Porter SB, Sande MA (1992). Toxoplasmosis of the central nervous system in the acquired immunodeficiency syndrome. N Engl J Med 327: 1643–1648.

Post MJ (1990). Neuroimaging in various stages of human immunodeficiency virus infection. Curr Opin Radiol 2: 73–79.

Post MJ, Chan JC, Hensley GT et al. (1983). Toxoplasma encephalitis in Haitian adults with acquired immunodeficiency syndrome: a clinical-pathologic-CT correlation. AJR Am J Roentgenology 140: 861–868.

Post MJ, Kursunoglu SJ, Hensley GT et al. (1985). Cranial CT in acquired immunodeficiency syndrome: spectrum of diseases and optimal contrast enhancement technique. AJR Am J Roentgenology 145: 929–940.

Post MJD, Berger JR, Hensley GT (1986). The radiology of central nervous system disease in acquired immunodeficiency syndrome. In: JM Taveras, JT Ferrucci, A Norman (Eds.), Radiology: Diagnosis, Imaging, Intervention, Lippincott, Philadelphia, PA, pp 1–26.

Post MJ, Tate LG, Quencer RM et al. (1988). CT, MR, and pathology in HIV encephalitis and meningitis. AJR Am J Roentgenology 151: 373–380.

Post MJ, Berger JR, Duncan R et al. (1993). Asymptomatic and neurologically symptomatic HIV-seropositive subjects: results of long-term MR imaging and clinical follow-up. Radiology 188: 727–733.

Post MJ, Thurnher MM, Clifford DB et al. (2012). CNS-immune reconstitution inflammatory syndrome in the setting of HIV infection, part 2: discussion of neuro-immune reconstitution inflammatory syndrome with and without other pathogens. AJNR Am J Neuroradiology 34: 1308–1318.

Post MJ, Thurnher MM, Clifford DB et al. (2013). CNS–immune reconstitution inflammatory syndrome in the setting of HIV infection, part 1: overview and discussion of progressive multifocal leukoencephalopathy–immune reconstitution inflammatory syndrome and cryptococcal–immune reconstitution inflammatory syndrome. AJNR Am J Neuroradiology 34: 1297–1307.

Prusiner SB (1986). Prions are novel infectious pathogens causing scrapie and Creutzfeldt–Jakob disease. BioEssays:

News and Reviews in Molecular, Cellular and Developmental Biology 5: 281–286.

Rahal Jr JJ, Hyams PJ, Simberkoff MS et al. (1974). Combined intrathecal and intramuscular gentamicin for gram-negative meningitis. Pharmacologic study of 21 patients. N Engl J Med 290: 1394–1398.

Rana S, Albayram S, Lin DD et al. (2002). Diffusion-weighted imaging and apparent diffusion coefficient maps in a case of intracerebral abscess with ventricular extension. AJNR Am J Neuroradiology 23: 109–112.

Restrepo BI, Llaguno P, Sandoval MA et al. (1998). Analysis of immune lesions in neurocysticercosis patients: Central nervous system response to helminth appears Th1-like instead of Th2. J Neuroimmunol 89: 64–72.

Riddell Jt, Shuman EK (2012). Epidemiology of central nervous system infection. Neuroimaging Clin N Am 22: 543–556.

Rodriguez S, Dorny P, Tsang VC et al. (2009). Detection of *Taenia solium* antigens and anti-*T. solium* antibodies in paired serum and cerebrospinal fluid samples from patients with intraparenchymal or extraparenchymal neurocysticercosis. J Infect Dis 199: 1345–1352.

Roos KL (1999). Encephalitis. Neurol Clin 17: 813–833.

Ruiz A, Ganz WI, Post MJ et al. (1994). Use of thallium-201 brain SPECT to differentiate cerebral lymphoma from toxoplasma encephalitis in AIDS patients. AJNR Am J Neuroradiology 15: 1885–1894.

Ruiz A, Post MJ, Bundschu C et al. (1997a). Primary central nervous system lymphoma in patients with AIDS. Neuroimaging Clin N Am 7: 281–296.

Ruiz A, Post MJ, Bundschu CC (1997b). Dentate nuclei involvement in AIDS patients with CNS cryptococcosis: imaging findings with pathologic correlation. J Comput Assist Tomogr 21: 175–182.

Rumboldt Z, Thurnher MM, Gupta RK (2007). Central nervous system infections. Semin Roentgenol 42: 62–91.

Saez-Llorens XJ, Umana MA, Odio CM et al. (1989). Brain abscess in infants and children. Pediatr Infect Dis J 8: 449–458.

Sage MR, Wilson AJ, Scroop R (1998). Contrast media and the brain. The basis of CT and MR imaging enhancement. Neuroimaging Clin N Am 8: 695–707.

Saigal G, Post MJ, Lolayekar S et al. (2005). Unusual presentation of central nervous system cryptococcal infection in an immunocompetent patient. AJNR Am J Neuroradiology 26: 2522–2526.

Samuel MA, Diamond MS (2006). Pathogenesis of West Nile Virus infection: a balance between virulence, innate and adaptive immunity, and viral evasion. J Virol 80: 9349–9360.

Schroeder PC, Post MJ, Oschatz E et al. (2006). Analysis of the utility of diffusion-weighted MRI and apparent diffusion coefficient values in distinguishing central nervous system toxoplasmosis from lymphoma. Neuroradiology 48: 715–720.

Sheth TN, Pillon L, Keystone J et al. (1998). Persistent MR contrast enhancement of calcified neurocysticercosis lesions. AJNR Am J Neuroradiology 19: 79–82.

Shukla R, Abbas A, Kumar P et al. (2008). Evaluation of cerebral infarction in tuberculous meningitis by diffusion weighted imaging. J Infect 57: 298–306.

Singh B, Garg RK, Singh MK et al. (2012). Computed tomography angiography in patients with tuberculous meningitis. J Infect 64: 565–572.

Sinha S, Sharma BS (2009). Neurocysticercosis: a review of current status and management. Journal of Clinical Neuroscience: Official Journal of the Neurosurgical Society of Australasia 16: 867–876.

Smirniotopoulos JG, Murphy FM, Rushing EJ et al. (2007). Patterns of contrast enhancement in the brain and meninges. Radiographics: a Review Publication of the Radiological Society of North America, Inc 27: 525–551.

Snider WD, Simpson DM, Nielsen S et al. (1983). Neurological complications of acquired immune deficiency syndrome: analysis of 50 patients. Ann Neurol 14: 403–418.

Solbrig MV, Hasso AN, Jay CA (2008). CNS viruses – diagnostic approach. Neuroimaging Clin N Am 18: 1–18. vii.

Spellberg B, Edwards Jr J, Ibrahim A (2005). Novel perspectives on mucormycosis: pathophysiology, presentation, and management. Clin Microbiol Rev 18: 556–569.

Starke JR (2010). Mycobacterial infections. Handb Clin Neurol 96: 159–177.

Steiner I, Budka H, Chaudhuri A et al. (2010). Viral meningoencephalitis: a review of diagnostic methods and guidelines for management. Eur J Neurol 17 (8): 999–1009, e55–e57.

Studahl M, Lindquist L, Eriksson BM et al. (2013). Acute viral infections of the central nervous system in immunocompetent adults: diagnosis and management. Drugs 73: 131–158.

Sze G, Zimmerman RD (1988). The magnetic resonance imaging of infections and inflammatory diseases. Radiol Clin North Am 26: 839–859.

Talmi YP, Goldschmied-Reouven A, Bakon M et al. (2002). Rhino-orbital and rhino-orbito-cerebral mucormycosis. Otolaryngology–Head and Neck Surgery: Official Journal of American Academy of Otolaryngology–Head and Neck Surgery 127: 22–31.

Tempkin AD, Sobonya RE, Seeger JF et al. (2006). Cerebral aspergillosis: radiologic and pathologic findings. Radiographics: a Review Publication of the Radiological Society of North America, Inc 26: 1239–1242.

Thurnher MM, Thurnher SA, Fleischmann D et al. (1997). Comparison of T2-weighted and fluid-attenuated inversion-recovery fast spin-echo MR sequences in intracerebral AIDS-associated disease. AJNR Am J Neuroradiology 18: 1601–1609.

Thurnher MM, Schindler EG, Thurnher SA et al. (2000). Highly active antiretroviral therapy for patients with AIDS dementia complex: effect on MR imaging findings and clinical course. AJNR Am J Neuroradiology 21: 670–678.

Thurnher MM, Post MJ, Rieger A et al. (2001). Initial and follow-up MR imaging findings in AIDS-related progressive multifocal leukoencephalopathy treated with highly active antiretroviral therapy. AJNR Am J Neuroradiology 22: 977–984.

Tien R, Dillon WP, Jackler RK (1990). Contrast-enhanced MR imaging of the facial nerve in 11 patients with Bell's palsy. AJR Am J Roentgenology 155: 573–579.

Tien RD, Chu PK, Hesselink JR et al. (1991). Intracranial cryptococcosis in immunocompromised patients: CT and MR findings in 29 cases. AJNR Am J Neuroradiology 12: 283–289.

Tien RD, Felsberg GJ, Osumi AK (1993). Herpesvirus infections of the CNS: MR findings. AJNR Am J Roentgenology 161: 167–176.

Trivedi R, Saksena S, Gupta RK (2009). Magnetic resonance imaging in central nervous system tuberculosis. Indian J Radiol Imaging 19: 256–265.

Tsuchiya K, Osawa A, Katase S et al. (2003). Diffusion-weighted MRI of subdural and epidural empyemas. Neuroradiology 45: 220–223.

Tung GA, Rogg JM (2003). Diffusion-weighted imaging of cerebritis. AJNR Am J Neuroradiology 24: 1110–1113.

Ukisu R, Kushihashi T, Kitanosono T et al. (2005). Serial diffusion-weighted MRI of Creutzfeldt–Jakob disease. AJNR Am J Roentgenology 184: 560–566.

van de Beek D, de Gans J, Spanjaard L et al. (2004). Clinical features and prognostic factors in adults with bacterial meningitis. N Engl J Med 351: 1849–1859.

Verma A, Madhavi, Patwari S (2011). Use of 3D CISS as part of a routine protocol for the evaluation of intracranial granulomas. The Indian Journal of Radiology & Imaging 21: 311–3026.90703.

Vossough A, Zimmerman RA, Bilaniuk LT et al. (2008). Imaging findings of neonatal herpes simplex virus type 2 encephalitis. Neuroradiology 50: 355–366.

Wallin MT, Kurtzke JF (2004). Neurocysticercosis in the United States: review of an important emerging infection. Neurology 63: 1559–1564.

Wehn SM, Heinz ER, Burger PC et al. (1989). Dilated Virchow-Robin spaces in cryptococcal meningitis associated with AIDS: CT and MR findings. J Comput Assist Tomogr 13: 756–762.

Weingarten K, Zimmerman RD, Becker RD et al. (1989). Subdural and epidural empyemas: MR imaging. AJNR Am J Roentgenology 152: 615–621.

White Jr AC (2000). Neurocysticercosis: Updates on epidemiology, pathogenesis, diagnosis, and management. Annu Rev Med 51: 187–206.

Whiteman ML, Post MJ, Berger JR et al. (1993). Progressive multifocal leukoencephalopathy in 47 HIV-seropositive patients: neuroimaging with clinical and pathologic correlation. Radiology 187: 233–240.

Wijdicks EF, Borleffs JC, Hoepelman AI et al. (1991). Fatal disseminated hemorrhagic toxoplasmic encephalitis as the initial manifestation of AIDS. Ann Neurol 29: 683–686.

Will RG, Ironside JW, Zeidler M et al. (1996). A new variant of Creutzfeldt–Jakob disease in the UK. Lancet 347: 921–925.

Wong J, Quint DJ (1999). Imaging of central nervous system infections. Semin Roentgenol 34: 123–143.

Wong AM, Zimmerman RA, Simon EM et al. (2004). Diffusion-weighted MR imaging of subdural empyemas in children. AJNR Am J Neuroradiology 25: 1016–1021.

World Health Organization (1998). Global surveillance, diagnosis and therapy of human Transmissible Spongiform Encephalopathies: Report of a WHO consultation. World Health Organization, Geneva, Switzerland.

Yikilmaz A, Taylor GA (2008). Sonographic findings in bacterial meningitis in neonates and young infants. Pediatr Radiol 38: 129–137.

Young GS, Geschwind MD, Fischbein NJ et al. (2005). Diffusion-weighted and fluid-attenuated inversion recovery imaging in Creutzfeldt–Jakob disease: high sensitivity and specificity for diagnosis. AJNR Am J Neuroradiology 26: 1551–1562.

Zinreich SJ, Kennedy DW, Malat J et al. (1988). Fungal sinusitis: diagnosis with CT and MR imaging. Radiology 169: 439–444.

Handbook of Clinical Neurology, Vol. 135 (3rd series)
Neuroimaging, Part I
J.C. Masdeu and R.G. González, Editors

Chapter 20

Multiple sclerosis

MASSIMO FILIPPI*, PAOLO PREZIOSA, AND MARIA A. ROCCA
Neuroimaging Research Unit, Institute of Experimental Neurology, Division of Neuroscience, San Raffaele Scientific Institute, Vita-Salute San Raffaele University, Milan, Italy

Abstract

Due to its sensitivity to the different multiple sclerosis (MS)-related abnormalities, magnetic resonance imaging (MRI) has become an established tool to diagnose MS and to monitor its evolution. MRI has been included in the diagnostic workup of patients with clinically isolated syndromes suggestive of MS, and *ad hoc* criteria have been proposed and are regularly updated. In patients with definite MS, the ability of conventional MRI techniques to explain patients' clinical status and progression of disability is still suboptimal. Several advanced MRI-based technologies have been applied to estimate overall MS burden in the different phases of the disease. Their use has allowed the heterogeneity of MS pathology in focal lesions, normal-appearing white matter and gray matter to be graded *in vivo*. Recently, additional features of MS pathology, including macrophage infiltration and abnormal iron deposition, have become quantifiable. All of this, combined with functional imaging techniques, is improving our understanding of the mechanisms associated with MS evolution. In the near future, the use of ultrahigh-field systems is likely to provide additional insight into disease pathophysiology. However, the utility of advanced MRI techniques in clinical trial monitoring and in assessing individual patients' response to treatment still needs to be assessed.

INTRODUCTION

Multiple sclerosis (MS) is the most common chronic inflammatory demyelinating disease affecting the central nervous system (CNS) of young adults in Western countries leading, in most cases, to severe and irreversible clinical disability. The clinical course of MS is extremely variable. In about 85% of MS cases, patients present with a clinically isolated syndrome (CIS) involving the optic nerve, brainstem, or spinal cord (Noseworthy et al., 2000). In these patients, symptoms and signs typically evolve over a period of several days, stabilize, and then often improve, resulting in a relapsing-remitting (RR) course. Persistent signs of CNS dysfunction may develop after a relapse, and the disease may progress between relapses (secondary progressive [SP] MS) (Lublin and Reingold, 1996). Patients with benign MS (BMS) represent 10–20% of patients with relapsing MS and are characterized by accumulation of modest or no disability over a long period of time (Hawkins and McDonnell, 1999). About 15% of patients have primary progressive (PP) MS, which is characterized by a steady progression of disability from clinical onset, without clear-cut relapses (Miller and Leary, 2007).

Magnetic resonance imaging (MRI) has a high sensitivity in revealing macroscopic tissue abnormalities in patients with MS. Conventional MR sequences, i.e., dual-echo, fluid-attenuated inversion recovery (FLAIR), and T1-weighted, both with and without gadolinium (Gd) contrast agent administration (Fig. 20.1), provide important pieces of information for diagnosing MS, understanding its natural history, and assessing treatment efficacy. Dual-echo and FLAIR imaging have a high sensitivity in detecting MS lesions, which appear as hyperintense focal areas on these scans. However, they

*Correspondence to: Massimo Filippi, Neuroimaging Research Unit, Institute of Experimental Neurology, Division of Neuroscience, San Raffaele Scientific Institute, Vita-Salute San Raffaele University, Via Olgettina, 60, 20132 Milan, Italy. Tel: +39-02-26433033, Fax: +39-02-26433031, E-mail: filippi.massimo@hsr.it

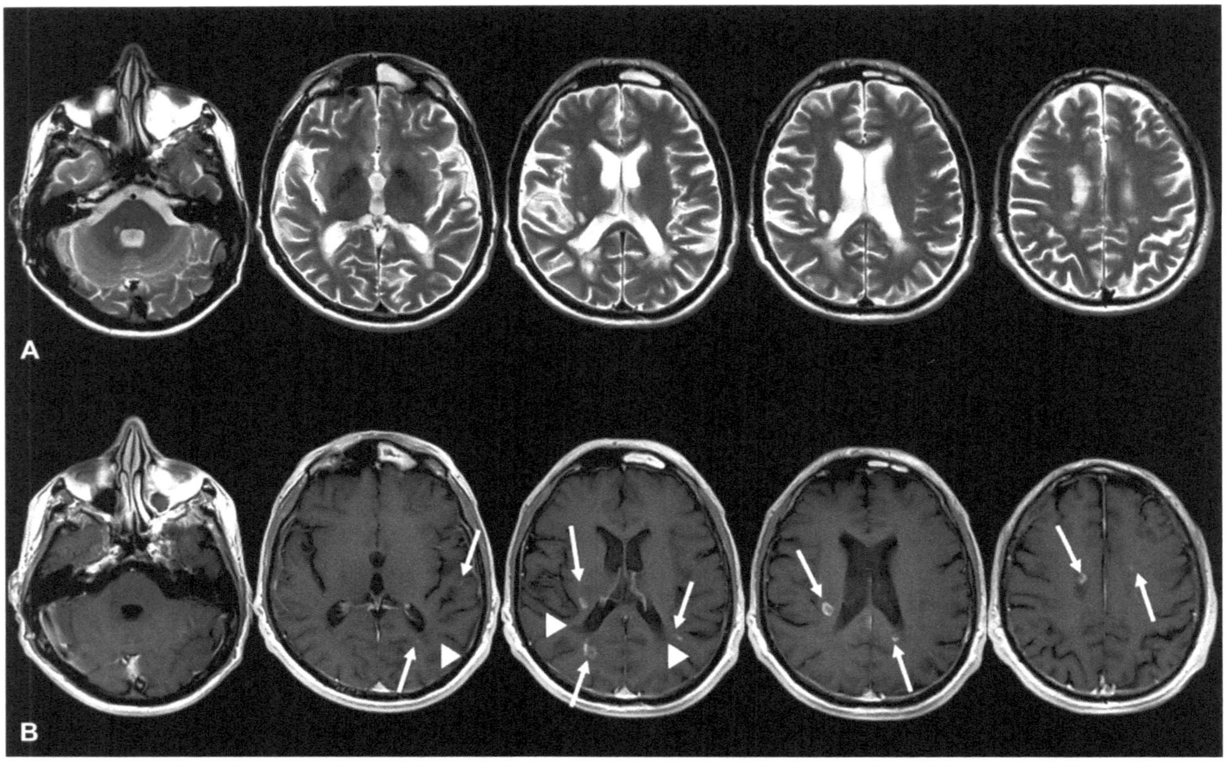

Fig. 20.1. Brain axial T2-weighted (**A**) and postcontrast T1-weighted (**B**) spin-echo magnetic resonance images from a 28-year-old patient with relapsing-remitting multiple sclerosis. In (**A**), multiple hyperintense lesions are visible, which suggest multifocal white-matter pathology, involving infratentorial regions, periventricular and juxtacortical white matter. In (**B**), several of these lesions (white arrows) are clearly contrast-enhanced, which indicates the presence of a local disruption of the blood–brain barrier, while others are hypointense, representing regions with irreversible axonal loss, demyelination, and gliosis (arrowhead).

lack specificity to the heterogeneous pathologic substrates of individual lesions. Gd-enhanced T1-weighted images allow active lesions to be distinguished from inactive lesions, since enhancement occurs as a result of increased blood–brain barrier permeability and corresponds to areas with ongoing inflammation. Finally, lesions that persistently appear dark on postcontrast T1-weighted images are associated with more severe tissue damage (both demyelination and axonal loss) compared to lesions that do not appear dark on such images (Fig. 20.1).

Disappointingly, the strength of the association between conventional MRI findings and the clinical manifestations of the disease remains modest in patients with MS. This is likely due to the relative lack of specificity of conventional MRI in the evaluation of the heterogeneous pathologic substrates of the disease, its inability to provide accurate estimates of damage outside focal lesions, and the fact that it cannot provide information on CNS functional reorganization after tissue injury has occurred. Structural, metabolic, and functional MRI (fMRI) techniques have allowed the identification of novel markers of the disease, more closely linked to its pathologic features, which may in part overcome the limitations of conventional MRI.

This chapter discusses the main insights derived from the application of MRI-based techniques to diagnose MS, define its pathophysiology, and monitor the efficacy of disease-modifying treatments.

MRI AND THE DIAGNOSIS OF MS

Features of MS lesions

The characterization of lesion features suggestive of MS on conventional MR scans is central in the diagnostic workup of patients suspected of having this condition. Brain MS lesions are frequently located, asymmetrically between the two hemispheres, in the periventricular and juxtacortical white matter (WM), the corpus callosum (CC) (where the so-called "Dawson's fingers" can be seen) and infratentorial areas (with the pons and cerebellum more frequently affected than the medulla and midbrain). Such lesions can have oval or elliptic shapes (Ormerod et al., 1987). Consensus has also been reached on criteria useful to identify T2-hyperintense (Filippi et al., 1998a) and T1-enhancing lesions (Barkhof et al., 1997c).

MRI diagnostic criteria

In 2001, MRI was formally included in the diagnostic workup of patients suspected of having MS by an

Table 20.1

Magnetic resonance imaging criteria for dissemination in space and dissemination in time of multiple sclerosis

	Dissemination in space	Dissemination in time
International Panel (IP) criteria 2001 (McDonald et al., 2001)	≥3 of the following: 9 T2 lesions or 1 Gd-enhancing lesion; ≥3 periventricular lesions; ≥1 juxtacortical lesion; ≥1 posterior fossa lesion 1 spinal cord lesion can replace 1 brain lesion	A Gd-enhancing lesion ≥3 months after CIS onset or A new T2 lesion with reference to a previous scan ≥3 months after CIS onset
Revised IP criteria 2005 (Polman et al., 2005)	≥3 of the following: 9 T2 lesions or 1 Gd-enhancing lesion; ≥3 periventricular lesions; ≥1 juxtacortical lesion; ≥1 posterior fossa lesion or spinal cord lesion A spinal cord lesion can replace an infratentorial lesion Any number of spinal cord lesions can be included in total lesion count	A Gd-enhancing lesion ≥3 months after CIS onset or A new T2 lesion with reference to a baseline scan obtained ≥30 days after CIS onset
Swanton et al. (2006)	≥1 lesion in each of ≥2 characteristic locations: periventricular, juxtacortical, posterior fossa, spinal cord All lesions in symptomatic region excluded in brainstem and spinal cord syndromes	A new T2 lesion on follow-up MRI irrespective of timing of baseline scan
Multicenter Collaborative Research Network for MRI in MS (MAGNIMS) 2010 (Montalban et al., 2010) and revised IP criteria 2010 (Polman et al., 2011)	≥1 lesion in each of ≥2 characteristic locations: periventricular, juxtacortical, posterior fossa, spinal cord All lesions in symptomatic regions excluded in brainstem and spinal cord syndromes	Simultaneous presence of asymptomatic Gd-enhancing and nonenhancing lesions at any time or A new T2 and/or Gd-enhancing lesion on follow-up MRI irrespective of timing of baseline scan

Gd, gadolinium; CIS, clinically isolated syndrome; MRI, magnetic resonance imaging.

International Panel (IP) of MS experts (McDonald et al., 2001). The definition of MRI criteria for a diagnosis of MS is based, on the one hand, on the demonstration of lesion dissemination in space (DIS) and time (DIT), and, on the other, on the exclusion of alternative neurologic conditions (Table 20.1). The original IP criteria for MS diagnosis were revised in 2005 (Polman et al., 2005) to simplify the approach, while maintaining adequate sensitivity and specificity (Table 20.1). The main changes introduced by such a revision pertain to the demonstration of DIT, that can be obtained by the detection of a new T2 lesion, if it appears at any time compared with a reference scan done at least 30 days after the onset of the first clinical event, and the clarification of the use of spinal-cord MRI to demonstrate DIS (Polman et al., 2005). Importance to clinical and imaging (brain or spinal cord) findings has been given for a diagnosis of PPMS, with less emphasis on cerebrospinal fluid assessment.

Meanwhile several other proposals have been made to simplify further the revised IP criteria and to make them easier to implement in clinical and research settings. According to the Swanton criteria (Swanton et al., 2006), at least one subclinical T2 lesion in at least two of the four locations defined as characteristic for MS in the revised IP criteria (i.e., juxtacortical, periventricular, infratentorial, and spinal cord) is required for DIS (Table 20.1). Rovira et al. (2009) suggested that a single brain MRI study performed early (i.e., < 3 months) after the onset of a CIS is highly predictive for the development of definite MS in the presence of both Gd-enhancing and nonenhancing lesions, which when occurring simultaneously are considered a marker of DIT. Both the previous criteria have been included in the criteria proposed by the European Multicenter Collaborative Research Network for MRI in MS (MAGNIMS) (Montalban et al., 2010), as well as in the most recent revision of the 2001 IP criteria (Table 20.1) (Polman et al., 2011). One aspect that has not been considered yet in the available sets of MRI diagnostic criteria is the role of cortical lesions (CL), some of which can be visualized using double-inversion recovery (DIR) sequences (Geurts et al., 2005) (Fig. 20.2). The sensitivity of such lesion detection in the context of MS diagnosis has been considered by Filippi and coworkers (2010), who proposed a model for DIS which includes the presence of at least one intracortical lesion, in addition to

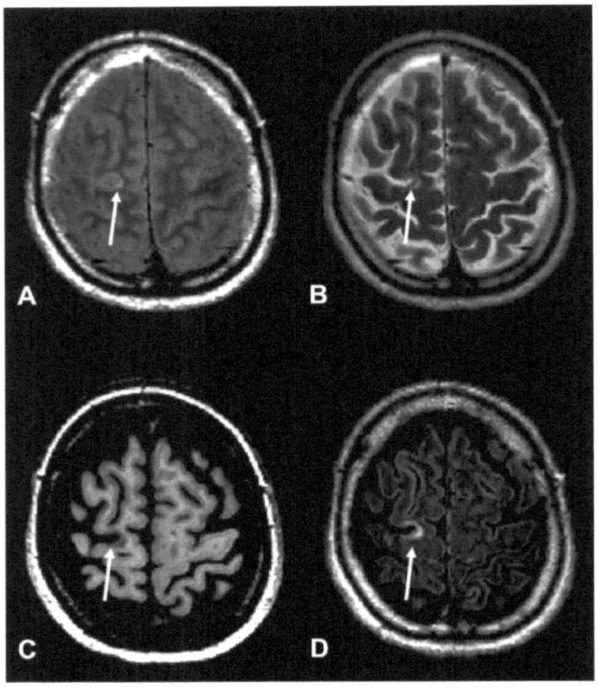

Fig. 20.2. Axial proton density-weighted (**A**), T2-weighted (**B**), T1-weighted (**C**) spin-echo, and double-inversion recovery (**D**) magnetic resonance images of the brain from a 44-year-old patient with relapsing-remitting multiple sclerosis. One cortical lesion (white arrow), hypointense on T1-weighted sequence and more visible on double-inversion recovery sequence, is evident.

the presence of at least one infratentorial and one spinal cord or Gd-enhancing lesion.

Another aspect that has been recently investigated is the contribution of spinal cord involvement in CIS patients in diagnosing MS, according to the revised 2010 IP criteria, and in predicting conversion to definite MS (Sombekke et al., 2013). The presence of spinal cord lesions facilitated the diagnosis of MS and was predictive of conversion to definite MS, especially in those patients without spinal CIS and who did not fulfill brain MRI criteria.

MRI and differential diagnosis

A series of MRI "red flags," derived from evidence-based findings and educated guesses, have been identified in the setting of clinically suspected MS, which should alert clinicians to prompt the performance of "nonroutine" tests and to reconsider a differential diagnosis more extensively (Charil et al., 2006b; Miller et al., 2008) (Fig. 20.3). The so-called classic MS variants consist of neuromyelitis optica (NMO), Balo's concentric sclerosis, Schilder's disease, acute MS (Marburg type), and acute disseminated encephalomyelitis. Conditions mimicking MS also include a broad spectrum of diseases, such as hypoxic-ischemic vasculopathies, cerebral autosomal-dominant arteriopathy with subcortical infarcts and leukoencephalopathy (CADASIL), primary and secondary vasculitides of the CNS, systemic inflammatory diseases (e.g., systemic lupus erythematosus and neuro-Behçet), progressive multifocal leukoencephalopathy, and other leukoencephalopathies. Although relatively rare, these conditions are clinically important as they can cause considerable diagnostic uncertainty.

The presence of symmetric, diffuse T2-weighted hyperintensities in the deep and periventricular WM is a typical MRI finding of dystrophies. NMO should be distinguished from MS for its different course, prognosis, presence of antibodies against aquaporin-4, and response to immunomodulatory therapy. In addition, most NMO patients have a normal brain MRI or only a few and nonspecific T2 hyperintensities that may have a predilection for regions with a high expression of aquaporin-4, including the hypothalamus, medulla, and other brainstem areas. Myelitis in this condition, unlike that which occurs in MS, is usually accompanied in the acute phase by a T2-weighted spinal cord lesion extending over three or more spinal segments, which may be hypointense on T1-weighted sequences and associated with varying degrees of Gd enhancement (Charil et al., 2006b; Miller et al., 2008). MRI and NMO-IgG have been formally included in the diagnostic criteria of NMO (Wingerchuk et al., 2006).

MRI and prognosis in CIS

In several studies, MRI findings at disease onset that showed the strongest predictive value for the subsequent development of definite MS were the number and extent of brain T2 lesions (Brex et al., 2002; Minneboo et al., 2004; Fisniku et al., 2008), the presence of infratentorial lesions (Minneboo et al., 2004), and the presence of Gd-enhancing lesions (Barkhof et al., 1997a). For patients with CIS and brain MRI lesions, the chance of developing definite MS was >80% over the subsequent 20 years, in the longest follow-up study to date (Brex et al., 2002; Fisniku et al., 2008). Baseline T2 lesion load and the accumulation of such lesions in the first 5 years after clinical onset are strong predictors of disability accumulation over time in these patients (Fisniku et al., 2008). In a longitudinal study (Summers et al., 2008a), baseline T1 hypointense lesion number and volume predicted the severity of executive deficits, and new T2 lesions at 3-month follow-up predicted slowed information processing 7 years later.

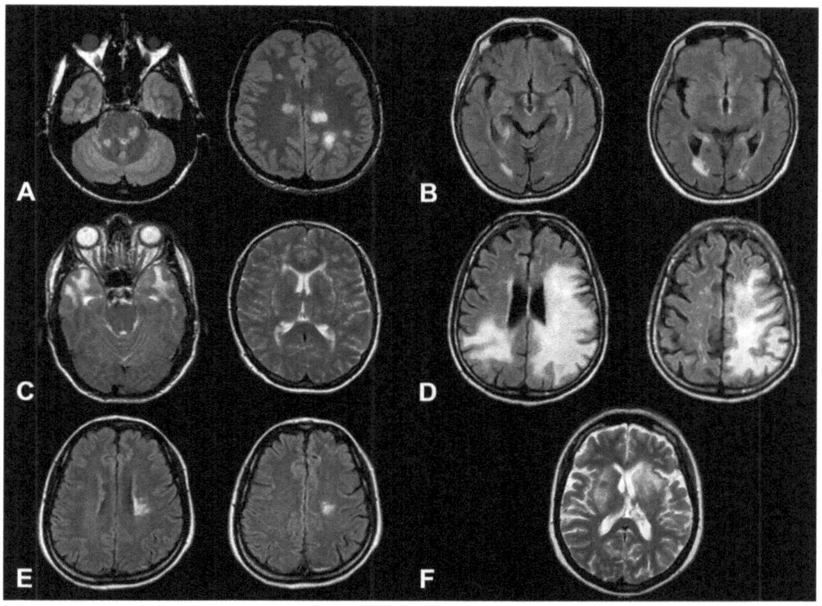

Fig. 20.3. Axial fluid-attenuated inversion recovery (FLAIR) (**A–F**) magnetic resonance images of six patients showing different and heterogeneous patterns of white-matter (WM) hyperintensities. In **A**, typical round lesions of a multiple sclerosis patient are visible. In **B**, several WM hyperintensities are located in regions with a high expression of aquaporin-4 in one patient affected by neuromyelitis optica. In **C**, T2 hyperintensity of the temporal pole, U-fibers at the vertex, external capsule, and insular region are visible in one patient with cerebral autosomal-dominant arteriopathy with subcortical infarcts and leukoencephalopathy. In **D**, an asymmetric and widespread WM hyperintensity is visible in one patient with progressive multifocal leukoencephalopathy. In **E**, one periventricular lesion following blood vessels is shown in one patient affected by neuro-Behçet disease. In **F**, a diffuse hyperintensity of deep gray matter and WM is seen in one patient affected by neurosystemic lupus erythematosus.

MRI AND PATHOPHYSIOLOGY OF MS

Conventional MRI

T2 LESIONS

Lesion burden on T2-weighted MRI scans of MS patients increases by about 5–10% per year. Several cross-sectional studies evaluated differences in T2 lesion load among different MS phenotypes. T2 lesion load is higher in SPMS in comparison to BMS, RRMS, and PPMS (Thompson et al., 1990). However, the magnitude of the correlation between T2 lesion burden and disability in cross-sectional studies remains disappointing. The presence of this so-called "clinicoradiologic paradox" might be due to the poor pathologic specificity of T2-hyperintense lesions which do not distinguish edema and inflammation from irreversible demyelination and axonal loss. This may also simply be a reflection of the fact that many T2 lesions are clinically silent (Goodin, 2006).

A plateauing relationship between T2 lesion load and disability has been suggested for Expanded Disability Status Scale (EDSS) scores higher than 4.5 (Li et al., 2006); however, this finding has not been confirmed by subsequent studies (Sormani et al., 2009b; Caramanos et al., 2012).

GD-ENHANCING LESIONS

Serial MRI studies have shown that enhancement occurs in virtually all new lesions in patients with RRMS or SPMS and can sometimes be detected even before the onset of clinical symptoms (Kermode et al., 1990). The frequency of MRI activity varies according to the clinical phenotype of the disease, being higher in RRMS (Thompson et al., 1992) and SPMS (Thompson et al., 1991) than in PPMS (Thompson et al., 1991) and BMS (Thompson et al., 1992). Severely disabled SPMS patients exhibit a substantially lower incidence of enhancing lesions when compared to those with RRMS (Filippi et al., 1997).

The number of enhancing lesions increases shortly before and during clinical relapses and predicts subsequent MRI activity. As noted for T2 lesions, contrast-enhancing lesions also show a relatively modest correlation with disability accumulation (Kappos et al., 1999).

Recently, using dynamic contrast-enhanced (DCE) MRI and ultrahigh-field magnets, different patterns of centrifugal and centripetal Gd enhancement have been described (Gaitan et al., 2011, 2013; Absinta et al., 2013), suggesting a possible replacement of the previously accepted definition of nodular and ring-like lesions based on single post-Gd T1-weighted scans in favor of a paradigm based on spatiotemporal enhancement dynamics. One of these studies (Absinta et al., 2013) showed that centrifugal DCE lesions appear isointense or hypointense on phase images, whereas centripetal DCE lesions have thin, hypointense phase rims that clearly colocalize with the initial site of contrast enhancement. This hypointense rim was found to disappear in most lesions once enhancement resolved. On the contrary, chronic lesions showed stable hypointense phase rims which were typically thicker and darker than those seen in acute lesions. These findings suggest different underlying pathologic processes in the two types of lesion.

T1-hypointense lesions

A subset of T2 lesions (around 30–40%) appears persistently dark on postcontrast T1-weighted images on serial scans and represents regions where irreversible axonal loss, demyelination, and gliosis have occurred (Filippi et al., 2012b). T1-hypointense lesions are only a few in the early stage of MS and increase over the course of the disease. Studies assessing the correlations between T1-hypointense lesion burden and disability provided conflicting results, since some found such a correlation to be stronger than for T2 lesions, while others did not.

New contrast agents

MRI contrast agents composed of iron particles, known as ultrasmall particles of iron oxide (USPIO) or superparamagnetic iron particles of oxide, have been assessed as another way to monitor the MS inflammatory process. These particles are taken up by cells of the monocyte/macrophage system. As a consequence, USPIO enhancement reflects cellular infiltration and may complement Gd enhancement (Vellinga et al., 2008; Tourdias et al., 2012). The pattern of enhancement might differ after USPIO and Gd administration, with some lesions enhancing only with Gd, others only with USPIO, and others with both (Vellinga et al., 2008). Furthermore, USPIO enhancement may precede by a few weeks Gd enhancement and may persist after Gd enhancement is ceased (Vellinga et al., 2008).

Cortical lesions

As previously discussed, DIR sequences (which use two inversion times to suppress the signal from both WM and cerebrospinal fluid) have improved the sensitivity of MRI to detect CLs *in vivo* (a gain of 538% has been reported vs the use of T2-weighted sequences) (Geurts et al., 2005). Using DIR sequences, CLs have been detected in all the major MS clinical phenotypes, including CIS patients (Calabrese et al., 2007, 2009b, c). CLs are more frequently seen in patients with SPMS than in those with CIS or RRMS (Calabrese et al., 2007), whereas in patients with BMS they are fewer than in those with early RRMS (Calabrese et al , 2009b). Such lesions have also been visualized in the hippocampus (Roosendaal et al., 2008). Longitudinal studies have shown that new CLs continue to form in patients with early RRMS (Calabrese et al., 2009b) and in those with the progressive disease phenotypes over 1–2-year periods of follow-up (Calabrese et al., 2008, 2009c, 2010; Roosendaal et al., 2009b). An association has been found between CL burden and progression of disability over the subsequent 2–5 years (Calabrese et al., 2009c, 2010) in patients with different MS phenotypes, as well as between CL burden and the severity of cognitive impairment (Calabrese et al., 2009a, 2010, 2012; Roosendaal et al., 2009b).

Compared to postmortem assessment, DIR imaging detects 18% of all CLs (Seewann et al., 2012). As a consequence, a set of new strategies has been proposed to improve *in vivo* MR sensitivity and allow a reliable classification of these lesions, including the combination of DIR with other sequences, such as phase-sensitive inversion recovery (Nelson et al., 2007) and 3D magnetization-prepared rapid acquisition with gradient echo (Nelson et al., 2008). An additional gain in CL detection and characterization is likely to be achieved thanks to the increased availability of ultra-high-field MR scanners (Kangarlu et al., 2007; Mainero et al., 2009).

Brain atrophy

In MS patients, brain volume decreases on average by about 0.7–1% yearly (Miller et al., 2002) (Fig. 20.4). Although brain atrophy measurements are more pathologically specific than T2 lesion load measurements, they are at best only moderately correlated with disability in RRMS and SPMS (Miller et al., 2002; Giorgio et al., 2008). The strength of such a correlation increases when neuropsychologic impairment is considered (Lanz et al., 2007) and in longitudinal studies (Fisher et al., 2002; Khaleeli et al., 2008b). A large-scale, 14-month follow-up study (De Stefano et al., 2010) of untreated MS patients showed that the progression of brain atrophy is independent of clinical phenotype, when such an assessment is corrected for brain volume at baseline. Recently, it has been demonstrated that a higher intellectual enrichment lessens the negative impact of brain atrophy on both learning and memory (Sumowski et al., 2010).

Improvements in methods of analysis have allowed measurement of the extent of tissue loss in the gray matter (GM) and WM, separately, and also to define the distribution of atrophy at a regional level. Cross-sectional and longitudinal studies showed that GM atrophy occurs from the early stages of the disease (Chard et al., 2002b;

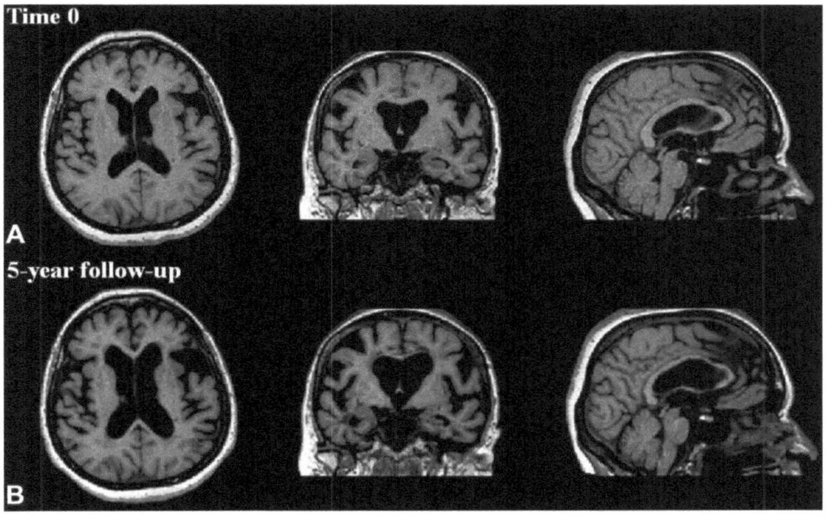

Fig. 20.4. 3D T1-weighted magnetic resonance images of the brain from a 42-year-old patient with relapsing-remitting multiple sclerosis acquired at two different times, at time 0 (**A**) and (**B**) after 5 years of follow-up. A significant diffuse atrophy is evident after 5 years, with a brain volume decrease of 15.6%.

De Stefano et al., 2003), is associated with MS clinical disability (Sanfilipo et al., 2005; Tedeschi et al., 2005; Prinster et al., 2010) and cognitive deterioration (Benedict et al., 2006; Amato et al., 2007), and tends to worsen over time (Valsasina et al., 2005). Chen et al. (2004) measured cortical thickness from patients with stable disease or progressing disability, and showed an increased rate of cortical tissue loss in the latter group. Fisher et al. (2008) compared atrophy rates over 4 years across the main MS clinical phenotypes and found that GM atrophy rate increases with disease stage, from 3.4-fold normal in CIS patients converting to RRMS to 14-fold normal in SPMS.

The topography of atrophy varies in the different brain structures and in different phases of the disease, as suggested by several voxel-based morphometry studies. In CIS patients, GM atrophy involves mainly the deep GM nuclei (Henry et al., 2008). In RRMS, atrophy of the frontotemporal lobes is typically detected (Bendfeldt et al., 2009). In SPMS patients, atrophy of deep GM structures, brainstem, cerebellum, and several cortical regions (virtually in all lobes) is observed (Ceccarelli et al., 2008). Compared to controls, BMS patients have GM atrophy in subcortical and frontoparietal regions (Mesaros et al., 2008). In comparison with BMS patients, those with SPMS have a significant GM loss in the cerebellum (Mesaros et al., 2008). More recently, Riccitelli et al. (2011) showed that the pattern of regional GM atrophy differs among cognitively impaired patients according to their clinical phenotype.

Assessment of atrophy of strategic GM structures could contribute to explain deficits in selective cognitive domains, as well as the occurrence of specific symptoms and disability progression. Hippocampal atrophy has been associated with deficits in memory encoding and retrieval (Sicotte et al., 2008); atrophy of the frontal and parietal lobes has been correlated with the presence and severity of fatigue (Sepulcre et al., 2009; Pellicano et al., 2010); and thalamic atrophy has been correlated with accumulation of disability after an 8-year follow-up period in patients with relapse-onset MS (Rocca et al., 2010b) and after a 5-year follow-up period in PPMS patients (Mesaros et al., 2011).

Despite these promising findings, brain atrophy has several important limitations that prevent this measure from being an optimal marker of MS progression. First, measurements of brain atrophy do not distinguish axonal injury from myelin loss. Second, reactive gliosis has the potential to mask considerable tissue loss. Third, brain atrophy fluctuates considerably with the amount of tissue water, which, in turn, can be affected by the presence of vasogenic edema from active inflammation, the administration of "anti-inflammatory" treatments such as steroids, and dehydration. Fourth, atrophy is an end-stage phenomenon. Although detection of atrophy may be considered as a robust endpoint, the ability to monitor MS at a stage prior to irreversible tissue loss would seem preferable to simply measuring its end result.

Quantitative structural and metabolic MRI techniques

Quantitative MR-based techniques, including magnetization transfer (MT) (Ropele and Fazekas, 2009) and diffusion tensor (DT) (Rovaris et al., 2009) MRI, can quantify the extent and improve the characterization of the nature of structural changes occurring within and outside focal MS lesions. Proton MR spectroscopy (^{1}H-MRS) (Sajja et al., 2009) can add information on the biochemical nature of such abnormalities. T2 hypointense areas and reduced T2 relaxation time are thought to reflect iron deposition, which is believed to be a sign of neurodegeneration.

MT MRI

MT MRI is based on the interactions between protons in free fluid and protons bound to macromolecules (Wolff and Balaban, 1994). MT MRI allows the calculation of an index, the MT ratio (MTR), which, when reduced, indicates a diminished capacity of the protons bound to the brain tissue matrix to exchange magnetization with the surrounding free water. As a consequence, this index provides an estimate of the extent of MS tissue disruption. Variable degrees of MTR reduction have been reported in acute and chronic MS lesions, with the most prominent changes found in T1-hypointense lesions. Several studies with serial scanning showed that at least in some lesions dramatic changes in normal-appearing (NA) WM areas can be seen days to weeks before the development of enhancing lesions (Filippi et al., 2011b). This observation suggests that, prior to the MRI-visible inflammatory activity, there are focal changes in the tissue, which precede the occurrence of lesion formation. Such abnormalities could include changes in the amount of unbound water caused by edema, astrocytic proliferation, early myelin injury, or axonal loss (Allen and McKeown, 1979; van Waesberghe et al., 1999; Evangelou et al., 2000).

Reduced MTR values have been found in NAWM and GM of MS patients, including those with CIS. Such MT MRI abnormalities are more severe in patients with the progressive clinical phenotypes and tend to worsen over time (Filippi et al., 2011b). MT MRI changes in the NAWM and GM correlate with the severity of clinical disability and cognitive impairment (Amato et al., 2008). In addition, in patients with relapse-onset MS, GM MTR was found to be an independent predictor of cognitive deterioration over the subsequent 13 years (Filippi et al., 2013a). In PPMS patients, GM MTR decline was shown to reflect the rate of clinical deterioration over 3 years (Khaleeli et al., 2008a) and it was the best predictor of poor cognitive performance after 5.5 years (Penny et al., 2010).

Voxel-wise procedures have been applied to track longitudinal changes of MTR values within individual, newly formed MS lesions, and to map the regional distribution of microscopic damage to the NAWM and GM. Chen et al. (2008) developed a method to monitor the evolution of MTR changes of individual lesion voxels and found significant changes of lesional MTR consistent with demyelination and remyelination that followed different temporal evolutions and which were still present in some lesions 3 years after their formation. Recently, a postmortem study reported the correlation between MTR values and focal cortical demyelination, supporting the notion that this technique is sensitive to demyelination/remyelination processes also in the cortex (Chen et al., 2013). MTR decreases in cortical regions are correlated with clinical disability and Paced Auditory Serial Addition Task (PASAT) performance in patients with PPMS (Khaleeli et al., 2007) and RRMS (Ranjeva et al., 2005).

DT MRI

Diffusion-weighted MRI is a quantitative technique that exploits the diffusion of water within biologic tissues (Le Bihan et al., 2001). The diffusion coefficient measures the ease of this translational motion of water. In biologic tissues this coefficient is lower than that in free water because the various structures of the tissues (e.g., membranes, macromolecules) impede the free movement of water molecules (Le Bihan et al., 2001). For this reason, the measured diffusion coefficient in biologic systems is referred to as the apparent diffusion coefficient (ADC) (Le Bihan et al., 2001). Pathologic processes that alter tissue integrity typically reduce the impediments to free-water motion and, as a result, these processes tend to increase the measured ADC values. A full characterization of diffusion can be provided in terms of a tensor (Pierpaoli et al., 2001), which has a principal axis and two smaller axes that describe its width and depth. The diffusivity along the principal axis is also called parallel or axial diffusivity, while the diffusivities in the two minor axes are often averaged to produce a measure of radial diffusivity. It is also possible to calculate the magnitude of diffusion, reflected by the mean diffusivity, and the degree of anisotropy, which is a measure of tissue organization that can be expressed by several indexes, including a dimensionless one, named fractional anisotropy (FA). Clearly, the different and heterogeneous pathologic elements of MS have the potential to alter the microarchitecture of brain tissue, influencing water diffusion in the CNS. In particular, axonal damage has been shown to alter predominantly FA and axial diffusivity (Pierpaoli et al., 2001), while myelin breakdown has been associated with an increased radial diffusivity (Pierpaoli et al., 2001; Wheeler-Kingshott and Cercignani, 2009).

In line with MT MRI findings, DT MRI studies confirmed the heterogeneity of MS-related damage to T2 lesions, NAWM, and GM, and showed that DT MRI abnormalities may precede lesion formation. In ring-enhancing lesions, a peripheral diffusion restriction (low ADC) is more common in MS lesion than in brain tumors/abscesses, which may reflect intramyelinic edema, myelin vacuolation, or water movement reduction due to the fiber tract organization disruption (Abou Zeid et al., 2012). Using DT MRI, an increased FA has been found in CLs of MS patients, suggesting local loss of dendrites and microglial activation (Poonawalla et al., 2008; Calabrese et al., 2011; Filippi et al., 2013c).

DT MRI abnormalities of the NAWM, cortex, and deep GM nuclei are present from the earliest stages of MS and become more pronounced with increasing disease duration and neurologic impairment (Rovaris et al., 2009). In addition, longitudinal DT MRI studies (Rovaris et al., 2002a, 2005, 2006; Oreja-Guevara et al., 2005) demonstrated a worsening of GM damage over time in patients with RRMS (Oreja-Guevara et al., 2005), SPMS, and PPMS (Rovaris et al., 2002a, 2005, 2006). The severity of GM damage has been correlated with the degree of cognitive impairment in mildly disabled RRMS patients (Rovaris et al., 2002b), and has been found to predict accumulation of disability over a 5-year period in patients with PPMS (Rovaris et al., 2006).

Several approaches have been developed to investigate damage to selected WM tracts, with the ultimate goal of improving the correlation with clinical measures. These approaches include the use of DT tractography, and the quantification of abnormalities at a voxel level, by means of voxel-based or tract-based spatial statistics (TBSS) analyses. In patients with CIS and definite MS, diffusivity measures of the corticospinal tract (CST) correlate with clinical measures of motor impairment (Wilson et al., 2003; Lin et al., 2005; Pagani et al., 2005). Using TBSS, FA (Giorgio et al., 2010), and radial diffusivity (Kern et al., 2011), abnormalities of the CC and CST have been related to clinical disability in RRMS patients. In patients with optic neuritis, reduced structural connectivity values in the optic radiations compared with controls have been shown (Ciccarelli et al., 2005). Reduced FA values in optic radiations correlate with retinal nerve fiber layer thinning (Reich et al., 2009; Dasenbrock et al., 2011). Diffusivity abnormalities in optic radiations have been related to transsynaptic degeneration secondary to optic nerve damage and Wallerian degeneration due to local lesions in a recent study in which patients were classified according to the presence of previous optic neuritis and lesions along these tracts (Rocca et al., 2013a). Another DT MRI study (Mesaros et al., 2009) showed that CC damage is more pronounced in BMS patients with cognitive impairment in comparison with those without (Fig. 20.5). Similarly, in a group of 69 MS patients with different clinical phenotypes, CC DT MRI abnormalities were related to the Multiple Sclerosis Functional Composite and PASAT scores (Ozturk et al., 2010). Two TBSS studies (Dineen et al., 2009; Roosendaal et al., 2009a) have found a correlation of impaired attention, working memory, and speed of information processing with decreased FA in the CC and other tracts mainly connecting prefrontal cortical regions.

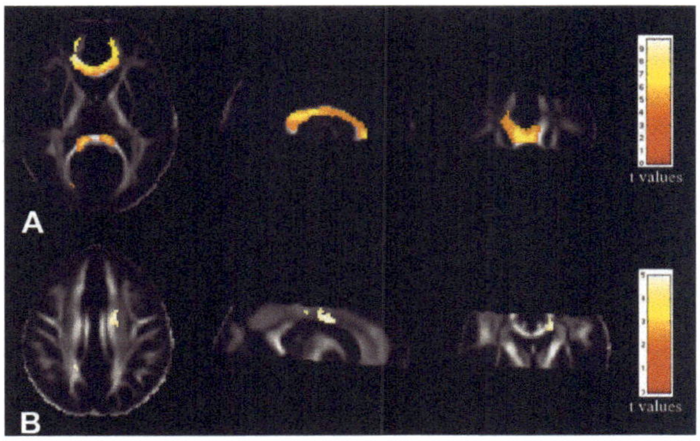

Fig. 20.5. Statistical parametric mapping analysis (color-coded for *t* values) of corpus callosum (CC) regions with increased mean diffusivity (MD) in: (**A**) benign multiple sclerosis (BMS) patients ($n=54$) vs healthy controls ($n=21$). Compared with controls, BMS patients showed a diffuse increase of CC MD, which was more pronounced in the genu; (**B**) BMS patients with ($n=9$) vs without ($n=45$) cognitive impairment. In comparison to patients with cognitive preservation, those cognitively impaired had significant clusters of increased MD in the body and left genu of the CC. Image orientation follows the neurologic convention. (Reproduced from Mesaros et al., 2009, with permission.)

Advances in DT MRI and tractography have spurred the development of brain neuroconnectivity techniques, which define and quantify anatomic links between remote brain regions by axonal fiber pathways (Guye et al., 2010). The use of these approaches has revealed reduced network efficiency in the WM structural networks of MS patients (Shu et al., 2011; Bozzali et al., 2013), including those at the earliest stages of the disease (Li et al., 2013).

^{1}H-MR SPECTROSCOPY

Water-suppressed, proton MR spectra of the healthy human brain at long echo times reveal four major resonances: choline-containing phospholipids (Cho), creatine and phosphocreatine (Cr), *N*-acetyl groups, mainly *N*-acetylaspartate (NAA), and lactate (Lac). Because NAA is a metabolite that is found almost exclusively in neurons and neuronal processes in the normal adult brain, a decrease in its concentration is thought to be secondary to axonal dysfunction, injury, or loss. By contrast, increases in Cho and Lac are thought to reflect acute inflammatory and demyelinating changes. ^{1}H-MRS with shorter echo times can detect additional metabolites, such as lipids and myo-inositol (mI), which are also thought to indicate ongoing myelin damage and glial proliferation, respectively.

Using ^{1}H-MRS, dynamic changes in metabolite profiles have been shown in NAWM areas which will become lesion (Narayana et al., 1998) and in acute MS lesions, extending from the first days of lesion formation over the subsequent months (Sajja et al., 2009). Several studies have found metabolite abnormalities, including reduced levels of NAA and Cho (a marker of membrane turnover), and increased levels of mI in the NAWM, cortex (Sharma et al., 2001; Chard et al., 2002a; Sarchielli et al., 2002), and subcortical GM tissue (Cifelli et al., 2002; Adalsteinsson et al., 2003; Inglese et al., 2004; Geurts et al., 2006) from MS patients, including those with CIS (Filippi et al., 2003; Fernando et al., 2004). A reduced concentration of glutamate-glutamine in the cortex of PPMS patients has also been detected, which was found to be significantly correlated with the EDSS score (Sastre-Garriga et al., 2005).

Significant correlations have also been found between NAA decrease in frontal regions and executive function performance (Staffen et al., 2005), as well as between decreased NAA in the pontine locus coeruleus and attentional deficits (Gadea et al., 2004). NAWM mI increase within 3 months of a CIS has been found to predict a poor performance on executive functions 7 years later (Summers et al., 2008b). A recent investigation (Tur et al., 2014) characterized metabolic abnormalities along the CST in MS patients using a novel application of chemical shift imaging and considering the spatial variation of metabolite levels. RRMS patients showed a higher CST Cho concentration than controls, and a higher CST mI concentration than PPMS, suggesting greater inflammation and glial proliferation in the RR than in the PP course. In RRMS, the association found between increased mI concentration and more severe disability suggested that gliosis may be relevant to the accumulation of disability. In PPMS, lower CST Cho and Cr concentrations correlated with more severe disability, suggesting that in the progressive stage of the disease, inflammation and energy metabolism are reduced.

A longitudinal study showed that whole-brain NAA declines significantly (5%/year) in RRMS patients over a 2-year time period (Rigotti et al., 2012). Another study (Kirov et al., 2013) assessed longitudinally for 3 years the metabolic abnormalities in the GM and WM from early RRMS, and found that WM Cr, Cho, and mI concentrations were higher while WM NAA was lower at all the time points in RRMS compared to controls. No difference was found in GM metabolites.

Inglese et al. (2010) showed the feasibility of sodium MRI at 3.0 T in RRMS patients. In this study, an increased sodium concentration in lesions, NAWM, and GM in MS patients compared to controls was found. Metabolic abnormalities were related to the extent of T2 lesions and the severity of clinical impairment. Recently, Steen et al. (2013) found a decreased axonal mitochondrial metabolism (NAA/Cr ratio) using ^{1}H-MRS and an increased astrocytic phosphocreatine metabolism (PCr/β-ATP ratio) using phosphorus (^{31}P) MRS in the centrum semiovale of 25 MS patients.

Imaging iron deposition

Abnormal iron deposition is thought to be the substrate of T2 hypointense areas and reduced T2 relaxation time seen in the basal ganglia, thalamus, dentate nucleus, and cortical regions of MS patients (Neema et al., 2007), including those with BMS (Ceccarelli et al., 2009) and CIS (Ceccarelli et al., 2010). In pediatric MS, T2 hypointensity seems to occur only in the head of the left caudate nucleus and is correlated with T2 lesion volume (Ceccarelli et al., 2011), suggesting that such an abnormality might be, at least partially, secondary to WM damage. In adult patients with MS, GM T2 hypointensities have been correlated with the severity of clinical disability and cognitive impairment (Bermel et al., 2005; Neema et al., 2007), as well as with clinical progression (Neema et al., 2009; Zhang et al., 2010).

The ability to detect abnormal iron deposition increased with the availability of 3.0 T scanners. Higher basal ganglia transverse relaxation rate (R2*) values were found in RRMS than in CIS patients (Khalil et al., 2009). Increased magnetic field correlation was demonstrated in the deep GM of RRMS patients, which was associated with the T2 lesion burden and severity of neuropsychologic deficits (Ge et al., 2007).

Susceptibility-weighted imaging has also been used to assess iron concentration in MS and confirmed the presence of an abnormal iron concentration in the deep GM nuclei of MS patients compared to healthy controls (Haacke et al., 2010; Zivadinov et al., 2010).

Functional imaging techniques

Functional imaging techniques allow the assessment of hemodynamic abnormalities in MS patients and are improving the understanding of the role of cortical reorganization following tissue injury.

Perfusion MRI

Brain tissue perfusion can be estimated using either exogenous tracers (e.g., Gd chelates) or endogenous arterial water (arterial spin labeling). While enhancing MS lesions typically show an increased perfusion, chronic lesions are characterized by a decreased perfusion (Holland et al., 2012). Reduced perfusion has also been recently detected in CLs of RRMS patients (Peruzzo et al., 2013). Several studies demonstrated a diffuse hypoperfusion in the NAWM, cortex, and deep GM of patients with different clinical phenotypes (Inglese et al., 2007), including CIS (Varga et al., 2009). Reduced cortical perfusion is strongly related with the volume of WM lesions (Amann et al., 2012). Hypoperfusion of cortical and subcortical GM has been correlated with locomotor disability (Adhya et al., 2006) and neuropsychologic impairment (Inglese et al., 2008; Aviv et al., 2012; Francis et al., 2013).

Functional MRI

fMRI is a noninvasive technique which allows the study of CNS function, and definition of abnormal patterns of activation and/or functional connectivity (FC) caused by injury or disease. The signal changes seen during fMRI studies depend on the blood oxygenation level-dependent (BOLD) mechanism (Vanzetta and Grinvald, 1999), which, in turn, involves changes of the transverse magnetization relaxation time – either T2* in a gradient-echo sequence, or T2 in spin-echo sequence. Local increases in neuronal activity result in a rise of blood flow and oxygen consumption. The increase in blood flow is greater than the oxygen consumption, thus determining an increased ratio between oxygenated and deoxygenated hemoglobin, which enhances the MRI signal (Ogawa et al., 1993). By analyzing these data with appropriate statistical methods, it is possible to obtain information about the location and extent of activation as well as connectivity of specific areas involved in the performance of a given task in healthy subjects and in patients with different neurologic conditions. Recently, a completely task-free approach, based on the assessment of functional correlations of neural networks at rest (resting-state fMRI) has been developed (for a review, see Biswal, 2012, and Filippi et al., 2013d).

Functional cortical abnormalities have been demonstrated consistently in all MS phenotypes using different active paradigms. The correlation found by the majority of these studies between measures of abnormal activations and quantitative MR metrics of disease burden suggests that, at least at some stages of the disease, functional reorganization might play an adaptive role which limits the clinical consequences of disease-related structural damage. The results of a cross-sectional study of the motor network in patients with different clinical MS phenotypes (Rocca et al., 2005) support the notion of a "natural history" of brain adaptive mechanisms in MS. Such a study showed, at the beginning of the disease, an increased recruitment of those areas "normally" devoted to the performance of a motor task, such as the primary sensorimotor cortex and the supplementary motor area. At a later stage, a bilateral activation of these regions is seen, followed by a widespread recruitment of additional areas, which are usually recruited in normal people to perform novel/complex tasks. The preservation of a focused and strictly lateralized movement-associated pattern of cortical activations has been suggested as a possible mechanism to explain the favorable clinical outcome of patients with pediatric MS (Rocca et al., 2009a) and BMS (Rocca et al., 2010a).

There is also evidence supporting a maladaptive role of cortical functional abnormalities in MS. In patients with progressive MS (Filippi et al., 2002; Rocca et al., 2002, 2010a), reduced activations of "classic" regions of the sensorimotor network and an increased recruitment of "high-order" regions, such as the superior temporal sulcus and the insula, have been found with motor tasks. In patients with cognitive decline, a "reallocation" of neuronal resources and an inefficiency of neuronal processes have been associated with the extent of structural damage. In RRMS patients, an abnormal recruitment of several areas of the motor network, including the thalamus and the cingulum, has been associated with the presence of fatigue (Fig. 20.6) (Rocca et al., 2007a).

The combination of measures of FC with measures of structural damage to specific WM tracts is likely to improve our understanding of the relationship between structural and functional abnormalities, as suggested by studies in patients with RRMS (Rocca et al., 2007b) and BMS (Rocca et al., 2009c).

Recently, the analysis of brain activity at rest has shown an increased synchronization of the majority of the resting-state networks in patients with CIS (Roosendaal et al., 2010), a reduced activity of the anterior regions of the default-mode network in patients with progressive MS (Bonavita et al., 2011) and cognitive impairment (Rocca et al., 2010c), and a complex reorganization of the visual network in normal-sighted patients who recovered from a previous optic neuritis (Gallo et al., 2012). Distributed abnormalities of resting-state FC within and between large-scale neuronal networks have been shown in RRMS patients and have been related to the extent of T2 lesions and severity of disability (Rocca et al., 2012).

Active and resting-state fMRI have also been applied to assess modifications of the patterns of activations and FC following cognitive rehabilitation in a few single-center studies (Sastre-Garriga et al., 2011; Filippi et al., 2012a). A recent study demonstrated that changes in resting-state FC of cognitive-related networks contribute to the persistence of the effects of cognitive rehabilitation after 6 months in RRMS patients (Parisi et al., 2014).

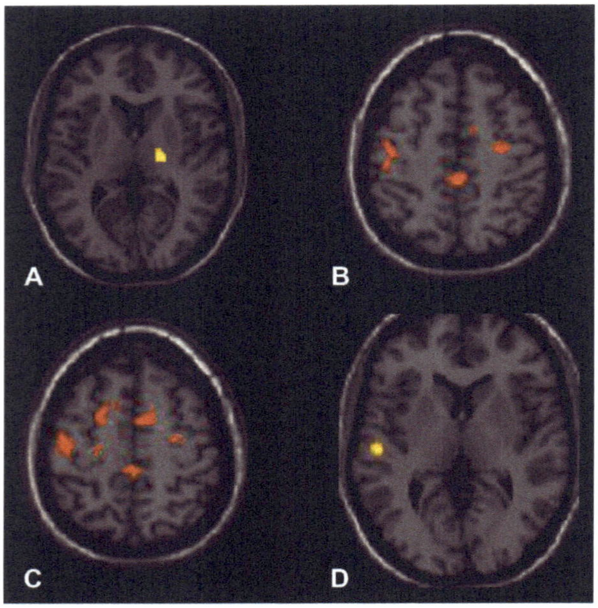

Fig. 20.6. Differences in cortical and deep gray-matter activations in multiple sclerosis (MS) patients with reversible fatigue following weekly interferon beta-1a administration vs MS patients treated with the same drug without fatigue, during the performance of a simple motor task with their clinically unimpaired, fully normal functioning, and dominant right hands. Compared to MS patients without fatigue (**A–C**), those complaining of reversible fatigue had an increased recruitment of the ipsilateral thalamus (**A**), cingulate motor area (**B** and **C**), bilateral middle frontal gyrus (**B** and **C**), primary sensorimotor cortex (**B** and **C**), and the supplementary motor area, bilaterally (**B** and **C**) when fatigue was present. Compared to MS patients with reversible fatigue (**D**), those without had an increased activation of the contralateral secondary sensorimotor cortex (**D**). The activations have been superimposed on a high-resolution T1-weighted scan obtained from a single, healthy subject and normalized into standard statistical parametric mapping space (neurologic convention). (Reproduced from Rocca et al., 2007a, with permission.)

Positron emission tomography

Positron emission tomography (PET) is an imaging technique that uses radiolabeled molecules to provide information about function and metabolism of different tissues. This technique is based on the detection and quantification of pairs of gamma rays emitted indirectly by a positron-emitting radionuclide (tracer), which is introduced into the body on a biologically active molecule. Three-dimensional images of tracer concentration within the body are then constructed by computer analysis. Many radiotracers are used in PET to image tissue concentration of many types of molecules of interest in different neurologic conditions.

Functional abnormalities in MS patients have also been investigated using PET (Kiferle et al., 2011). A seminal investigation (Pozzilli et al., 1992) showed an association between CC atrophy and decreased metabolic activity, especially in the association cortices of the left hemisphere. Sorensen et al. (2006) found a reduced cerebral metabolic rate of glucose in the cortex, putamen, thalamus, and hippocampus, which was correlated with cognitive impairment and T2 lesion load. A decreased metabolism of cerebral glucose in several frontal areas, the putamen, and caudate nuclei, as well as an increased glucose metabolism in the cerebellar vermis and anterior cingulate cortex, have been correlated to the severity of fatigue in MS (Roelcke et al., 1997). A 2-year longitudinal study (Blinkenberg et al., 1999) detected a decrease of global cortical metabolism, especially in frontal and parietal areas, which was not correlated with changes of T2 lesion load and clinical disability.

Other radioligands have been used to study patients with MS. Among them, [C11]-1(-2-chlorophenyl)-*N*-methyl-*N*-(-1methylpropyl)-3-isoquinolinecarboxamide (11C-PK11195), which binds specifically to translocator protein 18 kDa, a protein that is upregulated upon exposure to various insults, might be useful to evaluate neuroinflammation and microglia activation. A recent PK11195 PET study (Politis et al., 2012) found that MS patients have increased cortical GM PK11195 binding relative to controls. This increase was correlated with disability in patients with SPMS, but not in those with RRMS. No binding in the WM was detected. Interestingly, the binding patterns suggested the presence of regional pathology, with involvement detected in the postcentral, middle frontal, anterior orbital, fusiform, and parahippocampal gyri. Patients with SPMS showed additional binding in the precentral, superior parietal, lingual and anterior superior, medial, and inferior temporal gyri. A preliminary study in 9 RRMS patients has suggested the potential of this technique to monitor the effects of disease-modifying treatments, by showing a significant decrease of PK11195 uptake in cortical GM and WM after a year of treatment with glatiramer acetate (Ratchford et al., 2012).

Recently, in order to better define the microstructural tissue abnormalities in SPMS, a selective radioligand to adenosine A2A receptor ([C11]-TMSX), which is a potent regulator of inflammation, has been used (Rissanen et al., 2013). Compared to controls, patients showed increased NAWM [C11]-TMSX values, which were correlated with the EDSS score.

Imaging the spinal cord

MRI features of MS cord lesions have been identified (Lycklama et al., 2003). MS cord lesions are more frequently observed in the cervical than in other regions, are usually peripheral, limited to two vertebral segments in length or less, occupy less than half the cross-sectional area of the cord, and typically are not T1-hypointense (Fig. 20.7) (Lycklama et al., 2003). Asymptomatic spinal cord lesions have been described in 30–40% of CIS patients and in up to 90% of patients with definite MS (Lycklama et al., 2003). A set of new strategies has been proposed to improve the detection of spinal cord lesions, including the use of an axial 3D gradient-echo sequence with or without MT prepulse (Ozturk et al., 2013), and of an optimized T1 magnetization-prepared rapid-acquisition gradient-echo (MPRAGE) sequence (Nair et al., 2013).

Although a significant reduction of cervical cord size can be observed since the early phase of MS (Brex et al., 2001), cord atrophy is more severe in the progressive forms of the disease (Lycklama et al., 2003). Abnormalities at a given time point and changed time of cord cross-sectional area correlate better with clinical disability than changes of T2 lesion burden (Losseff et al., 1996). A new semiautomatic method (Horsfield et al., 2010), which allows segmentation of long portions of the cord, has been recently developed. The use of this method in a multicenter study of a large sample of MS patients has demonstrated that cord area differs significantly among the main MS clinical phenotypes and is correlated with the EDSS, with a differential effect among phenotypes: no association in either CIS or BMS patients; association in RRMS, SPMS, and PPMS (Rocca et al., 2011). A voxel-wise approach has also been applied to define the regional distribution of cervical cord damage of MS patients. While RRMS patients had a few clusters of regional atrophy, mainly located in the posterior and lateral columns, SPMS patients experienced a diffuse cord atrophy, which was significantly correlated with the EDSS score (Valsasina et al., 2013).

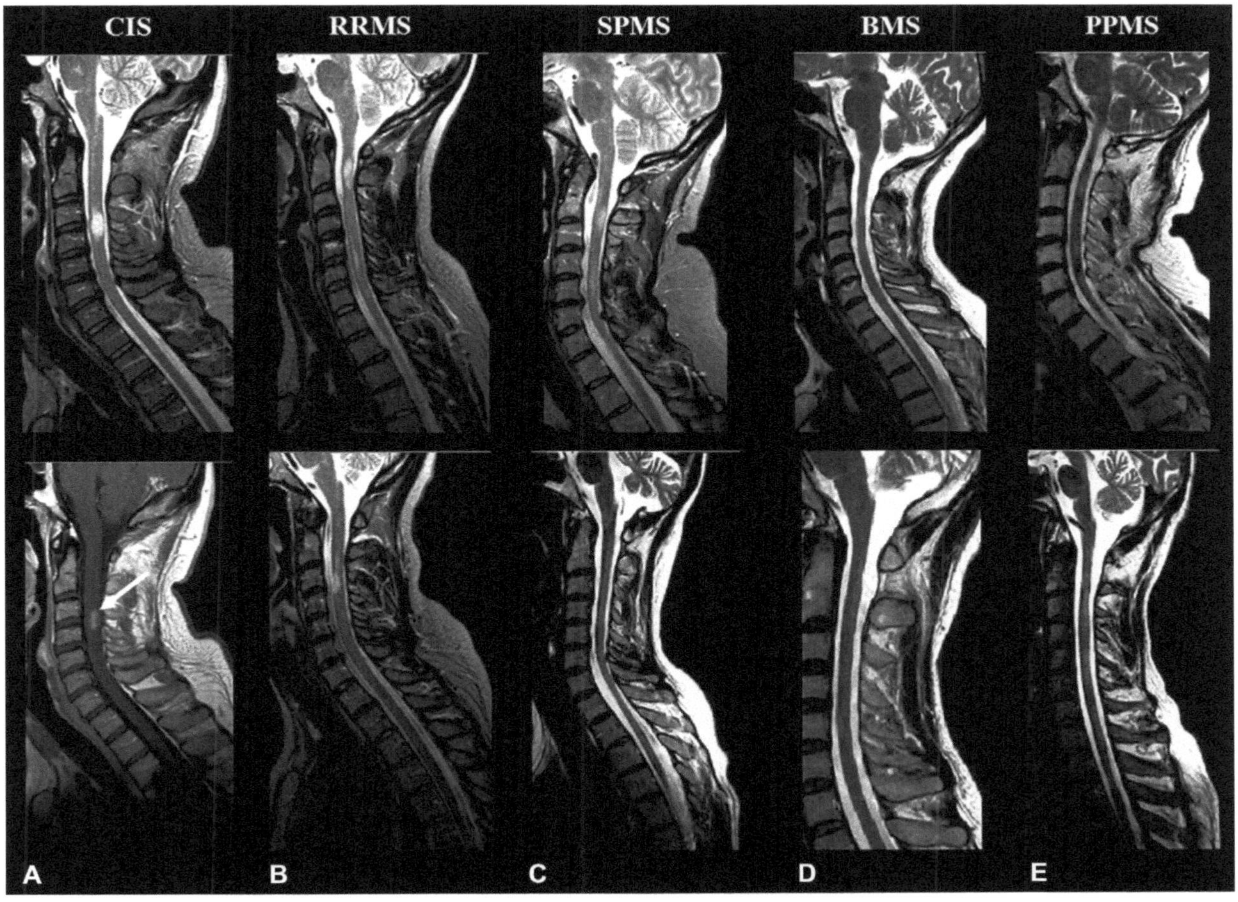

Fig. 20.7. Sagittal magnetic resonance images from the spinal cord of multiple sclerosis (MS) patients with different clinical phenotypes. (**A**) In a clinically isolated syndrome (CIS) patient, a focal, oval-shape lesion, hyperintense on T2-weighted scan and enhancing after gadolinium administration (white arrow) is visible at C3–C4. (**B**) In relapsing-remitting MS (RRMS), several oval-shape T2-hyperintense cervical cord lesions are visible. In both secondary progressive (SPMS: **C**) and primary progressive MS (PPMS: **E**), several T2 hyperintense lesions are evident, which are associated with some degree of spinal cord atrophy. In a patient with benign MS (BMS: **D**), no focal T2-hyperintense lesions are detectable.

A more recent study found no cord atrophy in CIS patients vs healthy controls, while PPMS had significant cord atrophy. Clusters of cord atrophy were found in BMS vs RRMS, and in SPMS vs RRMS, BMS, and PPMS patients, mainly involving the posterior and lateral cord segments. Cord lesion probability maps showed a significantly greater likelihood of cord abnormalities in RRMS, PPMS, and SPMS than in CIS and BMS patients. In progressive MS, regional cord atrophy was correlated with clinical disability and impairment of the pyramidal system (Rocca et al., 2013b; Valsasina et al., 2013).

MTR can also be measured in the cervical cord (Bozzali et al., 1999; Filippi et al., 2000; Rovaris et al., 2000, 2004; Bot et al., 2004; Charil et al., 2006a). A reduction of MTR of the cervical cord has been described in all phenotypes of the disease, except for CIS. These changes have been suggested to correlate with disability (Rovaris et al., 2001; Charil et al., 2006a). A study showed that MTR abnormalities located in the dorsal and lateral columns of the spinal cord correlate with deficits of vibration sensation and strength, respectively (Zackowski et al., 2009). In patients with RRMS, reduced cervical cord GM average MTR was correlated with the degree of disability (Agosta et al., 2007b).

Abnormal DT MRI quantities from the cervical cord have been shown in patients with definite MS, but not in those with CIS (Agosta and Filippi, 2007). A 2-year follow-up study of patients with relapse-onset MS found that baseline cord area and FA correlated with increased disability at follow-up (Agosta et al., 2007a). Compared to controls, MS patients with a cervical cord relapse have reduced NAA and lower structural connectivity in the lateral CST and posterior tracts, and such abnormalities were found to be correlated with disability (Ciccarelli et al., 2007). Recently, diffusional kurtosis imaging has been developed to assess non-Gaussian diffusion in cervical cord from MS patient. This approach provided a more comprehensive evaluation, in particular, of GM cord pathology (Raz et al., 2013). A cross-sectional study which combined different MR modalities (DT MRI, MTR, and atrophy) to quantify cervical cord damage in a large sample of MS patients showed that a multiparametric MR approach contributes to discriminate patients with high from those with low levels of disability (Oh et al., 2013).

An increased fMRI activation of the cervical cord has been demonstrated in all major MS clinical phenotypes and has been related to the severity of clinical disability and the extent of tissue damage (Agosta et al., 2009; Valsasina et al., 2010).

Imaging the optic nerve

In acute monophasic optic neuritis, the most sensitive conventional MR sequences are short tau inversion recovery, fast spin-echo T2-weighted, and spin-echo T1-weighted pre- and post-Gd fat-suppressed. Using these sequences, the causative lesion can be frequently identified (Glisson and Galetta, 2009). Additional typical findings include dilation of the optic nerve sheath immediately posterior to the globe on fat-saturated fast spin-echo sequences, and optic nerve sheath enhancement on T1-weighted postcontrast scans (Glisson and Galetta, 2009) (Fig. 20.8).

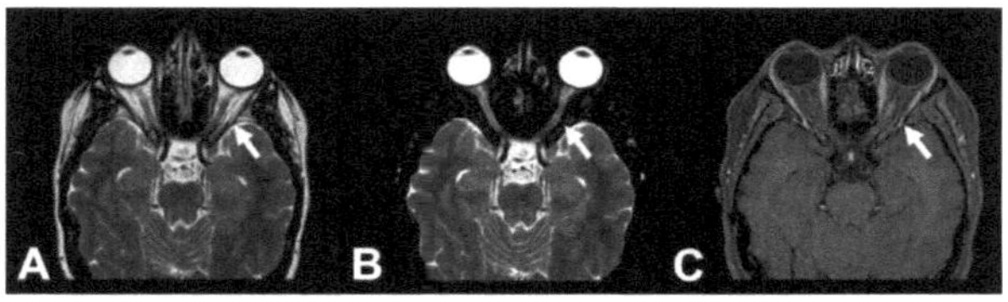

Fig. 20.8. Axial T2-weighted (**A**), T2-weighted with fat suppression (**B**) spin-echo and postcontrast T1-weighted (**C**) magnetic resonance images of the brain from a 25-year-old patient at presentation with clinically isolated syndrome suggestive of multiple sclerosis, characterized by left optic neuritis. In (**A**) and (**B**), a hyperintensity in the intraorbitary part of the left optic nerve is visible (white arrow). In (**B**), this portion of the optic nerve is contrast-enhanced (white arrow).

In a study of patients with an initial episode of unilateral optic neuritis, the mean cross-sectional area of the intraorbital portion of the optic nerve was lower in diseased eyes than in the fellow eyes and in the eyes of healthy controls (Hickman et al., 2001).

MTR can also be measured in the optic nerve and used to study longitudinally optic nerve damage (Thorpe et al., 1995; Inglese et al., 2002; Hickman et al., 2004; Melzi et al., 2007). MTR of the optic nerve correlates with the visual evoked potentials P100 latency (Thorpe et al., 1995) and with the degree of visual function recovery after an acute episode of optic neuritis (Inglese et al., 2002), even if there is no perfect agreement among studies (Hickman et al., 2004).

Full DT measurements from the optic nerve have been obtained (Hickman et al., 2005; Trip et al., 2006). In patients in the chronic phase following optic neuritis, mean diffusivity of the diseased optic nerve was significantly higher than in the healthy contralateral eye (Hickman et al., 2005). A multiparametric MRI study showed that, 4 years after a unilateral optic neuritis, MRI measures of optic nerve structural abnormalities (decreased FA and volume) are independently associated with visual dysfunction (Kolbe et al., 2009).

Ultrahigh-field imaging

Magnets operating at 3.0–4.0 T detect a greater number and volume of MS T2 and enhancing brain lesions than those operating at 1.5 T. However, one study compared the performance of the MRI diagnostic criteria for MS at 1.5 T and 3.0 T in CIS patients and found that, despite an increased lesion detection, 3.0 T imaging led only to a little gain in terms of showing DIS (Wattjes et al., 2008). The use of DIR imaging at 3.0 T has resulted in a higher detection of infratentorial lesions compared to FLAIR and T2-weighted sequences in patients with CIS and definite MS (Wattjes et al., 2007).

Ultrahigh-field MRI (7.0 T or more) provides a better definition of lesion location in the WM and GM, their morphology, and their association with vasculature (Ge et al., 2008; Hammond et al., 2008; Tallantyre et al., 2008). Using 7.0 T T2*-weighted MRI, the presence of a central vein in more than 40% of lesions contributed to discriminate patients with from those without definite MS (Tallantyre et al., 2011; Mistry et al., 2013). This finding was found to be more predictive of MS than the presence of subcortical or periventricular lesions (Tallantyre et al., 2011). Susceptibility-weighted imaging (examining both T2*-weighted magnitude and phase) has been used to detect features that may be more closely linked to important aspects of MS pathology. Myelin, iron, deoxyhemoglobin, and free radicals influence susceptibility due to their paramagnetic properties and can thereby determine image contrast. Several combined susceptibility MRI-pathologic studies have shown that the presence of a hypointense rim on T2*/phase contrast in chronic MS lesions appears to be influenced by the topography of iron-laden macrophages and ferritin at the lesion's edge (Pitt et al., 2010; Bagnato et al., 2011; Mehta et al., 2013). Another advantage of ultrahigh-field MRI is an increased susceptibility to local field shifts from iron, which has allowed the demonstration of an increased local field in the caudate, putamen, and globus pallidus of MS patients relative to control subjects (Hammond et al., 2008).

The cortical cyto- and myelo-architecture (Duyn et al., 2007; Cohen-Adad et al., 2012) as well as location and characteristics of CLs can also be visualized accurately at these field strengths in postmortem brain samples (Kangarlu et al., 2007; Pitt et al., 2010; Schmierer et al., 2010) and *in vivo* (Mainero et al., 2009; Tallantyre et al., 2010; Bluestein et al., 2012; de Graaf et al., 2012; Nielsen et al., 2012; Kilsdonk et al., 2013). Using a 7.0 T scanner, Mainero et al. (2009) were able to identify *in vivo* the three major CL patterns (type I: leukocortical; type II: intracortical, and type III/IV: subpial, extending partly or completely through the cortical layers) described histopathologically. Such a characterization of CL subtypes might contribute to identify novel biomarkers of MS clinical status, as suggested by the recent demonstration that leukocortical (type I) and subpial (III–IV) CLs are correlated with cognitive impairment and disability (Nielsen et al., 2013).

Ultrahigh-field MRI has also the potential to improve quantitative, metabolic, and fMRI studies of MS. A ^{1}H-MRS study at 7.0 T (Srinivasan et al., 2010) was able to quantify the concentration of glutathione, a marker of oxidative status, in the NAWM and GM from healthy controls and MS patients. In healthy controls, the concentration of glutathione was higher in the GM than the WM, and MS patients had a significant reduction of glutathione concentration in macroscopic lesions and the GM, but not in the NAWM, when compared to healthy individuals.

A novel approach, called diffusion tensor spectroscopy, which combines features of DT imaging and ^{1}H-MRS, has been developed to investigate the diffusion properties of intracellular, cell type-specific metabolites (Wood et al., 2012). A cross-sectional pilot study (Wood et al., 2012), which measured the diffusion of the NAA in the normal-appearing CC at 7.0 T, found that it was decreased in MS patients in comparison to healthy controls and that it was inversely correlated with clinical disability.

MRI IN THE MONITORING OF MS TREATMENT

In MS patients, disease activity is detected much more frequently on MRI scans than with clinical assessment of relapses. This is the main reason why MRI measures are used for monitoring response to treatment. In the context of clinical trials, MRI is used as a primary outcome measure in phase II studies, where serial scans (usually monthly) are acquired to detect disease activity (new or enlarged T2 lesions, total enhancing and new enhancing lesions, and enhancing lesion volume) (Barkhof et al., 1997b). In phase III trials, given the uncertainty of conventional MRI in predicting clinical evolution, imaging measures (absolute or percentage increases in total T2 lesion load) are used as secondary outcomes, and typically performed on yearly scans (Filippi et al., 1998b). Despite this, two studies showed that conventional MRI quantities are valid surrogate markers of clinical activity (Goodin, 2006; Sormani et al., 2009a). In addition, recent meta-analyses (Sormani and Bruzzi, 2013) of randomized, placebo-controlled clinical trials of RRMS found a strong correlation between treatment effect on relapse and MRI activity, which was weaker when considering EDSS worsening.

Because of its biologic and clinical relevance and its ease of measurement, brain atrophy has been proposed as a marker of neuroprotection in MS clinical trials (Barkhof et al., 2009). Most disease-modifying drugs seem to have a delayed effect on the rate of brain atrophy, and the optimal approach for use of atrophy measurements in trials and research studies is still under investigation. A recent meta-analysis of randomized clinical trials in RRMS lasting at least 2 years has found that the treatment effect on brain atrophy is correlated with the effect on disability progression over such a period of time. This effect is independent of the effect of active MRI lesions on disability. Importantly, the two MRI measures predicted treatment effect on disability more closely when used in combination, suggesting that they allow monitoring of different disease-related pathologic processes (Sormani et al., 2014). A measure that has been proposed as a tool to monitor neuroprotection is based on the assessment of the evolution of active lesions into permanent black holes (PBH), which correspond to areas of severe and irreversible tissue damage. While studies with glatiramer acetate, interferon, and natalizumab have shown that these treatments can modify, albeit with different magnitudes, the percentage of active lesions evolving into PBH (Filippi et al., 2001, 2011a; Dalton et al., 2004), BHT-3009, a DNA plasmid-encoding myelin basic protein that might induce antigen-specific tolerance, was found to have no effect on the evolution of new inflammatory lesions into PBH in RRMS patients (Papadopoulou et al., 2012).

Clearly, a rigorous and valid strategy for MR-based longitudinal monitoring of MS response to treatment requires the use of standardized imaging protocols (including consistency in slice thickness and imaging planes, field strength, and patient repositioning) and evaluation procedures. As a consequence, the definition of individual patient response to MS treatment based upon routine clinical MRI scanning remains a challenging task. Patients treated with interferon-beta who developed new MRI lesions after 2 years have a higher risk of poor treatment response than those who did not (Rudick et al., 2004). In patients with RRMS treated with interferon-beta, Rio et al. (2008) showed that the number of active MRI lesions detected on an MRI scan performed 12 months after treatment initiation was the most important factor related to the progression of disability after 2 years. In a subsequent study, the same group found that a combination of clinical and MRI measures of disease activity during the first year of treatment allows the identification of responders to interferon-beta treatment after 2 and 3 years (Rio et al., 2009). Tomassini et al. (2006) demonstrated that the formation of T1-hypointense and enhancing lesions during the first year of therapy with interferon-beta is associated with relapse rate and disability progression after 6 years. Based on the degree of clinical and MRI activity, guidelines have been proposed to identify responders to disease-modifying treatments (Freedman et al., 2004; Rio et al., 2009; Sormani and De Stefano, 2013).

The utility of advanced MR techniques in the context of clinical trial monitoring still needs to be validated. For instance, the acquisition of DIR sequences has not been standardized yet across different centers, and their performance has not been tested in the setting of MS clinical trials. MT MRI has been incorporated to provide additional outcome measures in limited subgroups of patients enrolled in trials. In particular, in patients with SPMS, a lack of effect of interferon-beta-1b (Inglese et al., 2003) on MT MRI quantities of the whole-brain tissue and NAWM was reported and the findings with intravenous immunoglobulins were equivocal (Filippi et al., 2004). One study used ^{1}H-MRS to assess the efficacy of glatiramer acetate in PPMS patients (Narayana et al., 2004), and at 3-year follow-up (Sajja et al., 2008) no significant difference in metabolite ratios between treated and placebo patients was found in lesions, NAWM, and GM. Only recently, the potential of DT MRI and fMRI in prospective multicenter studies has been assessed (Wegner et al., 2008; Rocca et al., 2009b; Pagani et al., 2010).

Laquinimod, a novel oral immunomodulator, is under study for treatment of MS. A recent investigation has evaluated several putative MR markers of brain tissue damage in patients treated with such a drug (Filippi et al., 2013b). Results of these exploratory study support the concept that laquinimod may reduce (at least in the initial phase of treatment) some of the most destructive pathologic processes in RRMS patients; compared with placebo, patients treated with laquinimod showed decreased rates of WM, GM, and thalamic atrophy, developed fewer PBH, and tended to accumulate less microscopic damage to the NABT, WM, and GM.

CONCLUSIONS

Conventional and advanced MR-based techniques have been applied extensively to the study of MS and such an effort has contributed to improve our ability to diagnose and monitor the disease, as well as our understanding of its pathophysiology and treatment efficacy. Nevertheless, many challenges remain. Quantitative, metabolic, and functional imaging techniques need to be optimized and standardized across multiple centers to monitor adequately disease evolution, either natural or modified by treatment. With the increased availability of high-field and ultrahigh-field MR scanners, such an issue is now becoming extremely critical. Furthermore, some of the MR approaches discussed here are in their infancy and their practical utility, from a research setting to daily-life clinical practice, still needs to be investigated.

References

Abou Zeid N, Pirko I, Erickson B et al. (2012). Diffusion-weighted imaging characteristics of biopsy-proven demyelinating brain lesions. Neurology 78: 1655–1662.

Absinta M, Sati P, Gaitan MI et al. (2013). Seven-tesla phase imaging of acute multiple sclerosis lesions: a new window into the inflammatory process. Ann Neurol 74: 669–678.

Adalsteinsson E, Langer-Gould A, Homer RJ et al. (2003). Gray matter N-acetyl aspartate deficits in secondary progressive but not relapsing-remitting multiple sclerosis. AJNR Am J Neuroradiol 24: 1941–1945.

Adhya S, Johnson G, Herbert J et al. (2006). Pattern of hemodynamic impairment in multiple sclerosis: dynamic susceptibility contrast perfusion MR imaging at 3.0 T. Neuroimage 33: 1029–1035.

Agosta F, Filippi M (2007). MRI of spinal cord in multiple sclerosis. J Neuroimaging 17: 46S–49S.

Agosta F, Absinta M, Sormani MP et al. (2007a). In vivo assessment of cervical cord damage in MS patients: a longitudinal diffusion tensor MRI study. Brain 130: 2211–2219.

Agosta F, Pagani E, Caputo D et al. (2007b). Associations between cervical cord gray matter damage and disability in patients with multiple sclerosis. Arch Neurol 64: 1302–1305.

Agosta F, Valsasina P, Absinta M et al. (2009). Primary progressive multiple sclerosis: tactile-associated functional MR activity in the cervical spinal cord. Radiology 253: 209–215.

Allen IV, McKeown SR (1979). A histological, histochemical and biochemical study of the macroscopically normal white matter in multiple sclerosis. J Neurol Sci 41: 81–91.

Amann M, Achtnichts L, Hirsch JG et al. (2012). 3D GRASE arterial spin labelling reveals an inverse correlation of cortical perfusion with the white matter lesion volume in MS. Mult Scler 18: 1570–1576.

Amato MP, Portaccio E, Goretti B et al. (2007). Association of neocortical volume changes with cognitive deterioration in relapsing-remitting multiple sclerosis. Arch Neurol 64: 1157–1161.

Amato MP, Portaccio E, Stromillo ML et al. (2008). Cognitive assessment and quantitative magnetic resonance metrics can help to identify benign multiple sclerosis. Neurology 71: 632–638.

Aviv RI, Francis PL, Tenenbein R et al. (2012). Decreased frontal lobe gray matter perfusion in cognitively impaired patients with secondary-progressive multiple sclerosis detected by the bookend technique. AJNR Am J Neuroradiol 33: 1779–1785.

Bagnato F, Hametner S, Yao B et al. (2011). Tracking iron in multiple sclerosis: a combined imaging and histopathological study at 7 Tesla. Brain 134: 3602–3615.

Barkhof F, Filippi M, Miller DH et al. (1997a). Comparison of MRI criteria at first presentation to predict conversion to clinically definite multiple sclerosis. Brain 120: 2059–2069.

Barkhof F, Filippi M, Miller DH et al. (1997b). Strategies for optimizing MRI techniques aimed at monitoring disease activity in multiple sclerosis treatment trials. J Neurol 244: 76–84.

Barkhof F, Filippi M, van Waesberghe JH et al. (1997c). Improving interobserver variation in reporting gadolinium-enhanced MRI lesions in multiple sclerosis. Neurology 49: 1682–1688.

Barkhof F, Calabresi PA, Miller DH et al. (2009). Imaging outcomes for neuroprotection and repair in multiple sclerosis trials. Nat Rev Neurol 5: 256–266.

Bendfeldt K, Radue EW, Borgwardt SJ et al. (2009). Progression of gray matter atrophy and its association with white matter lesions in relapsing-remitting multiple sclerosis. J Neurol Sci 285: 268–269. author reply 269.

Benedict RH, Bruce JM, Dwyer MG et al. (2006). Neocortical atrophy, third ventricular width, and cognitive dysfunction in multiple sclerosis. Arch Neurol 63: 1301–1306.

Bermel RA, Puli SR, Rudick RA et al. (2005). Prediction of longitudinal brain atrophy in multiple sclerosis by gray matter magnetic resonance imaging T2 hypointensity. Arch Neurol 62: 1371–1376.

Biswal BB (2012). Resting state fMRI: a personal history. Neuroimage 62: 938–944.

Blinkenberg M, Jensen CV, Holm S et al. (1999). A longitudinal study of cerebral glucose metabolism, MRI, and disability in patients with MS. Neurology 53: 149–153.

Bluestein KT, Pitt D, Sammet S et al. (2012). Detecting cortical lesions in multiple sclerosis at 7 T using white matter signal attenuation. Magn Reson Imaging 30: 907–915.

Bonavita S, Gallo A, Sacco R et al. (2011). Distributed changes in default-mode resting-state connectivity in multiple sclerosis. Mult Scler 17: 411–422.

Bot JC, Blezer EL, Kamphorst W et al. (2004). The spinal cord in multiple sclerosis: relationship of high-spatial-resolution quantitative MR imaging findings to histopathologic results. Radiology 233: 531–540.

Bozzali M, Rocca MA, Iannucci G et al. (1999). Magnetization-transfer histogram analysis of the cervical cord in patients with multiple sclerosis. AJNR Am J Neuroradiol 20: 1803–1808.

Bozzali M, Spano B, Parker GJ et al. (2013). Anatomical brain connectivity can assess cognitive dysfunction in multiple sclerosis. Mult Scler 19: 1161–1168.

Brex PA, Leary SM, O'Riordan JI et al. (2001). Measurement of spinal cord area in clinically isolated syndromes suggestive of multiple sclerosis. J Neurol Neurosurg Psychiatry 70: 544–547.

Brex PA, Ciccarelli O, O'Riordan JI et al. (2002). A longitudinal study of abnormalities on MRI and disability from multiple sclerosis. N Engl J Med 346: 158–164.

Calabrese M, De Stefano N, Atzori M et al. (2007). Detection of cortical inflammatory lesions by double inversion recovery magnetic resonance imaging in patients with multiple sclerosis. Arch Neurol 64: 1416–1422.

Calabrese M, Filippi M, Rovaris M et al. (2008). Morphology and evolution of cortical lesions in multiple sclerosis. A longitudinal MRI study. Neuroimage 42: 1324–1328.

Calabrese M, Agosta F, Rinaldi F et al. (2009a). Cortical lesions and atrophy associated with cognitive impairment in relapsing-remitting multiple sclerosis. Arch Neurol 66: 1144–1150.

Calabrese M, Filippi M, Rovaris M et al. (2009b). Evidence for relative cortical sparing in benign multiple sclerosis: a longitudinal magnetic resonance imaging study. Mult Scler 15: 36–41.

Calabrese M, Rocca MA, Atzori M et al. (2009c). Cortical lesions in primary progressive multiple sclerosis: a 2-year longitudinal MR study. Neurology 72: 1330–1336.

Calabrese M, Rocca M, Atzori M et al. (2010). A three-year MRI study of cortical lesions in relapse-onset multiple sclerosis. Ann Neurol 67: 376–383.

Calabrese M, Rinaldi F, Seppi D et al. (2011). Cortical diffusion-tensor imaging abnormalities in multiple sclerosis: a 3-year longitudinal study. Radiology 261: 891–898.

Calabrese M, Poretto V, Favaretto A et al. (2012). Cortical lesion load associates with progression of disability in multiple sclerosis. Brain 135: 2952–2961.

Caramanos Z, Francis SJ, Narayanan S et al. (2012). Large, nonplateauing relationship between clinical disability and cerebral white matter lesion load in patients with multiple sclerosis. Arch Neurol 69: 89–95.

Ceccarelli A, Rocca MA, Pagani E et al. (2008). A voxel-based morphometry study of grey matter loss in MS patients with different clinical phenotypes. Neuroimage 42: 315–322.

Ceccarelli A, Filippi M, Neema M et al. (2009). T2 hypointensity in the deep gray matter of patients with benign multiple sclerosis. Mult Scler 15: 678–686.

Ceccarelli A, Rocca MA, Neema M et al. (2010). Deep gray matter T2 hypointensity is present in patients with clinically isolated syndromes suggestive of multiple sclerosis. Mult Scler 16: 39–44.

Ceccarelli A, Rocca MA, Perego E et al. (2011). Deep grey matter T2 hypo-intensity in patients with paediatric multiple sclerosis. Mult Scler 17: 702–707.

Chard DT, Griffin CM, McLean MA et al. (2002a). Brain metabolite changes in cortical grey and normal-appearing white matter in clinically early relapsing-remitting multiple sclerosis. Brain 125: 2342–2352.

Chard DT, Griffin CM, Parker GJ et al. (2002b). Brain atrophy in clinically early relapsing-remitting multiple sclerosis. Brain 125: 327–337.

Charil A, Caputo D, Cavarretta R et al. (2006a). Cervical cord magnetization transfer ratio and clinical changes over 18 months in patients with relapsing-remitting multiple sclerosis: a preliminary study. Mult Scler 12: 662–665.

Charil A, Yousry TA, Rovaris M et al. (2006b). MRI and the diagnosis of multiple sclerosis: expanding the concept of "no better explanation". Lancet Neurol 5: 841–852.

Chen JT, Narayanan S, Collins DL et al. (2004). Relating neocortical pathology to disability progression in multiple sclerosis using MRI. Neuroimage 23: 1168–1175.

Chen JT, Collins DL, Atkins HL et al. (2008). Magnetization transfer ratio evolution with demyelination and remyelination in multiple sclerosis lesions. Ann Neurol 63: 254–262.

Chen JT, Easley K, Schneider C et al. (2013). Clinically feasible MTR is sensitive to cortical demyelination in MS. Neurology 80: 246–252.

Ciccarelli O, Toosy AT, Hickman SJ et al. (2005). Optic radiation changes after optic neuritis detected by tractography-based group mapping. Hum Brain Mapp 25: 308–316.

Ciccarelli O, Wheeler-Kingshott CA, McLean MA et al. (2007). Spinal cord spectroscopy and diffusion-based tractography to assess acute disability in multiple sclerosis. Brain 130: 2220–2231.

Cifelli A, Arridge M, Jezzard P et al. (2002). Thalamic neurodegeneration in multiple sclerosis. Ann Neurol 52: 650–653.

Cohen-Adad J, Polimeni JR, Helmer KG et al. (2012). T(2)* mapping and B(0) orientation-dependence at 7 T reveal cyto- and myeloarchitecture organization of the human cortex. Neuroimage 60: 1006–1014.

Dalton CM, Miszkiel KA, Barker GJ et al. (2004). Effect of natalizumab on conversion of gadolinium enhancing lesions to T1 hypointense lesions in relapsing multiple sclerosis. J Neurol 251: 407–413.

Dasenbrock HH, Smith SA, Ozturk A et al. (2011). Diffusion tensor imaging of the optic tracts in multiple sclerosis: association with retinal thinning and visual disability. J Neuroimaging 21: e41–e49.

de Graaf WL, Zwanenburg JJ, Visser F et al. (2012). Lesion detection at seven Tesla in multiple sclerosis using magnetisation prepared 3D-FLAIR and 3D-DIR. Eur Radiol 22: 221–231.

De Stefano N, Matthews PM, Filippi M et al. (2003). Evidence of early cortical atrophy in MS: relevance to white matter changes and disability. Neurology 60: 1157–1162.

De Stefano N, Giorgio A, Battaglini M et al. (2010). Assessing brain atrophy rates in a large population of untreated multiple sclerosis subtypes. Neurology 74: 1868–1876.

Dineen RA, Vilisaar J, Hlinka J et al. (2009). Disconnection as a mechanism for cognitive dysfunction in multiple sclerosis. Brain 132: 239–249.

Duyn JH, van Gelderen P, Li TQ et al. (2007). High-field MRI of brain cortical substructure based on signal phase. Proc Natl Acad Sci U S A 104: 11796–11801.

Evangelou N, Esiri MM, Smith S et al. (2000). Quantitative pathological evidence for axonal loss in normal appearing white matter in multiple sclerosis. Ann Neurol 47: 391–395.

Fernando KT, McLean MA, Chard DT et al. (2004). Elevated white matter myo-inositol in clinically isolated syndromes suggestive of multiple sclerosis. Brain 127: 1361–1369.

Filippi M, Rossi P, Campi A et al. (1997). Serial contrast-enhanced MR in patients with multiple sclerosis and varying levels of disability. AJNR Am J Neuroradiol 18: 1549–1556.

Filippi M, Gawne-Cain ML, Gasperini C et al. (1998a). Effect of training and different measurement strategies on the reproducibility of brain MRI lesion load measurements in multiple sclerosis. Neurology 50: 238–244.

Filippi M, Horsfield MA, Ader HJ et al. (1998b). Guidelines for using quantitative measures of brain magnetic resonance imaging abnormalities in monitoring the treatment of multiple sclerosis. Ann Neurol 43: 499–506.

Filippi M, Bozzali M, Horsfield MA et al. (2000). A conventional and magnetization transfer MRI study of the cervical cord in patients with MS. Neurology 54: 207–213.

Filippi M, Rovaris M, Rocca MA et al. (2001). Glatiramer acetate reduces the proportion of new MS lesions evolving into "black holes". Neurology 57: 731–733.

Filippi M, Rocca MA, Falini A et al. (2002). Correlations between structural CNS damage and functional MRI changes in primary progressive MS. Neuroimage 15: 537–546.

Filippi M, Bozzali M, Rovaris M et al. (2003). Evidence for widespread axonal damage at the earliest clinical stage of multiple sclerosis. Brain 126: 433–437.

Filippi M, Rocca MA, Pagani E et al. (2004). European study on intravenous immunoglobulin in multiple sclerosis: results of magnetization transfer magnetic resonance imaging analysis. Arch Neurol 61: 1409–1412.

Filippi M, Rocca MA, Calabrese M et al. (2010). Intracortical lesions: relevance for new MRI diagnostic criteria for multiple sclerosis. Neurology 75: 1988–1994.

Filippi M, Rocca MA, Camesasca F et al. (2011a). Interferon beta-1b and glatiramer acetate effects on permanent black hole evolution. Neurology 76: 1222–1228.

Filippi M, Rocca MA, De Stefano N et al. (2011b). Magnetic resonance techniques in multiple sclerosis: the present and the future. Arch Neurol 68: 1514–1520.

Filippi M, Riccitelli G, Mattioli F et al. (2012a). Effects of cognitive rehabilitation on structural and functional MRI measures in multiple sclerosis: an explorative study. Radiology 262: 932–940.

Filippi M, Rocca MA, Barkhof F et al. (2012b). Association between pathological and MRI findings in multiple sclerosis. Lancet Neurol 11: 349–360.

Filippi M, Preziosa P, Copetti M et al. (2013a). Gray matter damage predicts the accumulation of disability 13 years later. Neurology 81: 1759–1767.

Filippi M, Rocca MA, Pagani E et al. (2013b). Placebo-controlled trial of oral laquinimod in multiple sclerosis: MRI evidence of an effect on brain tissue damage. J Neurol Neurosurg Psychiatry 85: 851–858.

Filippi M, Preziosa P, Pagani E et al. (2013c). Microstructural MR imaging of cortical lesion in multiple sclerosis. Mult Scler 19: 418–426.

Filippi M, Agosta F, Spinelli EG et al. (2013d). Imaging resting state brain function in multiple sclerosis. J Neurol 260: 1709–1713.

Fisher E, Rudick RA, Simon JH et al. (2002). Eight-year follow-up study of brain atrophy in patients with MS. Neurology 59: 1412–1420.

Fisher E, Lee JC, Nakamura K et al. (2008). Gray matter atrophy in multiple sclerosis: a longitudinal study. Ann Neurol 64: 255–265.

Fisniku LK, Brex PA, Altmann DR et al. (2008). Disability and T2 MRI lesions: a 20-year follow-up of patients with relapse onset of multiple sclerosis. Brain 131: 808–817.

Francis PL, Jakubovic R, O'Connor P et al. (2013). Robust perfusion deficits in cognitively impaired patients with secondary-progressive multiple sclerosis. AJNR Am J Neuroradiol 34: 62–67.

Freedman MS, Patry DG, Grand'Maison F et al. (2004). Treatment optimization in multiple sclerosis. Can J Neurol Sci 31: 157–168.

Gadea M, Martinez-Bisbal MC, Marti-Bonmati L et al. (2004). Spectroscopic axonal damage of the right locus coeruleus relates to selective attention impairment in early stage relapsing-remitting multiple sclerosis. Brain 127: 89–98.

Gaitan MI, Shea CD, Evangelou IE et al. (2011). Evolution of the blood-brain barrier in newly forming multiple sclerosis lesions. Ann Neurol 70: 22–29.

Gaitan MI, Sati P, Inati S, Reich DS (2013). Initial investigation of the blood-brain barrier in MS lesions at 7 tesla. Mult Scler 19: 1068–1073.

Gallo A, Esposito F, Sacco R et al. (2012). Visual resting-state network in relapsing-remitting MS with and without previous optic neuritis. Neurology 79: 1458–1465.

Ge Y, Jensen JH, Lu H et al. (2007). Quantitative assessment of iron accumulation in the deep gray matter of multiple sclerosis by magnetic field correlation imaging. AJNR Am J Neuroradiol 28: 1639–1644.

Ge Y, Zohrabian VM, Grossman RI (2008). Seven-Tesla magnetic resonance imaging: new vision of microvascular abnormalities in multiple sclerosis. Arch Neurol 65: 812–816.

Geurts JJ, Pouwels PJ, Uitdehaag BM et al. (2005). Intracortical lesions in multiple sclerosis: improved detection with 3D double inversion-recovery MR imaging. Radiology 236: 254–260.

Geurts JJ, Reuling IE, Vrenken H et al. (2006). MR spectroscopic evidence for thalamic and hippocampal, but not cortical, damage in multiple sclerosis. Magn Reson Med 55: 478–483.

Giorgio A, Battaglini M, Smith SM et al. (2008). Brain atrophy assessment in multiple sclerosis: importance and limitations. Neuroimaging Clin N Am 18: 675–686. xi.

Giorgio A, Palace J, Johansen-Berg H et al. (2010). Relationships of brain white matter microstructure with clinical and MR measures in relapsing-remitting multiple sclerosis. J Magn Reson Imaging 31: 309–316.

Glisson CC, Galetta SL (2009). Nonconventional optic nerve imaging in multiple sclerosis. Neuroimaging Clin N Am 19: 71–79.

Goodin DS (2006). Magnetic resonance imaging as a surrogate outcome measure of disability in multiple sclerosis: have we been overly harsh in our assessment? Ann Neurol 59: 597–605.

Guye M, Bettus G, Bartolomei F et al. (2010). Graph theoretical analysis of structural and functional connectivity MRI in normal and pathological brain networks. MAGMA 23: 409–421.

Haacke EM, Garbern J, Miao Y et al. (2010). Iron stores and cerebral veins in MS studied by susceptibility weighted imaging. Int Angiol 29: 149–157.

Hammond KE, Metcalf M, Carvajal L et al. (2008). Quantitative in vivo magnetic resonance imaging of multiple sclerosis at 7 Tesla with sensitivity to iron. Ann Neurol 64: 707–713.

Hawkins SA, McDonnell GV (1999). Benign multiple sclerosis? Clinical course, long term follow up, and assessment of prognostic factors. J Neurol Neurosurg Psychiatry 67: 148–152.

Henry RG, Shieh M, Okuda DT et al. (2008). Regional grey matter atrophy in clinically isolated syndromes at presentation. J Neurol Neurosurg Psychiatry 79: 1236–1244.

Hickman SJ, Brex PA, Brierley CM et al. (2001). Detection of optic nerve atrophy following a single episode of unilateral optic neuritis by MRI using a fat-saturated short-echo fast FLAIR sequence. Neuroradiology 43: 123–128.

Hickman SJ, Toosy AT, Jones SJ et al. (2004). Serial magnetization transfer imaging in acute optic neuritis. Brain 127: 692–700.

Hickman SJ, Wheeler-Kingshott CA, Jones SJ et al. (2005). Optic nerve diffusion measurement from diffusion-weighted imaging in optic neuritis. AJNR Am J Neuroradiol 26: 951–956.

Holland CM, Charil A, Csapo I et al. (2012). The relationship between normal cerebral perfusion patterns and white matter lesion distribution in 1,249 patients with multiple sclerosis. J Neuroimaging 22: 129–136.

Horsfield MA, Sala S, Neema M et al. (2010). Rapid semi-automatic segmentation of the spinal cord from magnetic resonance images: application in multiple sclerosis. Neuroimage 50: 446–455.

Inglese M, Ghezzi A, Bianchi S et al. (2002). Irreversible disability and tissue loss in multiple sclerosis: a conventional and magnetization transfer magnetic resonance imaging study of the optic nerves. Arch Neurol 59: 250–255.

Inglese M, van Waesberghe JH, Rovaris M et al. (2003). The effect of interferon beta-1b on quantities derived from MT MRI in secondary progressive MS. Neurology 60: 853–860.

Inglese M, Liu S, Babb JS et al. (2004). Three-dimensional proton spectroscopy of deep gray matter nuclei in relapsing-remitting MS. Neurology 63: 170–172.

Inglese M, Park SJ, Johnson G et al. (2007). Deep gray matter perfusion in multiple sclerosis: dynamic susceptibility contrast perfusion magnetic resonance imaging at 3 T. Arch Neurol 64: 196–202.

Inglese M, Adhya S, Johnson G et al. (2008). Perfusion magnetic resonance imaging correlates of neuropsychological impairment in multiple sclerosis. J Cereb Blood Flow Metab 28: 164–171.

Inglese M, Madelin G, Oesingmann N et al. (2010). Brain tissue sodium concentration in multiple sclerosis: a sodium imaging study at 3 tesla. Brain 133: 847–857.

Kangarlu A, Bourekas EC, Ray-Chaudhury A et al. (2007). Cerebral cortical lesions in multiple sclerosis detected by MR imaging at 8 Tesla. AJNR Am J Neuroradiol 28: 262–266.

Kappos L, Moeri D, Radue EW et al. (1999). Predictive value of gadolinium-enhanced magnetic resonance imaging for relapse rate and changes in disability or impairment in multiple sclerosis: a meta-analysis. Gadolinium MRI Meta-analysis Group. Lancet 353: 964–969.

Kermode AG, Thompson AJ, Tofts P et al. (1990). Breakdown of the blood-brain barrier precedes symptoms and other MRI signs of new lesions in multiple sclerosis. Pathogenetic and clinical implications. Brain 113: 1477–1489.

Kern KC, Sarcona J, Montag M et al. (2011). Corpus callosal diffusivity predicts motor impairment in relapsing-remitting multiple sclerosis: a TBSS and tractography study. Neuroimage 55: 1169–1177.

Khaleeli Z, Cercignani M, Audoin B et al. (2007). Localized grey matter damage in early primary progressive multiple sclerosis contributes to disability. Neuroimage 37: 253–261.

Khaleeli Z, Altmann DR, Cercignani M et al. (2008a). Magnetization transfer ratio in gray matter: a potential surrogate marker for progression in early primary progressive multiple sclerosis. Arch Neurol 65: 1454–1459.

Khaleeli Z, Ciccarelli O, Manfredonia F et al. (2008b). Predicting progression in primary progressive multiple sclerosis: a 10-year multicenter study. Ann Neurol 63: 790–793.

Khalil M, Enzinger C, Langkammer C et al. (2009). Quantitative assessment of brain iron by R(2)* relaxometry in patients with clinically isolated syndrome and relapsing-remitting multiple sclerosis. Mult Scler 15: 1048–1054.

Kiferle L, Politis M, Muraro PA et al. (2011). Positron emission tomography imaging in multiple sclerosis-current status and future applications. Eur J Neurol 18: 226–231.

Kilsdonk ID, de Graaf WL, Soriano AL et al. (2013). Multicontrast MR Imaging at 7 T in Multiple sclerosis: highest lesion detection in cortical gray matter with 3D-FLAIR. AJNR Am J Neuroradiol 34: 791–796.

Kirov II, Tal A, Babb JS et al. (2013). Serial proton MR spectroscopy of gray and white matter in relapsing-remitting MS. Neurology 80: 39–46.

Kolbe S, Chapman C, Nguyen T et al. (2009). Optic nerve diffusion changes and atrophy jointly predict visual dysfunction after optic neuritis. Neuroimage 45: 679–686.

Lanz M, Hahn HK, Hildebrandt H (2007). Brain atrophy and cognitive impairment in multiple sclerosis: a review. J Neurol 254: II43–II48.

Le Bihan D, Mangin JF, Poupon C et al. (2001). Diffusion tensor imaging: concepts and applications. J Magn Reson Imaging 13: 534–546.

Li DK, Held U, Petkau J et al. (2006). MRI T2 lesion burden in multiple sclerosis: a plateauing relationship with clinical disability. Neurology 66: 1384–1389.

Li Y, Jewells V, Kim M et al. (2013). Diffusion tensor imaging based network analysis detects alterations of neuroconnectivity in patients with clinically early relapsing-remitting multiple sclerosis. Hum Brain Mapp 34: 3376–3391.

Lin X, Tench CR, Morgan PS et al. (2005). 'Importance sampling' in MS: use of diffusion tensor tractography to quantify pathology related to specific impairment. J Neurol Sci 237: 13–19.

Losseff NA, Kingsley DP, McDonald WI et al. (1996). Clinical and magnetic resonance imaging predictors of disability in primary and secondary progressive multiple sclerosis. Mult Scler 1: 218–222.

Lublin FD, Reingold SC (1996). Defining the clinical course of multiple sclerosis: results of an international survey. National Multiple Sclerosis Society (USA) Advisory Committee on Clinical Trials of New Agents in Multiple Sclerosis. Neurology 46: 907–911.

Lycklama G, Thompson A, Filippi M et al. (2003). Spinal-cord MRI in multiple sclerosis. Lancet Neurol 2: 555–562.

Mainero C, Benner T, Radding A et al. (2009). In vivo imaging of cortical pathology in multiple sclerosis using ultra-high field MRI. Neurology 73: 941–948.

McDonald WI, Compston A, Edan G et al. (2001). Recommended diagnostic criteria for multiple sclerosis: guidelines from the International Panel on the diagnosis of multiple sclerosis. Ann Neurol 50: 121–127.

Mehta V, Pei W, Yang G et al. (2013). Iron is a sensitive biomarker for inflammation in multiple sclerosis lesions. PLoS One 8: e57573.

Melzi L, Rocca MA, Marzoli SB et al. (2007). A longitudinal conventional and magnetization transfer magnetic resonance imaging study of optic neuritis. Mult Scler 13: 265–268.

Mesaros S, Rovaris M, Pagani E et al. (2008). A magnetic resonance imaging voxel-based morphometry study of regional gray matter atrophy in patients with benign multiple sclerosis. Arch Neurol 65: 1223–1230.

Mesaros S, Rocca MA, Riccitelli G et al. (2009). Corpus callosum damage and cognitive dysfunction in benign MS. Hum Brain Mapp 30: 2656–2666.

Mesaros S, Rocca MA, Pagani E et al. (2011). Thalamic damage predicts the evolution of primary-progressive multiple sclerosis at 5 years. AJNR Am J Neuroradiol 32: 1016–1020.

Miller DH, Leary SM (2007). Primary-progressive multiple sclerosis. Lancet Neurol 6: 903–912.

Miller DH, Barkhof F, Frank JA et al. (2002). Measurement of atrophy in multiple sclerosis: pathological basis, methodological aspects and clinical relevance. Brain 125: 1676–1695.

Miller DH, Weinshenker BG, Filippi M et al. (2008). Differential diagnosis of suspected multiple sclerosis: a consensus approach. Mult Scler 14: 1157–1174.

Minneboo A, Barkhof F, Polman CH et al. (2004). Infratentorial lesions predict long-term disability in patients with initial findings suggestive of multiple sclerosis. Arch Neurol 61: 217–221.

Mistry N, Dixon J, Tallantyre E et al. (2013). Central veins in brain lesions visualized with high-field magnetic resonance imaging: a pathologically specific diagnostic biomarker for inflammatory demyelination in the brain. JAMA Neurol: 1–6.

Montalban X, Tintore M, Swanton J et al. (2010). MRI criteria for MS in patients with clinically isolated syndromes. Neurology 74: 427–434.

Nair G, Absinta M, Reich DS (2013). Optimized T1-MPRAGE sequence for better visualization of spinal cord multiple sclerosis lesions at 3 T. AJNR Am J Neuroradiol 34: 2215–2222.

Narayana PA, Doyle TJ, Lai D et al. (1998). Serial proton magnetic resonance spectroscopic imaging, contrast-enhanced magnetic resonance imaging, and quantitative lesion volumetry in multiple sclerosis. Ann Neurol 43: 56–71.

Narayana PA, Wolinsky JS, Rao SB et al. (2004). Multicentre proton magnetic resonance spectroscopy imaging of primary progressive multiple sclerosis. Mult Scler 10: S73–S78.

Neema M, Stankiewicz J, Arora A et al. (2007). T1- and T2-based MRI measures of diffuse gray matter and white matter damage in patients with multiple sclerosis. J Neuroimaging 17: 16S–21S.

Neema M, Arora A, Healy BC et al. (2009). Deep gray matter involvement on brain MRI scans is associated with clinical progression in multiple sclerosis. J Neuroimaging 19: 3–8.

Nelson F, Poonawalla AH, Hou P et al. (2007). Improved identification of intracortical lesions in multiple sclerosis with phase-sensitive inversion recovery in combination with fast double inversion recovery MR imaging. AJNR Am J Neuroradiol 28: 1645–1649.

Nelson F, Poonawalla A, Hou P et al. (2008). 3D MPRAGE improves classification of cortical lesions in multiple sclerosis. Mult Scler 14: 1214–1219.

Nielsen AS, Kinkel RP, Tinelli E et al. (2012). Focal cortical lesion detection in multiple sclerosis: 3 Tesla DIR versus 7 Tesla FLASH-T2. J Magn Reson Imaging 35: 537–542.

Nielsen AS, Kinkel RP, Madigan N et al. (2013). Contribution of cortical lesion subtypes at 7 T MRI to physical and cognitive performance in MS. Neurology 81: 641–649.

Noseworthy JH, Lucchinetti C, Rodriguez M et al. (2000). Multiple sclerosis. N Engl J Med 343: 938–952.

Ogawa S, Menon RS, Tank DW et al. (1993). Functional brain mapping by blood oxygenation level-dependent contrast magnetic resonance imaging. A comparison of signal characteristics with a biophysical model. Biophys J 64: 803–812.

Oh J, Saidha S, Chen M et al. (2013). Spinal cord quantitative MRI discriminates between disability levels in multiple sclerosis. Neurology 80: 540–547.

Oreja-Guevara C, Rovaris M, Iannucci G et al. (2005). Progressive gray matter damage in patients with relapsing-remitting multiple sclerosis: a longitudinal diffusion tensor magnetic resonance imaging study. Arch Neurol 62: 578–584.

Ormerod IE, Miller DH, McDonald WI et al. (1987). The role of NMR imaging in the assessment of multiple sclerosis and isolated neurological lesions. A quantitative study. Brain 110: 1579–1616.

Ozturk A, Smith SA, Gordon-Lipkin EM et al. (2010). MRI of the corpus callosum in multiple sclerosis: association with disability. Mult Scler 16: 166–177.

Ozturk A, Aygun N, Smith SA et al. (2013). Axial 3D gradient-echo imaging for improved multiple sclerosis lesion detection in the cervical spinal cord at 3 T. Neuroradiology 55: 431–439.

Pagani E, Filippi M, Rocca MA et al. (2005). A method for obtaining tract-specific diffusion tensor MRI measurements in the presence of disease: application to patients with clinically isolated syndromes suggestive of multiple sclerosis. Neuroimage 26: 258–265.

Pagani E, Hirsch JG, Pouwels PJ et al. (2010). Intercenter differences in diffusion tensor MRI acquisition. J Magn Reson Imaging 31: 1458–1468.

Papadopoulou A, von Felten S, Traud S et al. (2012). Evolution of MS lesions to black holes under DNA vaccine treatment. J Neurol 259: 1375–1382.

Parisi L, Rocca MA, Mattioli F et al. (2014). Changes of brain resting state functional connectivity predict the persistence of cognitive rehabilitation effects in patients with multiple sclerosis. Mult Scler 20: 686–694.

Pellicano C, Gallo A, Li X et al. (2010). Relationship of cortical atrophy to fatigue in patients with multiple sclerosis. Arch Neurol 67: 447–453.

Penny S, Khaleeli Z, Cipolotti L et al. (2010). Early imaging predicts later cognitive impairment in primary progressive multiple sclerosis. Neurology 74: 545–552.

Peruzzo D, Castellaro M, Calabrese M et al. (2013). Heterogeneity of cortical lesions in multiple sclerosis: an MRI perfusion study. J Cereb Blood Flow Metab 33: 457–463.

Pierpaoli C, Barnett A, Pajevic S et al. (2001). Water diffusion changes in Wallerian degeneration and their dependence on white matter architecture. Neuroimage 13: 1174–1185.

Pitt D, Boster A, Pei W et al. (2010). Imaging cortical lesions in multiple sclerosis with ultra-high-field magnetic resonance imaging. Arch Neurol 67: 812–818.

Politis M, Giannetti P, Su P et al. (2012). Increased PK11195 PET binding in the cortex of patients with MS correlates with disability. Neurology 79: 523–530.

Polman CH, Reingold SC, Edan G et al. (2005). Diagnostic criteria for multiple sclerosis: 2005 revisions to the "McDonald Criteria". Ann Neurol 58: 840–846.

Polman CH, Reingold SC, Banwell B et al. (2011). Diagnostic criteria for multiple sclerosis: 2010 Revisions to the McDonald criteria. Ann Neurol 69: 292–302.

Poonawalla AH, Hasan KM, Gupta RK et al. (2008). Diffusion-tensor MR imaging of cortical lesions in multiple sclerosis: initial findings. Radiology 246: 880–886.

Pozzilli C, Fieschi C, Perani D et al. (1992). Relationship between corpus callosum atrophy and cerebral metabolic asymmetries in multiple sclerosis. J Neurol Sci 112: 51–57.

Prinster A, Quarantelli M, Lanzillo R et al. (2010). A voxel-based morphometry study of disease severity correlates in relapsing–remitting multiple sclerosis. Mult Scler 16: 45–54.

Ranjeva JP, Audoin B, Au Duong MV et al. (2005). Local tissue damage assessed with statistical mapping analysis of brain magnetization transfer ratio: relationship with functional status of patients in the earliest stage of multiple sclerosis. AJNR Am J Neuroradiol 26: 119–127.

Ratchford JN, Endres CJ, Hammoud DA et al. (2012). Decreased microglial activation in MS patients treated with glatiramer acetate. J Neurol 259: 1199–1205.

Raz E, Bester M, Sigmund EE et al. (2013). A better characterization of spinal cord damage in multiple sclerosis: a diffusional kurtosis imaging study. AJNR Am J Neuroradiol 34: 1846–1852.

Reich DS, Smith SA, Gordon-Lipkin EM et al. (2009). Damage to the optic radiation in multiple sclerosis is associated with retinal injury and visual disability. Arch Neurol 66: 998–1006.

Riccitelli G, Rocca MA, Pagani E et al. (2011). Cognitive impairment in multiple sclerosis is associated to different patterns of gray matter atrophy according to clinical phenotype. Hum Brain Mapp 32: 1535–1543.

Rigotti DJ, Inglese M, Kirov II et al. (2012). Two-year serial whole-brain N-acetyl-L-aspartate in patients with relapsing-remitting multiple sclerosis. Neurology 78: 1383–1389.

Rio J, Rovira A, Tintore M et al. (2008). Relationship between MRI lesion activity and response to IFN-beta in relapsing-remitting multiple sclerosis patients. Mult Scler 14: 479–484.

Rio J, Castillo J, Rovira A et al. (2009). Measures in the first year of therapy predict the response to interferon beta in MS. Mult Scler 15: 848–853.

Rissanen E, Virta JR, Paavilainen T et al. (2013). Adenosine A2A receptors in secondary progressive multiple sclerosis: a [(11)C]TMSX brain PET study. J Cereb Blood Flow Metab 33: 1394–1401.

Rocca MA, Matthews PM, Caputo D et al. (2002). Evidence for widespread movement-associated functional MRI changes in patients with PPMS. Neurology 58: 866–872.

Rocca MA, Colombo B, Falini A et al. (2005). Cortical adaptation in patients with MS: a cross-sectional functional MRI study of disease phenotypes. Lancet Neurol 4: 618–626.

Rocca MA, Agosta F, Colombo B et al. (2007a). fMRI changes in relapsing-remitting multiple sclerosis patients complaining of fatigue after IFNbeta-1a injection. Hum Brain Mapp 28: 373–382.

Rocca MA, Pagani E, Absinta M et al. (2007b). Altered functional and structural connectivities in patients with MS: a 3-T study. Neurology 69: 2136–2145.

Rocca MA, Absinta M, Ghezzi A et al. (2009a). Is a preserved functional reserve a mechanism limiting clinical impairment in pediatric MS patients? Hum Brain Mapp 30: 2844–2851.

Rocca MA, Absinta M, Valsasina P et al. (2009b). Abnormal connectivity of the sensorimotor network in patients with MS: a multicenter fMRI study. Hum Brain Mapp 30: 2412–2425.

Rocca MA, Valsasina P, Ceccarelli A et al. (2009c). Structural and functional MRI correlates of Stroop control in benign MS. Hum Brain Mapp 30: 276–290.

Rocca MA, Ceccarelli A, Rodegher M et al. (2010a). Preserved brain adaptive properties in patients with benign multiple sclerosis. Neurology 74: 142–149.

Rocca MA, Mesaros S, Pagani E et al. (2010b). Thalamic damage and long-term progression of disability in multiple sclerosis. Radiology 257: 463–469.

Rocca MA, Valsasina P, Absinta M et al. (2010c). Default-mode network dysfunction and cognitive impairment in progressive MS. Neurology 74: 1252–1259.

Rocca MA, Horsfield MA, Sala S et al. (2011). A multicenter assessment of cervical cord atrophy among MS clinical phenotypes. Neurology 76: 2096–2102.

Rocca M, Valsasina P, Martinelli V et al. (2012). Large-scle neuronal network dysfunction in relapsing-remitting multiple sclerosis. Neurology 79: 1449–1457.

Rocca MA, Mesaros S, Preziosa P et al. (2013a). Wallerian and trans-synaptic degeneration contribute to optic radiation damage in multiple sclerosis: a diffusion tensor MRI study. Mult Scler 19: 1610–1617.

Rocca MA, Valsasina P, Damjanovic D et al. (2013b). Voxel-wise mapping of cervical cord damage in multiple sclerosis patients with different clinical phenotypes. J Neurol Neurosurg Psychiatry 84: 35–41.

Roelcke U, Kappos L, Lechner-Scott J et al. (1997). Reduced glucose metabolism in the frontal cortex and basal ganglia of multiple sclerosis patients with fatigue: a 18 F-fluorodeoxyglucose positron emission tomography study. Neurology 48: 1566–1571.

Roosendaal SD, Moraal B, Vrenken H et al. (2008). In vivo MR imaging of hippocampal lesions in multiple sclerosis. J Magn Reson Imaging 27: 726–731.

Roosendaal SD, Geurts JJ, Vrenken H et al. (2009a). Regional DTI differences in multiple sclerosis patients. Neuroimage 44: 1397–1403.

Roosendaal SD, Moraal B, Pouwels PJ et al. (2009b). Accumulation of cortical lesions in MS: relation with cognitive impairment. Mult Scler 15: 708–714.

Roosendaal SD, Schoonheim MM, Hulst HE et al. (2010). Resting state networks change in clinically isolated syndrome. Brain 133: 1612–1621.

Ropele S, Fazekas F (2009). Magnetization transfer MR imaging in multiple sclerosis. Neuroimaging Clin N Am 19: 27–36.

Rovaris M, Filippi M, Minicucci L et al. (2000). Cortical/subcortical disease burden and cognitive impairment in patients with multiple sclerosis. AJNR Am J Neuroradiol 21: 402–408.

Rovaris M, Bozzali M, Santuccio G et al. (2001). In vivo assessment of the brain and cervical cord pathology of patients with primary progressive multiple sclerosis. Brain 124: 2540–2549.

Rovaris M, Bozzali M, Iannucci G et al. (2002a). Assessment of normal-appearing white and gray matter in patients with primary progressive multiple sclerosis: a diffusion-tensor magnetic resonance imaging study. Arch Neurol 59: 1406–1412.

Rovaris M, Iannucci G, Falautano M et al. (2002b). Cognitive dysfunction in patients with mildly disabling relapsing-remitting multiple sclerosis: an exploratory study with diffusion tensor MR imaging. J Neurol Sci 195: 103–109.

Rovaris M, Gallo A, Riva R et al. (2004). An MT MRI study of the cervical cord in clinically isolated syndromes suggestive of MS. Neurology 63: 584–585.

Rovaris M, Gallo A, Valsasina P et al. (2005). Short-term accrual of gray matter pathology in patients with progressive multiple sclerosis: an in vivo study using diffusion tensor MRI. Neuroimage 24: 1139–1146.

Rovaris M, Judica E, Gallo A et al. (2006). Grey matter damage predicts the evolution of primary progressive multiple sclerosis at 5 years. Brain 129: 2628–2634.

Rovaris M, Agosta F, Pagani E et al. (2009). Diffusion tensor MR imaging. Neuroimaging Clin N Am 19: 37–43.

Rovira A, Swanton J, Tintore M et al. (2009). A single, early magnetic resonance imaging study in the diagnosis of multiple sclerosis. Arch Neurol 66: 587–592.

Rudick RA, Lee JC, Simon J et al. (2004). Defining interferon beta response status in multiple sclerosis patients. Ann Neurol 56: 548–555.

Sajja BR, Narayana PA, Wolinsky JS et al. (2008). Longitudinal magnetic resonance spectroscopic imaging of primary progressive multiple sclerosis patients treated with glatiramer acetate: multicenter study. Mult Scler 14: 73–80.

Sajja BR, Wolinsky JS, Narayana PA (2009). Proton magnetic resonance spectroscopy in multiple sclerosis. Neuroimaging Clin N Am 19: 45–58.

Sanfilipo MP, Benedict RH, Sharma J et al. (2005). The relationship between whole brain volume and disability in multiple sclerosis: a comparison of normalized gray vs. white matter with misclassification correction. Neuroimage 26: 1068–1077.

Sarchielli P, Presciutti O, Tarducci R et al. (2002). Localized (1)H magnetic resonance spectroscopy in mainly cortical gray matter of patients with multiple sclerosis. J Neurol 249: 902–910.

Sastre-Garriga J, Ingle GT, Chard DT et al. (2005). Metabolite changes in normal-appearing gray and white matter are linked with disability in early primary progressive multiple sclerosis. Arch Neurol 62: 569–573.

Sastre-Garriga J, Alonso J, Renom M et al. (2011). A functional magnetic resonance proof of concept pilot trial of cognitive rehabilitation in multiple sclerosis. Mult Scler 17: 457–467.

Schmierer K, Parkes HG, So PW et al. (2010). High field (9.4 Tesla) magnetic resonance imaging of cortical grey matter lesions in multiple sclerosis. Brain 133: 858–867.

Seewann A, Kooi EJ, Roosendaal SD et al. (2012). Postmortem verification of MS cortical lesion detection with 3D DIR. Neurology 78: 302–308.

Sepulcre J, Masdeu JC, Goni J et al. (2009). Fatigue in multiple sclerosis is associated with the disruption of frontal and parietal pathways. Mult Scler 15: 337–344.

Sharma R, Narayana PA, Wolinsky JS (2001). Grey matter abnormalities in multiple sclerosis: proton magnetic resonance spectroscopic imaging. Mult Scler 7: 221–226.

Shu N, Liu Y, Li K et al. (2011). Diffusion tensor tractography reveals disrupted topological efficiency in white matter structural networks in multiple sclerosis. Cereb Cortex 21: 2565–2577.

Sicotte NL, Kern KC, Giesser BS et al. (2008). Regional hippocampal atrophy in multiple sclerosis. Brain 131: 1134–1141.

Sombekke MH, Wattjes MP, Balk LJ et al. (2013). Spinal cord lesions in patients with clinically isolated syndrome: a powerful tool in diagnosis and prognosis. Neurology 80: 69–75.

Sorensen PS, Jonsson A, Mathiesen HK et al. (2006). The relationship between MRI and PET changes and cognitive disturbances in MS. J Neurol Sci 245: 99–102.

Sormani MP, Bruzzi P (2013). MRI lesions as a surrogate for relapses in multiple sclerosis: a meta-analysis of randomised trials. Lancet Neurol 12: 669–676.

Sormani MP, De Stefano N (2013). Defining and scoring response to IFN-beta in multiple sclerosis. Nat Rev Neurol 9: 504–512.

Sormani MP, Bonzano L, Roccatagliata L et al. (2009a). Magnetic resonance imaging as a potential surrogate for relapses in multiple sclerosis: a meta-analytic approach. Ann Neurol 65: 268–275.

Sormani MP, Rovaris M, Comi G et al. (2009b). A reassessment of the plateauing relationship between T2 lesion load and disability in MS. Neurology 73: 1538–1542.

Sormani MP, Arnold DL, De Stefano N (2014). Treatment effect on brain atrophy correlates with treatment effect on disability in multiple sclerosis. Ann Neurol 75: 43–49.

Srinivasan R, Ratiney H, Hammond-Rosenbluth KE et al. (2010). MR spectroscopic imaging of glutathione in the white and gray matter at 7 T with an application to multiple sclerosis. Magn Reson Imaging 28: 163–170.

Staffen W, Zauner H, Mair A et al. (2005). Magnetic resonance spectroscopy of memory and frontal brain region in early multiple sclerosis. J Neuropsychiatry Clin Neurosci 17: 357–363.

Steen C, D'Haeseleer M, Hoogduin JM et al. (2013). Cerebral white matter blood flow and energy metabolism in multiple sclerosis. Mult Scler 19: 1282–1289.

Summers M, Fisniku L, Anderson V et al. (2008a). Cognitive impairment in relapsing-remitting multiple sclerosis can be predicted by imaging performed several years earlier. Mult Scler 14: 197–204.

Summers M, Swanton J, Fernando K et al. (2008b). Cognitive impairment in multiple sclerosis can be predicted by imaging early in the disease. J Neurol Neurosurg Psychiatry 79: 955–958.

Sumowski JF, Wylie GR, Chiaravalloti N et al. (2010). Intellectual enrichment lessens the effect of brain atrophy on learning and memory in multiple sclerosis. Neurology 74: 1942–1945.

Swanton JK, Fernando K, Dalton CM et al. (2006). Modification of MRI criteria for multiple sclerosis in patients with clinically isolated syndromes. J Neurol Neurosurg Psychiatry 77: 830–833.

Tallantyre EC, Brookes MJ, Dixon JE et al. (2008). Demonstrating the perivascular distribution of MS lesions in vivo with 7-Tesla MRI. Neurology 70: 2076–2078.

Tallantyre EC, Morgan PS, Dixon JE et al. (2010). 3 Tesla and 7 Tesla MRI of multiple sclerosis cortical lesions. J Magn Reson Imaging 32: 971–977.

Tallantyre EC, Dixon JE, Donaldson I et al. (2011). Ultra-high-field imaging distinguishes MS lesions from asymptomatic white matter lesions. Neurology 76: 534–539.

Tedeschi G, Lavorgna L, Russo P et al. (2005). Brain atrophy and lesion load in a large population of patients with multiple sclerosis. Neurology 65: 280–285.

Thompson AJ, Miller DH, MacManus DG et al. (1990). Patterns of disease activity in multiple sclerosis. BMJ 301: 44–45.

Thompson AJ, Kermode AG, Wicks D et al. (1991). Major differences in the dynamics of primary and secondary progressive multiple sclerosis. Ann Neurol 29: 53–62.

Thompson AJ, Miller D, Youl B et al. (1992). Serial gadolinium-enhanced MRI in relapsing/remitting multiple sclerosis of varying disease duration. Neurology 42: 60–63.

Thorpe JW, Barker GJ, Jones SJ et al. (1995). Magnetisation transfer ratios and transverse magnetisation decay curves in optic neuritis: correlation with clinical findings and electrophysiology. J Neurol Neurosurg Psychiatry 59: 487–492.

Tomassini V, Paolillo A, Russo P et al. (2006). Predictors of long-term clinical response to interferon beta therapy in relapsing multiple sclerosis. J Neurol 253: 287–293.

Tourdias T, Roggerone S, Filippi M et al. (2012). Assessment of disease activity in multiple sclerosis phenotypes with combined gadolinium- and superparamagnetic iron oxide-enhanced MR imaging. Radiology 264: 225–233.

Trip SA, Schlottmann PG, Jones SJ et al. (2006). Optic nerve atrophy and retinal nerve fibre layer thinning following optic neuritis: evidence that axonal loss is a substrate of MRI-detected atrophy Neuroimage 31: 286–293.

Tur C, Wheeler-Kingshott CA, Altmann DR et al. (2014). Spatial variability and changes of metabolite concentrations in the cortico-spinal tract in multiple sclerosis using coronal CSI. Hum Brain Mapp 35: 993–1003.

Valsasina P, Benedetti B, Rovaris M et al. (2005). Evidence for progressive gray matter loss in patients with relapsing-remitting MS. Neurology 65: 1126–1128.

Valsasina P, Agosta F, Absinta M et al. (2010). Cervical cord functional MRI changes in relapse-onset MS patients. J Neurol Neurosurg Psychiatry 81: 405–408.

Valsasina P, Rocca MA, Horsfield MA et al. (2013). Regional cervical cord atrophy and disability in multiple sclerosis: a voxel-based analysis. Radiology 266: 853–861.

van Waesberghe JH, Kamphorst W, De Groot CJ et al. (1999). Axonal loss in multiple sclerosis lesions: magnetic resonance imaging insights into substrates of disability. Ann Neurol 46: 747–754.

Vanzetta I, Grinvald A (1999). Increased cortical oxidative metabolism due to sensory stimulation: implications for functional brain imaging. Science 286: 1555–1558.

Varga AW, Johnson G, Babb JS et al. (2009). White matter hemodynamic abnormalities precede sub-cortical gray matter changes in multiple sclerosis. J Neurol Sci 282: 28–33.

Vellinga MM, Oude Engberink RD, Seewann A et al. (2008). Pluriformity of inflammation in multiple sclerosis shown by ultra-small iron oxide particle enhancement. Brain 131: 800–807.

Wattjes MP, Lutterbey GG, Gieseke J et al. (2007). Double inversion recovery brain imaging at 3 T: diagnostic value in the detection of multiple sclerosis lesions. AJNR Am J Neuroradiol 28: 54–59.

Wattjes MP, Harzheim M, Lutterbey GG et al. (2008). Does high field MRI allow an earlier diagnosis of multiple sclerosis? J Neurol 255: 1159–1163.

Wegner C, Filippi M, Korteweg T et al. (2008). Relating functional changes during hand movement to clinical parameters in patients with multiple sclerosis in a multi-centre fMRI study. Eur J Neurol 15: 113–122.

Wheeler-Kingshott CA, Cercignani M (2009). About "axial" and "radial" diffusivities. Magn Reson Med 61: 1255–1260.

Wilson M, Tench CR, Morgan PS et al. (2003). Pyramidal tract mapping by diffusion tensor magnetic resonance imaging in multiple sclerosis: improving correlations with disability. J Neurol Neurosurg Psychiatry 74: 203–207.

Wingerchuk DM, Lennon VA, Pittock SJ et al. (2006). Revised diagnostic criteria for neuromyelitis optica. Neurology 66: 1485–1489.

Wolff SD, Balaban RS (1994). Magnetization transfer imaging: practical aspects and clinical applications. Radiology 192: 593–599.

Wood ET, Ronen I, Techawiboonwong A et al. (2012). Investigating axonal damage in multiple sclerosis by diffusion tensor spectroscopy. J Neurosci 32: 6665–6669.

Zackowski KM, Smith SA, Reich DS et al. (2009). Sensorimotor dysfunction in multiple sclerosis and column-specific magnetization transfer-imaging abnormalities in the spinal cord. Brain 132: 1200–1209.

Zhang Y, Metz LM, Yong VW et al. (2010). 3 T deep gray matter T2 hypointensity correlates with disability over time in stable relapsing-remitting multiple sclerosis: a 3-year pilot study. J Neurol Sci 297: 76–81.

Zivadinov R, Schirda C, Dwyer MG et al. (2010). Chronic cerebrospinal venous insufficiency and iron deposition on susceptibility-weighted imaging in patients with multiple sclerosis: a pilot case-control study. Int Angiol 29: 158–175.

Handbook of Clinical Neurology, Vol. 135 (3rd series)
Neuroimaging, Part I
J.C. Masdeu and R.G. González, Editors

Chapter 21

Other noninfectious inflammatory disorders

ÁLEX ROVIRA[1]*, CRISTINA AUGER[1], AND ANTONI ROVIRA[2]

[1]*MR Unit, Department of Radiology, Hospital Universitari Vall d'Hebron, Autonomous University of Barcelona, Barcelona, Spain*

[2]*Corporació Sanitària Parc Taulí, CD-UDIAT, Sabadell, Spain*

Abstract

Idiopathic inflammatory-demyelinating diseases (IIDDs) represent a broad spectrum of central nervous system (CNS) disorders, including monophasic, multiphasic, and progressive disorders that range from highly localized forms to multifocal or diffuse variants. In addition to the classic multiple sclerosis (MS) phenotypes, several MS variants have been described, which can be differentiated on the basis of severity, clinical course, and lesion distribution. Other forms of IIDD are now recognized as distinct entities and not MS variants, such as acute disseminated encephalomyelitis, and neuromyelitis optica spectrum disorders.

The CNS can also be affected by a variety of inflammatory diseases. These include primary angiitis of the CNS (PACNS), a rare disorder specifically targeting the CNS vasculature, and various systemic conditions which, among other organs and systems, can also affect the CNS, such as systemic vasculitis and sarcoidosis. The diagnosis of PACNS is difficult, as this condition may be confused with reversible cerebral vasoconstriction syndrome (RCVS), a term comprising a group of conditions characterized by prolonged but reversible vasoconstriction of the cerebral arteries.

Magnetic resonance imaging of the brain and spine is the radiologic technique of choice for diagnosing these disorders, and, together with the clinical and laboratory findings, enables a prompt and accurate diagnosis.

IDIOPATHIC INFLAMMATORY-DEMYELINATING DISEASES OF THE CENTRAL NERVOUS SYSTEM

The term idiopathic inflammatory-demyelinating disease (IIDD) encompasses a broad spectrum of central nervous system (CNS) disorders that can be differentiated according to their severity, clinical course, and lesion distribution, as well as their imaging, laboratory, and pathological findings. The spectrum includes monophasic, multiphasic, and progressive disorders, ranging from highly localized forms to multifocal or diffuse variants (Cañellas et al., 2007).

Relapsing-remitting and secondary progressive MS are the two most common forms of IIDD. MS can also have a progressive course from onset (primary progressive MS). Some patients have a benign course with minimal or no disability years after onset (benign MS). Fulminant forms of IIDD include a variety of disorders that have in common the severity of the clinical symptoms, an acute clinical course, and atypical findings on magnetic resonance imaging (MRI). The classic fulminant IIDD is Marburg disease. Balo concentric sclerosis, Schilder disease, and acute disseminated encephalomyelitis (ADEM) can also present with severe, acute attacks.

Some IIDDs have a restricted topographic distribution, as is the case with neuromyelitis optica (NMO) and NMO-spectrum disorders, which can have a monophasic or, more often, a relapsing course. Other types of IIDD

*Correspondence to: Álex Rovira, Unitat de Ressonància Magnètica (IDI), Servei de Radiologia, Hospital Universitari Vall d'Hebron, Pg. Vall d'Hebron 119–129, 08035 Barcelona, Spain. Tel: +34 934286034, E-mail: alex.rovira@idi.gencat.cat

occasionally present as a focal lesion that may be clinically and radiologically indistinguishable from a brain tumor. It is difficult to classify these tumefactive or pseudotumoral lesions within the IIDD spectrum. Some cases have a monophasic, self-limited course, whereas in others the tumefactive plaque is the first manifestation or appears during a typical relapsing form of MS.

Multiple sclerosis variants

Marburg disease

Marburg disease (also termed malignant MS) is a rare, acute MS variant that occurs predominantly in young adults. It is characterized by a confusional state, headache, vomiting, gait unsteadiness, and hemiparesis. This entity has a rapidly progressive course with frequent, severe relapses leading to death or severe disability within weeks to months after onset of the clinical signs, mainly due to brainstem involvement or mass effect with herniation. Most patients who survive subsequently develop a relapsing form of MS. Because Marburg disease is often preceded by a febrile illness, it can also be considered a fulminant form of ADEM when it has a monophasic course. At the time of the clinical presentation, it may be difficult to find good predictors of whether the patient will have a fulminant course, develop mild or severe MS, or even develop MS at all.

Pathologically, Marburg lesions are more destructive than those of typical MS or ADEM and are characterized by massive macrophage infiltration, demyelination (not restricted to the perivascular areas), hypertrophic astrocytes, and severe axonal injury, features compatible with the histomorphologic diagnosis of a severe, acute demyelinating disease. Despite the destructive nature of these lesions, areas of remyelination are often observed (Popescu and Lucchinetti, 2012). Neuropathologic studies suggest that this fulminant form of MS is often associated with immunoglobulin deposition and pronounced complement activation at sites of active myelin destruction, which may support plasma exchange or mitoxantrone as treatment options when high-dose steroids are not effective.

In Marburg disease, MRI typically shows multiple focal T2 lesions of varying size, which may coalesce to form large white-matter plaques disseminated throughout the hemispheric white matter and brainstem (Fig. 21.1). Perilesional edema is often present, and enhancement is commonly seen. A similar imaging pattern is seen in ADEM.

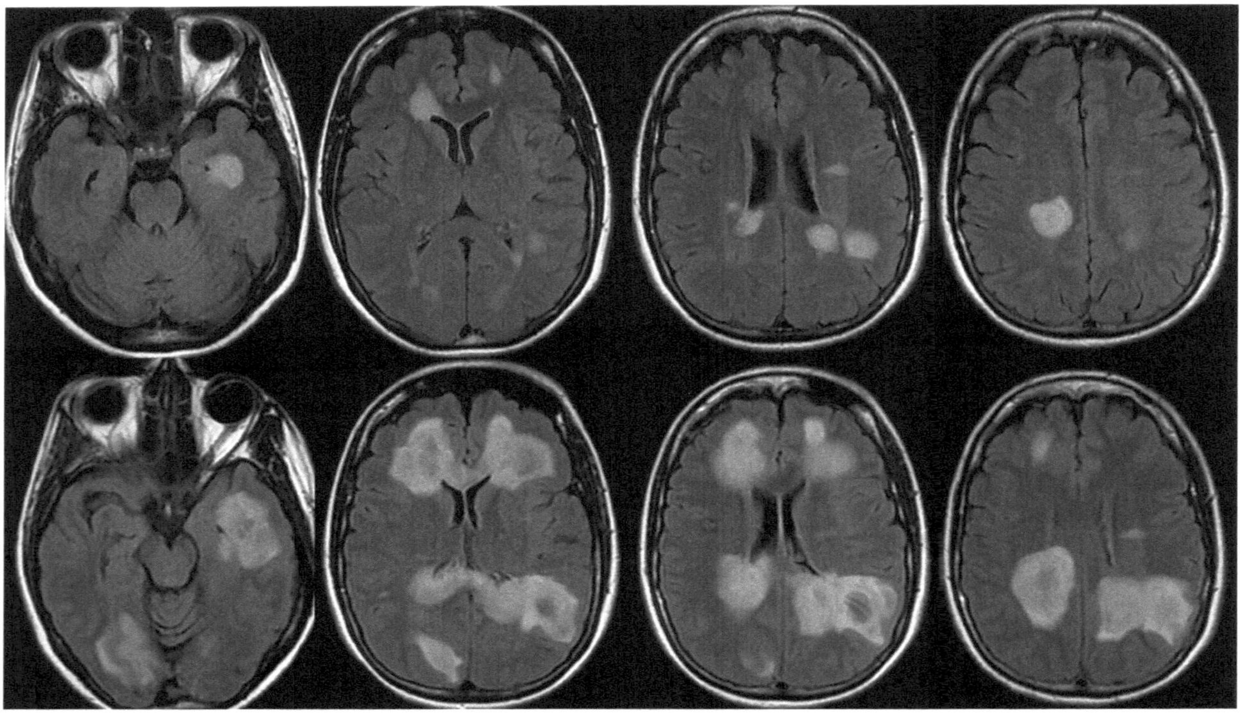

Fig. 21.1. Marburg disease in a 34-year-old woman with encephalopathic syndrome and rapidly progressive cognitive decline. T2 fluid-attenuated inversion recovery (FLAIR) images at admission show multiple focal demyelinating lesions affecting the cerebral hemispheric white matter (upper row). Despite aggressive steroid treatment, the lesions showed marked enlargement on a follow-up magnetic resonance imaging obtained 2 weeks later (lower row).

Schilder disease

Schilder disease is a rare acute or subacute disorder that can be defined as a specific clinical-radiologic presentation of MS. It commonly affects children and young adults. The clinical spectrum of Schilder disease includes psychiatric predominance, acute intracranial hypertension, intermittent exacerbations, and progressive deterioration. Imaging studies show large ring-enhancing lesions involving both hemispheres, sometimes symmetrically, and located preferentially in the parieto-occipital regions. These large, focal demyelinating lesions can resemble a brain tumor, an abscess, or even adrenoleukodystrophy. MRI features that suggest possible Schilder disease include large and relatively symmetric involvement of the brain hemispheres, incomplete ring enhancement, minimal mass effect, restricted diffusivity, and sparing of the brainstem (Fig. 21.2). (Mehler and Rabinowich, 1989; Cañellas et al., 2007). Histopathologically, Schilder disease consistently shows well-demarcated demyelination and reactive gliosis with relative sparing of the axons. Microcystic changes and even frank cavitation can occur. The clinical and imaging findings usually show a dramatic response to steroids.

Balo concentric sclerosis

Balo concentric sclerosis is a rare IIDD subtype, considered a variant of MS, with characteristic radiologic and pathologic features. Balo concentric sclerosis was formerly considered an aggressive MS variant, leading to death in weeks to months after onset, and in which the diagnosis was made on histopathologic findings at postmortem examination. However, with the widespread use of MRI, this MS variant is often identified in patients who later have a complete or almost complete clinical recovery (Hardy and Miller, 2014).

The pathologic hallmarks of the disease are large demyelinated lesions showing a peculiar pattern of alternating layers of preserved and destroyed myelin. One possible explanation for this pattern is that sublethal tissue injury is induced at the edge of the expanding lesion, which would then stimulate expression of neuroprotective proteins to protect the rim of periplaque tissue from damage, thereby resulting in alternating layers of preserved and nonpreserved myelinated tissue (Stadelmann et al., 2005). These alternating bands are best identified with T2-weighted sequences, which typically show thick concentric hyperintense bands corresponding to areas of demyelination and gliosis, alternating with thin isointense bands corresponding to normal myelinated white matter (Fig. 21.3). This pattern can be also identified on T1-weighted images as alternating isointense (preserve myelin) and hypointense (demyelinated) concentric rings. These bands, which may eventually disappear over time, can appear as multiple concentric layers (onion-skin lesion), as a mosaic, or as a "floral" configuration. The center of the lesion usually shows no layering because of massive demyelination (storm center). Contrast enhancement and decreased diffusivity are common in the outer rings (inflammatory edge) of the lesion (Fig. 21.4) (Hardy and Miller, 2014).

The Balo pattern can be isolated, multiple, or combined with typical MS-like lesions, and the lesion structure can vary from one or two to several alternating

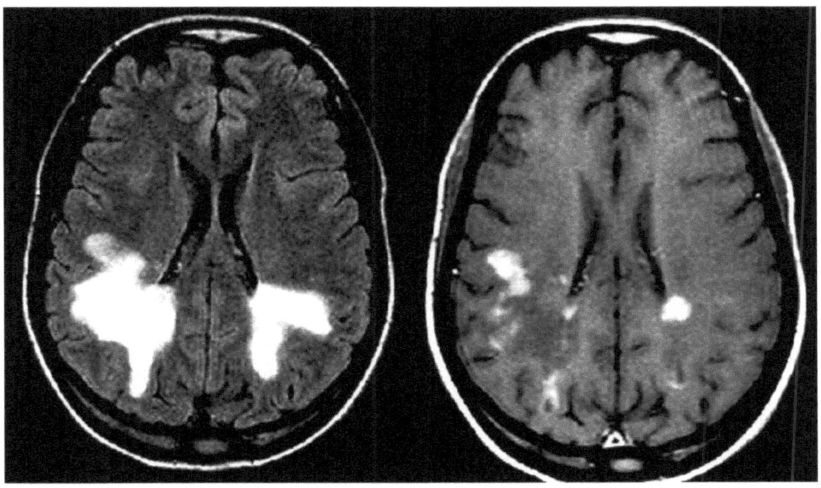

Fig. 21.2. Schilder disease. Brain magnetic resonance images in a 23-year-old woman who presented with encephalopathy and visual loss. Transverse T2 fluid-attenuated inversion recovery (FLAIR) images (left) and contrast-enhanced T1-weighted images (right) show large, bilateral, almost symmetric lesions in the posterior periventricular white matter with peripheral contrast uptake. Despite considerable extension of the lesions, there is no mass effect. (Reproduced from Cañellas et al. (2007) and Sastre-Garriga et al. (2003), with permission from Springer Science and Business Media.)

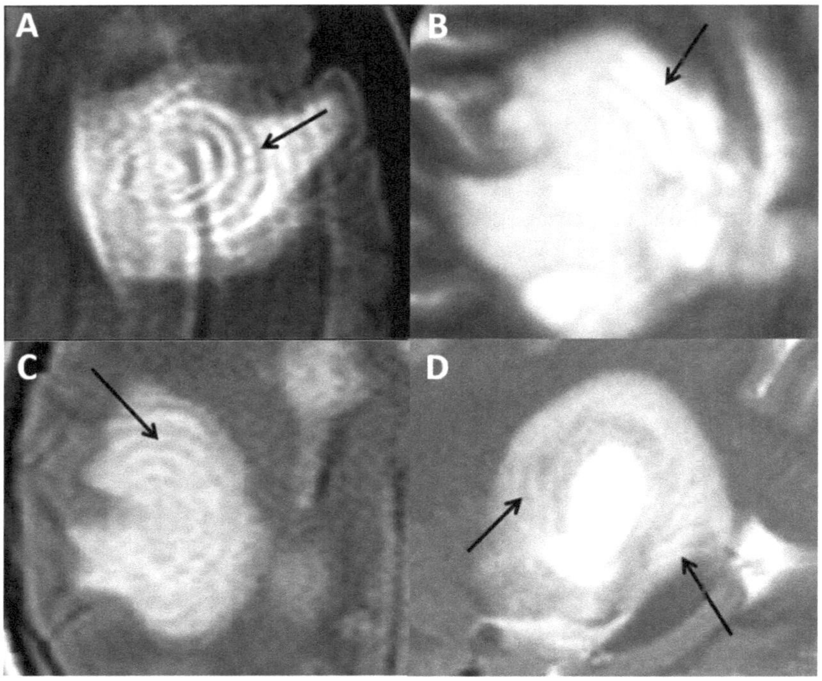

Fig. 21.3. Balo-like lesions from four different patients (**A–D**). Transverse T2-weighted brain magnetic resonance images of the brain show large, focal, white-matter lesions with a lamellated pattern of alternating bands of demyelination and relatively normal white matter, reflecting either spared or remyelinated regions (arrows). The center of the lesion in (**D**) shows no layering because of massive demyelination.

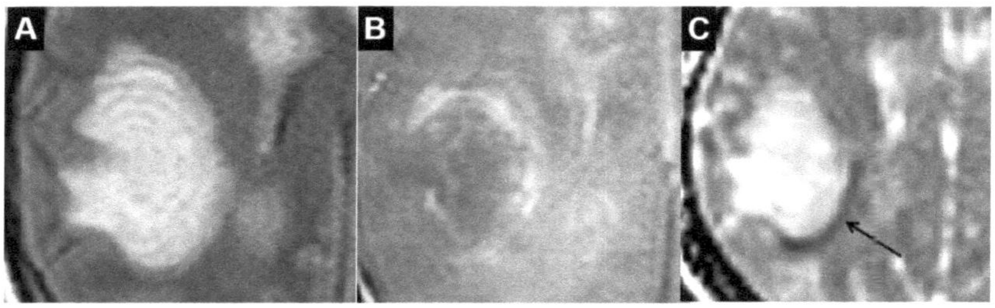

Fig. 21.4. Balo-like lesion in a 25-year-old man. (**A**) Transverse T2-weighted, (**B**) contrast-enhanced T1-weighted magnetic resonance images, and (**C**) apparent diffusion coefficient map. Note the alternating concentric bands, peripheral contrast uptake, and decreased peripheral diffusivity (arrow). (Reproduced from Cañellas et al. (2007), with permission from Springer Science and Business Media.)

bands, with a total size from one to several centimeters. Lesions occur predominantly in the cerebral white matter, although brainstem, cerebellum, and spinal cord involvement has also been reported.

Tumefactive or pseudotumoral IIDDs

IIDDs can present as single or multiple focal brain lesions that may be clinically and radiologically indistinguishable from tumors. Radiologically, pseudotumoral IIDD can be defined as demyelinating lesions of greater than 2 cm, usually showing a ring-enhancing or open-ring-enhancing pattern, but without the layering that defines Balo concentric sclerosis. These nonspecific features represent a diagnostic challenge and reasonably call for a biopsy, despite clinical suspicion of demyelination. However, even the biopsy specimen may resemble a brain tumor because of the hypercellular nature of the lesions, which are often associated with large protoplasmic glial cells with fragmented chromatin and abnormal mitosis (Creutzfeldt cells). On MRI, these pseudotumoral lesions usually present as large, single or multiple focal lesions located in the brain hemispheres (Masdeu et al., 2000). Clues that can help to differentiate these lesions from a brain tumor include a relatively minor mass effect or vasogenic edema, and incomplete ring

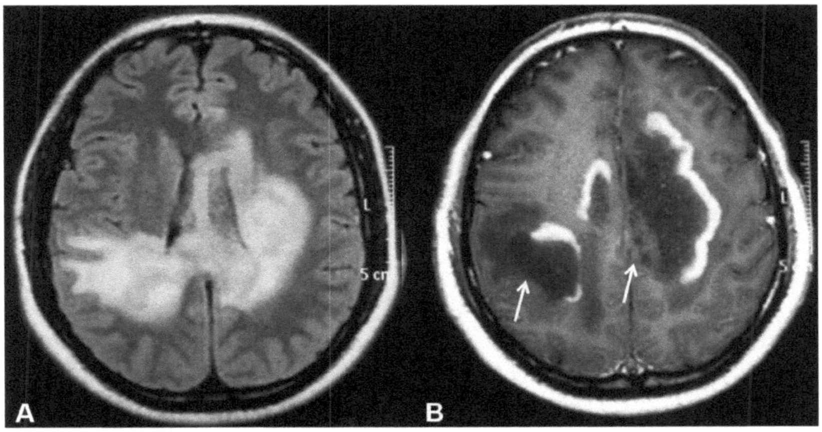

Fig. 21.5. Pseudotumoral inflammatory demyelinating lesions in an 18-year-old woman, who presented an acute episode of bilateral motor weakness, headache, and lethargy. (**A**) T2 fluid-attenuated inversion recovery (FLAIR) image shows multiple circumscribed lesions in the subcortical white matter of both frontoparietal regions with edema and an open-ring-enhancing pattern on contrast-enhanced T1-weighted sequence (arrows in **B**). (Courtesy of Dr. Patricia Orellana, Santiago de Chile.)

enhancement on T1-weighted gadolinium-enhanced images with the open border facing the cortical/subcortical gray matter (Fig. 21.5), sometimes associated with a rim of peripheral hypointensity on T2-weighted sequences (Masdeu et al., 2000). Nonetheless, the differential diagnosis between malignant gliomas and pseudotumoral demyelinating brain lesions may be impossible based solely on these conventional MRI features. Proton MR spectroscopy (^{1}H-MRS) can provide useful additional information, although reports on the diagnostic value of this technique in the differential diagnosis with high-grade gliomas have yielded conflicting results. The ^{1}H-MRS lesion pattern is characterized by the presence of lactate, macromolecules/lipids, and choline-containing compounds (Cho) with a marked decrease in *N*-acetyl aspartate (NAA), a spectral pattern showing similarities to that typically described in high-grade gliomas. However, it is reported that a glutamine/glutamate increase should suggest a pseudotumoral demyelinating lesion (Cianfoni et al., 2007; Saini et al., 2011), whereas high myo-inositol/NAA and Cho/NAA ratios should suggest a tumoral lesion (Majós et al., 2009).

Dynamic-susceptibility contrast MR perfusion imaging has also been used to differentiate active tumefactive demyelinating lesions from high-grade gliomas. Some studies have shown that this technique can distinguish grade IV gliomas from active tumefactive demyelinating lesions based on regional cerebral blood volume (rCBV) analysis. This ability is based on important biologic dissimilarities between the two types of lesions: grade IV gliomas are characterized by the presence of neoangiogenesis and vascular endothelial proliferation leading to a marked increase of rCBV, whereas tumefactive demyelinating lesions show intrinsically normal vessels or only mild inflammatory angiogenesis, with a normal or mildly increased rCBV (Fig. 21.6).

Neuromyelitis optica and NMO-spectrum disorders

NMO is an autoimmune inflammatory disorder of the CNS with a predilection for the optic nerves and spinal cord. The discovery of NMO-IgG and an NMO-specific autoantibody directed against aquaporin-4 (AQP4-Ab), the major water channel in the CNS, clearly identified NMO as a disease separate from MS (Wingerchuk et al., 2007).

This uncommon and topographically restricted form of IIDD is characterized by severe unilateral or bilateral optic neuritis and complete transverse myelitis, which occur simultaneously or sequentially over a varying period of time (weeks or years). AQP4-Ab has been also demonstrated in patients with conditions other than classic NMO, including isolated longitudinally extensive transverse myelitis, defined by lesions spanning over more than three segments; monophasic or recurrent isolated optic neuritis; and certain types of brainstem encephalitis (particularly if the diencephalon or medulla oblongata is affected) (Fig. 21.7). As most of these patients later develop NMO, various groups have suggested classifying these symptoms as high-risk syndromes for NMO when they occur in AQP4-Ab-seropositive patients. In addition, it has been proposed that AQP4-Ab-positive classic NMO and AQP4-Ab-positive high-risk syndromes be referred to as NMO-spectrum disorder or autoimmune AQP4 channelopathy (Trebst et al., 2014).

The incidence and prevalence of NMO are unknown, and there are important differences in its regional

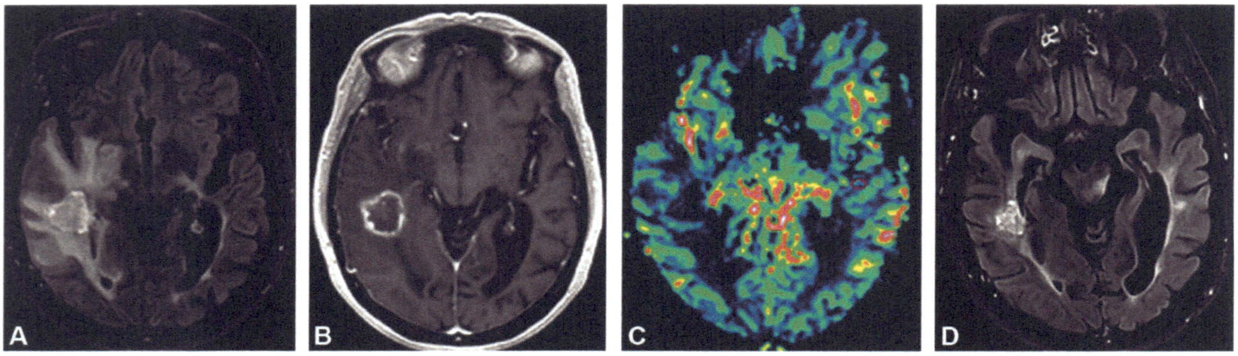

Fig. 21.6. Pseudotumoral inflammatory demyelinating lesion in a 47-year-old woman previously diagnosed with relapsing multiple sclerosis, who presented with an acute episode of left-sided motor weakness. (**A**) T2 fluid-attenuated inversion recovery (FLAIR) image shows a well-circumscribed focal lesion in the subcortical right temporal white matter with extensive edema and mild mass effect, and a closed-ring-enhancing pattern on contrast-enhanced T1-weighted image (**B**). (**C**) The colored cerebral blood volume (CBV) parametric map obtained from a dynamic susceptibility contrast sequence shows no CBV increase or only a mild increase in the enhancing areas of the lesion compared to the normal-appearing white matter. (**D**) A follow-up scan performed 1 month later after aggressive steroid treatment and plasma exchange demonstrates a reduction in lesion size and disappearance of perilesional edema, supporting the diagnosis of a tumefactive demyelinating lesion.

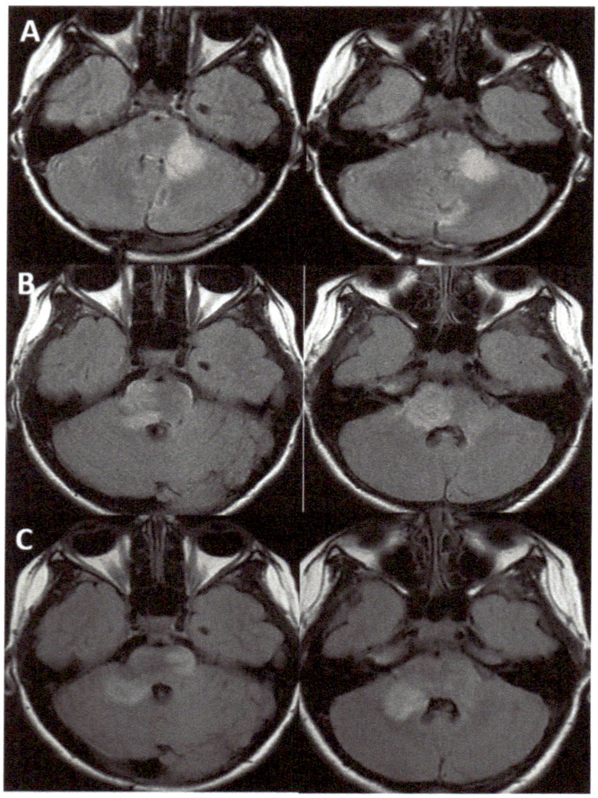

Fig. 21.7. High-risk syndrome for neuromyelitis optica in a 14-year-old boy with recurrent brainstem syndromes. Serial brain magnetic resonance imaging scans (T2 fluid-attenuated inversion recovery (FLAIR) sequences) performed at first admission (**A**), and at 2 (**B**) and 3 (**C**) years later show multiple recurrent focal lesions involving the brainstem and middle cerebellar peduncles. The patient was seropositive for aquaporin-4 antibody.

distribution worldwide. In a study performed in Thailand, the local IIDD cohort showed a high proportion of AQP4-Ab-positive patients (39%) in comparison to European and American cohorts (less than 10%) (Nagaishi et al., 2011). The median age at onset is late in the fourth decade, about 10 years later than typical MS. NMO appears to be a sporadic disease, although rare familial cases have been reported.

The index events of new-onset NMO are severe unilateral or bilateral optic neuritis, acute myelitis, or a combination of these symptoms. The myelitis attacks appear as complete transverse myelitis with severe bilateral motor deficits, sensory-level, bowel and bladder dysfunction, pain and significant residual neurologic injury. Optic neuritis attacks are generally more severe than those typically seen in MS. Approximately 85% of patients have a relapsing course with severe acute exacerbations and poor recovery, which leads to increasing neurologic impairment and a high risk of respiratory failure and death due to cervical myelitis (Wingerchuk and Weinshenker, 2003). Patients who experience acute optic neuritis and transverse myelitis simultaneously or within days of each other are much more likely to have a monophasic course. On the other hand, a relapsing course correlates with NMO-IgG seropositivity, a longer interval between attacks, older age at onset, female sex, and less severe motor impairment after the myelitic onset. Although the initial attacks are more severe in patients proven to have monophasic NMO, the long-term neurologic prognosis is somewhat better in this group because patients do not accumulate disability from recurrent attacks.

Clinical features alone are insufficient to diagnose NMO; cerebrospinal fluid (CSF) analysis and MRI are usually required to confidently exclude other disorders. CSF pleocytosis (>50 leukocytes/mm^3) is often present, while oligoclonal bands are seen less frequently (20–40%) than in MS patients (80–90%). AQP4-Ab detection is reported to have a sensitivity of 73% and a specificity of 91% for NMO. AQP4-Ab may be helpful to distinguish this form of IIDD from MS and it can predict relapse and conversion to NMO in patients presenting with a single attack of longitudinally extensive myelitis. NMO-IgG is positive in 52% of patients with relapsing transverse myelitis and in 25% of patients with recurrent idiopathic optic neuritis (Lennon et al., 2004). Wingerchuk et al. (2006) proposed a revised set of criteria for diagnosing NMO. These new criteria remove the absolute restriction on CNS involvement beyond the optic nerves and spinal cord, allow any interval between the first events of optic neuritis and transverse myelitis, and emphasize the specificity of longitudinally extensive spinal cord lesions on MRI and NMO-IgG-seropositive status. More recently the International Panel for NMO diagnosis developed new diagnostic criteria that define the unifying term NMO-spectrum disorders, which is stratified by serologic testing (with or without AQP4-IgG) (Table 21.1). These new criteria require, in patients with AQP4-IgG, core clinical and MRI findings related to optic nerve, spinal cord, area postrema, other braistem, diencephalic, or cerebral presentations. However, more stringent clinical and MRI criteria are required for diagnosis of NMO-spectrum disorders without AQP4-IgG or when serologic testing is unavailable (Wingerchuk et al., 2015).

A possible explanation for selective involvement of the spinal cord and optic nerve in this condition may be that these structures are particularly vulnerable to antibody-mediated injury due to the inherent weakness of the blood–brain barrier at these sites (Papadopoulos and Verkman, 2011).

The increased blood–brain barrier permeability in the spinal cord may also be a result of its vascular properties, with larger capillaries than those in the brain. Thus, on a background of an inflammatory process in the presence of extremely high antibody titers, lesions might preferentially, but not exclusively, affect the spinal cord and optic nerve.

MRI of the affected optic nerve demonstrates swelling and loss of blood–brain barrier integrity with gadolinium enhancement that can extend into the optic chiasm (Fig. 21.8). The cord lesions in NMO typically extend over three or more contiguous vertebral segments and occasionally the entire spinal cord (longitudinally extensive spinal cord lesions); they are centrally located (preferential central gray-matter involvement) and affect much of the cross-section on axial images (Fig. 21.9). During the acute and subacute phase, the

Table 21.1

Neuromyelitis optica (NMO)-spectrum disorders diagnostic criteria for adults

Diagnostic criteria for NMO-spectrum disorders with AQP4-IgG

1. At least one core clinical characteristic
2. Positive test for AQP4-IgG using best available detection method (cell-based assay strongly recommended)
3. Exclusion of alternative diagnoses

Diagnostic criteria for NMO-spectrum disorders without AQP4-IgG or NMO-spectrum disorders with unknown AQP4-IgG status

1. At least two core clinical characteristics occurring as a result of one or more clinical attacks and meeting all of the following requirements:
   a. At least one core clinical characteristic must be optic neuritis, acute myelitis with LETM, or area postrema syndrome
   b. Dissemination in space (two or more different core clinical characteristics)
   c. Fulfillment of additional MRI requirements, as applicable
2. Negative tests for AQP4-IgG using best available detection method, or testing unavailable
3. Exclusion of alternative diagnoses

Core clinical characteristics

1. Optic neuritis
2. Acute myelitis
3. Area postrema syndrome: episode of otherwise unexplained hiccups or nausea and vomiting
4. Acute brainstem syndrome
5. Symptomatic narcolepsy or acute diencephalic clinical syndrome with NMO-spectrum disorders typical diencephalic MRI lesions
6. Symptomatic cerebral syndrome with NMO-spectrum disorders typical brain lesions

Additional MRI requirements for NMO-spectrum disorders without AQP4-IgG and NMO-spectrum disorders with unknown AQP4-IgG status

1. Acute optic neuritis: requires brain MRI showing: (a) normal findings or only nonspecific white-matter lesions, or (b) optic nerve MRI with T2-hyperintense lesion or T1-weighted gadolinium enhancing lesion extending over >1/2 optic nerve length or involving optic chiasm
2. Acute myelitis: requires associated intramedullary MRI lesion extending over $\geq$3 contiguous segments (LETM) or $\geq$3 contiguous segments of focal spinal cord atrophy in patients with history compatible with acute myelitis
3. Area postrema syndrome: requires associated dorsal medulla/area postrema lesions
4. Acute brainstem syndrome: requires associated periependymal brainstem lesions

Reproduced from Wingerchuk et al. (2015).

AQP4, aquaporin-4; LETM: longitudinal extensive transverse myelitis; MRI, magnetic resonance imaging.

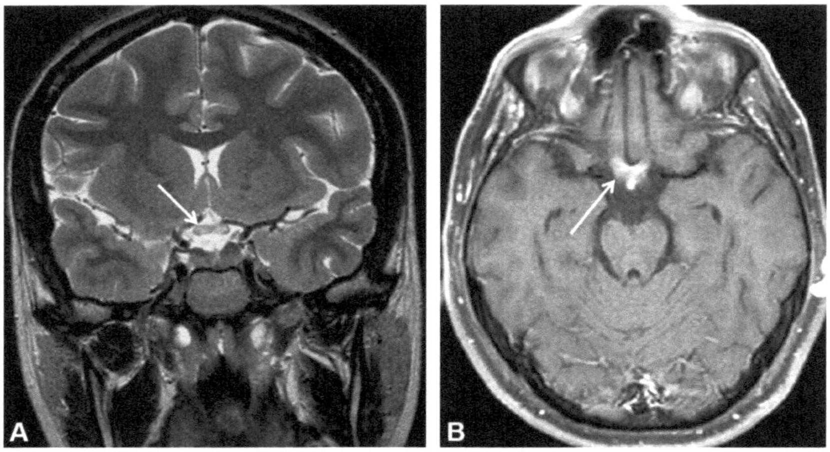

Fig. 21.8. Devic neuromyelitis optica (NMO) in a 24-year-old woman presenting with acute, bilateral visual loss. Coronal T2-weighted (**A**) and transverse contrast-enhanced T1-weighted (**B**) magnetic resonance images demonstrate an enhancing demyelinating lesion affecting the optic chiasm (arrows).

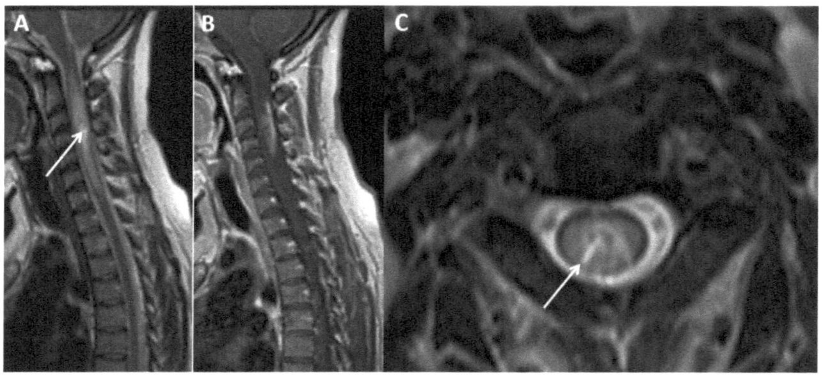

Fig. 21.9. Devic neuromyelitis optica (NMO). (**A**) Sagittal T2-, (**B**) contrast-enhanced T1-, and (**C**) transverse T2-weighted magnetic resonance images of the cervical spinal cord depict a large, tumefactive cord lesion with peripheral contrast uptake, affecting most of the transverse cord area. Observe the bright spotty lesion in the sagittal and transverse T2-weighted images (arrows).

lesions are tumefactive and show contrast uptake. In some cases, the spinal cord lesions are small at the onset of symptoms, mimicking those of MS, and then progress in extent over time. The presence of very hyperintense spotty lesions on T2-weighted images ("bright spotty sign") is a specific feature that helps differentiate NMO from MS, particularly in patients without longitudinally extensive spinal cord lesions (Yonezu et al., 2014), and likely reflects the highly destructive component of the inflammatory lesion (Fig. 21.9). Spinal cord lesions can progress to atrophy and necrosis, and may lead to syrinx-like cavities on T1-weighted images.

NMO was long considered a disease without brain involvement, and a negative brain MRI at disease onset was considered a major supportive criterion for the diagnosis of NMO. However, various studies have shown that brain MRI abnormalities exist in a significant proportion (50–85%) of patients. Brain MRI lesions are often asymptomatic, but sometimes are associated with symptoms even at disease onset. The brain lesions are commonly nonspecific. They can be dot-like or patchy, <3 cm in diameter, and located in the deep white matter, brainstem, or cerebellum. Nonetheless, some brain MRI features appear to be quite characteristic and distinct from MS lesions. These abnormalities may parallel sites with high AQP4 expression adjacent to the ventricular system at any level, such as the hypothalamus, periependymal areas surrounding the third and lateral ventricles, cerebral aqueduct, corpus callosum, and dorsal brainstem adjacent to the fourth ventricle (Fig. 21.10).

The appearance of periventricular lesions in NMO is quite characteristic. In contrast to MS, where periventricular lesions are discrete, oval-shaped, and perpendicular to the ependymal lining due to their perivenular distribution (Dawson's fingers), NMO lesions are not oval-shaped, located immediately adjacent to the lateral

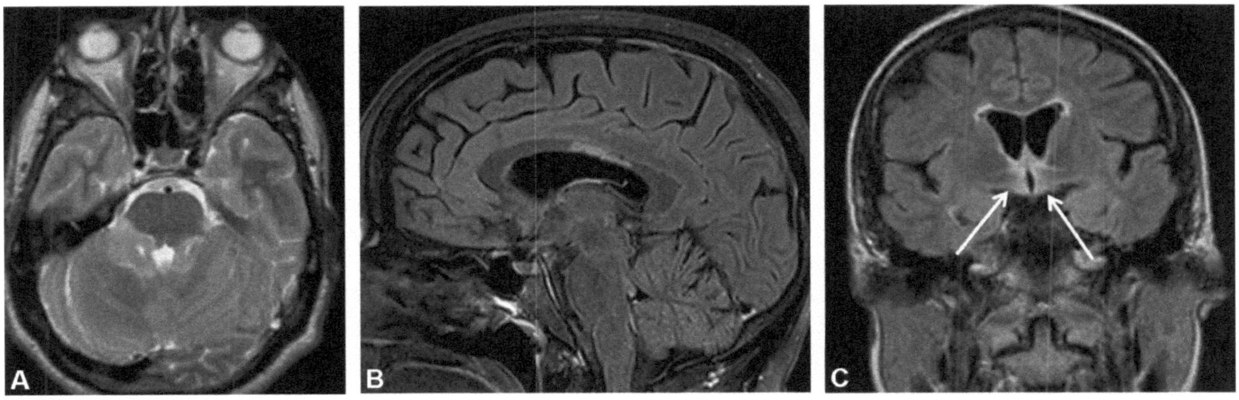

Fig. 21.10. Devic neuromyelitis optica (NMO). Different types of brain involvement. T2-weighted images show hyperintense lesions involving the brainstem and upper cerebellar peduncles (surrounding the fourth ventricle) (**A**), the entire width of the middle segment of the corpus callosum (**B**), and the hypothalamic region (arrows in **C**).

ventricles following the ependymal lining in a disseminated pattern, and are often edematous and heterogeneous (Kim et al., 2010). As opposed to what occurs in MS, NMO lesions do not affect the cortical gray matter.

Involvement of the corpus callosum has been described in 18% of AQP4-seropositive NMO patients. The lesions are multiple, large, and edematous, show heterogeneous signal intensity on T2-weighted images, and sometimes affects the entire thickness of the corpus callosum (Fig. 21.10).

Lesions may also affect areas where AQP4 expression is not particularly high, such as the corticospinal tracts. These lesions, which can be unilateral or bilateral and may affect the posterior limb of the internal capsule and cerebral peduncle of the midbrain, are contiguous and often longitudinally extensive (Kim et al., 2010).

Other brain MRI findings described in NMO include extensive and confluent hemispheric white-matter lesions and radial hemispheric lesions (sometimes corresponding to an extension of periventricular lesions), which are likely related to vasogenic edema involving the white-matter tracts. These lesions usually do not show mass effect or contrast enhancement, but there may be a "cloud-like" pattern of enhancement, defined as multiple patches of enhancing lesions with blurred margins (Kim et al., 2010).

Some of the typical brain MRI findings may be specific to clinical presentations, such as intractable vomiting and hiccup (linear dorsal medullary lesions involving the area postrema and nucleus tractus solitarius) (Fig. 21.11), or a syndrome of inappropriate antidiuretic hormone secretion (hypothalamic and periaqueductal lesions) (Misu et al., 2005).

As distinct from MS, MR spectroscopy findings in NMO are normal in normal-appearing brain tissue (gray and white matter), with no NAA decreases or Cho

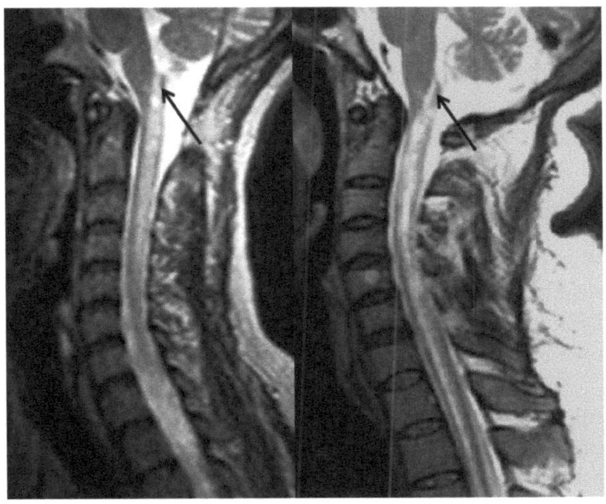

Fig. 21.11. Devic neuromyelitis optica (NMO). Magnetic resonance imaging features in 2 patients presenting with intractable hiccup and vomiting. Sagittal T2-weighted magnetic resonance images demonstrate longitudinally extensive myelitis involving the cervical cord connected to the tegmentum of the lower medulla oblongata (area postrema region in the brainstem) (arrows). (Reproduced from Cañellas et al. (2007), with permission from Springer Science and Business Media.)

increases. These normal findings occur both in patients with and without brain abnormalities on conventional MRI, indicating that brain tissue is not diffusely affected in NMO (de Seze et al., 2010).

Distinguishing NMO from MS is critical, particularly in the early stages, since the treatment and prognosis of these disorders differ. In fact, some evidence suggests that MS-modifying treatments such as interferon-ß, natalizumab, and laquinimod exacerbate NMO. By contrast, several immunosuppressants (e.g., azathioprine, rituximab, mitoxantrone) seem to help in preventing NMO relapses.

NMO-spectrum disorders can be associated with systemic autoimmune diseases such as systemic lupus erythematosus (SLE) and Sjögren's syndrome (SS). Whether the neurologic manifestations are solely due to NMO-spectrum disorder or are a manifestation of these diseases is controversial, although optic neuritis and transverse myelitis are rare presentations of them, and several studies have shown that patients with systemic autoimmune diseases and NMO-IgG-positive antibodies always have optic neuritis, myelitis, or NMO.

Acute disseminated encephalomyelitis and variants

Acute disseminated encephalomyelitis

ADEM is a severe, immune-mediated inflammatory disorder of the CNS that predominantly affects the white matter of the brain and spinal cord. In the absence of specific biologic markers, the diagnosis of ADEM is based on clinical and radiologic features. This disorder affects children more commonly than adults, and, in contrast to MS, shows no sex preponderance. The estimated incidence is 0.8 per 100 000 population per year. In most cases, the clinical onset of disease is preceded by viral or bacterial infections, usually nonspecific upper-respiratory-tract infections. ADEM may also develop following a vaccination (postimmunization encephalomyelitis) (Menge et al., 2005).

Patients commonly present with nonspecific multifocal symptoms, which developed subacutely over a period of days, frequently associated with encephalopathy (relatively uncommon in MS), defined as an alteration in consciousness (e.g., stupor, lethargy) or a behavioral change unexplained by fever, systemic illness, or postictal symptoms.

Although ataxia, encephalopathy, and brainstem symptoms are frequently present in both pediatric and adult cases, certain signs and symptoms appear to be age-related. In childhood ADEM, long-lasting fever and headaches occur more frequently, while in adult cases, motor and sensory deficits predominate. In general, the disease is self-limiting and the prognostic outcome favorable.

Although ADEM usually has a monophasic course, multiphasic forms have been reported, raising diagnostic difficulties in distinguishing these cases from MS. This multiphasic form, which accounts for less than 4% of ADEM cases, is defined as a new encephalopathic event consistent with ADEM, separated by 3 months after the initial illness but not followed by any further events. The second ADEM event can involve either new or re-emergence of prior neurologic symptoms, signs, and MRI findings. Relapsing disease following ADEM that occurs beyond a second encephalopathic event is no longer consistent with multiphasic ADEM but rather indicates a chronic disorder, most often leading to the diagnosis of MS or NMO (Krupp et al., 2013).

An ADEM event as the first manifestation of the classic relapsing form of MS occurs in 2–10%. According to the International Pediatric Multiple Sclerosis Study Group, the diagnosis of MS is met if, after the initial ADEM, a second clinical event meets the following three requirements: (1) it is nonencephalopathic; (2) it occurs 3 months or more after the incident neurologic illness; and (3) it is associated with new MRI findings consistent with the 2010 McDonald criteria for dissemination in space (Krupp et al., 2013). The presence of hypointense lesions and two or more periventricular lesions are MRI features that predict an MS diagnosis in children with acute CNS demyelination (Verhey et al., 2011).

Unlike the lesions in MS, ADEM lesions are often large, patchy, and poorly marginated on MRI (Fig. 21.12). There is usually asymmetric involvement of the subcortical and central white matter and cortical gray–white junction of the cerebral hemispheres, cerebellum, brainstem, and spinal cord. Lesions confined to the periventricular white matter and corpus callosum are less common than in MS. The gray matter of the thalamus and basal ganglia is often affected, particularly in children, and typically in a symmetric pattern (Tenembaum et al., 2002). However, the frequency of thalamus involvement in adult ADEM does not differ from that of adult MS. This can be explained by the fact that involvement of this structure is less common in adult ADEM than in childhood ADEM. The main radiologic differences between ADEM and MS are described in Table 21.2.

Four patterns of cerebral involvement have been proposed to describe the MRI findings in ADEM (Tenembaum et al., 2002): (1) ADEM with small lesions (less than 5 mm); (2) ADEM with large, confluent, or tumefactive lesions, and frequent extensive perilesional edema and mass effect (Fig. 21.12); (3) ADEM with additional symmetric deep gray-matter involvement; and (4) acute hemorrhagic encephalomyelitis. Gadolinium enhancement of one or more lesions occurs in 14–30% of cases (Krupp et al., 2013). The pattern of enhancement varies and can be complete or incomplete ring-shaped, nodular, gyral, or spotty. Although ADEM is usually a monophasic disease, new lesions may be seen on follow-up MRI within the first month of the initial attack.

Most MRI lesions appear early in the course of the disease, supporting the clinical diagnosis of ADEM. Nonetheless, in some cases there may be a delay of more

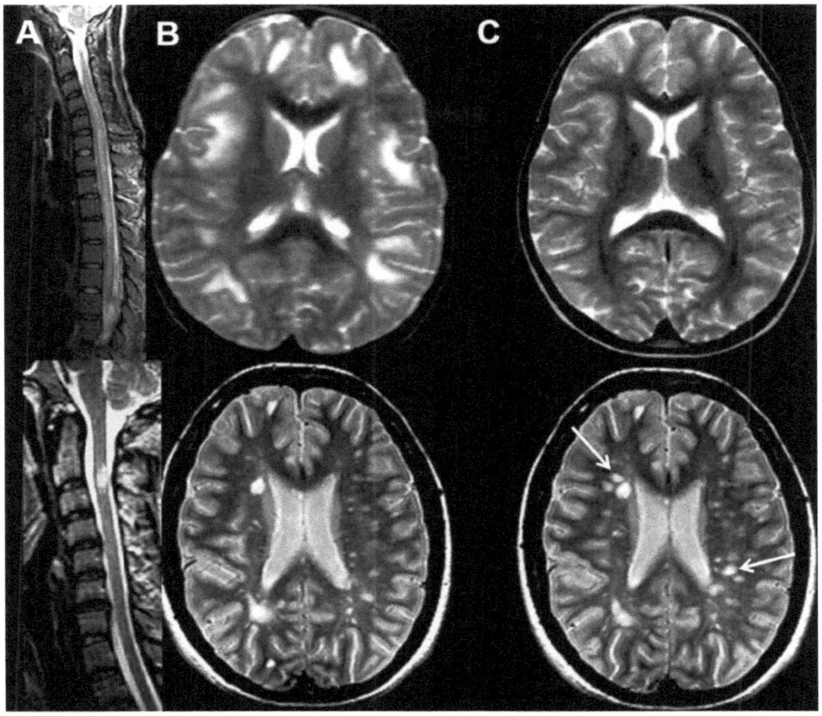

Fig. 21.12. Magnetic resonance imaging differences between acute disseminated encephalomyelitis (ADEM) (upper row) and multiple sclerosis (MS) (lower row). Initial spinal cord sagittal (**A**), and initial (**B**) and follow-up (**C**) brain transverse T2-weighted magnetic resonance images. In ADEM, spinal cord lesions are extensive and usually associated with large, poorly defined subcortical white-matter lesions on brain magnetic resonance imaging. In MS, symptomatic cord lesions are usually small and commonly associated with subclinical brain white-matter lesions of the type seen in MS. In ADEM, longitudinal studies usually show resolution of lesions (**C**), while in MS, new lesions frequently appear over time (arrows in **C**). (Reproduced from Cañellas et al. (2007), with permission from Springer Science and Business Media.)

Table 21.2

Radiologic differences between acute disseminated encephalomyelitis (ADEM) and multiple sclerosis (MS)

	ADEM	MS
Periventricular lesions	+	+++
Isolated subcortical lesions	++	–
Deep gray-matter lesions	++	+/–
Poorly marginated lesions	++	+
Contrast enhancement	+	++
Symmetric white-matter lesions	+	++
Symmetric gray-matter lesions	++	–
New lesions on follow-up	+	+++
Hemorrhagic lesions	+	–
Same-appearance lesions	++	+
Large and confluent lesions	++	+
Resolution of lesions	++	+
Hypointense (T1) nonenhancing lesions	–	++

than 1 month between the onset of symptoms and the appearance of lesions on MRI. Therefore, a normal brain MR scan obtained within the first days after the onset of neurologic symptoms suggestive of ADEM does not exclude this diagnosis.

The spinal cord is affected in less than 30% of ADEM patients (Tenembaum et al., 2002), predominantly in the thoracic region. The cord lesion is typically large, causes swelling of the cord, and shows variable enhancement. In most ADEM patients, partial or complete resolution of the MRI abnormalities occurs within a few months of treatment. This course is positively associated with a final diagnosis of ADEM.

Bickerstaff encephalitis

Bickerstaff encephalitis (BE) is a rare acute syndrome considered a subgroup of ADEM or a subtype of Miller–Fischer syndrome (MFS), in which inflammation appears to be confined to the brainstem. The syndrome consists of localized encephalitis of the brainstem, commonly preceded by a febrile illness, and has a benign prognosis. Because of the clinical similarities between BE and MFS, some authors believe they are both within the same autoimmune disorder with a broad spectrum of symptoms, which include ataxia, ocular paresis, and

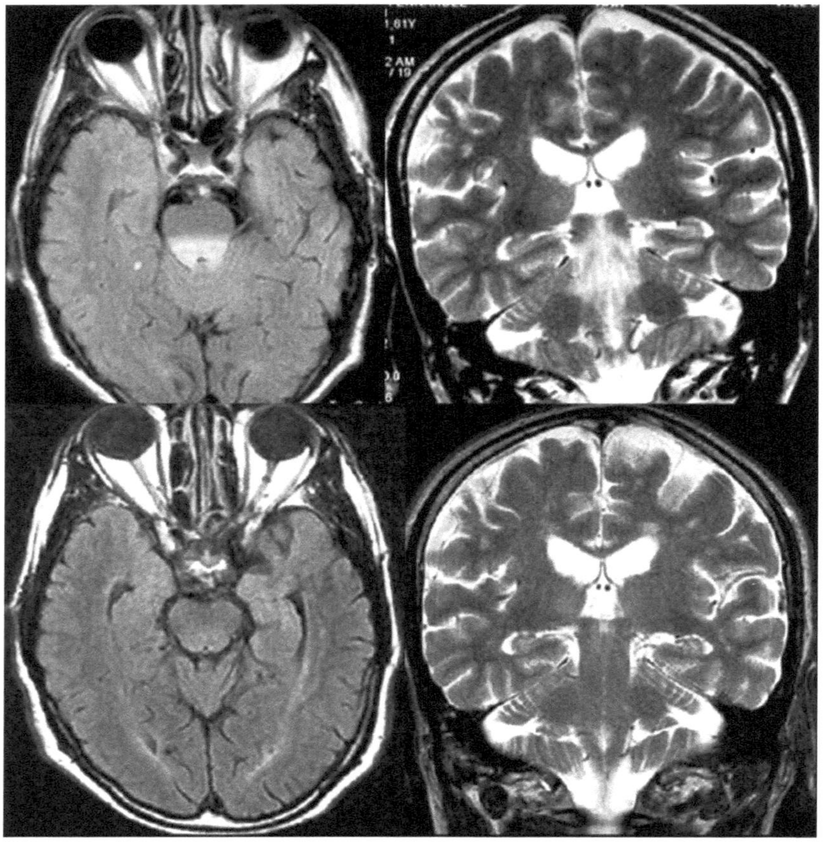

Fig. 21.13. Bickerstaff encephalitis. Initial brain magnetic resonance imaging (transverse T2 fluid-attenuated inversion recovery (FLAIR)-weighted and coronal T2-weighted magnetic resonance images) shows an extensive brainstem lesion (upper row) that had completely resolved on a follow-up study obtained 2 months later (lower row).

impaired reflexes (markedly reduced or absent in MFS, and variable in BE). However, in contrast to MFS (which is a peripheral nervous system process), BE is a CNS disease. The MRI findings in BE, which are nonspecific, include an extensive high-signal intensity lesion on T2-weighted images affecting the midbrain and pons, and sometimes the thalamus and basal ganglia. The clinical outcome is good and parallels resolution of the MRI lesions (Fig. 21.13) (Mondejar et al., 2002). The pathogenesis of BE is uncertain; however, the absence of CSF oligoclonal bands and resolution of the clinical symptoms and MRI lesions suggest an inflammatory origin and make demyelination unlikely.

Acute disseminated necrohemorrhagic leukoencephalitis

Acute disseminated necrohemorrhagic leukoencephalitis (acute hemorrhagic encephalomyelitis or Hurst disease) is an uncommon condition that has been observed in patients of all ages. It is thought to be a hyperacute form, or the most severe variant of ADEM. This usually fatal disease manifests clinically with abrupt onset of fever, neck stiffness, and hemiplegia or other focal signs, seizures, and decreasing level of consciousness (Menge et al., 2005). At autopsy, the brain is congested and swollen, sometimes asymmetrically, and herniation is frequent. Multiple petechial hemorrhages are distributed diffusely throughout the brain. The perivascular lesions chiefly consist of ball-like or ring hemorrhages surrounding necrotic venules, sometimes with fibrinous exudates within the vessel wall or extending into adjacent tissue. Perivenous demyelinating lesions, identical to those occurring in ADEM, may also be present. Perivascular cuffs of mononuclear cells are seen, often with neutrophils. T2*-weighted or susceptibility-weighted MR sequences show large regions of demyelination and petechial hemorrhages in peripheral white matter of the cerebral hemispheres.

CENTRAL NERVOUS SYSTEM VASCULITIS

Primary vasculitis restricted to the central nervous system

Primary CNS vasculitis (PACNS) is an uncommon and poorly understood vasculitis restricted to the brain and spinal cord and representing less than 2% of vasculitis cases involving the CNS. PACNS occurs at the same frequency in men as in women, with a median age at diagnosis of about 50 years, although it may affect children and the elderly. The pathogenesis of PACNS is unknown, but, similarly to other chronic or autoimmune diseases, is thought to be triggered by infection. Nonetheless, in most patients this relationship cannot be demonstrated.

Typically, PACNS involves small to medium-sized vessels (both arteries and veins), mainly those in a leptomeningeal and subcortical location, with a focal and segmental distribution. Three main histopathologic patterns have been described (Miller et al., 2009) – granulomatous, lymphocytic, and necrotizing vasculitis – which are not closely linked to specific clinical manifestations. The granulomatous pattern is the most common (58%) and is defined by vasculocentric mononuclear inflammation and well-formed granulomas. Lymphocytic vasculitis (28%), which is characterized by lymphocytic infiltration with occasional vessel destruction, is typically reported in children with angiography-negative PACNS. Finally, necrotizing vasculitis, accounting for only 4% of PACNS, is characterized by transmural fibrinoid necrosis that may be associated with intracranial hemorrhage.

The diagnosis of PACNS is a challenge because of the wide variety of clinical findings, which are nonspecific and related to the CNS areas affected, and the absence of highly sensitive and specific diagnostic tests.

The majority of patients present with subacute manifestations of diffuse CNS dysfunction, with the most frequent initial manifestations being headache and cognitive impairment. Focal symptoms usually appear later in the disease course and include hemiparesis, aphasia, dysarthria, ataxia, seizures, and blurred vision or decreased visual acuity. Intracranial hemorrhage, which is the presenting feature in 11–12% of patients, and spinal cord syndrome are infrequent manifestations. By contrast with systemic vasculitis, constitutional symptoms such as fever and weight loss are uncommon.

Three major clinical phenotypes have been proposed to facilitate clinical recognition and early diagnosis of PACNS (Molloy and Hajj-Ali, 2007):

1. acute or subacute encephalopathy, presenting as a confusional syndrome with progression to stupor and coma
2. disease presentation resembling atypical MS with a variety of focal symptoms
3. intracranial mass lesions with headache, drowsiness, focal signs, and elevated intracranial pressure.

Results of blood tests are usually normal, while CSF analysis is abnormal in 80–90% of patients (mild increase in leukocyte count and total protein concentration). Cerebral angiography supports the diagnosis of PACNS when biopsy is not undertaken or results are negative. Characteristic angiographic findings include alternating segments of stenosis with normal or dilated intervening segments, and arterial occlusions (Figs 21.14 and 21.15). Microaneurysms are rarely seen. These abnormalities, which usually affect several arteries bilaterally, are nonspecific and might be encountered in several other nonvasculitic disorders such as vasospasm, CNS infection, reversible cerebral vasoconstriction syndrome (RCVS), and atherosclerosis. Therefore, a diagnosis of PACNS should not be based on positive angiography alone, and angiography results should always be interpreted in conjunction with clinical, laboratory, and MRI findings (Salvarani et al., 2012). False-negative results are also common, and can be

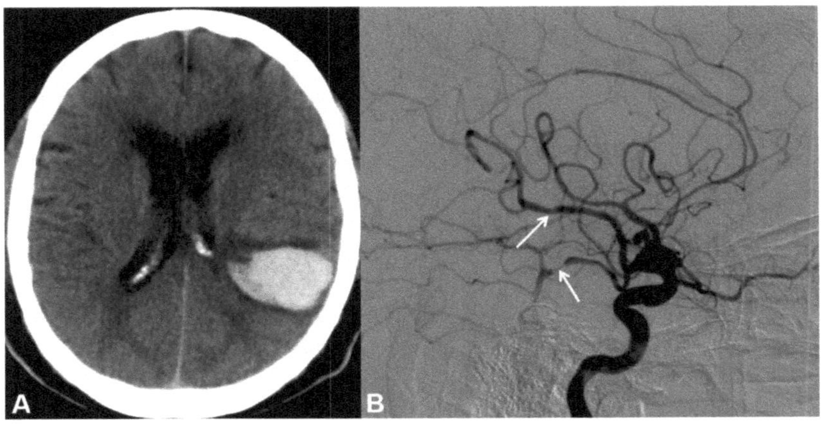

Fig. 21.14. (**A**) Primary angiitis of the central nervous system in a 55-year-old man with known chronic arterial hypertension who developed a left parietal hematoma. (**B**) X-ray angiography (selective injection in the left internal carotid artery) performed 2 months later depicts multiple stenoses involving the middle and posterior cerebral arteries (arrows).

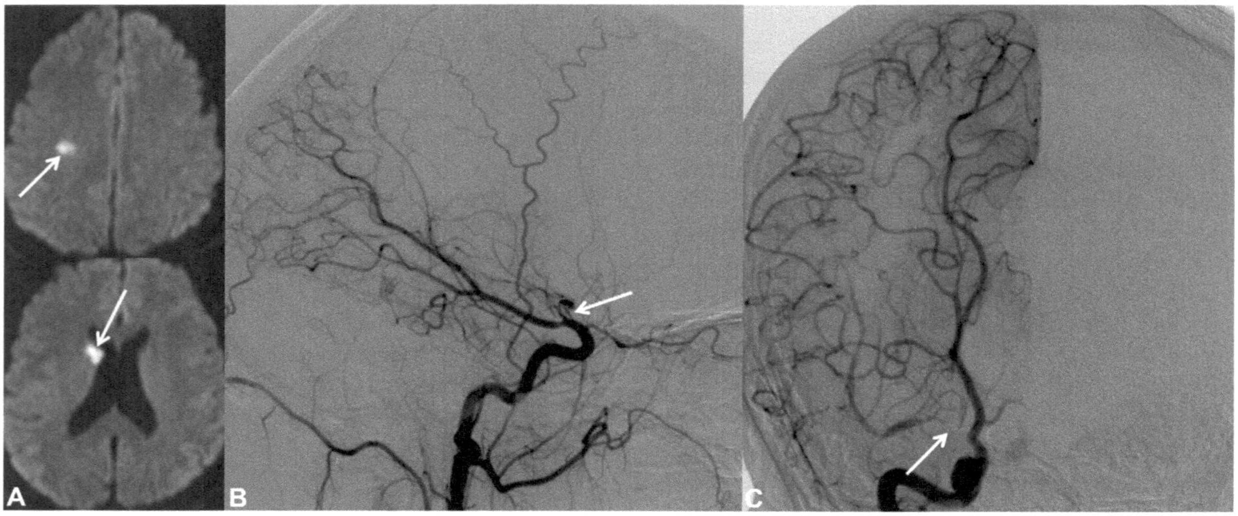

Fig. 21.15. Primary angiitis of the central nervous system in a 28-year-old patient with various minor stroke episodes and transient ischemic attacks involving several arterial territories. (**A**) Diffusion-weighted images show two small acute infarcts affecting the deep territory of the middle cerebral artery (MCA). (**B, C**) X-ray angiography (selective injection in the right internal carotid artery, ICA) performed a few days later shows multiple severe stenoses involving the supraclinoid segment of the ICA and proximal segment of the MCA (arrows).

explained by involvement of brain arteries smaller than can be detected on cerebral angiography. Such patients often present with cognitive dysfunction, have meningeal or parenchymal enhancing lesions on MRI, and respond favorably to treatment. MR angiography has been considered an alternative to cerebral angiography for supporting the diagnosis of PACNS. However this technique is less sensitive in detecting arterial lesions mainly involving the posterior circulation and distal vessels.

The diagnosis of PACNS is unlikely if MRI is normal, as the sensitivity of this technique is close to 100%. However MRI findings are nonspecific and include cortical and subcortical infarctions (Fig. 21.15), parenchymal and leptomeningeal enhancement (Fig. 21.16), intracranial hemorrhages (intracerebral and subarachnoid) (Fig. 21.14), tumor-like lesions (Fig. 21.16), and areas of increased signal intensity on T2-weighted images. Concentric vessel wall thickening and intramural enhancement of large arteries are specific to PACNS, and are better demonstrated with high-resolution fat-suppressed T1-weighted images (Obusez et al., 2014).

Reversible cerebral vasoconstriction syndrome

The most common mimicker of PACNS is RCVS. RCVS is a recently proposed term to describe a group of conditions characterized by prolonged but reversible vasoconstriction of the cerebral arteries (Calabrese et al., 2007). This syndrome may occur spontaneously, but is usually associated with precipitating factors such as the use of vasoactive substances (ergotamine derivatives, amphetamines, and nasal decongestants), contraceptives, recreational drugs (cannabis, ecstasy, LSD, cocaine, alcohol), late pregnancy or puerperium, sexual intercourse, and catecholamine-producing tumors. Clinical manifestations are characterized by hyperacute severe and recurrent headache, sometimes associated with neurologic symptoms and signs (Calabrese et al., 2007). Brain MRI is usually normal unless complicated by intracerebral (6%) or cortical subarachnoid hemorrhage (22%) (Fig. 21.17), cerebral infarct (4%), or posterior reversible encephalopathy syndrome (9%) (Ducros et al., 2007).

The pathophysiology of RVCS is unknown, but the most widely accepted hypothesis considers that there is a transient disturbance in control of the cerebral vascular tone (Calabrese et al., 2007). In the absence of validated diagnostic criteria, Calabrese et al. (2007) have proposed a set of key clinical, laboratory, and imaging characteristics that may be useful to distinguish RVCS from PACNS (Table 21.3). This distinction is important because the prognosis and treatment requirements differ in these conditions. The overall outcome of RVCS is good, with no relapses and a low rate of persistent neurologic deficits. Cerebral angiography typically demonstrates multifocal segmental cerebral artery vasoconstriction with no evidence of aneurysmal subarachnoid hemorrhage, which, by definition, substantially or completely reverses within approximately 3 months (Fig. 21.17).

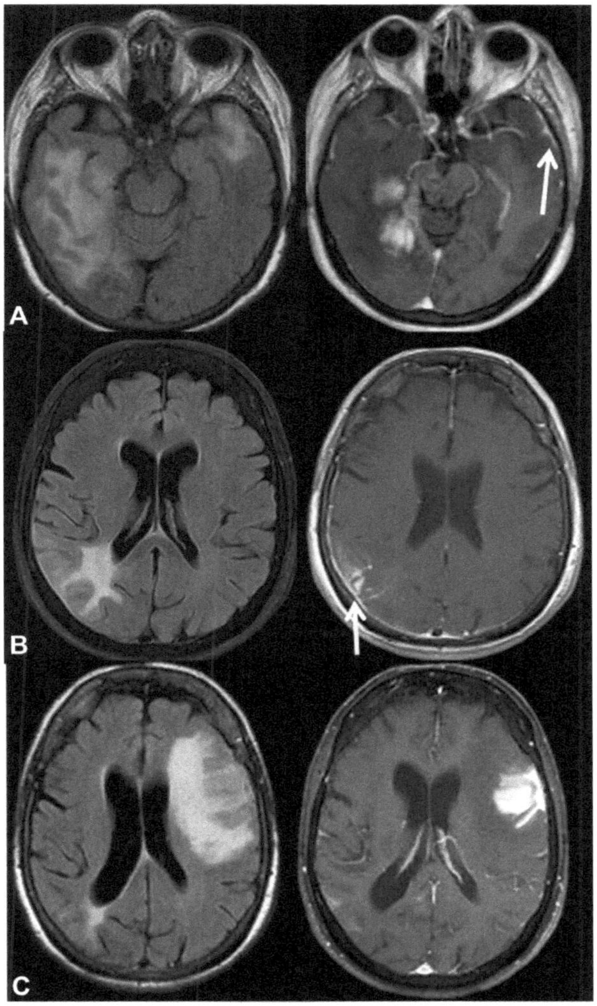

Fig. 21.16. Recurrent pseudotumoral lesions in a 45-year-old woman with primary angiitis of the central nervous system. T2 fluid-attenuated inversion recovery (FLAIR) and contrast-enhanced brain magnetic resonance imaging obtained at the onset of the first clinical episode revealed multiple contrast-enhancing lesions in temporal lobes, with edema (**A**). Brain biopsy revealed evidence of necrotizing lymphocytic vasculitis. The patient showed clinical and magnetic resonance imaging evidence of recurrence at 5 (**B**) and 18 (**C**) months after her initial presentation, with new pseudotumoral lesions involving the right parietal lobe and left frontal lobe. Note the leptomeningeal enhancement of some lesions (arrows).

Vasculitis associated with systemic disease

Systemic lupus erythematosus

SLE is a multisystem autoimmune disease that can affect many organs, including the skin, joints, lungs, and kidneys. It is overrepresented in Afro-Caribbean populations and has a female preponderance. SLE commonly affects the CNS, and numerous related neurologic and psychiatric syndromes are recognized. Neuropsychiatric SLE (NPSLE), which occurs in 25–70% of patients with SLE, is associated with a poorer prognosis and more cumulative damage than occurs in patients with SLE alone. The underlying reasons behind why patients develop NPSLE are uncertain. Investigators speculate that CNS damage is secondary to autoantibody production, noninflammatory vasculopathy of small arterioles and capillaries, atherosclerosis, or intrathecal production of proinflammatory cytokines (Hanly, 2005). Histopathologically, patients with NPSLE may show multifocal microinfarcts, cortical atrophy, gross infarcts, hemorrhage, ischemic demyelination, or patchy MS-like areas of demyelination. The clinical manifestations of NPSLE include psychosis, stroke, and epilepsy, in addition to more subtle symptoms such as headache and neurocognitive dysfunction. Patients with concomitant antiphospholipid antibodies (APLA) are at additional risk for neuropsychiatric events. CNS vasculitis and/or cerebritis represent a potentially severe form of NPSLE, in which patients may present with seizures, movement disorders, altered consciousness, stroke, or coma.

Although clinical assessment is the keystone in the diagnosis of NPSLE, the diagnosis is often difficult and remains presumptive in some patients. Brain MRI abnormalities are common in both SLE and NPSLE patients and range from nonspecific small, punctate, focal lesions in the subcortical and periventricular white matter (present in the majority of NPSLE patients, but not specific) (Fig. 21.18) to more severe findings, such as diffuse brain atrophy (present in about 43% of patients) (Fig. 21.19), cerebral edema, cerebral infarcts (large territorial infarcts, lacunar infarcts in the deep white matter, localized cortical infarcts in the territory of the middle cerebral arteries, bilateral borderzone infarcts, anterior basal ganglia lesions), and intracranial hemorrhage (parenchymal or subarachnoid hemorrhage, hemorrhagic infarcts, subdural hematoma). These abnormalities are more common in SLE patients with concomitant APLA (Kaichi et al., 2014).

Angiographic studies show signs of vasculitis, with reduced diameter or occlusion of the intracranial carotid arteries (Sibbitt et al., 2010). Spinal cord involvement has been described in 1–3% of patients in the form of longitudinal extensive myelitis with variable contrast enhancement. These findings are attributed to different mechanisms, including thrombosis, small-vessel vasculitis, and antibody-mediated neuronal injury.

Brain MRI abnormalities in NPSLE are sometimes indistinguishable from those of MS. The predominance of lesions located at the cortical or subcortical junction, as well as the concomitant finding of brain infarcts, calcification, or hemorrhages, should always raise the

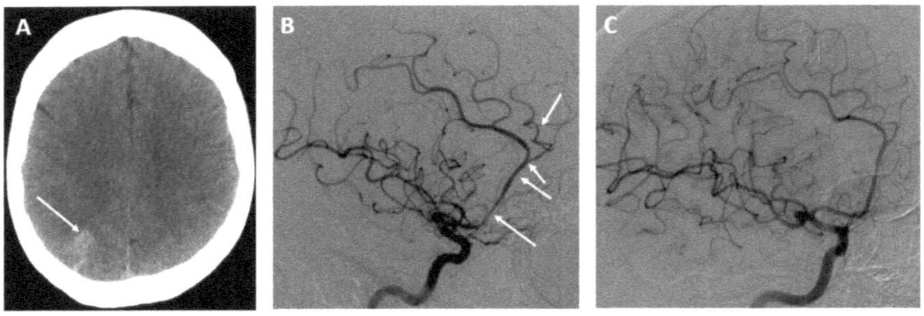

Fig. 21.17. Reversible cerebral vasoconstriction syndrome. A 58-year-old woman who presented with severe headache and vomiting. (**A**) Unenhanced brain computed tomography scan demonstrates parietal subarachnoid hemorrhage (arrow). (**B**) X-ray angiography in a right internal carotid artery lateral projection demonstrates areas of narrowing in proximal and distal segments of the anterior cerebral artery (arrows). (**C**) On follow-up X-ray angiography performed 3 months later the vessel caliber has normalized.

Table 21.3

Clinical, laboratory, imaging, and histopathologic characteristics useful to differentiate reversible cerebral vasoconstriction syndrome (RVCS) from primary angiitis of the central nervous system (PACNS)

	RVCS	PACNS
Clinical data		
Age	20–40 years	40–60 years
Sex	Primarily women	More frequent in men
Trigger	Frequently identified	Absent
Headache	Acute and severe	Insidious
Cognitive impairment	Unusual	Frequent
Cerebrospinal fluid analysis	Normal or minimal protein increase	Abnormal (increased protein concentration and mild pleocytosis)
Magnetic resonance imaging	Normal (>70%), unless complicated by stroke, PRES, or hemorrhage	Abnormal in >90%
Angiography	Multiple, diffuse areas of stenosis and dilatation that must reverse in 6–12 weeks	May be normal Single or multiple abnormalities
Central nervous system/ leptomeningeal biopsy	Normal	Vasculitis
Treatment	Calcium-channel blockers Glucocorticoids	Glucocorticoids Immunosuppressants

PRES, posterior reversible encephalopathy syndrome.

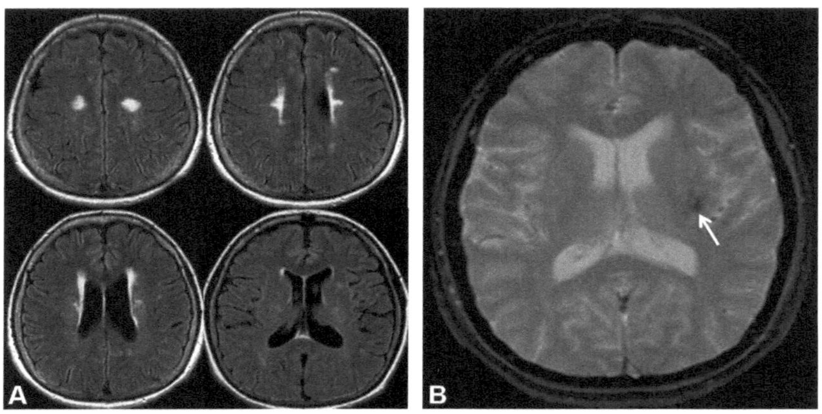

Fig. 21.18. A 39-year-old woman with neuropsychiatric systemic lupus erythematosus. (**A**) Transverse T2 fluid-attenuated inversion recovery (FLAIR) magnetic resonance images depict multiple small, white-matter hyperintensities, mainly involving the periventricular region and mimicking multiple sclerosis lesions. Note the microbleed in the left subinsular region on the T2* gradient-echo image (arrow in **B**). (Courtesy of Dr. Nuria Bargalló, Hospital Clinic Barcelona.)

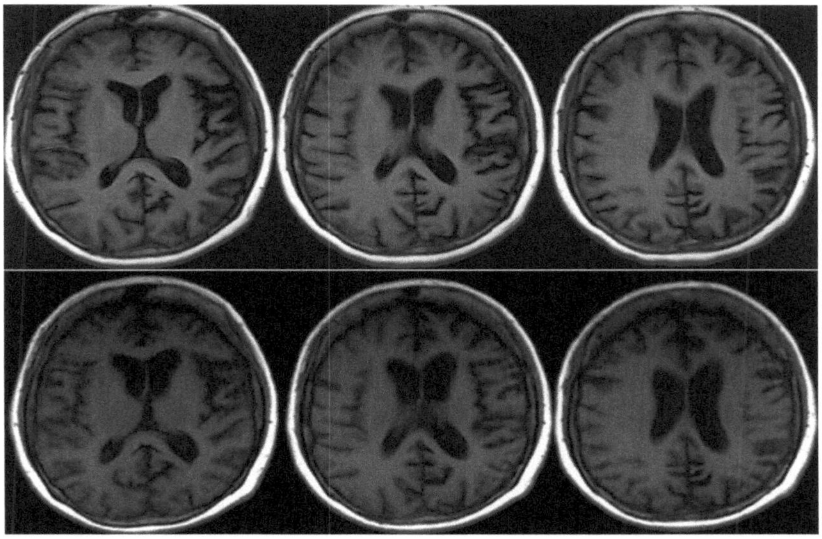

Fig. 21.19. A 55-year-old woman with neuropsychiatric systemic lupus erythematosus (cognitive decline and extrapyramidal symptoms). Serial transverse T1-weighted brain magnetic resonance images at admission (upper row) and 13 months later (lower row) demonstrate progressive volume loss, predominantly affecting the left-brain hemisphere.

suspicion of NPSLE or APLA syndrome (either primary or secondary to systemic immune-mediated diseases). Enhancing lesions and T1 black holes are much less common than in MS and can be discriminating features. In contrast to MS, asymptomatic spinal cord lesions are rare in SLE.

Neuro-Behçet's disease

Behçet's disease is a multisystemic, inflammatory vascular disease of unknown origin that affects small and medium-sized vessels and may present with a classic triad of oral and genital ulcerations with uveitis. The disease mainly occurs in young adults, and is more common in men. Patients present with various focal or multifocal neurologic problems. The most common neurologic symptom, which appears in up to one-third of patients, is severe headache; other common symptoms are weakness and cognitive and behavioral changes. Isolated optic neuritis, aseptic meningitis, and intracranial hemorrhage secondary to ruptured aneurysms are rare manifestations of the disease. Neurologic involvement in Behçet's disease is a cause of major morbidity; approximately 50% of patients are moderately or severely disabled 10 years after the onset.

Behçet's disease with CNS involvement can be divided into two groups: the parenchymal group (80%), which includes hemispheric meningoencephalitis, rhombencephalitis, and involvement of the cranial nerves and spinal cord; and the nonparenchymal type (20%), which includes intracranial venous thrombosis, and arterial occlusion or aneurysm (Razek et al., 2014). MRI is very sensitive in demonstrating the typical isolated or confluent reversible inflammatory parenchymal lesions, generally located within the brainstem and occasionally extending to the diencephalon, or within the basal ganglia, periventricular and subcortical white matter, spinal cord, and cranial nerves (Akman-Demir et al., 2003) (Fig. 21.20). In rare cases, the lesions may resemble those seen in MS, although Behçet's disease lesions are usually larger and more extensive. Leptomeningeal enhancement is present in patients presenting with cranial nerve palsy or meningoencephalitis. Brainstem atrophy is seen in chronic cases. Spinal cord involvement has been described in Behçet's disease, although it is rarely the presenting symptom.

Sjögren syndrome

SS is an autoimmune disease that characteristically causes xerophthalmia and xerostomia due to lymphocytic infiltration and malfunction of salivary and lacrimal glands. It is more common in women and usually manifests in middle age. It may occur as an isolated condition (primary SS) or be accompanied by a variety of connective tissue diseases and autoimmune disorders, such as SLE, rheumatoid arthritis, and scleroderma (secondary SS).

Extraglandular complications can occur in SS, including involvement of the central and peripheral nervous systems, which is reported to occur in in 25–30% of patients. Presenting symptoms include peripheral neuropathy (symmetric sensorimotor polyneuropathy, mononeuritis multiplex, and trigeminal

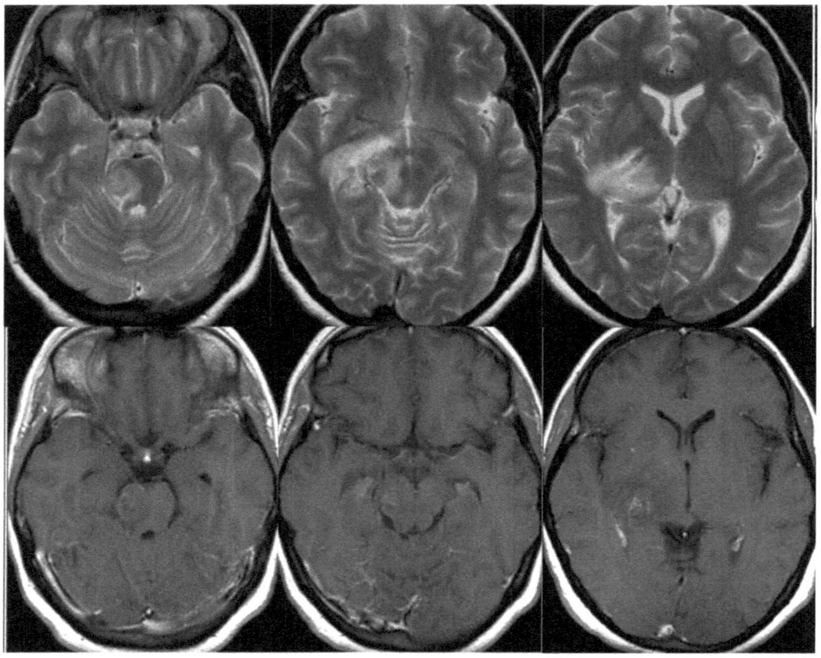

Fig. 21.20. Neuro-Behçet's disease in a 36-year-old man with fever of unknown origin, who presented with acute left-sided hemianopsia and hemiparesis. Clinical examination showed oral aphthas. Transverse T2- (upper row) and contrast-enhanced T1-weighted (lower row) brain magnetic resonance images demonstrate focal enhancing lesions with edema involving the mesencephalopontine region of the brainstem, and the capsulothalamic region on the right side.

sensory neuropathy), seen in 10–35% of patients with primary SS. CNS involvement is less common in primary SS and its manifestations may be localized (optic neuropathy, hemiparesis, transverse myelitis) or diffuse (encephalopathy, recurrent aseptic meningoencephalitis, and dementia) (Hasiloglu et al., 2012). In SS, optic neuritis and myelitis are usually associated with AQP4 antibodies and probably represent coexisting NMO, since Sjögren's patients lacking these features are AQP4-Ab-negative.

Occasionally, SS can present with acute, extensive focal or multifocal hemispheric white- and gray-matter stroke-like lesions and microbleeds. The white-matter lesions may resemble MS, although the corpus callosum and posterior fossa are rarely affected, and there may be involvement of deep gray-matter structures, particularly the basal ganglia. Angiographic studies sometimes show multiple arterial narrowing. Lesions in the spinal cord are rare, and may present with acute transverse myelitis or, less often, with progressive myelopathy that mimics MS. In patients presenting with acute myelitis, spinal cord MRI may demonstrate a longitudinally extensive spinal cord lesion, mimicking NMO, with predominant involvement of the dorsal columns.

Antiphospholipid antibody syndrome

APLA syndrome is a relatively common autoimmune disorder characterized by arterial and/or venous thrombosis and pregnancy morbidity as well as antibodies against several plasma proteins with affinity for anionic phospholipids (APLAs). These antibodies are present in up to 5% of the general population, and can also be found in infections, neoplasms, or following administration of certain drugs. In these cases, the antibodies are usually transient and are not associated with increased cardiovascular risk. Primary APLA syndrome occurs in patients with no predisposing conditions, whereas secondary APLA syndrome is found in 30–50% of patients with SLE and up to 30% of patients with human immunodeficiency virus infection.

Antiphospholipid syndrome is strongly associated with recurrent transient ischemic attacks, and strokes in young adults, secondary to arterial or venous thrombosis and thrombocytopenia. Other neurologic manifestations include migraine, seizures, chorea, and MS-like lesions. In fact, a proportion of MS patients are reported to be positive for APLAs. These patients often have optic neuritis and myelitis and therefore some of them may actually have NMO with coexistent APLA syndrome. Overall, it seems that APLA syndrome and MS are distinct entities, although the former can mimic the latter. Hence, atypical features in MS patients should prompt screening for APLAs. Unfortunately, clinical symptoms, examination findings, and MRI appearance cannot differentiate between the two conditions. However, a

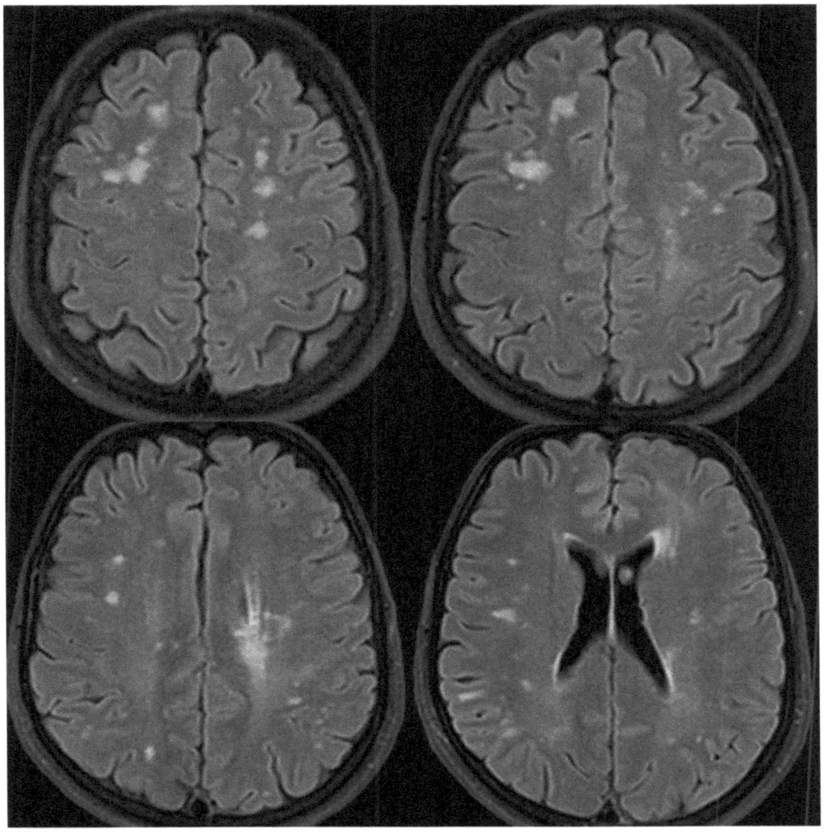

Fig. 21.21. A 45-year-old woman with antiphospholipid syndrome. Transverse T2 fluid-attenuated inversion recovery (FLAIR) brain magnetic resonance images demonstrate multiple hyperintense foci in the subcortical and deep white matter.

history of thrombosis, pregnancy loss, or the presence of livedo reticularis should prompt testing for APLAs.

Brain MRI shows white-matter abnormalities suggesting small-vessel disease, including acute infarcts and microhemorrhages (Muscal and Brey, 2010) (Fig. 21.21). APLA syndrome has been described as a common cause of RCVS.

NEUROSARCOIDOSIS

Sarcoidosis is a systemic granulomatous disease of unknown origin, characterized by the presence of noncaseating granulomas with proliferation of epithelioid cells in affected organs. Lesions are commonly seen in the lungs, lymphatic system, eyes, skin, liver, spleen, salivary glands, heart, nervous system, muscles, and bones.

Clinical signs and symptoms are nonspecific and include fatigue, weight loss, general malaise, and, less commonly, fever. About one-half of patients remain asymptomatic. Bilateral hilar lymphadenopathy is the most common radiologic finding. Adenopathy in the right paratracheal nodes, left aortic-pulmonary window, and subcarinal nodes can also be seen, often with associated pulmonary infiltrates. However, extrathoracic involvement is an initial manifestation in one-half of symptomatic patients. Asymptomatic CNS involvement is seen in up to 25% of patients at autopsy, whereas clinically recognizable involvement is estimated in 5–15% of patients. Manifestations of CNS sarcoidosis are variable, and depend on the site and extent of involvement, and its clinical presentation varies from a monophasic to a recurrent course, and from an acute explosive onset to a slow, progressive, chronic evolution (Hoitsma et al., 2004).

Although the radiologic features of CNS sarcoidosis may simulate those of infectious, inflammatory, or neoplastic disorders, mild clinical manifestations and laboratory data from CSF analysis, such as increased angiotensin-converting enzyme titer, CD4:CD8 ratio, and soluble interleukin-2 receptor may be helpful to distinguish sarcoidosis from these other disorders (Koyama et al., 2004; Petereit et al., 2010).

Several studies have shown that in most patients with neurosarcoidosis (70%), neurologic symptoms are the first manifestation of the disease (Dumas et al., 2000; Shah et al., 2009). These data emphasize the relevance

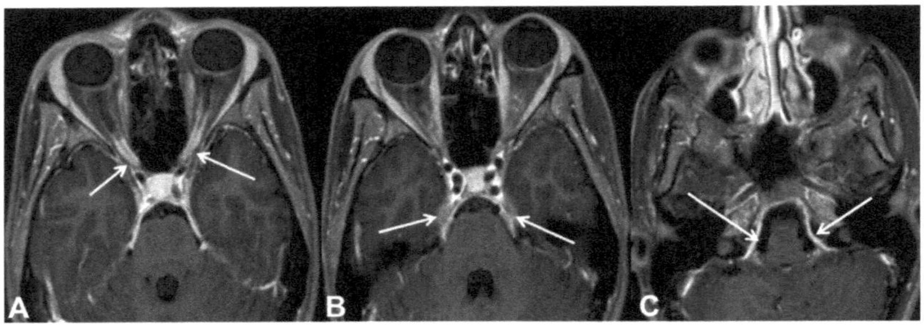

Fig. 21.22. Neurosarcoidosis in a 32-year-old woman presenting with subacute visual impairment. Contrast-enhanced transverse T1-weighted magnetic resonance images show bilateral enhancement of the distal segment of optic nerve (arrows in **A**), the trigeminal nerve (arrows in **B**), and the dura mater of the posterior fossa (arrows in **C**). (Courtesy of Dr. Ana Ramos, Hospital 12 de Octubre, Madrid.)

of recognizing neurosarcoidosis on the basis of radiologic findings in the absence of a history of systemic sarcoidosis at the time of presentation.

The most common radiologic finding in neurosarcoidosis is dural involvement (29–50%) (Shah et al., 2009) (Fig. 21.22). Epidural masses can mimic meningiomas, but the presence of noncontiguous dural enhancement may help in differentiating dural sarcoidosis from these tumors (Shah et al., 2009). A hypointense appearance on T2-weighted images may also be helpful in suggesting dural sarcoidosis, though T2-hypointensity is not specific for sarcoidosis and can be seen in a variety of other conditions, such as calcified meningiomas, dural metastases, lymphomas, idiopathic hypertrophic cranial pachymeningitis, Wegener granulomatosis, and rheumatoid nodulosis (Shah et al., 2009). Although most of these lesions affect the supratentorial compartment, infratentorial involvement has also been described (Shah et al., 2009). The low signal intensity of intracranial sarcoid lesions on T2-weighted sequences has been correlated with fibrocollagenous/gliotic tissue, and likely represents a reparative tissue reaction that has a poor response to immunosuppressive therapy. Cranial nerve lesions may be seen in 34–50% of patients with CNS sarcoidosis (Shah et al., 2009). These lesions have a weak correlation with clinical symptoms and rapidly respond to immunosuppressive therapy. Brain MRI typically shows an enlarged enhancing nerve trunk, predominantly involving the optic nerve, followed by the trigeminal and oculomotor nerves (Figs 21.22 and 21.23). Optic nerve involvement produces an optic neuropathy that may resemble a demyelinating disease, particularly in young patients.

From the clinical viewpoint, the peripheral facial nerve is most commonly affected, and is the most common neurologic manifestation of sarcoidosis overall (Hoitsma et al., 2004). However this clinical manifestation is mainly due to entrapment in affected meninges or parotid gland lesions.

Leptomeningeal involvement is less frequent, appearing in almost one-third of the patients (Fig. 21.23). Radiologically, these lesions manifest as thickening and enhancement of the leptomeninges with predominant involvement of the suprasellar and frontobasal regions. The disease may spread from these areas along the Virchow–Robin spaces, resulting in intraparenchymal involvement. This imaging pattern resembles the features observed in tuberculosis, Wegener granulomatosis, fungal meningitis, lymphoma, and leptomeningeal carcinomatosis (Shah et al., 2009). Single or multiple intraparenchymal masses representing granulomas and commonly associated with leptomeningeal involvement are uncommon, but their presence poses a diagnostic challenge, as they mimic primary or metastatic neoplasms. However, the absence of central necrosis is a constant feature in intraparenchymal neurosarcoidosis (Shah et al., 2009).

Granulomatous lesions are commonly found in the hypothalamus or pituitary gland (Hoitsma et al., 2004) (Fig. 21.23). This may cause endocrine manifestations, such as diabetes insipidus, adenopituitary failure, and amenorrhea-galactorrhea syndrome, which can appear alone or in various combinations. Hypothalamic granulomatous lesions producing diabetes insipidus are associated with disappearance of the normally hyperintense signal of the posterior pituitary lobe on T1-weighted images.

Asymptomatic periventricular and subcortical nonenhancing multifocal hyperintense lesions on T2-weighted images, mimicking those seen in MS, have been commonly described in patients with neurosarcoidosis. However, the presence of such asymptomatic white-matter lesions in patients older than 50 years is likely not caused by sarcoidosis and can be regarded as age-related small-vessel disease (Hoitsma et al., 2004).

Spinal cord involvement is not uncommon, particularly in the early phases of the disease, although it is rarely the first manifestation. Lesions have a fusiform

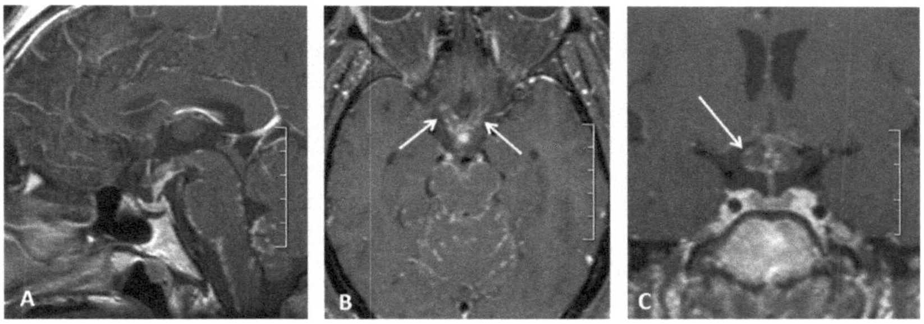

Fig. 21.23. Neurosarcoidosis. A 45-year-old man presenting with endocrine insufficiency and multiple cranial nerve dysfunction (visual impairment and diplopia). Contrast-enhanced (**A**) sagittal, (**B**) transverse, and (**C**) coronal T1-weighted images demonstrate diffuse nodular leptomeningeal enhancement in the basilar cisterns and posterior fossa. Observe the leptomeningeal enhancement surrounding the prechiasmatic segment of both optic nerves and chiasm (arrows). (Courtesy of Dr. Rafael Glikstein and Dr. Carlos Torres, University of Ottawa.)

appearance and tend to affect the cervical or upper thoracic segments (Fig. 21.24). As opposed to intracranial lesions, spinal cord lesions have high signal intensity on T2-weighted images, which likely reflects a predominant inflammatory pathologic substrate, which will have a good response to steroids and immunosuppressive therapy. Less frequently, CNS sarcoidosis presents with spinal arachnoiditis, and extradural and intradural extramedullary lesions, representing the leptomeningeal and dural lesions described intracranially.

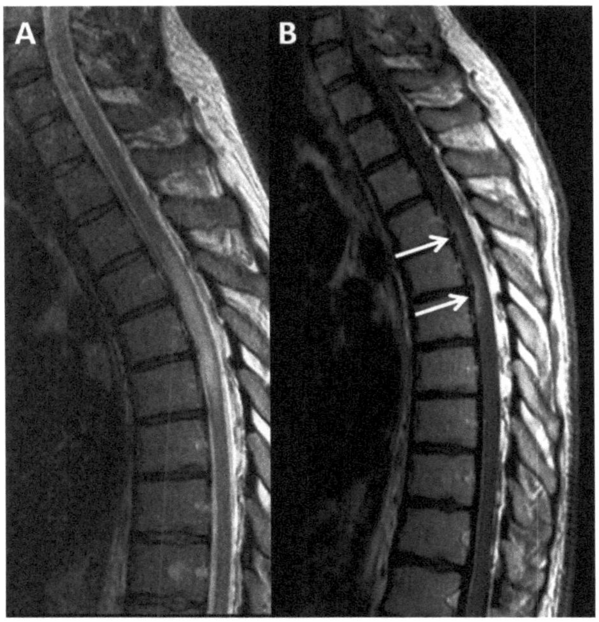

Fig. 21.24. Spinal cord involvement in sarcoidosis in a 23-year-old man presenting with acute incomplete transverse myelitis. (**A**) Sagittal T2-weighted and (**B**) enhanced transverse T1-weighted images of the thoracic cord show longitudinally extensive myelitis with marginal anterior enhancement (arrows), suggesting leptomeningeal involvement.

CONCLUSIONS

Several neuroradiologic imaging techniques have been extensively applied to the study of IIDDs and other inflammatory disorders that affect the CNS. These examinations play an important role in narrowing the differential diagnosis of this heterogeneous group of disorders. Due to the lack of specificity of imaging findings in many of these conditions, the imaging features should be correlated with clinical manifestations and laboratory results to improve their diagnostic value. Although computed tomography and conventional MRI provide most of the information needed to establish or suggest a diagnosis, X-ray angiography is still required for this purpose in specific diseases involving the intracranial vessels. High-resolution vessel wall imaging may play a more relevant role in diagnosing these conditions in the near future.

References

Akman-Demir G, Bahar S, Coban O et al. (2003). Cranial MRI in Behçet's disease: 134 examinations of 98 patients. Neuroradiology 45: 851–859.

Calabrese LH, Dodick DW, Schwedt TJ et al. (2007). Narrative review: reversible cerebral vasoconstriction syndromes. Ann Intern Med 146: 34–44.

Cañellas AR, Gols AR, Izquierdo JR et al. (2007). Idiopathic inflammatory-demyelinating diseases of the central nervous system. Neuroradiology 49: 393–409.

Cianfoni A, Niku S, Imbesi SG (2007). Metabolite findings in tumefactive demyelinating lesions utilizing short echo time proton magnetic resonance spectroscopy. AJNR Am J Neuroradiol 28: 272–277.

de Seze J, Blanc F, Kremer S et al. (2010). Magnetic resonance spectroscopy evaluation in patients with neuromyelitis optica. J Neurol Neurosurg Psychiatry 81: 409–411.

Ducros A, Boukobza M, Porcher R et al. (2007). The clinical and radiological spectrum of reversible cerebral vasoconstriction syndrome. A prospective series of 67 patients. Brain 130: 3091–3101.

Dumas JL, Valeyre D, Chapelon-Abric C et al. (2000). Central nervous system sarcoidosis: follow-up at MR imaging during steroid therapy. Radiology 214: 411–420.

Hanly JG (2005). Neuropsychiatric lupus. Rheum Dis Clin North Am 31: 273–298.

Hardy TA, Miller DH (2014). Baló's concentric sclerosis. Lancet Neurol 13: 740–746.

Hasiloglu ZI, Albayram S, Tasmali K et al. (2012). A case of primary Sjögren's syndrome presenting primarily with central nervous system vasculitic involvement. Rheumatol Int 32: 805–807.

Hoitsma E, Faber CG, Drent M et al. (2004). Neurosarcoidosis: a clinical dilemma. Lancet Neurol 3: 397–407.

Kaichi Y, Kakeda S, Moriya J et al. (2014). Brain MR findings in patients with systemic lupus erythematosus with and without antiphospholipid antibody syndrome. AJNR Am J Neuroradiol 35: 100–105.

Kim W, Park MS, Lee SH et al. (2010). Characteristic brain magnetic resonance imaging abnormalities in central nervous system aquaporin-4 autoimmunity. Mult Scler 16: 1229–1236.

Koyama T, Ueda H, Togashi K et al. (2004). Radiologic manifestations of sarcoidosis in various organs. Radiographics 24: 87–104.

Krupp LB, Tardieu M, Amato MP et al. (2013). International Pediatric Multiple Sclerosis Study Group criteria for pediatric multiple sclerosis and immune-mediated central nervous system demyelinating disorders: revisions to the 2007 definitions. Mult Scler 19: 1261–1267.

Lennon VA, Wingerchuk DM, Kryzer TJ et al. (2004). A serum autoantibody marker of neuromyelitis optica: distinction from multiple sclerosis. Lancet 364: 2106–2112.

Majós C, Aguilera C, Alonso J et al. (2009). Proton MR spectroscopy improves discrimination between tumor and pseudotumoral lesion in solid brain masses. AJNR Am J Neuroradiol 30: 544–551.

Masdeu JC, Quinto C, Olivera C et al. (2000). Open-ring imaging sign: highly specific for atypical brain demyelination. Neurology 54: 1427–1433.

Mehler MF, Rabinowich L (1989). Inflammatory myelinoclastic diffuse sclerosis (Schilder's disease): neuroradiologic findings. AJNR Am J Neuroradiol 10: 176–180.

Menge T, Hemmer B, Nessler S et al. (2005). Acute disseminated encephalomyelitis: an update. Arch Neurol 62: 1673–1680.

Miller DV, Salvarani C, Hunder GG et al. (2009). Biopsy findings in primary angiitis of the central nervous system. Am J Surg Pathol 33: 35–43.

Misu T, Fujihara K, Nakashima I et al. (2005). Intractable hiccup and nausea with periaqueductal lesions in neuromyelitis optica. Neurology 65: 1479–1482.

Molloy ES, Hajj-Ali RA (2007). Primary angiitis of the central nervous system. Curr Treat Options Neurol 9: 169–175.

Mondejar RR, Santos JM, Villalba EF (2002). MRI findings in a remitting-relapsing case of Bickerstaff encephalitis. Neuroradiology 44: 411–414.

Muscal E, Brey RL (2010). Antiphospholipid syndrome and the brain in pediatric and adult patients. Lupus 19: 406–411.

Nagaishi A, Takagi M, Umemura A et al. (2011). Clinical features of neuromyelitis optica in a large Japanese cohort: comparison between phenotypes. J Neurol Neurosurg Psychiatry 82: 1360–1364.

Obusez EC, Hui F, Hajj-Ali RA et al. (2014). High-resolution MRI vessel wall imaging: spatial and temporal patterns of reversible cerebral vasoconstriction syndrome and central nervous system vasculitis. AJNR Am J Neuroradiol 35: 1527–1532.

Papadopoulos MC, Verkman AS (2011). Aquaporin 4 and neuromyelitis optica. Lancet Neurol 11: 535–544.

Petereit HF, Reske D, Tumani H et al. (2010). Soluble CSF interleukin 2 receptor as indicator of neurosarcoidosis. J Neurol 257: 1855–1863.

Popescu BF, Lucchinetti CF (2012). Pathology of demyelinating diseases. Annu Rev Pathol 7: 185–217.

Razek AA, Alvarez H, Bagg S et al. (2014). Imaging spectrum of CNS vasculitis. Radiographics 34: 873–894.

Saini J, Chatterjee S, Thomas B et al. (2011). Conventional and advanced magnetic resonance imaging in tumefactive demyelination. Acta Radiol 52: 1159–1168.

Salvarani C, Brown Jr RD, Hunder GG (2012). Adult primary central nervous system vasculitis. Lancet 380 (9843): 767–777.

Sastre-Garriga J, Rovira A, Rio J et al. (2003). Clinically definite multiple sclerosis after radiological Schilder-like onset. J Neurol 250: 871–873.

Shah R, Roberson GH, Curé JK (2009). Correlation of MR imaging findings and clinical manifestations in neurosarcoidosis. AJNR Am J Neuroradiol 30: 953–961.

Sibbitt Jr WL, Brooks WM, Kornfeld M et al. (2010). Magnetic resonance imaging and brain histopathology in neuropsychiatric systemic lupus erythematosus. Semin Arthritis Rheum 40: 32–52.

Stadelmann C, Ludwin S, Tabira T et al. (2005). Tissue preconditioning may explain concentric lesions in Baló's type of multiple sclerosis. Brain 128: 979–987.

Tenembaum S, Chamoles N, Fejerman N (2002). Acute disseminated encephalomyelitis: a long-term follow-up study of 84 pediatric patients. Neurology 59: 1224–1231.

Trebst C, Jarius S, Berthele A et al. (2014). Update on the diagnosis and treatment of neuromyelitis optica: recommendations of the Neuromyelitis Optica Study Group (NEMOS). J Neurol 261: 1–16.

Verhey LH, Branson HM, Shroff MM et al. (2011). MRI parameters for prediction of multiple sclerosis diagnosis in children with acute CNS demyelination: a prospective national cohort study. Lancet Neurol 10: 1065–1073.

Wingerchuk DM, Weinshenker BG (2003). Neuromyelitis optica: clinical predictors of a relapsing course and survival. Neurology 60: 848–853.

Wingerchuk DM, Lennon VA, Pittock SJ et al. (2006). Revised diagnostic criteria for neuromyelitis optica. Neurology 66: 1485–1489.

Wingerchuk DM, Lennon VA, Lucchinetti CF et al. (2007). The spectrum of neuromyelitis optica. Lancet Neurol 6: 805–815.

Wingerchuk DM, Banwell B, Bennett JL et al. (2015). International consensus diagnostic criteria for neuromyelitis optica spectrum disorders. Neurology 14: 177–189.

Yonezu T, Ito S, Mori M et al. (2014). "Bright spotty lesions" on spinal magnetic resonance imaging differentiate neuromyelitis optica from multiple sclerosis. Mult Scler 20: 331–337.

Handbook of Clinical Neurology, Vol. 135 (3rd series)
Neuroimaging, Part I
J.C. Masdeu and R.G. González, Editors

Chapter 22

Imaging of head trauma

SANDRA RINCON[1]*, RAJIV GUPTA[1,2], AND THOMAS PTAK[1,3]

[1]*Division of Neuroradiology, Massachusetts General Hospital, Boston, MA, USA*

[2]*Division of Neuroradiology and Cardiac Radiology, Massachusetts General Hospital, Boston, MA, USA*

[3]*Division of Emergency Radiology, Massachusetts General Hospital, Boston, MA, USA*

Abstract

Imaging is an indispensable part of the initial assessment and subsequent management of patients with head trauma. Initially, it is important for diagnosing the extent of injury and the prompt recognition of treatable injuries to reduce mortality. Subsequently, imaging is useful in following the sequelae of trauma. In this chapter, we review indications for neuroimaging and typical computed tomography (CT) and magnetic resonance imaging (MRI) protocols used in the evaluation of a patient with head trauma. We review the role of CT), the imaging modality of choice in the acute setting, and the role of MRI in the evaluation of patients with head trauma. We describe an organized and consistent approach to the interpretation of imaging of these patients. Important topics in head trauma, including fundamental concepts related to skull fractures, intracranial hemorrhage, parenchymal injury, penetrating trauma, cerebrovascular injuries, and secondary effects of trauma, are reviewed. The chapter concludes with advanced neuroimaging techniques for the evaluation of traumatic brain injury, including use of diffusion tensor imaging (DTI), functional MRI (fMRI), and MR spectroscopy (MRS), techniques which are still under development.

INTRODUCTION

Traumatic brain injury (TBI) is a leading cause of morbidity and mortality both in the USA and worldwide (Faul et al., 2010). The Centers for Disease Control and Prevention (CDC) estimate that TBI affects approximately 1.7 million Americans each year, generating approximately 1 365 000 emergency department visits in the USA per year (CDC, 2003). While a majority of these 1.7 million cases present with minor trauma, about 1 in 5 patients are severely affected, resulting in 275 000 hospitalizations and 52 000 deaths in the USA alone (CDC, 2003; Faul et al., 2010). TBI is a contributing factor to a third of all injury-related deaths in the USA (Faul et al., 2010). Imaging plays a key role in the management of TBI, including detection, triage, surgical guidance, and prognostication.

Young children, older adolescents, and adults aged 65 years and older are most likely to sustain a TBI. In every age group, TBI rates are higher for males than females (Faul et al., 2010). Falls are the leading cause of TBI, with rates highest for young children and adults aged 75 years and older. Motor vehicle accidents are the leading cause of TBI-related deaths, with rates highest for adults aged 20–24 years (Faul et al., 2010). Severe TBI not only impacts the life of an individual and the individual's family, but it also has a large societal and economic toll. The estimated economic cost of TBI in 2010, including direct and indirect medical costs, is estimated to be approximately $76.5 billion (Teasdale and Jennett, 1974).

The Glasgow Coma Scale (GCS) is one of the most commonly used tools for the clinical assessment of patients with TBI (Iverson et al., 2000; Cushman et al., 2001; Servadei et al., 2001). It is a reliable and objective way of assessing the initial and subsequent level of consciousness in a person after a brain injury. The GCS score

*Correspondence to: Sandra Rincon, MD, Massachusetts General Hospital, 55 Fruit St, Gray 2-B285, Boston MA 02114, USA. Tel: +1-617-726-8320, E-mail: srincon@mgh.harvard.edu

is based on the sum of the best eye-opening response (Teasdale and Jennett, 1974; CDC, 2003; Finkelstein et al., 2006; Faul et al., 2010), best verbal response (Teasdale and Jennett, 1974; Iverson et al., 2000; CDC, 2003; Finkelstein et al., 2006; Faul et al., 2010), and best motor response (Teasdale and Jennett, 1974; Iverson et al., 2000; Cushman et al., 2001; CDC, 2003; Finkelstein et al., 2006; Faul et al., 2010). The GCS, therefore, ranges between 3 and 15, 3 being the worst score and 15 the best score. A GCS score of 13 or higher correlates with mild brain injury, 9–12 is a moderate injury, and 8 or less a severe brain injury.

Concussion, or mild TBI (mTBI), is stratified clinically according to symptoms such as confusion, amnesia, and loss of consciousness, and has a GCS > 13 (National Center for Injury Prevention and Control, 2003). A World Health Organization study estimates that mTBI comprises 75–90% of all head injuries that receive treatment annually. Concussion is fairly common, representing nearly 10% of all sports injuries, and is the second leading cause of brain injury in young people aged 15–24 years behind motor vehicle accidents.

In general, there should be a low threshold for imaging patients with a history of amnesia, headache, vomiting, focal neurologic deficit, visible head trauma, seizure, or bleeding diathesis. It is especially important in patients in the age groups with the highest frequency of mTBI: 0–4, 15–19, and >65 years. Imaging should certainly be performed where drug or alcohol intoxication interferes with the clinical exam. Symptoms of somnolence, nausea, and vomiting when associated with head trauma are worrisome, as they may indicate increased intracranial pressure. Follow-up imaging is indicated in patients who experience a change in mental status.

This chapter describes an overall approach to the imaging of head trauma. We first describe the indications for neuroimaging and describe typical computed tomography (CT) and magnetic resonance imaging (MRI) protocols. The next section provides guidelines on how to avoid pitfalls when analyzing imaging studies on trauma patients. Subsequent sections describe individual pathologies, such as fractures, intracranial hemorrhage, parenchymal injury, penetrating head trauma, cerebrovascular injuries, and secondary effects of trauma. The last section is devoted to some advanced neuroimaging techniques that are still under development.

INDICATIONS AND IMAGING PROTOCOLS

Indications for head CT

A noncontrast head CT (NCCT) is the standard of care for moderate and severe TBI; its use in mTBI is not well established and multiple guidelines (Cushman et al., 2001; Jagoda et al., 2008; Tavender et al., 2011), such as the New Orleans Criteria, the Canadian CT Head Rules, and the National Emergency X-ray Utilization Study-II studies, provide patient selection guidelines for the use of NCCT in the setting of mTBI.

NCCT has a high sensitivity and specificity for demonstrating intracranial hemorrhage, extra-axial collections, edema, swelling, midline shift, herniation, and fracture (National Collaborating Centre for Acute Care, 2007). Its widespread availability, speed of acquisition, and lack of contraindications make it the first-line modality in the management of TBI. Nonetheless, when subjecting pediatric patients to an NCCT, the risks and benefits should be carefully considered because of the radiation exposure.

Head CT protocol

A typical trauma head CT is performed helically at 120 kVp, 200 mAs, with a fast rotation time (e.g., 0.5 seconds), and a pitch of 1 or 0.5. Many times, a cervical spine CT is acquired in conjunction with the head CT to rule out a concomitant cervical spine fracture or dislocation. The optimal protocol for detecting fractures, in the calvaria or the spine, requires thin axial slices constructed using a sharp kernel (e.g., the bone kernel for a GE scanner, or H50-sharp kernel for a Siemens scanner). The axial slices must be at least 1.25 mm or thinner in slice thickness, with about 50% overlap (Fig. 22.1A). These may be augmented by coronal, sagittal, multiplanar oblique, or three-dimensional (3D) images to aid visualization (Fig. 22.1B). Multiplanar reconstructions are useful to the reviewing radiologist to assess bony asymmetry and alignment, as well as to access certain structures that are optimally visualized in the coronal or sagittal imaging planes. All images should be visualized in predefined window/level settings such as "brain," "subdural," "bone," and "soft-tissue" to optimize detection of different pathologies (Fig. 22.1C). 3D reconstructions are useful to the referring physician for preoperative planning and intraoperative image guidance.

Some institutions prefer axial (or step-and-shoot) rather than helical scanning. Axial scans reduce the windmill artifact. One can also use a customized technique such as a higher-kV scan for the posterior fossa and a lower-kV scan for the supratentorial brain. Helically acquired scans, however, can be retrospectively reconstructed into multiple different formats and spacings. For example, with a helical or spiral protocol, thinner image slices can be retrospectively generated with any desired spacing and/or overlap. This can be done as long as the raw projection data is still available. Operationally, it is therefore mandatory that the raw projection data be saved, for at least a few days after the

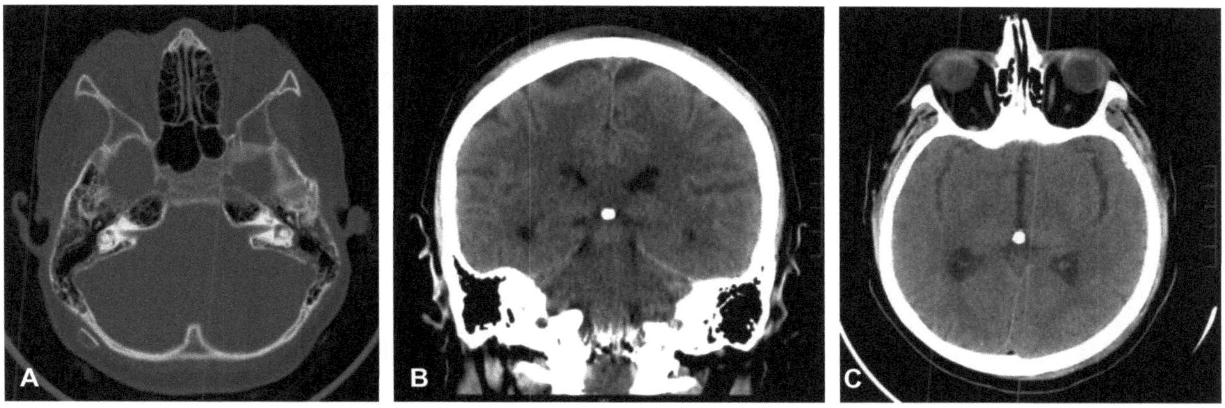

Fig. 22.1. A thin axial CT image in bone kernel (**A**), a coronal CT image reconstructed from an axial helical acquisition (**B**), and an axial CT image in a subdural window/level setting (**C**).

scan, while clinical questions during the acute care of a patient are still being addressed.

Indications for MRI

While considerable research is being conducted in the use of MRI for characterizing TBI, it is not the primary tool for investigation of acute TBI. An MRI is more sensitive in demonstrating certain pathologies such as diffuse axonal injury (DAI) as compared to NCCT. However, there are no studies that confirm the clinical utility of MRI in terms of patient management in the acute setting. However, MRI should be obtained in a patient where the CT findings fail to explain the neurologic deficits. MRI may also provide prognostic information about long-term outcome (Galanaud et al., 2012). MRI is also better suited for grading stages of intracranial hemorrhage and for detecting contusions, DAI, microhemorrhages, edema, and brainstem injuries (Anon et al., 2008).

Major drawbacks of MRI include multiple contraindications such as pacemakers, need for careful patient screening in an acute setting, long exam times, and the relative unavailability of MRI compared to CT.

MRI PROTOCOL

A typical MRI protocol for evaluating TBI may include T1W, T2W, T2W-fluid-attenuated inversion recovery (FLAIR), T2*-gradient-recalled echo (GRE), and diffusion-weighted imaging (DWI) sequences. Susceptibility-weighted images (SWI) may also be included (perhaps in lieu of T*-GRE), as they increase the conspicuity of microhemorrhages (Davis et al., 2000; Le and Gean, 2009). Generally, there is no need to administer intravenous contrast for the evaluation of TBI.

Approach to image evaluation

The initial imaging of head trauma is important for diagnosing the extent of injury and the prompt recognition of treatable injuries to reduce mortality. For example, neuroimaging is indispensable for early recognition of treatable injuries such as an epidural hematoma (EDH), a large subdural hematoma, or significantly depressed skull fracture. CT is the imaging modality of choice to triage patients with acute head trauma because of its widespread availability, speed, and compatibility with life support and monitoring devices. CT is very sensitive in the detection of acute hemorrhage and in the evaluation of skull fractures. The limitations of CT are related to metallic streak artifacts, patient motion, partial volume averaging, and beam-hardening artifact in the posterior fossa, inferior temporal, and inferior frontal regions.

MRI is an alternative initial imaging modality which provides multiplanar capability. It is helpful for the characterization and timing of hemorrhage, and is better for the evaluation of intraparenchymal injury such as intraparenchymal hematoma, contusion, DAI, and cerebral edema. Unlike CT, MRI provides excellent visualization of the inferior frontal and temporal lobes and the posterior fossa. SWI is a newer imaging technique that maximizes sensitivity to magnetic susceptibility effects, and is more sensitive than conventional gradient echo images for the detection of blood products. In uncooperative, unstable, or claustrophobic patients, ultrafast sequences may provide answers to crucial questions in the shortest time possible. Limitations of MRI are related to the long imaging time, the cumbersome nature of imaging and monitoring the trauma patient, and the location of most MRIs outside of the emergency department. MRI is also less sensitive than CT in detecting fractures.

Patients with TBI have abnormalities that are attributable to primary and secondary brain injury. A primary injury occurs at the time of injury and secondary brain injury evolves and complicates the primary injury. Primary or immediate injuries include intracranial hemorrhage, intraparenchymal injuries, including DAI and contusions, cerebral edema, fractures, and extracranial soft-tissue injury/lacerations. Secondary injuries consist of hypoxia/ischemia, increased intracranial pressure, hydrocephalus, and infection.

The details of the head trauma are crucial. Particular emphasis should be placed on the location and force of impact, as this information will help in the search for expected findings given the nature and severity of the trauma. For example, a patient who has sustained a fall and has focal soft-tissue swelling may also have an underlying fracture with an associated EDH. If the patient's history is not known, however, a careful search of the extracranial soft tissues for evidence of trauma may guide the search for an intracranial abnormality (Fig. 22.2). The pattern of a skull fracture may show the direction, location, and force of the impact producing the injury.

An organized and consistent approach to the evaluation of a head CT of a trauma patient is essential. The images should be viewed with variable window widths and levels to accentuate differences in the CT attenuation between different structures. Window widths refer to the Hounsfield unit (HU) range selected for gray-scale display, whereas the window level refers to the center point about which the range is displayed (Grossman and Yousem, 2003). The images should be viewed in brain (window 80, level 40), subdural (window 200, level 80), stroke (window 36, level 30), bone (window 2500, level 575), and soft-tissue (window 400, level 40) "windows" to evaluate for parenchymal, extra-axial, ischemic, osseous, and soft-tissue injuries, respectively. Subdural windows are particularly useful in detecting superficial hemorrhage, shallow contusions, and small extra-axial collections, where the acute hyperdense hemorrhage may be obscured by the adjacent high attenuation bone (Fig. 22.3). Coronal reformatted images are very useful in looking for small extra-axial collections over the cerebral convexities at the vertex, as well as along the falx cerebri and tentorium cerebelli. In addition, coronal reformatted images are helpful in the

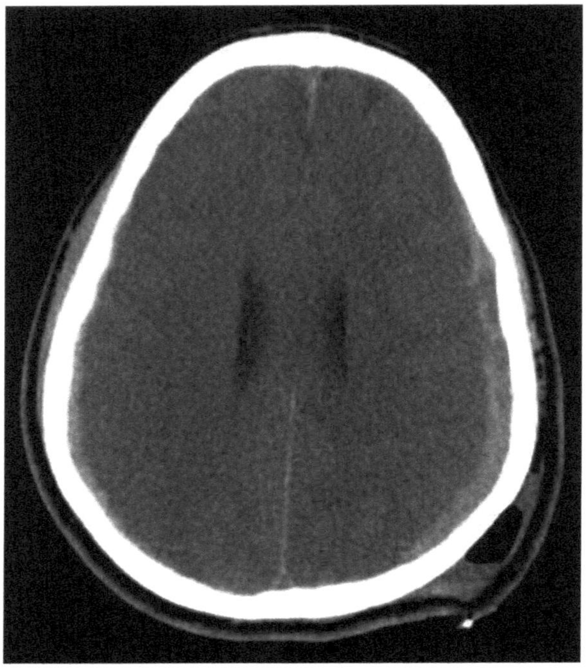

Fig. 22.3. Axial image from a noncontrast computed tomography in subdural windows shows bilateral subdural hematomas, left larger than right.

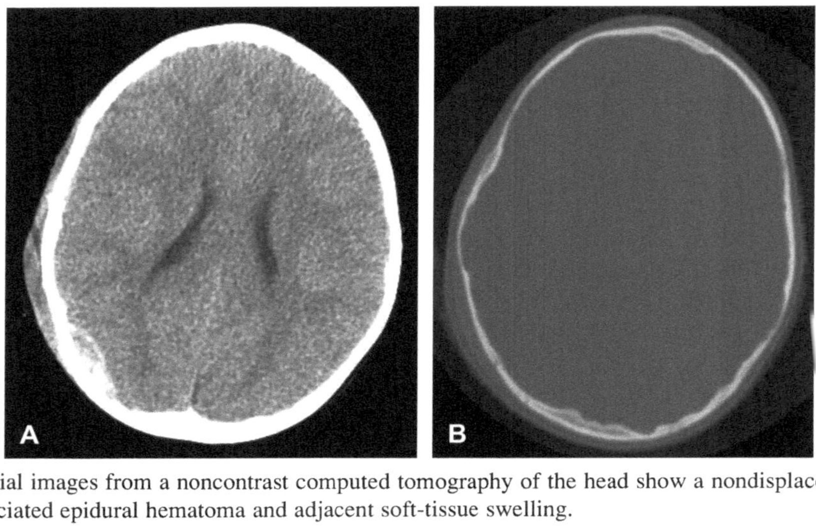

Fig. 22.2. (**A, B**) Axial images from a noncontrast computed tomography of the head show a nondisplaced right parietal bone fracture with an associated epidural hematoma and adjacent soft-tissue swelling.

evaluation of the inferior frontal and temporal lobes, which can be difficult to evaluate on the axial images due to beam-hardening streak artifact. Soft-tissue injury over the vertex is also better appreciated on coronal images. Thin-section bone algorithm images are essential for the evaluation of fractures. A combination of axial and coronal reformatted images is important in evaluating the integrity of the skull base, temporal bones, orbits, and face. It is important to review the scout image from the CT for evidence of a subtle linear fracture that may not be apparent on axial images because it is oriented parallel to the scan plane. Familiarity with anatomy of the skull is necessary so that a suture is not mistakenly called a fracture.

SKULL FRACTURES

Assessing for skull fractures can seem a tedious undertaking with at times dubious value. Many of the common fractures encountered will not require treatment, but, more importantly, serve as indicators of injury mechanism, and in many cases give clues to underlying brain injury.

Anatomy

The skull is comprised of two main components: the skull base and the calvaria or vault. Note that while calvaria (singular; = skull) and calvariae (plural) are the original Latin terms, the more common usage of calvarium (singular) and calvaria (plural) are accepted. The calvaria and overlying scalp provide protection and a controlled environment for the brain from the surrounding outside world. The skull base, in addition to providing physical and structural support for the calvaria and brain, is invested with an intricate network of canals and channels for the passage of nerves and blood vessels to and from the brain. The skull base also contains compartments dedicated to housing the special senses. Attention to the intricate anatomic detail of each compartment is important in differentiating fractures from normal structures and in anticipating injury.

The calvaria is comprised of a set of broadly curved plates of bone that are joined at junctions called sutures. These plates of bone fit together to form an inverted bowl-shaped structure. The bony plates have a bilayer structure with two thin sheets of compact bone (outer thicker than inner) separated by a porous cancellous bone compartment, which provides strength to the complex and is home to blood-forming elements, vessels, and fat. This bilayered arrangement is not uniform at all points around the skull. The diploic space is thickest over the vertex, frontal, occipital, and lateral convexities, and thinnest at points of muscular attachment, making some calvarial regions more vulnerable to injury than others. The temporalis muscle, for example, arises from a broad attachment across the junction of the frontal, parietal, and squamous temporal bones in the infratemporal fossa. As a result, this segment of skull has a thin diploic space and is a common site for fractures. The scalp provides additional physical support as well as nutrition to the underlying skull. It has been estimated that the skull covered by an intact scalp can withstand an impact of up to 10 times that of one with the scalp removed (Cantu, 1995).

Imaging

CT is the first-line imaging modality for evaluating the skull. It is fast, commonly available, and sensitive for evaluating dense bony structures. Recent advances in imaging allow for very thin imaging sections and arrangement of images into multiple planes. Common skull-imaging protocols can include images in thick (e.g., 2.5 mm) sections as well as submillimeter (e.g., 0.625 mm) sections. Images are acquired using high spatial frequency reconstruction algorithms to provide fine trabecular detail. Thin-section axial images are also often reformatted into coronal and sagittal planes and in some cases 3D renderings. Examining these images using bone window and level settings (e.g., W1300: L600) provides exquisite detail of the cortical mantle as well as diploic space.

Fracture characteristics

Skull fractures can be separated into two large categories: linear and depressed. This is a useful delineation in that linear or hairline fractures are often treated conservatively, whereas depressed fractures portend more severe intracranial injury and often require surgery. Linear fractures result from a broad, low-energy impact, resulting in a shear force established at the point of contact that propagates in a wave-like fashion parallel to the long axis of the offending blunt object. Depressed fractures result from an impact concentrated on a small area which fails in compression with concentric waves of force extending radially from the impact point. Low-energy-point impacts result in a radial concentric set of fracture lines, producing a comminuted "dent" in the skull (Fig. 22.4).

A similar fracture is seen in the skeletally immature neonate, where the skull is in the early stages of formation. The neonatal skull consists of a higher proportion of nonossified cartilaginous elements, resulting in a more plastic fracture akin to the greenstick fracture seen in the extremities. The concentric radial fracture lines in the neonatal skull are more continuous rather than comminuted, giving the appearance of a dent, as might be seen in a ping-pong ball (Fig. 22.5). High-energy

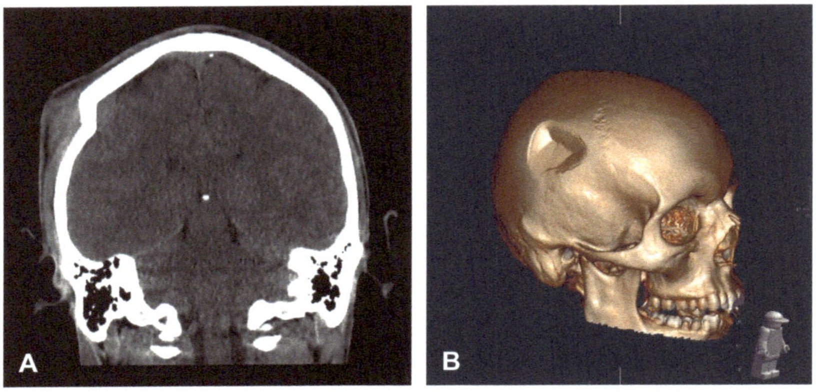

Fig. 22.4. (**A, B**) A depressed fracture from brick to head.

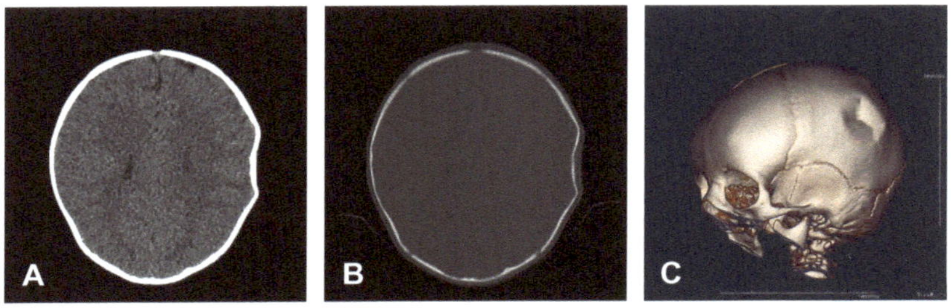

Fig. 22.5. (**A–C**) Ping-pong ball fracture.

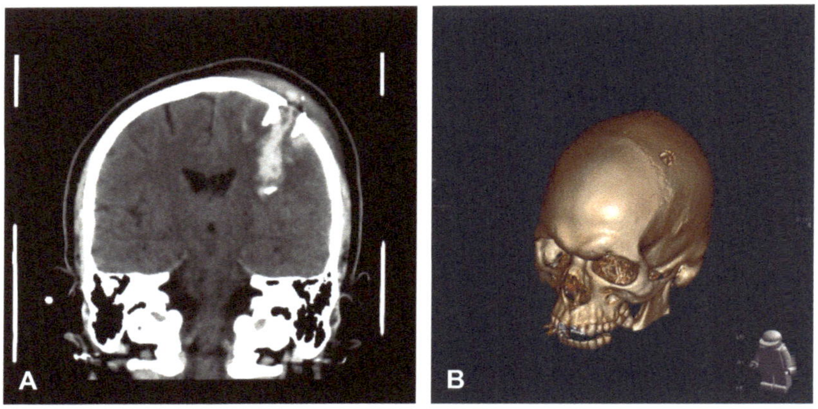

Fig. 22.6. (**A, B**) Stiletto-heel fracture.

point impacts (e.g. hammer blow or bullet) produce a "punched-out" defect with sharp margins and typically smaller fracture fragments, often propelled into the underlying brain tissue (Fig. 22.6).

In addition to the fracture, it is important to take note of the overlying scalp. A penetrating fracture accompanied by a deep laceration or complete disruption of the scalp constitutes an open fracture and is susceptible to infection. Fractures extending through air cells such as the frontal sinuses with an intact overlying scalp may be treated conservatively without antibiotics (Ali and Ghosh, 2002; Adalarasan et al., 2010). Fractures through the mastoid segment of the temporal bone however should be considered, not for the likelihood of infection from communication with air cell contents, but rather for the possibility that the fracture line lies in close proximity to the groove for the transverse or sigmoid venous sinus, raising the possibility of vessel injury or thrombosis (Burlew et al., 2012).

A schema for evaluating skull fractures with potential complications is provided in Figure 22.7.

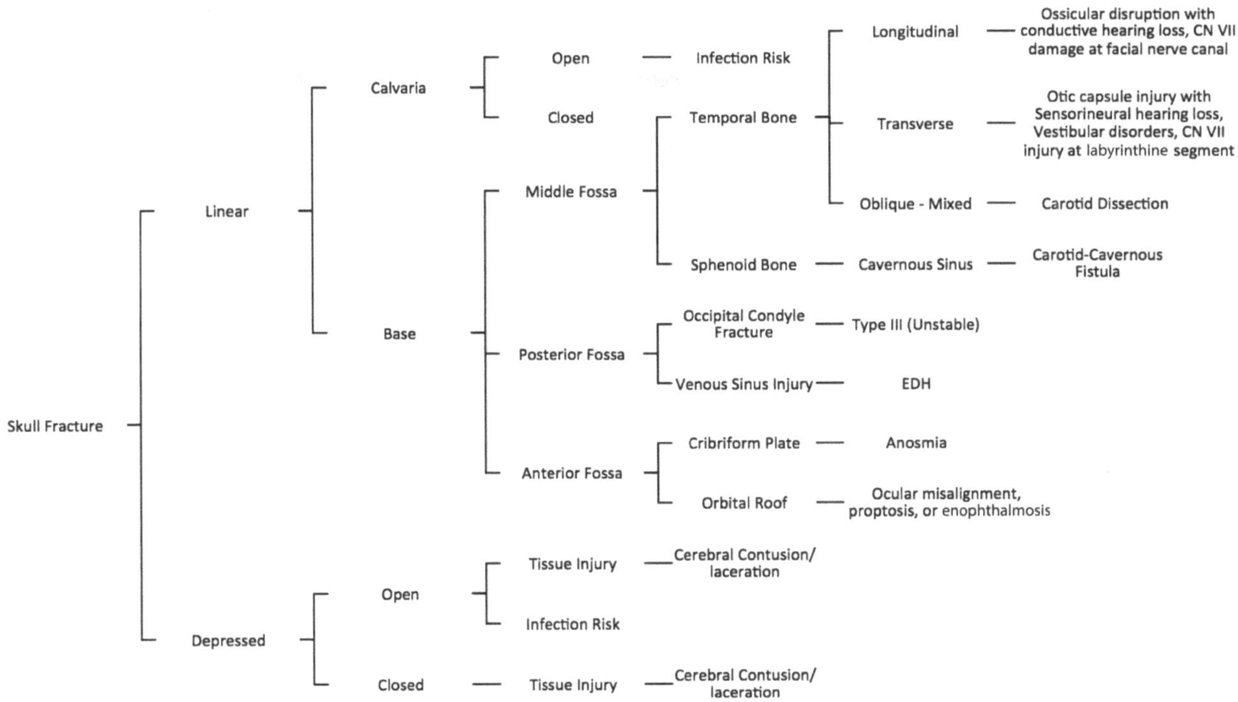

Fig. 22.7. Skull fracture schema. EDH, epidural hematoma; CN, cranial nerve.

Table 22.1

Differentiation of a linear fracture from normal structures

Attribute	Fracture	Vessel	Suture
Wall margins	Sharp, imperceptible	Thick, sclerotic	Imperceptible (child) Fused (adult)
Course	Nonbranching	Branching	May branch
Appearance	Linear	May curve	Zigzag (child)
Thickness	Varies, often <2 mm	>2 mm	<2 mm
Location	Point of impact	Some characteristic	Characteristic
Skull layers	Inner and outer	One, usually inner	Inner and outer

Analyzing the skull for fractures requires a detailed evaluation of the suspicious lucent line found on imaging. A reviewer can organize the inquiry around a set of questions: How wide is it? Through what portion of skull does it pass? Does it conform to the course of a known fissure, vessel canal, or suture? Is the course smooth or tightly zigzagged? Are the margins of the lucent line thick and sclerotic, or barely perceptible and sharp? Does the line branch? A list of useful identifying attributes can be found in Table 22.1.

Imaging and interpretation

In evaluating the bone for fracture, in general, more is better. While linear calvarial fractures can be any width, the vast majority are less than 2 mm in thickness (so-called "hairline"), and many are on the order of 1 mm. These hairline fractures may easily be averaged into a 2.5- or 1-mm thick CT slice, making detection virtually impossible, especially when the long axis of the fracture lies parallel to the CT acquisition plane (Collins et al., 2012). Keeping this in mind, consider some options that offer a more circumspect assessment. In theory, a two-view plain film series would be a good answer, giving the best overall general view of the skull. Since CT provides the detail we need for an indepth analysis, we can use all aspects of the CT examination to help guide our evaluation. For example, the scout view used for setting up the scan can be used as a skull study, providing the same images as a plain film series. This scout can be magnified and windowed to optimize visualization of fracture lucencies and provide a good overall look at the calvaria. Another option is the coronal and sagittal reformatted view. Off-axis reformations can provide two additional orthogonal imaging planes so that fractures lost in the axial plane may be seen *en face*. Also, these views may be reformatted at a larger slice thickness than the original axial series, and may even be rendered in maximum-intensity projection format, providing optimal contrast in defining fracture lines, especially in "hairline fractures," where there is little separation defining the fracture defect (Fig. 22.8). Lastly, do not overlook 3D volume rendering. The shaded surface display may help to define the course and character of fracture lines and give the best view of fracture continuity.

Potential complications of fractures

In general, uncomplicated minimally displaced and nondepressed fractures heal without issue. In 2–3% of cases, a tear in the dura at the site of the fracture may result in a cerebrospinal fluid (CSF) leak. This number may rise as high as 25% if the skull fracture is accompanied by facial fractures (Eljamel, 1994). CSF leaks from traumatic injury generally are established and diagnosed immediately following the incident, while iatrogenic CSF leaks may present after a delay. Duraplasty with or without craniotomy or autologous bone cranioplasty may be required to close the underlying dural defect (Liu et al., 2012).

The growing fracture or leptomeningeal cyst is a rare, delayed complication of skull fracture occurring predominantly in children and infants (Fig. 22.9). In this complication, the dura and its closely apposed arachnoid membrane may become entrapped in the fracture defect. Over time, the pulsatile force transferred by CSF in the subarachnoid space erodes at the margins of the free fracture edges, causing loss of bony cortex with widening of the original fracture defect. Patients may present with a deformity of the scalp that on CT imaging shows a smoothly marginated defect in the calvaria with interposed CSF density.

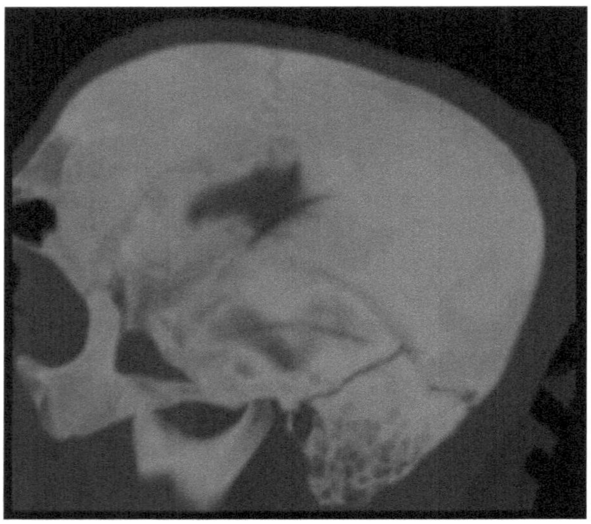

Fig. 22.8. Thick maximum-intensity projection (MIP) rendering of the bone.

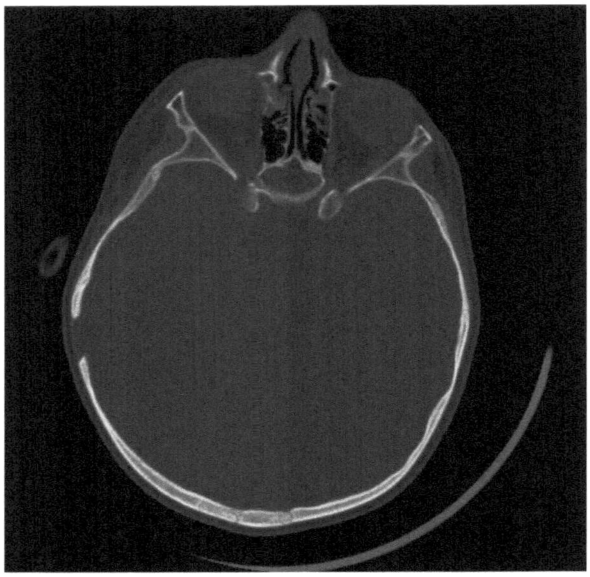

Fig. 22.9. Growing fracture.

HEMORRHAGE

Intracranial hemorrhage is commonly seen in the setting of trauma and is readily detected on neuroimaging studies. On CT, there is a linear relationship between the CT attenuation (density) of hemorrhage and the patient's hematocrit value. In the acute phase, intracranial hemorrhage is hyperdense, with an attenuation coefficient in the range of 80–90 HU, primarily due to the protein concentration of the blood (mostly hemoglobin). After the initial extravasation of blood, clot formation and retraction occur, with a progressive increase in density, over approximately 72 hours (Grossman and Yousem, 2003). After the third day, the attenuation values of the clot begin to decrease and the hemorrhage becomes isodense to brain over the next few weeks (subacute phase). After the first week, the amount of hemorrhage also diminishes, as does the associated mass effect and edema. Eventually, the hemorrhage becomes similar in density to CSF (chronic phase).

It is important to remember that acute hemorrhage may appear isodense to the adjacent cortex in an anemic patient (hemoglobin value less than 8–10 g/dL) or a coagulopathic patient. Patients with deficient coagulation, those with clotting disorders or on anticoagulants, can also demonstrate a hematocrit fluid–fluid level as the blood does not form a clot and the red cells settle dependently (Brant and Helms, 2007).

On MRI, the imaging characteristics of parenchymal hemorrhage are variable and change with the age of the blood. There are five stages of hemorrhage: hyperacute, acute (1–2 days), early subacute (2–7 days), late subacute (1 week to months), and chronic (months–years). Table 22.2 summarizes the salient features of the MRI appearance of intracranial hemorrhage.

SWI is a new imaging method that maximizes sensitivity to magnetic susceptibility effects and is extremely sensitive for the detection of microhemorrhage. As a result, it is particularly useful in the evaluation of TBI and has been shown to be more sensitive than conventional gradient-echo techniques for the detection of blood products.

Extra-axial hemorrhage

Subdural hematoma

Subdural hematomas are seen in 10–20% of patients with head trauma (Young and Destian, 2002). A subdural hematoma results from the stretching and tearing of bridging cortical veins in the subdural space, a potential space between the pia arachnoid and the dura (Figs 22.10–22.13). The bridging cortical veins rupture because of trauma-induced rotational movement of the brain, which shears the cortical veins where they are fixed and drain into the adjacent dural sinus. About 95% of subdural hematomas occur in the frontoparietal regions because of the tearing of these bridging veins. Approximately 10–15% of subdural hematomas are bilateral.

Use of an intermediate window width may enhance the sensitivity for detecting a small SDH, which can be difficult to differentiate from the adjacent calvarium (Fig. 22.14). Using "subdural windows" should be a routine part of every head CT evaluation for increased conspicuity of subtle subdural hematomas.

Subdural hematomas are seen in approximately 30% of patients with severe closed head trauma (Grossman and Yousem, 2003). They may or may not be associated with a brain parenchymal injury. When associated with a brain parenchymal injury, a subdural hematoma is associated with a 35–50% mortality rate (Grossman and

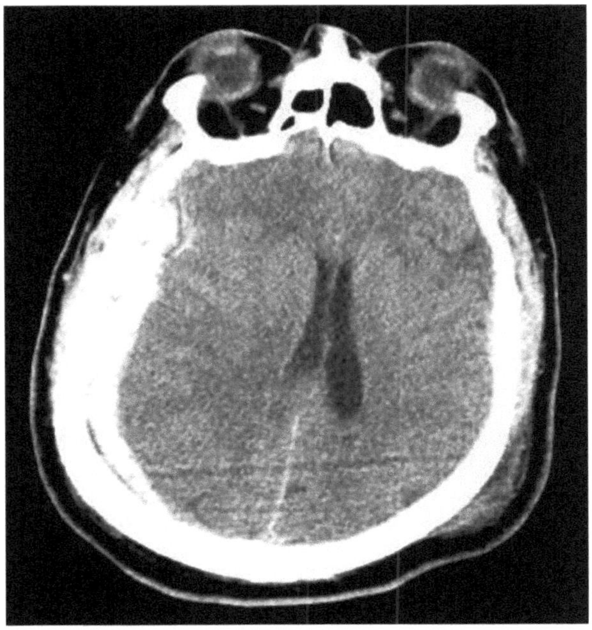

Fig. 22.10. Axial noncontrast computed tomography image shows a large acute right cerebral convexity subdural hematoma and smaller left cerebral convexity subdural hematoma.

Table 22.2

Magnetic resonance imaging appearance of intracranial hemorrhage

	Age	T1-weighted	T2-weighted
Hyperacute	Hours old, mainly oxyhemoglobin with surrounding edema	Hypointense	Hyperintense
Acute	Days old, mainly deoxyhemoglobin with surrounding edema	Hypointense	Hypointense, surrounded by hyperintense margin
Subacute	Weeks old, mainly methemoglobin	Hyperintense	
Early			Hypointense: early subacute with predominantly intracellular methemoglobin
Late			Hypointense: late subacute with predominantly extracellular methemoglobin
Chronic	Years old, hemosiderin slit or hemosiderin margin surrounding cavity	Hypointense	Hypointense slit, or hypointense margin surrounding cavity

Yousem, 2003). Subdural hematomas may also be seen in the setting of minor trauma, particularly in the elderly. In older patients, a subdural hematoma tends to be larger because of generalized parenchymal volume loss. In some patients, a history of trauma may be lacking.

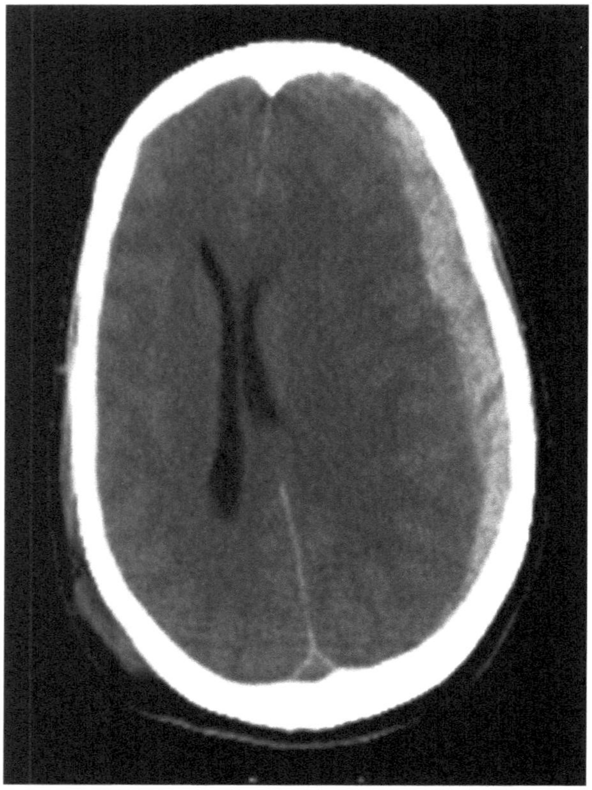

Fig. 22.11. Axial noncontrast computed tomography image shows a left cerebral convexity subdural hematoma with associated mass effect on the left cerebral hemisphere, effacement of the left lateral ventricle and mild midline shift.

The appearance of a subdural hematoma on CT varies with clot age and organization of the hemorrhage. Acute subdural hematomas are usually hyperdense, typically crescent-shaped, are not limited by the cranial sutures, but are limited by dural reflections, such as the falx cerebri, tentorium, and falx cerebelli. Up to 40% of acute subdural hematomas have a heterogeneous appearance with both hyperattenuating and hypoattenuating areas that reflect acute unclotted blood, serum extruded

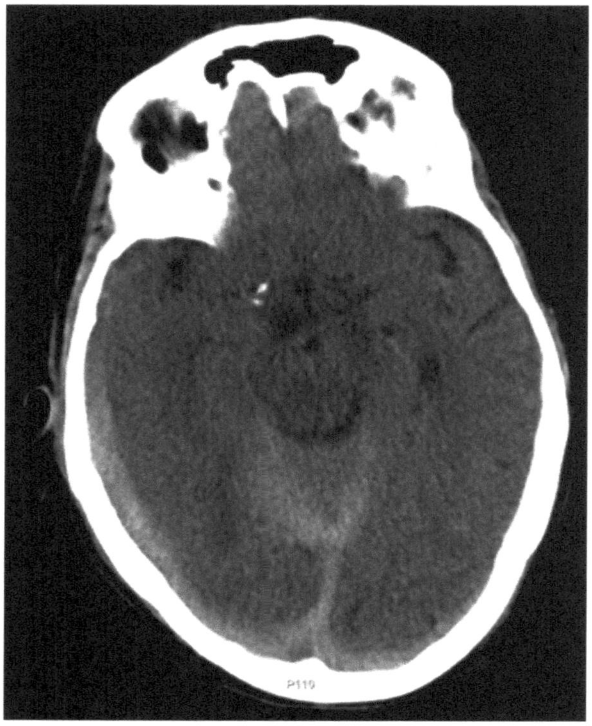

Fig. 22.12. Axial noncontrast computed tomography image shows bilateral acute subdural hematomas extending along the tentorium cerebelli.

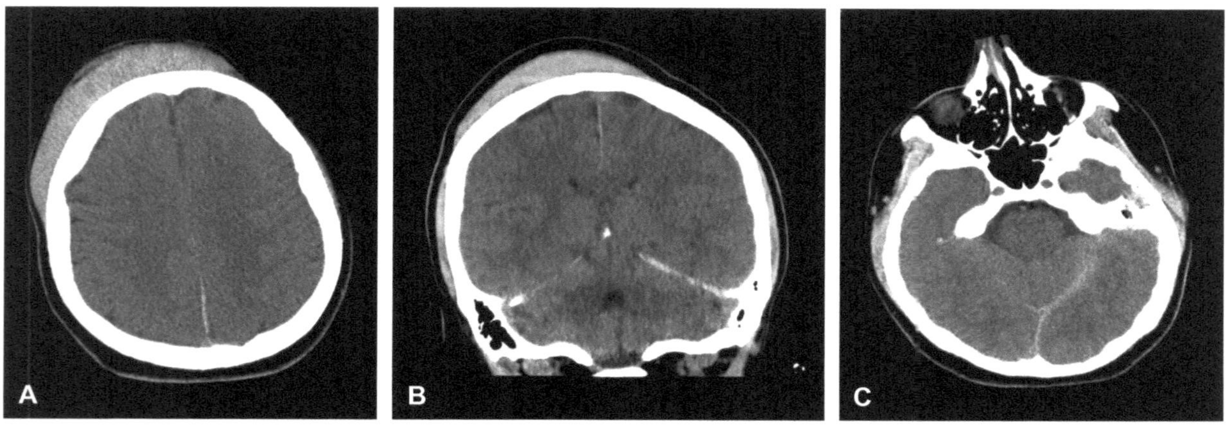

Fig. 22.13. (A–C) Axial noncontrast computed tomography images show a small acute subdural hematoma along the posterior aspect of the falx and left tentorial leaflet.

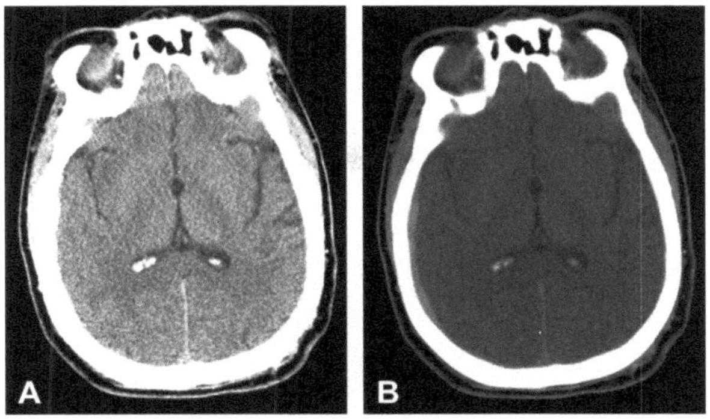

Fig. 22.14. (**A, B**) Axial noncontrast computed tomography images show a small subdural hematoma along the right cerebral convexity. The subdural hematoma is better visualized on image (**B**) because of subdural windows.

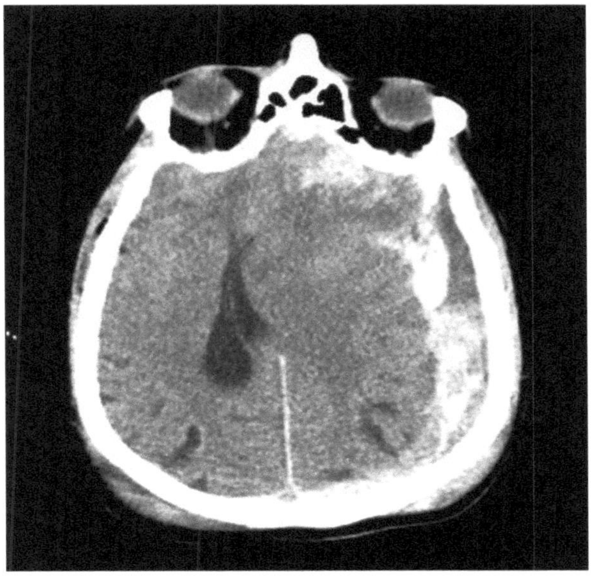

Fig. 22.15. Axial noncontrast computed tomography image shows an acute heterogeneous subdural hematoma with significant mass effect on the left cerebral convexity, effacement of the left lateral ventricle, and subfalcine herniation.

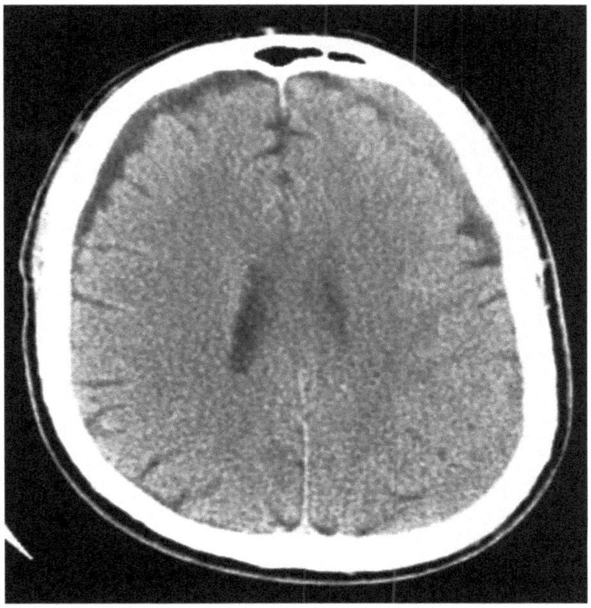

Fig. 22.16. Axial noncontrast computed tomography image shows an isodense subacute left cerebral convexity subdural hematoma and chronic right frontal subdural hematoma.

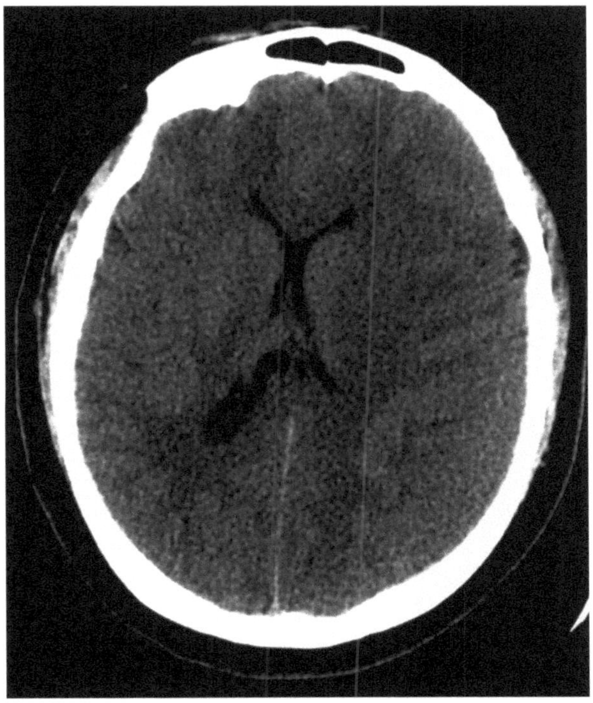

Fig. 22.17. Axial noncontrast computed tomography image shows a large isodense subacute left cerebral convexity subdural hematoma with associated mass effect on the left cerebral hemisphere, effacement of the left lateral ventricle, and minimal midline shift.

during clot retraction, or mixing with CSF from an arachnoid tear (Fig. 22.15).

In the hyperacute phase, a subdural hematoma may appear isodense to the adjacent cortex, with a swirled appearance due to a mixture of serum with clotted and unclotted blood (Brant and Helms, 2007). A subacute subdural hematoma may appear isodense or hypodense to the adjacent brain and may be apparent only by the attendant mass effect (Figs 22.16 and 22.17). On imaging, an isodense subdural hematoma may result in effacement of the ipsilateral sulci, inward displacement of the cortical veins and gray–white matter junction, effacement of the ventricles, and midline shift.

Identification of isodense subdural hematomas may be difficult, especially if they are bilateral.

A chronic subdural hematoma is usually hypodense on CT. It typically appears as a crescent-shaped, multiseptated extra-axial collection encapsulated by enhancing membranes. A subdural hygroma, by contrast, is a CSF collection in the subdural space caused by an arachnoid tear. A subdural hygroma will have no evidence of hemorrhage and no enhancing membranes. A subdural hygroma, however, can be indistinguishable from a chronic subdural hematoma on imaging.

An acute on chronic subdural hematoma refers to acute hemorrhage into a pre-existing chronic subdural hematoma. It typically appears as a hypodense extra-axial collection with a dependent hematocrit level (Fig. 22.18). A recurrent, mixed-density subdural hematoma in a child raises suspicion for nonaccidental trauma and shaking injury. MRI is extremely useful in the evaluation of children suspected of nonaccidental trauma, because it can better characterize blood products of different ages. The MRI appearance of a subdural hematoma is variable and changes with the age of the blood products, as described earlier in the chapter (Fig. 22.19).

Epidural hematoma

Only 1–4% of patients with acute head trauma present with an EDH (Young and Destian, 2002; Osborn, 2005). An EDH occurs in the potential space between the inner table of the skull and the dura mater. Ninety percent of EDHs are arterial, related to the middle meningeal artery, and 10% are venous in origin, associated with the dural venous sinuses – the transverse or sigmoid sinus in the posterior fossa and superior sagittal sinus. Nearly all EDHs occur at the site of impact and 85–95% are associated with a skull fracture. Approximately of 90–95% of EDHs are supratentorial and 5–10% occur in the posterior fossa (Osborn, 2005).

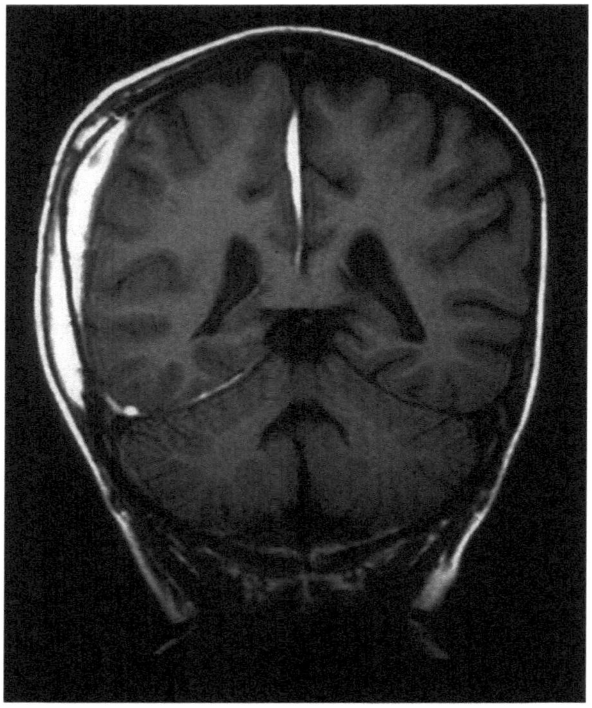

Fig. 22.19. Coronal T1-weighted magnetic resonance image shows T1 hyperintense subdural hemorrhage along the right cerebral convexity, falx, and right tentorial leaflet, consistent with subacute hemorrhage.

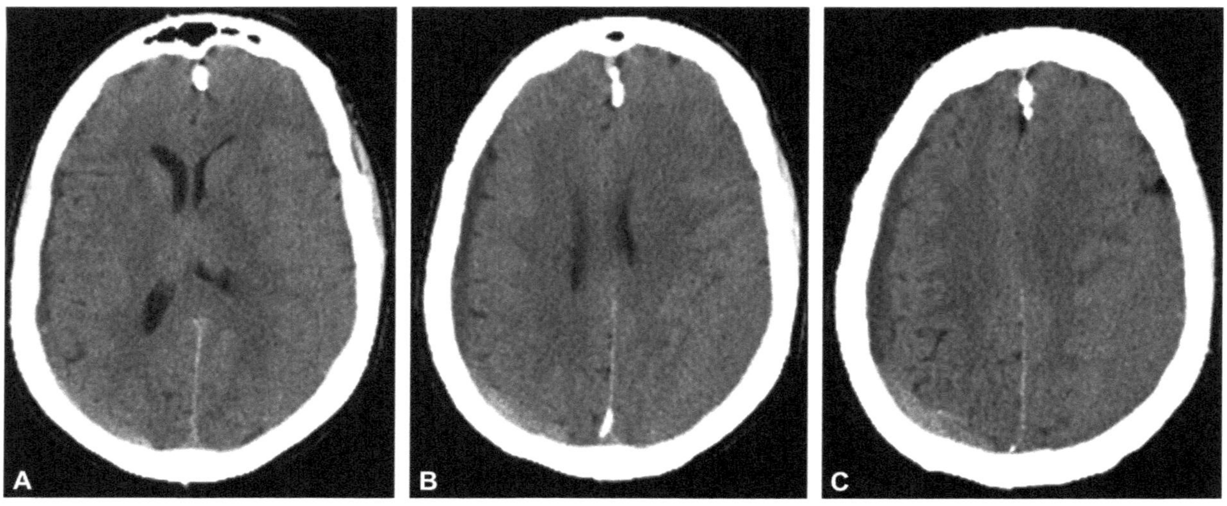

Fig. 22.18. (A–C) Axial noncontrast computed tomography images show an acute on chronic right cerebral convexity subdural hematoma with a layering hyperdense component representing acute hemorrhage. There is also a large isodense subacute left cerebral convexity subdural hematoma with associated mass effect on the left cerebral hemisphere and left lateral ventricle.

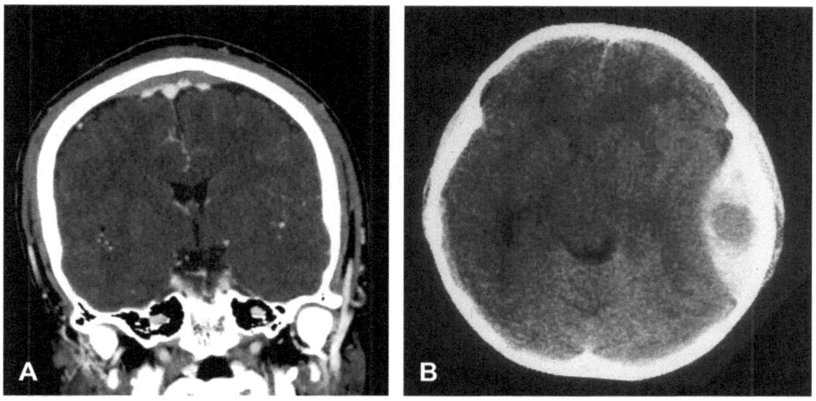

Fig. 22.20. (**A**) An epidural hematoma at the vertex crossing the midline and displacing the superior sagittal sinus; (**B**) axial noncontrast computed tomography image shows a large left cerebral convexity epidural hematoma with a "swirl sign" consistent with active hemorrhage.

EDHs are more common in younger patients, aged 20–40 years (Osborn, 2005). Clinically, the classic lucid interval after the injury with later loss of consciousness is seen in approximately 50% of patients.

On imaging, an EDH is biconvex in shape, due to the strong attachment of the dura to the inner table of the skull. Unlike a subdural hematoma, an EDH does not cross sutures but can cross the midline or into the posterior fossa by lifting the dural venous sinus off the inner table of the skull (Fig. 22.20A). In cases where this is seen, a CT venogram (CTV) may help define any resulting venous sinus obstruction. The presence of a swirl sign, areas of low attenuation within the hematoma, suggests active bleeding at the time of the CT scan (Fig. 22.20B).

Prompt recognition and appropriate treatment are essential as EDHs may enlarge rapidly (Fig. 22.21). EDHs nearly always require surgical evacuation; the major exception is the small EDH in the anterior aspect of the middle cranial fossa. A small EDH may be managed conservatively and followed with serial imaging to assess for interval change.

Subarachnoid hemorrhage

The most common cause of subarachnoid hemorrhage (SAH) is trauma. Most patients with significant head trauma have SAH on imaging or lumbar puncture, or at autopsy. SAH occurs in the subarachnoid spaces between the pia and arachnoid membranes. It is rarely space-occupying and is usually self-limited. Traumatic SAH is often associated with other intracranial injuries.

On imaging, there is high density on CT and FLAIR hyperintensity on MRI in the sulci and basal cisterns, in the setting of trauma (Fig. 22.22). The SAH may appear as a localized clot or may be distributed more diffusely throughout the CSF spaces. A small amount of SAH in the interpeduncular cistern may be the only manifestation of SAH. Complications of SAH include hydrocephalus (Fig. 22.23) and vasospasm, which is an uncommon cause of posttraumatic infarct (Osborn, 2005).

Intraventricular hemorrhage (IVH) occurs in 2.8% of all patients with blunt head trauma (Young and Destian, 2002). Isolated IVH is relatively uncommon. More often, it results from extension of a parenchymal hematoma or SAH. Minimal layering hemorrhage in the occipital horns of the lateral ventricles may be the only sign of IVH (Fig. 22.24). Alternatively, extensive IVH may clot, forming a cast of the ventricles and resulting in outflow obstruction of CSF, causing noncommunicating hydrocephalus (Fig. 22.25).

PARENCHYMAL INJURY

Parenchymal contusion

A parenchymal contusion results from blunt trauma to the brain parenchyma (Fig. 22.26). It involves the superficial gray matter and occurs in characteristic locations adjacent to a bony protuberance or dural fold. Nearly 50% of parenchymal contusions involve the temporal lobes, 33% involve the inferior frontal lobes, and 25% involve the parasagittal white matter of the frontal lobes ("gliding" contusions) (Osborn, 2005). A focal contusion may occur at the site of a depressed fracture (Fig. 22.27). Multiple, bilateral contusions are seen in 90% of cases.

Contusions have traditionally been described as coup or contrecoup. A coup contusion occurs at the site of impact and may be associated with a calvarial fracture. A contrecoup contusion occurs opposite the site of impact, frequently involving the inferior frontal and anterior temporal lobes.

Parenchymal contusions evolve over time. Initially, a contusion may not be apparent by CT. However, as it evolves, a contusion may appear as a patchy and

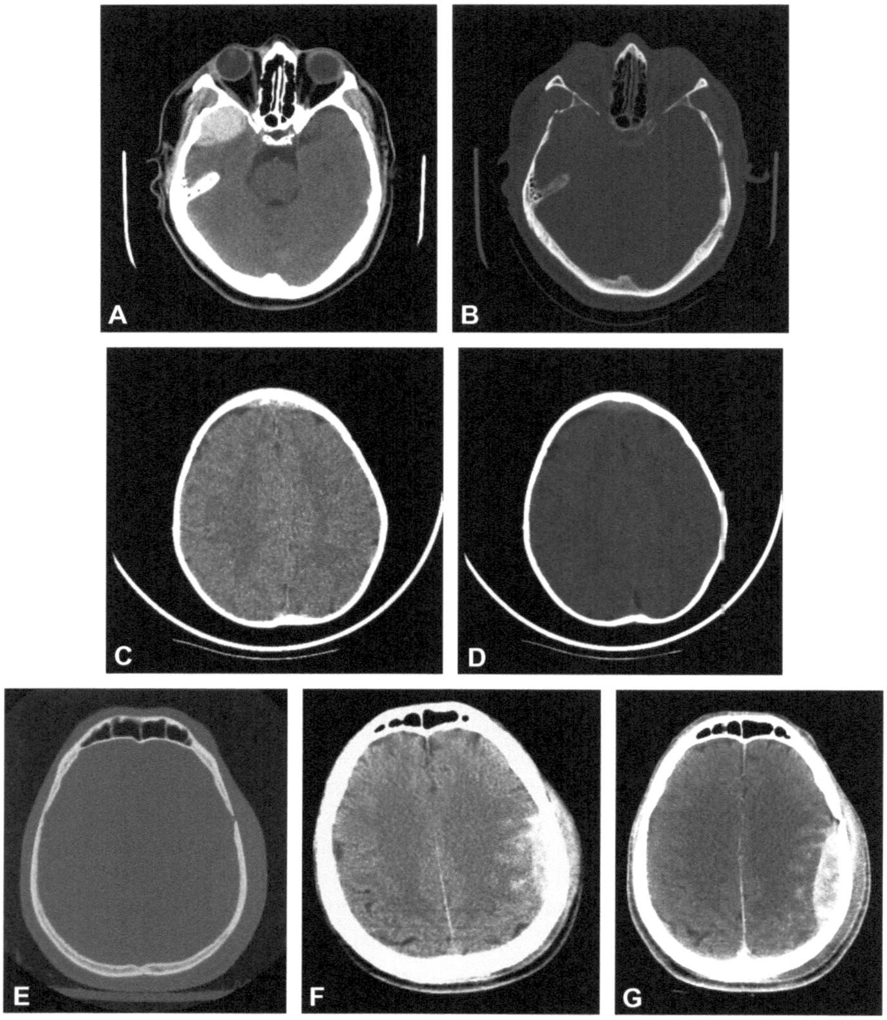

Fig. 22.21. Examples of epidural hematomas. Right temporal-bone fracture with an associated epidural hematoma (top row; images **A** and **B**); small epidural hematoma crossing the midline (middle row; images **C** and **D**); and enlargement of a left cerebral convexity epidural hematoma over a 1-hour time period with an associated fracture (bottom row; images **E**, **F** and **G**).

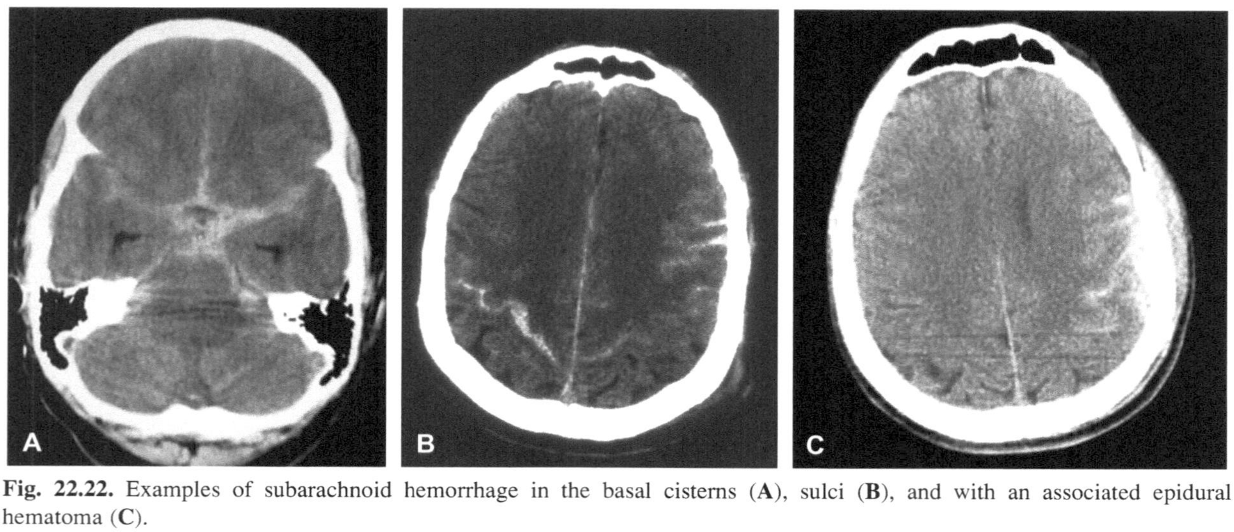

Fig. 22.22. Examples of subarachnoid hemorrhage in the basal cisterns (**A**), sulci (**B**), and with an associated epidural hematoma (**C**).

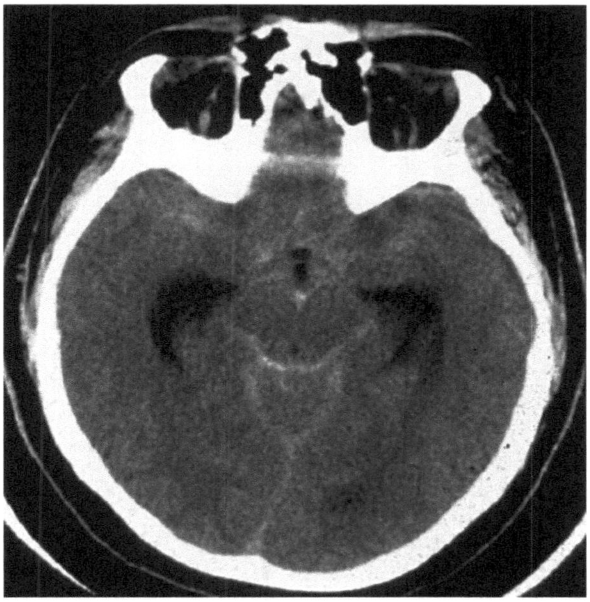

Fig. 22.23. Axial noncontrast computed tomography image shows subarachnoid hemorrhage and enlargement of the temporal horns of the lateral ventricles reflecting hydrocephalus.

ill-defined hypodense lesion with small foci of hemorrhage. Over the next 24–48 hours, multiple new hypodense lesions may appear and lesions may enlarge with worsening edema and mass effect (Fig. 22.28). Delayed hemorrhages may develop and petechial hemorrhages may coalesce into larger hematomas. Chronically, a contusion will evolve into a focal area of encephalomalacia with parenchymal volume loss.

While findings related to evolving contusions may become more conspicuous on CT over time, these findings are easily demonstrated on MRI, which is a more sensitive examination for the detection of a parenchymal injury and delineating the extent of injury. FLAIR images are particularly helpful in evaluating the extent of edema. GRE or SWI is very sensitive for the detection of hemorrhage in a parenchymal hematoma (Fig. 22.29).

Subcortical injury

Subcortical injuries are traumatic injuries of the brainstem, basal ganglia, thalamus, and regions around the third ventricle. Patients also present with IVH and choroidal hemorrhage (Osborn, 2005). The parenchymal findings are better appreciated on MRI than CT, whereas early extraparenchymal blood is better demonstrated on CT.

Hematoma expansion and "spot sign"

The CT angiographic (CTA) spot sign refers to a focus or foci of enhancement within an acute primary intracranial hemorrhage visible on CTA images. It corresponds to a site of active hemorrhage and is an independent predictor of intracranial hemorrhage growth and poor outcome. Of those patients scanned within 6 hours of symptom onset, about 30% will demonstrate the spot sign (Wada et al., 2007; Demchuk et al., 2012). The spot sign is more commonly seen in spontaneous intracerebral hemorrhage, and morbidity and mortality are correlated with hematoma progression.

Diffuse axonal injury

DAI results from the differential motion that occurs between gray matter and white matter during rapid rotational acceleration or deceleration due to their differences in density. This type of injury results from axonal stretching, which occurs when the overlying cortex moves at a different speed than the white matter. DAI is the injury responsible for coma and poor outcome

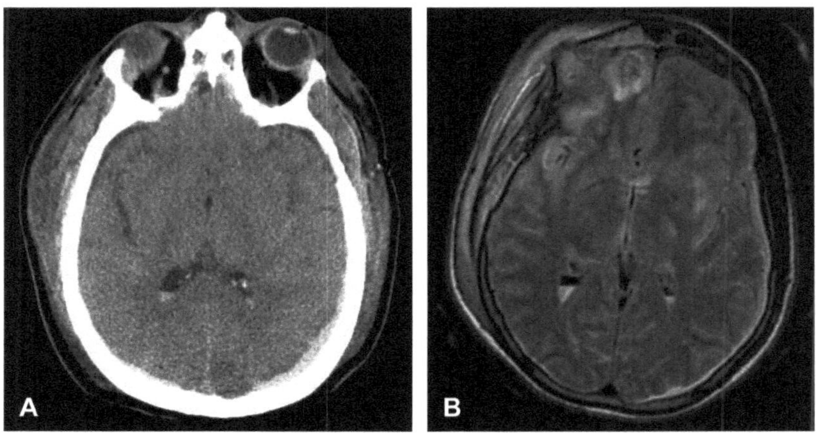

Fig. 22.24. Axial noncontrast computed tomography and axial fluid-attenuated inversion recovery (FLAIR) magnetic resonance images showing minimal-layering intraventricular hemorrhage.

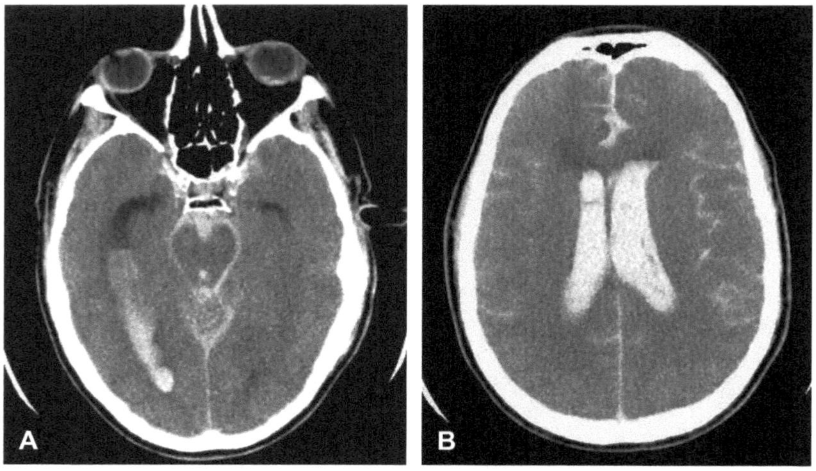

Fig. 22.25. Axial computed tomography images from two different patients showing intraventricular hemorrhage and subarachnoid hemorrhage in the basal cisterns (**A**) and sulci (**B**).

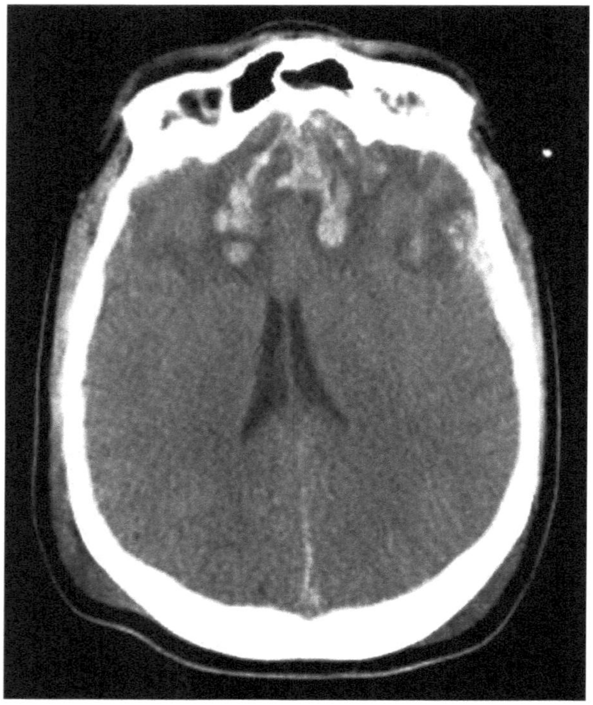

Fig. 22.26. Axial noncontrast computed tomography image shows large bilateral frontal parenchymal contusions.

in most patients with significant closed head injury (Grossman and Yousem, 2003). Clinically, a patient with DAI will lose consciousness at the moment of impact. Depending on the severity of the injury, a patient may remain in a persistent vegetative state.

DAI occurs at characteristic locations in the brain. Typical locations include the gray–white matter junction, especially in the frontotemporal regions, splenium and posterior body of the corpus callosum, and brainstem, especially the dorsolateral midbrain and upper pons (Fig. 22.30).

In a patient with nonhemorrhagic DAI, the initial noncontrast CT may be normal (50–80%) (Osborn, 2005), or, the CT may demonstrate multiple small hypodense foci corresponding to edema at the sites of shear injury, with or without associated hemorrhage. These lesions are usually ovoid with the long axis parallel to the axonal direction. As these lesions evolve over time, they become more conspicuous. DAI should be suspected when the patient's clinical findings are significantly discrepant from the imaging findings.

MRI is the modality of choice for assessing suspected DAI. Thirty percent of patients with a negative CT will have a positive MRI (Osborn, 2005). The SWI (or GRE) sequence is exquisitely sensitive to blood products and may demonstrate small regions of susceptibility artifact at the gray–white matter junction, in the corpus callosum or the brainstem, corresponding to DAI (Fig. 22.31). Some lesions may be entirely nonhemorrhagic and these lesions will be visible as regions of FLAIR hyperintense signal. On DWI, shear injury may appear as foci of restricted diffusion (Fig. 22.32).

PENETRATING TRAUMA

Although less common than closed head injury, penetrating head trauma presents a more complicated range of injuries, requiring a more detailed and sometimes specialized workup. In penetrating head trauma, the protective enclosure of the skull is breached by a foreign body. While the evaluation is largely similar, the degree and character of injury expected vary widely.

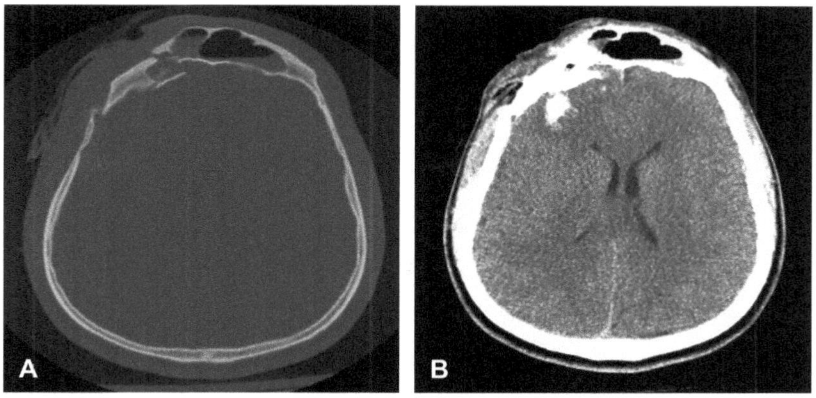

Fig. 22.27. (**A, B**) Right frontal lobe parenchymal contusion at the site of a comminuted depressed fracture.

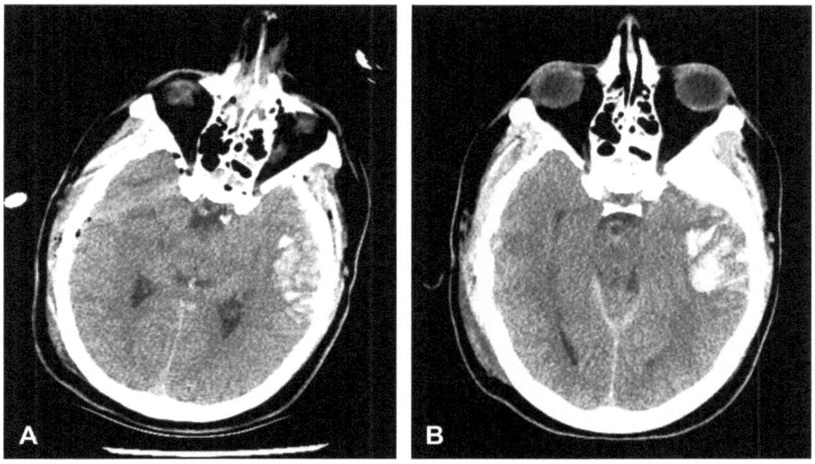

Fig. 22.28. Left temporal parenchymal contusion (**A**) shows enlargement and increased mass effect on a follow-up CT (**B**).

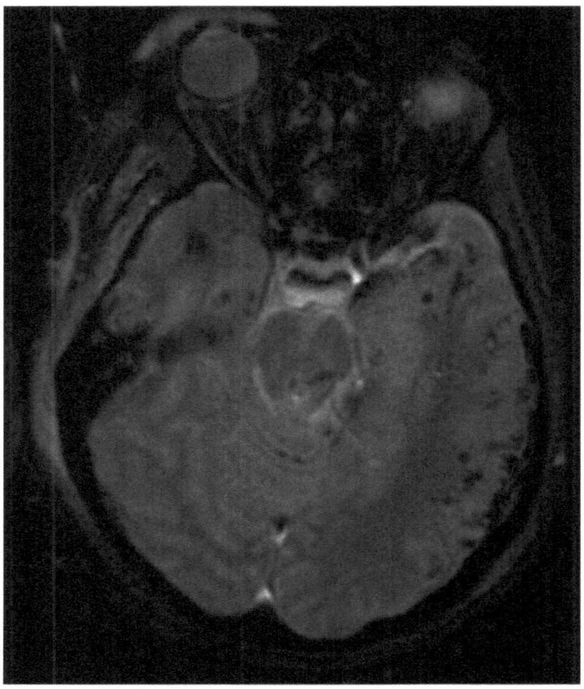

Fig. 22.29. Axial gradient-recalled echo image shows multiple foci of susceptibility effect in the left temporal lobe, right temporal lobe, and brainstem.

Penetrating injury by a low-velocity, sharp object such as a knife causes injury by traversing the brain, its vessels, and support structures. The degree of injury expected relates essentially to the width of the blade, the depth and path traveled, and the specific structures traversed. The act of cutting a path through vessels, nerves, and fiber bundles as the blade advances through the brain is considered the primary injury.

In contrast to the somewhat static event of a single knife pass, a penetrating projectile becomes much more complicated. The relatively high energy of even a low- to moderate-velocity projectile creates extensive injury. Consider a bullet fired from a handgun. The missile travels to the target, penetrates the skull, and encounters the brain. The bullet then impacts on the elastic brain tissue, crushing the tissue as it advances. As the tissue compresses and then tears at the nose of the bullet, the pressure wave created by deposition of the bullet's kinetic energy expands concentrically away from the bullet (Fig. 22.33). Energy from the expanding pressure wave pushes the brain away from the bullet's path, creating an expanded cavity many times larger than the diameter of the bullet. After a short period, determined by the energy of the bullet and the elasticity of the target, the cavity collapses back to nearly the diameter of the bullet.

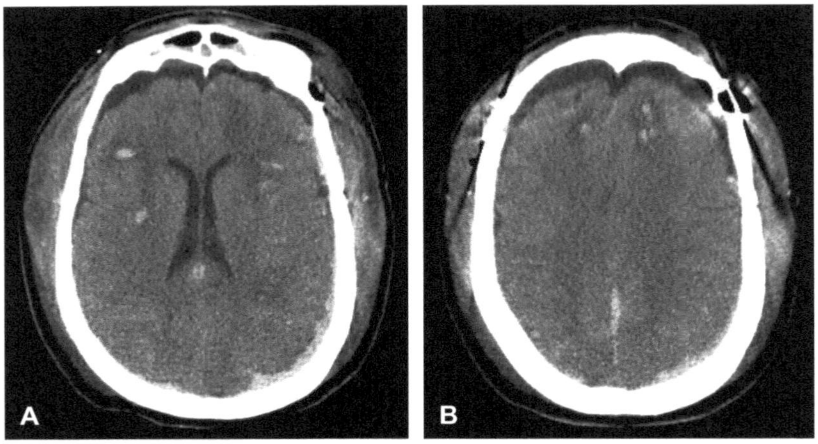

Fig. 22.30. (**A, B**) Axial noncontrast computed tomography images show diffuse axonal injury (DAI) involving the gray–white matter junction bilaterally as well as the splenium of the corpus callosum. There are also bilateral heterogeneous subdural hematomas, with subdural hemorrhage extending along the falx.

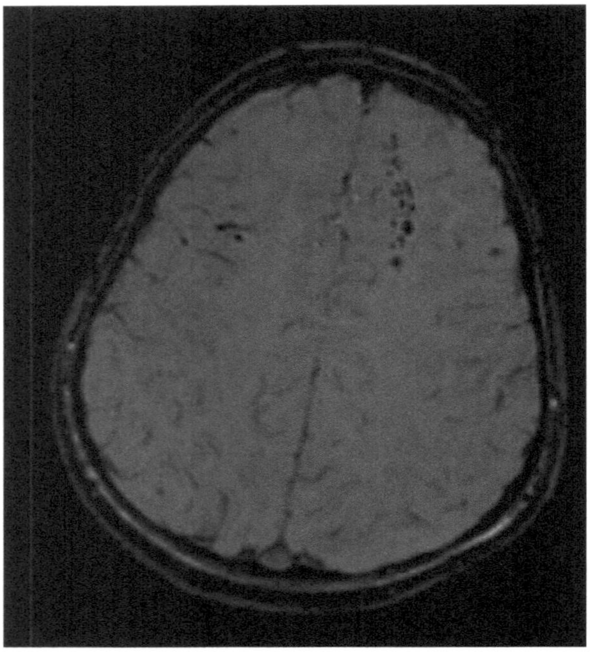

Fig. 22.31. Axial susceptibility-weighted image shows multiple foci of susceptibility effect at the gray–white matter junction of both frontal lobes, representing diffuse axonal injury.

In this scenario, the path that the bullet physically cut by crushing through the tissue is termed the permanent cavity. The short-lived, wide cavity created by the bullet's pressure wave is termed the temporary cavity. It is thought that the temporary cavity imparts tissue damage by stretching and tearing the expanded tissue, although this is somewhat controversial and in part depends on the tissue in question (Karger, 1995). It is clear, however, when looking at imaging of penetrating brain injury, that substantial damage does occur. The permanent cavity may be filled with hemorrhagic debris or show closely apposed brain across a line of edema. Although the temporary cavity cannot be seen directly, the effects of the transient pressure wave can be noted as widespread parenchymal injury. Swelling, edema, hemorrhage, gas, and residual debris may be seen (Fig. 22.34A). Widespread injury may be manifest simply as a featureless brain showing monotonous density from loss of gray and white matter distinction.

The imaging workup of penetrating head injury is tailored to the injury question. First things first: In general, it is not recommended that MRI be performed on penetrating missile injuries. This is reasonable on many

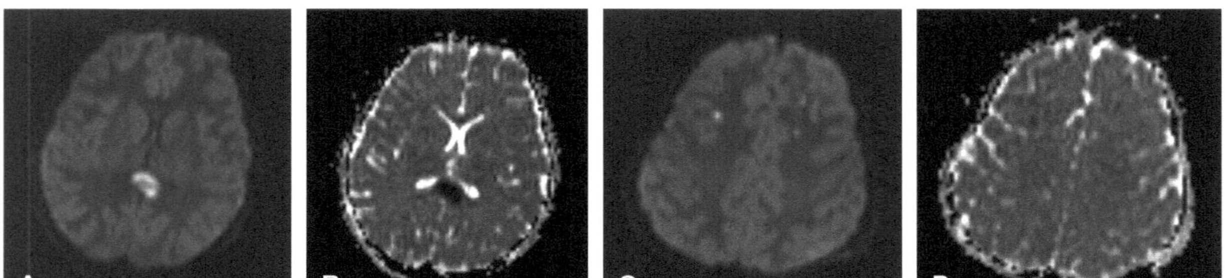

Fig. 22.32. (**A–D**) Axial diffusion-weighted images show foci of restricted diffusion in the splenium of the corpus callosum and at the gray–white matter junction in the frontal lobes bilaterally, consistent with diffuse axonal injury.

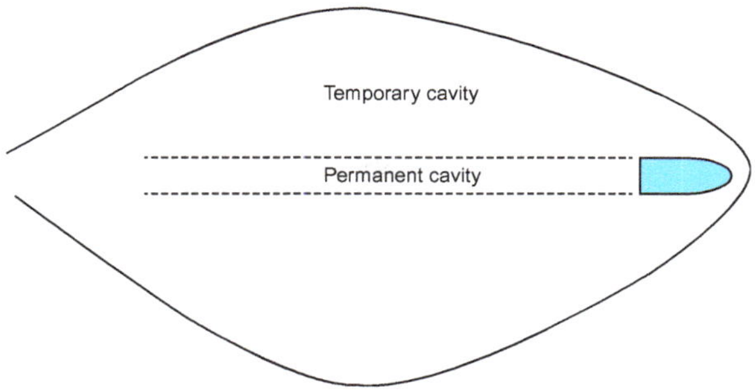

Fig. 22.33. Schematic representation of a bullet traveling through brain parenchyma.

grounds. First and foremost, metal is never a good thing in a magnetic field. In addition to the deflection and heating potential, which is always the first consideration, metal fragments disturb the static field and significantly hinder image formation.

CT scanning is appropriately suited to answer the initial questions required for surgical planning. The degree of injury, missile path, structures involved, and retained fragments can all be assessed adequately. Consideration should be given to the dense metals used in bullet manufacture and the beam-hardening artifact created. This will obviously hinder evaluation but cannot be avoided.

A critical consideration in evaluating intracranial missile injury is vascular damage. Injury to cerebral arteries and veins, whether from direct interaction with the missile or as a consequence of the temporary cavity wave, is an issue. CTA can give an initial assessment of the vasculature and, if further detail is needed or if artifact from metal in the field diminishes image quality beyond use, conventional digital subtraction angiography may be performed (Wellwood et al., 2002).

CEREBROVASCULAR INJURY

Traumatic vascular injury to the intracranial and extracranial circulation can be the sequelae of blunt or penetrating trauma to the head or neck. These injuries can be difficult to recognize because of the frequent coexistence of traumatic brain injury that can obscure the diagnosis. It is important to identify those patients who may be at risk for a vascular injury, if a stroke is to be prevented.

Blunt extracranial vascular injuries occur most commonly from motor vehicle accidents, mostly involving young patients. The most common mechanism of injury postulated results from stretching of the artery because of rapid deceleration, producing an intimal tear. Some tears probably heal spontaneously, but others lead to dissection, with or without pseudoaneurysm formation, and some thrombose (Larsen, 2002). Other mechanisms of injury include direct blows to the head, neck, or face; strangulation injuries, basilar skull fractures, falls, blunt intraoral trauma, and hyperextension of the neck. A penetrating injury, such as a gunshot wound or stabbing, may injure the common carotid artery, internal carotid artery, or vertebral artery.

Various types of vascular injuries have been identified and include occlusion or thrombosis, dissection, complete transection, pseudoaneurysm, arteriovenous fistula, or a combination of injuries. Bilateral dissections have been reported in up to 45% of patients (Larsen, 2002). A stroke in a patient with a head and neck injury should raise the possibility of a dissection and requires further evaluation.

With a dissection, there is hemorrhage within the vascular wall, typically within the media, that can produce luminal irregularity, stenosis, occlusion, and/or aneurysmal dilatation. Vascular dissection is responsible for 1%

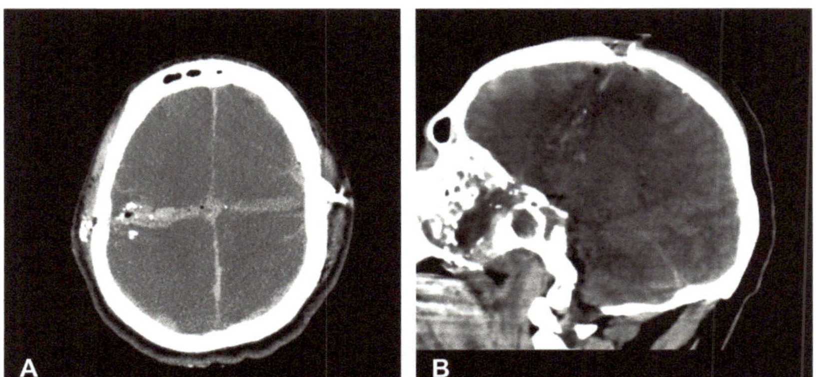

Fig. 22.34. Axial gunshot wound (**A**), and, in a different patient, sagittally oriented gunshot wound entering the oral cavity and exiting the vertex (**B**).

of strokes overall, but is responsible for 20% of strokes in young adults (Osborn, 2005).

Traumatic dissections more commonly affect the extracranial vasculature than the intracranial vasculature. In the neck, the internal carotid artery is more frequently involved than the vertebral artery. A dissection of the internal carotid artery can occur a few centimeters above the carotid bifurcation, ending at the skull base (Osborn, 2005). A vertebral artery dissection occurs commonly at the C1–C2 level, where it is most mobile after exiting the foramen transversarium.

Evaluation of a trauma patient suspected of having a cervical dissection includes a noncontrast CT to assess the brain for any associated intracranial injury as well as identify ischemic or embolic sequelae of a vascular injury. Subsequently, a CTA could be performed to evaluate for an abnormal vessel contour, generally considered highly specific and sensitive (Leclerc et al., 1996). Findings of a dissection on CTA include irregular vessel narrowing $\pm$ occlusion, tapered stenosis, fusiform aneurysmal dilatation/pseudoaneurysm, "string sign" (long-segment stenosis), intimal flap/double lumen – specific, but rarely seen, and evidence of distal emboli (Fig. 22.35). In the setting of a known cervical spine fracture which can be easily seen on CTA, a careful search should be conducted for an associated vascular injury (Fig. 22.36). Similarly, a CTV could be performed to assess for a dural sinus injury if there is an adjacent fracture. If necessary, the findings on CTA/CTV can be corroborated on conventional angiography.

MRI, magnetic resonance angiography (MRA), and magnetic resonance venography (MRV) are also useful in the detection of an acute infarct or vascular injury in the setting of trauma. MRI findings of a dissection include a T1 hyperintense intramural hematoma, usually eccentric but sometimes circumferential, that surrounds and may narrow the flow void (Figs 22.37

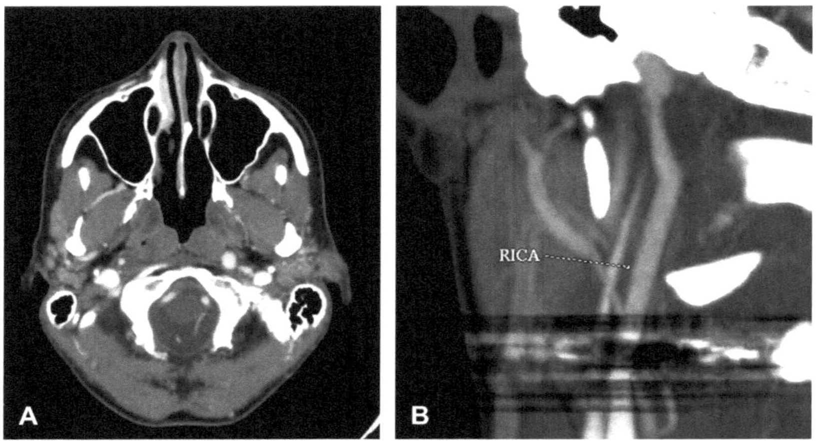

Fig. 22.35. (**A, B**) Axial and oblique coronal reformatted images from a computed tomography angiogram (CTA) demonstrate a dissection of the distal cervical right internal carotid artery (RICA) with narrowing of the true lumen.

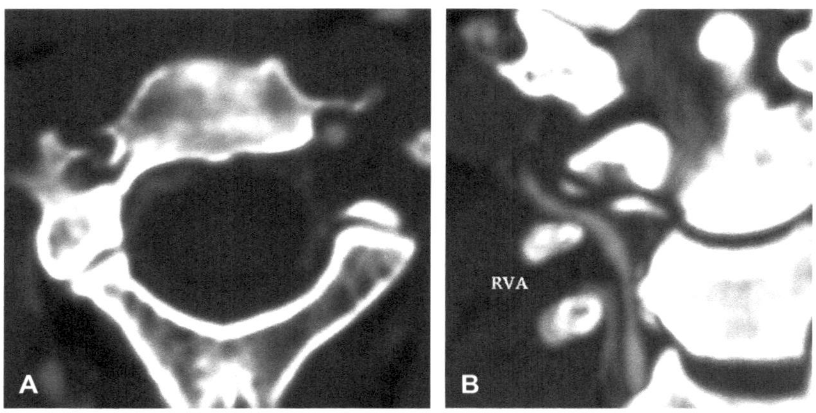

Fig. 22.36. (**A, B**) Axial and coronal reformatted images from a computed tomography angiogram (CTA) demonstrate a displaced fracture involving the right foramen transversarium with an associated dissection of the right vertebral artery (RVA).

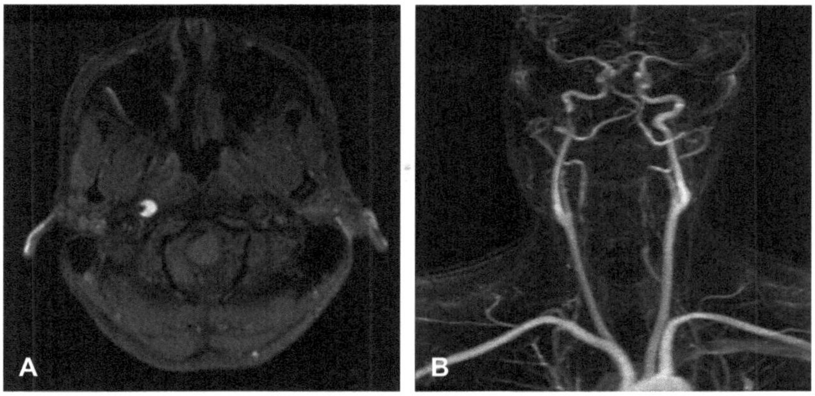

Fig. 22.37. Axial T1 fat-suppressed image (**A**) shows a T1 hyperintense intramural hematoma with severe narrowing of the distal cervical right internal carotid artery, also seen on the coronal MRA maximum-intensity projection image (**B**).

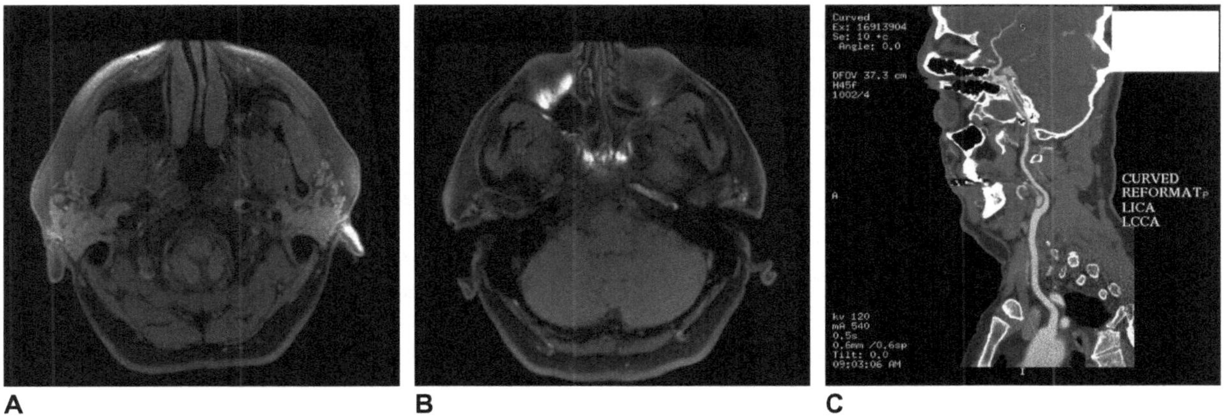

Fig. 22.38. Axial T1-weighted images show a T1 hyperintense intramural hematoma associated with the distal cervical (**A**) and intracranial (**B**) left internal carotid artery, consistent with a dissection. A corresponding curved reformatted CTA image (**C**) shows irregularity and moderate narrowing of the left cervical and intracranial internal carotid artery caused by this dissection.

and 22.38). Other findings include the presence of an intimal flap, a thin partition separating the true and false lumens, and a diminished/absent flow void. Like CTV, MRV can assess the integrity of the dural venous sinuses if an adjacent fracture is present. Limitations of MRI are related to the long imaging time and the need for close monitoring of a critically ill trauma patient.

Intracranial vascular trauma may be due to a closed head injury or penetrating skull injury, and may present in a delayed fashion. Traumatic injuries of the intracranial arteries include dissections, aneurysms, and fistulas. These may present individually, or in combination (Larsen, 2002). Traumatic aneurysms account for 1% of intracranial aneurysms.

Carotid-cavernous fistulas (CCFs) are spontaneous or acquired connections between the internal carotid artery and the cavernous sinus. A direct or traumatic CCF is created by a direct connection between the internal carotid artery and the cavernous sinus, resulting from a basal skull fracture with associated laceration of the internal carotid artery or penetrating injury to the head and orbit. Motor vehicle accidents represent the most common cause of traumatic CCFs, followed by trauma from falls and penetrating injuries (Larsen, 2002). Patients with a direct CCF may present with a bruit, pulsating exophthalmos, orbital edema/erythema, decreased vision, glaucoma, and headache. Clinically, these patients may have focal deficits related to cranial nerves III–VI. DSA is required for definitive diagnosis and treatment. However, CT and MRI may suggest the diagnosis. Imaging findings include proptosis, enlargement of the superior ophthalmic vein, cavernous sinus, and extraocular muscles, and reticulation of the intraorbital fat secondary to edema (Fig. 22.39). CT may demonstrate a skull base fracture that may compromise the carotid canal or optic canal. Magnetic resonance angiography may demonstrate increased flow-related signal in the

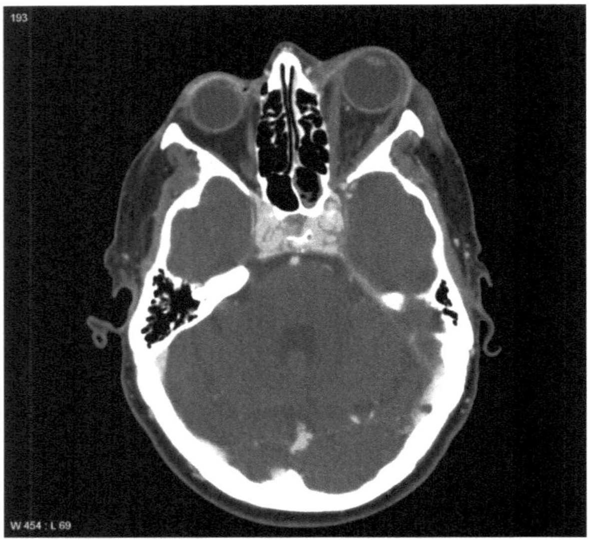

Fig. 22.39. Axial CTA image shows left proptosis, asymmetric enlargement of the left extraocular muscles, as well as left cavernous sinus, consistent with a left carotid-cavernous fistula.

affected cavernous sinus and superior ophthalmic vein, and loss of flow-related signal in the internal carotid artery.

SECONDARY EFFECTS OF TRAUMA

Introduction and general physiology

Pressure, volume, and CSF physiology

Throughout any discussion of head injury, it is best to keep in mind that morbidity and mortality result chiefly as a result of increased intracranial pressure. The volume of the intact skull is fixed. Since skull formation is the result of induction from the neural tissue, intracranial volume occupied by neural elements is included in the fixed intracranial volume. The dura mater, a tough fibrous bag, lines the intact skull. In all, 150–250 cc of CSF is created at a rate of 0.2–0.7 cc/min (or 600–700 cc/day) at multiple points throughout the brain. CSF is created from choroid plexi located within the lateral, third and fourth ventricles, which together can contain 25–50 cc of the total CSF volume at any given time. CSF flows through the ventricles and then out through the foramina of Magendie and Luschka into the subarachnoid space, filling the remaining recesses in this closed, watertight intracranial and intraspinal volume. Acting as a water bath, the CSF helps structurally buffer forces transmitted by the skull and cushion the intracranial contents.

Within this closed system, CSF provides a buffer for small changes in volume. For example, the brain increases and decreases in size slightly with each systolic impulse of blood from the heart, but otherwise maintains a constant volume. The pressure we measure across the calvaria as intracranial pressure is largely mediated by the CSF. Although the total volume is fixed, CSF is dynamic in that the entire volume is exchanged once every 5–8 hours, with fresh fluid being created at the choroid plexi, and resorbed at the Pacchionian (arachnoid) granulations in the venous sinuses. Alteration in either the rate of production or absorption of CSF would result in an overall increase in CSF volume, and subsequently in increased intracranial pressure.

In reviewing posttraumatic imaging, always keep in mind: do I see any additional volume elements that might add to the already fixed intracranial volume, and as a result increase intracranial pressure?

Brain injury is not a static event. It is a process that begins with the initial injury, whether a direct impact with a solid object, or when an indirect application of force to the brain via a pressure wave, as in blast injury, serves as the starting point in a cascade of events. Extravasated blood from torn vessels collects in potential spaces, creating volume elements not previously present in the closed intracranial space. Free blood in the subarachnoid space mixes with CSF, increasing overall volume. Solid elements of blood and debris in the CSF space obstruct CSF flow pathways. Interruption of CSF flow through the ventricles results in enlargement proximal to the occlusion. Fouling of Pacchionian granulations with proteinaceous debris increases intracranial pressure by blocking CSF resorption.

Tissue edema vs swelling

Gross expansion of cerebral tissue may occur as a result of an increase in volume because of capillary congestion and transmural flow of plasma filtrate into the interstitial space (Miller, 1982). Additionally, injured or dying cells lose the ability to maintain their membrane integrity. As a result, fluid accumulates within the cell body. Tissue swelling as a result of cell swelling is termed cytotoxic edema and is identified in the swelling and diminished radiographic density in gray-matter regions. Debris, whether blood products or cytoplasmic elements, activates a series of cytokine networks that initiate an inflammatory response. The inflammatory cascade initiates a series of events, from fenestration of existing vessels to inducing the formation of neovascularity. The eventual outcome is filtration of plasma volume across the vessel wall and increasing intravascular blood volume at the site of injury respectively. Once in the interstitial space, the free fluid is free to track along white-matter fiber bundles, expanding the space and allowing macrophage and glial cell migration to aid in the healing process. Macroscopically at imaging, expansion and a slight increase in radiographic density in the white matter regions are termed vasogenic edema.

In cerebral swelling, extracellular fluid is not an issue. Pressure exerted by a hematoma or injured tissue may cause obstruction of a draining cortical vein or sinus. The resulting obstruction of venous outflow from the brain produces congestion of the more proximal tissue capillary beds. These compliant vessels expand in size in an attempt to accommodate backed-up venous drainage. In doing so, the overall cerebral blood volume of the tissue increases, as the engorged vessels take up more space than if they were in their usual collapsed form, thus contributing to overall tissue expansion. In this instance, the density of the gray or white matter does not necessarily change individually, although the density of the overall brain may appear reduced (Kontos et al., 1978).

Compensatory mechanisms

In the normal functioning or compensated intracranial system, intracranial pressure remains relatively stable, at about 10–14 mmHg above atmospheric pressure. Any perturbation in the intracranial contents threatens the stability of the intracranial pressure. The Monro-Kellie doctrine asserts that the sum of the volume of each component that makes up the intracranial contents (brain tissue, CSF volume, and cerebral blood volume) is constant. An increase in any one of the volume elements has to be accompanied by a corresponding reduction in one or both of the remaining volume elements in order to keep intracranial pressure constant. Compliance in the system allows for a certain amount of buffering of pressure changes in the system, but when the buffering capacity is overcome, intracranial pressure rises exponentially (Marmarou et al., 1978).

An increase in brain volume by either edema or swelling (neural tissue volume), for example, may be compensated for by a reduction of the extra-axial spaces (CSF volume). Effacement of sulci, fissures, ventricles, or cisterns displaces CSF, eventually resulting in increased CSF resorption until intracranial pressure normalizes. Similarly, compression of brain parenchyma results in compression of capillary beds (cerebral blood volume), forcing blood into the venous system and out of the intracranial compartment.

Pressure may be able to normalize in a situation with very slowly changing addition of additional volume (e.g., meningioma), but in a situation of rapid volume change (e.g., EDH), the increased intracranial volume occurs too quickly. Some compensation can occur quickly, such as displacement of the capillary blood pool of the compressed brain segment into the venous sinuses and to the heart. Ventricles may be effaced, forcing their CSF into connecting ventricles or the subarachnoid space, but this only mitigates pressure local to the offending volume element. That is, intracranial pressure may be partially normalized in the hemispheric compartment of the mass or hematoma, but results in displacement of CSF volume (and hence pressure) to other compartments. A left parietal EDH, for example, might increase the pressure greatly in the left hemispheric supratentorial compartment (Thuomas et al., 1993). Displaced brain compresses the left lateral ventricle, reducing its volume and displacing CSF to the third and, to a lesser degree, the right lateral and fourth ventricles. As a result, the intracranial pressure in the left hemispheric supratentorial compartment will be high, but not as high as if uncompensated. The third ventricle will contribute its increased volume to the right lateral and fourth ventricles, resulting in relatively increased pressure in the central, right hemispheric supratentorial and infratentorial compartments. Most importantly, this behavior allows for the establishment of a CSF pressure gradient, greatest in the left hemispheric compartment, lesser in the right hemispheric compartment, and least in the infratentorial and spinal extra-axial compartments. The last intracranial volume element to shift its position is the densest and best anchored of the three, the neural tissue, as will be discussed in the section on herniation syndromes, below.

Dangers of increased intracranial pressure

If intracranial pressure is increased uniformly throughout all intracranial compartments, intracranial pressure effects will be exerted greatest against forces seeking to introduce new volume to the closed compartment. The best example of this notion is the resistance to arterial blood flow into the skull produced by increased intracranial pressure. The heart forces blood into the skull at systemic mean arterial pressures. In order for a net movement of blood into the skull, systemic pressure must exceed intracranial pressure. To understand the balance of forces, we introduce cerebral perfusion pressure (CPP). CPP is proportional to the mean arterial pressure (MAP), supplied by the system in opposition to intracranial pressure (ICP), or CPP = MAP – ICP. When monitoring pressures clinically, in general we aim to maintain CPP between 75 and 90 mmHg (Lewelt et al., 1980). A diminished CPP may ultimately result in tissue hypoperfusion, ischemia, and eventually infarct. Resulting cerebral injury incurs further edema and contributes to a further increase in ICP.

On the other side of the capillary bed, tissue expansion may also contribute to effacement of cortical veins and dural sinuses. This impedes venous outflow, resulting in venous congestion, increasing cerebral blood volume. To make matters worse, increased venous capillary pressure results in transmural plasma flow, contributing to congestive (vasogenic) edema, all of which eventually contribute to increased neural tissue volume and hence intracranial pressure.

Imaging

Imaging in the acute phase of head trauma has two goals: Firstly, to define areas of primary closed head injury such as brain contusion, cerebral hemorrhage, extra-axial hematomas, skull integrity, and hydrocephalus, and then to anticipate progression of the primary injuries that may contribute to change in each of the three principal volume elements and hence increased intracranial pressure.

Imaging features of edema and swelling

Alteration of gray and white matter density may provide clues as to accumulation of edema. One cardinal feature is that of loss of the differentiation of gray and white matter structures. Gray matter is normally of higher density than white matter and as such the interface between the two is clearly demarcated on CT images. Accumulation of intracellular water produces an overall decrease in the density of gray-matter structures, such as the cortical mantle or deep nuclei. As edema accumulates, differentiation of the newly low-density gray matter and the native low-density white matter becomes less apparent. Conversely, white matter, which is less dense due to the myelinated axons within its cellular elements, has an overall aggregate lower density (23–26 HU) than the densely cellular gray matter (32–35 HU). Infiltration of water into the interstices of this already low-attenuation environment produces a further reduction in the overall density. This reveals itself as an expanded white-matter region with pronounced differentiation between the now very-low-density white matter and dense gray matter (Fig. 22.40). Cerebral swelling, produced by increasing the blood volume percent of brain tissue volume, may retain the differentiation of the gray and white matter, but show a reduction in the density of the volume as a whole.

Observations that arise from both brain edema and whole-brain swelling with reduced overall density include the hyperdense cerebellum sign and the hyperdense vessel sign.

The hyperdense cerebellum, or white cerebellum sign is evoked in diffuse cerebral swelling or edema, as might be seen in global anoxia (e.g., global hypoperfusion in asystole). Here, the posterior fossa is viewed at the level of the tentorium and shows the normally dense cerebellum juxtaposed against the adjacent supratentorial parenchyma of the temporal and occipital lobes (Fig. 22.41) (Chalela et al., 2013).

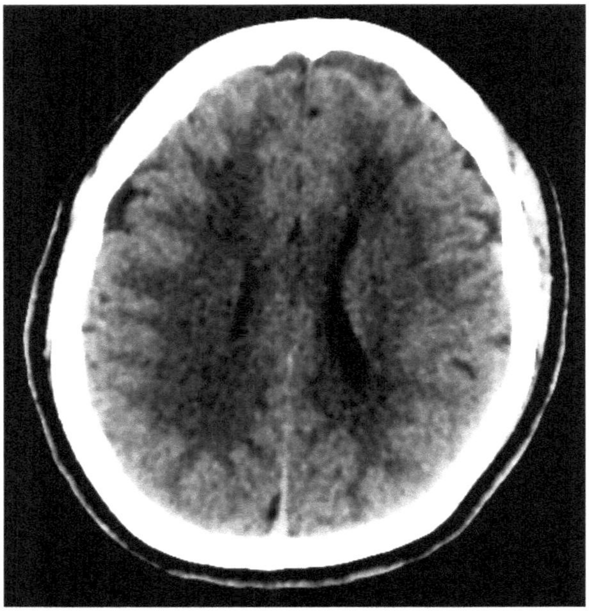

Fig. 22.40. Axial CT image shows vasogenic edema in the right cerebral hemisphere with accentuation of the gray–white matter junction and partial effacement of the right lateral ventricle.

The hyperdense vessel sign is seen typically at the level of the middle cerebral artery (MCA) as it passes in the Sylvian cistern to the Sylvian fissure. In cerebral swelling/edema, the expanded low-density tissue crowds and displaces the CSF space that normally lies between it and the vessel. Direct contact between the low-density brain parenchyma and the vessel of normal density gives the impression of accentuated contrast between the two structures (Fig. 22.42).

Mitigation of volume displacement by CSF volume elements on imaging

As noted previously, swelling and edema both result in expansion of the brain parenchyma, displacing the CSF spaces. This can be a focal or regional response or may involve the entire brain (Thuomas et al., 1993). One of the most important observations in assessing the brain is that of the normal overall architecture. Definition of the gyri against the CSF density sulci of the subarachnoid space provides for recognition of the normal lobar architecture. Loss of the water density CSF space reduces the ability to differentiate between adjacent gyri. Effacement of the sulcal markings due to regional or global tissue expansion can then be used as a sensitive marker for swelling and edema. Displacement of swollen brain tissue into the sulci, cisterns, fissures, and even ventricles is an important compensatory mechanism for mitigating increased intracranial volume and intracranial pressure, but is not without cost. Encroachment on the normal

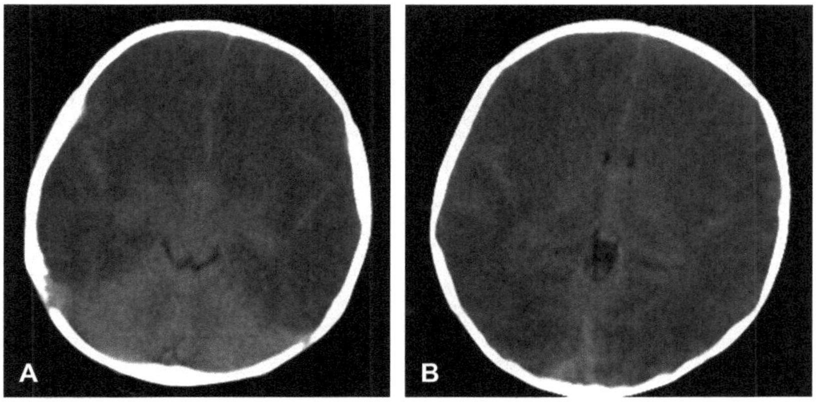

Fig. 22.41. (**A, B**) White cerebellum sign.

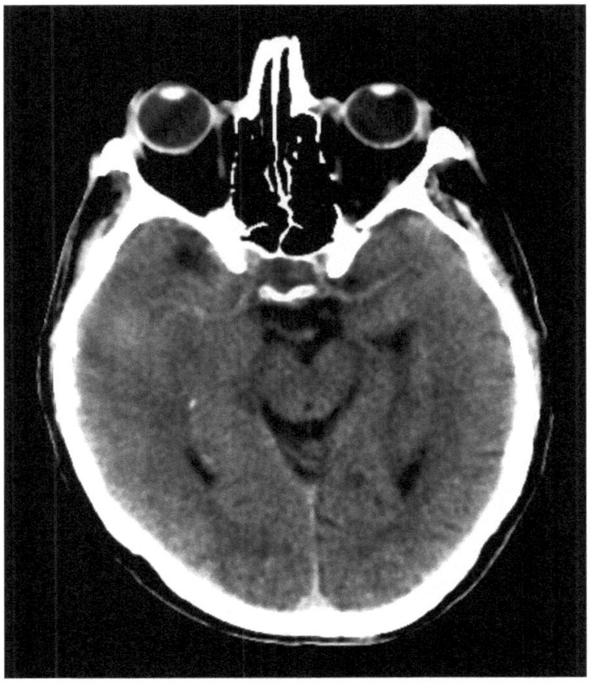

Fig. 22.42. Dense vessels.

channels to CSF flow may result in entrapment. For example, effacement of the foramen of Monro resulting from medially displaced brain parenchyma impedes CSF flow from the lateral to the third ventricle and results in compensatory enlargement of the lateral ventricle. The ventriculomegaly created then contributes further to increased intracranial pressure.

Herniation syndromes

Compartmentalization of the calvaria

Within the closed-brain case, the volume is further divided into three main compartments. The tentorium cerebelli divides the anterior cranial fossa and middle cranial fossa from the posterior cranial fossa, and the falx cerebri divides the supratentorial compartment into left and right subcompartments. The three compartments communicate through two openings: the tentorial hiatus or notch, between the posterior cranial fossa and bilateral supratentorial compartments, and the open space under the free edge of the falx, between the left and right supratentorial compartments. The presence of a pressure gradient between compartments creates an environment where the contents of the high-pressure compartment could become displaced into the lower-pressure compartment through a path of least resistance.

Forms of cerebral herniation

Subfalcine (cingulate) herniation

In the case of increased pressure in one of the supratentorial compartments, there is motivation for the lobe occupying that high-pressure compartment to move into a lower-pressure compartment. A large EDH, for instance, in the left high lateral convexity would exert direct pressure on the left frontal and parietal lobes. The brain would respond by compressing toward the right. The open space under the free edge of the falx provides a low-resistance pathway for the brain to shift across the midline from left to right. The subfalcine opening is arched higher anteriorly than posteriorly. As a result, the anterior cingulate gyrus and corpus callosum are free to squeeze under the free edge of the falx and cross the midline. The earliest indicator of movement of brain parenchyma from one side to the other across the subfalcine opening is a shift of the septum pellucidum. This thin membranous structure is loosely anchored and lies directly in the subfalcine opening, making it susceptible to easy displacement across the midline at lower intercompartmental pressures. As pressure increases, more of the cingulate gyrus is forced under the anterior free edge of the falx (Fig. 22.43). Remember that the anterior cerebral arteries lie to either side of the falx along the body of the corpus callosum just above the free edge of the falx. As the cingulate

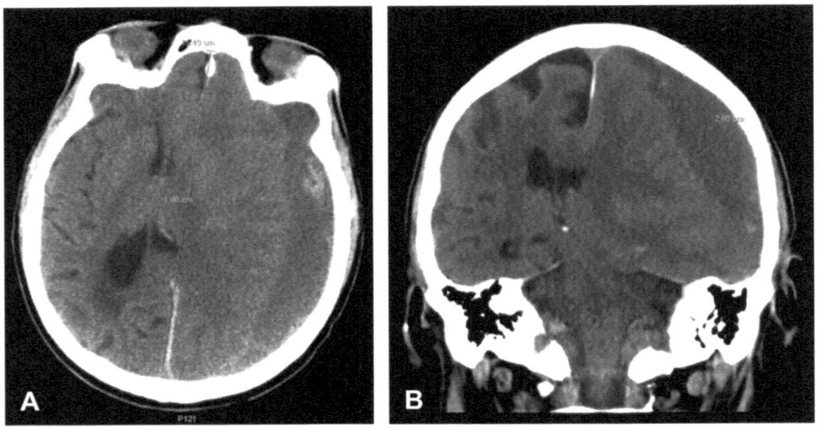

Fig. 22.43. (A) Axial and (B) coronal CT images show subfalcine and transtentorial herniation related to a large left cerebral convexity subdural hematoma.

and corpus callosum are drawn across the midline, the ipsilateral anterior cerebral artery is drawn with them. The artery eventually becomes compressed between the free edge of the falx and the crossing brain parenchyma and carries a risk of infarct in the distal anterior cerebral artery territory.

The subfalcine herniation is the most frequently encountered of the herniation syndromes and should be evaluated in each case of intracranial trauma. The neurosurgeon should be made aware of any midline shift. Depending on the clinical circumstances, surgical intervention may be warranted for shifts of over 5 mm (Zwienenberg and Muizelaar, 2003).

Transtentorial (uncal) herniation

Increased pressure on the temporal lobe from the lateral convexity toward the midline will result in migration of the anteriormost medial portion of the temporal lobe, the uncas (mostly hippocampal formation and amygdala) toward the midline and over the tentorial free edge. Once over the free edge and into the tentorial hiatus, the brain parenchyma tends to follow the low-resistance path, usually into the lower-pressure posterior cranial fossa. Although less frequent in occurrence than the subfalcine form, transtentorial herniation carries more dangerous complications.

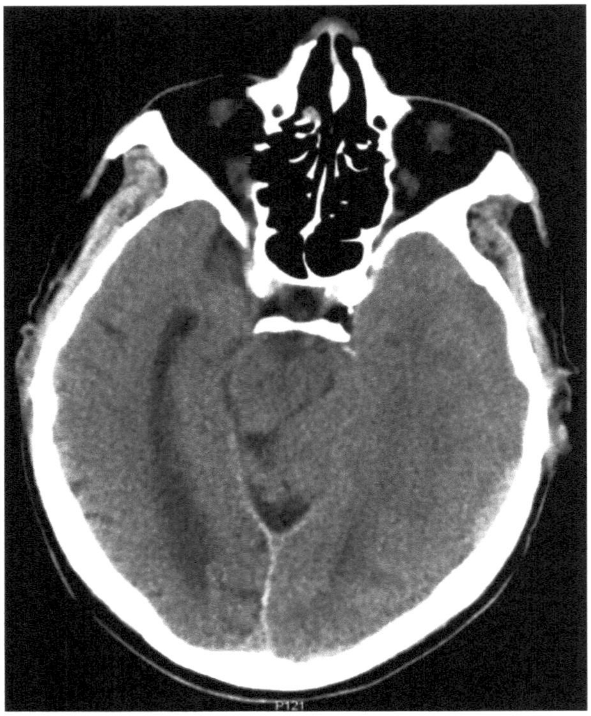

Fig. 22.44. Axial image showing transtentorial herniation of the left temporal lobe.

Movement of brain from one of the supratentorial compartments into the tentorial hiatus results in severe crowding of the midbrain (Fig. 22.44). The midbrain is displaced laterally toward the tentorial free edge opposite the herniating temporal lobe. In addition, because of the herniating temporal lobe's anterior position and downward momentum, the midbrain experiences a rotational force around its brainstem axis away from the herniating tissue. This creates two dangerous situations: impingement of the midbrain on the contralateral tentorial free edge, and torsion and kinking of the small perforating arteries that supply the midbrain originating from the basilar artery. Impingement and pressure necrosis of the contralateral cerebral peduncle and midbrain carve a groove into those structures, known as Kernohan's notch. Interruption of the descending corticospinal fibers results in contralateral or bilateral hemiparesis or hemiplegia, depending on severity. Although the exact mechanism is not known, it is thought that with increasing torsion from the

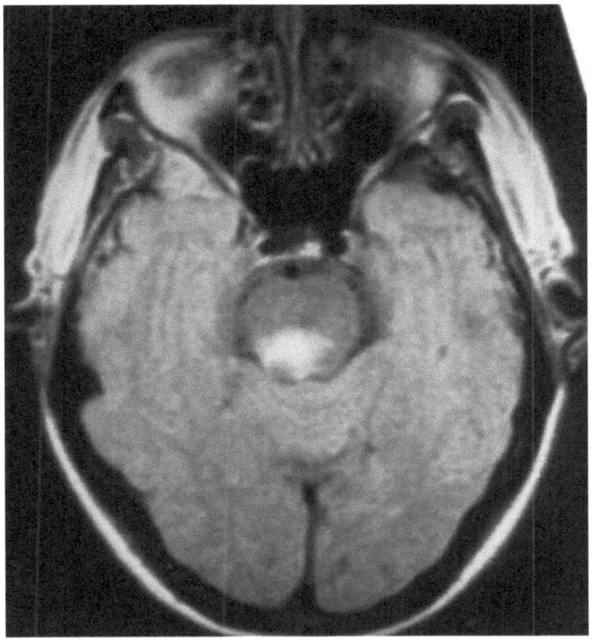

Fig. 22.45. Duret hemorrhage in the brainstem.

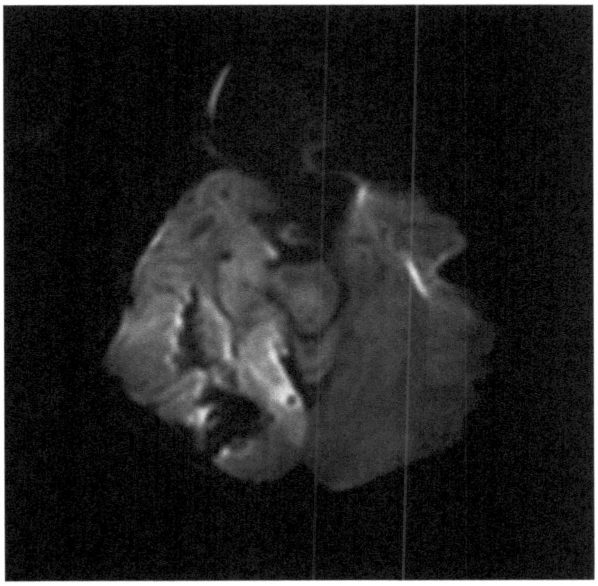

Fig. 22.46. Diffusion-weighted image shows a large right temporo-occipital hemorrhage and transtentorial herniation. Note the acute right medial occipital lobe infarct.

herniating temporal lobe, the kinked perforating arteries that supply the midbrain become severely narrowed or occluded, causing ischemia and eventually infarct in the midbrain. Hemorrhage into this infarcted segment is termed Duret hemorrhage and is a poor prognostic sign (Fig. 22.45).

Movement of the more posterior portion of the inferomedial temporal lobe across the tentorial free edge can impinge upon the posterior cerebral artery. Compression of the posterior cerebral artery against the tentorial free edge results in compromised blood flow and occipital infarcts (Fig. 22.46). Entrapment of cranial nerve III (oculomotor nerve) by herniating brain tissue results in an ipsilateral dilated pupil.

Transalar (sphenoidal) herniation

Although less frequently encountered, increased pressure in either the anterior or middle cranial fossae can result in movement of either frontal or temporal lobe across the sphenoid ridge. Downward transalar herniation describes a situation in which the frontal lobe is forced downward across the sphenoid ridge into the middle cranial fossa. This can occur either with severe frontal lobe swelling or a large extra-axial hematoma overlying the frontal convexity. Moderate forms of downward transalar herniation will involve mainly the orbital gyri, but severe forms will involve the gyrus rectus. Severe downward herniation of the frontal lobe can result in impingement of the MCA on the sphenoid ridge, with a subsequent MCA territory infarct.

Upward transalar herniation involves severe anterior temporal edema or infratemporal hematoma, resulting in movement of the temporal lobe superiorly into the anterior cranial fossa. Severe upward transalar herniation can cause impingement of the supraclinoid internal carotid artery on the anterior clinoid process, with a subsequent infarcts in both the MCA and anterior cerebral artery (ACA) territories.

Transforaminal (tonsillar) and upward herniation

With hematomas of the posterior cranial fossa, severe cerebellar swelling or occlusion of CSF drainage from the fourth ventricle, the cerebellum and brainstem can be forced either downward through the foramen magnum, or upward through the tentorial hiatus. In mild cases, transforaminal or tonsillar herniation results in crowding of the foramen magnum. In more severe cases, tissue descent and crowding can result in obstruction of CSF outflow from the fourth ventricle, worsening elevated intracranial pressure in the posterior fossa and, in extreme cases, compression of the medullary respiratory centers may cause respiratory arrest. Less commonly, upward movement of posterior fossa contents through the tentorial notch can be observed. Symptoms attributable to upward herniation are not well delineated, but are thought to include somnolence and confusion, progressing to obtundation.

ADVANCED NEUROIMAGING FOR TBI

Advanced neuroimaging for acute TBI is an active area of research. Advanced CT techniques, including dual-energy CT and iterative reconstruction algorithms, have been discussed previously. In this section we will review the following advanced MRI techniques that may be applied to imaging of head trauma: diffusion tensor imaging (DTI), blood oxygen-level dependent (BOLD) functional MRI, and MR spectroscopy (MRS).

Diffusion tensor imaging

DTI enables measurement of diffusion properties of water molecules in the cerebral tissue. Since water diffusion is relatively free along the length of a white-matter tract, while it is restricted by myelination in the perpendicular direction, one can use DTI to assess integrity of neural tracts. While DTI has been in use for some time, many new variants, such as high angular resolution diffusion imaging (HARDI), diffusion kurtosis imaging (DKI), and diffusion spectrum imaging (DSI) are currently under investigation. HARDI acquires diffusion parameters in many more directions, typically 32 or more, in order to assess diffusion properties of crossing fibers. DKI uses multiple b-values to assess a property known as kurtosis. Use of multiple b-values is sometimes referred to as multiple "shells." DSI can model voxel-to-voxel heterogeneities in diffusion directions and can more accurately map white matter tracts.

In traditional DTI, it is customary to model the diffusion tensor by a single ellipsoid (i.e., single "shell"), whose long axis is oriented along the major diffusion direction (i.e., the length of the white-matter tract). The lengths of the three axes of this ellipsoid denote the three principal diffusivities of the diffusion tensor. Commonly, it is assumed that the two minor axes have the same length denoting the transverse diffusivity (L_t) of a white-matter bundle; the major axis represents the longitudinal diffusivity (L_1) of a white-matter bundle (Fig. 22.47). From the L_1 and L_t parameters of the diffusion tensor, one can also compute the mean diffusivity and the fractional anisotropy (FA). FA can be thought of as an index of white matter organization. The mean diffusivity, or the related quantity, called apparent diffusion coefficient, represents the global ease of water diffusivity.

The fact that trauma induces changes in diffusion tensor is well known (Wilde et al, 2008; Chu et al., 2010; Davenport et al., 2012; Mayer et al., 2010, 2012; Ling et al., 2012). For example, Figure 22.48 shows FA maps for two patients after severe TBI. Both patients were in coma and were imaged in the neurologic intensive care unit in the acute stage. The patient on the left shows a relatively preserved FA map, at both axial levels shown, as compared to the patient on the right. In fact, the patient on the right had an unfavorable outcome (defined as death or persistent vegetative state) while the patient on the left survived with motor disabilities but no long-term cognitive deficits.

While multiple studies have documented changes in diffusion tensor, the direction of change (i.e., increase vs decrease) is somewhat variable and may depend on the time of imaging with respect to the original insult.

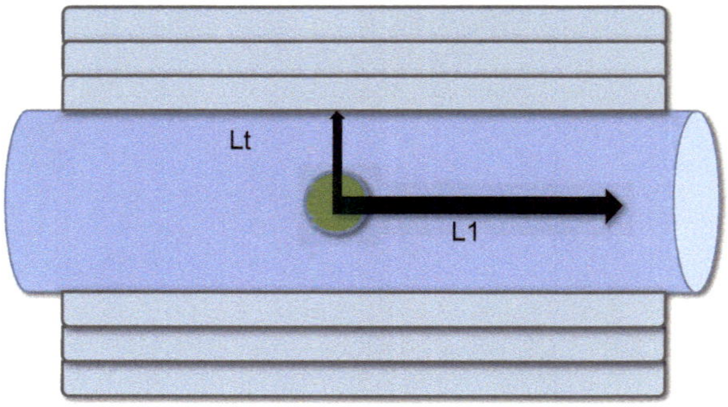

Fig. 22.47. A schematic view of the diffusion tensor along a white matter tract, where L1 denotes the diffusivity along the long axis of the tract and Lt denotes the diffusivity along the short axis.

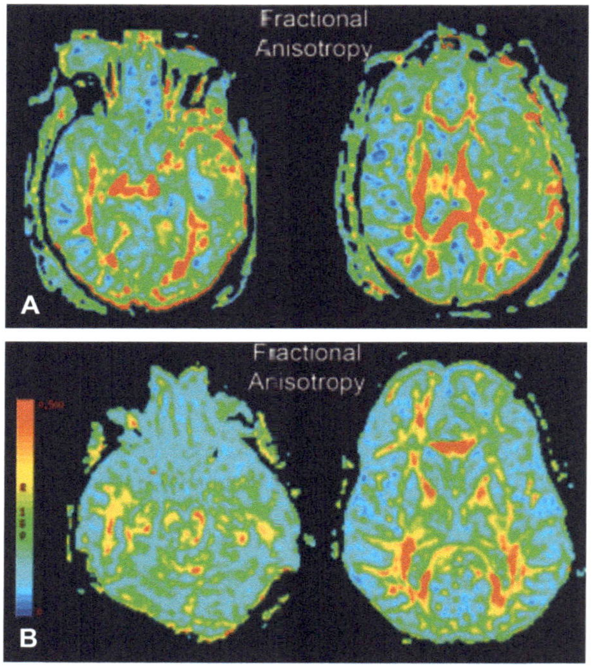

Fig. 22.48. Fractional anisotropy maps for two patients after severe traumatic brain injury who were imaged during the acute stage. The fractional anisotropy maps are shown at two, approximately matched, levels. The FA map for Patient A, who had a favorable outcome, is relatively intact while the FA map for Patient B, who had a poor outcome, is severely altered.

Most studies in this field, however, report a decrease in the FA value. One can think of this as degradation of myelin, resulting in a breakdown of the normal anisotropy associated with an axonal tract, even though the exact process underlying these changes is unknown. Despite intense research activity, no guidelines exist on how to interpret the DTI images. A part of the difficulty lies in lack of standardization in the numeric values associated with the diffusion tensor. Sensitivity of these numeric parameters to patient motion, artifacts, field strength, age, and the echo time poses another problem in determining a standardized algorithm. Due to these difficulties, at the current time, DTI in the setting of trauma remains a research topic and its routine use is not recommended.

Functional MRI (fMRI)

fMRI, sometimes referred to as BOLD imaging, relies on changes in blood flow in response to increased neuronal activity (Logothetis et al., 2001; Arthurs and Boniface, 2002; Heeger and Ress, 2002; Jantzen, 2010). As the neuronal activity increases and if the standard physiologic response of the brain is preserved, the cerebral blood flow increases in response to increased metabolic demand. This increase in cerebral blood flow, which is regional, outstrips the metabolic demand. In fact, the ratio of oxyhemoglobin to deoxyhemoglobin increases in the areas of the brain where there is increased demand and consumption of oxygen. This change in oxy/deoxyhemoglobin can be detected and mapped by MRI, because these two states of hemoglobin affect the local magnetic environment differently. Hence the name, "BOLD" imaging. The temporal resolution of BOLD fMRI imaging is slow because the hemodynamic processes it is trying to measure are slow. The changes, however, can be plotted on a fine grid with millimeter-scale resolution.

One can sequentially acquire BOLD signal in all parts of the brain, while the brain is at "rest," i.e., when no active motor, memory, visual, or other paradigm is prescribed. These datasets consist of time-series data points of BOLD signal over a certain time period. This task-free resting-state paradigm is attractive for TBI studies, as it does not require any active participation from the patient. It relies on the low-frequency fluctuations in the resting brain that reflect the underlying sequence of neuronal activity. It turns out that this so-called resting-state fMRI, rs-fMRI for short, is far from random. There are repeatable and reliable activation patterns and sequences that can be found in this time-series of BOLD data. Researchers have defined the concept of "functional connectivity" between regions of brain where there is high interregional correlation in the BOLD waveform. This has given rise to the concept of functional networks within the brain that are comprised of spatially distributed regions that have highly correlated BOLD activity pattern. A variety of research techniques have been applied to identify and characterize these networks from a graph theoretic point of view.

In addition to rs-fMRI, task-based paradigms have been studied. These paradigms require active participation from the subject. During fMRI acquisition, simple tasks are prescribed to the patient, and the BOLD signal in response to the prescribed task (e.g., finger tapping) is recorded. This paradigm can be used to activate individual portions or circuits within the brain. Both task-based and task-free fMRI paradigms are being actively studied and a number of brain networks have been identified. The data to date, however, is inconclusive and routine use of fMRI in the setting of acute TBI is not recommended.

Magnetic resonance spectroscopy

MRI provides anatomic maps of T1 and T2 relaxation times; MRS, unlike MRI, gives a spectrum of the signal intensities of different metabolites within the brain as a function of their Larmor resonance frequency. This can be done for a single voxel, a matrix of voxels in two or three dimensions (designated as single-voxel spectroscopy and 2D/3D multivoxel chemical shift imaging, respectively). The brain metabolites that are commonly imaged include *N*-acetyl aspartate for neuronal integrity, creatine for cellular energy/density, choline for membrane turnover, and lactate for anaerobic metabolism. By varying the echo times, other metabolites, such as glutamate/glutamine (excitatory amino acids released after TBI: Bullock et al., 1998), and myo-inositol, a marker of astroglial proliferation (Garnett et al., 2000), can also be quantified. Because TBI is a heterogeneous disease, there is considerable heterogeneity in the published MRS studies on TBI. The sensitivity and specificity of MRS in TBI have never been confirmed by any large, prospective controlled trial. Ample evidence exists that TBI affects the underlying metabolic mix and the metabolites. However, MRS remains an experimental tool and is not recommended for routine workup of TBI patients.

References

Adalarasan S, Mohan A, Pasupathy S (2010). Prophylactic antibiotics in maxillofacial fractures: a requisite? J Craniofac Surg 21 (4): 1009–1011.

Ali B, Ghosh A (2002). Antibiotics in compound depressed skull fractures. Emerg Med J 19 (6): 552–553.

Anon J, Remonda L, Spreng A et al. (2008). Traumatic extra-axial hemorrhage: correlation of postmortem MSCT, MRI, and forensic-pathological findings. J Magn Reson Imaging 28: 823–836.

Arthurs OJ, Boniface S (2002). How well do we understand the neural origins of the fMRI BOLD signal? Trends Neurosci 25: 27–31.

Brant WE, Helms CA (2007). Fundamentals of Diagnostic Radiology, Lippincott Williams & Wilkins, Philadelphia.

Bullock R, Zauner A, Woodward JJ et al. (1998). Factors affecting excitatory amino acid release following severe human head injury. J Neurosurg 89: 507–518.

Burlew CC, Biffl WL, Moore EE et al. (2012). Blunt cerebrovascular injuries: redefining screening criteria in the era of noninvasive diagnosis. J Trauma Acute Care Surg 72 (2): 330–335. discussion 336–337, quiz 539.

Cantu RC (1995). Head and spine injuries in youth sports. Clin Sports Med 14 (3): 517–532.

Centers for Disease Control and Prevention (2003). Report to congress on mild traumatic brain injury in the United States: Steps to prevent a serious public health problem, CDC, National Center for Injury Prevention and Control, Atlanta.

Chalela JA, Rothlisberger J, West B et al. (2013). The white cerebellum sign: an under recognized sign of increased intracranial pressure. Neurocrit Care 18 (3): 398–399.

Chu Z, Wilde EA, Hunter JV et al. (2010). Voxel-based analysis of diffusion tensor imaging in mild traumatic brain injury in adolescents. AJNR Am J Neuroradiol 31: 340–346.

Collins JM, Krishnamoorthy AK, Kubal WS et al. (2012). Multidetector CT of temporal bone fractures. Semin Ultrasound CT MR 33 (5): 418–431.

Cushman JG, Agarwal N, Fabian TC et al. (2001). Practice management guidelines for the management of mild traumatic brain injury: the east practice management guidelines work group. J Trauma 51: 1016–1026.

Davenport ND, Lim KO, Armstrong MT et al. (2012). Diffuse and spatially variable white matter disruptions are associated with blast-related mild traumatic brain injury. Neuroimage 59: 2017–2024.

Davis PC, Drayer BP, Anderson RE et al. (2000). Head trauma. American College of Radiology. ACR appropriateness criteria. Radiology 215 (Suppl): 507–524.

Demchuk AM, Dowlatshahi D, Rodriguez-Luna D et al. (2012). Prediction of haematoma growth and outcome in patients with intracerebral haemorrhage using the CT-angiography spot sign (PREDICT): a prospective observational study. Lancet Neurol 11 (4): 307–314.

Eljamel MS (1994). Fractures of the middle third of the face and cerebrospinal fluid rhinorrhoea. Br J Neurosurg 8: 289–293.

Faul M, Xu L, Wald MM et al. (2010). Traumatic Brain Injury in the United States: Emergency Department Visits, Hospitalizations and Deaths 2002–2006. Centers for Disease Control and Prevention, National Center for Injury Prevention and Control, Atlanta (GA).

Finkelstein E, Corso P, Miller T et al. (2006). The Incidence and Economic Burden of Injuries in the United States, Oxford Unity Press, New York (NY).

Galanaud D, Perlbarg V, Gupta R et al. (2012). Neuro Imaging for Coma Emergence and Recovery Consortium. Assessment of white matter injury and outcome in severe brain trauma: a prospective multicenter cohort. Anesthesiology 117 (6) 1300–1310.

Garnett MR, Blamire AM, Rajagopalan B et al. (2000). Evidence for cellular damage in normal-appearing white matter correlates with injury severity in patients following traumatic brain injury: a magnetic resonance spectroscopy study. Brain 123 (Pt 7): 1403–1409.

Grossman RI, Yousem DM (2003). Neuroradiology: The Requisites, 2nd edn. Mosby, Philadelphia PA.

Heeger DJ, Ress D (2002). What does fMRI tell us about neuronal activity? Nat Rev Neurosci 3: 142–151.

Iverson GL, Lovell MR, Smith S et al. (2000). Prevalence of abnormal CT-scans following mild head injury. Brain Inj 14: 1057–1061.

Jagoda AS, Bazarian JJ, Bruns JJ et al. (2008). Clinical policy: neuroimaging and decision making in adult mild traumatic brain injury in the acute setting. Ann Emerg Med 52: 714–748.

Jantzen KJ (2010). Functional magnetic resonance imaging of mild traumatic brain injury. J Head Trauma Rehabil 25: 256–266.

Karger B (1995). Penetrating gunshots to the head and lack of immediate incapacitation. I Wound ballistics and mechanisms of incapacitation. Int J Legal Med 108 (2): 53–61.

Kontos HA, Wei EP, Navari RM et al. (1978). Responses of cerebral arteries and arterioles to acute hypotension and hypertension. Am J Physiol 234 (4): H371–H383.

Larsen DW (2002). Traumatic vascular injuries and their management. Neuroimaging Clin N Am 12: 249–269.

Le TH, Gean AD (2009). Neuroimaging of traumatic brain injury. Mt Sinai J Med 76: 145–162.

Leclerc X, Godefroy O, Salhi A et al. (1996). Helical CT for the diagnosis of extracranial internal carotid artery dissection. Stroke 27 (3): 461–466.

Lewelt W, Jenkins LW, Miller JD (1980). Autoregulation of cerebral blood flow after experimental fluid percussion injury of the brain. J Neurosurg 53 (4): 500–511.

Ling JM, Peña A, Yeo RA et al. (2012). Biomarkers of increased diffusion anisotropy in semi-acute mild traumatic brain injury: a longitudinal perspective. Brain 135: 1281–1292.

Liu XS1, You C, Lu M et al. (2012). Growing skull fracture stages and treatment strategy. J Neurosurg Pediatr 9 (6): 670–675.

Logothetis NK, Pauls J, Augath M et al. (2001). Neurophysiological investigation of the basis of the fmri signal. Nature 412: 150–157.

Marmarou A, Shulman K, Rosende RM (1978). A nonlinear analysis of the cerebrospinal fluid system and intracranial pressure dynamics. J Neurosurg 48 (3): 332–344.

Mayer AR, Ling J, Mannell MV et al. (2010). A prospective diffusion tensor imaging study in mild traumatic brain injury. Neurology 74: 643–650.

Mayer AR, Ling JM, Yang Z et al. (2012). Diffusion abnormalities in pediatric mild traumatic brain injury. J Neurosci 32: 17961–17969.

Miller JD (1982). Physiology of trauma. Clin Neurosurg 29: 103–130.

National Center for Injury Prevention and Control (2003). Report to Congress on Mild Traumatic Brain Injury in the United States: Steps to Prevent a Serious Public Health Problem. Centers for Disease Control and Prevention, Atlanta, GA.

National Collaborating Centre for Acute Care (2007). Head injury: Triage, assessment, investigation and early management of head injury in infants, children and adults. NCCfA, London.

Osborn A (2005). Diagnostic Imaging: Brain, Amirsys, Salt Lake City, UT.

Servadei F, Teasdale G, Merry G et al. (2001). Defining acute mild head injury in adults: a proposal based on prognostic factors, diagnosis, and management. J Neurotrauma 18: 657–664.

Tavender EJ, Bosch M, Green S et al. (2011). Quality and consistency of guidelines for the management of mild traumatic brain injury in the emergency department. Acad Emerg Med 18: 880–889.

Teasdale G, Jennett B (1974). Assessment of coma and impaired consciousness: a practical scale. Lancet 2: 81–84.

Thuomas KA, Vlajkovic S, Ganz JC et al. (1993). Progressive brain compression. Changes in vital physiological variables, correlated with brain tissue water content and brain tissue displacement. Experimental MR imaging in dogs. Acta Radiol 34 (3): 289–295.

Wada R, Aviv RI, Fox AJ et al. (2007). CT angiography "spot sign" predicts hematoma expansion in acute intracerebral hemorrhage. Stroke 38 (4): 1257–1262.

Wellwood J, Alcantara A, Michael DB (2002). Neurotrauma: the role of CT angiogram. Neurol Res 24 (Suppl 1): S13–S16.

Wilde EA, McCauley SR, Hunter JV et al. (2008). Diffusion tensor imaging of acute mild traumatic brain injury in adolescents. Neurology 70: 948–955.

Young RJ, Destian S (2002). Imaging of traumatic intracranial hemorrhage. Neuroimaging Clin N Am 12: 189–204.

Zwienenberg M, Muizelaar JP (2003). Imaging of Head Trauma. In: J Youmans (Ed.), Clinical Pathophysiology of Traumatic Brain Injury, 5th edn. WB Saunders, Philadelphia, pp. 5039–5054.

Handbook of Clinical Neurology, Vol. 135 (3rd series)
Neuroimaging, Part I
J.C. Masdeu and R.G. González, Editors

Chapter 23

Cerebellar disorders: clinical/radiologic findings and modern imaging tools

MARIO MANTO[1]* AND CHRISTOPHE HABAS[2]

[1]*Department of Neurology, Université Libre de Bruxelles Erasme, Brussels, Belgium*

[2]*Neuroimaging Service, Centre National d'Ophtalmologie des Quinze-Vingts, Paris, France*

Abstract

Cerebellar disorders, also called cerebellar ataxias, comprise a large group of sporadic and genetic diseases. Their core clinical features include impaired control of coordination and gait, as well as cognitive/behavioral deficits usually not detectable by a standard neurologic examination and therefore often overlooked. Two forms of cognitive/behavioral syndromes are now well identified: (1) the cerebellar cognitive affective syndrome, which combines an impairment of executive functions, including planning and working memory, deficits in visuospatial skills, linguistic deficiencies such as agrammatism, and inappropriate behavior; and (2) the posterior fossa syndrome, a very acute form of cerebellar cognitive affective syndrome occurring essentially in children. Sporadic ataxias include stroke, toxic causes, immune ataxias, infectious/parainfectious ataxias, traumatic causes, neoplasias and paraneoplastic syndromes, endocrine disorders affecting the cerebellum, and the so-called "degenerative ataxias" (multiple system atrophy, and sporadic adult-onset ataxias). Genetic ataxias include mainly four groups of disorders: autosomal-recessive cerebellar ataxias, autosomal-dominant ataxias (spinocerebellar ataxias and episodic ataxias), mitochondrial disorders, and X-linked ataxias. In addition to biochemical studies and genetic tests, brain imaging techniques are a cornerstone for the diagnosis, clinicoanatomic correlations, and follow-up of cerebellar ataxias. Modern radiologic tools to assess cerebellar ataxias include: functional imaging studies, magnetic resonance spectroscopy, volumetric studies, and tractography. These complementary methods provide a multimodal appreciation of the whole long-range cerebellar network functioning, and allow the extraction of potential biomarkers for prognosis and rating level of recovery after treatment.

INTRODUCTION

Cerebellar disorders, also called cerebellar ataxias, represent a large and heterogeneous group of diseases, often considered as a complex spectrum (Manto, 2010). This chapter has two objectives. First, we aim to provide an overview of the main cerebellar disorders encountered in daily practice, with a focus on clinical and radiologic findings. Second, we discuss the recent advances in imaging techniques used in the field of cerebellar disorders.

Anatomic background

Cellular anatomy of the cerebellum

Cerebellar cortex is organized in a triple layer: the Purkinje cells form the ganglionic layer, which is intermediate between the granular layer (internal, made of granule cells which send a centrifugal ascending axon divided in two parallel fibers crossing the dendritic trees of Purkinje cells) and the outer molecular layer composed of inhibitory interneurons (basket cells and stellate cells) (Ito and Yoshida, 1964; Manto and Habas, 2013).

*Correspondence to: Prof. Mario Manto, FNRS ULB Erasme, 808 Route de Lennik, 1070 Brussels, Belgium. Tel/fax: +32-2-555-39-92, E-mail: mmanto@ulb.ac.be

Lugaro cells and Golgi cells are inhibitory interneurons located in the granular layer. Purkinje neurons project to cerebellar nuclei and vestibular nuclei, and receive projections from the contralateral inferior olive (climbing fibers) and a large number of brainstem nuclei (mossy fibers). Several tracts project to the inferior olive, mainly from spinal cord, motor cortex, sensory root of the trigeminal nerve, red nucleus, and cerebellar nuclei themselves (inhibitory nucleo-olivary pathway) (Colin et al., 2002). Afferent tracts enter the cerebellum via the inferior peduncle (restiform body), the large middle peduncle (brachium pontis), and the superior peduncle (brachium conjunctivum), whereas efferent tracts leave the cerebellar circuitry mainly via the superior and inferior peduncles.

Cerebellar lobes and cerebellar zones

Our current division of the cerebellum into three lobes (the anterior lobe, the posterior lobe, and the paraflocculus/flocculus) and three parasagittal zones comes from the works of Jansen (1969). The parasagittal division is based on the mossy fiber projections to the cerebellar cortex. The flocculonodulus corresponds to the vestibulocerebellum, the vermal portion of anterior/posterior lobes with mainly spinal connections is the paleocerebellum, and the corticopontocerebellar connections define the neocerebellum, located laterally. Both pontocerebellar and spinocerebellar afferents contribute to the intermediate zone. There is a segregation of the connections between the cerebellum and the cerebral cortex into parallel multiple loops. In terms of corticonuclear arrangements, the vermis projects to the fastigial nucleus, the intermediate cerebellar cortex projects to the interpositus nucleus (globosus and emboliformis), and the lateral cerebellar cortex projects to the dentate nucleus.

Cerebellar motor deficits: the classic cerebellar syndrome

The classic cerebellar syndrome comprises the following.

Oculomotor deficits

Oculomotor deficits include instability of gaze and nystagmus, hypermetria/hypometria of saccades, saccadic pursuit, ocular misalignment (skew deviation), disorders of vestibulo-ocular reflex, and optokinetic responses. The key structures involved in the smoothness and calibration of ocular movements are the dorsal vermis, the fastigial nucleus, the flocculus and paraflocculus, and the uvula and nodulus (Waterson et al., 1992; Lewis and Zee, 1993). There is a clinicoanatomic correlation between the oculomotor deficits and the location of the lesion in the cerebellum (Table 23.1).

Table 23.1

Oculomotor deficits and localization of cerebellar lesion(s)

Oculomotor disorders	Localization of the lesion
Dysmetria of saccades	Dorsal vermis/fastigial nucleus
Saccadic pursuit	
Nystagmus:	Flocculus/paraflocculus
Gaze-evoked	
Rebound	
Downbeat	
Saccadic pursuit	
Abnormal gain of vestibulo-ocular responses	
Periodic alternating nystagmus	Nodulus, ventral uvula

Speech deficits

Speech in cerebellar patients is typically slow with slurring. Very often, words become unintelligible when the cerebellar disorder progresses over time, as a result of the temporal dysregulation of muscle contractions (Kent et al., 1997). When speech takes a scanning aspect (scanning speech is characterized by hesitations and pauses and is "explosive," with a greater intensity over some syllables), it becomes highly suggestive of a cerebellar ataxia. Lesions of the superior paravermal region are commonly associated with speech deficits (Lechtenberg and Gilman, 1978). Cerebellar mutism is discussed below (under posterior fossa syndrome).

Impaired coordination of limb movements lateralized to the side of the lesion

Dysmetria, dysdiadochokinesia, kinetic and/or action tremor, decomposition of movements, loss of check and rebound affect the upper and lower limbs.

Ataxia of gait and posture

Stance is broad-based and postural sway is increased. Midline cerebellar lesions are usually associated with deficits in sitting, stance, and gait performances. Cerebellar patients have a high risk of falls.

Impaired muscle tone

Hypotonia is observed in patients with extensive cerebellar lesions. Children are more prone to develop hypotonia than adults. Cerebellar fits designate spasms associated with intermittent opisthotonos, related to a disinhibition of extensor muscle tone (Stewart and Holmes, 1904). They occur in patients with posterior fossa tumors, Chiari malformations, and stroke involving the cerebellar cortex but sparing the nuclei.

Cognitive/behavioral syndromes

The cerebellar cognitive affective syndrome (CCAS)

CCAS, also called Schmahmann's syndrome (Manto and Mariën, 2015), is demonstrated by a comprehensive neuropsychologic evaluation. It includes impairment of executive functions, including planning and working memory, deficits in visuospatial skills, linguistic deficiencies such as agrammatism, and inappropriate behavior (Schmahmann and Sherman, 1998). Intellectual decline is typically observed in spinocerebellar ataxia type 17 (SCA 17) and dentatorubral-pallidoluysian atrophy, two forms of dominant ataxias. CCAS is caused by a disruption of the cerebellar contribution in the neural circuits that link prefrontal, posterior parietal, superior temporal, and limbic structures, including the amygdala, hippocampus, and septum (Schutter and van Honk, 2005). Behavioral changes seem more common in lesions of the posterior cerebellar lobe and the vermis. Attention errors and abnormal visuospatial skills are encountered in these patients. Visuospatial deficits may be more common in left-sided lesions.

The posterior fossa syndrome

This syndrome occurs mainly after surgery of the posterior fossa in children, developing within 48 hours of surgery in most cases (Rekate et al., 1985). A typical mutism with absence of speech develops subacutely. It will be followed by a phase of dysarthria and behavioral disturbances. Buccal and lingual apraxia, apathy, and poverty of movements are observed (Riva and Giorgi, 2000). There is still a debate regarding the pathogenesis of posterior fossa syndrome: some authors argue for hydrocephalus and postsurgical edema, whereas others believe that mutism is due to a lesion within the cerebellum itself.

Table 23.2

Sporadic ataxias: main causes

Stroke
Arterial origin
Ischemia
Hemorrhage
Venous origin
Toxic causes
Alcohol
Drugs
Solvent
Immune ataxias
Multiple sclerosis
Gluten ataxia
Lupus erythematosus
Miller–Fisher syndrome (ataxia, ophthalmoplegia, tendon areflexia)
Infectious/parainfectious ataxias
Cerebellitis
Bickerstaff encephalitis
Traumatic causes
Neoplasias and paraneoplastic syndromes
Endocrine disorders
Thyroiditis
Superficial siderosis
"Degenerative ataxias"
Multiple system atrophy
Sporadic adult-onset ataxias

Table 23.3

Causes of acute ataxia

Neurovascular
Migraine
Stroke
Immune ataxia
Infection
Intoxication
Paraneoplastic
Traumatism
Psychogenic

SPORADIC ATAXIAS

Table 23.2 summarizes the main causes of sporadic ataxias encountered in daily practice. Trying to obtain details on the course of ataxia is very useful. The causes of acute ataxias are listed in Table 23.3. Subacute ataxia in adults is associated with an infection, an immune disorder, or a paraneoplastic syndrome in most cases. So-called "degenerative ataxias" have a slowly progressive course and tend to involve both sides, although an asymmetry of deficits may be found. Brain magnetic resonance imaging (MRI) is particularly informative to distinguish the various forms of sporadic ataxias (Table 23.4). An acute cerebellar syndrome in a context of cardiovascular risk factors such as diabetes mellitus or hypertension points towards a vascular cause (Fig. 23.1). Follow-up of a vascular lesion may be associated with atrophy of a portion of the cerebellar parenchyma (Fig. 23.2). In adults, pancerebellar atrophy is one of the most common radiologic patterns observed on MRI. Figure 23.3 illustrates an example of cerebellar atrophy as a consequence of a paraneoplastic cerebellar syndrome. Figure 23.4 shows cerebellar atrophy associated with a systemic immune disorder. Specific radiologic signs, such as a hypointense rim around the brainstem in T2-weighted images, as observed in superficial siderosis

Table 23.4

Radiologic clues for the differential diagnosis of sporadic or genetic ataxias

Magnetic resonance imaging findings	Suggestive of
Mass effect	Tumor Infection (abscess; acute stage of cerebellitis) Malformation
Lesion in a cerebellar vessel territory	Stroke Vasculitis
Abnormal signal in cerebral white matter	Multiple sclerosis Acute disseminated encephalomyelitis (ADEM) Leukodystrophy Intoxication (heroin)
Cerebellar cortical atrophy	Sporadic adult-onset ataxias Multiple system atrophy (early stage) Immune ataxia Intoxication (alcohol) Spinocerebellar ataxia type 6
Olivopontocerebellar atrophy	Multiple system atrophy (advanced stage) Spinocerebellar ataxia types 1, 2, 3, 7
Impaired signal in middle cerebellar peduncles	Multiple system atrophy (MSA) Atrophy in the recessive ataxia of Charlevoix-Saguenay (ARSACS) Fragile X tremor-ataxia syndrome (FXTAS) Metabolic disease Human immunodeficiency virus (HIV) infection
Impaired signal in cerebellar nuclei	Metabolic disease Intoxication (metronidazole)
Cerebellar calcifications	Histiocytosis Infection Calcified tumor
Spinal cord atrophy	Friedreich ataxia Ataxia with deficiency in vitamin E Spinocerebellar ataxia type 3

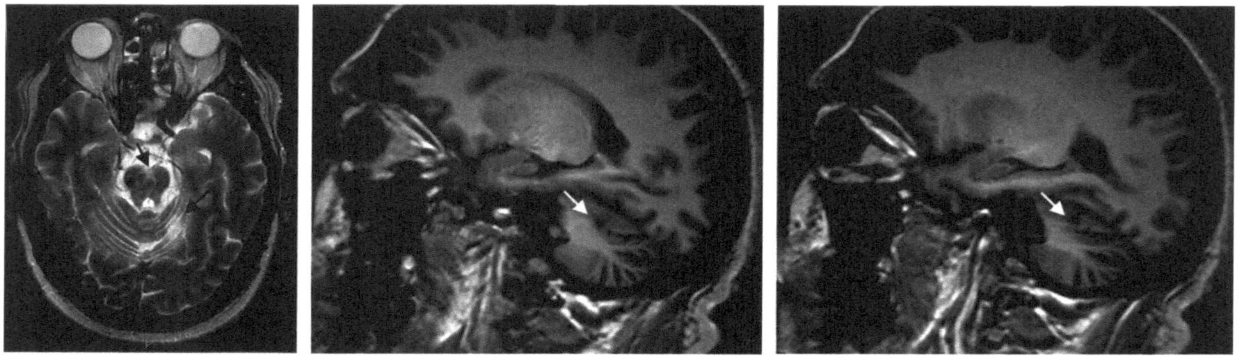

Fig. 23.1. Multiple stroke in the posterior fossa in a patient with multiple cardiovascular risk factors. Left: hyperintense signals (arrows) in the brainstem and the cerebellar parenchyma (T2-weighted sequence). Middle and right: hypointense area (T1-weighted sagittal; arrows).

(Fig. 23.5), may confirm the diagnosis immediately. Irreversible cerebellar sequelae are common following removal of a primary tumor and their extent can be clearly delineated with structural imaging (Fig. 23.6). In a context of dysautonomia associated with cerebellar ataxia, the main cause is the cerebellar form of multiple system atrophy (Fig. 23.7). The presence of a "cross sign" in the pons is very suggestive, although not specific (Fig. 23.8).

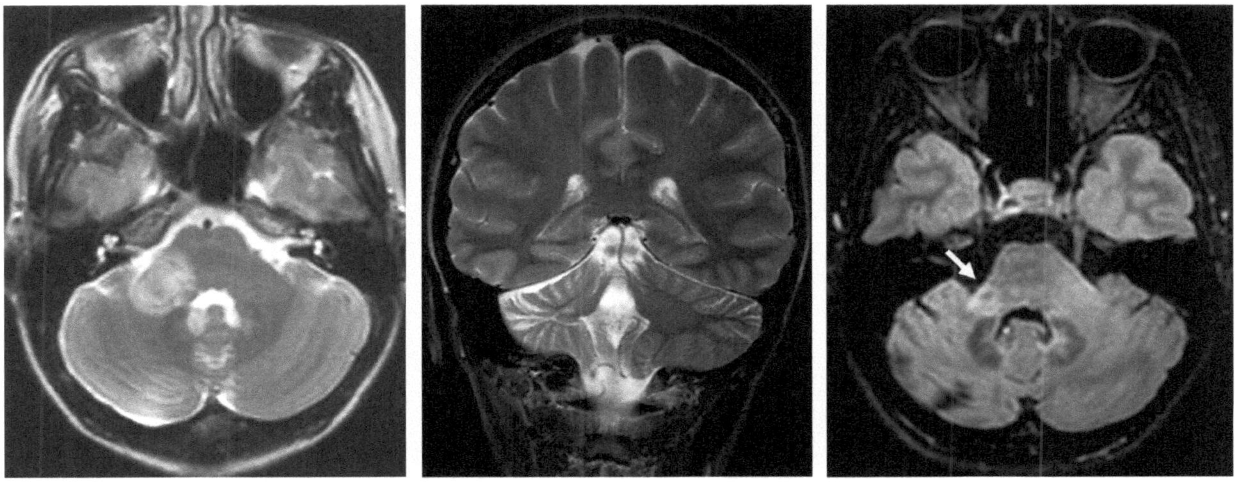

Fig. 23.2. Acute vascular lesion of the right middle cerebellar peduncle (left: T2-weighted). Middle: coronal T2-weighted image showing atrophy of the ipsilateral cerebellar hemisphere (predominating in crus I/II) 8 years later. Right: atrophic middle cerebellar peduncle (arrow) with abnormal signal and atrophy 9 years after the vascular insult (axial fluid-attenuated inversion recovery (FLAIR) sequence).

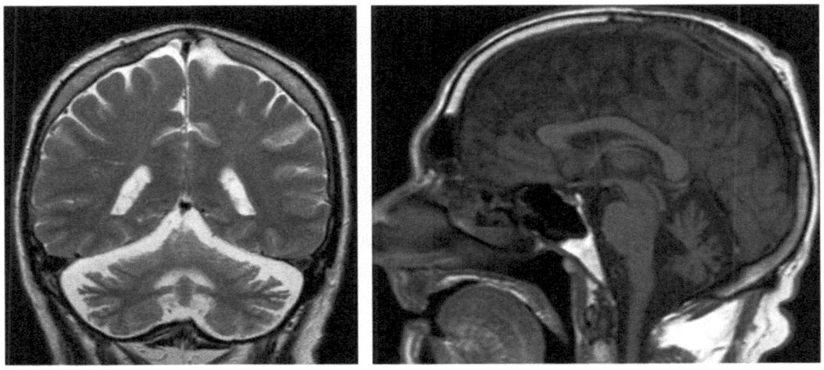

Fig. 23.3. Marked pancerebellar atrophy associated with a paraneoplastic cerebellar syndrome. The patient had a history of subacute cerebellar syndrome with subsequent discovery of a malignant thymoma. Left: coronal T2-weighted image. Right: T1-weighted sagittal.

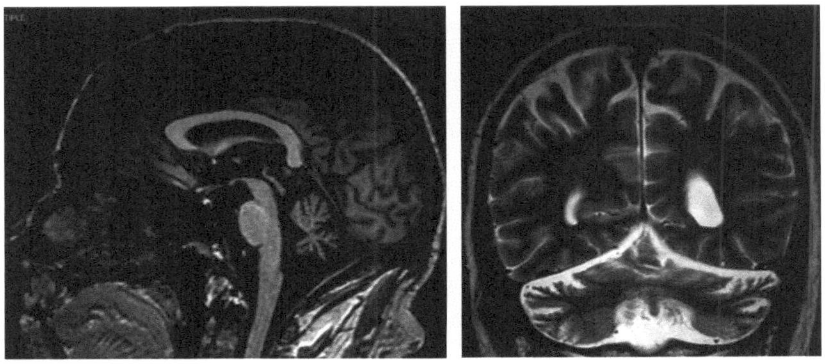

Fig. 23.4. Marked cerebellar atrophy associated with an autoimmune polyglandular syndrome. Left: T1-weighted sagittal magnetic resonance imaging showing atrophy of the vermis. Right: coronal T2-weighted image showing a widening of cerebellar sulci.

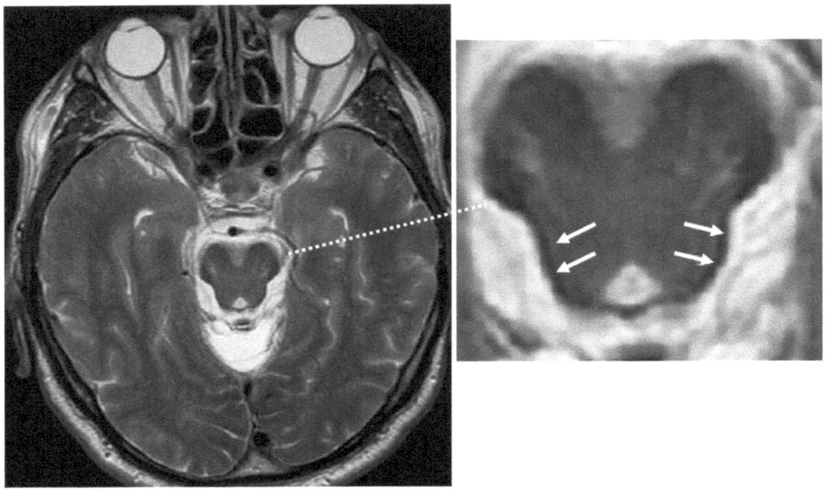

Fig. 23.5. Superficial siderosis in a patient exhibiting cerebellar ataxia. Hypointense rim (arrows) of the brainstem in T2-weighted sequence.

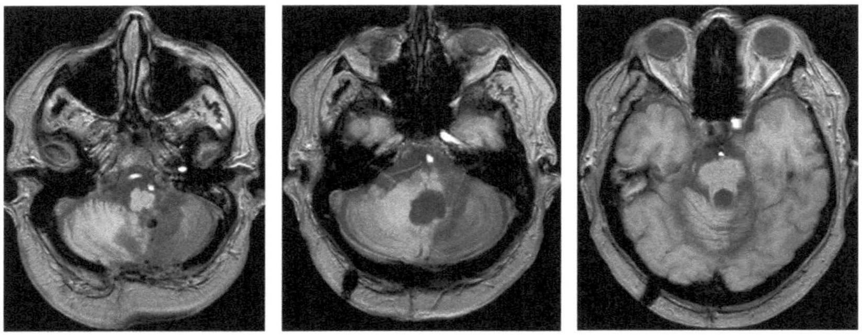

Fig. 23.6. Cerebellar and brainstem sequelae following surgical removal of an ependymoma. T1-weighted axial sequence.

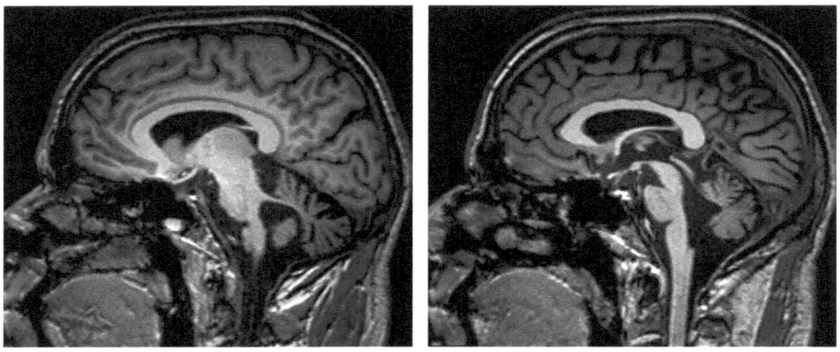

Fig. 23.7. Cerebellar form of multiple system atrophy. Marked cerebellar atrophy (T1-weighted sagittal images).

GENETIC ATAXIAS

The four principal groups of genetic ataxias are summarized in Table 23.5. Cerebellar atrophy is common amongst the four groups. Figure 23.9 illustrates cerebellar atrophy in the recessive ataxia of Charlevoix-Saguenay (ARSACS). Figure 23.10 shows an example of cerebellar atrophy associated with a mitochondrial disease. Movement disorders such as tremor and the presence of a Kayser–Fleischer ring should prompt the diagnosis of Wilson disease (Fig. 23.11). A pattern of progressive olivopontocerebellar atrophy evolves in most forms of SCAs (Figs 23.12 and 23.13).

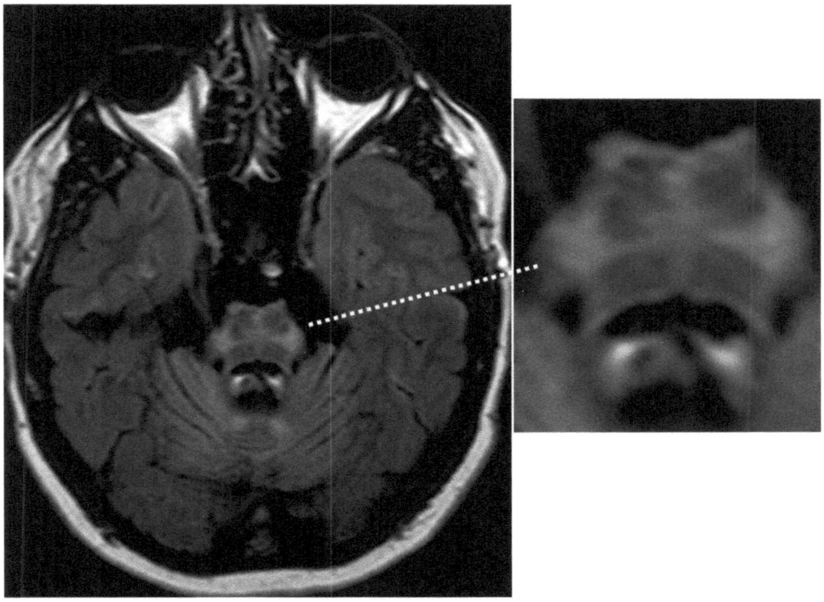

Fig. 23.8. "Cross sign" (hot-cross bun sign) in multiple system atrophy. Axial fluid-attenuated inversion recovery (FLAIR) sequence. Enlargement of the pons on the right panel. The cruciform hyperintensity is due to neuronal loss of pontine raphe nuclei and pontocerebellar fibers.

MODERN TOOLS TO ASSESS CEREBELLAR ATAXIAS

Brain imaging, especially MRI, is indicated for: (1) anatomic and morphologic characterization of the lesion; (2) differential diagnosis; and (3) follow-up of the course of the disease. Besides the classic MRI sequences (T1, T2, proton density, and fluid-attenuated inversion recovery (FLAIR)), unconventional sequences can be used to identify thoroughly the disease process and determine: (1) associated biochemical abnormalities with spectroscopy; (2) white-matter (WM) and gray-matter (GM) microstructural disorganization (diffusion, diffusion tensor imaging), axonal and neuronal loss (morphometry), and cerebellar network alterations from an anatomic (tractography) or functional (functional MRI) point of view (Maschalchi and Vella, 2012; Currie et al., 2013). Other sequences such as magnetization transfer or T2 relaxometry are used to track brain structural alterations. Therefore, these complementary methods offer a potential multimodal appreciation of the whole long-range cerebellar network functioning. Moreover, some parameters can be extracted as biomarkers of the clinical disability and can be used for the prognosis and rating the level of recovery after a given therapy. Lastly, probabilistic cerebellar atlases (cerebellum and deep cerebellar nuclei) based on ultrahigh-field MRI have been developed (Diedrichsen et al., 2009, 2011). Such atlases allow an anatomic segmentation of the cerebellum into lobules as well as vermis/hemispheres, and, thus, an accurate localization of lesions. Individual cerebellar nuclei are demarcated.

Functional imaging studies

Blood oxygenation level-dependent functional magnetic resonance imaging (BOLD-fMRI)

BOLD-fMRI enables the delineation of brain areas specifically recruited during an experimental task and therefore allows a functional network to be composed. Alterations of anatomic brain activity and of glioneuronal metabolism may cause disturbed activation maps and may be correlated with specific clinical deficiencies and disease severity. It should be pointed out that relatively few fMRI studies have been performed with ataxic patients. In SCA 1 patients performing alternate pronation and supination, no significant activity in the motor cerebellum was found, showing a functional disconnection between cerebellum and thalamocortical sensorimotor areas (Jayakumar et al., 2008). In fragile X-associated tremor/ataxia syndrome (FXTAS), hypoactivation was specifically recorded in the right premotor/dorsal inferior prefrontal cortex during a verbal working-memory task, and negative correlation was shown between right ventral inferior frontal cortex and the level of fragile X mental retardation 1 gene expression (Hashimoto et al., 2011).

Table 23.5

Commonest genetic ataxias

Autosomal-recessive cerebellar ataxias (ARCAs)
Friedreich ataxia
Ataxia-telangiectasia
Ataxia with deficiency in vitamin E (AVED)
Atrophy in the recessive ataxia of Charlevoix-Saguenay (ARSACS)
Ataxia with oculomotor apraxia type 1 (AOA1)
Ataxia with oculomotor apraxia type 2 (AOA2)
Abetalipoproteinemia
Cerebellar ataxia with deficiency in coenzyme Q10
Cerebrotendinous xanthomatosis
Refsum disease
Autosomal-recessive ataxia type 1 (ARCA-1)
Early-onset cerebellar ataxia with retained tendon reflexes (EOCARR)
Cerebellar ataxia with hypogonadism
Dysequilibrium syndrome
Wilson disease
Aceruloplasminemia
Lysosomal storage diseases
Autosomal-dominant ataxias
Spinocerebellar ataxias (SCAs)
Episodic ataxias (EAs)
Mitochondrial disorders
Kearns–Sayre syndrome
Progressive external ophthalmoplegia
Mitochondrial encephalopathy, lactic acidosis, stroke-like episodes (MELAS)
Myoclonic epilepsy with ragged-red fibers (MEERF)
Neuropathy, ataxia, and retinitis pigmentosa (NARP)
Leber hereditary optic neuropathy
Sensorineural deafness
X-linked ataxias
Fragile X tremor-ataxia syndrome (FXTAS)
X-linked adrenoleukodystrophy (X-ALD)
Arts syndrome
Congenital ataxia
Rett syndrome
Pelizaeus–Merzbacher variant
Ataxia-dementia

Resting-state functional connectivity

This technique relies on temporal correlation of spontaneous low-frequency oscillation of the BOLD signal (0.01–0.1 Hz) at rest between brain areas participating in the same functional network. Two main methods are used to compute synchronization maps. First, independent component analysis generates a set of maps representing networks spatially maximally independent as well as noisy data. Second, specific maps can be generated by linear regression of a region of interest against the other brain region. Functional links between two brain areas are rated by their coefficient of correlation. In normal subjects, independent component analysis has identified several circuits passing through the cerebellum, such as: left and right executive fronto-parietal, limbic "salience," default-mode, and sensorimotor networks (Habas et al., 2009). Linear regression has clarified the functional relations between cerebellar lobules, and brain cortex and thalamus (reviewed in Habas et al., 2012). These methods are promising tools to decipher ataxia-related functional alterations. Interestingly, they do not require active participation of the patients, as in fMRI. One study conducted with SCA 17 patients using voxel-based morphometry first demonstrated specific atrophy in anterior lobule V and posterior lobulesVIIb/VII/IX (Reetz et al., 2012). Second, the authors utilized these two cerebellar loci as seeds in a meta-analytic, task-driven connectivity analysis and in a task-free, resting-state functional group analysis of normal subjects in order to model networks passing through these atrophic lobules and to point out their functional role. The authors found that the anterior seed was associated with motor and somatosensory systems whereas the posterior seed was connected with the areas implicated in cognition and emotion that may explain neuropsychiatric signs observed in SCA 17.

A second study was devoted to intrinsic functional connectivity not between but within brain areas (lateral cerebellum and thalamus). Coefficient correlations were measured between voxels of regions of interest; the resulting functional voxels and their distribution were visualized and a comparison was drawn between normal volunteers and SCA 1 patients. Symptomatic SCA 1 patients exhibited an increase in the absolute value of the correlation coefficients in the lateral cerebellum and, more lately, in the thalamus (Solodkin et al., 2011). A patchy distribution of the neocerebellar functional clusters is found in patients whereas these clusters appear parasagittally oriented in normal subjects (stripes). Thalamic changes linearly vary with disease severity and duration. This study not only reveals an intracerebellar functional disorganization – probably caused by bulbar olivary impairment – but also cerebellothalamic functional disconnections and thalamic correlation coefficients as biomarkers of SCA clinical progression.

MR spectroscopy

Mono- or multivoxel ^{1}H spectroscopy detects specific biochemical alterations in the WM and GM of the cerebellar system: cerebellum, cerebellar peduncles, brainstem (especially, the basis pontis). Five molecules are most often targeted by this method: *N*-acetyl-aspartate (NAA: a neuronal and axonal biomarker), choline (Cho: a neuronal membrane biomarker), creatine (Creat: an energetic

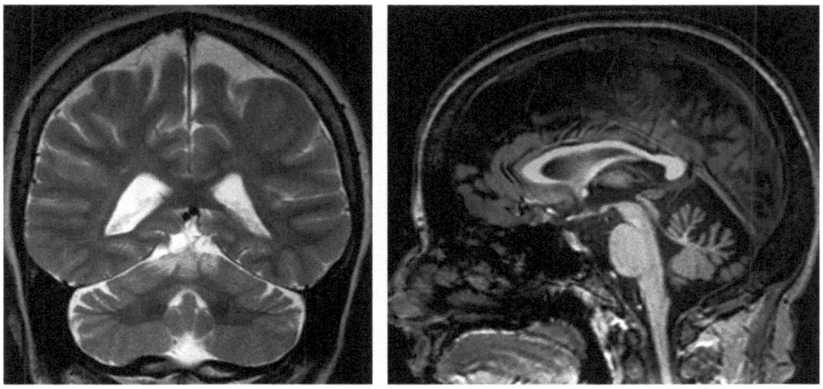

Fig. 23.9. Cerebellar atrophy associated with the recessive ataxia of Charlevoix-Saguenay (ARSACS). Left: coronal T2-weighted image; right: sagittal T1-weighted.

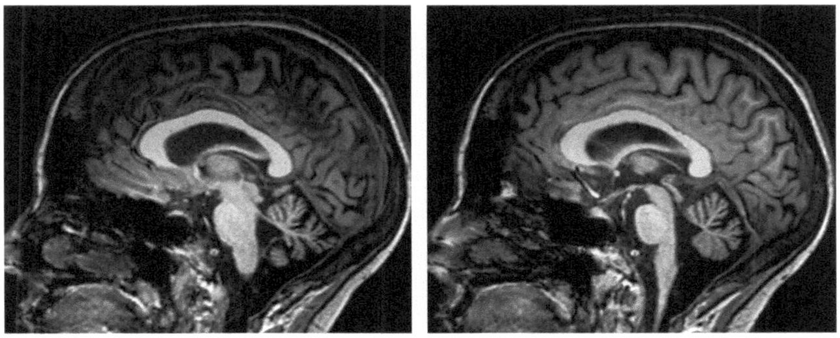

Fig. 23.10. Cerebellar vermal atrophy associated with a mitochondrial disease, as demonstrated by brain magnetic resonance imaging (T1-weighted sagittal images).

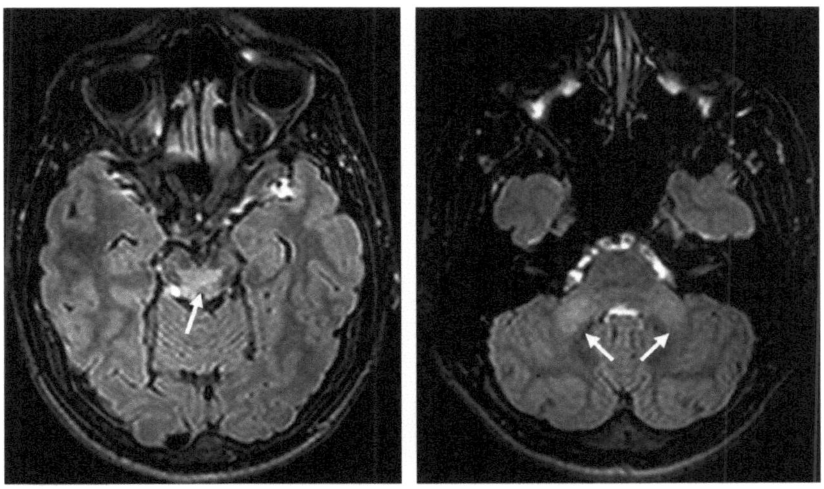

Fig. 23.11. Hyperintense signals (arrows) in the tectum and middle cerebellar peduncles in Wilson's disease. Axial fluid-attenuated inversion recovery (FLAIR) images.

biomarker), myo-inositol (Myo: an astrocytic biomarker), and lactate (Lac: a marker of the glycolytic cycle devoted to cellular energetic metabolism in anaerobic conditions). More precisely, variations of these biomarkers/Creat ratios usually refer to: (1) neuronal and axonal loss for NAA/Creat decrease; (2) membrane turnover for Cho/Creat decrease (destruction and, consequently, also neuronal loss) or increase (synthesis); and (3) gliosis for Myo/Creat increase. Other molecules can also be identified, such as, for instance, amino acids, free lipids, and ethanol. The measurement of these ratios must be done with two echo lengths: short (Myo, Lac) and long

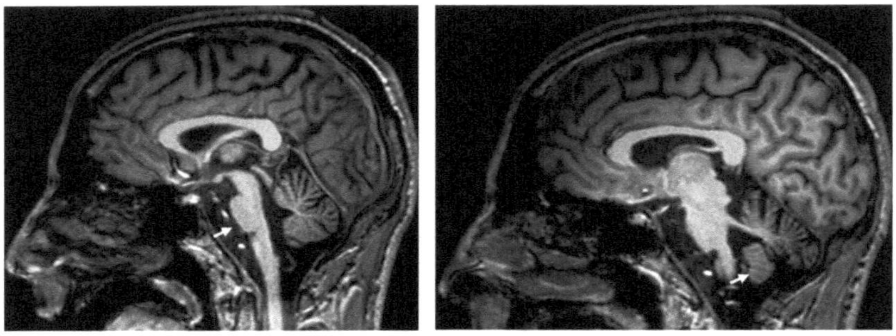

Fig. 23.12. Cerebellar atrophy associated with spinocerebellar ataxia type 2 (SCA2), demonstrated by sagittal magnetic resonance imaging (T1-weighted images). Note the slight flattening of the pons (arrow, left) and the preservation of the cerebellar tonsil (arrow, right).

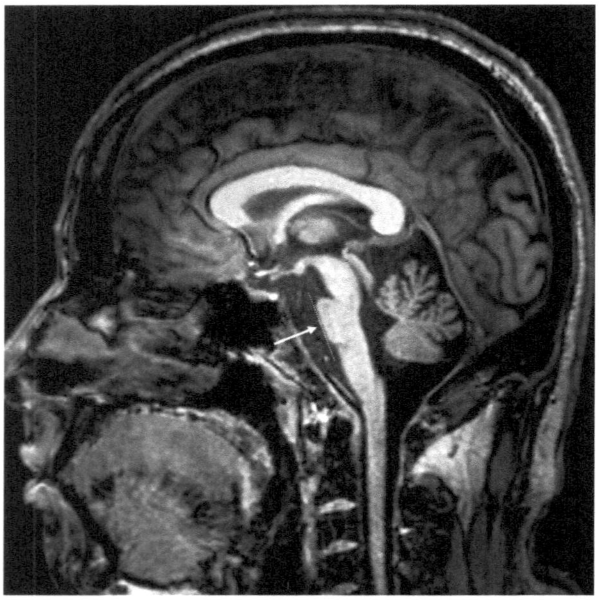

Fig. 23.13. Radiologic picture of cerebellum plus brainstem atrophy in spinocerebellar ataxia type 2. Vermal atrophy and flattening of the pons (arrow). Possible shrinkage of the spinal cord. T1-weighted sagittal image.

(NAA, Cho, Lac): for example: echo time (TE) = 35 ms and TE = 144 ms with a PRESS sequence.

Examples of clinical results

Spectroscopy can be applied to inflammatory, infectious, metabolic, neoplastic, and neurodegenerative cerebellar ataxias in order to characterize the lesional process. The major alteration observed in SCA 1, 2, 3, 6, and 7 is an NAA decrease in the cerebellum; a decrease of this marker is also seen in the pons for SCA 1. However, other spectroscopic modifications are more inconstantly found, such as Myo increase (SCA 1), Creat decrease (SCA 1 and 2), Cho decrease (SCA 2), Lac increase (SCA 1, SCA 2, type 2 episodic ataxia and mitochondropathy), and lipid increase (cerebrotendinous xanthomatosis). Of interest, decrease in NAA is correlated with the severity of the neurologic deficit in SCA 1 but not in SCA 2, and with the age of the disease in SCA 2, 3, and 6. SCAs and multiple system atrophy share a common spectroscopic profile, with decrease affecting NAA/Creat, Cho/Creat, and NAA/Cho in the hemispheric and vermian parts of cerebellum, but slight differences exist between the different genotypes of SCAs. Therefore, spectroscopy data may help to differentiate the various forms of ataxias, to evaluate the degree of severity, and to predict age onset of the neurologic deficits.

Volumetric studies

The specific pattern of cerebellar, brainstem, and brain atrophy due to cellular degeneration (mostly, Purkinje cell in neurodegenerative ataxias) can be assessed by manual (operator-dependent), morphometric, or automated (operator-independent) volumetric measurements. The most frequently used automated method corresponds to voxel-based volumetry (VBM), based upon statistical parametric analysis. Voxel-based volumetry provides tissue segmentation separating white WM, GM, and ventricles, and investigates focal volumetric differences within these structures. It is noteworthy that discrepant results are obtained between distinct volumetric methods (Schulz et al., 2010). The most studied areas are the cerebellum as a whole (and normalized), cerebellar lobules, the cerebellar peduncles, and the pons.

For example, SCA 1, 2, 3, 6, and 17, type 2 episodic ataxia, Friedreich ataxia, and ataxia-telangiectasia are characterized by different atrophic patterns of cerebellum and associated structures (Maschalchi and Vella, 2012; Currie et al., 2013). Atrophy was observed in: (1) vermis and cerebellar hemispheres and pons in SCA 1 and 2, especially in lobules VI, VIIA, and uvula in SCA 2 (Jung et al., 2012); (2) vermis and pons in SCA 3; (3) vermis and cerebellar hemispheres and likely brainstem and pons in SCA 6 (Schulz et al., 2010); (4) cerebellum (lobules V bilaterally and left lobules VIIB/VIII/IX) in SCA 17 (Reetz et al., 2012); (5) cerebellum in episodic ataxia 2; (6) cervical cord, dorsal medulla, cerebellar hemisphere, and rostral vermis in Friedreich ataxia; and (7) cerebellum, most often the vermis, in ataxia-telangiectasia. Atrophy can differentially affect WM or GM. For instance, atrophy is restricted to GM in SCA 6, whereas pontine, cerebellopeduncular, or peridentate WM can be affected in SCA 1, 2, and 3.

Again, some specific atrophic areas can be correlated with clinical deficits (and, sometimes, disease duration) such as: pons in SCA 1 and 2, total brainstem in SCA 3, cerebellum in SCA 6, and cerebellum and spinal cord in Friedreich ataxia. Jung et al. (2012) reported presymptomatic atrophy and specific correlation between duration/age/severity of ataxia and cerebellar subregion atrophy.

Diffusion-weighted imaging (DWI) and diffusion tensor imaging (DTI)

Diffusion-weighted imaging

This method tracks the random microscopic displacement of water molecules inside tissues and cells. Water mobility is greatly constrained by the environmental anisotropy relying, in particular, on cellular density/orientation and membrane integrity, and myelin. DWI deals only with the global mean water movement regardless of its direction, and can quantify the apparent diffusion coefficient (ADC: also called mean diffusivity and expressed in mm^2/s). Hyperintensity on diffusion-weighted images and decrease in ADC occur during water movement restriction mainly caused by ischemic stroke and by neoplasms because of cytotoxic edema and high cellularity, respectively. An augmented ADC can correspond to an augmentation of water mobility linked to a tissue disorganization and cellular loss. In SCA 1 and 2, ADC is increased and is correlated with the clinical dysfunction.

Diffusion tensor imaging

This variant reconstructs anatomic fascicles and thus allows WM to be segmented. DTI detects preferential directions of water displacement, which is highly constrained by the microstructural tissue architecture. In particular, water molecules preferentially move along the axonal main (longitudinal) axis, which permits the invidualization of tracts of parallel axons composing fascicles. These motion directions correspond to the nonco-linear gradients applied in the DTI sequence (at least, six). Tractography refers to the algorithmic method which computes smooth axonal trajectories by interpolating pixel encoding local water displacement according to *a priori* geometric and anisotropic parameters. DTI enables: (1) measurement of the degree of tissue anisotropy, for instance, with the fractional anisotropy (FA) parameter; and (2) visualization of anatomic tracts between their origin and their target. Of course, this latter has some limitations, such as spatial resolution, and the difficulty in clearly discriminating fiber crossings and fiber kissings, which may entail false tracking. Other methods may be preferable to overcome these limitations, such as multicompartmental probabilistic tractography, model-free diffusion spectrum imaging or Q-ball imaging. DTI not only tracks one fascicle of interest but also all the ones involved in the interconnections between nodes of anatomic networks passing through the cerebellum. These data complement functional ones obtained with functional imaging with or without stimulation (brain resting state). Moreover, these data provide the means of quantifying topologic characteristics of these networks, such as internodal path length or degree of clustering, for example.

FA measurements

Tissue disorganization and cellular loss are generally accompanied by a decreased FA, as there are fewer obstacles against water motion. SCA 1 and, more extensively, SCA 2 display FA decrease not only in the cerebellar peduncles and pontine transverses fibers, but also in the lemniscus, corticospinal tract, and corpus callosum. In SCA 1, the FA value of the superior cerebellar peduncle linearly depends on the duration and severity of the disease. FA decrease is also observed in SCA 7 and in multiple system atrophy with, in this latter case, a correlation with severity of some symptoms, age, and duration of the disease. During adult-onset ataxia, an alteration of the corticopontocerebellar pathway was noticed by severity-related reduction of FA in the internal capsule, pons, and middle cerebellar peduncle. It ensures that the cerebellar peduncles is a good location for evaluating structural degeneration by FA, and that this parameter is often correlated with severity of ataxia.

Network evaluation

Help in diagnosis

Developmental disorders can lead to abnormal cerebellar WM organization. DTI not only visualizes abnormal fascicular wiring but also helps to confirm or infer the occurrence of two distinct pathologies. For instance, DTI allowed researchers to conclude that a patient was affected by both rhombencephalosynapsis and Chiari type 2 malformations, as these methods showed specific signs of these two malformations: vertical mediocerebellar fibers and scarce fibers in the middle cerebellar peduncles, respectively (Merlini et al., 2012).

White-matter structural evaluation

Axonal degeneration and loss induce a diminished number and volume of fibers composing the anatomic fascicles calculated by tractography. It is thus possible to precisely estimate the degree of interconnections between the cerebellum and other specific brain structures, and eventually, their correlation with clinical impairments. It was shown that, after medulloblastoma removal, children suffering from cerebellar mutism had a lower volume of frontocerebellar fibers compared to controls (Soelva et al., 2013). This case illustrates the role of this method in identifying altered circuitry underlying motor or cognitive/affective cerebellar symptoms. Furthermore, this method can be extended to a more widespread cerebellar network, which allows the study of topologic alterations using parameters stemming from graph theory. Anatomic networks are assimilated to graphs with nodes (neural relays) and edges (interareal/nodal fascicles; note that edge can also consist of functional links, as measured by correlation coefficient in fMRI). The topology of this network/graph can be represented and quantified with an index, such as clustering coefficient (density of internodal connections) related to local functional integration or segregation in modules, shortest path length (the shortest length or the least number of edges connecting to given nodes) related to global integration, or nodal efficiency (the average of the inverse of the between-pair distance matrix). This coefficient is used to classify networks from random ones to highly regular ones passing through intermediary small-word networks, where any pair of nodes can be connected by a few edges. Brain networks seem to be configured in a small-word fashion, which optimizes signal integration and propagation. This approach was applied to the whole-brain network of cerebellar-type multiple atrophy system patients (Lu et al., 2013). Lower WM network efficiency was demonstrated in the cerebellum and cerebrum. Cerebellar nodal alterations were present in lobules III, IX, and X, and in vermis III, VI, VII, VIII, IX, and X. In the cerebellum, correlations were found between truncal ataxia and strength in vermis III and IX and adjacent hemispheres (negatively), and between lobular modal efficiency and ataxia handicap (positively). Therefore, this method can estimate the remote effect of cerebellar WM degeneration, and its potential impact upon long-range signal integration.

Help in therapy

Delineation of WM bundles could be an important parameter for stereotactical neurostimulation therapy. For instance, DTI determination of the dentate-rubrothalamic pathway was carried out in a patient suffering from dystonic head tremor (Coenen et al., 2011). This fascicle was specifically targeted by electrodes to relieve tremor. Of course, this method can be extended to more fundamental approaches in order to decipher the *in vivo* functional role of cerebellar tracts.

References

Coenen VA, Allert N, Mädler B (2011). A role of diffusion tensor imaging fiber tracking in deep brain stimulation surgery: DBS of the dentate-rubro-thalamic tract (drt) for the treatment of treatment-refractory tremor. Acta Neurochirg 153: 1579–1585.

Colin F, Ris L, Godaux E (2002). Neuroanatomy of the cerebellum. In: MU Manto, M Pandolfo (Eds.), The cerebellum and its disorders, Cambridge University Press, Cambridge, UK, pp. 6–29.

Currie S, Hadjivassiliou M, Craven IJ et al. (2013). Magnetic resonance imaging biomarkers in patients with progressive ataxia: current status and future directions. Cerebellum 29: 245–266.

Diedrichsen J, Balster JH, Flavell J et al. (2009). A probabilistic MR atlas of the human cerebellum. Neuroimage 46: 39–46.

Diedrichsen J, Maderwald S, Küper M et al. (2011). Imaging the deep cerebellar nuclei: a probabilistic atlas and normalization procedure. Neuroimage 54: 1786–1794.

Habas C, Kamdar N, Nguyen D et al. (2009). Distinct cerebellar contributions to intrinsic connectivity networks. J Neurosci 29 (26): 8586–8594.

Habas C, Shirer WR, Greicius MD (2012). Delineation of the cerebro-cerebellar networks with MRI measures of functional and structural connectivity. In: M Manto, DI Gruol, JD Schmahmann et al. (Eds.), Handbook of Cerebellum, Springer Verlag, Berlin, pp. 571–585.

Hashimoto R, Backer KC, Tassone KC et al. (2011). A fMRI study of the prefrontal activity during the performance of a working task in premutation carriers of the fragile X-associated tremor/ataxia syndrome (FXTAS). J Psychiatr Res 45: 36–43.

Ito M, Yoshida M (1964). The cerebellar-evoked monosynaptic inhibition in Deiters' neurones. Experientia 20: 515–516.

Jansen J (1969). On cerebellar evolution and organization, from the point of view of a morphologist. In: E Llinas (Ed.), Neurobiology of Cerebellar Evolution and Development, AMA-ERF Inst Biomed RES, Chicago, pp. 881–893.

Jayakumar PN, Desai S, Pal PK et al. (2008). Functional correlates of incoordination in patients with spinocerebellar ataxia 1: a preliminary fMRI study. J Clin Neurosci 15 (3): 269–277.

Jung BC, Choi SI, Du AX et al. (2012). MRI shows a region-specific pattern of atrophy in spinocerebellar ataxia type 2. Cerebellum 11: 272–279.

Kent RD, Kent JF, Rosenbek JC et al. (1997). A speaking task analysis of the dysarthria in cerebellar disease. Folia Phoniatr Logop 49 (2): 63–82.

Lechtenberg R, Gilman S (1978). Speech disorders in cerebellar disease. Ann Neurol 3: 285–290.

Lewis RF, Zee DS (1993). Ocular motor disorders associated with cerebellar lesions: pathophysiology and topical localization. Rev Neurol (Paris) 149 (11): 665–677.

Lu C-F, Soong B-W, Wu H-M et al. (2013). Disrupted cerebellar connectivity reduces whole-brain network efficiency in multiple system atrophy. Mov Disord 28: 362–369.

Manto M (2010). Cerebellar disorders. A practical approach to diagnosis and management, Cambridge University Press, Cambridge.

Manto M, Habas C (2013). Le cervelet. De l'anatomie et la physiologie à la Clinique humaine, Springer, Paris.

Manto M, Mariën P (2015). Schmahmann's syndrome - identification of the third cornerstone of clinical ataxiology. Cerebellum Ataxias 27 (2): 2.

Maschalchi M, Vella A (2012). Magnetic resonance and nuclear medicine imaging in ataxias. In: SH Subramony, A Durr (Eds.), Handbook of Clinical Neurology, Vol 103, Ataxic disorders, Elsevier, Amsterdam.

Merlini L, Fluss J, Korff C et al. (2012). Partial rhombencephalosynapsis and Chiari type II malformation in a child: a true association supported by DTI tractography. Cerebellum 11: 227–232.

Reetz K, Dogan I, Rolfs A et al. (2012). Investigating function and connectivity of morphometric findings – Examplified on cerebellar atrophy in spinocerebellar ataxia 17 (SCA 17). Neuroimage 62: 1354–1366.

Rekate HL, Grubb RL, Aram DM et al. (1985). Muteness of cerebellar origin. Arch Neurol 42 (7): 697–698.

Riva D, Giorgi C (2000). The cerebellum contributes to higher functions during development: evidence from a series of children surgically treated for posterior fossa tumours. Brain 123: 1051–1061.

Schmahmann JD, Sherman JC (1998). The cerebellar cognitive affective syndrome. Brain 121: 561–579.

Schulz JB, Borkert J, Wolf S et al. (2010). Visualization, quantification and correlation of brain atrophy with clinical symptoms in spinocerebellar ataxia type 1, 3 and 6. Neuroimage 49: 158–168.

Schutter DJLG, van Honk J (2005). The cerebellum on the rise of human emotion. Cerebellum 4: 290–294.

Soelva V, Hernáiz Driever P, Abbushi A et al. (2013). Frontocerebellar fiber tractography in pediatric following posterior fossa tumor surgery. Child Nerv Syst 29: 597–607.

Solodkin A, Peri E, Chen EE et al. (2011). Loss of intrinsic organization of cerebellar networks in spinocerebellar ataxia type 1: correlates with disease severity and duration. Cerebellum 10: 218–232.

Stewart TG, Holmes G (1904). Symptomatology of cerebellar tumors: a study of forty cases. Brain 27: 522–591.

Waterson JA, Barnes GR, Grely MA (1992). A quantitative study of eye and head movements during smooth pursuit in patients with cerebellar disease. Brain 115 (5): 1343–1358.

Handbook of Clinical Neurology, Vol. 135 (3rd series)
Neuroimaging, Part I
J.C. Masdeu and R.G. González, Editors

Chapter 24

Imaging of genetic and degenerative disorders primarily causing Parkinsonism

DAVID J. BROOKS*
Department of Medicine, Imperial College London, London, UK

Abstract

In this chapter the structural and functional imaging changes associated with both genetic causes of Parkinson's disease and the sporadic condition are reviewed. The role of imaging for supporting diagnosis and detecting subclinical disease is discussed and the potential use and drawbacks of using imaging biomarkers for monitoring disease progression are debated. Additionally, the use of imaging for differentiating atypical parkinsonian syndromes from Parkinson's disease is presented.

PARKINSON'S DISEASE

The pathology of Parkinson's disease (PD) targets the dopamine cells in the substantia nigra compacta. In late-onset idiopathic PD and dominantly inherited genetic variants, the cell loss occurs in association with the formation of intraneuronal Lewy inclusion bodies. Serotonergic cells in the median raphe, noradrenergic cells in the locus ceruleus, and cholinergic cells in the nucleus basalis are also involved to a lesser extent, as are other pigmented and brainstem nuclei. In later-stage disease Lewy bodies are found in limbic and association cortical areas. The condition typically presents as progressive asymmetric limb rigidity, bradykinesia, and rest tremor with later postural instability and nonmotor complications, such as depression, dementia, daytime somnolence, and autonomic dysfunction.

While the majority of PD is idiopathic, up to 10% of PD cases are genetic in origin and both autosomal-dominant and recessive susceptibility genes have now been identified. Surprisingly, it is mutations of the glucocerebrosidase (GBA) gene that are the most common genetic determinant of PD and up to 30% of "sporadic" cases are heterozygous carriers of a GBA mutation depending on the population ascertained. Homozygous GBA mutation carriers develop Gaucher's disease, a lysosomal storage disorder. The G2019S mutation of the lysine-rich repeat kinase 2 (LRRK2) gene is the second most common genetic cause of dominantly inherited PD. LRRK2 disease typically mimics late-onset sporadic PD and 40% of North African Arab PD cases, but less than 5% of Causcasian cases carry the G2019S mutation. Mutations of the alpha-synuclein (SNCA) gene were the first identified genetic cause of PD. Alpha-synuclein is concentrated in nerve terminals and regulates synaptic plasticity but abnormally aggregated alpha-synuclein is a principal component of the Lewy body, and SNCA mutations are associated with early-onset autosomal-dominant PD and Lewy-body dementia. SNCA mutations are very rare compared to LRRK2 and GBA mutations.

Autosomal-recessive PD is generally early-onset and is rarely associated with Lewy-body pathology. The most common cause is homozygous or compound heterozygous mutations of the parkin gene and patients typically present in their teens or 20s with lower-limb dystonia and parkinsonism. Levodopa-induced

*Correspondence to: David J. Brooks, MD DSc FRCP FMedSci, Hartnett Professor of Neurology, Department of Medicine, Imperial College London; Hammersmith Hospital, Du Cane Rd, London W12 0NN, UK. Tel: +44-20-8383-3172, Fax: +44-20-8383-1783/2029, E-mail: david.brooks@imperial.ac.uk

dyskinesias occur early on and are severe, while nonmotor problems are less frequent than in late-onset sporadic disease. Other causes of recessive PD include homozygous or compound heterozygous mutations of the PINK1 or DJ1 genes.

IMAGING THE PRESYNAPTIC DOPAMINERGIC SYSTEM

Integrity of the substantia nigra can be imaged structurally with both magnetic resonance imaging (MRI) and transcranial sonography (TCS) or functionally with positron emission tomography (PET) and single-photon emission computed tomography (SPECT). With the advent of 7 T MRI it is now possible to see altered susceptibility in the ventrolateral nigra in cases of established PD (Lotfipour et al., 2012). These changes are not evident at lower field strengths, but diffusion tensor imaging (DTI) at 3 T has been reported to detect reduced directionality (fractional anisotropy) of water flow in the lateral nigra of PD cases (Fig. 24.1). The sensitivity of this approach is still being established – an initial series has claimed 100% discrimination of early PD cases from controls (Vaillancourt et al., 2009) but, while later series have found mean lateral nigral fractional anisotropy values for PD are significantly reduced compared with healthy controls, some overlap between the individual ranges of values has been reported. A recent report has suggested that magnetization transfer sequences with 3 T MRI, sensitive to melanin levels, can detect increased melanin in PD nigra (Schwarz et al., 2011).

TCS detects increased midbrain echogenicity in both sporadic and genetic variants of PD (Berg et al., 2001). Over 90% of patients with established PD showed midbrain hyperechogenicity (Fig. 24.2), which may represent increased iron deposition in the substantia nigra (Berg et al., 2002). This finding is not specific for PD, however, as 10% of elderly normal individuals and 15% of essential tremor cases have also been reported to show increased midbrain echogenicity. TCS has also been reported to be abnormal in clinically affected GBA mutation carriers (Saunders-Pullman et al., 2010) and homozygous or compound heterozygote symptomatic parkin gene carriers (Walter et al., 2004). In a 5-year follow-up study of PD cases, however, it was noted that no significant change in TCS signal occurred (Berg et al., 2005). This suggests that the presence of midbrain hyperechogenicity is a trait rather than state biomarker, indicating a susceptibility to parkinsonism.

The function of dopamine terminals in PD can be examined *in vivo* with PET and SPECT (Brooks et al., 2003):

1. The availability of presynaptic dopamine transporters (DAT) can be assessed with tracers which are usually tropane-based, such as ^{123}I-beta-CIT, ^{123}I-FP-CIT, or ^{123}I-altropane for SPECT, and ^{18}F-CFT or ^{18}F-FP-CIT for PET.
2. ^{18}F-dopa PET is a marker of terminal dopadecarboxylase activity which converts dopa to dopamine.
3. Vesicle monoamine transporter (VMAT2) density in dopamine terminals can be examined with ^{11}C- or ^{18}F-dihydrotetrabenazine PET.

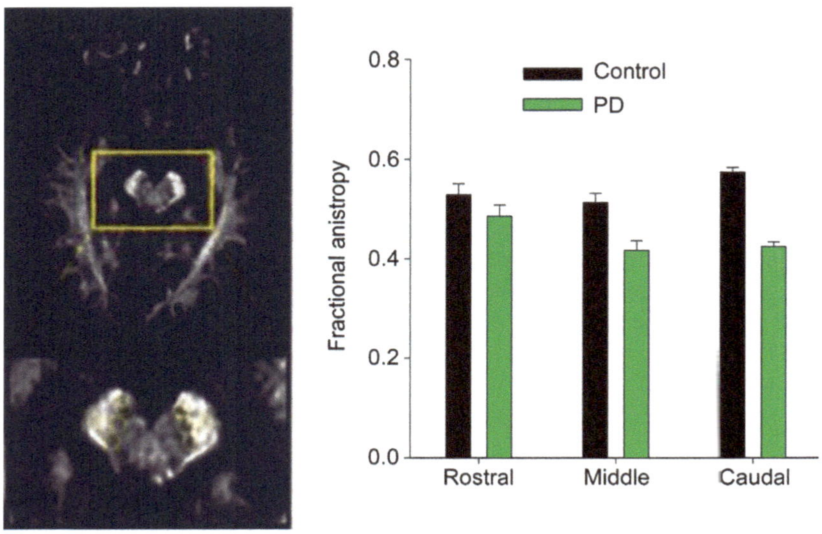

Fig. 24.1. (**A, B**) Fractional anisotropy (FA) of the midbrain. Nigral FA is reduced in a rostral caudal gradient in Parkinson's disease (PD). (Reproduced from Vaillancourt et al., 2009, with permission from Wolters Kluwer.)

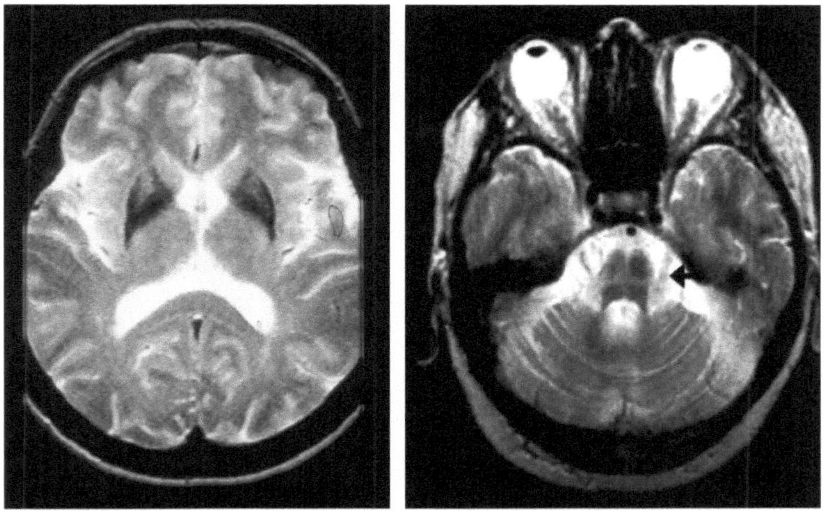

Fig. 24.2. (**A**) T2-weighted magnetic resonance imaging (MRI) showing low lateral putamen signal at the same level as the pallidum in multiple system atrophy (MSA). (**B**) T2-weighted MRI showing the pontine hot-cross bun sign in MSA (arrow).

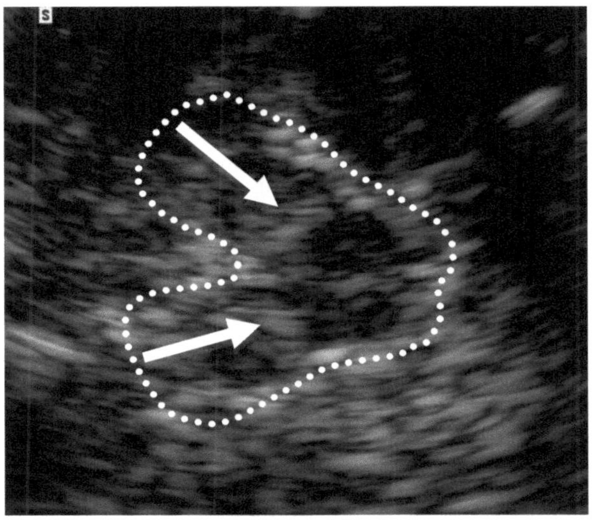

Fig. 24.3. Transcranial sonography showing hyperechogenicity from the lateral midbrain (substantia nigra) in Parkinson's disease. (Reproduced from Berg et al., 2001, with permission from Springer Science and Business Media.)

Early hemiparkinsonian cases all show bilaterally reduced putamen dopaminergic function; activity is most depressed in the putamen contralateral to the affected limbs, while head of caudate and ventral striatal function is relatively spared (Fig. 24.3). This is true for both idiopathic late-onset PD and dominant genetic causes of the disorder, such as LRRK2 (Adams et al., 2005) and GBA mutations (Goker-Alpan et al., 2012). Recessive causes of PD tend to show severe loss of striatal dopamine terminal function compared with the degree of disability present and the loss is more symmetric, involving the head of caudate to a greater degree (Khan et al., 2001). PET and SPECT are able to detect subclinical disease in late-onset asymmetric PD, evidenced as involvement of the "asymptomatic" putamen contralateral to the clinically unaffected limbs. It has been estimated that in late-onset disease clinical parkinsonism occurs when PD patients have lost around 50% of their posterior putamen dopamine terminal function, the most targeted region (Morrish et al., 1998).

In series where clinically probable PD and essential tremor cases have been compared, imaging the dopamine system with PET and SPECT has been shown to differentiate these conditions with a sensitivity and specificity greater than 90% (Brooks et al., 1992; Benamer et al., 2000). Given this, an abnormal PET or SPECT scan can be valuable for supporting a diagnosis of PD where there is diagnostic doubt. Several studies have now examined the role of DAT imaging in influencing the management of cases with uncertain parkinsonism (CUPS). All have reported that the management of such cases is influenced and confidence in diagnosis increased by including DAT SPECT in the workup (Booij et al., 2001; Catafau and Tolosa, 2004; Jennings et al., 2004). While the pathology of these cases was not established, in the CUPS study baseline SPECT findings were found to concord well with the clinical diagnosis made after 2 years of clinical disease onset, whereas the baseline clinical diagnosis had changed in 50% of cases (Tolosa et al., 2007).

What still remains unclear is whether the finding of normal dopaminergic function with PET or SPECT fully excludes a diagnosis of PD. Long-term follow-up studies on patients clinically thought to have PD but with normal ^{18}F-dopa PET or DAT SPECT imaging generally show little clinical progression or change in imaging findings. In one series where 150 cases of possible PD with normal FP-CIT SPECT at baseline were followed up, only 3% of these subjects were still felt to have PD 2 years later (Marshall et al., 2006). A number of these subjects were reclassified as having a benign essential or dystonic tremor, while other diagnoses included small-vessel disease and drug-induced syndromes. In general, a finding of normal presynaptic dopaminergic function on imaging is associated with a good prognosis in a case of suspected PD, whatever the ultimate diagnosis.

Putamen uptake of PET and SPECT dopaminergic tracers shows an inverse correlation with the severity of limb bradykinesia and rigidity in PD, though interestingly, not rest tremor severity (Vingerhoets et al., 1997; Benamer et al., 2000). This finding suggests that loss of nigrostriatal dopaminergic function is not directly responsible for tremor onset in PD and may help to explain the variable response of tremor to dopaminergic replacement. While all markers of dopamine terminal function are reduced in PD putamen, ^{18}F-dopa uptake is relatively upregulated and binding of the DAT marker ^{11}C-methylphenidate relatively downregulated relative to the dopamine vesicle transporter marker, ^{11}C-DHTBZ (Lee et al., 2000). This finding makes physiologic sense, as relatively increased levels of dopa-decarboxylase will promote dopamine turnover in the remaining terminals of the dopamine-depleted PD striatum, while relatively decreased DAT availability will act to preserve synaptic transmitter levels.

DETECTION OF SUBCLINICAL DISEASE

Postmortem studies suggest that, for every patient who develops clinical PD, there are at least 10 subclinical cases with incidental brainstem Lewy-body disease. While the greatest risk factor for PD remains aging, other factors increasing the risk of developing PD include a family history or carriage of known susceptibility genes, late-onset idiopathic hyposmia, rapid-eye-movement (REM) sleep behavior disorder, and severe late-onset constipation.

Ten percent of elderly normal individuals show midbrain hyperechogenicity on TCS, and this can be associated with the presence of soft signs of parkinsonism (Berg et al., 2011). However, the positive predictive value of abnormal TCS in healthy elderly subjects for subsequent development of PD has been estimated to be only 3%. Increased midbrain echogenicity has been reported in asymptomatic parkin gene carriers, but only one-third of these were found to also have reduced striatal ^{18}F-dopa uptake (Walter et al., 2004). Subjects who developed idiopathic hyposmia have been investigated with TCS. Eleven out of 30 such cases showed midbrain hyperechogenicity and five of these 11 had reduced striatal FP-CIT binding (Sommer et al., 2004). While increased nigral echogenicity can be detected in up to one-third of subjects with risk factors for PD, this is associated with reduced dopamine terminal function in less than 50% of these cases.

In a Dutch series, 40 elderly relatives of PD patients who had no overt parkinsonism but who manifested hyposmia on olfactory screening were investigated with baseline beta-CIT SPECT and then followed clinically. Seven of these 40 relatives showed reduced ^{123}I-beta-CIT uptake in one or more striatal subregions and the four with lowest DAT binding subsequently converted to clinical PD over a 2-year follow-up period (Ponsen et al., 2004). These findings suggest that, while ^{123}I-DAT SPECT is capable of detecting preclinical dopaminergic dysfunction when present in at-risk subjects for PD, it has a positive predictive value of only around 10%.

Asymptomatic carriers of LRRK2 and GBA gene mutations have been investigated with PET. DAT imaging proved the most sensitive marker of subclinical disease in LRRK2 disease, ^{11}C-methylphendiate PET detected significant reductions in putamen signal in two of three asymptomatic carriers of the gene where ^{18}F-dopa PET was normal (Adams et al., 2005). However, ^{18}F-dopa PET has detected subclinical disease in other series of asymptomatic adult LRRK2 (Nicholl et al., 2002), GBA (Goker-Alpan et al., 2012), parkin mutation carriers (Khan et al., 2002), and relatives in kindreds with known familial PD (Piccini et al., 1997). Three of eight asymptomatic relatives in PD kindreds who were found to have reduced putamen ^{18}F-dopa uptake were reported to subsequently develop clinical parkinsonism over a 5-year follow-up period.

^{18}F-dopa PET has been used to study the role of inheritance in apparently sporadic disease. Thirty-four asymptomatic co-twins of PD patients with apparently idiopathic sporadic disease aged 23–67 years were recruited – 18 co-twins were monozygotic (MZ) while 16 were dizygotic (DZ) (Piccini et al., 1999). Fifty-five percent of the MZ but only 18% of the DZ co-twins showed reduced putamen ^{18}F-dopa uptake. This significantly higher concordance for dopaminergic dysfunction in MZ compared with DZ PD co-twins supports a genetic contribution towards apparently sporadic disease. Over 7 years of follow-up, four MZ co-twins became clinically concordant for PD between

2 and 20 years after the onset of PD in their co-twin, resulting in a clinical concordance of 22.2% at follow-up. None of the DZ twin pairs became clinically concordant.

FOLLOWING PARKINSON'S DISEASE PROGRESSION

Imaging biomarkers can in principle be used to objectively monitor PD progression and, more importantly, examine the effects of putative neuroprotective and restorative agents on the course of the disorder. A limitation is that these biomarkers give information about only one aspect of the disease, such as levels of dopaminergic function or glucose metabolism. Additionally, the use of such biomarkers assumes that therapeutic interventions have no direct effects on the imaging itself. This has proved to be problematic in practice as chronic exposure to dopaminergic drugs can potentially influence uptake and binding of dopaminergic imaging agents.

Initial studies using ^{18}F-dopa PET and DAT SPECT reported a 5–10% annual decline in putamen dopamine terminal function in early PD patients over 2–4 years (Morrish et al., 1998; Marek et al., 2001). These PD cases were all exposed to dopamine agonists and levodopa during the course of these series and, more recently, a slower rate of decline has been reported for placebo-treated cases (Parkinson Study Group, 2007). As a result of these initial observations a series of studies followed, using ^{18}F-dopa PET and DAT SPECT as biomarkers of efficacy of drugs with potential neuroprotective properties. The REAL-PET (^{18}F-dopa PET) (Whone et al., 2003) and CALM-PD (beta-CIT SPECT) (Parkinson Study Group, 2000) trials compared clinical and imaging rates of disease progression in early PD cases randomized to either levodopa or a dopamine agonist (ropinirole in REAL-PET and pramipexole in CALM-PD). Both trials concluded that imaging measures of dopamine terminal function were reduced relatively more slowly in patients receiving an agonist compared with levodopa. However, clinically the patients were managed better when taking levodopa.

The ELLDOPA trial used beta-CIT SPECT to examine the relative rates of progression of *de novo* PD patients randomized to placebo, 150 mg, 300 mg, or 600 mg daily doses of levodopa (Fahn, 1999). Higher doses of levodopa were associated with faster reductions in striatal beta-CIT uptake over 9 months but greater clinical benefit. These trials highlight the difficulties of employing imaging biomarkers to follow PD progression. It seems probable that levodopa has a direct depressant effect on striatal uptake of ^{18}F-dopa and beta-CIT when administered over months, thus erroneously giving the impression that disease is progressing faster (Ahlskog, 2003).

Other neuroprotective studies using imaging biomarkers have been negative. The JNK inhibitor CEP1347, the vitamin coenzyme Q10 that promotes mitochondrial aerobic respiration, the neuroimmunophylline GPI1845, and the glutamate release inhibitor riluzole have all failed to influence disease progression either clinically or with imaging measures in PD. Interestingly, CEP1347 had a mild and unsuspected depressant effect on striatal beta-CIT uptake (Parkinson Study Group, 2007).

Restorative approaches to PD have been monitored with functional imaging. Several small open series and two larger double-blind control trials have examined the efficacy of striatal implants of fetal midbrain cells. ^{18}F-dopa PET has consistently showed graft function, increases in striatal dopamine storage capacity being seen in actively treated cases within 6–12 months of surgery (Lindvall, 2003). Response to transplantation, however, was disappointing in the two double-blind control trials (Freed et al., 2001; Olanow et al., 2003). Both failed to meet their primary endpoints, though in one of the trials younger cases showed a significant improvement by 12 months after engraftment and by 36 months all patients had improved when rated with the Unified Parkinson's Disease Rating Scale (UPDRS) motor scale (Ma et al., 2010). A problem, however, was the development of continuous dyskinesias in a significant minority of these cases, even when their oral medication was withdrawn.

An alternative restorative approach trialed was direct putamen infusions of glial-derived neurotrophic factor (GDNF). This agent stimulates neural progenitor cells to become dopamine cells *in vitro*, promotes terminal sprouting of neurons, and protects dopamine cells against nigral toxins, such as 6-hydroxydopamine and 1-methyl-4-phenyl-1,2,3,6-tetrahydropyridine (MPTP). A small open pilot study reported that intraputamen infusions of GDNF were effective in reversing disability and this was associated with a 25% increase in putamen ^{18}F-dopa uptake (Gill et al., 2003). In a larger double-blind controlled study, however, the clinical responses to intraputamen infusions of GDNF were variable: some patients derived no benefit, despite the consistent demonstration by ^{18}F-dopa PET that putamen dopamine storage capacity was increased in the actively treated patients (Lang et al., 2006). The GDNF and transplant trials both suggest that it is not enough simply to implant dopamine-producing cells or encourage terminal sprouting in the denervated PD striatum. The production of dopamine will need to be linked to appropriate postsynaptic receptors and its release will need to be physiologically regulated for it to be effective.

MECHANISMS OF MOTOR COMPLICATIONS IN PD

Within 2–3 years of beginning oral dopaminergic replacement therapy PD patients begin to experience motor complications. Progressive loss of striatal dopamine terminal function reduces capacity of cases to convert exogenous levodopa into dopamine, store it in vesicles, and release it physiologically. As a consequence patients feel doses of levodopa wearing off. One series has reported that mean putamen ^{18}F-dopa uptake was 28% lower in PD patients with motor fluctuations compared to those without this problem, though individual values overlapped, suggesting loss of dopamine storage capacity cannot be the only factor involved (De La Fuente-Fernandez et al., 2000).

An inability to store dopamine and loss of dopamine transporters can lead to swings in brain extracellular dopamine levels with overstimulation of postsynaptic receptors and breakthrough of involuntary movements (dyskinesias). It has been reported that levels of postsynaptic dopamine D2 receptor binding are similar in dyskinetic and nondyskinetic PD patients (Turjanski et al., 1997). Some radioligands that bind reversibly to the D2 site, such as the benzamides ^{11}C-raclopride and ^{123}I iodobenzamide, compete with endogenous dopamine and so levels of their striatal uptake are influenced by levels of brain dopamine. Using ^{11}C-raclopride PET it has been shown that, in patients with a sustained response to oral doses of levodopa, there is a progressive slow increase in brain synaptic dopamine levels over 4 hours after taking this agent (de la Fuente-Fernandez et al., 2004). In contrast, after oral levodopa, patients with motor fluctuations show higher rises of brain dopamine that peak at 1 hour and then fall back to baseline by 4 hours due to reduced storage capacity. In another study with dyskinetic patients it was reported that severity of peak dose dyskinesias induced by levodopa correlated with the increases in brain levels of dopamine induced by this agent (Pavese et al., 2006).

While excessive dopaminergic stimulation explains aspects of dykinesia induction, postsynaptic mechanisms are also important. Adenosine A2A sites on the striatum regulate the response to dopamine of the "indirect" pathway connecting the striatum, external pallidum, subthalamus, and thalamus. It has been shown that, while levels of A2A binding measured with ^{11}C-SCH442416 PET are normal in nondyskinetic PD patients, those with dyskinesias show increased A2A availability (Ramlackhansingh et al., 2011). Increased adenosine transmission could potentially dampen indirect pathway activity. The striatum and subthalamus also contain glutamate *N*-methyl-D-aspartate (NMDA) ion channels which are voltage-gated and contain a phencyclidine site only available to ligands when the ion channel is open and active. The PET tracer ^{11}C-CNS5161 binds to the phencyclidine site and it has been reported that, when PD patients are experiencing mild dyskinesias, striatal uptake of ^{11}C-CNS5161 is abnormally increased (Ahmed et al., 2011).

SEROTONERGIC AND NORADRENERGIC DYSFUNCTION

In PD, the Lewy-body pathology affects not only dopaminergic but also serotoninergic, noradrenergic, and cholinergic projections. These transmitter systems have a profound influence on mood, cognition, and sleep patterns.

Serotonergic function can be assessed either by measuring median raphe serotonin HT_{1A} binding in the midbrain or availability of serotonin transporters (SERT) in the brainstem and cortex. ^{11}C-WAY100635 PET is a marker of HT_{1A} sites, which are found postsynaptically in limbic cortex, but are also autoreceptors on serotonergic cell bodies in the median raphe. In PD, ^{11}C-WAY100635 PET has shown a 25% loss of median raphe HT_{1A} binding. While individual levels of raphe ^{11}C-WAY100635 uptake did not correlate with levels of rigidity or bradykinesia, interestingly, they correlated inversely with severity of rest tremor (Doder et al., 2003). This suggests that midbrain tegmentum pathology may be more relevant than nigrostriatal projection loss to the etiology of PD tremor.

It has been suggested that a potential mechanism promoting development of dyskinesias involves the serotonergic system. Serotonergic terminals are capable of taking up levodopa and converting it to dopamine, but then release the transmitter in an unregulated fashion as vesicular storage is not available. As dopaminergic terminals are lost in PD, this unregulated release of dopamine by serotonergic nerves becomes more important and results in inappropriate stimulation of motor pathways. The level of serotonin terminal function is reflected by transporter (SERT) availability, which can be measured with the selective marker ^{11}C-DASB PET. It has been reported that PD patients who develop dyskinesias after striatal implantation with fetal midbrain cells have higher striatal SERT binding than nondyskinetic cases (Politis et al., 2011).

It is conventional to treat depression in PD with selective serotonin reuptake inhibitors (SSRIs), though evidence that reduced serotonergic transmission underlies this depression is lacking. An ^{11}C-WAY100635 PET study failed to find differences in raphe HT_{1A} binding between depressed and nondepressed PD cases. Beta-CIT binds to SERT in the pons and midbrain, but a SPECT study with this agent found no correlation between midbrain levels of tracer uptake and depressive symptoms in PD (Kim et al., 2003). ^{11}C-RTI 32 PET is a marker of both norepinephrine and dopamine terminal function. Depressed patients with PD have been reported to show loss of thalamic and locus ceruleus ^{11}C-RTI 32 uptake relative to those equivalently disabled but without depression. Lower ^{11}C-RTI 32 uptake was also seen in amygdala and ventral striatum, both limbic areas (Remy et al., 2005). These findings suggest that depression in PD is associated with dysfunction of noradrenergic and limbic monoaminergic projections rather than of the serotonergic system. This could explain why some patients experience relief of depression after taking levodopa.

While depression in PD shows no clear correlation with serotonergic dysfunction, a subset of PD patients experience disabling tiredness reminiscent of chronic fatigue syndrome, although their locomotor disability is no greater than that of nonfatigued cases. Such fatigued cases have been studied with ^{11}C-DASB PET and it was found that patients with fatigue had significantly reduced ^{11}C-DASB binding in caudate, putamen, ventral striatum and thalamus, cingulate, and amygdala (Pavese et al., 2010). In contrast, there was no correlation between levels of fatigue and dopaminergic function. This suggests that fatigue in PD is associated with reduced serotoninergic rather than dopaminergic function in basal ganglia and limbic structures.

IMAGING MECHANISMS OF DEMENTIA IN PD

The majority of older PD patients will eventually develop dementia due to a combination of cortical Lewy-body disease, degeneration of dopaminergic and cholinergic projections to cortical areas, small-vessel disease, and concomitant Alzheimer pathology. ^{18}F-2-fluoro-2-deoxyglucose (FDG) is taken up by brain regions and phosphorylated by hexokinase. Its uptake provides a measure of regional cerebral glucose metabolism (rCMRGlc), which primarily reflects neuronal synaptic activity (Fig. 24.4). In nondemented PD patients rCMRGlc is generally within normal limits, but covariance analysis reveals an abnormal profile of relatively increased lentiform nucleus and reduced frontoparietal metabolism (Eidelberg et al., 1990). This has been labeled the "PD-related profile (PDRP)," and its degree of expression correlates with levels of motor disability rated with the UPDRS. Successful treatment with either dopaminergic replacement therapy or deep-brain stimulation acts to normalize the PDRP (Feigin et al., 2001; Hilker et al., 2004; Lin et al., 2008).

Frankly demented PD patients show an Alzheimer pattern of impaired brain glucose utilization; the posterior cingulate, parietal, and temporal association areas are targeted (Kuhl et al., 1985). This pattern of glucose hypometabolism in demented PD patients primarily reflects cortical Lewy-body disease, but concomitant

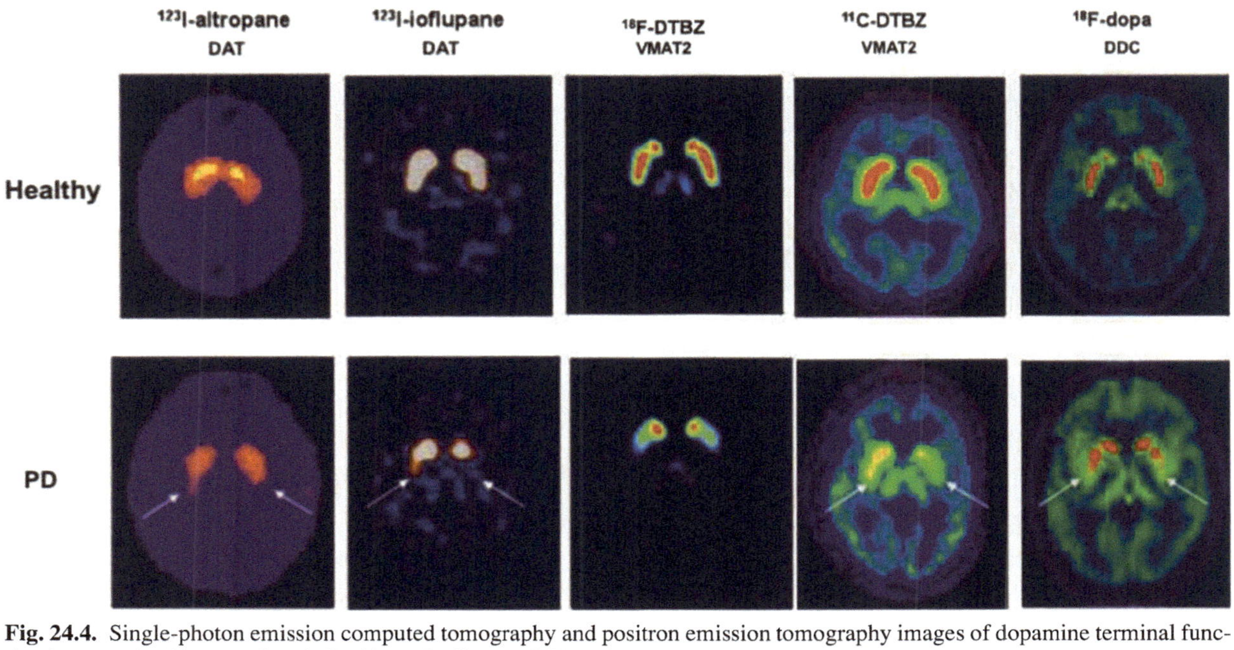

Fig. 24.4. Single-photon emission computed tomography and positron emission tomography images of dopamine terminal function in normal subjects and early Parkinson's disease (PD) patients.

Alzheimer pathology, loss of cholinergic projections, and vascular disease can also be contributors. In cases later proven pathologically to have cortical Lewy-body disease there is a greater degree of occipital cortex hypometabolism than is seen in Alzheimer patients (Albin et al., 1996).

^{11}C-NMP4A and ^{11}C-PMP PET are both markers of acetylcholine esterase activity and their uptake reflects cholinergic terminal function. Nondemented PD patients show reduced cholinergic function in parietal and occipital cortex and this spreads to involve all the cortex when dementia is present (Hilker et al., 2005). Levels of cortical ^{11}C-PMP uptake in PD do not correlate with locomotor disability in PD but correlate with Mini Mental State Examination scores and performance on executive tests such as card sorting and trail making (Bohnen et al., 2006). These results suggest progressive cognitive impairment in PD is, at least in part, a consequence of cholinergic deficit. Presynaptic cholinergic terminal function can also be assessed with SPECT using the vesicular transporter marker ^{123}I-benzovesamicol (Kuhl et al., 1996). As with markers of acetylcholine esterase activity, nondemented PD patients show focally reduced ^{123}I-benzovesamicol uptake in parietal and occipital cortex, which becomes global when dementia is present. These findings suggest that loss of cholinergic projections contributes to development of dementia. The onset of falls has also been associated with loss of cholinergic function, possibly reflecting loss of projections from the pedunculopontine nucleus to the thalamus (Bohnen and Albin, 2011).

The PET ligand, ^{11}C-PIB, is a neutral analog of the histologic dye thioflavin-T, which has been developed to image ß-amyloid plaques in Alzheimer's disease. ^{11}C-PIB PET has been used to search for evidence of raised beta-amyloid deposition in PD patients with later-onset dementia (PDD). To date, under half the reported PDD cases have shown increased ^{11}C-PIB uptake, suggesting that amyloid pathology is not the major contributor to their cognitive problems (Edison et al., 2007; Gomperts et al., 2008). In contrast, a majority of dementia with Lewy-body (DLB) patients, where onset of dementia has coincided with parkinsonism, show increased cortical ^{11}C-PIB signal. This suggests

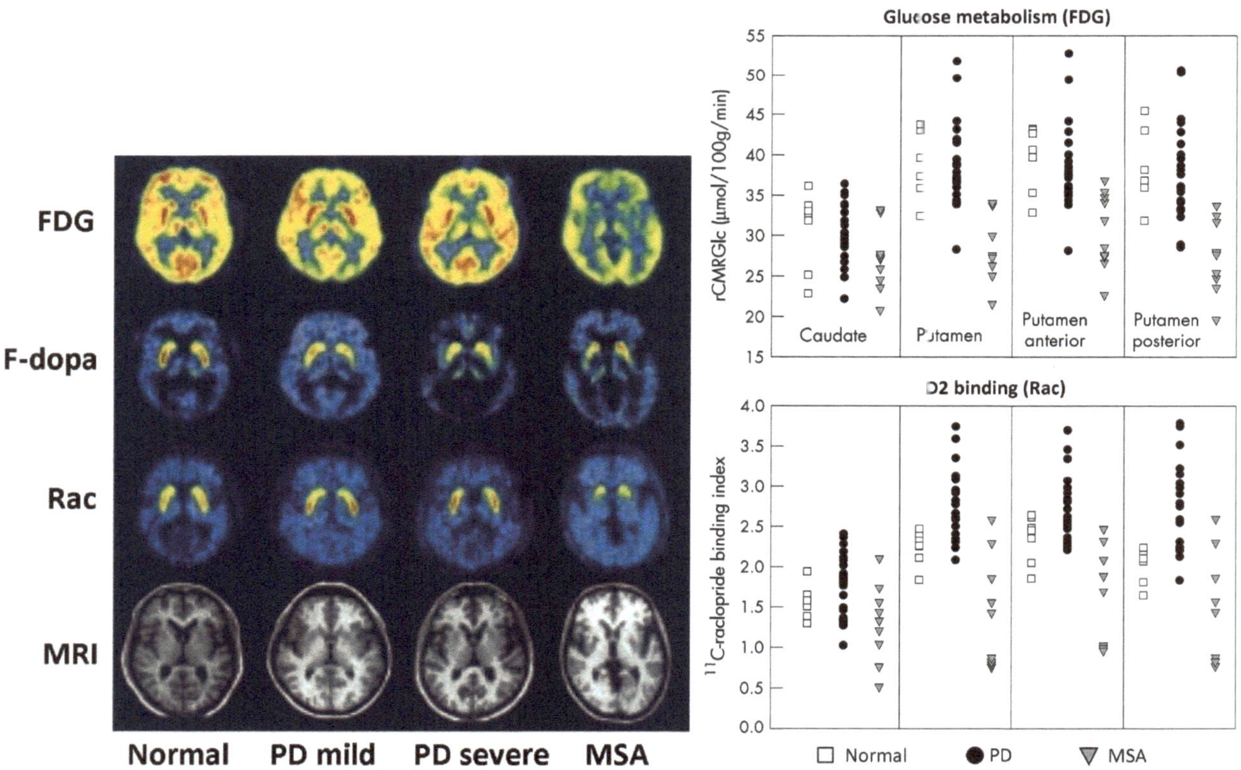

Fig. 24.5. Glucose metabolism, dopamine storage capacity, and D2 receptor binding in parkinsonian syndromes. FDG, ^{18}F-2-fluoro-2-deoxyglucose; Rac, ^{11}C-raclopride; MRI, magnetic resonance imaging; PD, Parkinson's disease; MSA, multiple system atrophy; rCMRGlc, regional cerebral metabolic rates of glucose. (Reproduced from Ghaemi et al., 2002, with permission from BMJ Publishing Group.)

that two pathologies, Lewy body and amyloid, underlie the entity commonly labelled as DLB, explaining its aggressive nature.

ATYPICAL PARKINSONIAN SYNDROMES

Multiple system atrophy

Multiple system atrophy (MSA) is an atypical sporadic form of degenerative parkinsonism which is associated with autonomic failure and ataxia. The pathology is characterized by argyrophilic inclusions containing alpha-synuclein and ubiquitin, which target the nigra and the striatum along with brainstem and cerebellar nuclei and the intermediolateral columns of the spinal cord.

As the putamen is pathologically targeted in MSA, patients may show reduced signal on T_2-weighted MRI when iron deposition is present (Fig. 24.5A). This can be accompanied by a lateral rim of increased signal due to gliosis and, if degeneration of the pons has occurred, the lateral as well as longitudinal pontine fibers become evident as high signal, manifesting as the "hot-cross bun" sign (Fig. 24.5B) (Schrag et al., 2000; Brooks and Seppi, 2009). In advanced MSA cerebellar and pontine atrophy becomes visually obvious on MRI. While these MRI changes are all helpful for discriminating MSA from other parkinsonian syndromes, they are only present in around half the cases and so lack sensitivity. DTI has now increased the sensitivity on MRI for detecting changes specific for MSA. Increased putamen water diffusion and reduced directionality "anisotropy" of flow are seen in the putamen and middle cerebellar peduncles in a majority of cases, whereas DTI is normal in these regions in PD (Seppi et al., 2003; Nicoletti et al., 2006).

^{18}FDG PET studies in MSA show reduced levels of striatal, brainstem, and cerebellar glucose metabolism, in contrast to PD, where these are preserved (Antonini et al., 1998; Spetsieris et al., 2009). The presynaptic dopaminergic system is impaired in a similar way to PD so that, while ^{18}F-dopa PET, VMAT2, and DAT imaging can separate PD and MSA from normal, they cannot reliably discriminate these two parkinsonian conditions (Brooks, 2010). Unlike PD, MSA is associated with loss of putamen dopamine D2 binding, but this can be mild, so does not provide a sensitive discriminator of MSA from PD. In one series ^{123}I iodobenzamide SPECT detected reduced striatal D2 binding in only two-thirds of *de novo* parkinsonian patients who had a negative apomorphine response and were thought to have early MSA (Schwarz et al., 1998).

^{123}I-MIBG SPECT is a marker of adrenergic terminal function and can be used to study functional integrity of cardiac sympathetic innervation in PD. Mediastinal ^{123}I-MIBG signal is reduced in the majority of PD cases, even if no clinical evidence of autonomic failure is present (Fig. 24.6). However, 50% of stage 1 PD cases still show normal cardiac MIBG uptake, so this approach is not as sensitive a marker as DAT imaging for discriminating early PD from healthy subjects (Nagayama et al., 2005). ^{123}I-MIBG SPECT is normal in most cases of MSA, as here the autonomic dysfunction results from loss of pre- rather than postsynaptic innervation (Druschky et al., 2000). Use of ^{123}I-MIBG SPECT can, thus, help differentiate MSA from PD.

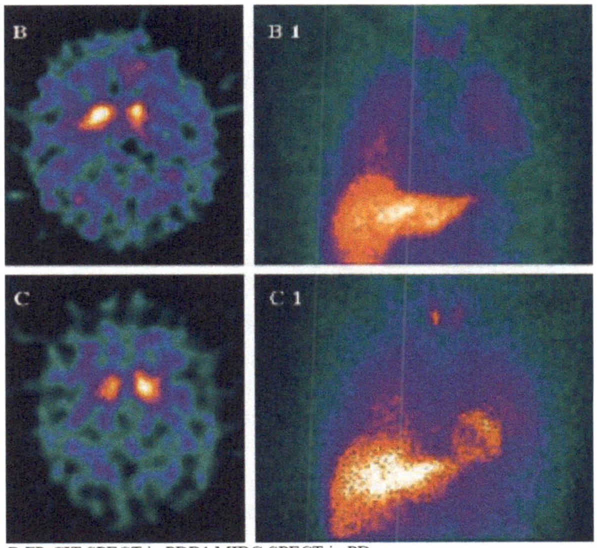

B FP-CIT SPECT in PDB1 MIBG SPECT in PD
B FP-CIT SPECT in MSAB1 MIBG SPECT in MSA

Fig. 24.6. FP-CIT single-photon emission computed tomography and ^{123}I-MIBG images of cardiac sympathetic function in (top) Parkinson's disease and (bottom) multiple system atrophy. (Reproduced from Novellino et al., 2009, with permission from John Wiley.)

Progressive supranuclear palsy

Progressive supranuclear palsy (PSP) is an atypical sporadic parkinsonian syndrome characterized clinically by early axial rigidity, postural instability, and falls along with impairment of voluntary eye movements. The pathology is associated with globose neurofibrillary tangles containing 4-repeat tau in the substantia nigra, basal ganglia, oculomotor nuclei, superior colliculi, brainstem nuclei, and the periaqueductal gray matter.

The MRIs of PSP patients do not show the reduced putamen T2 signal changes that characterize MSA, but established cases have third ventricular widening and midbrain atrophy evident on sagittal views – sometimes known as the "humming bird" sign (Schrag et al., 2000). These MRI changes are only evident on well-established cases, but sensitivity can be improved for the detection of PSP by the use of DTI. As with MSA, DTI detects reduced fractional anisotropy in the putamen of a majority of PSP cases (Seppi et al., 2003). However, in contrast to MSA, it is the superior rather than the middle cerebellar peduncle that shows increased diffusivity in PSP, so discriminating these conditions (Paviour et al., 2007).

FDG PET reveals depressed frontal cortex, basal ganglia, cerebellar, and thalamic glucose metabolism in PSP which correlates with disease duration and performance on psychometric tests of frontal function (Brooks, 2010). The presence of reduced striatal metabolism sensitively discriminates 90% of PSP cases from PD; however, as striatal hypometabolism is also a feature of MSA, FDG PET cannot reliably discriminate between these atypical conditions (Eckert et al., 2005). As with MSA, striatal D2 binding is reduced in more advanced PSP cases and this can be detected with ^{11}C-raclopride PET or iodobenzamide SPECT (Brooks, 2010).

CONCLUSIONS

Structural changes can be detected in the substantia nigra of both sporadic and genetic PD cases with TCS and diffusion tensor MRI. The presence of midbrain hyperechogenicity, however, appears to reveal a susceptibility to PD rather than correlating with the severity of disease, so cannot be used to track its progression. Atypical parkinsonian syndromes, such as MSA and PSP, can be sensitively discriminated from typical PD by the presence of abnormal putamen water diffusivity seen with DTI or abnormal lentiform nucleus echogenicity detectable with TCS. Additionally, DTI can discriminate MSA from PSP, as the middle cerebellar peduncles show increased diffusivity in MSA while the superior cerebellar peduncles are targeted in PSP.

PET and SPECT imaging both provide a sensitive and objective means of detecting dopamine terminal dysfunction in PD and so can help rationalize trials of dopaminergic medication where clinical diagnostic doubt exists. Individual levels of dopaminergic dysfunction in PD cases correlate with their degree of locomotor disability. Loss of striatal dopaminergic function in dominantly inherited genetic forms of PD, such as those associated with GBA or LRRK2 mutations, mimics that seen in late-onset sporadic disease, being asymmetric and targeting the putamen. In recessively inherited PD, however, dopamine terminal dysfunction is more severe, symmetric, and less selective, also targeting head of caudate. FDG PET can detect lentiform nucleus hypometabolism in 90% of suspected atypical PD variants, so sensitively discriminating them from PD, where lentiform nucleus metabolism is normal or raised. MIBG SPECT can detect reduced cardiac adrenergic innervation in a majority of PD cases, even in the absence of altered cardiovascular reflexes, but this is not seen in MSA or PSP cases.

When present, subclinical dopamine terminal dysfunction can be detected with PET and SPECT in subjects at risk for PD. At-risk subjects include GBA, LRRK2, and parkin mutation carriers, subjects with a family history, cases of late-onset hyposmia, and patients with REM sleep behavior disorder. Identification of subclinical disease could potentially help identify cases for neuroprotective approaches if a successful and safe therapy is identified.

Imaging potentially enables progression of parkinsonian syndromes to be objectively monitored and the efficacy of putative neuroprotective and restorative approaches to be evaluated. However, direct effects of interventions on imaging modalities have proven to be a confound in the interpretation of past trials.

Finally, imaging can help understand the mechanisms underlying nonmotor complications of PD, such as dementia and depression, and so help rationalize therapeutic approaches.

REFERENCES

Adams JR, van Netten H, Schulzer M et al. (2005). PET in LRRK2 mutations: comparison to sporadic Parkinson's disease and evidence for presymptomatic compensation. Brain 128: 2777–2785.

Ahlskog JE (2003). Slowing Parkinson's disease progression: recent dopamine agonist trials. Neurology 60: 381–389.

Ahmed I, Bose SK, Pavese N et al. (2011). Glutamate NMDA receptor dysregulation in Parkinson's disease with dyskinesias. Brain 134: 979–986.

Albin RL, Minoshima S, D'Amato CJ et al. (1996). Fluorodeoxyglucose positron emission tomography in diffuse Lewy body disease. Neurology 47: 462–466.

Antonini A, Kazumata K, Feigin A et al. (1998). Differential diagnosis of parkinsonism with [18 F]Fluorodeoxyglucose and PET. Mov Disord 13: 268–274.

Benamer TS, Pat J, Grosset DG et al. (2000). Accurate differentiation of parkinsonism and essential tremor using visual assessment of [123I]-FP-CIT imaging: The [123I]-FP-CIT Study Group. Mov Disord 15: 503–510.

Berg D, Siefker C, Becker G (2001). Echogenicity of the substantia nigra in Parkinson's disease and its relation to clinical findings. J Neurol 248: 684–689.

Berg D, Roggendorf W, Schroder U et al. (2002). Echogenicity of the substantia nigra: association with increased iron content and marker for susceptibility to nigrostriatal injury. Arch Neurol 59: 999–1005.

Berg D, Merz B, Reiners K et al. (2005). Five-year follow-up study of hyperechogenicity of the substantia nigra in Parkinson's disease. Mov Disord 20: 383–385.

Berg D, Seppi K, Behnke S et al. (2011). Enlarged substantia nigra hyperechogenicity and risk for Parkinson disease: a 37-month 3-center study of 1847 older persons. Arch Neurol 68: 932–937.

Bohnen NI, Albin RL (2011). The cholinergic system and Parkinson disease. Behav Brain Res 221: 564–573.

Bohnen NI, Kaufer DI, Hendrickson R et al. (2006). Cognitive correlates of cortical cholinergic denervation in Parkinson's disease and parkinsonian dementia. J Neurol 253: 242–247.

Booij J, Speelman JD, Horstink MW et al. (2001). The clinical benefit of imaging striatal dopamine transporters with [123I]FP-CIT SPET in differentiating patients with presynaptic parkinsonism from those with other forms of parkinsonism. Eur J Nucl Med 28: 266–272.

Brooks DJ (2010). Imaging approaches to Parkinson disease. J Nucl Med 51: 596–609.

Brooks DJ, Seppi K (2009). Proposed neuroimaging criteria for the diagnosis of multiple system atrophy. Mov Disord 24: 949–964.

Brooks DJ, Playford ED, Ibanez V et al. (1992). Isolated tremor and disruption of the nigrostriatal dopaminergic system: an 18 F-dopa PET study. Neurology 42: 1554–1560.

Brooks DJ, Frey KA, Marek KL et al. (2003). Assessment of neuroimaging techniques as biomarkers of the progression of Parkinson's disease. Exp Neurol 184: S68–S79.

Catafau AM, Tolosa E (2004). Impact of dopamine transporter SPECT using 123I-Ioflupane on diagnosis and management of patients with clinically uncertain Parkinsonian syndromes. Mov Disord 19: 1175–1182.

De La Fuente-Fernandez R, Pal PK, Vingerhoets FJG et al. (2000). Evidence for impaired presynaptic dopamine function in parkinsonian patients with motor fluctuations. J Neural Transm 107: 49–57.

de la Fuente-Fernandez R, Sossi V, Huang Z et al. (2004). Levodopa-induced changes in synaptic dopamine levels increase with progression of Parkinson's disease: implications for dyskinesias. Brain 127: 2747–2754.

Doder M, Rabiner EA, Turjanski N et al. (2003). Tremor in Parkinson's disease and serotonergic dysfunction: an (11) C-WAY 100635 PET study. Neurology 60: 601–605.

Druschky A, Hilz MJ, Platsch G et al. (2000). Differentiation of Parkinson's disease and multiple system atrophy in early disease stages by means of I-123-MIBG-SPECT. J Neurol Sci 175: 3–12.

Eckert T, Barnes A, Dhawan V et al. (2005). FDG PET in the differential diagnosis of parkinsonian disorders. Neuroimage 26: 912–921.

Edison P, Rowe CC, Rinne J et al. (2007). Amyloid load in Lewy body dementia (LBD), Parkinson's disease dementia (PDD) and Parkinson's disease (PD) measured with C-11-PIB PET. Neurology 68: A98.

Eidelberg D, Moeller JR, Dhawan V et al. (1990). The metabolic anatomy of Parkinson's disease: complementary [18 F]fluorodeoxyglucose and [18 F]fluorodopa positron emission tomographic studies. Mov Disord 5: 203–213.

Fahn S (1999). Parkinson Disease, the effect of levodopa, and the ELLDOPA trial. Arch Neurol 56: 529–535.

Feigin A, Fukuda M, Dhawan V et al. (2001). Metabolic correlates of levodopa response in Parkinson's disease. Neurology 57: 2083–2088.

Freed CR, Greene PE, Breeze RE et al. (2001). Transplantation of embryonic dopamine neurons for severe Parkinson's disease. N Engl J Med 344: 710–719.

Ghaemi M, Hilker R, Rudolf J et al. (2002). Differentiating multiple system atrophy from Parkinson's disease: contribution of striatal and midbrain MRI volumetry and multitracer PET imaging. J Neurol Neurosurg Psychiatry 73: 517–523.

Gill SS, Patel NK, Hotton GR et al. (2003). Direct brain infusion of glial cell line-derived neurotrophic factor in Parkinson disease. Nat Med 9: 589–595.

Goker-Alpan O, Masdeu JC, Kohn PD et al. (2012). The neurobiology of glucocerebrosidase-associated parkinsonism: a positron emission tomography study of dopamine synthesis and regional cerebral blood flow. Brain 135: 2440–2448.

Gomperts SN, Rentz DM, Moran E et al. (2008). Imaging amyloid deposition in Lewy body diseases. Neurology 71: 903–910.

Hilker R, Voges J, Weisenbach S et al. (2004). Subthalamic nucleus stimulation restores glucose metabolism in associative and limbic cortices and in cerebellum: evidence from a FDG-PET study in advanced Parkinson's disease. J Cereb Blood Flow Metab 24: 7–16.

Hilker R, Thomas AV, Klein JC et al. (2005). Dementia in Parkinson disease: functional imaging of cholinergic and dopaminergic pathways. Neurology 65: 1716–1722.

Jennings DL, Seibyl JP, Oakes D et al. (2004). (123I) beta-CIT and single-photon emission computed tomographic imaging vs clinical evaluation in Parkinsonian syndrome: unmasking an early diagnosis. Arch Neurol 61: 1224–1229.

Khan NL, Pavese N, Wood NW et al. (2001). An 18 F-dopa PET study of disease progression and subclinical nigrostriatal dysfunction in a parkin kindred. Neurology 56 (Supp 3): A249.

Khan NL, Scherfler C, Graham EA et al. (2002). Nigrostriatal dysfunction in asymptomatic subjects with a single parkin mutation. Mov Disord 17: P560.

Kim SE, Choi JY, Choe YS et al. (2003). Serotonin transporters in the midbrain of Parkinson's disease patients: a study with 123I-beta-CIT SPECT. J Nucl Med 44: 870–876.

Kuhl DE, Metter EJ, Benson DF et al. (1985). Similarities of cerebral glucose metabolism in Alzheimer's and Parkinsonian dementia. J Cereb Blood Flow Metabol 5 (suppl 1): S169–S170.

Kuhl DE, Minoshima S, Fessler JA et al. (1996). In vivo mapping of cholinergic terminals in normal aging, Alzheimer's disease, and Parkinson's disease. Ann Neurol 40: 399–410.

Lang AE, Gill S, Patel NK et al. (2006). Randomized controlled trial of intraputamenal glial cell line-derived

neurotrophic factor infusion in Parkinson disease. Ann Neurol 59: 459–466.
Lee CS, Samii A, Sossi V et al. (2000). In vivo positron emission tomographic evidence for compensatory changes in presynaptic dopaminergic nerve terminals in Parkinson's disease. Ann Neurol 47: 493–503.
Lin TP, Carbon M, Tang C et al. (2008). Metabolic correlates of subthalamic nucleus activity in Parkinson's disease. Brain 131: 1373–1380.
Lindvall O (2003). Stem cells for cell therapy in Parkinson's disease. Pharmacol Res 47: 279–287.
Lotfipour AK, Wharton S, Schwarz ST et al. (2012). High resolution magnetic susceptibility mapping of the substantia nigra in Parkinson's disease. J Magn Reson Imaging 35: 48–55.
Ma Y, Tang C, Chaly T et al. (2010). Dopamine cell implantation in Parkinson's disease: long-term clinical and (18)F-FDOPA PET outcomes. J Nucl Med 51: 7–15.
Marek K, Innis R, van Dyck C et al. (2001). [123I]beta-CIT SPECT imaging assessment of the rate of Parkinson's disease progression. Neurology 57: 2089–2094.
Marshall VL, Patterson J, Hadley DM et al. (2006). Two-year follow-up in 150 consecutive cases with normal dopamine transporter imaging. Nucl Med Commun 27: 933–937.
Morrish PK, Rakshi JS, Sawle GV et al. (1998). Measuring the rate of progression and estimating the preclinical period of Parkinson's disease with [18 F]dopa PET. J Neurol Neurosurg Psychiatry 64: 314–319.
Nagayama H, Hamamoto M, Ueda M et al. (2005). Reliability of MIBG myocardial scintigraphy in the diagnosis of Parkinson's disease. J Neurol Neurosurg Psychiatry 76: 249–251.
Nicholl DJ, Vaughan JR, Khan NL et al. (2002). Two large British kindreds with familial Parkinson's disease: a clinico-pathological and genetic study. Brain 125: 44–57.
Nicoletti G, Lodi R, Condino F et al. (2006). Apparent diffusion coefficient measurements of the middle cerebellar peduncle differentiate the Parkinson variant of MSA from Parkinson's disease and progressive supranuclear palsy. Brain 129: 2679–2687.
Novellino F, Arabia G, Bagnato A et al. (2009). Combined use of DAT-SPECT and cardiac MIBG scintigraphy in mixed tremors. Mov Disord 24: 2242–2248.
Olanow CW, Goetz CG, Kordower JH et al. (2003). A double-blind controlled trial of bilateral fetal nigral transplantation in Parkinson's disease. Ann Neurol 54: 403–414.
Parkinson Study Group (2000). Pramipexole vs levodopa as initial treatment for Parkinson's disease: a randomized controlled trial. JAMA 284: 1931–1938.
Parkinson Study Group (2007). Mixed lineage kinase inhibitor CEP-1347 fails to delay disability in early Parkinson disease. Neurology 69: 1480–1490.
Pavese N, Evans AH, Tai YF et al. (2006). Clinical correlates of levodopa-induced dopamine release in Parkinson disease: a PET study. Neurology 67: 1612–1617.
Pavese N, Metta V, Bose SK et al. (2010). Fatigue in Parkinson's disease is linked to striatal and limbic serotonergic dysfunction. Brain 133: 3434–3443.
Paviour DC, Thornton JS, Lees AJ et al. (2007). Diffusion-weighted magnetic resonance imaging differentiates Parkinsonian variant of multiple-system atrophy from progressive supranuclear palsy. Mov Disord 22: 68–74.
Piccini P, Morrish PK, Turjanski N et al. (1997). Dopaminergic function in familial Parkinson's disease: a clinical and 18 F-dopa PET study. Ann Neurol 41: 222–229.
Piccini P, Burn DJ, Ceravalo R et al. (1999). The role of inheritance in sporadic Parkinson's disease: evidence from a longitudinal study of dopaminergic function in twins. Ann Neurol 45: 577–582.
Politis M, Oertel WH, Wu K et al. (2011). Graft-induced dyskinesias in Parkinson's disease: high striatal serotonin/dopamine transporter ratio. Mov Disord 26: 1997–2003.
Ponsen MM, Stoffers D, Booij J et al. (2004). Idiopathic hyposmia as a preclinical sign of Parkinson's disease. Ann Neurol 56: 173–181.
Ramlackhansingh AF, Bose SK, Ahmed I et al. (2011). Adenosine 2A receptor availability in dyskinetic and non-dyskinetic patients with Parkinson disease. Neurology 76: 1811–1816.
Remy P, Doder M, Lees AJ et al. (2005). Depression in Parkinson's disease: loss of dopamine and noradrenaline innervation in the limbic system. Brain 128: 1314–1322.
Saunders-Pullman R, Hagenah J, Dhawan V et al. (2010). Gaucher disease ascertained through a Parkinson's center: imaging and clinical characterization. Mov Disord 25: 1364–1372.
Schrag A, Good CD, Miszkiel K et al. (2000). Differentiation of atypical parkinsonian syndromes with routine MRI. Neurology 54: 697–702.
Schwarz J, Tatsch K, Gasser T et al. (1998). 123I-IBZM binding compared with long-term clinical follow up in patients with de novo parkinsonism. Mov Disord 13: 16–19.
Schwarz ST, Rittman T, Gontu V et al. (2011). T1-Weighted MRI shows stage-dependent substantia nigra signal loss in Parkinson's disease. Mov Disord 26: 1633–1638.
Seppi K, Schocke MF, Esterhammer R et al. (2003). Diffusion-weighted imaging discriminates progressive supranuclear palsy from PD, but not from the Parkinson variant of multiple system atrophy. Neurology 60: 922–927.
Sommer U, Hummel T, Cormann K et al. (2004). Detection of presymptomatic Parkinson's disease: combining smell tests, transcranial sonography, and SPECT. Mov Disord 19: 1196–1202.
Spetsieris PG, Ma Y, Dhawan V et al. (2009). Differential diagnosis of parkinsonian syndromes using PCA-based functional imaging features. Neuroimage 45: 1241–1252.
Tolosa E, Borght TV, Moreno E (2007). Accuracy of DaTSCAN ((123)I-ioflupane) SPECT in diagnosis of patients with clinically uncertain parkinsonism: 2-Year

follow-up of an open-label study. Mov Disord 22: 2346–2351.

Turjanski N, Lees AJ, Brooks DJ (1997). PET studies on striatal dopaminergic receptor binding in drug naive and L-dopa treated Parkinson's disease patients with and without dyskinesia. Neurology 49: 717–723.

Vaillancourt DE, Spraker MB, Prodoehl J et al. (2009). High-resolution diffusion tensor imaging in the substantia nigra of de novo Parkinson disease. Neurology 72: 1378–1384.

Vingerhoets FJG, Schulzer M, Calne DB et al. (1997). Which clinical sign of Parkinson's disease best reflects the nigrostriatal lesion? Ann Neurol 41: 58–64.

Walter U, Klein C, Hilker R et al. (2004). Brain parenchyma sonography detects preclinical parkinsonism. Mov Disord 19: 1445–1449.

Whone AL, Watts RL, Stoessl J et al. (2003). Slower progression of PD with ropinirol versus L-dopa: the REAL-PET study. Ann Neurol 54: 93–101.

Handbook of Clinical Neurology, Vol. 135 (3rd series)
Neuroimaging, Part I
J.C. Masdeu and R.G. González, Editors

Chapter 25

Genetic and degenerative disorders primarily causing other movement disorders

NICOLA PAVESE[1,2]* AND YEN F. TAI[1]
[1]*Division of Brain Sciences, Imperial College London, UK*
[2]*Aarhus University, Denmark*

Abstract

In this chapter, we will discuss the contributions of structural and functional imaging to the diagnosis and management of genetic and degenerative diseases that lead to the occurrence of movement disorders. We will mainly focus on Huntington's disease, Wilson's disease, dystonia, and neurodegeneration with brain iron accumulation, as they are the more commonly encountered clinical conditions within this group.

HUNTINGTON'S DISEASE

Huntington's disease (HD) is an autosomal-dominantly inherited neurodegenerative disease caused by a CAG-repeat expansion in the IT15 gene of chromosome 4 (The Huntington's Disease Collaborative Research Group, 1993). This is translated into a mutant huntingtin protein with an elongated N-terminal polyglutamine chain, which in turn leads to the formation of abnormal intraneuronal inclusions (DiFiglia et al., 1997). The pathologic hallmark of HD is progressive and severe atrophy of the striatum (caudate nucleus and putamen). Medium spiny neurons of the striatum, which correspond to 90–95% of the striatal neuronal population, are preferentially lost in HD. The cerebral cortex is affected later on in the disease and the areas involved are widespread (Vonsattel et al., 1985). Clinically, HD manifests as a clinical triad of movement disorders, particularly chorea, cognitive impairment, and psychiatric disturbances.

Structural magnetic resonance imaging

Magnetic resonance imaging (MRI) brain findings in HD patients reflect the underlying pathology, namely striatal and, to a lesser extent, cortical atrophy (Fig. 25.1A). Striatal atrophy is predominantly caused by the loss of medium spiny neurons in the striatum (Guo et al., 2012). Striatal atrophy in premanifest HD gene carriers (pre-HD) can be detected using volumetric MRI up to 20 years before predicted disease onset (Paulsen et al., 2008). At the time of diagnosis, the striatal volume loss may be as much as 50% (Aylward et al., 1994). Compared to aged matched healthy controls, the annual whole-brain atrophy rates were 0.20% higher in pre-HD and 0.60% higher in early HD; whereas the caudate atrophy rates were 1.37% higher in pre-HD and 2.86% higher in early HD (Tabrizi et al., 2011).

Striatal atrophy in HD correlated with the disease burden as estimated with age and length of the CAG repeat (Tabrizi et al., 2011) and the degree of motor and cognitive, but not psychiatric, impairment (Aylward et al., 2013). Two large-scale prospective multicenter studies, PREDICT-HD and TRACK-HD, have both shown that striatal volume strongly correlated with the likelihood of disease onset in pre-HD (Tabrizi et al., 2012; Paulsen et al., 2014).

An MRI-based morphometric study found widespread degeneration in early to mid-HD involving virtually all brain structures, including basal ganglia, cerebral cortex, total white matter, amygdala, brainstem, and cerebellum (Rosas et al., 2003). Using cortical MRI

*Correspondence to: Dr. Nicola Pavese, MD, PhD, FRCP, Clinical Senior Lecturer and Consultant in Neurology, Division of Brain Sciences, Imperial College London, Hammersmith Campus, Du Cane Road, London W12 0NN, UK. Tel: +44-20-3313-3766, Fax: +44-20-3313-4320, E-mail: nicola.pavese@imperial.ac.uk

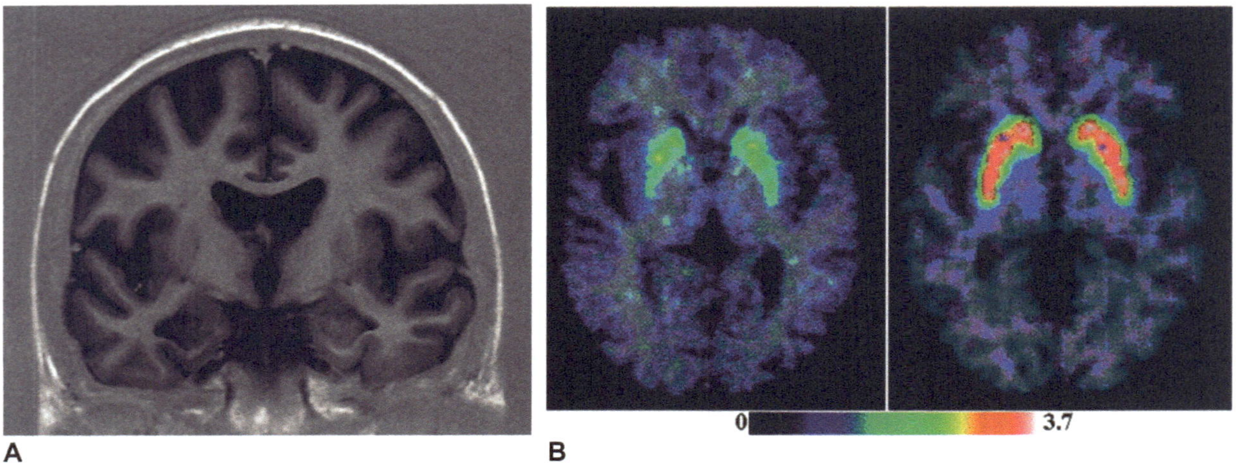

Fig. 25.1. (**A**) T1-weighted volumetric magnetic resonance imaging (MRI) of a Huntington's disease patient with disease duration of 3 years showing marked caudate atrophy with relative preservation of cortical volume. (**B**) [^{11}C]-raclopride positron emission tomography binding potential map of a Huntington's disease patients (left) and a normal subject (right) superimposed on their respective MRI. The color bar indicates binding potential values for [^{11}C]-raclopride PET. The Huntington's disease patient showed significantly reduced striatal [^{11}C]-raclopride binding potential compared to the normal subject.

morphometry, the same group showed that cortical thinning in patients with early HD was heterogeneous and topographically selective, with greater volume loss seen in the sensorimotor and primary visual cortices, while anterior frontal and temporal regions were relatively spared. They also demonstrated that distinct motor phenotypes and cognitive impairments in HD are associated with discrete patterns of cortical thinning. For example, HD subjects with prominent parkinsonian motor phenotype demonstrated greater atrophy over the anterior frontal cortical regions compared with those with prominent chorea phenotype, but there was no difference in the striatal volume between the two groups (Rosas et al., 2008). These findings were corroborated in another study which demonstrated cortical atrophy in the superior and posterior regions of the cerebrum in pre-HD, with the subjects closest to predicted disease onset demonstrating greater volume loss (Nopoulos et al., 2010). A longitudinal study showed that the rate of atrophy was faster in the frontal and parietal regions, and earlier disease onset appeared to be associated with a greater rate of cortical atrophy (Rosas et al., 2011). Gray-matter volume was also shown to be strongly associated with the likelihood of disease onset in pre-HD in the TRACK-HD study (Tabrizi et al., 2013).

Diffusion tensor imaging (DTI) studies also identified early and progressive involvement of pyramidal and extrapyramidal tracts (Rosas et al., 2006; Weaver et al., 2009) and white-matter microstructure in the corpus callosum (Rosas et al., 2010). A longitudinal MRI study in pre-HD showed that measures of volume change in striatum and white matter, particularly in the frontal lobe, are particularly sensitive markers of disease progression (Aylward et al., 2011). In a multimodal MRI study investigating longitudinal macrostructural (regional and voxel-wide volumetric changes) and microstructural (diffusivity) changes in HD, the authors concluded that the former are more sensitive than the latter in detecting longitudinal group changes between pre-HD, early HD, and controls. In particular, caudate atrophy was the most sensitive marker of early neurodegeneration and could detect changes in pre-HD over 15 years prior to predicted disease onset (Dominguez et al., 2013).

Functional MRI

Numerous activation studies using functional MRI (fMRI) have been performed in HD (Paulsen, 2009). Many of them have confirmed/corroborated the findings of impaired frontostriatal circuitry, as shown in previous $H_2{}^{15}O$ positron emission tomography (PET) activation studies (discussed further in the section on PET, below), but further insights were gained regarding longitudinal fMRI changes and default mode network (DMN) abnormalities, especially in pre-HD.

It is hypothesized that striatal neuronal dysfunction may precede cell death in pre-HD, and hence functional imaging, including fMRI and PET, may be more sensitive than structural imaging in detecting earliest subclinical changes in pre-HD. One study investigated fMRI changes while performing a verbal working-memory task in pre-HD. The working-memory scores were similar between pre-HD and healthy controls, but the former demonstrated reduced activation in the left dorsolateral prefrontal cortex, even though morphometric study showed that the area had not been affected by cortical atrophy. Pre-HD closer to predicted onset of motor symptoms had increased activation in the left inferior parietal lobule and right superior frontal gyrus compared with pre-HD further away from predicted disease onset and healthy controls, suggesting compensatory neural response in these pre-HD individuals (Wolf et al., 2007). However, a follow-up study 2 years later did not show progressive loss of activity in the left dorsolateral prefrontal cortex (Wolf et al., 2011).

Using resting-state fMRI to study the integrity of DMN, one group showed that pre-HD exhibited reduced connectivity in the anterior medial prefrontal cortex, left inferior parietal, and posterior cingulate cortex, but there was increased connectivity between the anterior and posterior DMN subsystems (Wolf et al., 2012). This disturbed connectivity became more widespread in symptomatic HD, which correlated with the degree of cognitive impairment (Quarantelli et al., 2013).

Magnetic resonance spectroscopy (MRS)

A number of MRS studies have been carried out in HD, though sometimes with contradictory findings. An MRS study of pre-HD and early HD patients showed that most subjects demonstrated various combinations of reduced *N*-acetylaspartate (marker of neuronal integrity), enhanced glutamate/glutamine and lactate (a reflection of bioenergetics) activities, and reduced creatine levels (measure of metabolism) (Reynolds et al., 2005). However, there was significant heterogeneity in the findings between HD patients. For example, low creatine level was found in pre-HD but not in symptomatic patients. Another group found that there was no difference in the putamen metabolite levels of *N*-acetylaspartate, choline (an indicator of membrane synthesis), and creatine between pre-HD and controls (van Oostrom et al., 2007).

A more recent MRS study has shown that the level of total *N*-acetylaspartate in the putamen was 8% lower in pre-HD and 17% lower in early HD compared to healthy controls, whereas the myo-inositol level, a glial cell marker, was 50% higher in early HD compared to pre-HD (Sturrock et al., 2010). At 24 months, these metabolite levels were stable (Sturrock et al., 2015), which suggests that MRS might not be sensitive enough to be employed as a marker of disease progression in HD.

Positron emission tomography

The striatal medium spiny neurons, which bear the brunt of HD pathology, express dopamine, opioid, and cannabinoid receptors on their cell surface so their functions can be imaged with a variety of PET tracers.

^{18}F-fluorodeoxyglucose (FDG) PET, which reflects cellular and synaptic glucose utilization, showed severely decreased striatal glucose metabolism in early symptomatic HD. The cortical uptake was normal initially, but as the disease progressed, impairment of frontal metabolism became apparent (Kuhl et al., 1982; Kuwert et al., 1990). A significant proportion of asymptomatic adult relatives at risk for HD also showed reduced striatal hypometabolism, though, as many of these studies were performed prior to the identification of HD gene, they were likely to have included some non-HD gene carriers (Hayden et al., 1987; Grafton et al., 1990; Kuwert et al., 1993). Network analysis of FDG PET showed a discrete pattern of metabolic abnormality in pre-HD compared to controls, with hypometabolism in the caudate, putamen, and mediotemporal regions and hypermetabolism in the occipital region (Feigin et al., 2001).

[^{11}C]-SCH23390 and [^{11}C]-raclopride PET have been used to image striatal dopamine D1 and D2 binding respectively. Contrary to the classical basal ganglia circuit model which predicts preferential involvement of D2 receptor-expressing striatal neurons of the indirect pathway in choreic HD (Albin et al., 1989), PET studies have shown a parallel reduction in striatal D1 and D2 receptor binding in HD patients and many pre-HD (Turjanski et al., 1995; Weeks et al., 1996). Striatal [^{11}C]-raclopride binding correlated cross-sectionally with motor and functional scores on the Unified Huntington's Disease Rating Scale (Andrews et al., 1999). Striatal D2 binding also correlated with cognitive dysfunction, including frontal executive domain, in both manifest HD patients and pre-HD (Backman et al., 1997; Lawrence et al., 1998). [^{11}C]-raclopride PET has also detected progressive frontal, temporal, and hypothalamic loss of D2 binding in HD (Pavese et al., 2003; Politis et al., 2008). However, using a different D2 tracer [^{11}C]-FLB457, another group did not detect reduced extrastriatal D2 binding in early to mid-stage HD (Esmaeilzadeh et al., 2011).

FDG and [^{11}C]-raclopride PET have been evaluated as markers of disease progression in HD. One [^{11}C]-raclopride PET study reported that early to mid-stage HD showed a linear progression over 5 years, with striatal D2 receptor binding falling by approximately 5% of the baseline value per annum (Pavese et al., 2003) (Fig. 25.1B). A second group reported an annual reduction of 6.3% (Antonini et al., 1996) and suggested that the progression in striatal [^{11}C]-raclopride binding is nonlinear over the whole course of the disease, later striatal degeneration being preceded by a period of relatively preserved neuronal function in pre-HD (Antonini et al., 1998). Studies of pre-HD have shown on average an annual decline in striatal [^{11}C]-raclopride binding of

2.7–6.5% and FDG metabolism of 2.3–7.6% (Antonini et al., 1996; Andrews et al., 1999; Ciarmiello et al., 2006; Feigin et al., 2007). Comparing the three imaging modalities, one group reported that [^{11}C]-raclopride PET, which reflects striatal neuronal dysfunction in addition to striatal cell loss, was more sensitive than either FDG PET or volumetric MRI in detecting subclinical abnormalities in pre-HD (van Oostrom et al., 2005). However, a longitudinal study of pre-HD showed that the FDG network abnormalities, which increased linearly over 7 years, were more sensitive than regional glucose metabolism in detecting HD progression. Its rate of increase was greater than the rates of decline of caudate [^{11}C]-raclopride binding or caudate volume, indicating that FDG network analysis could be a sensitive marker of disease progression in HD (Tang et al., 2013).

Several studies investigating the efficacy of fetal striatal transplantation in HD have been carried out, with mixed outcomes. In two of the studies, where a proportion of implanted patients had demonstrated clinical improvement/stabilization, there was an accompanying improvement in their FDG uptake and [^{11}C]-raclopride binding at the implantation sites, indicating graft survival and functional differentiation (Bachoud-Levi et al., 2006; Reuter et al., 2008).

[^{11}C]-dihydrotetrabenazine binds to vesicular monoamine transporter type-2 (VMAT2) and reflects the functional integrity of monoaminergic terminals in brain. One group reported reduced striatal ^{11}C-dihydrotetrabenazine binding in HD, particularly in patients with akinetic-rigid rather than choreic phenotype. The reduction was most marked in the posterior putamen, a pattern similar to that seen in Parkinson's disease. This suggests that nigrostriatal pathology is a feature of HD, particularly in those with akinetic-rigid phenotype (Bohnen et al., 2000).

[^{11}C]-diprenorphine PET is a marker of mu, kappa, and delta opioid receptors and is influenced by synaptic levels of endorphins. One study has reported reduced opioid receptor binding in the striatum and cingulate in HD while prefrontal and thalamic signals were increased (Weeks et al., 1997b). The increased opioid receptor availability in frontal and thalamic areas could reflect reduced endorphin levels. More recently, using a novel type 1 cannabinoid receptor (CB1) PET tracer, one study reported marked early and widespread reduction of CB1 binding in HD (Van Laere et al., 2010). This is felt to be due to the repression of CB1 transcription by mutant huntingtin. How this relates to neuronal injury in HD is yet to be fully elucidated, but it may represent a new avenue for therapeutic intervention.

Preclinical studies have suggested that microglial activation may play an important role in the pathogenesis of HD (Sapp et al., 2001). Using [^{11}C]-(R)-PK11195 (PK) PET to image activated microglia, we have shown that HD patients demonstrated increased microglial activation in the striatum, which correlated with the degree of striatal neuronal dysfunction as measured with [^{11}C]-raclopride PET (Pavese et al., 2006). Similar findings were also documented in pre-HD, where the degree of striatal microglial activation also correlated with a higher likelihood of developing HD in 5 years (Tai et al., 2007). The findings suggested that microglial activation is an early process in HD pathogenesis. The close spatial and temporal relationships between microglial activation and neuronal dysfunction in HD lend further support to the pathogenic link between the two processes (Tai et al., 2007).

Cerebral activation studies using $H_2{}^{15}O$ PET to measure regional cerebral blood flow will be briefly reviewed here. Motor tasks such as paced sequential finger opposition movements or paced joystick movements in freely chosen directions in HD patients have revealed impaired activation of the striatum and its frontal motor projection areas, with compensatory hyperactivity of insular and parietal areas (Bartenstein et al., 1997; Weeks et al., 1997a). When vibrotactile stimulation was applied to the index fingers to investigate integrity of sensory processing in HD, one study demonstrated reduced activation of contralateral sensory cortex, parietal areas 39 and 40, basal ganglia and bilateral prefrontal cortex, with enhanced activation of ipsilateral sensory cortical areas. This suggests that central gating of sensory impulses is altered with compensatory recruitment of associative sensory areas in the presence of basal ganglia dysfunction (Boecker et al., 1999). Motor sequence learning is also impaired in pre-HD individuals, who showed abnormally increased activation responses in the left mediodorsal thalamus and orbitofrontal cortex during motor tasks, possibly to compensate for caudate degeneration (Feigin et al., 2006).

NEUROACANTHOCYTOSIS

Neuroacanthocytosis syndromes refer to a group of rare genetically defined neurodegenerative disorders where underlying erythrocyte membrane abnormalities result in acanthocytosis. Within this group of disorders, they are subdivided into the "core" disorders, which include autosomal-recessive chorea-acanthocytosis (due to *VPS13A* mutation which encodes Chorein), X-linked McLeod syndrome (*XK* gene mutation), Huntington's disease-like 2 (HDL2), and pantothenate kinase-associated neurodegeneration (or PKAN, which will be discussed in the section on neurodegeneration with brain iron accumulation (NBIA), below). Acanthocytosis is only occasionally seen in the latter two conditions. The second group of neuroacanthocytosis disorders are characterized by lipoprotein abnormalities and they include abetalipoproteinemia and hypobetalipoproteinemia (Walker et al., 2011). The "core" group of disorders often manifest clinically with choreic movement disorders, cognitive and psychiatric impairments, hence representing phenocopies of HD. There are further clinical features that help to distinguish these conditions. For example, patients with choreoacanthocytosis tend to develop marked orofaciolingual dystonia which can lead to involuntary tongue/lip biting, but this is an unusual finding in patients with McLeod syndrome.

Patients with choreoacanthocytosis and McLeod syndrome both showed marked striatal atrophy on MRI and striatal hypometabolism on FDG PET (Jung et al., 2001), though, unlike HD, the cortical volume is usually preserved (Henkel et al., 2006). Significant periventricular and corpus callosum white-matter signal abnormalities have also been reported in cases of McLeod syndrome (Nicholl et al., 2004). The MRI findings of HDL-2 showed striatal and cortical atrophy and are indistinguishable from HD (Margolis, 1993).

WILSON'S DISEASE

Wilson's disease (WD) is an autosomal-recessive disorder of copper metabolism, caused by mutations in the copper-transporting ATPase ATP7B (Bull et al., 1993). The impaired biliary copper excretion leads to the accumulation of copper in a number of organs, particularly brain, liver, and cornea. Neurologic manifestations of WD include dysarthria, dystonia, ataxia, chorea, parkinsonism, and myoclonus (Lorincz, 2010).

There are a number of characteristic MRI changes in WD. In an MRI study of 100 WD patients, signal abnormalities in the putamen, caudate, thalamus, and midbrain were found in 49–72% of patients (Fig. 25.2A). Most patients also exhibited widespread atrophy involving the cerebrum, cerebellum, and brainstem (Sinha et al., 2006). Globus pallidus hypointensity on T2-weighted MRI brain was seen in 34% of patients. The midbrain "face of the giant panda" sign on T2-weighted MRI (Fig. 25.2B) is caused by hyperintensity in the tegmentum and hypointensity in the superior colliculi, while sparing the red nuclei and lateral portion of the pars reticulata of substantia nigra (Shivakumar and Thomas, 2009). It is present in 12–16% of WD patients and is considered pathognomonic for the condition. Another characteristic T2-weighted MRI finding in the pontine tegmentum of WD patients, often termed "face of the panda cub" sign (Fig. 25.2C), is caused by relative hypointensity of the medial longitudinal fasciculi and central tegmental tract, and hyperintensity of the aqueductal opening to fourth ventricle (Jacobs et al., 2003). In a study comparing the MRI findings of 56 WD cases versus 44 other early-onset extrapyramidal disorders, tectal-plate hyperintensity (76%), central pontine myelinolysis-like abnormalities (62.5%), concurrent signal changes in basal ganglia, brainstem, and thalamus (55.3%) and "face of the giant panda" sign (14.3%) were seen only in WD but not in other movement disorders (Prashanth et al., 2010), hence are helpful to establish radiologic diagnosis of WD.

FDG PET has shown severe reduction in regional glucose metabolism in the striatum and cortex of WD

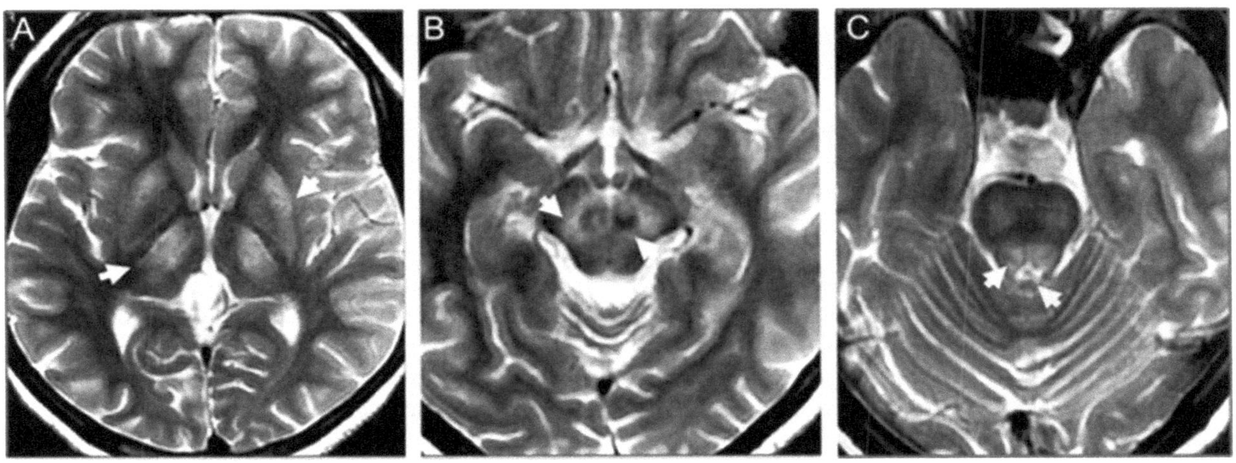

Fig. 25.2. Magnetic resonance imaging (MRI) findings in Wilson's disease. T2-weighted MRI findings of a patient's with Wilson's disease, showing (**A**) symmetric hyperintensity of the putamen and thalami; (**B**) the midbrain "face of the giant panda" sign is caused by hyperintensity in the tegmentum and hypointensity in the superior colliculi, while sparing the red nuclei and lateral portion of the pars reticulata of substantia nigra. (**C**) The pontine tegmentum "face of the panda cub" sign is caused by relative hypointensity of the medial longitudinal fasciculi and central tegmental tract, and hyperintensity of the aqueductal opening to fourth ventricle. (Reproduced from Shivakumar and Thomas, 2009.) With permission from Wolters Kluwer Publishers.

patients with neurologic symptoms, with the striatum being particularly affected. WD patients without neurologic symptoms had normal FDG PET (Hermann, 2014). ^{123}I-β-CIT, which binds to presynaptic dopamine transporters, and ^{123}I-IBZM (benzamide), which binds to dopamine D2 receptors on single-photon emission computed tomography (SPECT), have detected both pre- and postsynaptic disruption of the nigrostriatal dopaminergic pathways in WD patients with neurologic symptoms. Similar to their FDG PET findings, the pre- and postsynaptic dopaminergic SPECT binding in WD patients without neurologic symptoms was normal (Barthel et al., 2003).

The reduced striatal D2 binding and glucose metabolism and abnormal MRI signals in Wilson's disease have been shown to improve after successful treatment with copper chelation therapy (Roh et al., 1994; Schlaug et al., 1994; Schwarz et al., 1994) and liver transplantation (Wu et al., 2000).

DYSTONIA

The term dystonia refers to a group of movement disorders that vary in symptoms, causes, and progression but are characterized by the presence of dystonic movements. The definition of dystonia has recently been revised by an international panel of dystonia experts. Consensus was reached that dystonia is a movement disorder characterized by sustained or intermittent muscle contractions causing abnormal, often repetitive, movements, postures, or both. Dystonic movements are typically patterned, twisting, and may be tremulous. Dystonia is often initiated or worsened by voluntary action and associated with overflow muscle activation (Albanese et al., 2013).

The consensus committee also updated the classification system for dystonia, basing it upon clinical characteristics (axis I) and etiology (axis II). The clinical characteristics (axis I) include age at onset, body distribution, temporal pattern, associated features, and coexistence of other neurologic or systemic manifestations. In axis I, the term isolated or combined refers to the clinical phenomenology, with no implications about the underlying etiology. "Isolated dystonia" encompasses all conditions where dystonia is the only motor feature, with the exception of tremor, whereas "combined dystonia" is used to classify forms of dystonia occurring in combination with other movement disorders, previously classified under "dystonia plus" or "heredodegenerative."

The etiologic characteristics (axis II) are the presence or absence of identifiable anatomic changes and pattern of inheritance. It is suggested that the term "primary" should no longer be used to indicate genetic or idiopathic cases where dystonia is isolated and there is no consistent pathologic change. In the proposed classification, the two components of the etiologic axis are, in fact, considered separately. Idiopathic and acquired forms of dystonia include all forms of dystonia due to unknown or known specific causes, respectively, whereas inherited dystonia includes all dystonia forms of proven genetic origin. The DYT classification is still used for designating subtypes of inherited dystonia but not as a classification system. There are currently 25 locus symbols with a numeric DYT designation; some of them, however, still need independent confirmation (recently reviewed by Klein (2014)).

Conventional structural MRI sequences can be used to investigate anatomic causes of dystonia. A wide range of degenerative and destructive disorders of the nervous system, including tumors, arteriovenous malformations, head trauma, cerebral anoxia, infarction, and hemorrhage, can lead to the development of dystonia. Acquired brain lesions that cause dystonia typically affect the putamen, thalamus, and/or globus pallidus, resulting in hemidystonia in the contralateral side of the body (Marsden et al., 1985; Munchau et al., 2000). The development of dystonia after basal ganglia lesions, however, is not predictable, as most individuals with such lesions do not develop dystonia. In a large neuroimaging study, dystonia was observed in only about a third of patients with basal ganglia lesions (Bhatia and Marsden, 1994).

In patients with combined dystonia, conventional structural MRI can often show abnormalities related to the coexisting neurologic or systemic condition. WD, a disorder where dystonia is combined with other neurologic and psychiatric symptoms and liver disease, and dystonia with NBIA are described elsewhere in this chapter.

In patients with idiopathic or inherited isolated dystonia ("primary dystonia" in previous classifications), conventional MRI sequences, in line with postmortem studies, have shown no obvious degenerative changes or structural abnormalities. However, recent neuroimaging studies in these patients using more advanced MRI techniques, including voxel-based morphometry (VBM) for gray-matter assessment, DTI for white-matter assessment and structural connectivity (tractography), have consistently revealed subtle abnormalities in several brain regions, including the basal ganglia, thalamus, brainstem, cerebellum, and cerebral cortex. However, it remains to be established whether the reported brain structural changes are primary or secondary to "primary" focal dystonia. More longitudinal studies in larger cohorts with homogeneous participants are required.

VBM has been used to assess structural changes in gray matter in patients with several forms of focal dystonia, including cervical dystonia, blepharospasm, and focal hand dystonia. Patients with generalized dystonia have been less investigated.

In general, VBM abnormalities have been found in the basal ganglia, particularly in the putamen, the thalamus, the sensorimotor cortex, and the cerebellum (Zoons et al., 2011). However, there is a large variability in the different studies, which may be due to differences in the imaging sequences and/or population studied. A large meta-analysis has recently been performed to assess consistency of gray-matter changes in patients with "primary" focal dystonia (Zheng et al., 2012). The final analysis included 11 comparisons between "primary" focal dystonia patients and healthy subjects (199 patients and 247 healthy subjects in total). Gray-matter volume was found to be greater in the caudate and in sensorimotor areas including postcentral area (BA2, 3, 40) and primary motor cortex, and smaller in the thalamus and putamen. These findings provide evidence that structures in the sensorimotor network are abnormal in patients with "primary" focal dystonia. It should be noticed that the authors report that each significant cluster in the analysis was only contributed by two to four studies, suggesting that the results had high sensitivity but low robustness.

One study has assessed VBM changes in 9 patients with "primary" generalized dystonia, 11 patients with "primary" cervical dystonia, 11 patients with "primary" focal hand dystonia, and 31 age- and gender-matched controls. Interestingly, all three dystonia subtypes showed similar, although not identical, pattern of gray-matter changes compared to healthy controls, suggesting that different subtypes of "primary" dystonia may share common pathophysiologic features (Egger et al., 2007).

White matter in patients with "primary" dystonia also shows some abnormalities. DTI studies have shown a number of abnormalities in the fiber tracks connecting basal ganglia, cortex, and cerebellum. Compared to controls, patients with cervical dystonia have been reported to have higher fractional anisotropy (FA) values in both putaminal nuclei and lower FA values in the genu and in the body of the corpus callosum. The same patients also had lower mean diffusivity (MD) values in the left pallidum, left putamen, and caudate, bilaterally (Colosimo et al., 2005). Another study found that FA in patients with cervical dystonia was significantly reduced in corpus callosum (body) and bilateral putamen, whereas MD was reduced in the right caudate, left putamen, bilateral prefrontal cortex, and left supplementary area (Fabbrini et al., 2008). The authors suggest that increased FA and decreased MD values in these patients could reflect increased cellularity, increased fiber coherence, and more ordered tissue containing a large number of similarly aligned neurons in the basal ganglia, whereas decreased FA in the prefrontal cortical areas, supplementary motor area, and corpus callosum could reflect reduced cell number and decreased number of axons connecting cortical regions of the two hemispheres (Colosimo et al., 2005; Fabbrini et al., 2008).

Disrupted thalamic-prefrontal pathways and altered connection between pallidal output and brainstem have also been reported in patients with cervical dystonia (Bonilha et al., 2009; Blood et al., 2012). Patients with blepharospasm had similar FA and MD values as the healthy volunteers (Fabbrini et al., 2008; Horovitz et al., 2012). However, corticobulbar tract volume and peak tract connectivity appeared to be decreased in patients compared with controls (Horovitz et al., 2012). Patients with writer's cramp had shown increased FA values bilaterally in the white matter of the posterior limb of the internal capsule and adjacent structure, involving fiber tracts connecting the primary sensorimotor areas with subcortical structures (Delmaire et al., 2009).

Interestingly, botulinum toxin treatment seems to normalize some of the white-matter abnormalities seen in dystonic patients. Blood and colleagues (2006) found that 4 patients with cervical dystonia and 2 with hand dystonia exhibited an abnormal hemispheric asymmetry in a focal region between the pallidum and the thalamus. This asymmetry disappeared after botulinum toxin treatment, suggesting that it could have been an expression of activity-dependent white-matter plasticity in these patients.

FA abnormalities in the subgyral white matter of the sensorimotor cortex have been reported in both manifesting and nonmanifesting DYT1 carriers compared to controls (Carbon et al., 2004) (Fig. 25.3). Additional FA reductions were found in the dorsal brainstem in the vicinity of the pedunculopontine nucleus and cerebellar outflow pathways as a characteristic of manifesting subjects (Carbon et al., 2008). A more recent DTI study with diffusion tractography has revealed reduced integrity of cerebellothalamocortical fiber tracts, likely developmental in origin, in both manifesting (7 DYT1 and 5 DYT6) and clinically nonmanifesting (4 DYT1 and 4 DYT6) dystonia mutation carriers (Argyelan et al., 2009). In these subjects, reductions in cerebellothalamic connectivity correlated with increased motor activation responses, consistent with loss of inhibition at the cortical level. Nonmanifesting mutation carriers, however, were characterized by an additional area of fiber tract disruption situated distally along the thalamocortical segment of the pathway, in tandem with the proximal cerebellar outflow abnormality. In individual gene carriers, clinical penetrance was determined by the difference in connectivity measured at these two sites. The authors proposed this tandem-lesion model as a possible explanation for the differences in clinical expression in carriers of dystonia mutation (Argyelan et al., 2009).

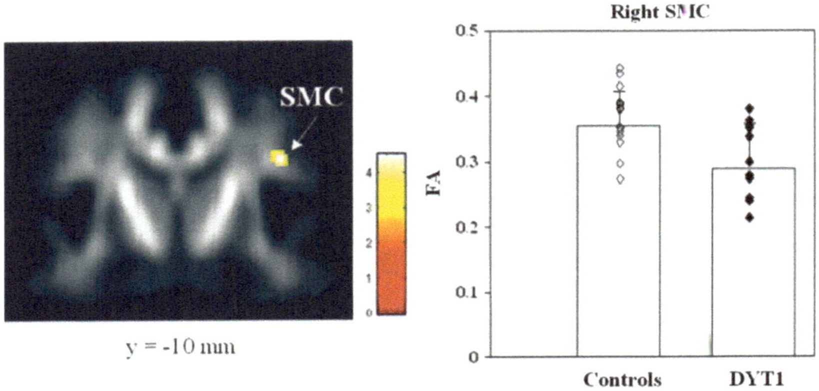

Fig. 25.3. Left: Statistical parametric map analysis showing declines in fractional anisotropy (FA) in DYT1 gene carriers compared to age-matched controls superimposed on the mean group FA map. The color scale represents T-scores at a threshold of 2.9, p less than 0.005. Right: Bar chart showing significant reduction in FA values in the subgyral white matter of the primary sensorimotor cortex (SMC) of DYT1 gene carriers (filled symbols) relative to controls (open symbols). Bars indicate standard errors. (Reproduced from Carbon et al., 2004.) With permission from John Wiley and Sons.

Briefly, reduced connectivity in the proximal segment of cerebellothalamocortical fiber tracts, present in all carriers, would result in symptom manifestation due to reduced cortical inhibition, unless this transmission was disrupted by a second lesion in the distal segment of the tract, as seen in nonmanifesting carriers. This model could also explain the variability in phenotype and clinical severity in acquired dystonias. However, this has not been investigated yet.

Studies of regional cerebral glucose metabolism with FDG PET and cerebral blood flow with $H_2{}^{15}O$ PET, and, more recently, fMRI have revealed widespread changes in cortical and subcortical activity in patients with different types of dystonia both at rest and on action (van Eimeren and Siebner, 2006; Neychev et al., 2011). Using FDG PET and network analysis, Eidelberg and colleagues (1995) reported that idiopathic torsion dystonia was characterized by relative metabolic overactivity of the lentiform nucleus and premotor cortices (Fig. 25.4), suggesting that dystonia may arise through excessive activity of the direct putaminopallidal inhibitory pathway. An abnormal pattern of regional glucose utilization, characterized by hypermetabolism of the basal ganglia, cerebellum, and supplementary motor area, has been reported in affected and unaffected DYT1 carriers (Eidelberg et al., 1998). This distinct metabolic topography has also been identified in affected and unaffected DYT6 carriers (Trost et al., 2002), suggesting that the reported metabolic changes are not genotype-specific and overactivity of these regions is an important trait feature of dystonia.

Activation studies with $H_2{}^{15}O$ PET and fMRI in both idiopathic and acquired dystonia have demonstrated abnormal activation patterns during motor tasks and on exposure to tactile stimuli (van Eimeren and Siebner, 2006; Neychev et al., 2011; Zoons et al., 2011). The most common activation finding reported in these studies is the overactivity of premotor and parietal cortices during performances of motor tasks, particularly those inducing dystonia, which has been interpreted as evidence of cortical disinhibition. Abnormalities in movement imagination have also been reported. Compared with healthy controls, patients with writer's cramp showed deficient activation of the left primary sensorimotor cortex, mesial and left dorsal premotor cortex, bilateral putamen, and bilateral thalamus during motor imagery (Castrop et al., 2012)

Several lines of evidence suggest that abnormalities of dopaminergic pathways contribute to the pathophysiology of dystonia. A cohort of patients with idiopathic dystonia showed reduced dopamine D_2 binding in the striatum, compatible with underfunctioning of the indirect basal ganglia pathway (Carbon et al., 2009). It has recently been suggested that a defect in D3, rather than D2, receptor expression may be associated with primary focal dystonia (Karimi et al., 2011). Disturbances in task-induced endogenous dopamine release as measured by changes in [^{11}C]-raclopride binding have been reported in patients with writer's cramp, suggesting abnormal dopaminergic neurotransmission in these patients (Berman et al., 2013).

Several studies have assessed striatal function in patients with dopa-responsive dystonia, which is linked to a mutation in the DYT5 gene coding for GTP cyclohydrolase 1 (Calne et al., 1997; van Eimeren and Siebner, 2006). [^{18}F]-dopa uptake, a marker of dopamine synthesis and storage, in the striatum is generally normal in these patients, while striatal [^{11}C]-dihydrotetrabenazine binding can be mildly increased, possibly reflecting upregulation of VMAT2 expression. Increased dopamine D_2

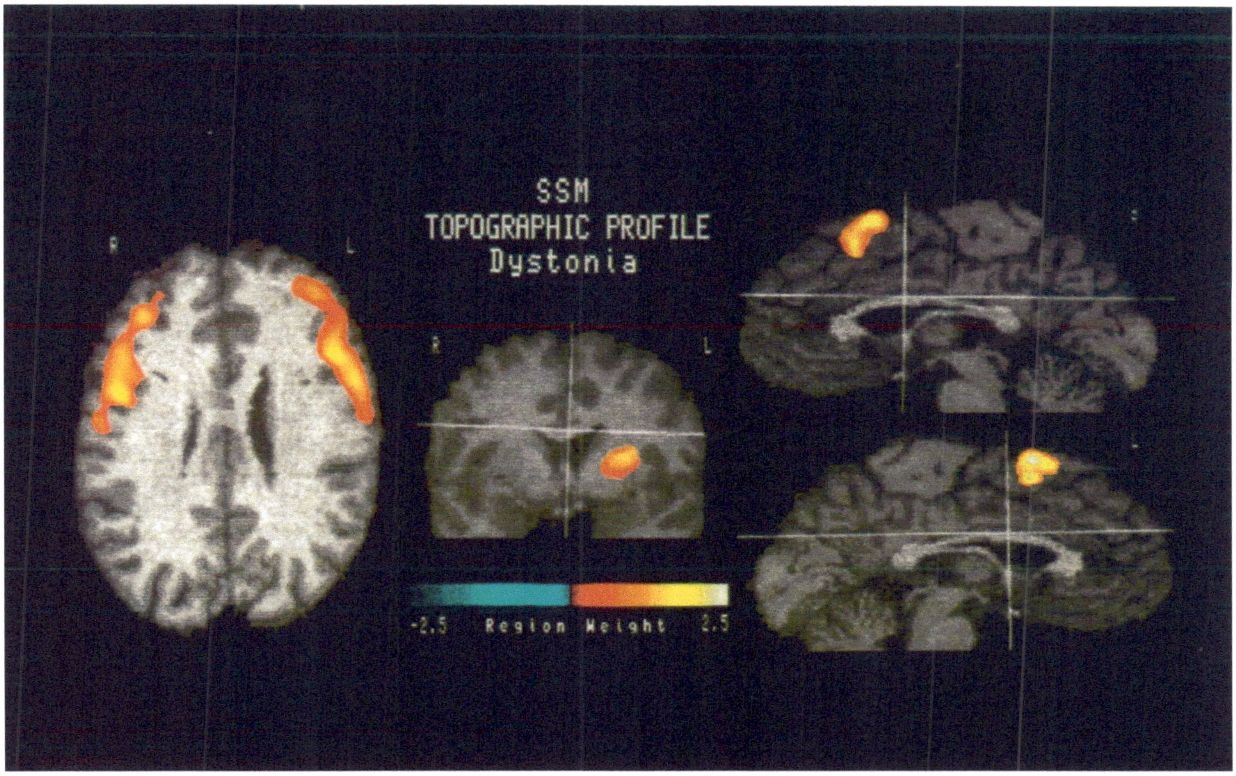

Fig. 25.4. Topographic profile of [^{18}F]-fluorodeoxyglucose changes associated with asymmetric idiopathic torsion dystonia overlaid on a normal magnetic resonance imaging scan. Relative hypermetabolism of the contralateral lentiform nucleus (coronal) is associated with covariate metabolic increases in the lateral frontal cortex (transverse) and paracentral regions (sagittal), corresponding respectively to the lateral premotor cortex and supplementary motor areas. (Reproduced from Eidelberg et al., 1995.) With permission from Oxford University Press.

receptor availability has also been reported in these patients (Rinne et al., 2004). Finally, FDG PET has shown a specific pattern of regional metabolic covariation consisting of increases in the dorsal midbrain, cerebellum, and supplementary motor area and reductions in the motor and lateral premotor cortex and basal ganglia (Asanuma et al., 2005). Gamma-aminobutyric acid (GABA) transmission also appears to be impaired in primary dystonia, as indicated by reduced cortical [^{11}C]-flumazenil in carriers of DYT1 mutation and sporadic cases (Garibotto et al., 2011). Taken together, these studies support the view that dystonia is associated with reduced inhibitory basal ganglia output and abnormalities in cortical processing. Failure of cortical inhibition, abnormal sensorimotor integration, and maladaptive plasticity seem to be the key contributors to the pathogenesis of this movement disorder.

NEURODEGENERATION WITH BRAIN IRON ACCUMULATION

NBIA is a group of disorders characterized by accumulation of iron in several brain regions, but more consistently in the basal ganglia. Other pathologic findings include widespread alpha-synuclein-positive Lewy pathology, accumulation of hyperphosphorylated tau protein in neuronal cell bodies and cellular projections, axonal swelling, and cerebral and cerebellar atrophy, depending on NBIA subtype (Schneider et al., 2012). Clinically, these conditions manifest with a combination of movement disorders, including dystonia, parkinsonism, choreoathetosis, and spasticity. Oculomotor abnormalities and a spectrum of visual problems, including progressive blindness, due to retinal degeneration and optic atrophy, can also occur. Cognitive decline may occur in some types of NBIA. Onset of NBIA ranges from infancy to adulthood. Progression can be rapid or slow with long periods of stability. The factors that influence disease severity and the rate of progression are still unknown.

Most NBIA types are genetically determined. To date, mutations in nine genes have been associated with NBIA (Arber et al., 2015). These include pantothenate kinase 2 (*PANK2*), phospholipase A_2 group 6 (*PLA2G6*), fatty acid hydroxylase 2 (*FA2H*), coenzyme a synthase (*COASY*), ceruloplasmin (*Cp*), ferritin light chain

(*FTL*), C19orf12, WDR45, and DCAF17 (*C2orf37*). Some patients, however, particularly those with onset of neurologic symptoms in mid to late life, have sporadic disorders of uncertain origin.

Structural imaging with conventional MRI sequences and with more recently developed iron-sensitive MRI sequences, such as gradient recall echo (GRE) and susceptibility-weighted imaging (SWI), have a valuable role in diagnosing NBIA (McNeill et al., 2008; Amaral et al., 2015). In fact, excessive iron deposition in the brain is clearly detectable on MRI images, appearing as isointense areas on T1-weighted sequences and hypointense areas on GRE, SWI, and T2-weighted sequences. Additionally, in combination with clinical findings, specific MRI findings can help to distinguish the different subtypes of NBIA, although the presence of the specific mutation is required for the final diagnosis. The imaging findings in the most common NBIA subtypes will be summarized below.

Pantothenic kinase-associated neurodegeneration

PKAN, previously known as Hallervorden–Spatz disease – terminology now abandoned as both physicians were involved in the Nazi euthanasia program – is an autosomal-recessive disease caused by mutations in the *PANK2* gene on chromosome 20p13. PKAN is the most common form of NBIA, making up 35–50% of the NBIA population. The *PANK2* gene encodes pantothenate kinase, a key enzyme in the biosynthesis of coenzyme A from vitamin B_5.

PKAN can manifest itself in the classic form, characterized by early onset and more rapid progression of symptoms; or in the atypical form with late onset and slow disease over several years, and sometimes decades. Some people, however, have characteristics that place them between these two categories.

Children with PKAN typically manifest with gait or postural problems around age 3 and later develop progressive dystonia, dysarthria, rigidity, and pyramidal symptoms. Visual symptoms and retinal degeneration are common in these patients. Individuals with later-onset PKAN generally present with speech difficulty and neurocognitive symptoms and less severe motor symptoms.

The most common MRI finding in PKAN patients is bilateral area of hypointensity localized in the globi pallidi containing a central area of hyperintensity on GRE, SWI, and T2-weighted images. While the marked low signal intensity of the globi pallidi is due to the paramagnetic effects of excessive iron accumulation, the central high signal is attributed to neuronal loss, gliosis, and cavitation of the neuropil (Guillerman, 2000). These symmetric pallidal hypointensities with the central area of increased MRI signal create a peculiar visual effect on axial and coronal MRI images that recalls the appearance of a pair of eyes. This is known as "the eye of the tiger" sign (Sethi et al., 1988) and has been reported to have a sensitivity for PKAN close to 100% (Hayflick et al., 2003) (Figs 25.5 and 25.6A). However, this

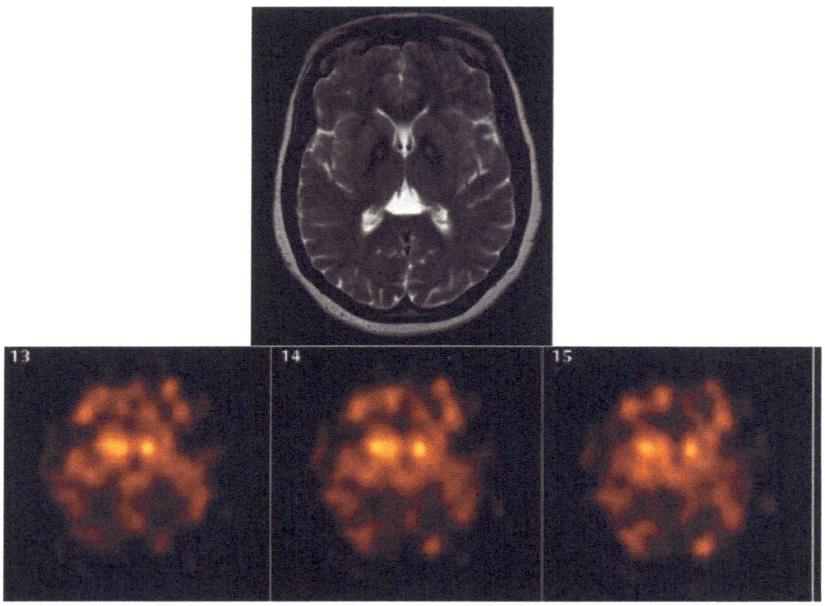

Fig. 25.5. T2-weighted magnetic resonance imaging image (top) and ^{123}ioflupane single-photon emission computed tomography images (bottom) of a 50-year-old woman with *PANK2* mutation showing the "the eye of the tiger" sign and reduced striatal ^{123}ioflupane binding, respectively. Clinically, the patient presented with oromandibular dystonia and mild parkinsonism.

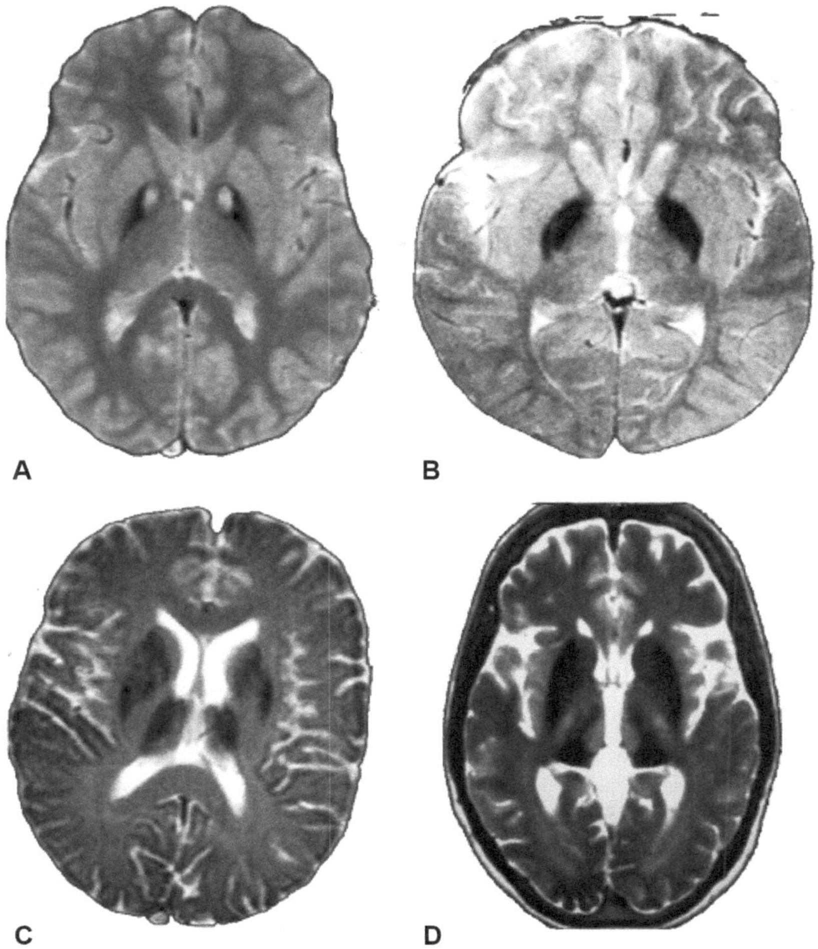

Fig. 25.6. (**A**) T2* magnetic resonance imaging (MRI) scan from a 17-year-old boy with pantothenate kinase-associated neurodegeneration. Note bilateral "eye of the tiger" sign in globus pallidus. (**B**) T2* MRI scan from a 9-year-old girl with infantile neuroaxonal dystrophy. Note bilateral hypointensity of globus pallidus. (**C**) T2* MRI scan from a 69-year-old woman with neuroferritinopathy. Note hypointensity of globus pallidus, putamen, caudate, and thalamus. (**D**) T2* MRI scan from a 55-year-old man with aceruloplasminemia. Note hypointensity of globus pallidus, putamen, caudate, and thalamus. (Reproduced from McNeill et al., 2008.) With permission from Wolters Kluwer Publishers.

characteristic MRI finding does not seem to be pathognomonic of *PANK2* mutation and it has been described in patients with other NBIA (neuroferritinopathy) (McNeill et al., 2008), as well as in patients with multiple system atrophy (Strecker et al., 2007) and cortical basal degeneration (Molinuevo et al., 1999). Recently, the "eye of the tiger" sign has also been reported as an incidental finding in a healthy research control subject and negative genetic testing for *PKAN2* and *FTL* gene mutation (van den Bogaard et al., 2014).

The "eye of the tiger" sign can be found in premanifest gene carriers, suggesting that significant brain iron may accumulate before clinical symptoms appear (Hayflick et al., 2001). On the other hand, the sign may be not fully visible in later stages of the disease, but without necessarily indicating a devastating course. Delgado and colleagues (2012) have recently reported 6 patients with a genetically proven *PANK2* mutation with absence of the complete "eye of the tiger" on MRI images. This might be explained, at least in some cases, by an excessive accumulation of iron deposits obscuring the central hyperintensity. Another abnormality commonly observed on iron-sensitive sequences in these patients is T2 hypointensity in the substantia nigra (McNeill et al., 2008). There is also variable atrophy in the affected structures.

Recent MRI studies have assessed gray- and white-matter changes in PKAN patients.

VBM has shown that, compared to controls, children with PKAN have increased gray-matter density in the putamen and caudate nucleus, whereas affected adults have increased gray-matter density in the ventral part of the anterior cingulate cortex. Multiple regression analyses with dystonia score and age as predictors showed gray-matter reduction in several cortical and subcortical regions. The authors suggest that gray-matter increases represent secondary phenomena compensating the increased activity of the motor system due to a reduced inhibitory output of the globus pallidus. Gray-matter reduction of cortical midline structures combined with increasing age, on the other hand, might contribute to the progression of dystonic symptoms due to loss of compensatory control (Rodriguez-Raecke et al., 2014).

A recent study in patients with dystonia due to PKAN has shown reductions of FA values in the periventricular substance surrounding the third ventricle, the medial part of putamen bilaterally, the frontal white matter, including the anterior limbs of the internal capsules, the corpus callosum, the cerebellar white matter and dorsal parts of pons and medulla, suggesting the occurrence of both gray-matter changes and microstructural white-matter alterations in these patients (Stoeter et al., 2015).

At variance with this, Delgado and colleagues (2012) found that, with the exception of the frontobasal tracts, white matter was well preserved.

Dopaminergic function of the basal ganglia, including dopamine D2 receptor, as measured with PET and SPECT, is generally reported to be normal (Hermann et al., 2000). However, a case of a patient with confirmed single mutation in the *PANK2* gene, MRI evidence of "eye of the tiger" sign and reduced striatal ^{123}ioflupane uptake has been reported (Kang and Minoshima, 2014) (Fig. 25.5), suggesting heterogeneity in these patients. Interestingly, in one study, PET measurement of cerebral blood flow using [^{15}O]-labeled water found significant hypoperfusion of the head of the right caudate nucleus, pons, and cerebellar vermis but no pallidal abnormalities (Castelnau et al., 2001).

PLA2G6-associated neurodegeneration

PLA2G6-associated neurodegeneration (PLAN) is an autosomal-recessive disease named after the responsible gene, *PLA2G6*, located on chromosome 22q13. This gene encodes the calcium-independent phospholipase A_2 (iPLA2) beta, which contributes to membrane homeostasis and energy metabolism (Murakami et al., 2011). The clinical presentation of PLAN is age-dependent and three different subtypes have been identified: (1) infantile neuroaxonal dystrophy (INAD) with typical onset between 6 months and 3 years of age and rapid progression; (2) atypical neuroaxonal dystrophy (ANAD), which starts a few years later; and (3) an adult form of dystonia-parkinsonism in which onset occurs in the second to third decade.

The first sign in children with classic INAD is developmental delay, followed by progressive occurrence of hypotonia, ataxia, pyramidal symptoms, optic atrophy, sensorimotor axonal neuropathy, and seizures. ANAD typically starts during early childhood or, less frequently, during the second decade. It has a slower progression and a different variety of symptoms than INAD, including dystonia-parkinsonism, pyramidal signs, and cognitive and psychiatric features. Ataxia and sensory abnormalities are absent in ANAD. Patients with *PLA2G6*-related dystonia-parkinsonism usually present with dystonia, parkinsonism, abnormal eye movements, pyramidal signs, and marked neuropsychiatric changes.

On iron-sensitive MRI sequences, excessive iron deposition in the globi pallidi is seen in up 50% of PLAN cases but the central T2 hyperintensity observed in PKAN is absent in these patients (Fig. 25.6B) (Gregory et al., 2008; McNeill et al., 2008). Iron deposition in the substantia nigra and the subthalamic nucleus can also been seen in INAD patients but is not common in ANAD patients (Schneider et al., 2012). However, the most common MRI finding in PLAN patients is the severe cerebellar atrophy affecting both cerebellar hemispheres and the vermis (Gregory et al., 2008). This is an early finding in INAD patients and may precede iron deposition, but occurs in later stages in ANAD patients. The presence of severe cerebellar atrophy in combination with the clinical phenotype described above is strongly suggestive of *PLA2G6* mutation. Other characteristic MRI findings of PLAN patients include optic atrophy and reduced optic chiasm volume, thinning of the posterior part of the corpus callosum with a vertical orientation, and the occurrence of T2 hyperintensities in cerebellum and putamen (Gregory et al., 2008; Kurian et al., 2008).

Kim and colleagues (2015) have recently reported MRI and PET findings in siblings of a Korean PLAN family showing intrafamilial phenotypic variability. Two brothers, one with adult-onset dystonia-parkinsonism and one with childhood-onset ANAD, were assessed with MRI and [^{18}F]-FP-CIT PET, a dopamine transporter marker. The patient with adult-onset dystonia-parkinsonism showed markedly reduced [^{18}F]-FP-CIT uptake in the whole putamen, but fluid-attenuated inversion recovery and GRE MRI studies revealed mild hypointensities in the substantia nigra and putamen and severe hypointensities in the globus pallidus. Conversely, the patient with childhood-onset ANAD had severe hypointensities in the substantia nigra and the pallidum, but the [^{18}F]-FP-CIT PET was normal. These findings suggest that dopaminergic neuronal degeneration in PLAN may occur independently from iron accumulation.

Other NBIA subtypes

Less common NBIA subtypes include aceruloplasminemia (*CP*), neuroferritinopathy (*FTL*), beta-propeller protein-associated neurodegeneration (*WDR45*), Woodhouse–Sakati syndrome (*DCAF17*), CoA synthase protein-associated neurodegeneration (*COASY*), fatty acid hydroxylase-associated neurodegeneration (*FA2H*), and mitochondrial membrane protein-associated neurodegeneration (C19orf12).

In most patients with these less common NBIA subtypes, the globus pallidus is uniformly hypointense on iron-sensitive MRI sequences without the central T2 hyperintensity characteristic of the "eye of the tiger" sign. Iron deposition in the substantia nigra, red nucleus, and dentate nucleus with cerebellar atrophy is also common in patients with these conditions. Additionally, specific MRI findings have been reported in these subtypes of NBIA (McNeill et al., 2008; Amaral et al., 2015). McNeill and colleagues (2008) reported a consistent involvement of the dentate nuclei, globus pallidus, and putamen in neuroferritinopathy (Fig. 25.6C). Fifty-two percent of patients had confluent areas of hyperintensity, probably due to cavitation, involving globus pallidus and putamen, and a subset of patients had similar lesions in caudate nuclei and thalami. Conversely, patients with aceruloplasminemia have a more uniform involvement of all basal ganglia and the thalami but without cavitation (Fig. 25.6D).

Patients with beta-propeller protein-associated neurodegeneration show a characteristic bilateral and symmetric T1 hyperintensity in the substantia nigra, probably due to neuromelanin, with a band of central T1 hypointensity. In these patients, the earliest and most prominent iron accumulation occurs in the substantia nigra rather than globus pallidus. Patients with fatty acid hydroxylase-associated neurodegeneration show moderate to severe white-matter abnormalities, prominent cerebellum and brainstem atrophy, and thinning of the corpus callosum (Kruer et al., 2010; Tonelli et al., 2012). Finally, patients with mitochondrial membrane protein-associated neurodegeneration have a characteristic T2 hyperintensity involving the medial medullary lamina between globus pallidus interna and externa and mild diffuse brain atrophy.

In conclusion, different NBIA subtypes have specific MRI findings that, along with the clinical phenotype, can help in the differential diagnosis of these conditions and facilitate molecular diagnosis.

References

Albanese A, Bhatia K, Bressman SB et al. (2013). Phenomenology and classification of dystonia: a consensus update. Mov Disord 28 (7): 863–873.

Albin RL, Young AB, Penney JB (1989). The functional anatomy of basal ganglia disorders. Trends Neurosci 12 (10): 366–375.

Amaral LL, Gaddikeri S, Chapman PR et al. (2015). Neurodegeneration with brain iron accumulation: clinicoradiological approach to diagnosis. J Neuroimaging 25: 539–551.

Andrews TC, Weeks RA, Turjanski N et al. (1999). Huntington's disease progression. PET and clinical observations. Brain 122: 2353–2363.

Antonini A, Leenders KL, Spiegel R et al. (1996). Striatal glucose metabolism and dopamine D2 receptor binding in asymptomatic gene carriers and patients with Huntington's disease. Brain 119 (Pt 6): 2085–2095.

Antonini A, Leenders KL, Eidelberg D (1998). [11C] raclopride-PET studies of the Huntington's disease rate of progression: relevance of the trinucleotide repeat length. Ann Neurol 43 (2): 253–255.

Arber C, Li A, Houlden H et al. (2015). Insights into molecular mechanisms of disease in neurodegeneration with brain iron accumulation; unifying theories. Neuropathol Appl Neurobiol. http://dx.doi.org/10.1111/nan.12242.

Argyelan M, Carbon M, Niethammer M et al. (2009). Cerebellothalamocortical connectivity regulates penetrance in dystonia. J Neurosci 29: 9740–9747.

Asanuma K, Ma Y, Huang C et al. (2005). The metabolic pathology of dopa-responsive dystonia. Ann Neurol 57 (4): 596–600.

Aylward EH, Brandt J, Codori AM et al. (1994). Reduced basal ganglia volume associated with the gene for Huntington's disease in asymptomatic at-risk persons. Neurology 44 (5): 823–828.

Aylward EH, Nopoulos PC, Ross CA et al. (2011). Longitudinal change in regional brain volumes in prodromal Huntington disease. J Neurol Neurosurg Psychiatry 82 (4): 405–410.

Aylward EH, Harrington DL, Mills JA et al. (2013). Regional atrophy associated with cognitive and motor function in prodromal Huntington disease. J Huntingtons Dis 2: 477–489.

Bachoud-Levi AC, Gaura V et al. (2006). Effect of fetal neural transplants in patients with Huntington's disease 6 years after surgery: a long-term follow-up study. Lancet Neurol 5 (4): 303–309.

Backman L, Robins-Wahlin TB, Lundin A et al. (1997). Cognitive deficits in Huntington's disease are predicted by dopaminergic PET markers and brain volumes. Brain 120: 2207–2217.

Bartenstein P, Weindl A, Spiegel S et al. (1997). Central motor processing in Huntington's disease. A PET study. Brain 120: 1553–1567.

Barthel H, Hermann W, Kluge R et al. (2003). Concordant pre- and postsynaptic deficits of dopaminergic neurotransmission in neurologic Wilson disease. AJNR Am J Neuroradiol 24 (2): 234–238.

Berman BD, Hallett M, Herscovitch P et al. (2013). Striatal dopaminergic dysfunction at rest and during task performance in writer's cramp. Brain 136: 3645–3658.

Bhatia KP, Marsden CD (1994). The behavioural and motor consequences of focal lesions of the basal ganglia in man. Brain 117: 859–876.

Blood AJ, Tuch DS, Makris N et al. (2006). White matter abnormalities in dystonia normalize after botulinum toxin treatment. Neuroreport 17: 1251–1255.

Blood AJ, Kuster JK, Woodman SC et al. (2012). Evidence for altered basal ganglia-brainstem connections in cervical dystonia. PLoS One 7: e31654.

Boecker H, Ceballos-Baumann A, Bartenstein P et al. (1999). Sensory processing in Parkinson's and Huntington's disease: investigations with 3D H(2)(15)O-PET. Brain: 1221651–1221665.

Bohnen NI, Koeppe RA, Meyer P et al. (2000). Decreased striatal monoaminergic terminals in Huntington disease. Neurology 54 (9): 1753–1759.

Bonilha L, de Vries PM, Hurd MW et al. (2009). Disrupted thalamic prefrontal pathways in patients with idiopathic dystonia. Parkinsonism Relat Disord 15: 64–67.

Bull PC, Thomas GR, Rommens JM et al. (1993). The Wilson disease gene is a putative copper transporting P-type ATPase similar to the Menkes gene. Nat Genet 5 (4): 327–337.

Calne DB, de la Fuente-Fernandez R, Kishore A (1997). Contributions of positron emission tomography to elucidating the pathogenesis of idiopathic parkinsonism and dopa responsive dystonia. J Neural Transm Suppl 50: 47–52.

Carbon M, Kingsley PB, Su S et al. (2004). Microstructural white matter changes in carriers of the DYT1 gene mutation. Ann Neurol 56 (2): 283–286.

Carbon M, Kingsley PB, Tang C et al. (2008). Microstructural white matter changes in primary torsion dystonia. Mov Disord 23 (2): 234–239.

Carbon M, Niethammer M, Peng S et al. (2009). Abnormal striatal and thalamic dopamine neurotransmission: genotype-related features of dystonia. Neurology 72: 2097–2103.

Castelnau P, Zilbovicius M, Ribeiro MJ et al. (2001). Striatal and pontocerebellar hypoperfusion in Hallervorden-Spatz syndrome. Pediatr Neurol 25: 170–174.

Castrop F, Dresel C, Hennenlotter A et al. (2012). Basal ganglia-premotor dysfunction during movement imagination in writer's cramp. Mov Disord 27 (11): 1432–1439.

Ciarmiello A, Cannella M, Lastoria S et al. (2006). Brain white-matter volume loss and glucose hypometabolism precede the clinical symptoms of Huntington's disease. J Nucl Med 47 (2): 215–222.

Colosimo C, Pantano P, Calistri V et al. (2005). Diffusion tensor imaging in primary cervical dystonia. J Neurol Neurosurg Psychiatry 76: 1591–1593.

Delgado RF, Sanchez PR, Speckter H et al. (2012). Missense PANK2 mutation without "eye of the tiger" sign: MR findings in a large group of patients with pantothenate kinase-associated neurodegeneration (PKAN). J Magn Reson Imaging 35 (4): 788–794.

Delmaire C, Vidailhet M, Wassermann D et al. (2009). Diffusion abnormalities in the primary sensorimotor pathways in writer's cramp. Arch Neurol 66: 502–508.

DiFiglia M, Sapp E, Chase KO et al. (1997). Aggregation of huntingtin in neuronal intranuclear inclusions and dystrophic neurites in brain. Science 277 (5334): 1990–1993.

Dominguez DJ, Egan GF, Gray MA et al. (2013). Multi-modal neuroimaging in premanifest and early Huntington's disease: 18 month longitudinal data from the IMAGE-HD study. PLoS One 8: e74131.

Egger K, Mueller J, Schocke M et al. (2007). Voxel based morphometry reveals specific gray matter changes in primary dystonia. Mov Disord 22 (11): 1538–1542.

Eidelberg D, Moeller JR, Ishikawa T et al. (1995). The metabolic topography of idiopathic torsion dystonia. Brain 118: 1473–1484.

Eidelberg D, Moeller JR, Antonini A et al. (1998). Functional brain networks in DYT1 dystonia. Ann Neurol 44 (3): 303–312.

Esmaeilzadeh M, Farde L, Karlsson P et al. (2011). Extrastriatal dopamine D(2) receptor binding in Huntington's disease. Hum Brain Mapp 32 (10): 1626–1636.

Fabbrini G, Pantano P, Totaro P et al. (2008). Diffusion tensor imaging in patients with primary cervical dystonia and in patients with blepharospasm. Eur J Neurol 15: 185–189.

Feigin A, Leenders KL, Moeller JR et al. (2001). Metabolic network abnormalities in early Huntington's disease: an [(18)F]FDG PET study. J Nucl Med 42 (11): 1591–1595.

Feigin A, Ghilardi MF, Huang C et al. (2006). Preclinical Huntington's disease: compensatory brain responses during learning. Ann Neurol 59 (1): 53–59.

Feigin A, Tang C, Ma Y et al. (2007). Thalamic metabolism and symptom onset in preclinical Huntington's disease. Brain 130 (Pt 11): 2858–2867.

Garibotto V, Romito LM, Elia AE et al. (2011). In vivo evidence for GABA(A) receptor changes in the sensorimotor system in primary dystonia. Mov Disord 26 (5): 852–857.

Grafton ST, Mazziotta JC, Pahl JJ et al. (1990). A comparison of neurological, metabolic, structural, and genetic evaluations in persons at risk for Huntington's disease. Ann Neurol 28 (5): 614–621.

Gregory A, Westaway SK Holm IE et al. (2008). Neurodegeneration associated with genetic defects in phospholipase A(2). Neurology 71: 1402–1409.

Guillerman RP (2000). The eye-of-the-tiger sign. Radiology 217 (3): 895–896.

Guo Z, Rudow G, Pletnikova O et al. (2012). Striatal neuronal loss correlates with clinical motor impairment in Huntington's disease. Mov Disord 27 (11): 1379–1386.

Hayden MR, Hewitt J, Stoessl AJ et al. (1987). The combined use of positron emission tomography and DNA polymorphisms for preclinical detection of Huntington's disease. Neurology 37 (9): 1441–1447.

Hayflick SJ, Penzien JM, Michl W et al. (2001). Cranial MRI changes may precede symptoms in Hallervorden-Spatz syndrome. Pediatr Neurol 25: 166–169.

Hayflick SJ, Westaway SK, Levinson B et al. (2003). Genetic, clinical, and radiographic delineation of Hallervorden-Spatz syndrome. N Engl J Med 348: 33–40.

Henkel K, Danek A, Grafman J et al. (2006). Head of the caudate nucleus is most vulnerable in chorea-acanthocytosis: a

voxel-based morphometry study. Mov Disord 21 (10): 1728–1731.
Hermann W (2014). Morphological and functional imaging in neurological and non-neurological Wilson's patients. Ann N Y Acad Sci 1315: 24–29.
Hermann W, Barthel H, Reuter M et al. (2000). Hallervorden-Spatz disease: findings in the nigrostriatal system. Nervenarzt 71 (8): 660–665.
Horovitz SG, Ford A, Najee-Ullah MA et al. (2012). Anatomical correlates of blepharospasm. Transl Neurodegener 1: 12.
Jacobs DA, Markowitz CE, Liebeskind DS et al. (2003). The "double panda sign" in Wilson's disease. Neurology 61 (7): 969.
Jung HH, Hergersberg M, Kneifel S et al. (2001). McLeod syndrome: a novel mutation, predominant psychiatric manifestations, and distinct striatal imaging findings. Ann Neurol 49 (3): 384–392.
Kang A, Minoshima S (2014). 123I-ioflupane SPECT findings of pantothenate kinase-associated neurodegeneration. Clin Nucl Med 39 (9): 849–851.
Karimi M, Moerlein SM, Videen TO et al. (2011). Decreased striatal dopamine receptor binding in primary focal dystonia: a D2 or D3 defect? Mov Disord 26 (1): 100–106.
Kim YJ, Lyoo CH, Hong S et al. (2015). Neuroimaging studies and whole exome sequencing of PLA2G6-associated neurodegeneration in a family with intrafamilial phenotypic heterogeneity. Parkinsonism Relat Disord 21 (4): 402–406.
Klein C (2014). Genetics in dystonia. Parkinsonism Relat Disord 20 (Suppl 1): S137–S142.
Kruer MC, Paisan-Ruiz C, Boddaert N et al. (2010). Defective FA2H leads to a novel form of neurodegeneration with brain iron accumulation (NBIA). Ann Neurol 68 (5): 611–618.
Kuhl DE, Phelps ME, Markham CH et al. (1982). Cerebral metabolism and atrophy in Huntington's disease determined by 18FDG and computed tomographic scan. Ann Neurol 12 (5): 425–434.
Kurian MA, Morgan NV, MacPherson L et al. (2008). Phenotypic spectrum of neurodegeneration associated with mutations in the PLA2G6 gene (PLAN). Neurology 70: 1623–1629.
Kuwert T, Lange HW, Langen KJ et al. (1990). Cortical and subcortical glucose consumption measured by PET in patients with Huntington's disease. Brain 113 (Pt 5): 1405–1423.
Kuwert T, Lange HW, Boecker H et al. (1993). Striatal glucose consumption in chorea-free subjects at risk of Huntington's disease. J Neurol 241 (1): 31–36.
Lawrence AD, Weeks RA, Brooks DJ et al. (1998). The relationship between striatal dopamine receptor binding and cognitive performance in Huntington's disease. Brain 121: 1343–1355.
Lorincz MT (2010). Neurologic Wilson's disease. Ann N Y Acad Sci 1184: 173–187.
Margolis RL (1993). Huntington disease-like 2. In: RA Pagon, MP Adam, HH Ardinger (Eds.), GeneReviews, University of Washington, Seattle, WA.
Marsden CD, Obeso JA, Zarranz JJ et al. (1985). The anatomical basis of symptomatic hemidystonia. Brain 108: 463–483.
McNeill A, Birchall D, Hayflick SJ et al. (2008). T2* and FSE MRI distinguishes four subtypes of neurodegeneration with brain iron accumulation. Neurology 70: 1614–1619.
Molinuevo JL, Munoz E, Valldeoriola F et al. (1999). The eye of the tiger sign in cortical-basal ganglionic degeneration. Mov Disord 14 (1): 169–171.
Munchau A, Mathen D, Cox T et al. (2000). Unilateral lesions of the globus pallidus: report of four patients presenting with focal or segmental dystonia. J Neurol Neurosurg Psychiatry 69 (4): 494–498.
Murakami M, Taketomi Y, Miki Y et al. (2011). Recent progress in phospholipase A(2) research: from cells to animals to humans. Prog Lipid Res 50: 152–192.
Neychev VK, Gross RE, Lehericy S et al. (2011). The functional neuroanatomy of dystonia. Neurobiol Dis 42: 185–201.
Nicholl DJ, Sutton I, Dotti MT et al. (2004). White matter abnormalities on MRI in neuroacanthocytosis. J Neurol Neurosurg Psychiatry 75: 1200–1201.
Nopoulos PC, Aylward EH, Ross CA et al. (2010). Cerebral cortex structure in prodromal Huntington disease. Neurobiol Dis 40 (3): 544–554.
Paulsen JS (2009). Functional imaging in Huntington's disease. Exp Neurol 216: 272–277.
Paulsen JS, Langbehn DR, Stout JC et al. (2008). Detection of Huntington's disease decades before diagnosis: the Predict-HD study. J Neurol Neurosurg Psychiatry 79 (8): 874–880.
Paulsen JS, Long JD, Ross CA et al. (2014). Prediction of manifest Huntington's disease with clinical and imaging measures: a prospective observational study. Lancet Neurol 13 (12): 1193–1201.
Pavese N, Andrews TC, Brooks DJ et al. (2003). Progressive striatal and cortical dopamine receptor dysfunction in Huntington's disease: a PET study. Brain 126 (Pt 5): 1127–1135.
Pavese N, Gerhard A, Tai YF et al. (2006). Microglial activation correlates with severity in Huntington disease: a clinical and PET study. Neurology 66 (11): 1638–1643.
Politis M, Pavese N, Tai YF et al. (2008). Hypothalamic involvement in Huntington's disease: an in vivo PET study. Brain 131: 2860–2869.
Prashanth LK, Sinha S, Taly AB et al. (2010). Do MRI features distinguish Wilson's disease from other early onset extrapyramidal disorders? An analysis of 100 cases. Mov Disord 25 (6): 672–678.
Quarantelli M, Salvatore E, Giorgio SM et al. (2013). Default-mode network changes in Huntington's disease: an integrated MRI study of functional connectivity and morphometry. PLoS One 8: e72159.
Reuter I, Tai YF, Pavese N et al. (2008). Long-term clinical and positron emission tomography outcome of fetal striatal transplantation in Huntington's disease. J Neurol Neurosurg Psychiatry 79: 948–951.

Reynolds Jr NC, Prost RW, Mark LP (2005). Heterogeneity in 1H-MRS profiles of presymptomatic and early manifest Huntington's disease. Brain Res 1031: 82–89.

Rinne JO, Iivanainen M, Metsahonkala L et al. (2004). Striatal dopaminergic system in dopa-responsive dystonia: a multitracer PET study shows increased D2 receptors. J Neural Transm 111 (1): 59–67.

Rodriguez-Raecke R, Roa-Sanchez P, Speckter H et al. (2014). Grey matter alterations in patients with pantothenate kinase-associated neurodegeneration (PKAN). Parkinsonism Relat Disord 20 (9): 975–979.

Roh JK, Lee TG, Wie BA et al. (1994). Initial and follow-up brain MRI findings and correlation with the clinical course in Wilson's disease. Neurology 44 (6): 1064–1068.

Rosas HD, Koroshetz WJ, Chen YI et al. (2003). Evidence for more widespread cerebral pathology in early HD: an MRI-based morphometric analysis. Neurology 60 (10): 1615–1620.

Rosas HD, Tuch DS, Hevelone ND et al. (2006). Diffusion tensor imaging in presymptomatic and early Huntington's disease: Selective white matter pathology and its relationship to clinical measures. Mov Disord 21 (9): 1317–1325.

Rosas HD, Salat DH, Lee SY et al. (2008). Cerebral cortex and the clinical expression of Huntington's disease: complexity and heterogeneity. Brain 131 (Pt 4): 1057–1068.

Rosas HD, Lee SY, Bender AC et al. (2010). Altered white matter microstructure in the corpus callosum in Huntington's disease: implications for cortical "disconnection". Neuroimage 49 (4): 2995–3004.

Rosas HD, Reuter M, Doros G et al. (2011). A tale of two factors: what determines the rate of progression in Huntington's disease? A longitudinal MRI study. Mov Disord 26 (9): 1691–1697.

Sapp E, Kegel KB, Aronin N et al. (2001). Early and progressive accumulation of reactive microglia in the Huntington disease brain. J Neuropathol Exp Neurol 60 (2): 161–172.

Schlaug G, Hefter H, Nebeling B et al. (1994). Dopamine D2 receptor binding and cerebral glucose metabolism recover after D-penicillamine-therapy in Wilson's disease. J Neurol 241 (10): 577–584.

Schneider SA, Hardy J, Bhatia KP (2012). Syndromes of neurodegeneration with brain iron accumulation (NBIA): an update on clinical presentations, histological and genetic underpinnings, and treatment considerations. Mov Disord 27 (1): 42–53.

Schwarz J, Antonini A, Kraft E et al. (1994). Treatment with D-penicillamine improves dopamine D2-receptor binding and T2-signal intensity in de novo Wilson's disease. Neurology 44 (6): 1079–1082.

Sethi KD, Adams RJ, Loring DW et al. (1988). Hallervorden-Spatz syndrome: clinical and magnetic resonance imaging correlations. Ann Neurol 24 (5): 692–694.

Shivakumar R, Thomas SV (2009). Teaching NeuroImages: Face of the giant panda and her cub: MRI correlates of Wilson disease. Neurology 72 (11): e50.

Sinha S, Taly AB, Ravishankar S et al. (2006). Wilson's disease: cranial MRI observations and clinical correlation. Neuroradiology 48 (9): 613–621.

Stoeter P, Roa-Sanchez P, Speckter H et al. (2015). Changes of cerebral white matter in patients suffering from pantothenate kinase-associated neurodegeneration (PKAN): a diffusion tensor imaging (DTI) study. Parkinsonism Relat Disord 21 (6): 577–581.

Strecker K, Hesse S, Wegner F et al. (2007). Eye of the tiger sign in multiple system atrophy. Eur J Neurol e1–e2.

Sturrock A, Laule C, Decolongon J et al. (2010). Magnetic resonance spectroscopy biomarkers in premanifest and early Huntington disease. Neurology 75: 1702–1710.

Sturrock A, Laule C, Wyper K et al. (2015). A longitudinal study of magnetic resonance spectroscopy Huntington's disease biomarkers. Mov Disord 30 (3): 393–401.

Tabrizi SJ, Scahill RI, Durr A et al. (2011). Biological and clinical changes in premanifest and early stage Huntington's disease in the TRACK-HD study: the 12-month longitudinal analysis. Lancet Neurol 10: 31–42.

Tabrizi SJ, Reilmann R, Roos RA et al. (2012). Potential endpoints for clinical trials in premanifest and early Huntington's disease in the TRACK-HD study: analysis of 24 month observational data. Lancet Neurol 11: 42–53.

Tabrizi SJ, Scahill RI, Owen G et al. (2013). Predictors of phenotypic progression and disease onset in premanifest and early-stage Huntington's disease in the TRACK-HD study: analysis of 36-month observational data. Lancet Neurol 12 (7): 637–649.

Tai YF, Pavese N, Gerhard A et al. (2007). Microglial activation in presymptomatic Huntington's disease gene carriers. Brain 130: 1759–1766.

Tang CC, Feigin A, Ma Y et al. (2013). Metabolic network as a progression biomarker of premanifest Huntington's disease. J Clin Invest 123 (9): 4076–4088.

The Huntington's Disease Collaborative Research Group (1993). A novel gene containing a trinucleotide repeat that is expanded and unstable on Huntington's disease chromosomes. Cell 72 (6): 971–983.

Tonelli A, D'Angelo MG, Arrigoni F et al. (2012). Atypical adult onset complicated spastic paraparesis with thin corpus callosum in two patients carrying a novel FA2H mutation. Eur J Neurol 19 (11): e127–e129.

Trost M, Carbon M, Edwards C et al. (2002). Primary dystonia: is abnormal functional brain architecture linked to genotype? Ann Neurol 52 (6): 853–856.

Turjanski N, Weeks R, Dolan R et al. (1995). Striatal D1 and D2 receptor binding in patients with Huntington's disease and other choreas. A PET study. Brain 118: 689–696.

van den Bogaard SJ, Kruit MC, Dumas EM et al. (2014). Eye-of-the-tiger-sign in a 48 year healthy adult. J Neurol Sci 336: 254–256.

van Eimeren T, Siebner HR (2006). An update on functional neuroimaging of parkinsonism and dystonia. Curr Opin Neurol 19: 412–419.

Van Laere K, Casteels C, Dhollander I et al. (2010). Widespread decrease of type 1 cannabinoid receptor availability in Huntington disease in vivo. J Nucl Med 51: 1413–1417.

van Oostrom JC, Maguire RP, Verschuuren-Bemelmans CC et al. (2005). Striatal dopamine D2 receptors, metabolism, and volume in preclinical Huntington disease. Neurology 65 (6): 941–943.

van Oostrom JC, Sijens PE, Roos RA et al. (2007). 1H magnetic resonance spectroscopy in preclinical Huntington disease. Brain Res 1168: 67–71.

Vonsattel JP, Myers RH, Stevens TJ et al. (1985). Neuropathological classification of Huntington's disease. J Neuropathol Exp Neurol 44 (6): 559–577.

Walker RH, Jung HH, Danek A (2011). Neuroacanthocytosis. In: Handbook of Clinical Neurology, Elsevier, Amsterdam, pp. 141–151.

Weaver KE, Richards TL, Liang O et al. (2009). Longitudinal diffusion tensor imaging in Huntington's disease. Exp Neurol 216 (2): 525–529.

Weeks RA, Piccini P, Harding AE et al. (1996). Striatal D1 and D2 dopamine receptor loss in asymptomatic mutation carriers of Huntington's disease. Ann Neurol 40 (1): 49–54.

Weeks RA, Ceballos-Baumann A, Piccini P et al. (1997a). Cortical control of movement in Huntington's disease. A PET activation study. Brain 120 (Pt 9): 1569–1578.

Weeks RA, Cunningham VJ, Piccini P et al. (1997b). 11C-diprenorphine binding in Huntington's disease: a comparison of region of interest analysis with statistical parametric mapping. J Cereb Blood Flow Metab 17 (9): 943–949.

Wolf RC, Vasic N, Schonfeldt-Lecuona C et al. (2007). Dorsolateral prefrontal cortex dysfunction in presymptomatic Huntington's disease: evidence from event-related fMRI. Brain 130: 2845–2857.

Wolf RC, Sambataro F, Vasic N et al. (2011). Longitudinal functional magnetic resonance imaging of cognition in preclinical Huntington's disease. Exp Neurol 231: 214–222.

Wolf RC, Sambataro F, Vasic N et al. (2012). Default-mode network changes in preclinical Huntington's disease. Exp Neurol 237: 191–198.

Wu JC, Huang CC, Jeng LB et al. (2000). Correlation of neurological manifestations and MR images in a patient with Wilson's disease after liver transplantation. Acta Neurol Scand 102 (2): 135–139.

Zheng Z, Pan P, Wang W et al. (2012). Neural network of primary focal dystonia by an anatomic likelihood estimation meta-analysis of gray matter abnormalities. J Neurol Sci 316: 51–55.

Zoons E, Booij J, Nederveen AJ et al. (2011). Structural, functional and molecular imaging of the brain in primary focal dystonia – a review. Neuroimage 56: 1011–1020.

Handbook of Clinical Neurology, Vol. 135 (3rd series)
Neuroimaging, Part I
J.C. Masdeu and R.G. González, Editors

Chapter 26

Genetic and degenerative disorders primarily causing dementia

JOSEPH C. MASDEU* AND BELEN PASCUAL
Department of Neurology, Houston Methodist Hospital, Houston, TX, USA

Abstract

Neuroimaging comprises a powerful set of instruments to diagnose the different causes of dementia, clarify their neurobiology, and monitor their treatment. Magnetic resonance imaging (MRI) depicts volume changes with neurodegeneration and inflammation, as well as abnormalities in functional and structural connectivity. MRI arterial spin labeling allows for the quantification of regional cerebral blood flow, characteristically altered in Alzheimer's disease, diffuse Lewy-body disease, and the frontotemporal dementias. Positron emission tomography allows for the determination of regional metabolism, with similar abnormalities as flow, and for the measurement of β-amyloid and abnormal tau deposition in the brain, as well as regional inflammation. These instruments allow for the quantification *in vivo* of most of the pathologic features observed in disorders causing dementia. Importantly, they allow for the longitudinal study of these abnormalities, having revealed, for instance, that the deposition of β-amyloid in the brain can antecede by decades the onset of dementia. Thus, a therapeutic window has been opened and the efficacy of immunotherapies directed at removing β-amyloid from the brain of asymptomatic individuals is currently being tested. Tau and inflammation imaging, still in their infancy, combined with genomics, should provide powerful insights into these disorders and facilitate their treatment.

INTRODUCTION[1]

Dementia has been defined as an acquired loss of intellectual abilities of sufficient severity to interfere with social or occupational functioning (American Psychiatric Association, 1994). The somewhat pejorative term "dementia," still very useful in scientific writing and widely used by the public, is being replaced in the psychiatric literature by the less threatening "major neurocognitive disorder" (American Psychiatric Association, 2013). More relevant to the scope of this chapter, dementia refers to cognitive deterioration due to diffuse or disseminated disease of the cerebral hemispheres (Petersen, 2004). Bilateral hemispheric lesions identified by imaging can belong to any of a number of categories reviewed in this volume: vascular, autoimmune, infectious, traumatic, metabolic, or even neoplastic. This chapter focuses on the most frequent cause of dementia, namely neurodegenerative disorders.

The landscape of imaging of neurodegenerative disorders causing dementia is changing rapidly. Until the 2012 approval by the Food and Drug Administration of florbetapir to image brain β-amyloid (abeta) deposition (Johnson et al., 2013b), neuroimaging in patients with slowly progressive cognitive impairment leading to dementia was being used in the clinic mostly to detect tumors, hydrocephalus, or vascular lesions, all quite apparent on magnetic resonance imaging (MRI) simply by inspecting images, without the need to quantify them. Neurodegenerative disorders, however, cause subtle changes on MRI, but remarkable changes on positron

[1]Abbreviations used in the chapter are listed at the end of the chapter before References Section.

*Correspondence to: Joseph C. Masdeu, M.D., Ph.D., Graham Distinguished Chair in Neurological Sciences, Houston Methodist Institute for Academic Medicine, Professor of Neurology, Weill Medical College of Cornell University, 6560 Fannin Street, Scurlock 802, Houston TX 77030, USA. Voice cell: +1-202-255-7899, E-mail: jcmasdeu@houstonmethodist.org

emission tomography (PET), using amyloid or metabolism markers. Now these tools are not infrequently used in the clinic to define the presence of early Alzheimer changes in patients with mild cognitive impairment (MCI) or to differentiate Alzheimer's disease (AD) from frontotemporal dementia (FTD) (Johnson et al., 2013a; Sanchez-Juan et al., 2014). PET imaging of hyperphosphorylated tau (or, simply, tau) became of age in 2013, with the discovery of several new tau imaging agents (Villemagne et al., 2015).

A better understanding of the neurobiology of dementia has also derived from the advances in neuroimaging, increasingly combined with genetic studies (Whitwell et al., 2012b). Neurodegenerative disorders are caused by genetic factors or by still incompletely understood environmental risk factors playing on a predisposing genetic background. The genetics of dementia have advanced prodigiously in the last few years, alongside the explosion in knowledge of the human genome (Lambert et al., 2013). An impressive body of work in the past 15 years, which is accelerating vertiginously at present, has led to a much clearer picture of the heterogeneity of what is still referred to as neurodegenerative dementia and of its evolution over time, as well as to the frequency of the varieties in the different age groups. Imaging findings confirm and define well-established neuropathologic findings in the dementias (Nelson et al., 2012). Incidence of dementia in the adult is positively correlated with age, with very few cases manifesting in people in their fourth decade of life or earlier but then increasing with each passing decade (Fig. 26.1) (Nelson et al., 2011, 2012). In the fourth and fifth decades, dementia stems from cerebrovascular disease, particularly of the microvascular type, from frontotemporal processes, from diffuse Lewy-body disease (DLB), and from autosomal-dominant AD, as caused by presenilin or *APP* mutations (Nelson et al., 2012). Later in life, AD, hippocampal sclerosis, and cerebrovascular disease are the main neuropathologically defined causes of dementia.

However, more important than the changes found at the end of life are the brain abnormalities that antecede the first symptoms, because treatment at this stage may prevent or delay the clinical onset (Sperling et al., 2014). Neuroimaging has provided essential information on the preclinical evolution of AD, regularly associated with the deposition of abeta in the brain. The new insights led to the promulgation of a set of research guidelines for the diagnosis of the preclinical stages of AD (Sperling et al., 2011a). These guidelines will probably soon permeate the thinking of clinicians and eventually become commonplace in the clinic.

An important environmental risk factor for neurodegeneration is traumatic brain injury (TBI): people who

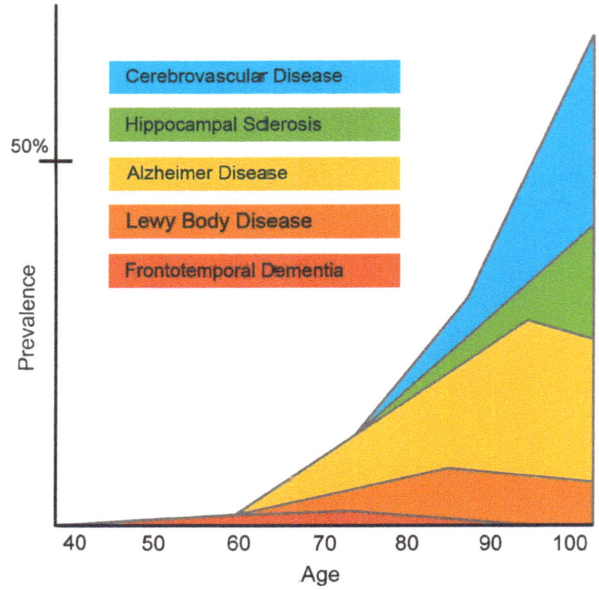

Fig. 26.1. Neuropathology of dementia. Most frequent predominant neuropathologic diagnoses at each age group (Nelson et al., 2011). In each single individual a mixture of several pathologies is common.

have sustained TBI are more likely to develop dementia later in life (Barnes et al., 2014). Furthermore, even repeated mild TBI may predispose to dementia, associated with tau deposition on neuropathologic studies (McKee et al., 2013). The neurodegeneration that follows TBI may provide important information to understand the genesis of other dementias. For this reason, although TBI is discussed extensively in Chapter 22, a brief section will be devoted to it in this chapter as it is relevant for a type of dementia, chronic traumatic encephalopathy (CTE). Similarly, vascular brain disease has been described in Chapters 16–18. However, aspects of vascular disease that specifically relate to dementia will be discussed briefly here. The characteristic MRI findings of Creutzfeldt–Jakob disease, a rare cause of dementia, are discussed in Chapter 19.

CHRONIC TRAUMATIC ENCEPHALOPATHY

Cognitive impairment has been described after repeated mild TBI (McKee et al., 2013; Barnes et al., 2014). It may be progressive in the absence of additional traumatic events, and therefore an ongoing neurodegenerative process is likely (Fig. 26.2). Clinically, the patients may have a syndrome resembling Parkinson disease with dementia, such as the typical dementia pugilistica of boxers, or a dementia with executive function loss, more typically seen with war or football injuries (Stern et al., 2013).

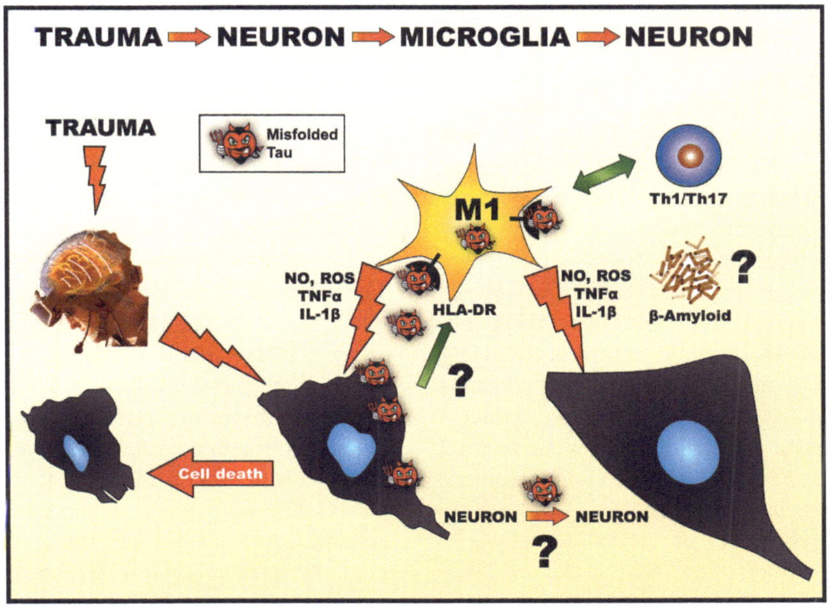

Fig. 26.2. Cellular events after mild traumatic brain injury. Acceleration–deceleration forces would injure neurons, inducing abnormal tau deposition within them. Either while injured neurons are still viable or after neuronal death, tau would be presented to microglia, setting up an inflammatory cascade involving peripheral T cells and the production of cytokines, which would cause oxidative stress not only to the damaged neurons, inducing their death, but also involving intact nearby neurons. Furthermore, tau could propagate from damaged to intact neurons, causing disease progression, independent from additional traumatic events. Similar events, with a trigger other than trauma, could be postulated in other neurodegenerative brain disorders. HLA-DR, human leukocyte antigen (class II); IL-1β, interleukin 1 beta; NO, nitrous oxide; ROS, reactive oxygen species; Th1, T-helper 1 immune cells; Th17, T-helper 17 immune cell; TNFα, tumor necrosis factor-alpha.

Pathologically, CTE is defined by the abnormal accumulation of tau, with a preference for the depths of the cortical sulci as compared to the gyral crests, a unique pattern that is distinct from other tauopathies, including AD (McKee et al., 2013). Using ^{18}F-FDDNP, a tau imaging compound, increased uptake was detected in the upper brainstem, thalami, and amygdala of a group of 14 retired football players with some degree of cognitive impairment (Barrio et al., 2015).

Although tau pathology has been described as the neuropathologic hallmark of CTE (McKee et al., 2013), the development of tau pathology in mild TBI has been hypothetically linked to both axonal damage, which can be studied with diffusion tensor imaging (DTI), and neuroinflammation (McKee et al., 2013). Supporting the role of inflammation is the presence of perivascular microgliosis in close proximity to abnormal tau in the brains of individuals with postconcussion syndromes. Brain inflammation in people after mild TBI has been documented not only neuropathologically but also using inflammation markers for PET (Folkersma et al., 2011; Ramlackhansingh et al., 2011). It is remarkable that the two available studies, both performed with a PET tracer described in the early 1990s, ^{11}C-PK1195, were positive, because this tracer has poor brain uptake and has yielded negative findings in other disorders with an important inflammatory component, such as AD (Groom et al., 1995; Schuitemaker et al., 2013). Second-generation inflammation markers, recently available, are much more sensitive to activated microglia. For instance, in monkey, ^{11}C-PBR28 has an 80-fold higher specific binding than ^{11}C-PK1195 to the protein expressed by activated microglia, an 18-kDa translocator protein (TSPO) (Kreisl et al., 2010). However, depending on a single-nucleotide polymorphism (*rs6971*) within the human *TSPO* gene, about 15% of individuals do not bind second-generation TSPO PET markers and therefore cannot be studied with these compounds (Owen et al., 2012; Kreisl et al., 2013a). Among the ones that bind them, one genotype binds about 30% less than the other and this differential binding has important effects on PET data analysis (Yoder et al., 2013), but, knowing the genotype of each study subject, it can be adequately accounted for (Kreisl et al., 2013a). At the time of this writing, there were no extant studies of second-generation PET inflammation markers in CTE, but abundant activity in this area heralds forthcoming publications.

Brain metabolism, measured with ^{18}F-2-deoxy-2-fluoro-D-glucose (^{18}F-FDG) PET, has been reported to be reduced in boxers with cognitive impairment and in war veterans exposed to blast during deployment (Koerte et al., 2015). The regions most affected have not been defined, but the cerebellum has shown decreased metabolism in several studies (Koerte et al., 2015).

In mild TBI or concussion, acute MRI is typically unremarkable by visual inspection. Decreased signal at the crown of a gyrus on susceptibility-weighted imaging (Fig. 26.3) would indicate a focal hemorrhage, characteristic of a contusion, and therefore would not qualify the event as a pure concussion. However, in concussion, careful comparison with control scans using susceptibility-weighted imaging may show decreased signal in the depth of the sulci, corresponding to microhemorrhages (Hahnel et al., 2008). In repetitive mild TBI, which may lead to cognitive impairment, a number of subtle MRI findings have been reported (Koerte et al., 2015), including hippocampal or frontal atrophy and white-matter abnormalities. On DTI, decreased fractional anisotropy and increased radial diffusivity have been detected in the corpus callosum and posterior limb of the internal capsule, or even more widespread in the white matter of the hemispheres (Koerte et al., 2015). Using blood oxygen level-dependent (BOLD) functional MRI (fMRI), increased connectivity of the default network and increased activation during memory or visual tasks have been detected in subjects exposed to multiple mild TBI, suggesting that these subjects need to recruit a larger area of the brain to accomplish the same task as the controls (Koerte et al., 2015).

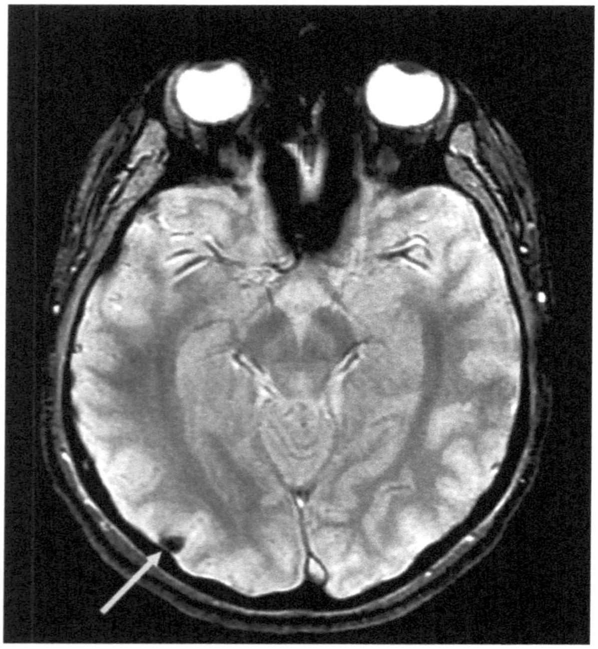

Fig. 26.3. Contusion. Gradient-echo magnetic resonance imaging from a 15-year-old young woman who sustained a contusion (arrow) in the inferior temporal gyrus during a soccer game.

VASCULAR COGNITIVE IMPAIRMENT

Cognitive impairment to the point of dementia can result from multiple bi-hemispheric strokes (multi-infarct dementia). Bilateral ischemic lesions in Papez circuit may present as isolated memory loss (Fig. 26.4), but the sudden onset differentiates them from AD. Successive ischemic lesions in the hemispheres may mimic one of the FTDs, particularly primary progressive aphasia (PPA). While ischemic lesions do not spare the primary cortices (paracentral, auditory), neurodegenerative disorders manifesting as dementia typically do (Fig. 26.5). However, autopsy studies in a general population have shown that dementia is seldom associated with large ischemic lesions: it is much more often associated with small or even microinfarcts, related to small-artery disease (Esiri et al., 1997) and with white-matter changes on MRI (Fig. 26.6). White-matter damage is more likely when the lesions are visible on T1-weighted images; enlarged perivascular spaces can give rise to marked changes on T2 images, including FLAIR (Kirkpatrick and Hayman, 1987), but have little clinical significance. Several arteriolar disorders, discussed in Chapter 17, are characterized by dementia, such as cerebral autosomal-dominant arteriopathy with subcortical infarcts and leukoencephalopathy (CADASIL) (Viswanathan et al., 2007) and cerebral amyloid angiopathy (Johnson et al., 2007; Gurol et al., 2013; Reijmer et al., 2015) (Fig. 26.7).

The role of vascular versus neurodegenerative factors in the genesis of cognitive impairment in older people is currently a matter of some controversy (Chui and Ramirez-Gomez, 2015). Vascular lesions are very frequent in the brain of patients with neurodegenerative diseases, particularly in the older age groups (Schneider et al., 2007; Savva et al., 2009). These neuropathologic studies have highlighted the difficulty in attributing the cognitive impairment characteristic of dementia to either AD changes or vascular injury. Even more challenging is making a clinical differential diagnosis between vascular dementia and AD (Knopman et al., 2001; Ballard et al., 2004). The presence of white-matter changes or lacunar strokes on MRI or CT, required by the National Institute of Neurological Disorders and Stroke-Association Internationale pour la Recherche et l'Enseignement en Neurosciences (NINDS-AIREN) diagnostic criteria for vascular dementia (Roman et al., 1993), is of limited value, as patients with extensive changes on MRI may not be demented (de Leeuw et al., 2001). Some have speculated that progressive vascular dementia, as associated with small-vessel disease, is

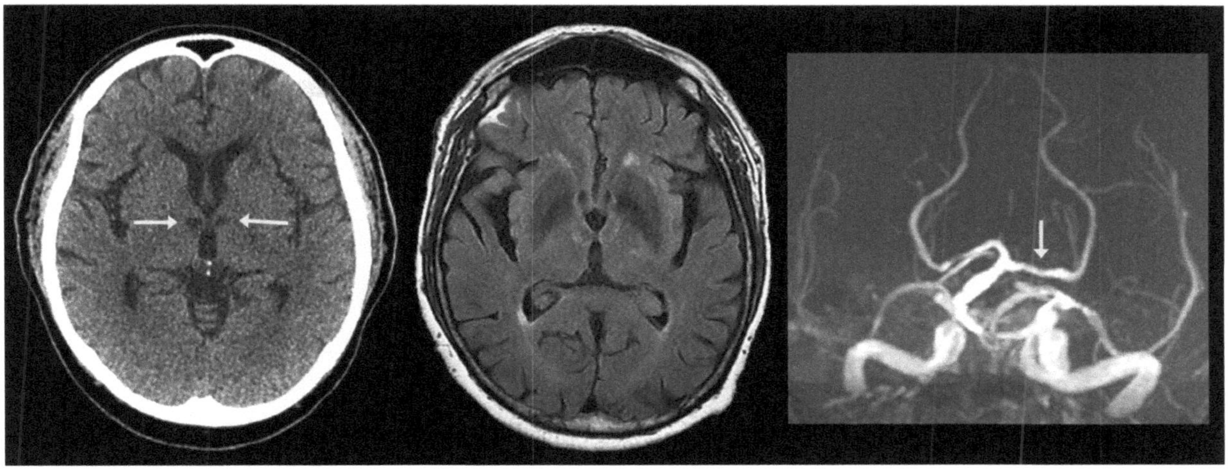

Fig. 26.4. Critical-location-infarct dementia. This 74-year-old man had sustained a silent infarction of the right dorsomedial-anterior nuclei of the thalamus, affecting the mammillothalamic tract of Vic D'Azyr. He became symptomatic, with loss of episodic memory for recent events and impaired executive function, after the second infarction, almost symmetric to the first, on the left side. The chronic infarctions (arrows) are more apparent on computed tomography (CT) than on fluid-attenuated inversion recovery (FLAIR) imaging. Note the arteriosclerotic changes in the proximal segment of the posterior cerebral artery (arrow). MRA, magnetic resonance angiography.

simply vascular brain disease plus AD (Nolan et al., 1998). By contrast, AD has been postulated to be a vascular disorder (de la Torre, 2002). As both disorders increase in prevalence in the 70–90-years age group, it is difficult to separate their effects in studies showing an association between cognitive impairment and vascular disease on MRI (van der Flier et al., 2005). By contrast, using MRI as a marker of vascular disease and PET imaging of AD, the contribution of these two pathologies can be elucidated. Patients with dementia and a large vascular load on MRI may not show the characteristic metabolic pattern of AD, but show frontal and thalamic hypometabolism on ^{18}F-FDG PET (Pascual et al., 2010) (Fig. 26.8) Likewise, vascular MRI features and amyloid deposition, the latter characteristic of AD, seem to be independent predictors of cognitive impairment (Marchant et al., 2013) and of the risk of developing cognitive decline (Vemuri et al., 2015). Vascular and neurodegenerative disorders are probably additive for the causation of dementia (Chui and Ramirez-Gomez, 2015; Vemuri et al., 2015).

ALZHEIMER DISEASE

A rather long time, estimated in decades, witnesses the evolution of neurobiologic events leading to, but preceding, the cognitive impairment characteristic of AD (Jack et al., 2013; Villemagne et al., 2013). In autosomal-dominant AD, where the timing of the onset of dementia can be predicted with a certain accuracy, cerebrospinal fluid (CSF) Aβ1–42 declined 25 years before onset, followed by amyloid deposition as measured by PET imaging 15 years before onset, along with increased CSF tau and hippocampal atrophy. This was followed by cerebral hypometabolism on ^{18}F-FDG PET about 10 years before onset (Bateman et al., 2012). A similar sequence seems to be present with abeta deposition in sporadic, late-onset AD, although the etiologic mix in the more advanced age group yields more complex biomarker results (Villemagne et al., 2013). Research AD diagnostic guidelines issued in 2011 distinguish a preclinical stage (Sperling et al., 2011a), an MCI stage (Albert et al., 2011), and an AD stage (McKhann et al., 2011). The neurobiologic cascade is likely to consist of distinct processes, still only partially understood, but the clinical progression is smooth, such that, for instance, the clinical differentiation between MCI and mild AD is far from clear-cut (Morris, 2012). Neuroimaging, with or without CSF biomarkers, is needed to detect preclinical changes (Fig. 26.9) (Sperling et al., 2011a; Jack et al., 2012; Villemagne et al., 2013; Vos et al., 2013). It also helps in the process of staging the evolution of the disorder once the patient begins to manifest cognitive impairment (Jack et al., 2010a). Recent data suggest that abeta deposition begins early in the AD process but may be one of the markers of neurodegeneration, although not the only one and perhaps not the most important (Jack et al., 2013). To study the evolution of AD, progressive atrophy from neuronal loss and loss of anisotropy in the white matter have been measured with MRI and

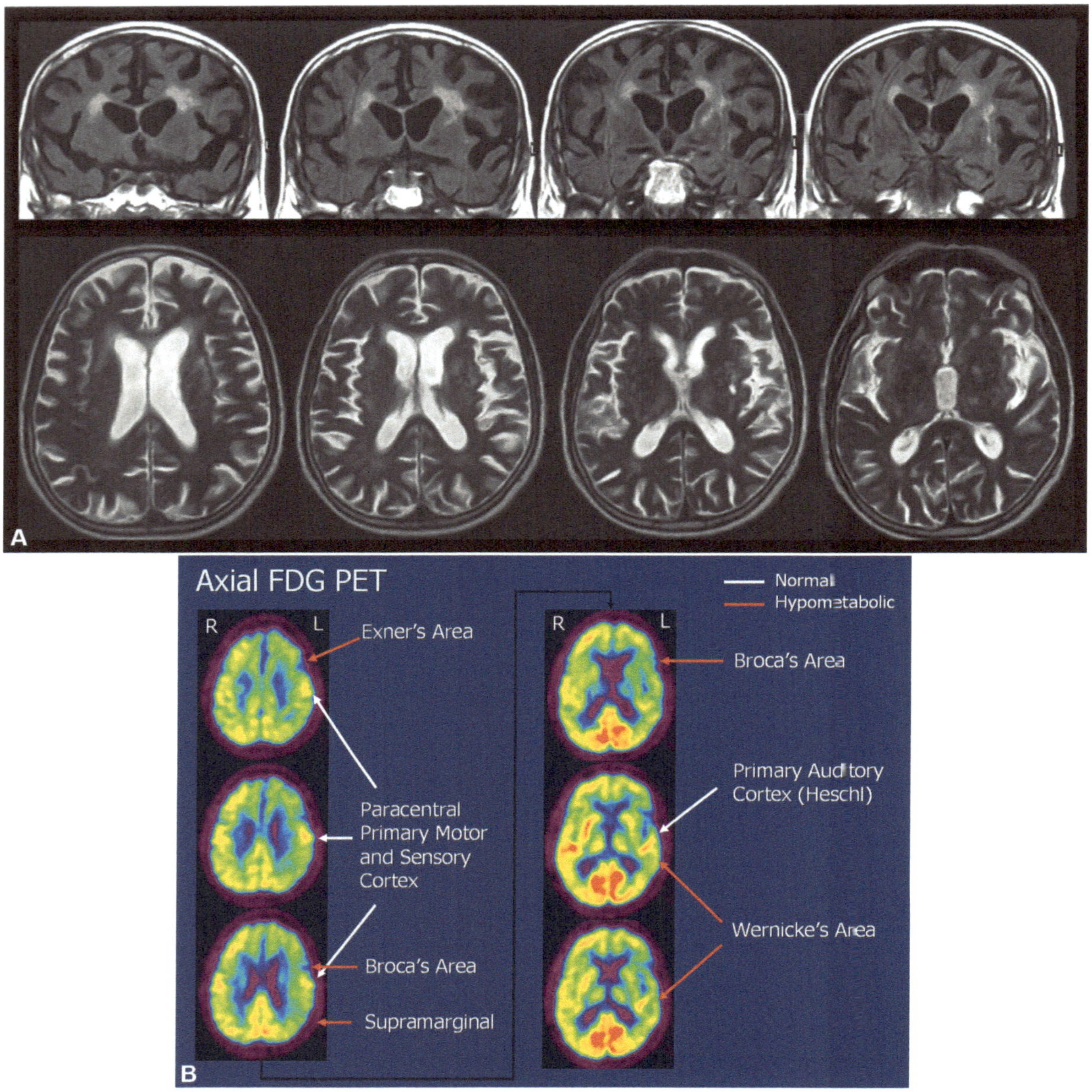

Fig. 26.5. Primary progressive aphasia, nonfluent type. An 80-year-old man with progressive impairment of language fluency for about 2 years before these images were obtained. (**A**) Coronal fluid-attenuated inversion recovery and axial T2-weighted magnetic resonance imaging images showing mild to moderate leukoaraiosis of the frontal periventricular white matter and lacunar infarctions in the left putamen, globus pallidus, pulvinar, and internal and extreme capsules. (**B**) Axial 2-deoxy-2-fluoro-D-glucose positron emission tomography (FDG-PET) showing hypometabolism in the perisylvian association cortex of the frontal, parietal, and temporal lobes of the left hemisphere. The primary auditory and motor-sensory cortices are spared. (Reproduced from Masdeu, 2008.)

fMRI respectively, synaptic dysfunction leading to an abnormal BOLD signal with fMRI (Logothetis, 2008), and to impaired metabolism with ^{18}F-FDG (Rocher et al., 2003), and fibrillary abeta deposition in the brain with several compounds, of which ^{11}C-PIB has been applied to the largest number of patients. Much less experience exists with specific tau markers, of which ^{18}F-AV-1415 is the first reported, originally as ^{18}F-T807 (Chien et al., 2013). ^{18}F-FDG, amyloid, and tau studies are carried out using PET. Because metabolism and brain perfusion are coupled in AD, perfusion studies with ^{15}O water PET or single-photon emission computed tomography (SPECT) provide information similar to ^{18}F-FDG PET (Fox et al., 1988). SPECT brain perfusion studies

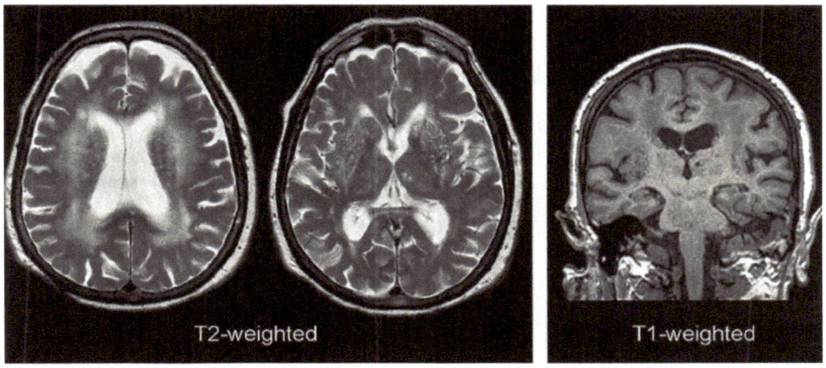

Fig. 26.6. Vascular dementia. Axial T2-weighted and coronal T1-weighted images from an 80-year-old woman with impairment of cognition and gait. Note the thalamic infarctions and the large areas of altered signal (increased on T2 and decreased on T1) in the centrum semiovale. (Reproduced from Masdeu, 2008.)

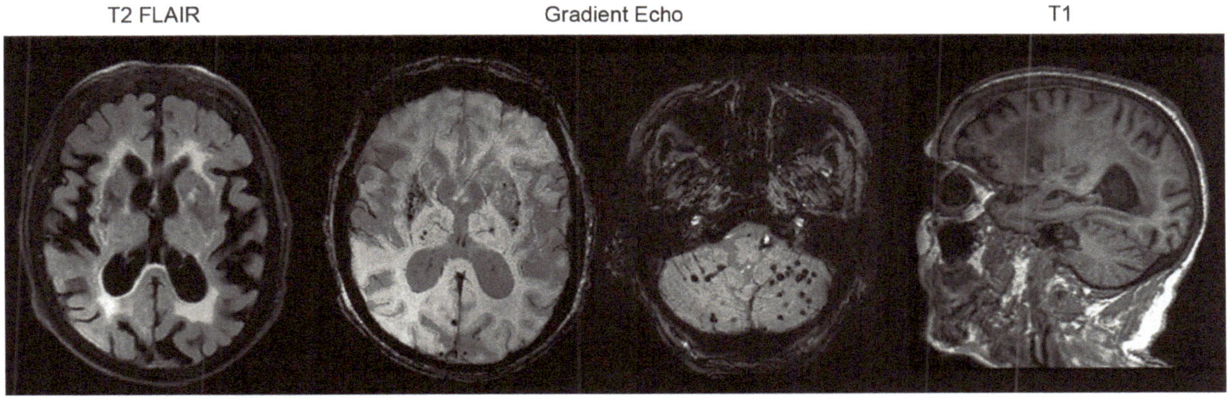

Fig. 26.7. Cerebral amyloid angiopathy (CAA). Magnetic resonance images from a 72-year-old woman with dementia and CAA. The white matter contains many abnormal areas, which appear hyperintense on the transverse fluid-attenuated inversion recovery (FLAIR) image and hypointense on the sagittal T1-weighted image. Multiple lacunar infarcts are present in the lenticular nuclei and few in the thalami. Microbleeds, best seen on the gradient-echo images, dot the lenticular nuclei, thalami, and the cerebellum. Scattered microbleeds can also be seen in the cortex or subcortical white matter. (Reproduced from Masdeu, 2008.)

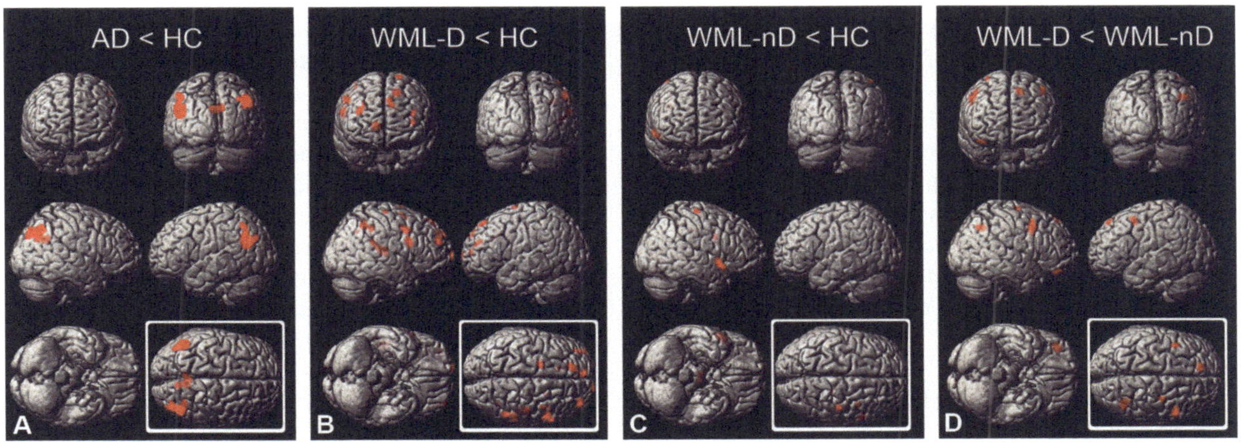

Fig. 26.8. Metabolism in Alzheimer's disease (AD) and vascular dementia. From **A** to **D**: four panels, each showing in red the regions of the brain with reduced metabolism in the first, as compared to the second, of two comparison groups. In **A** to **C** each of the patient groups, AD, vascular disease and dementia (WML-D), and vascular disease without dementia (WML-nD), is compared to a healthy control group (HC). In **D**, WML-D is compared to WML-nD. The height thresholds for the comparisons are as follows: **A**, $T = 4.07$ (voxel-level significance, $p < 0.01$, false discovery rate corrected); **B** and **C**, $T = 3.29$ (voxel-level, $p < 0.001$); and **D**, $T = 2.12$ (voxel-level, $p < 0.02$). In AD (**A**), note the classic pattern of bilaterally decreased metabolism in the parietotemporal association cortex and precuneus. The pattern in vascular disease with dementia resembles more the pattern in vascular disease without dementia than the pattern in AD. In vascular disease, patients with dementia have a reduction primarily in frontal metabolism, as compared to those who are not demented (**D**). Group patterns are most obvious on the superior aspect of the brain, highlighted with a frame in each panel of the figure. (Reproduced from Pascual et al., 2010.)

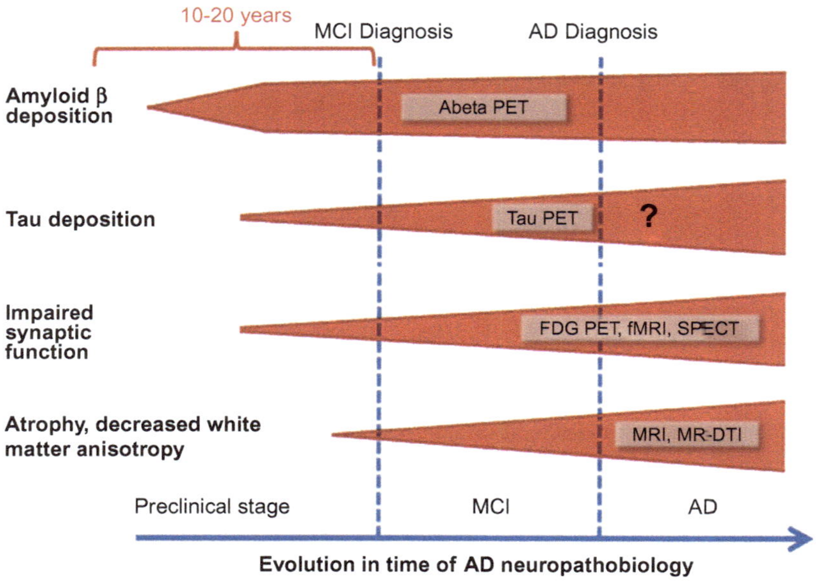

Fig. 26.9. Evolution of imaging findings in Alzheimer's disease (AD). Neurobiologic changes in the various stages in the development of AD, illustrated by specific neuroimaging techniques. A wider area in red indicates a greater degree of the neurobiologic disorder (abeta or tau deposition, impaired synaptic function or atrophy, and decreased white-matter anisotropy). Please note that the sequence of tau deposition is only an estimate, because studies are still sparse. MCI, mild cognitive impairment; amyloid PET, ^{11}C-PIB positron emission tomography (PET); FDG PET, ^{18}F fluoro-deoxy-glucose PET; fMRI, functional magnetic resonance imaging; SPECT, single-photon emission computed tomography; MR-DTI, diffusion tensor imaging performed with functional MRI.

are easier to perform and less expensive than PET studies (Masdeu and Arbizu, 2008). However, because they have less spatial resolution, SPECT studies have less sensitivity and specificity, particularly at early stages of the disease (Silverman, 2004; Yuan et al., 2009). More recently, arterial spin labeling has been applied to the study of brain perfusion in AD using MRI (Chen et al., 2011b). To follow the currently most conventional approach, from the older to the newer findings, we first review atrophy, followed by impaired metabolism and finally abeta deposition. However, as the disease evolves, abeta deposition antecedes the other two, and atrophy is the last to develop (Fig. 26.9). Abnormally phosphorylated tau deposition occurs in AD, but its timing in relation to abeta deposition or to the onset of clinical symptoms has not been determined by *in vivo* studies. Tau is closely associated with neuronal damage and cognitive impairment (Braak et al., 2011; Nelson et al., 2012; Monsell et al., 2013). Finally we will touch upon another feature of the AD brain, inflammation, now amenable to imaging.

Atrophy and white-matter anisotropy loss

Atrophy

In familial autosomal-dominant AD, as caused by mutations in the presenilin and amyloid precursor protein genes, genotyping allows for the determination, with a high degree of certainty, of who will develop the disease (Apostolova et al., 2011). Serial MRIs performed in presymptomatic individuals have suggested that atrophy in some regions, particularly the precuneus and medial temporal areas, may start as early as 4 years before the onset of cognitive impairment (Knight et al., 2011). This finding has only been determined with automated methods and has not been observed by all investigators (Ringman et al., 2010; Apostolova et al., 2011). One group has even reported increased cortical thickness in presymptomatic individuals (Fortea et al., 2010), which could suggest that an acceleration of cortical inflammatory changes before atrophy, associated with neuronal loss and increased phospho-tau in CSF, supervenes (Fortea et al., 2014). Another genetically at-risk group, cognitively intact apoliprotein E (*APOE*) ϵ4 homozygotes, has been reported to have an increased rate of cortical thinning (Crivello et al., 2010) or, for *APOE* ϵ4 carriers, preferential atrophy of some hippocampal subregions (Burggren et al., 2008; Mueller and Weiner, 2009; Donix et al., 2010). In cognitively normal elderly individuals, cortical thinning in precuneus and medial temporal regions has been found to correlate with subsequent cognitive decline as much as a decade later (Chiang et al., 2011; Dickerson et al., 2011; Kantarci et al., 2013) or with amyloid deposition and reduced

CSF abeta (Becker et al., 2011; Chetelat et al., 2012b; Dickerson and Wolk, 2012), again, suggesting that atrophy may antedate the onset of cognitive decline. The pattern of cortical thinning in people who will develop AD differs from that associated with cognitive loss of healthy aging (Bakkour et al., 2013) (Fig. 26.10). Cortical thinning associated with other AD-related changes, such as abeta deposition (Becker et al., 2011) or increased hippocampal activation during episodic memory tasks (Putcha et al., 2011), has been also been explored as a marker of early AD changes in cognitively normal older individuals. Regional atrophy correlates with regional abeta deposition, particularly in posterior cingulate cortex, in presymptomatic people or those with subjective cognitive complaints, but not in MCI or AD, suggesting that the damaging effect of abeta occurs in the presymptomatic or very mildly symptomatic stages, when abeta-reducing therapies should be applied (Chetelat et al., 2010, 2012b).

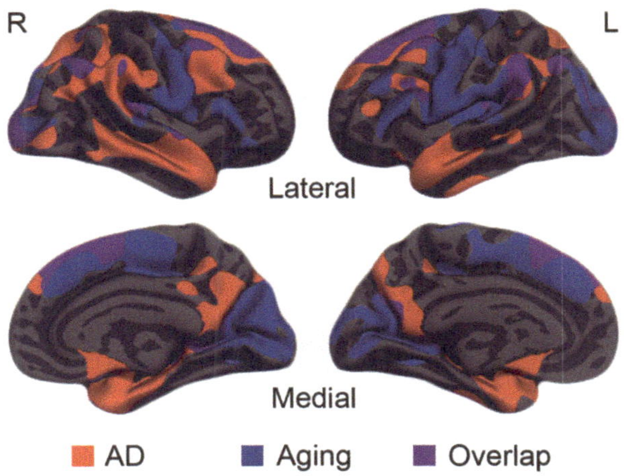

Fig. 26.10. Atrophy in healthy aging and Alzheimer's disease (AD). Areas of the brain in which progressive atrophy is detected in healthy aging (blue), AD (red), or an overlap of either (violet). (Reproduced from Bakkour et al., 2013.)

In patients with MCI, thinning of the temporal cortex and precuneus is a predictor of worsening to AD, particularly when combined with neuropsychologic, PET, and CSF markers (Hua et al., 2008; Chen et al., 2011a; Heister et al., 2011; Wolz et al., 2011). Although atrophy can be appreciated visually (Fig. 26.11) (Scheltens et al., 2002; Urs et al., 2009), automated methods are more precise and facilitate longitudinal follow-up (McEvoy et al., 2009; Morra et al., 2009; Wang et al., 2009). The accuracy of software that classifies clinically appropriate cases has been compared favorably with the accuracy of trained readers (Kloppel et al., 2008). MRI end-points compared across healthy individuals and those in various stages of the AD continuum have included hippocampal volume, tensor-based morphometry, cortical thickness, and a novel technique based on manifold learning (Hua et al., 2008; Wolz et al., 2011). The best results are usually achieved combining all features, in one longitudinal clinical study yielding 67% sensitivity and 69% specificity to separate stable MCI from MCI worsening to AD, 86% and 82% to separate healthy controls from MCI worsening to AD, and 93% sensitivity and 85% specificity to separate healthy controls from AD (Wolz et al., 2011). In another longitudinal study with a 3-year follow-up (Heister et al., 2011), the combination of greater learning impairment and increased medial temporal atrophy was associated with the highest risk: 85% of patients with both risk factors converted to AD within 3 years, vs 5% of those with neither. Medial temporal atrophy was associated with the shortest median dementia-free period (Heister et al., 2011).

In autopsy series, containing more advanced AD, medial temporal atrophy, even judged with a visual scale (Scheltens et al., 2002), has shown a sensitivity of 91% and specificity of 94% for autopsy-confirmed AD

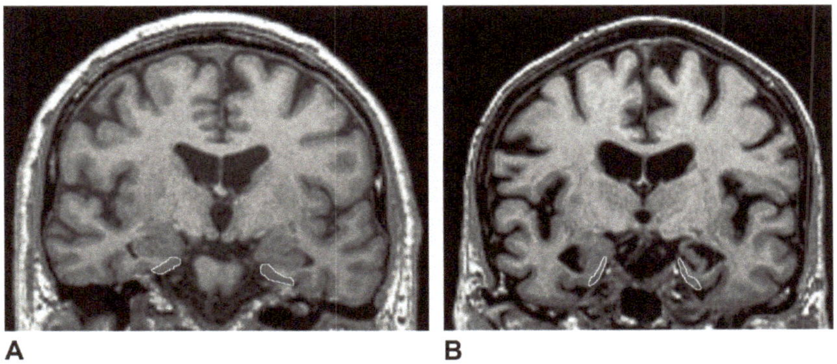

Fig. 26.11. Temporal atrophy in Alzheimer's disease (AD). Coronal magnetic resonance imaging at the level of the mammillary bodies. The entorhinal cortex has been outlined in a normal control (**A**) and a person with mild cognitive impairment of the amnesic type (**B**). Note the dilation of the temporal horns of the person with mild cognitive impairment corresponding to hippocampal atrophy. (Reproduced from Masdeu, 2008.)

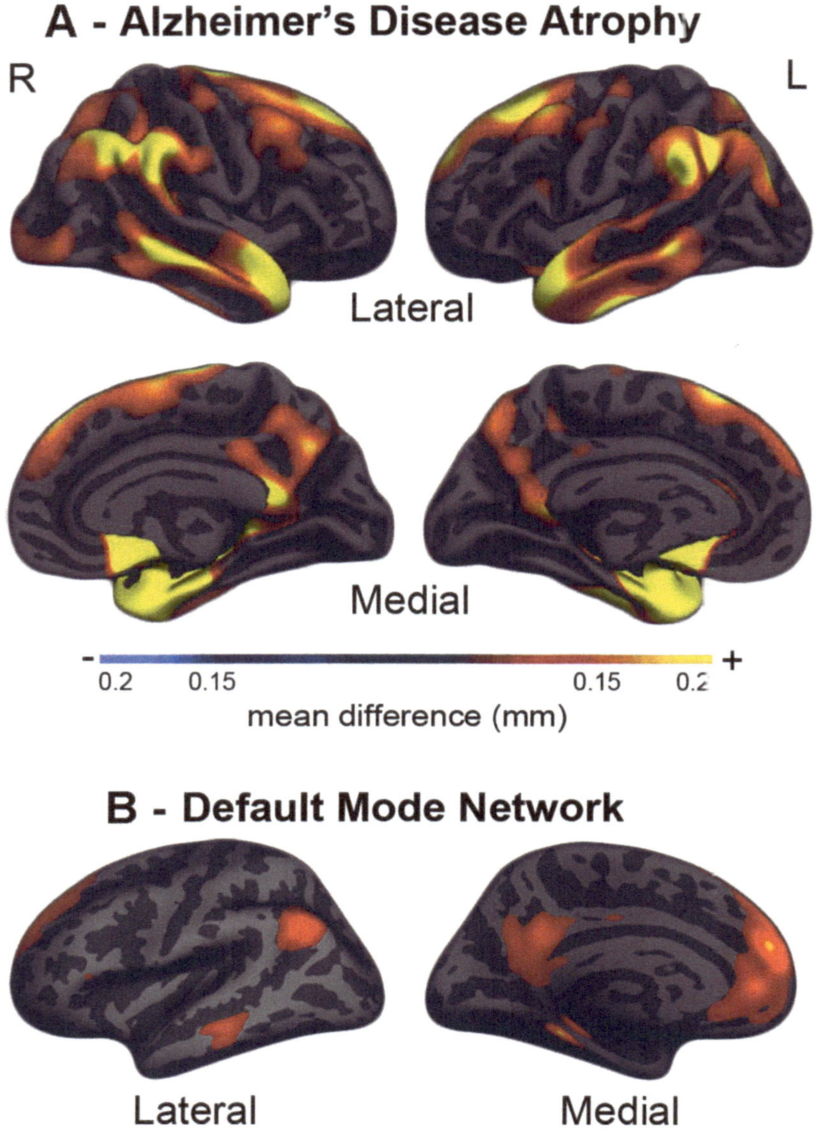

Fig. 26.12. Atrophy in Alzheimer's disease (AD). (**A**) Areas of the brain characteristically atrophied in AD. Note that they involve many of the same regions as the resting-state or default network (**B**). (**A**, Reproduced from Dickerson et al., 2009.) With permission from Oxford University Press.

(Burton et al., 2009). Regional atrophy correlates with tangle density and therefore with Braak neurofibrillary tangle stage, rather than with amyloid plaque deposition (Vemuri et al., 2008; Whitwell et al., 2008; Burton et al., 2009). Atrophy typically extends from limbic structures to neocortex at a rate of 2–5% per year (Thompson et al., 2003). The pattern of atrophy reflects preferential involvement of the parietotemporal components of the resting-state or default network (Dickerson et al., 2009) (Fig. 26.12). Atrophy shows striking network properties: when the medial temporal lobe is more atrophied, as are other regions of the ventral default network (Fig. 26.13); when the inferior parietal lobule has more atrophy, as do other regions of the dorsal default network and frontoparietal executive systems (Dickerson et al., 2009) (Fig. 26.14). Hippocampal atrophy affects mostly the CA1 subfield, a pattern that differs from healthy aging (Chetelat et al., 2008b) (Fig. 26.15).

Atrophy on MRI correlates well with the degree of regional neuronal loss (Brun and Englund, 1981). Another approach to measure neuronal loss is to quantify the regional density of neuronal receptors such as the gamma-aminobutyric acid (GABA)-A receptor, which is abundant in neurons and widespread in the brain. Binding to GABA-A receptors by ^{11}C-flumazenil, a PET tracer, has been reported to be reduced in early AD (Pascual et al.,

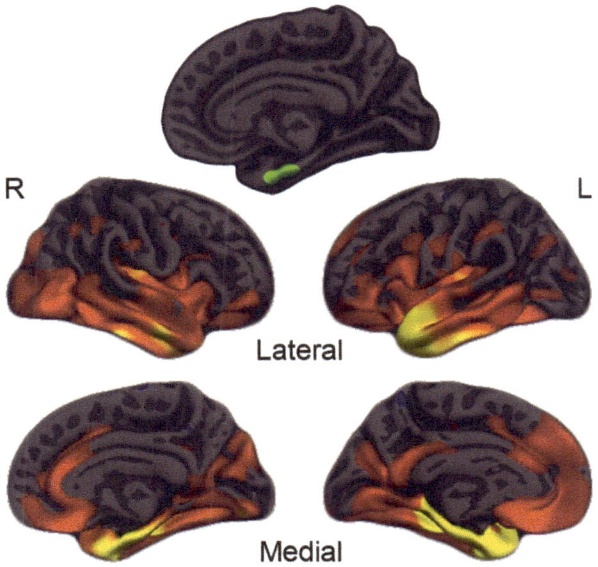

Fig. 26.13. Ventral network degeneration in Alzheimer's disease. Greater atrophy in the anteromedial temporal region (seed in green) correlates with greater atrophy in the temporal lobes and anteromedial prefrontal cortex. (Reproduced from Dickerson et al., 2009.) With permission from Oxford University Press.

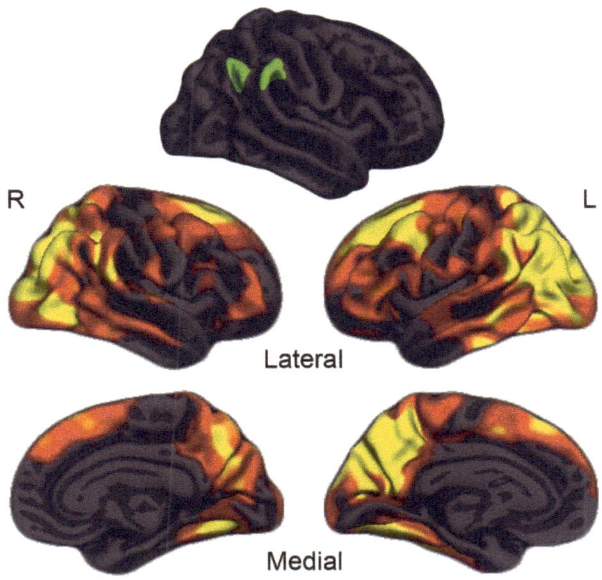

Fig. 26.14. Dorsal network degeneration in Alzheimer's disease. Greater atrophy in the inferior parietal lobule (seeds in green) correlates with greater atrophy in the precuneus and lateral temporoparietal association cortex. (Reproduced from Dickerson et al., 2009.) With permission from Oxford University Press.

2012a). The anatomy of reduction paralleled the distribution of neuronal loss in early AD described in neuropathologic studies (Brun and Englund, 1981) (Fig. 26.16).

By correlating postmortem findings with the pattern of atrophy on MRI, three distinct atrophy patterns have been found in patients with typical AD neuropathology, including abeta deposition: typical AD (about 70% of cases), limbic-predominant AD (20%), and hippocampal-sparing AD (10%) (Whitwell et al., 2012a) (Fig. 26.17). Most patients with typical and limbic-predominant AD initially present with an amnestic syndrome, but only about 40% of those with hippocampal-sparing AD do. Medial temporal atrophy is most severe in patients with limbic-predominant AD, followed closely by typical AD, and milder in those with hippocampal-sparing AD. Conversely, the most severe cortical atrophy was noted in patients with hippocampal-sparing AD, followed by those with typical disease, and then limbic-predominant AD. The ratio of hippocampal to cortical volumes allowed the best discrimination between subtypes (Whitwell et al., 2012a). In addition, some AD patients present with a profound disorder of visual perception, including one or several components of Balint's syndrome and even field defects on confrontation testing (Rosenbloom et al., 2011; Lehmann et al., 2013a; Ossenkoppele et al., 2015). This disorder, associated with severe bilateral atrophy of the angular gyri, is called posterior cortical atrophy (Fig. 26.18).

White-matter anisotropy loss

White-matter abnormalities in the fornix (Ringman et al., 2007) or in fronto-occipital and inferior temporal fasciculi, the splenium of the corpus callosum, subcallosal white matter, and the cingulum bundle (Smith et al., 2010) have been found with the use of DTI in healthy individuals at risk for AD, either with autosomal-dominant mutations (Ringman et al., 2007; Fortea et al., 2010) or carrying the *APOE* ϵ4 allele (Smith et al., 2010). In affected areas, DTI shows decreased functional anisotropy (Ringman et al., 2007) or increased mean diffusivity (Fortea et al., 2010). However, higher anisotropy can be found in white-matter volumes where a disrupted tract, such as the superior longitudinal fasciculus, crosses an intact one, such as the corticospinal tract, effectively increasing volume anisotropy (Douaud et al., 2011). In agreement with the anatomy of cortical atrophy, neocortical white-matter changes are more pronounced in late-myelinating fiber pathways, while sparing the corticospinal tract, originating in paracentral cortex (Stricker et al., 2009). White-matter abnormalities are also present in MCI, affecting to the greatest degree the cingulum bundle, the uncinate fasciculus, the corpus callosum, and the superior longitudinal fasciculus (Fellgiebel et al., 2004; Kiuchi et al., 2009; Mielke et al., 2009; Kantarci et al., 2010; Agosta et al., 2011; Douaud et al., 2011). Changes in the parahippocampal cingulum may separate best MCI from healthy controls (Clerx et al., 2012). For

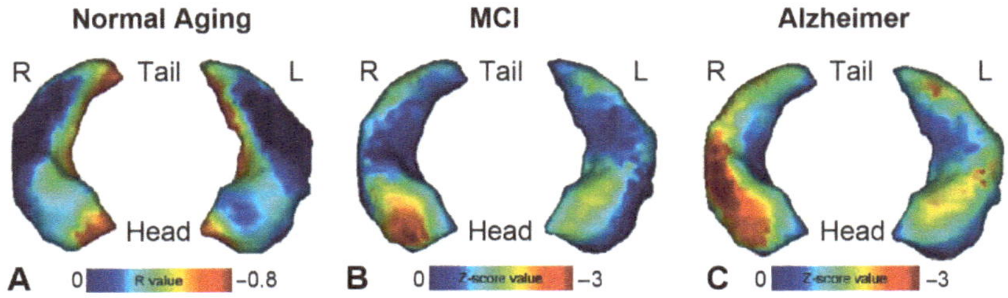

Fig. 26.15. Hippocampal atrophy in Alzheimer's disease. Areas of the hippocampus characteristically atrophied in (**A**) healthy aging, (**B**) mild cognitive impairment (MCI), and (**C**) Alzheimer's disease. (Reproduced from Chetelat et al., 2008b.)

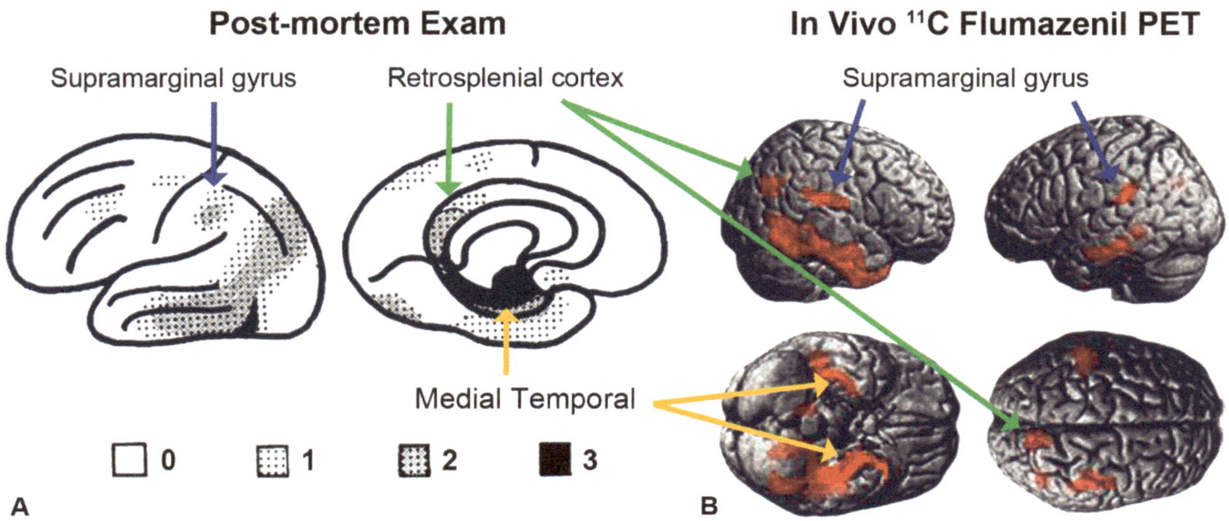

Fig. 26.16. Flumazenil positron emission tomography (PET) to detect neuronal loss in Alzheimer's disease (AD). Areas showing neuronal loss in AD had a similar distribution in our flumazenil PET study (Pascual et al., 2012b) and in the classic histologic study of early AD by Brun and Englund (1981). In a whole-brain histologic survey of neuronal loss (**A**), from 0 (no neuronal loss) to 3 (most neuronal loss), the regions most affected were the temporal lobes, particularly in their medial aspect, the retrosplenial cortex and the supramarginal-angular gyri, which were the regions involved on flumazenil PET (**B**). (Reproduced from Pascual et al., 2012a.)

DTI, discrimination values higher than 90% have been achieved comparing MCI to healthy controls using support vector machine classifiers (O'Dwyer et al., 2012; Wee et al., 2012). However, these optimistic outcomes need to be validated in independent samples. The value of DTI to predict worsening from MCI to AD is still to be determined.

Impaired synaptic function

Impaired synaptic function across the various AD stages can be gauged with techniques measuring the fMRI BOLD signal, regional metabolism, and regional perfusion. Findings are concordant, but each technique is amenable to different applications. Metabolism has been studied most extensively, but the most recent developments are the increasing use of resting-state BOLD fMRI to assess functional connectivity changes and of arterial spin labeling to measure regional perfusion using noninvasive MRI.

Metabolism

Regional cerebral metabolism studies with PET have used ^{18}F-FDG as a metabolic marker (Jagust et al., 2007; Herholz, 2014; O'Brien et al., 2014). The most typical pattern found in early AD is decreased metabolism bilaterally in the parietotemporal association cortex and posterior cingulate gyrus (Chen et al., 2011a) (Fig. 26.19). A similar pattern has been described by one group in asymptomatic, even young, *APOE* ε4 carriers (Reiman et al., 1996, 2004). Metabolism reflects synaptic activity and therefore is most affected early in the regions to which medial temporal neurons project Miettinen et al., 2011; Bozoki et al., 2012), and may reflect impaired connectivity even in presymptomatic subjects (Drzezga et al., 2011). As atrophy corresponds to neuronal loss, it is no surprise that the regions most affected on volumetric MRI and metabolic PET do not coincide early in the disease (Chetelat et al., 2008a), but they partially overlap as the disease progresses (La Joie et al., 2012)

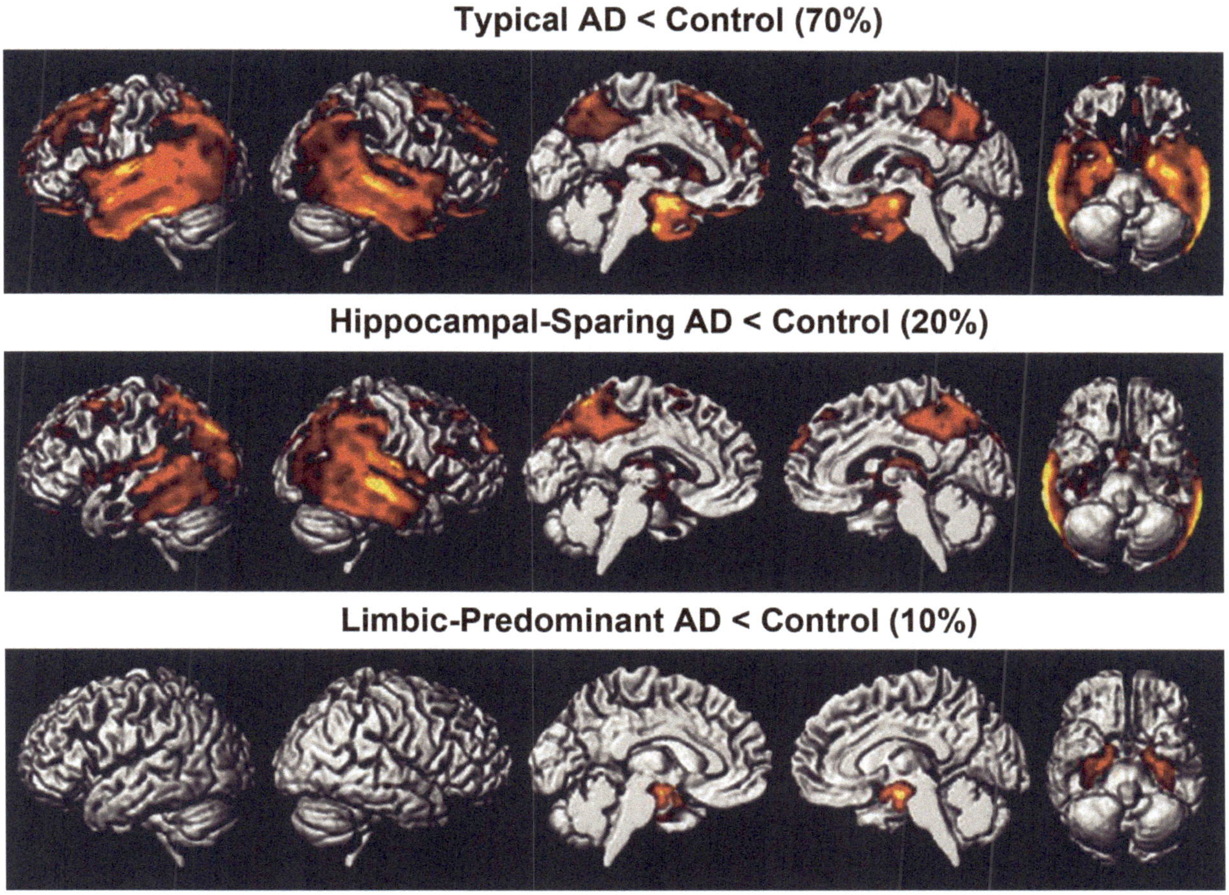

Fig. 26.17. Imaging and pathology types of Alzheimer's disease (AD). On standard templates, regions of atrophy on magnetic resonance imaging performed during life in patients who at autopsy were found to have each of three different pathologic types of AD. The percentages indicate the frequency of each type in this sample of 177 patients. (Modified from Whitwell et al., 2012a.)

(Fig. 26.20). As the disease progresses, some areas of the frontal association cortex become hypometabolic, while the paracentral cortex (primary motor-sensory areas) remains preserved (Fig. 26.19). The specificity and sensitivity of these findings continue to be debated. In studies with neuropathologic confirmation, the sensitivity (84–95%) has been higher than the specificity (71–74%); that is, a normal study is seldom associated with AD (Silverman et al., 2001; Jagust et al., 2007). Using consensus diagnosis, in an area under the receiver operating characteristic (ROC) analysis for three automated approaches to mild AD diagnosis, the specificity approximates 85% when the sensitivity is pegged at 80% (Caroli et al., 2012). Depending on the approach and the sample studied, the accuracy for predicting the evolution of MCI to AD varies from 0.774 to 0.983 (Caroli et al., 2012). Among persons with MCI, those most likely to progress to AD have metabolic findings similar to AD (Mosconi et al., 2007). ^{18}F-FDG PET may predict better than structural MRI or SPECT the worsening from MCI to AD (Yuan et al., 2009).

Perfusion

Initially studied with $H_2{}^{15}O$ PET (Boles Ponto et al., 2006), in current clinical practice brain perfusion is most often studied with SPECT because the performance of $H_2{}^{15}O$ PET is both cumbersome and expensive. Arterial spin labeling could facilitate perfusion data at the same time that other MRI parameters are obtained, but it requires further validation (Chen et al., 2011b). The most commonly used tracers for studying cerebral perfusion with SPECT are Tc-99m hexamethyl propylamine oxime (Ceretec), a lipid-soluble macrocyclic amine, and Tc-99m ethyl cysteinate dimer (Neurolite). The pattern of decreased regional perfusion in parietotemporal cortex, hippocampus, anterior and posterior cingulum, and dorsomedial and anterior nucleus of the thalamus had a sensitivity of 86% and a specificity of 80% comparing AD to normal controls (Johnson et al., 1998; Masdeu et al., 2005). In a group of 70 patients with dementia and 14 controls, all with autopsy, SPECT was most useful when the clinical diagnosis was of possible AD, with a

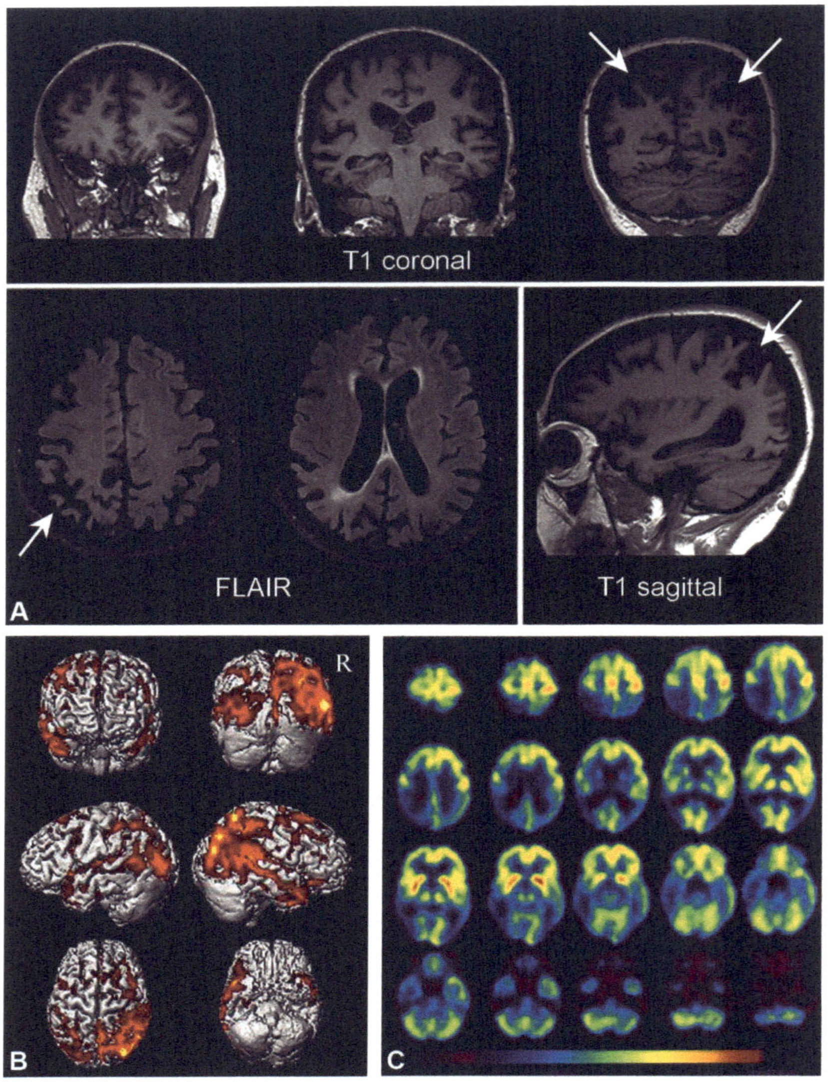

Fig. 26.18. Posterior cortical atrophy in Alzheimer's disease. (**A**) Conventional magnetic resonance imaging (MRI), (**B**) volumetric MRI on a rendered image, and (**C**) positron emission tomography (PET) studies from a 61-year-old woman with a 3-year history of progressive reading difficulties, agraphia, and dressing apraxia. On examination she had a Balint syndrome with simultanagnosia, apraxia of eye movements, optic ataxia, and "tunnel vision." Note in (**A**) the marked atrophy in the lateral parietal lobe, with dilation of the intraparietal sulcus (arrows). There is also hippocampal atrophy, albeit less prominent. (**B**) Voxels with significant atrophy (compared with statistical parametric mapping to 48 controls, $p < 0.05$ uncorrected; $k > 20$) are displayed in red. Note that in (**B**) the right side of the brain is displayed on the right side of the image, opposite to the radiologic convention on the conventional MRI (**A**) and PET (**C**). Areas of decreased metabolism on PET (**C**) most closely match the clinical picture.

probability of a diagnosis of AD of 67% without SPECT, of 84% with a positive SPECT, and of 52% with a negative SPECT (Jagust et al., 2001). However, to predict progression from MCI to AD, SPECT has been reported to have 41.9% sensitivity and 82.3% specificity (Devanand et al., 2010b), although a meta-analysis assigned to SPECT a similar predictive value as MRI measurements (Yuan et al., 2009). A head-to-head comparison of perfusion SPECT with metabolism PET has shown a much better sensitivity and specificity of PET over SPECT in AD and DLB (O'Brien et al., 2014).

BOLD signal

Activation

The great variety of methods, including different activation paradigms, has yielded disparate results among various groups. For instance, both increased

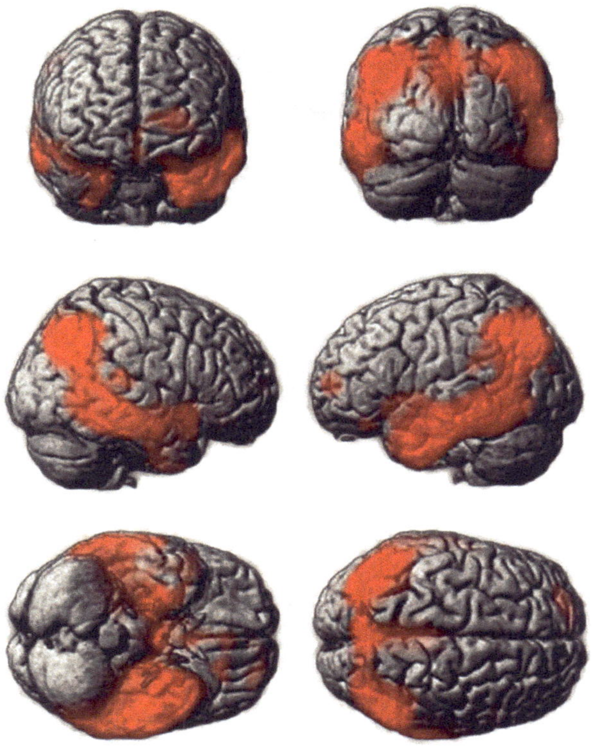

Fig. 26.19. Deoxy-2-fluoro-D-glucose positron emission tomography (FDG PET) group findings in Alzheimer's disease. Projected on a rendered magnetic resonance imaging and shown in red are areas with low metabolism in a group of 28 patients with early Alzheimer's disease, compared with 28 healthy controls. Note sparing of the paracentral (primary motor-sensory) cortex. (Reproduced from Masdeu, 2008.)

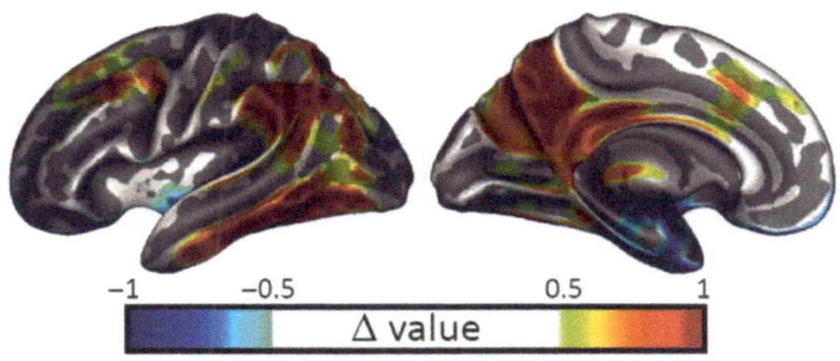

Fig. 26.20. Areas of greatest atrophy and lowest metabolism in Alzheimer's disease. Projected on surface templates are areas of the brain with greatest atrophy (in blue) and greatest metabolic loss (in red). (Courtesy of Dr. Renaud La Joie, Institut National de la Santé et de la Recherche Médicale (Inserm), Unité, 1077 Caen, France.)

(Bondi et al., 2005; Bookheimer et al., 2000; Fleisher et al., 2005; Trivedi et al., 2008) and decreased (Johnson et al., 2006; Mondadori et al., 2007) medial temporal-lobe activation has been reported in *APOE* ϵ4 carriers. Some apparent differences may reflect still unclear underlying biology. For instance, the apparent discrepancy in activation in *APOE* ϵ4 carriers may be explained by their failure to experience a decrease in activation with age, as other *APOE* genotypes do (Nichols et al., 2012). Then, *APOE* ϵ4 carriers will be likely to show decreased activation compared to other *APOE* genotypes in young samples (Johnson et al., 2006; Mondadori et al., 2007), but increased activation in older samples (Bookheimer et al., 2000; Bondi et al., 2005; Fleisher et al., 2005; Trivedi et al., 2008). Despite the complexity of activation results, a bimodal pattern seems consistent. Medial temporal activation, increased in asymptomatic at-risk subjects (Quiroz et al., 2010; Putcha et al., 2011; Braskie et al., 2012; but see Ringman et al., 2011), tends to decrease as the AD process worsens and cognition deteriorates (Dickerson et al., 2004; O'Brien et al., 2010). Indeed, increased activation in mildly symptomatic, or even asymptomatic, individuals may predict their worsening (Dickerson et al., 2004; O'Brien et al., 2010).

Functional connectivity

Abnormalities in functional connectivity have been found consistently in the different stages of AD and correspond to abnormal DTI, volumetric and metabolic findings (Sperling et al., 2010; Filippi and Agosta, 2011). Most of the recent studies have explored resting BOLD, easier and faster to obtain than activation paradigms. This potentially powerful technique depends heavily on careful data recording and analysis; even in the best hands it can yield results that reflect nonbiologic variables, such as greater movement in the scanner on the part of one of the study groups (Power et al., 2012). As with other neuroimaging findings, abnormal connectivity may already be detected in presymptomatic, at-risk individuals, particularly to and from areas, like the posterior cingulate gyrus, precuneus, and medial temporal regions, known to be affected early in the disease (Hedden et al., 2009; Dennis et al., 2010; Sheline et al., 2010; Gour et al., 2011; Machulda et al., 2011; Jacobs et al., 2012). Unlike atrophy, impaired functional connectivity reflects synaptic dysfunction, not neuronal loss. For this reason it tends to be affected in areas with low metabolism (Drzezga et al., 2011) and amyloid deposition (Hedden et al., 2009; Drzezga et al., 2011). Different precuneus connectivity patterns have been reported in AD and DLB (Galvin et al., 2011; Kenny et al., 2012) and across *APOE* genotypes (Sheline et al., 2010).

Abeta deposition

Undoubtedly, abeta imaging, accomplished for the first time in humans in February 2002 (Kadir et al., 2011), has been the greatest boon yet for early-stage AD imaging (Fig. 26.21). Brain abeta has been imaged most

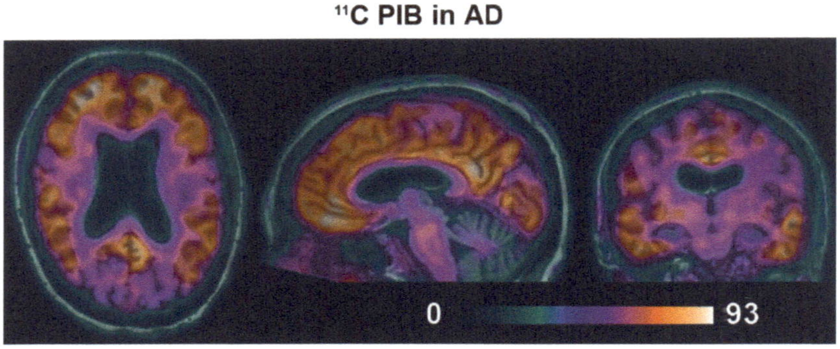

Fig. 26.21. Pittsburgh compound B (^{11}C-PIB)-positive scan in Alzheimer's disease (AD). In yellow, areas of the brain with abeta deposition, displayed on the magnetic resonance imaging of this 65-year-old woman. Note the distribution of amyloid binding, predominantly in the frontal and temporal lobes, as well as precuneus. There is slight binding to white matter, but not as pronounced as in the ^{18}F-florbetapir scan (Fig. 26.22).

extensively with "Pittsburgh compound B" (^{11}C-PIB) (Rowe and Villemagne, 2011), helping separate the dementias with marked abeta deposition from the rest (Table 26.1). PIB is only available bound to ^{11}C, a positron-emitting isotope with a half-life of 20.4 minutes, but since 2012 there are abeta-imaging compounds bound to ^{18}F, with a half-life of 109.8 minutes (Table 26.2). The longer half-life allows for the radiotracer to be synthesized at a facility with a cyclotron and then shipped to institutions with PET cameras, a process much less expensive than having an on-site cyclotron and one that is also potentially available at many health care settings. Good concordance with histologically measured abeta load has been shown for three PET abeta binding agents, ^{18}F-florbetapir (Choi et al., 2012), ^{18}F-flutemetamol (Wolk et al., 2011), and ^{18}F-florbetaben (Sabri et al., 2015). All of them are approved by the Food and Drug Administration for use in the clinical setting. Newer ^{18}F compounds are on the way (Rowe et al., 2013), attempting to correct the marked nonspecific white-matter binding of currently available ^{18}F abeta compounds. In early AD, ^{11}C-PIB binds mostly to frontoparietotemporal association cortex, sparing the paracentral regions and primary sensory cortex. It also binds to striatum. The regional retention of PIB-like compounds reflects the regional density of abeta plaques (Bacskai et al., 2007; Ikonomovic et al., 2008; Kadir et al., 2011; Choi et al., 2012).

Like another biomarker of AD, decreased CSF abeta 42 (Jack et al., 2011), abeta brain deposition begins in the preclinical stages of AD, increases during the MCI stage and, by the time of the AD diagnosis, remains relatively stable as the disease progresses (Fig. 26.9) (Jack et al., 2008; Villemagne et al., 2011b; Ossenkoppele et al., 2012). Thus, it is a marker of the preclinical stages of the disease and correlates with the degree of cognitive impairment only in the preclinical stages and MCI, not during AD (Koivunen et al., 2011; Villemagne et al., 2011b; Chetelat et al., 2012a; Perrotin et al., 2012), while atrophy and synaptic dysfunction continue to increase and spread as clinical AD worsens and cognition deteriorates (Jack et al., 2008; Mormino et al., 2009; Devanand et al., 2010a; Koivunen et al., 2011). In asymptomatic individuals of a similar age, abeta deposition has been found more often among *APOE*4 carriers (Castellano et al., 2011; Vlassenko et al., 2011). Lifetime cognitive engagement has been found to protect from preclinical abeta deposition in some studies (Landau et al., 2012) but not in others (Vemuri et al., 2012). Also in asymptomatic individuals, a more sedentary lifestyle has been associated with higher abeta levels, but only among *APOE4* carriers (Head et al., 2012). Furthermore, longitudinal imaging allows for the evaluation of the natural history of abeta deposition among at-risk genotypes (Vlassenko et al., 2011), and it has the potential to be a marker of effectiveness in studies carried out during the preclinical stage of AD, as it has helped elucidate brain changes during AD therapy (Sperling et al., 2012). Although more data are needed, abeta deposition could be the strongest and earliest neuroimaging predictor of worsening to AD. In a 2-year follow-up of MCI patients, 19 of 30 ^{11}C-PIB-positive patients worsened to AD, whereas only one among the ^{11}C-PIB-negative patients did (Okello et al., 2009b; Wolk et al., 2009). Among the ^{11}C-PIB-negative MCI patients, 3 regained normal cognition and others developed non-AD dementias (Okello et al., 2009b; Wolk et al., 2009), providing a specificity for AD possibly superior to other imaging biomarkers at a very early stage of the AD spectrum. In addition, ^{11}C-PIB deposition predicts time to conversion to AD (Jack et al., 2010b). Another PET amyloid marker, ^{18}F-FDDNP, has also been reported to predict worsening from MCI to AD (Small et al., 2012; but see Ossenkoppele et al., 2012).

Table 26.1

Clinical, imaging, and genetic findings associated with the neurodegenerative dementias

Dementia type	Clinical findings	Atrophy (MRI)	Decreased metabolism (PET) or perfusion (SPECT, ASL)	β-amyloid (PET)	Tau (PET)	Predisposing gene variants or mutations
AD	Memory loss, language, or visuospatial function impairment	Medial temporal, precuneus, lateral temporoparietal association cortex	Precuneus, lateral parietotemporal association cortex	+	+	*APOE4, TREM2, TOMM40, APP, PS1/2*
lvPPA	Impaired repetition of sentences and phrases, phonologic errors in speech	Left posterior perisylvian or parietal association cortex	Left posterior perisylvian or parietal association cortex	+>>−	+	*APOE, TREM2, TOMM40, APP, PS1/2, MAPT*
nfvPPA	Nonfluent speech, agrammatism	Left posterior frontoinsular association cortex	Left posterior frontoinsular association cortex	−	+>−	*MAPT, GRN*
svPPA	Anomic aphasia, loss of comprehension, surface dyslexia	Left or right anterior temporal lobe	Left or right anterior temporal lobe	−>>+	−>>+	*GRN, MAPT, C9orf72*
bvFTD	Behavioral and personality changes, executive dysfunction	Symmetric to moderately right predominant frontal or anterior temporal regions	Anterior frontal and temporal cortex association cortex	−	+≈−	*MAPT, GRN, C9orf72, FUS, CHMP2B*
CBD	Apraxia, rigidity	Superior parietal lobule	Superior parietal lobule, premotor cortex, putamen	−	+	*MAPT, GRN*
PSP	Supranuclear palsy, executive function loss, parkinsonism	Midbrain	Frontal association cortex	−	+	*MAPT*
DLB	Memory loss, visual hallucinations, parkinsonism	Similar to AD, but less medial temporal atrophy	Posterior parieto-occipital association cortex, putamen	+	+	*APOE4, GBA*

MRI, magnetic resonance imaging; PET, positron emission tomography; SPECT, single-photon emission computed tomography; ASL, arterial spin labeling; AD, Alzheimer's disease; lvPPA, logopenic aphasia; nfvPPA, nonfluent primary progressive aphasia; svPPA, semantic variant of primary progressive aphasia; bvFTD, behavioral variant of frontotemporal dementia; CBD, corticobasal degeneration; PSP, progressive supranuclear palsy; DLB, diffuse Lewy-body dementia.

Abeta, MRI, and ^{18}F-FDG abnormalities in healthy people with mean or median age in the decade of the 70s have been determined by two separate groups in the USA using either PET ($n = 430$) or CSF ($n = 311$), yielding remarkably concordant results (Knopman et al., 2012; Petersen, 2013; Vos et al., 2013). The National Institute on Aging–Alzheimer's Association research criteria for preclinical AD were used to stage individual participants, according to results (Sperling et al., 2011a; Jack et al., 2012). About 40% of the subjects were in stage 0, without abnormal abeta or other preclinical markers; about 15% were in stage 1, with only abeta abnormality; about 12% in stage 2, with abeta plus MRI or ^{18}F-FDG markers of AD; about 5% in stage 3, having in addition subtle cognitive decline; about 23% had MRI or ^{18}F-FDG abnormalities characteristic of AD, but no abeta deposition (suspected non-Alzheimer pathology or SNAP); and about 5% were difficult to classify (Knopman et al., 2012; Petersen, 2013; Vos et al., 2013). These groupings had significant prognostic value, quite similar in the two studies: at 1 or 5 years, the progression rate to MCI or dementia was 2–5% for participants classed as normal, 11% for stage 1, 21–26% for stage 2, 43–56% for stage 3, and 5–10% for SNAP (Knopman et al., 2012;

Table 26.2

Properties of most commonly available abeta positron emission tomography (PET) tracers

		Requires cyclotron at site		Allows for two PET studies in same visit*		Radiation exposure (in mSv)		Number of PubMed listings†		Signal-to-noise ratio
^{11}C PIB	†	Yes	✓	Yes	✓	2.93	✓	299	✓	‡
^{18}F Florbetaben	✓	No		No		5.8		16		
^{18}F Florbetapir	✓	No		No		7.00		44		
^{18}F Flutemetamol	✓	No		No		5.92		11		
^{18}F AZD4694 (NAV4694)	✓	No		No		?		2		Same as PIB?

^{11}C PIB, Pittsburgh compound B.

PET tracers are listed in the left column by publication date. Checkmarks (✓) indicate the most advantageous tracer(s) for each property (listed in the top row).

*[^{11}C] but not [^{18}F], compounds allow for the performance of two different scans the same day.

†As of December, 2014.

‡Regarding image quality, see Rowe et al. (2013) and Landau et al. (2014).

Vos et al., 2013). Remarkably, in the abeta PET study, the SNAP group did not differ from the groups with amyloid deposition in MRI and ^{18}F-FDG characteristics (Knopman et al., 2013a), leading to the conclusion that these changes may be independent of abeta deposition in the brain. However, groups 2 and 3, with abnormal abeta, had a greater rate of worsening to dementia and progressive worsening of MRI and ^{18}F-FDG parameters, not observed in the SNAP group, in a 15-month follow-up (Knopman et al., 2013b). The proportion of abeta-negative MCI may climb to about 30% for patients aged 82 or older (Mathis et al., 2013). A few autopsies in the SNAP group have yielded inconclusive neuropathology (Vos et al., 2013). However, over a 14-year follow-up, the progression to dementia of the SNAP group is only slightly higher than that of abeta-negative, MRI-normal participants and lower than those with abeta on PET and normal MRI (Vos et al., 2013).

The effect of abeta deposition on cognitive impairment in early stages of the AD continuum may be modulated by some common genetic variants. For instance, healthy *APOE4* carriers not only have greater abeta deposition, but worse memory and visuospatial skills for the same amount of ^{11}C-PIB binding (Kantarci et al., 2012a). This finding may reflect a longer period of time with abeta deposition in the *APOE4* carriers. Healthy, abeta-positive carriers of the Met genotype of the brain-derived neurotrophic factor *Val66Met* allele have a greater worsening on follow-up in episodic memory, language, and executive function than the Val homozygotes despite similar abeta PET binding in both groups (Lim et al., 2013).

Abeta imaging is also a powerful tool to separate the dementias characterized by abeta deposition, such as AD and DLB, from the FTDs, which course without abeta deposition (Table 26.1). Separating patient samples of AD and FTD validated clinically, areas under the ROC curve for ^{11}C-PIB (0.888) and ^{18}F-FDG (0.910) were similar (Rabinovici et al., 2011). ^{11}C-PIB slightly outperformed ^{18}F-FDG in patients with known histopathology (Rabinovici et al., 2011). In this study, patients had symptoms suggestive of either disorder. More important is to define how often abeta PET is negative in patients with dementia of the AD type. In a clinical trial of early AD, 8/123 (6.5%) of *APOE4* carriers and 22/61 (36.1%) of noncarriers had negative ^{11}C-PIB studies, for a combined rate of 14% abeta-negative patients among 214 with AD symptomatology (Vellas et al., 2013). This proportion is very similar to the 14% abeta-negative in a population sample of 154 amnesic MCI patients and 16% of 58 MCI patients from the Alzheimer's Disease Neuroimaging Initiative (Petersen et al., 2013) and may rise to 30% when the patients studied are older than 82 years (Mathis et al., 2013). It may reflect the smaller subset of patients with dementia who do not have elevated abeta or tau at autopsy, which would correspond to imaging findings about 10 years earlier (Monsell et al., 2013). Thus, these imaging findings could reflect the rather mixed pathology found in the oldest old (Nelson et al., 2011, 2012) (Fig. 26.1). However, even with a careful neuropathologic exclusion of other etiologies, clinical and neuropathologic findings are occasionally dissociated: individuals with marked abeta and neurofibrillary pathology may be cognitively intact (Monsell et al., 2013). In these individuals there is less abeta deposition in the form of fibrillar plaques and intimately related oligomeric abeta assemblies, less hyperphosphorylated soluble tau species localized in synapses, and less glial activation (Perez-Nievas et al., 2013).

Tau deposition

In the healthy brain the protein tau stabilizes neurotubules and is therefore essential for normal neural function (Villemagne et al., 2015). However, in AD and other neurodegenerative disorders, tau becomes abnormally hyperphosphorylated, dysfunctional, and misfolded, constituting the tangles observed neuropathologically in AD and other tauopathies. The imaging compounds that we mention here do not bind to the healthy, native form of tau, but to the abnormally folded tau, using the folding properties of this protein for binding. For this reason these imaging compounds are helpful to study pathologic tau, separating it from the normal tau, which is not bound by the imaging agents and therefore not visible with them. As has become the common usage, we are referring to hyperphosphorylated tau simply as "tau." The first compound shown to bind to tau is ^{18}F-FDDNP (Shin et al., 2011), which binds also to abeta, but with less imaging sensitivity and specificity than the PIB-like compounds (Tolboom et al., 2010). It has shown increased binding in regions likely to have high tau, such as the medial temporal regions (Shin et al., 2010; Ercoli et al., 2012), which show relatively low ^{11}C-PIB binding (Rowe and Villemagne, 2011). In initial stages of use in humans are several tau-binding compounds that seem to have imaging characteristics superior to FDDNP (Table 26.3). These compounds include ^{11}C-PBB3 (Maruyama et al., 2013), ^{18}F-T807, most recently known as ^{18}F-AV-1451 (Chien et al., 2013, 2014), and ^{18}F-THK5117 (Villemagne et al., 2015). ^{11}C-PBB3 is photosensitive and therefore difficult to use in practice; it also has a high uptake in the superior sagittal sinus. The most experience exists with ^{18}F-AV-1451, which shows highly specific uptake in areas known neuropathologically to contain a large amount of tau in AD (Ossenkoppele et al., 2015) (Fig. 26.22). It has acceptable white-matter uptake but, in older individuals, even those cognitively intact, there is uptake in the lenticular nucleus, choroid plexus or its vicinity, red nucleus, and the region of the substantia nigra and subthalamic nucleus (Fig. 26.22). The reason for this uptake pattern is still unclear, but it does not seem to be related to tau deposition in these regions.

Inflammation

Inflammatory changes are prominent in AD: it is debated whether they are pathogenic, or simply reflect scavenging of neurons and neuronal processes, or even have a neuroprotective effect (Ferretti and Cuello, 2011; Hoozemans et al., 2011; Serrano-Pozo et al., 2011). Animal models of tau-induced neuronal loss have shown earlier and more severe inflammation than models of increased abeta (Maeda et al., 2011). However, data in humans are essential to understand the role of inflammation in the dementias. PET imaging allows *in vivo* quantification of neuroinflammation by measuring the density of the 18-kDa translocator protein (TSPO) in activated microglia and, to a lesser extent, in astrocytes. Activated brain microglia in AD has been largely imaged with ^{11}C-PK11195, not an ideal compound due to its low affinity for the receptor (Kropholler et al., 2007; Okello et al., 2009a), and a low ratio of specific-to-nonspecific binding (Kreisl et al., 2010). However, even ^{11}C-PK11195 has shown moderately increased binding in AD (Cagnin et al., 2001; Schuitemaker et al., 2013) and in some patients with MCI (Okello et al., 2009a). A correlation with cognitive performance was documented in one study (Edison et al., 2008), which used also ^{11}C-PIB to select the AD sample. The limitations of ^{11}C-PK11195 have prompted the development of second-generation radioligands for imaging activated microglia (Chauveau et al., 2008) (Fig. 26.23 and Table 26.4). ^{11}C-PBR28 is a second-generation radioligand with high affinity to TSPO, favorable *in vivo* kinetics, and greater signal-to-noise ratio than ^{11}C-PK11195 in monkey brain (Kreisl et al., 2010). Unfortunately, the affinity of this and other

Table 26.3

Properties of available p-tau positron emission tomography (PET) tracers*

	Requires cyclotron at site	Allows for two PET studies in same visit†	Radiation exposure (in mSv)	Specificity (binds to tau, not to abeta)	Photosensitive (requires dark-room handling)
^{18}F FDDNP	✓ No	No	?	Poor	✓ No
^{18}F AV1451	✓ No	No	8.92	✓ Good	✓ No
^{11}C PBB3	Yes	✓ Yes	?	✓ Good	Yes
^{18}F THK5117	✓ No	No	?	?	✓ No

PET tracers are listed in the left column by publication date. Checkmarks (✓) indicate the most advantageous tracer(s) for each property (listed in the top row).

*As of May 2015.

†^{11}C but not ^{18}F, compounds allow for the performance of two different scans the same day.

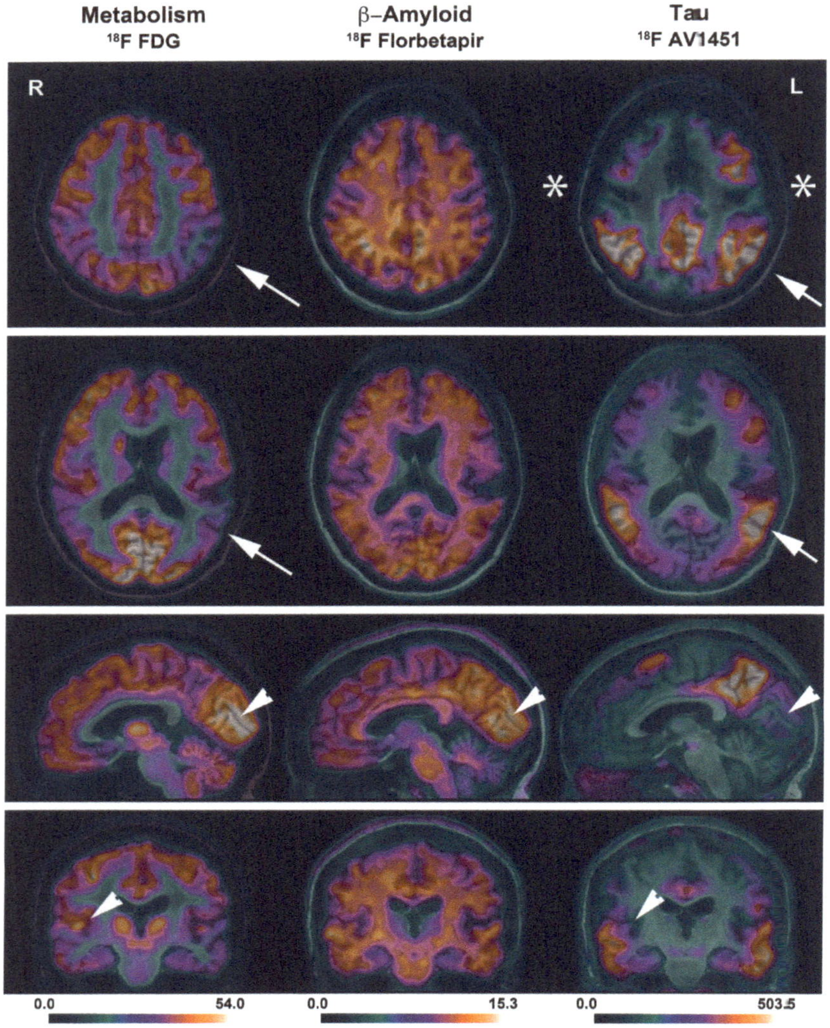

Fig. 26.22. Imaging findings in a patient with Alzheimer's disease (logopenic aphasia). Metabolism, abeta, and tau imaging from a 57-year-old woman with the logopenic-aphasia variety of Alzheimer's disease. The primary sensory-motor areas (asterisks), as well as the primary visual (striatal cortex) and auditory (Heschl's gyrus) regions (arrowheads), have normal metabolism and no tau deposition. By contrast, areas with high tau deposition (e.g., inferior parietal lobule, arrows) tend to have decreased metabolism. In some areas, high amyloid deposition corresponds to low metabolism and increased tau (e.g., the precuneus). However, there are areas with high amyloid load and normal metabolism, such as the medial occipital region. Uptake in the region of the substantia nigra does not correspond to tau deposition.

TSPO-binding compounds is strongly determined by the rs6971 polymorphism on the TSPO gene, leading to high- and low-affinity groups, as well as an intermediate phenotype. However, using a technique to determine binding in the intermediate phenotype, Kreisl et al. (2013b) have shown increased binding in regions typically affected in AD, particularly inferior-medial temporal regions, the inferior parietal lobule, and precuneus, but only a trend for hippocampus and precuneus in MCI. There was correlation with atrophy on MRI but not with abeta deposition when partial-volume correction was not used. Furthermore, binding correlated with several relevant cognitive measures (Kreisl et al., 2013b), suggesting that inflammation does not precede the disorder, but accompanies progressive neuronal loss as the clinical disease progresses. Findings in AD have been less impressive with another second-generation TSPO radioligand, ^{11}C-DAA1106 (Yasuno et al., 2012). Increased astrocytosis has been detected in AD with ^{11}C-DED PET (Carter et al., 2012).

Imaging in the evaluation of new AD therapies

Recent therapeutic trials with anti-abeta antibodies have benefited from the use of abeta imaging to determine the target effect of the medication (Sperling et al., 2011b).

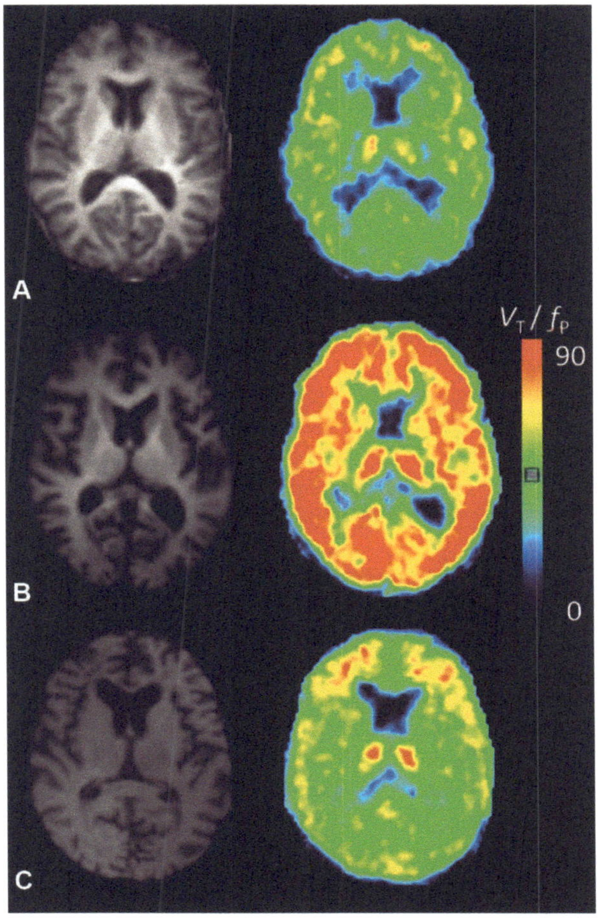

Fig. 26.23. Microglial activation imaged with ^{11}C-PBR28. From (**A**) a healthy control, (**B**) Alzheimer's disease, and (**C**) frontotemporal dementia. Note that the patient with Alzheimer's disease demonstrates diffuse increase in ^{11}C-PBR28 binding, whereas the frontotemporal dementia patient demonstrates increased binding localized to prefrontal cortex, where atrophy on magnetic resonance imaging is maximal. VT/fP, distribution volume corrected for plasma free fraction of radioligand. (Reproduced from Masdeu et al., 2012.)

Although improving or arresting the AD cognitive decline is the main goal of the new therapies, a more immediate need is to know whether abeta-removing therapies indeed remove abeta from the brain of the participants. Results from ^{11}C-PIB imaging have been reported for at least two therapeutic trials of abeta-removing antibodies (Ostrowitzki et al., 2012; Sperling et al., 2012) and abeta imaging has been built into protocols targeting abeta in the presymptomatic stages of AD (Sperling et al., 2014). Combined with MRI, abeta imaging has shown that some antibodies may remove abeta from the brain and that, in regions where the original concentration of abeta was higher, focal edema and microhemorrhages are more likely to develop (Sperling et al., 2012) (Fig. 26.24). These findings suggest that abeta is cleared at least in part through the vascular system of the brain, promoting increased vascular permeability and arteriolar wall fragility. Abeta deposition in arteriolar walls, causing increased fragility, was one of the neuropathologic observations from an earlier trial using an abeta vaccine (Ferrer et al., 2004). It is possible that immunotherapy in the preclinical stages, when amyloid levels may be lower, could minimize this untoward side effect, detectable by imaging (Fig. 26.24). As amyloid imaging has provided a powerful tool to evaluate target engagement, tau imaging may be used to evaluate therapies directed to tau spreading. Furthermore, the amount of tau load, measured with tau PET, could be used as an endpoint in trials testing the efficacy of abeta-removing therapies to arrest or slow down the deposition of abnormal tau in the brain of individuals at the presymptomatic stages of AD.

DIFFUSE LEWY-BODY DEMENTIA

Considered as the second most common neurodegenerative dementia (Graff-Radford et al., 2014), DLB is clinically characterized by progressive, but fluctuating, cognitive impairment accompanied by visual hallucinations, parkinsonism and, in many cases, rapid eye movement sleep disorder (McKeith et al., 2005). DLB is associated with Lewy-body pathology not restricted to the substantia nigra and nucleus locus coeruleus, as in classical Parkinson's disease (see Chapter 24), but widespread throughout the cortex. In addition to Lewy bodies, the neuropathology of DLB includes diffuse amyloid plaques (Kantarci et al., 2012b), rather than the rounded, circumscribed plaques of AD (Montine et al., 2012). Both types of plaques bind ^{11}C-PIB (Kantarci et al., 2012b). In about half of the cases, Alzheimer-type pathology is present in the same patient, complicating the nosology of clinical DLB (Nedelska et al., 2015). Many of the imaging features of AD are also present in DLB, namely, atrophy, decreased metabolism, and abeta deposition (Rowe et al., 2007). However, unlike in AD, in pure DLB there is little medial temporal atrophy (Nedelska et al., 2015). Furthermore, compared to AD, DLB is associated with decreased occipital metabolism on ^{18}F-FDG PET (Fig. 26.25) and with less total abeta deposition on ^{11}C-PIB PET, although about 80% of patients have abnormal ^{11}C-PIB PET (Kantarci et al., 2012b). In one study (Kantarci et al., 2012b), the combination of volumetry, metabolism, and abeta imaging distinguished well DLB from AD (area under the ROC = 0.98).

On studies of metabolism (^{18}F-FDG PET) or perfusion ($H_2{}^{15}O$ PET, SPECT, arterial spin labeling), the posterior cingulate island sign is helpful to distinguish DLB from AD. Whereas the posterior cingulate gyrus, by the

Table 26.4

Properties of translocator protein positron emission tomography (PET) tracers used in clinical studies

	Requires cyclotron at site	Allows for two PET studies in same visit*	Radiation exposure (in mSv)	Number of PubMed listings[†]	Signal-to-noise ratio
^{11}C PK1195	Yes	✓ Yes	✓ 5.1	✓ 92	Poor
^{11}C PBR28	Yes	✓ Yes	✓ 2.4	✓ 19	✓
^{11}C DAA1106	Yes	✓ Yes	?	5	✓
^{11}C Vinpocetine	Yes	✓ Yes	?	7	?
^{11}C DPA713	Yes	✓ Yes	?	3	?
^{18}F DPA714	✓ No	No	?	3	?
^{18}F FEDAA1106	✓ No	No	36	5	?
^{18}F FEPPA	✓ No	No	20.2	5	?
^{18}F PBR111	✓ No	No	?	4	?

PET tracers are listed in the left column by publication date. Checkmarks (✓) indicate the most advantageous tracer(s) for each property (listed in the top row).

*^{11}C, but not ^{18}F, compounds allow for the performance of two different scans the same day.

[†]As to December, 2014.

splenium of the corpus callosum, is uniformly hypometabolic or hypoperfused in AD, it is less so in DLB (Goker-Alpan et al., 2012; Graff-Radford et al., 2014) (Fig. 26.26). Dopaminergic markers, such as ^{18}F-FDOPA PET or ^{123}I-beta-CIT SPECT, are likely to show decreased striatal uptake in DLB disease (Fig. 26.27), but not in AD (Lim et al., 2009). Characteristically, the decrease is greatest at the tail of the putamen and less pronounced in anterior putamen and caudate (Goker-Alpan et al., 2012) (Fig. 26.27).

FRONTOTEMPORAL DEMENTIA

FTD or frontotemporal lobar degeneration is a group of diseases accounting for about 10–20% of all dementias worldwide. It affects a younger age group than AD: FTD occurs in about 3–15 per 100 000 individuals aged between 55 years and 65 years (Ferrari et al., 2014). Atrophy and white-matter abnormalities on MRI, decreased metabolism on FDG PET, and decreased perfusion on SPECT or arterial spin labeling tend to be regional and correspond well to the area preferentially affected by the pathology (Table 26.1) (Sapolsky et al., 2010; Kirshner, 2012; Zhang et al., 2013; Kerklaan et al., 2014; Agosta et al., 2015). Except for rare cases with motor neuron involvement, FTD, like AD, tends to affect association cortex, rather than primary motor or sensory cortices (Figs 26.5 and 26.18). Unlike AD, which tends to affect posterior brain regions, FDT tends to affect the anterior portion of the brain (Herholz, 2014). Hippocampal volume alone differentiates poorly AD from FTD; hippocampal sclerosis associated with FTD could explain the overlap (de Souza et al., 2013). Frontotemporal abnormalities on FDG PET/SPECT may antedate the atrophy that eventually becomes obvious on MRI (Fig. 26.28) (Foster et al., 2007; Mendez et al., 2007). For this reason, PET has been approved for FTD diagnosis by the US Centers for Medicare and Medicaid Services. Amyloid imaging is generally negative in the FTDs (Rowe et al., 2007). Tau imaging should be very helpful, but is only starting to be applied to FTD.

Clinically, anatomically, neuropathologically, and genetically, FTD comprises a heterogeneous set of disorders (Rascovsky et al., 2011) (Table 26.1). The clinical presentation depends on the region of the brain earliest and most affected by the disease (Sapolsky et al., 2010; Kirshner, 2012; Zhang et al., 2013; Agosta et al., 2015). It can present with a frontal-lobe syndrome, characterized by impulsivity and disinhibition, the so-called behavioral variant of FTD (bvFTD or classic Pick's disease, affecting the frontotemporal poles; Fig. 26.28) (Liscic et al., 2007; Whitwell et al., 2009), with an aphasic syndrome, named PPA (with left hemispheric involvement) (Gorno-Tempini et al., 2011), or with progressive prosopagnosia, when the anterior portion of the right temporal lobe is affected (Josephs et al., 2009). PPA can be either semantic (svPPA, involving predominantly the left temporal tip; Fig. 26.29) or nonfluent (nfvPPA, involving the left anterior perisylvian area; Fig. 26.5). There is a third PPA variant, termed logopenic aphasia (lvPPA, involving the left posterior perisylvian area; Fig. 26.22) (Gorno-Tempini et al., 2004) which is most often associated with AD, rather than FTD, pathology (Mesulam et al., 2014). FTD can also co-occur with motor neurone disease, and atypical parkinsonian disorders,

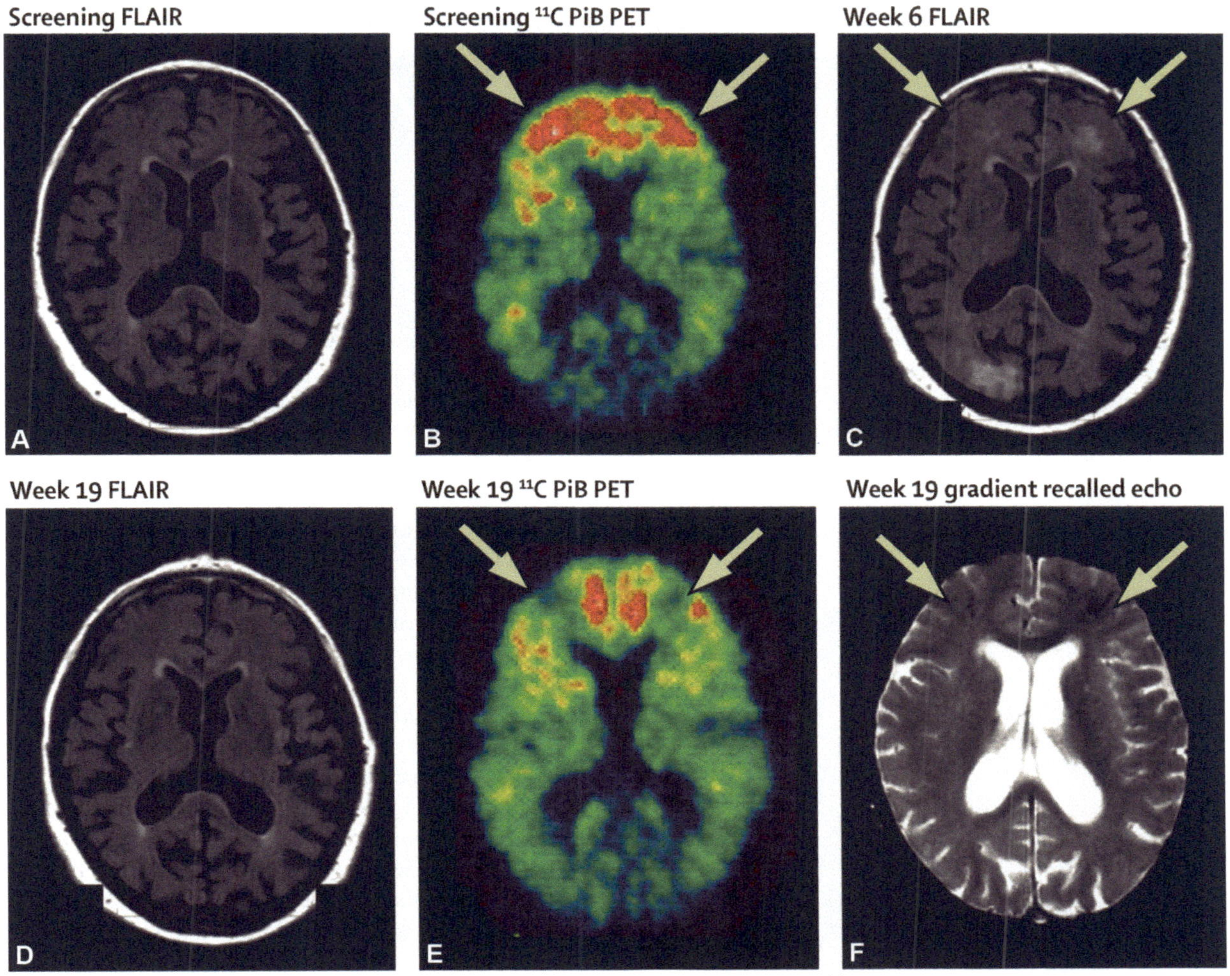

Fig. 26.24. Imaging in Alzheimer's disease therapy. Magnetic resonance imaging and ^{11}C Pittsburgh compound B (PIB) positron emission tomography scans of an apolipoprotein E ε4 heterozygote given bapineuzumab (2.0 mg/kg). The times indicated in the images represent time from bapineuzumab administration. (**A**) Baseline fluid-attenuated inversion recovery (FLAIR) image without evidence of ARIA-E. FLAIR sequence obtained at week 6 (**C**) shows bifrontal parenchymal hyperintensity (arrows: ARIA-E), which resolved by week 19 (**D**). Additionally, week 19 gradient-echo T2*-weighted sequence (**F**) shows the development of bifrontal microhemorrhages (ARIA-H: arrows) not present on previous images (not shown). A corresponding week 19 ^{11}C PIB scan (**E**) shows reduced ^{11}C PIB uptake (arrows) compared with that at baseline in regions with ARIA-E and ARIA-H (arrows: **B**). ARIA-E, amyloid-related imaging abnormalities thought to be parenchymal vasogenic edema and sulcal effusions; ARIA-H, amyloid-related imaging abnormalities thought to be a result of microhemorrhages and hemosiderosis. (Reproduced from Sperling et al., 2012.)

DLB

AD

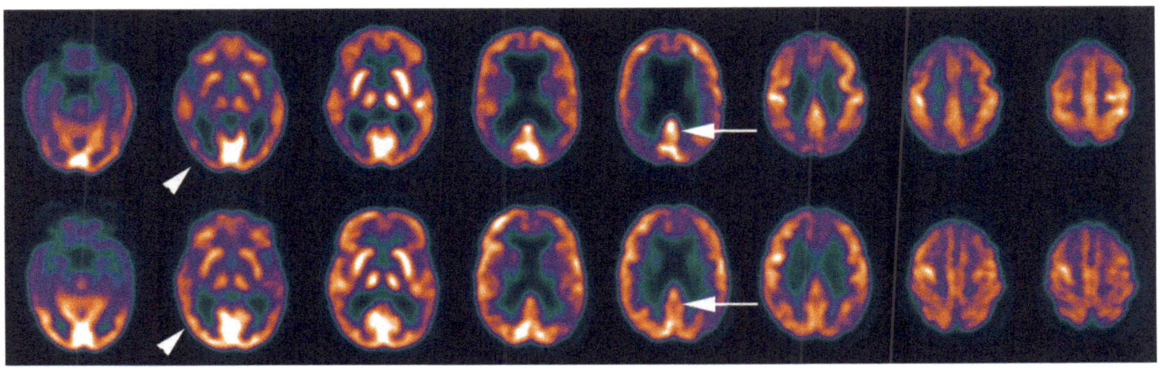

Fig. 26.25. Metabolism in diffuse Lewy-body disease (DLB). ^{18}F-2-deoxy-2-fluoro-D-glucose positron emission tomography from a 75-year-old man with DLB showing decreased metabolism in the lateral aspect of the occipital lobes (arrowheads) while having greater metabolism than the patient with Alzheimer's disease (AD) in the posterior cingulate region (arrows).

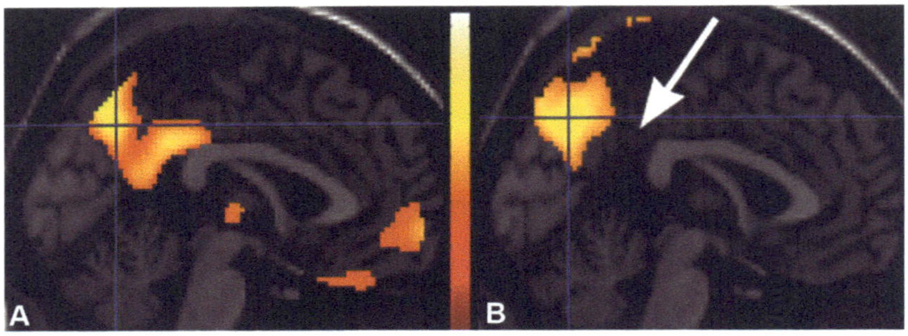

Fig. 26.26. "Island sign" in diffuse Lewy-body disease (DLB). On magnetic resonance imaging templates of the medial aspect of the brain, areas of decreased metabolism (^{18}F-2-deoxy-2-fluoro-D-glucose positron emission tomography) in Alzheimer's disease (AD) and decreased perfusion ($H_2{}^{15}O$-PET) in DLB. Metabolism and perfusion are coupled in AD and DLB. Note involvement of the posterior cingulate gyrus in AD, but sparing of this region (arrow) in DLB. (Modified from Goker-Alpan et al., 2012.)

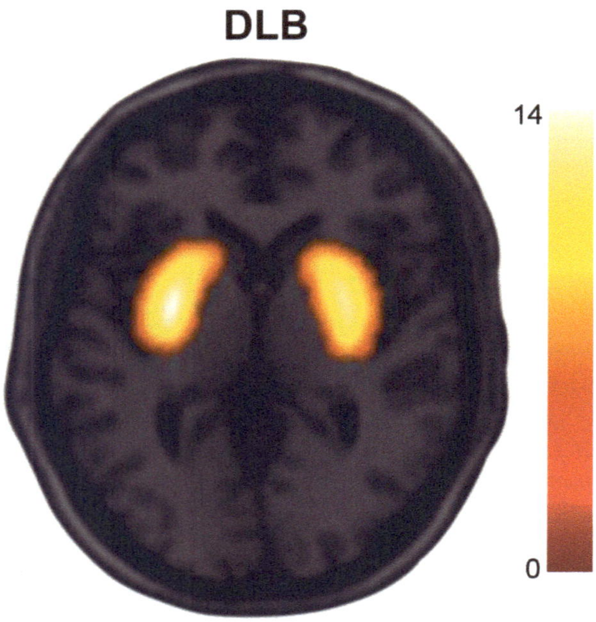

Fig. 26.27. Decreased presynaptic dopamine in diffuse Lewy-body disease (DLB). On an axial magnetic resonance imaging template, areas of decreased presynaptic dopamine (^{18}F-FDOPA-PET) in a sample of patients with DLB. (Reproduced from Goker-Alpan et al., 2012.)

such as corticobasal degeneration and progressive supranuclear palsy. These two disorders are associated to tau pathology, and their clinical and pathologic features overlap: the clinical syndrome of progressive supranuclear palsy can be associated with corticobasal degeneration pathology, and vice versa (Josephs et al., 2011; Whitwell et al., 2013). The clinical syndromes correspond to well-defined neuroimaging. At stages beyond the initial gait impairment, progressive supranuclear palsy is relatively easy to diagnose clinically by the characteristic parkinsonism associated with markedly impaired postural reflexes and downward-gaze palsy; frank dementia, of a frontal-lobe type, only supervenes as the disease advances. MRI shows minimal frontal atrophy (Agosta et al., 2015) but remarkable midbrain atrophy (hummingbird sign; Fig. 26.30), such that a decreased midbrain to pons area ratio on sagittal images distinguishes well this disorder (Massey et al., 2013). Corticobasal degeneration is characterized by progressive apraxia, accompanied by apractic agraphia when the left hemisphere is affected. Typically, both atrophy and decreased metabolism affect the superior parietal lobule (Fig. 26.31). This is the area of representation of the hand: thus corticobasal degeneration causes apraxia, while PPA, involving the perisylvian cortex, which subserves the mouth region of the motor strip (Fig. 26.5), is associated with aphasia.

FTD pathology is heterogeneous and based on the type of neuronal lesions and protein inclusions: 40% or more of patients have tau pathology, about 50% have TAR DNA-binding protein 43 (TDP-43) pathology, and the remaining 10% have inclusions positive for fused-in sarcoma (FUS) or ubiquitin/p62 (Ferrari et al., 2014). There is a loose correspondence between the underlying pathology and the cortical location of the damage, which determines the clinical and imaging findings (Josephs et al., 2011) (Fig. 26.32). While bvFTD is associated with tau and TDP, as well as, rarely, FUS, semantic dementia and any motor syndrome are more often associated with TDP. All the other types of FTD are associated more often, but not always, with tau (Fig. 26.32). The advent of tau imaging should greatly help characterize the neuropathology in a given case, although it is to be determined whether ^{18}F-AV-1451 and similar compounds bind to all types of tau tangles or miss some of them, such as the globose tangles of progressive supranuclear palsy. The importance of developing a TDP-43 PET ligand becomes clear from these data and from the recent studies emphasizing the correlation of TDP-43 pathology with cognitive impairment in AD (Josephs et al., 2014b).

Mutations in three main genes are commonly associated with FTD: the microtubule-associated protein tau

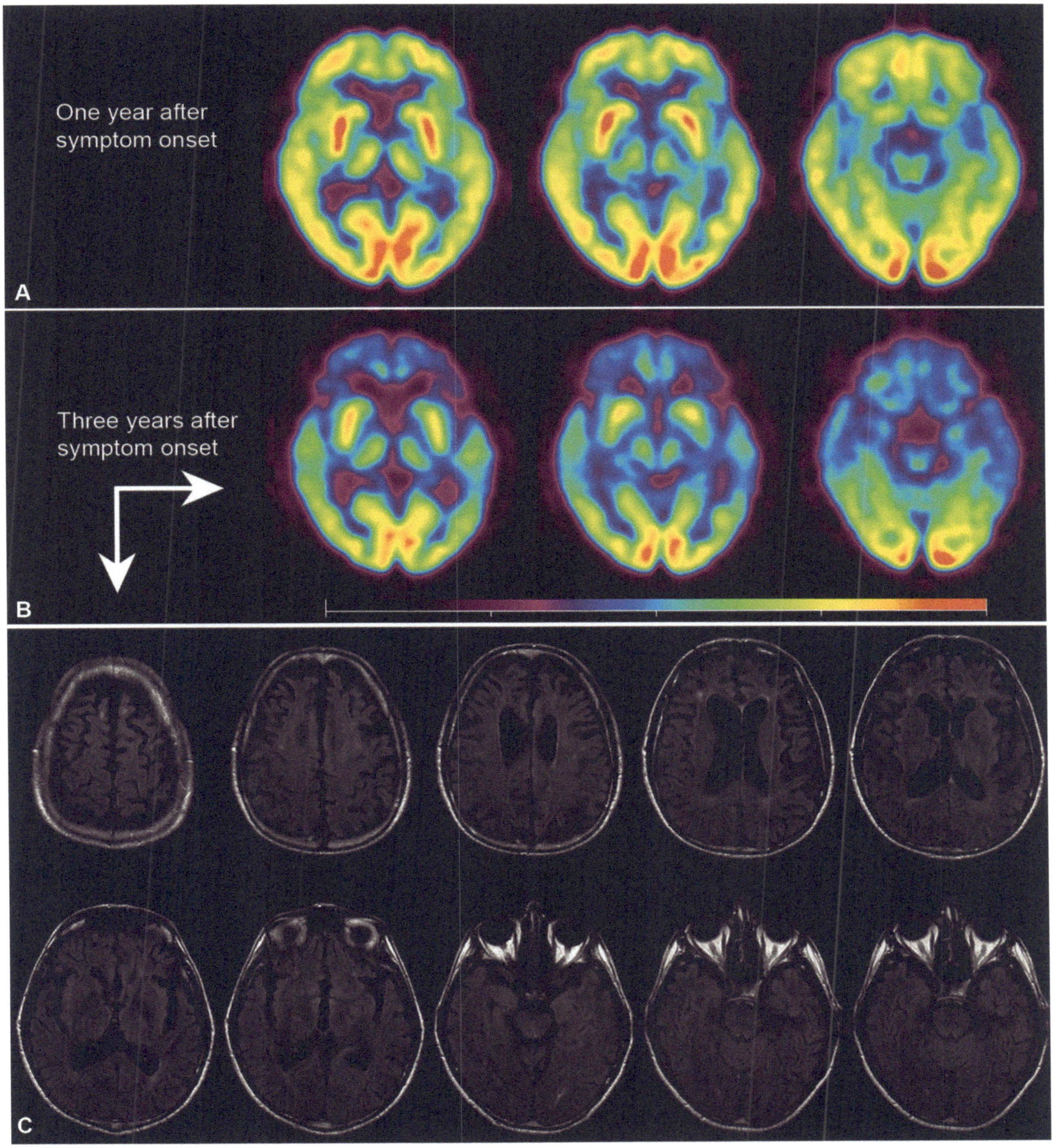

Fig. 26.28. Behavioral form of frontotemporal dementia. Shown are ^{18}F-2-deoxy-2-fluoro-D-glucose positron emission tomography (FDG)-positron emission tomography (PET) (**A, B**) and fluid-attenuated inversion recovery magnetic resonance imaging (MRI) (**C**) studies from a 51-year-old man with progressive speech apraxia and impaired planning, to the point of mutism and complete dependency for activities of daily living when studies **B** and **C** were obtained, on the same day. Metabolism was already decreased on the initial PET study, particularly on the frontal opercula and temporal tips, but it is much more obvious on the follow-up study, showing extensive frontotemporal hypometabolism. Note that the frontotemporal abnormality is much more obvious on the PET study (**A, B**) than on the MRI study (**C**), which shows frontal atrophy. (Reproduced from Masdeu, 2008.)

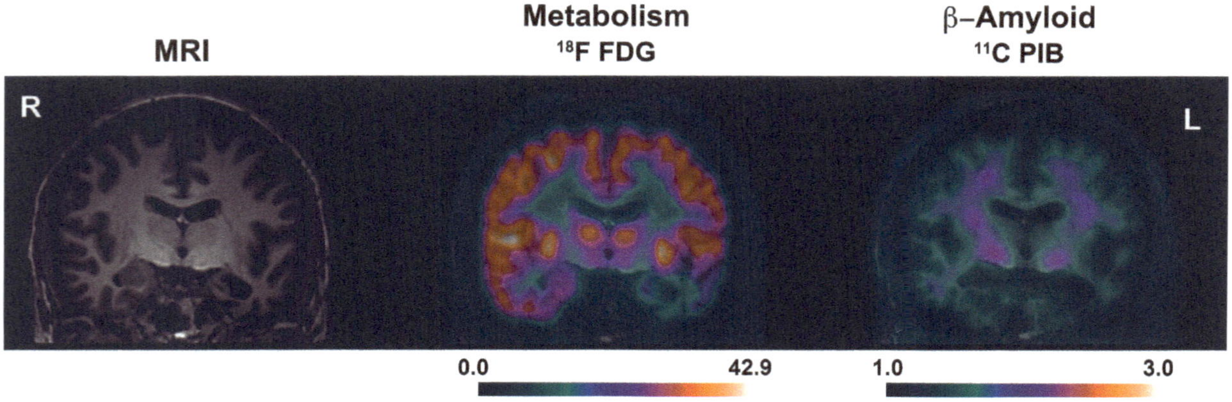

Fig. 26.29. Semantic dementia. Metabolism (^{18}F-2-deoxy-2-fluoro-D-glucose positron emission tomography: FDG) and abeta (^{11}C-PIB) positron emission tomography data superimposed to the magnetic resonance imaging (MRI) of a 65-year-old man with marked anomia, but preserved repetition. Note the marked left anterior temporal atrophy. Metabolism is markedly decreased on the left, but also, to a lesser degree, on the right temporal tip.

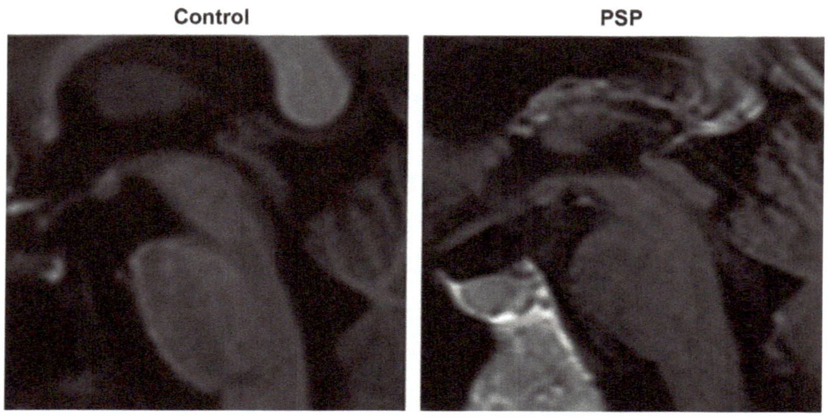

Fig. 26.30. Midbrain atrophy in progressive supranuclear palsy (PSP). Sagittal T1-weighted magnetic resonance imaging from a 79-year-old woman with PSP shows marked atrophy of the midbrain, which has the appearance of a hummingbird (hummingbird sign). Compare with the morphology of the midbrain at the same level in a healthy individual of a similar age.

(*MAPT*), granulin (*GRN*), and *C9orf72* (Ferrari et al., 2014). Mutations in the charged multivesicular body protein 2B (*CHMP2B*), the valosin-containing protein (*VCP*), and ubiquilin 2 (*UBQLN2*) genes are rare causes of FTD. However, less than 20% of patients have identified mutations; this proportion may change as deeper genetic studies are conducted. Predisposing to FTD are variants of some genes, such as *TMEM106B*, *RAB38/CTSC*, and a gene at the human leukocyte antigen locus, implicating the immune system (Ferrari et al., 2014). Unfortunately, there is little correspondence between the cortical location of the damage –and thus the clinical and imaging findings – and the type of mutation, suggesting that the damage is mediated by still poorly understood neurobiologic mechanisms. However, *MAPT* mutations have been associated with greater anteromedial temporal atrophy, and *GRN* mutations with greater parietal atrophy, while *C9ORF72* mutations were associated with symmetric atrophy predominantly involving dorsolateral, medial, and orbitofrontal lobes, with additional loss in anterior temporal lobes, parietal lobes, occipital lobes, and cerebellum (Whitwell et al., 2012b) (Fig. 26.33). In a longitudinal follow-up, whole-brain atrophy progressed faster with *GRN* mutations than with those in *C9ORF72* or *MAPT*. *C9ORF72* mutations showed greater rates of atrophy in the left cerebellum and right occipital lobe than *MAPT* (Whitwell et al., 2015a).

Altered connectivity

As in AD, connectivity in FTD has been studied with BOLD fMRI and with techniques that use diffusion imaging on MR, such as DTI and kurtosis.

Functional connectivity (BOLD fMRI)

Pathologic and compensatory mechanisms in FTD result in abnormal functional connectivity across networks. Specific network changes depend on the cortical regions most

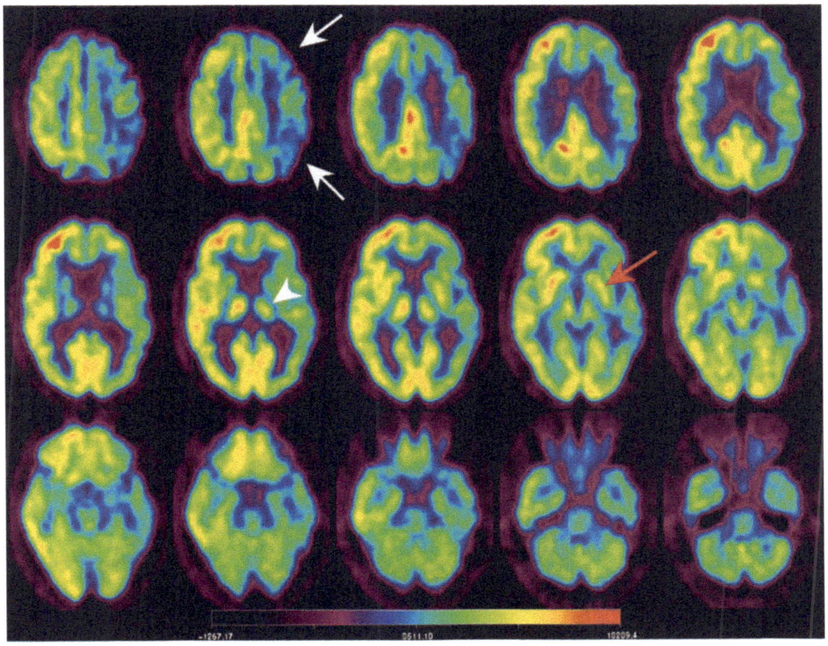

Fig. 26.31. Metabolism in corticobasal degeneration. Axial sections of an ^{18}F-2-deoxy-2-fluoro-D-glucose (FDG) positron emission tomography (PET) study from a 47-year-old man with progressive agraphia and apraxia, as well as right-sided parkinsonism. Metabolism in the association cortex of the frontal and parietal lobe is decreased (white arrows), as well as in the ipsilateral thalamus (arrowhead) and lenticular nucleus (red arrow). Note that the greatest decrease in metabolism is in the higher sections, corresponding to the area of representation of the hand in the motor strip. (Reproduced from Masdeu, 2008.)

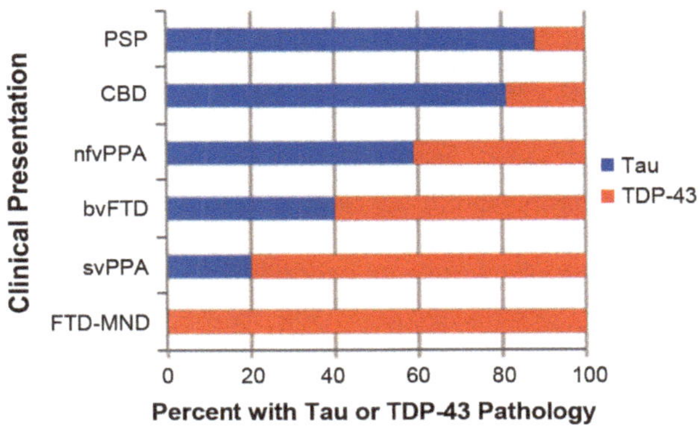

Fig. 26.32. Misfolded tau or TAR DNA-binding protein 43 (TDP-43) in the frontotemporal dementias. Percentages of cases with each of the clinical syndromes that have either tau or TDP-43 as the predominant brain pathology. PSP, progressive supranuclear palsy; CBD, corticobasal degeneration; nfvPPA, nonfluent primary progressive aphasia; bvFTD, behavioral variant of frontotemporal dementia; svPPA, semantic variant of primary progressive aphasia; FTD-MND, frontotemporal dementia– motor neuron disease. (Data from Josephs et al., 2011.)

affected by a given variety of FTD. Thus, bvFTD affects the emotional salience network, while svPPA affects the anterior portion of the semantic network, corresponding to a temporal pole–subgenual cingulate–ventral striatum–amygdala network (Guo et al., 2013). nfvPPA affects the frontal operculum, primary and supplementary motor cortices, and inferior parietal lobule bilaterally, linking the language and motor systems that enable speech fluency (Seeley et al., 2009). Asymmetric degeneration of this system may reflect its accentuated functional and connectional asymmetry in healthy humans.

lvPPA shows reduced connectivity in left temporal language network and inferior parietal and prefrontal regions of the left working-memory network compared with controls and typical AD (Whitwell et al., 2015c). Both groups show reduced connectivity in the parietal regions of the right working-memory network compared with controls. Only typical AD shows reduced ventral default-mode network connectivity compared with controls (Whitwell et al., 2015c).

Diffusion tensor imaging or kurtosis

In FTD, decreased fractional anisotropy or increased radial diffusivity is identified in tracts that interconnect the gray-matter regions that are atrophic, supporting the hypothesis that varieties of FTD involve different and specific brain networks (Whitwell et al., 2010). In FTD, white-matter changes involve the superior longitudinal fasciculus, uncinate fasciculus, cingulum bundle, and corpus callosum (Mahoney et al., 2014). When compared to AD, FTD is associated with greater fractional anisotropy reduction in frontal brain regions, as well as in the

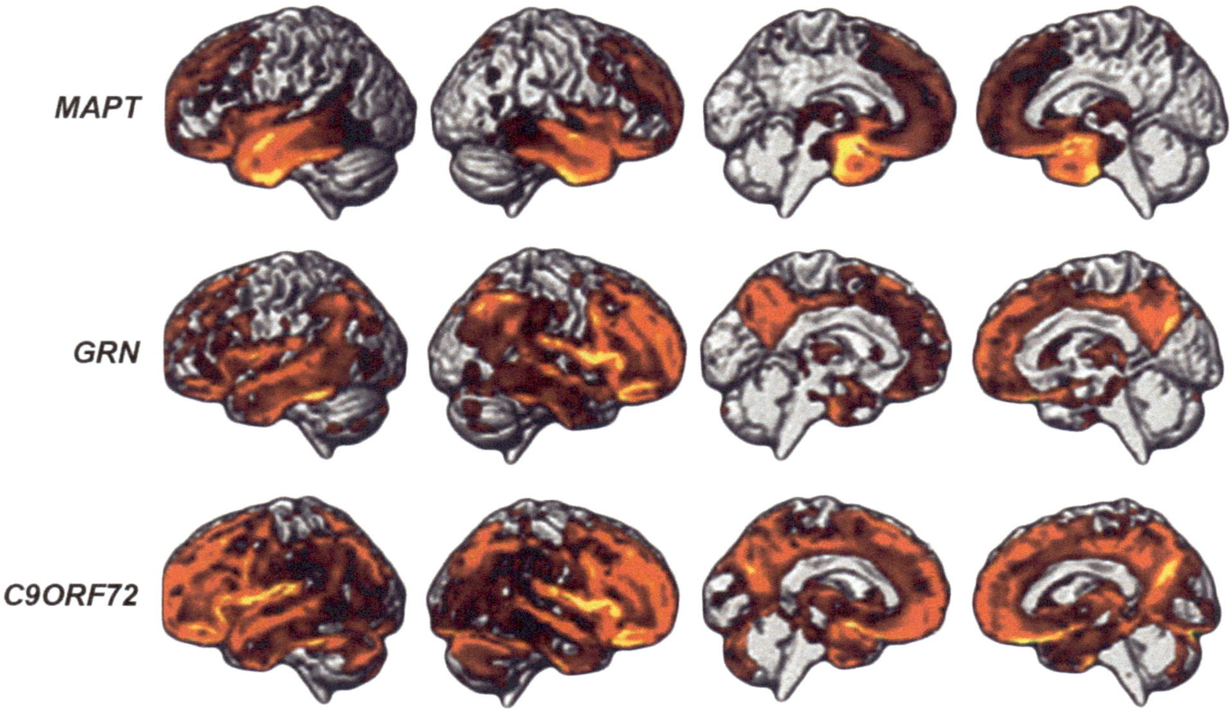

Fig. 26.33. Brain atrophy patterns associated with mutations in *MAPT*, *GRN*, and *C9ORF72*. In yellow-red and projected on rendered images, areas of the brain with significant atrophy in groups of patients with mutations in each of the three genes. (Reproduced from Whitwell et al., 2012b.) With permission from Oxford University Press.

anterior corpus callosum (Zhang et al., 2009; McMillan et al., 2012).

In bvFTD, abnormal white-matter diffusivity is observed in frontal white matter (Whitwell et al., 2010; Agosta et al., 2012; Maruyama et al., 2013), and the orbitofrontal and anterior temporal tracts (Lam et al., 2014), as well as the anterior cingulum bundle (Santillo et al., 2013).

Main language tracts are affected in the three variants of PPA. In nfvPPA, white-matter changes are observed in the pathways connecting the speech production network, with tract abnormalities observed in the superior longitudinal fasciculus, and reductions of fractional anisotropy and increased mean diffusivity in the left inferior frontal lobe, insula, supplementary motor area, and striatal regions (Whitwell et al., 2010; Galantucci et al., 2011; Zhang et al., 2013; Mandelli et al., 2014). The frontal aslant tract, connecting Broca's region with the anterior cingulate and presupplementary motor area, is affected in nfvPPA but not in svPPA, and seems to be involved in verbal fluency, more than in grammatic or repetition processes (Catani et al., 2013). In svPPA, the main changes are identified in the pathways connecting the semantic processing network, with tract abnormalities observed in the inferior longitudinal fasciculus and uncinate fasciculus, predominantly in the left anterior temporal lobe (Whitwell et al., 2010; Agosta et al., 2012; Galantucci et al., 2011; Catani et al., 2013; Zhang et al., 2013; Mandelli et al., 2014). Language tracts are more preserved in patients with lvPPA and the principal white-matter changes are observed in the temporoparietal component of the cingulum bundle (Galantucci et al., 2011).

Progression of white-matter diffusivity changes over time may be more pronounced and specific than progression of gray-matter changes in FTD (Sajjadi et al., 2013; Lam et al., 2014). In one study (Lam et al., 2014) mean diffusivity was most sensitive in detecting baseline changes while fractional anisotropy and radial diffusivity revealed greatest changes over time. Disease progression involved posterior temporal and occipital white matter in bvFTD, right frontotemporal white matter in nfvPPA, and bilateral frontotemporal tracts in svPPA (Lam et al., 2014). In another study with 1-year follow-up, all patients with nfvPPA evolved to either corticobasal degeneration or progressive supranuclear palsy, and showed white-matter abnormalities involving the entire cerebrum, suggesting a diffuse pathologic process in the white matter of these tauopathies and not merely a function of disease severity, since gray-matter analysis consisting of group-level voxel-based morphometry revealed only focal areas of atrophy (Sajjadi et al., 2013). Patients with AD and svPPA did not show this degree of white-matter changes.

According to analyses based on small numbers of genetic cases of bvFTD, *MAPT* mutation shows consistent alterations in left uncinate fasciculus across diffusivity metrics (Lam et al., 2014; Mahoney et al., 2014, 2015). Alterations detected in the *C9ORF72* mutation are less extensive and involve the corpus callosum and cingulum bundle. On direct comparison of *MAPT* with *C9ORF72,* those with *MAPT* showed alterations in white matter within the left anterior temporal pole, as measured by reduced fractional anisotropy. However, there are not differences between patients with *MAPT* and *C9ORF72* mutations and those with sporadic bvFTD (Mahoney et al., 2014, 2015).

Metabolism

Memory test performance may not distinguish between AD and FTD dementia syndromes (Frisch et al., 2013). In clinical practice, this may lead to misdiagnosis of FTD patients with poor memory performance. However, whereas in AD patients memory test performance correlates with ^{18}F-FDG PET changes in precuneus, performance in FTD patients correlates with changes in frontal cortex, with little overlap between the two disorders (Piolino et al., 2007; Frisch et al., 2013). In FTD, many studies have found decreased metabolic activity in frontal and temporal regions of the cortex, as well as some subcortical regions, such as the caudate nucleus or thalamus (Salmon et al., 2003; Diehl et al., 2004; Jeong et al., 2005; Foster et al., 2007; Kanda et al., 2008; Mosconi et al., 2008; Teune et al., 2010) (Figs 26.5, 26.28, 26.29, and 26.31). As the disease worsens, from the frontal and anterotemporal regions the metabolic changes spread into the parietal and posterior temporal cortices (Diehl-Schmid et al., 2007).

In the clinic, ^{18}F-FDG PET in FTD is commonly reserved for patients with suspected FTD without characteristic structural neuroimaging results. Nearly half of the patients with early bvFTD, but a normal MRI, have an abnormal ^{18}F-FDG PET, thus helping to exclude psychiatric and other neurodegenerative disorders (Kerklaan et al., 2014). Language phenotype in PPA is closely related to metabolic changes that are focal and anatomically distinct among subtypes (Rabinovici et al., 2008). Most patients with nfvPPA show asymmetric left frontal and insular hypometabolism (Fig. 26.5), sdPPA patients show prominent bilateral anterior temporal hypometabolism, left greater than right (Fig. 26.29), and finally, patients with lvPPA show the greatest metabolic decrements in the left parietal and posterolateral temporal lobes, but also in the left frontal lobe (Fig. 26.22). In lvPPE, there is greater left laterotemporal hypometabolism, and less right temporomedial and posterior cingulate hypometabolism than in overall AD (Madhavan et al., 2013). Focal decreased metabolism correlates well with focal atrophy and their severity correlates well with the severity of language impairment (Gorno-Tempini et al., 2011). To date, mutations associated with FTD have failed to show a pattern of metabolism helpful to discriminate different genotypes, possibly because the sample sizes were small (Jacova et al., 2013; Josephs et al., 2014a). However, ^{18}F-FDG PET may be useful to detect brain changes in subjects carrying a FTD-obligatory mutation (Deters et al., 2014).

Amyloid deposition

Because pathologic abeta deposition is a key component of AD but not a feature of FTD, amyloid PET is a valuable clinical tool to differentiate AD from FTD, especially in young patients in whom age-related amyloid deposition is less common. Studies on amyloid PET have shown very low rates of ^{11}C-PIB, ^{18}F-florbetapir, or ^{18}F-florbetaben positivity in most FTD patients, providing good discrimination from AD (Rabinovici et al., 2007, 2011; Villemagne et al., 2011a; Kobylecki et al., 2015). However, visual rating of FTD scans is challenging, with a higher rate of discordance between raters than when they have to separate AD from control subjects (Kobylecki et al., 2015). For this reason, software packages are being built to facilitate the comparison of individual scans with reference data, as has been done with ^{18}F-FDG PET (Thiele et al., 2013; Herholz, 2014).

In patients with PPA, the level of abeta burden varies considerably across different variants (Rabinovici et al., 2008; Leyton et al., 2011; Ikeda et al., 2014). Abnormal ^{11}C-PIB retention can be identified in most patients with lvPPA (Rabinovici et al., 2008; Leyton et al., 2011; Whitwell et al., 2015b), confirming that this variant represents a common presentation of AD. Abeta distribution across cortical regions is identical in lvPPA and in typical AD, although the total load is lower in the aphasic cases (Leyton et al., 2011). Among the small proportion of patients with lvPPA who do not have abeta deposition, up to 50% may have *GRN* mutations (Josephs et al., 2014a).

Increased ^{11}C-PIB is uncommon in patients with the nonfluent or semantic variants, confirming that these PPA variants are rarely associated with AD pathology (Drzezga et al., 2008; Mormino et al., 2009; Leyton et al., 2011). Occasional ^{11}C-PIB-positive scans of patients with nfvPPA and svPPA present amyloid deposition patterns similar to AD, but with lesser amounts of amyloid (Rabinovici et al., 2008; Leyton et al., 2011). However, these patients had metabolism studies characteristic of their type of FTD, not AD. It is possible that the amyloid deposition was an age-related phenomenon, not linked to the disease (Rabinovici et al., 2008, 2011).

Inflammation

Inflammation has seldom been imaged in FTD (Fig. 26.22), but both genetic studies (Ferrari et al., 2014) and studies looking at associations with autoimmune disease (Miller et al., 2013) suggest that immune mechanisms may be important in the sporadic form of FTD, particularly in TDP-43 FTD. In a small pilot study (Cagnin et al., 2004), ^{11}C-PK11195 PET showed increased binding in the typically affected frontotemporal brain regions.

NETWORK ABNORMALITIES IN FTD AND AD

It is likely that a better understanding of their neurobiology will change the nosologic understanding of AD and FTD. Using MRI and PET, a key step in this direction has been taken by disclosing network properties in these disorders. AD and other neurodegenerative dementias are characterized by cortex thinning, more profound and extensive as the disease worsens (Dickerson et al., 2009). This thinning is not uniform across the brain, but involves areas that are highly specific for each disorder, so much so that "cortical signatures" have been described for AD and each of the FTD disorders (Fig. 26.34)

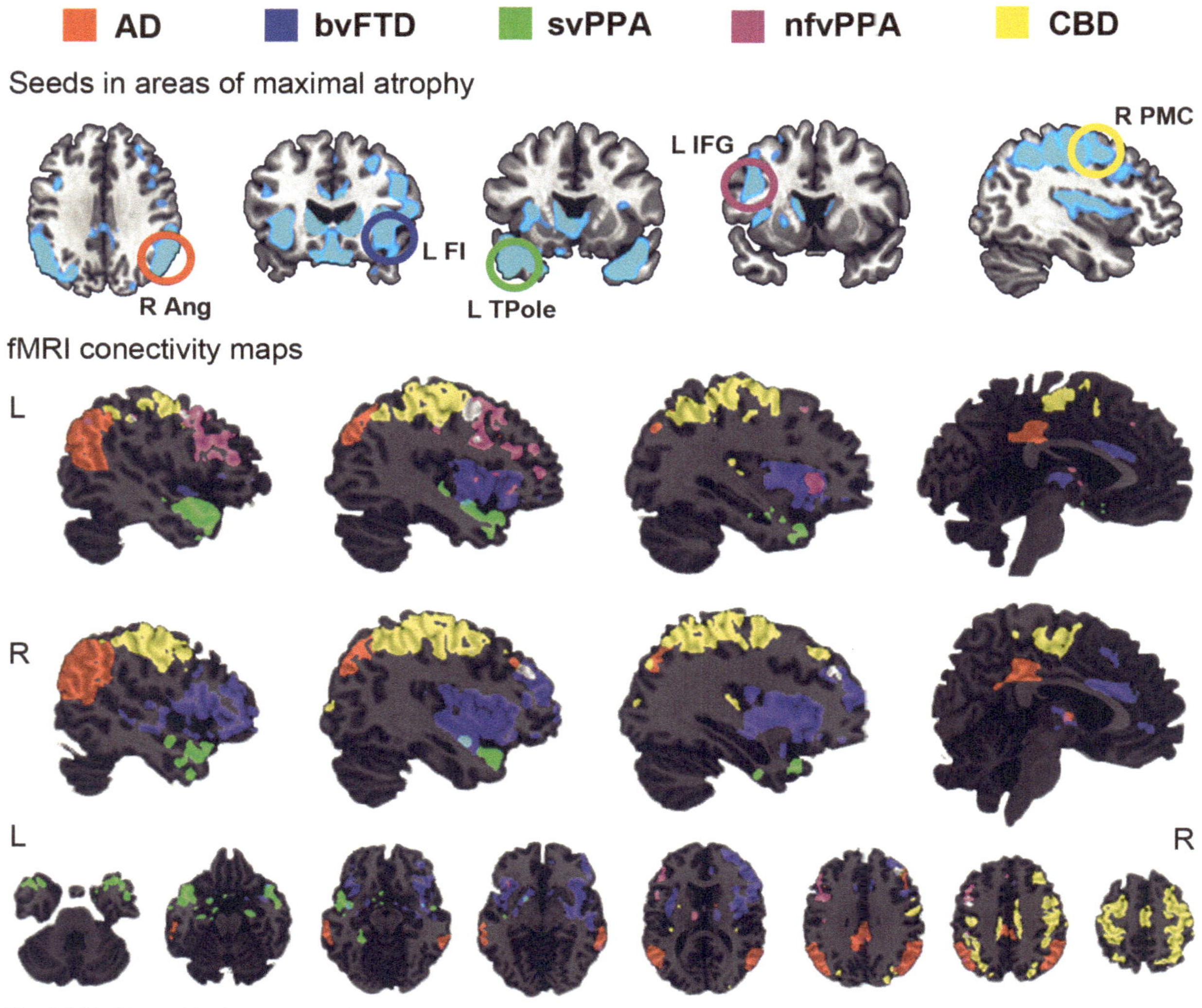

Fig. 26.34. Natural brain networks affected in each neurodegenerative phenotype. Seeds in areas of early and maximal atrophy in each dementia phenotype (top row) have predominant functional connectivity on blood oxygen level-dependent magnetic resonance imaging to distinct and characteristic brain networks, which become progressively affected as the disease worsens. AD, Alzheimer's disease; bvFTD, behavioral variant of frontotemporal dementia; svPPA, semantic variant of primary progressive aphasia; nfvPPA, nonfluent primary progressive aphasia; CBD, corticobasal degeneration; R Ang, right angular gyrus; R FI, right inferior frontal gyrus; L TPole, left temporal pole; L IFG, left inferior frontal gyrus; R PMC, right premotor cortex; fMRI, functional magnetic resonance imaging. (Reproduced from Seeley et al., 2009.)

(Dickerson et al., 2009; Seeley et al., 2009). Remarkably, when the area first developing thinning in each dementing disorder is used as a seed to study with fMRI its physiologic resting functional connectivity with the rest of the brain, it turns out that it connects most strongly with those areas which will be subsequently affected in the same disorder (Fig. 26.34) (Seeley et al., 2009; Zhou et al., 2012; Lehmann et al., 2013b). More recently, similar network relationships have been shown with amyloid imaging in AD (Sepulcre and Masdeu, 2015). Thus, the Hebbian principle, "neurons that fire together, wire together" (Hebb, 1961) has been extended to say: "neurons that wire together, die together" (Sepulcre et al., 2012). This finding, coupled with animal data showing that abnormal tau (de Calignon et al., 2012; Liu et al., 2012) or α-synuclein (Luk et al., 2012) can propagate transsynaptically from neuron to neuron in a prion-like fashion, has strengthened the hypothesis that neurodegenerative dementias are disorders of misfolded proteins propagating across brain networks and causing neuronal death (Prusiner, 2013).

In this scenario, inflammatory cells could be targeting neurons headed for apoptosis, or apoptotic byproducts, but they could also be pathogenetic (Fig. 26.2). For instance, through a prion-like mechanism misfolded proteins could change the antigenic properties of healthy neurons, making them the target of autoimmune attack (Franklin et al., 2014). Imaging tau and inflammation using PET compounds in patients being treated with immune therapy could help clarify these processes.

CONCLUSION

In the past few years, neuroimaging has provided powerful data on the neurobiologic changes associated with the disorders causing dementia. Imaging is emerging as a powerful biomarker to define target engagement in therapeutic trials. However, much work remains. Only recently, the correlation of imaging changes with gene variants or mutations predisposing to the various disorders has been undertaken on a large scale. Epistatic effects should now be evaluated more extensively, and work should continue on epigenetic factors influencing the development of abeta deposition and markers of neurodegeneration. Studies with PET markers of inflammation, combined with abeta, tau, and morphometric imaging, should provide data on the likelihood that inflammation in AD and other disorders is reactive or causal. The effect of therapies aimed at reducing abeta deposition or tau spread in the preclinical stages of the disease, when cognition is normal, needs to be monitored with neuroimaging.

FUNDING

This work was supported by the Nantz National Alzheimer Center, Houston Methodist Neurological Institute, and the Houston Methodist Research Institute.

ACKNOWLEDGMENTS AND POTENTIAL CONFLICTS OF INTEREST

Dr. Masdeu is a consultant for the General Electric Company. During the writing of this chapter he was the Editor-in-Chief of the *Journal of Neuroimaging.*

ABBREVIATIONS

^{18}F-FDG ^{18}F-2-deoxy-2-fluoro-D-glucose; AD Alzheimer's disease; APOE apoliprotein E; ASL arterial spin labeling; BOLD blood oxygenation level-dependent; bvFTD behavioral variant of frontotemporal dementia; CADASIL cerebral autosomal-dominant arteriopathy with subcortical infarcts and leukoencephalopathy; CBD corticobasal degeneration; CSF cerebrospinal fluid; CT computed tomography; CTE chronic traumatic encephalopathy; DLB diffuse Lewy-body dementia; DTI diffusion tensor imaging; DWI diffusion-weighted imaging; FLAIR fluid-attenuated inversion recovery; fMRI functional magnetic resonance imaging; FTD frontotemporal dementia; *GRN* progranulin gene; lvPPA logopenic aphasia; MCI mild cognitive impairment; MND-FTD frontotemporal dementia with motor neuron disease findings; MRI magnetic resonance imaging; nfvPPA nonfluent primary progressive aphasia; PET positron emission tomography; PPA primary progressive aphasia; PSP progressive supranuclear palsy; ROC receiver operating characteristic; SPECT single-photon emission computed tomography; svFTD semantic variant of frontotemporal dementia; TBI traumatic brain injury; TSPO translocator protein

References

Agosta F, Pievani M, Sala S et al. (2011). White matter damage in Alzheimer disease and its relationship to gray matter atrophy. Radiology 258: 853–863.

Agosta F, Scola E, Canu E et al. (2012). White matter damage in frontotemporal lobar degeneration spectrum. Cereb Cortex 22: 2705–2714.

Agosta F, Galantucci S, Magnani G et al. (2015). MRI signatures of the frontotemporal lobar degeneration continuum. Hum Brain Mapp 36: 2602–2614.

Albert MS, DeKosky ST, Dickson D et al. (2011). The diagnosis of mild cognitive impairment due to Alzheimer's disease: recommendations from the National Institute on Aging-Alzheimer's Association workgroups on diagnostic guidelines for Alzheimer's disease. Alzheimers Dement 7: 270–279.

American Psychiatric Association (1994). Diagnostic and statistical manual of mental disorders: DSM-IV. American Psychiatric Association, Washington, DC.

American Psychiatric Association (2013). Diagnostic and statistical manual of mental disorders: DSM-5. American Psychiatric Association, Washington, DC.

Apostolova LG, Hwang KS, Medina LD et al. (2011). Cortical and hippocampal atrophy in patients with autosomal dominant familial Alzheimer's disease. Dement Geriatr Cogn Disord 32: 118–125.

Bacskai BJ, Frosch MP, Freeman SH et al. (2007). Molecular imaging with Pittsburgh Compound B confirmed at autopsy: a case report. Arch Neurol 64: 431–434.

Bakkour A, Morris JC, Wolk DA et al. (2013). The effects of aging and Alzheimer's disease on cerebral cortical anatomy: specificity and differential relationships with cognition. Neuroimage 76: 332–344.

Ballard CG, Burton EJ, Barber R et al. (2004). NINDS AIREN neuroimaging criteria do not distinguish stroke patients with and without dementia. Neurology 63: 983–988.

Barnes DE, Kaup A, Kirby KA et al. (2014). Traumatic brain injury and risk of dementia in older veterans. Neurology 83: 312–319.

Barrio JR, Small GW, Wong KP et al. (2015). In vivo characterization of chronic traumatic encephalopathy using [F-18]FDDNP PET brain imaging. Proc Natl Acad Sci U S A 112: E2039–E2047.

Bateman RJ, Xiong C, Benzinger TL et al. (2012). Clinical and biomarker changes in dominantly inherited Alzheimer's disease. N Engl J Med 367: 795–804.

Becker JA, Hedden T, Carmasin J et al. (2011). Amyloid-beta associated cortical thinning in clinically normal elderly. Ann Neurol 69: 1032–1042.

Boles Ponto LL, Magnotta VA, Moser DJ et al. (2006). Global cerebral blood flow in relation to cognitive performance and reserve in subjects with mild memory deficits. Mol Imaging Biol 8: 363–372.

Bondi MW, Houston WS, Eyler LT et al. (2005). fMRI evidence of compensatory mechanisms in older adults at genetic risk for Alzheimer disease. Neurology 64: 501–508.

Bookheimer SY, Strojwas MH, Cohen MS et al. (2000). Patterns of brain activation in people at risk for Alzheimer's disease. N Engl J Med 343: 450–456.

Bozoki AC, Korolev IO, Davis NC et al. (2012). Disruption of limbic white matter pathways in mild cognitive impairment and Alzheimer's disease: a DTI/FDG-PET study. Hum Brain Mapp 33: 1792–1802.

Braak H, Thal DR, Ghebremedhin E et al. (2011). Stages of the pathologic process in Alzheimer disease: age categories from 1 to 100 years. J Neuropathol Exp Neurol 70: 960–969.

Braskie MN, Medina LD, Rodriguez-Agudelo Y et al. (2012). Increased fMRI signal with age in familial Alzheimer's disease mutation carriers. Neurobiol Aging 33 (424): e411–e421.

Brun A, Englund E (1981). Regional pattern of degeneration in Alzheimer's disease: neuronal loss and histopathological grading. Histopathology 5: 549–564.

Burggren AC, Zeineh MM, Ekstrom AD et al. (2008). Reduced cortical thickness in hippocampal subregions among cognitively normal apolipoprotein E e4 carriers. Neuroimage 41: 1177–1183.

Burton EJ, Barber R, Mukaetova-Ladinska EB et al. (2009). Medial temporal lobe atrophy on MRI differentiates Alzheimer's disease from dementia with Lewy bodies and vascular cognitive impairment: a prospective study with pathological verification of diagnosis. Brain 132: 195–203.

Cagnin A, Brooks DJ, Kennedy AM et al. (2001). In-vivo measurement of activated microglia in dementia. Lancet 358: 461–467.

Cagnin A, Rossor M, Sampson EL et al. (2004). In vivo detection of microglial activation in frontotemporal dementia. Ann Neurol 56: 894–897.

Caroli A, Prestia A, Chen K et al. (2012). Summary metrics to assess Alzheimer disease-related hypometabolic pattern with ^{18}F-FDG PET: head-to-head comparison. J Nucl Med 53: 592–600.

Carter SF, Scholl M, Almkvist O et al. (2012). Evidence for astrocytosis in prodromal Alzheimer disease provided by ^{11}C-deuterium-L-deprenyl: a multitracer PET paradigm combining ^{11}C-Pittsburgh compound B and ^{18}F-FDG. J Nucl Med 53: 37–46.

Castellano JM, Kim J, Stewart FR et al. (2011). Human apoE isoforms differentially regulate brain amyloid-beta peptide clearance. Sci Transl Med 3. 89ra57.

Catani M, Mesulam MM, Jakobsen E et al. (2013). A novel frontal pathway underlies verbal fluency in primary progressive aphasia. Brain 136: 2619–2628.

Chauveau F, Boutin H, Van Camp N et al. (2008). Nuclear imaging of neuroinflammation: a comprehensive review of [^{11}C]PK11195 challengers. Eur J Nucl Med Mol Imaging 35: 2304–2319.

Chen K, Ayutyanont N, Langbaum JB et al. (2011a). Characterizing Alzheimer's disease using a hypometabolic convergence index. Neuroimage 56: 52–60.

Chen Y, Wolk DA, Reddin JS et al. (2011b). Voxel-level comparison of arterial spin-labeled perfusion MRI and FDG-PET in Alzheimer disease. Neurology 77: 1977–1985.

Chetelat G, Desgranges B, Landeau B et al. (2008a). Direct voxel-based comparison between grey matter hypometabolism and atrophy in Alzheimer's disease. Brain 131: 60–71.

Chetelat G, Fouquet M, Kalpouzos G et al. (2008b). Three-dimensional surface mapping of hippocampal atrophy progression from MCI to AD and over normal aging as assessed using voxel-based morphometry. Neuropsychologia 46: 1721–1731.

Chetelat G, Villemagne VL, Bourgeat P et al. (2010). Relationship between atrophy and beta-amyloid deposition in Alzheimer disease. Ann Neurol 67: 317–324.

Chetelat G, Villemagne VL, Pike KE et al. (2012a). Relationship between memory performance and beta-amyloid deposition at different stages of Alzheimer's disease. Neurodegener Dis 10: 141–144.

Chetelat G, Villemagne VL, Villain N et al. (2012b). Accelerated cortical atrophy in cognitively normal elderly with high beta-amyloid deposition. Neurology 78: 477–484.

Chiang GC, Insel PS, Tosun D et al. (2011). Identifying cognitively healthy elderly individuals with subsequent memory decline by using automated MR temporoparietal volumes. Radiology 259: 844–851.

Chien DT, Bahri S, Szardenings AK et al. (2013). Early clinical PET imaging results with the novel PHF-tau radioligand [F-18]-T807. J Alzheimers Dis 34: 457–468.

Chien DT, Szardenings AK, Bahri S et al. (2014). Early clinical PET imaging results with the novel PHF-tau radioligand [F18]-T808. J Alzheimers Dis 38: 171–184.

Choi SR, Schneider JA, Bennett DA et al. (2012). Correlation of amyloid PET ligand florbetapir F 18 binding with abeta aggregation and neuritic plaque deposition in postmortem brain tissue. Alzheimer Dis Assoc Disord 26: 8–16.

Chui HC, Ramirez-Gomez L (2015). Clinical and imaging features of mixed Alzheimer and vascular pathologies. Alzheimers Res Ther 7: 21.

Clerx L, Visser PJ, Verhey F et al. (2012). New MRI markers for Alzheimer's disease: a meta-analysis of diffusion tensor imaging and a comparison with medial temporal lobe measurements. J Alzheimers Dis 29: 405–429.

Crivello F, Lemaitre H, Dufouil C et al. (2010). Effects of ApoE-epsilon4 allele load and age on the rates of grey matter and hippocampal volumes loss in a longitudinal cohort of 1186 healthy elderly persons. Neuroimage 53: 1064–1069.

de Calignon A, Polydoro M, Suarez-Calvet M et al. (2012). Propagation of tau pathology in a model of early Alzheimer's disease. Neuron 73: 685–697.

de la Torre JC (2002). Alzheimer disease as a vascular disorder: nosological evidence. Stroke 33: 1152–1162.

de Leeuw FE, de Groot JC, Achten E et al. (2001). Prevalence of cerebral white matter lesions in elderly people: a population based magnetic resonance imaging study. The Rotterdam Scan Study. J Neurol Neurosurg Psychiatry 70: 9–14.

de Souza LC, Chupin M, Bertoux M et al. (2013). Is hippocampal volume a good marker to differentiate Alzheimer's disease from frontotemporal dementia? J Alzheimers Dis 36: 57–66.

Dennis NA, Browndyke JN, Stokes J et al. (2010). Temporal lobe functional activity and connectivity in young adult APOE varepsilon4 carriers. Alzheimers Dement 6: 303–311.

Deters KD, Risacher SL, Farlow MR et al. (2014). Cerebral hypometabolism and grey matter density in MAPT intron 10+3 mutation carriers. Am J Neurodegener Dis 3: 103–114.

Devanand DP, Mikhno A, Pelton GH et al. (2010a). Pittsburgh compound B ((11)C-PIB) and fluorodeoxyglucose ((18)F-FDG) PET in patients with Alzheimer disease, mild cognitive impairment, and healthy controls. J Geriatr Psychiatry Neurol 23: 185–198.

Devanand DP, Van Heertum RL, Kegeles LS et al. (2010b). (99m)Tc hexamethyl-propylene-aminoxime single-photon emission computed tomography prediction of conversion from mild cognitive impairment to Alzheimer disease. Am J Geriatr Psychiatry 18: 959–972.

Dickerson BC, Wolk DA (2012). MRI cortical thickness biomarker predicts AD-like CSF and cognitive decline in normal adults. Neurology 78: 84–90.

Dickerson BC, Salat DH, Bates JF et al. (2004). Medial temporal lobe function and structure in mild cognitive impairment. Ann Neurol 56: 27–35.

Dickerson BC, Bakkour A, Salat DH et al. (2009). The cortical signature of Alzheimer's disease: regionally specific cortical thinning relates to symptom severity in very mild to mild AD dementia and is detectable in asymptomatic amyloid-positive individuals. Cereb Cortex 19: 497–510.

Dickerson BC, Stoub TR, Shah RC et al. (2011). Alzheimer-signature MRI biomarker predicts AD dementia in cognitively normal adults. Neurology 76: 1395–1402.

Diehl J, Grimmer T, Drzezga A et al. (2004). Cerebral metabolic patterns at early stages of frontotemporal dementia and semantic dementia. A PET study. Neurobiol Aging 25: 1051–1056.

Diehl-Schmid J, Grimmer T, Drzezga A et al. (2007). Decline of cerebral glucose metabolism in frontotemporal dementia: a longitudinal ^{18}F-FDG-PET-study. Neurobiol Aging 28: 42–50.

Donix M, Burggren AC, Suthana NA et al. (2010). Longitudinal changes in medial temporal cortical thickness in normal subjects with the APOE-4 polymorphism. Neuroimage 53: 37–43.

Douaud G, Jbabdi S, Behrens TE et al. (2011). DTI measures in crossing-fibre areas: increased diffusion anisotropy reveals early white matter alteration in MCI and mild Alzheimer's disease. Neuroimage 55: 880–890.

Drzezga A, Grimmer T, Henriksen G et al. (2008). Imaging of amyloid plaques and cerebral glucose metabolism in semantic dementia and Alzheimer's disease. Neuroimage 39: 619–633.

Drzezga A, Becker JA, Van Dijk KR et al. (2011). Neuronal dysfunction and disconnection of cortical hubs in non-demented subjects with elevated amyloid burden. Brain 134: 1635–1646.

Edison P, Archer HA, Gerhard A et al. (2008). Microglia, amyloid, and cognition in Alzheimer's disease: an ^{11}C (R) PK11195-PET and ^{11}C PIB-PET study. Neurobiol Dis 32: 412–419.

Ercoli LM, Small GW, Siddarth P et al. (2012). Assessment of dementia risk in aging adults using both FDG-PET and FDDNP-PET imaging. Int J Geriatr Psychiatry 27: 1017–1027.

Esiri MM, Wilcock GK, Morris JH (1997). Neuropathological assessment of the lesions of significance in vascular dementia. J Neurol Neurosurg Psychiatry 63: 749–753.

Fellgiebel A, Wille P, Muller MJ et al. (2004). Ultrastructural hippocampal and white matter alterations in mild cognitive impairment: a diffusion tensor imaging study. Dement Geriatr Cogn Disord 18: 101–108.

Ferrari R, Hernandez DG, Nalls MA et al. (2014). Frontotemporal dementia and its subtypes: a genome-wide association study. Lancet Neurol 13: 686–699.

Ferrer I, Boada Rovira M, Sanchez Guerra ML et al. (2004). Neuropathology and pathogenesis of encephalitis following amyloid-beta immunization in Alzheimer's disease. Brain Pathol 14: 11–20.

Ferretti MT, Cuello AC (2011). Does a pro-inflammatory process precede Alzheimer's disease and mild cognitive impairment? Curr Alzheimer Res 8: 164–174.

Filippi M, Agosta F (2011). Structural and functional network connectivity breakdown in Alzheimer's disease studied

with magnetic resonance imaging techniques. J Alzheimers Dis 24: 455–474.
Fleisher AS, Houston WS, Eyler LT et al. (2005). Identification of Alzheimer disease risk by functional magnetic resonance imaging. Arch Neurol 62: 1881–1888.
Folkersma H, Boellaard R, Yaqub M et al. (2011). Widespread and prolonged increase in (R)-(11)C-PK11195 binding after traumatic brain injury. J Nucl Med 52: 1235–1239.
Fortea J, Sala-Llonch R, Bartres-Faz D et al. (2010). Increased cortical thickness and caudate volume precede atrophy in PSEN1 mutation carriers. J Alzheimers Dis 22: 909–922.
Fortea J, Vilaplana E, Alcolea D et al. (2014). Cerebrospinal fluid beta-amyloid and phospho-tau biomarker interactions affecting brain structure in preclinical Alzheimer disease. Ann Neurol 76: 223–230.
Foster NL, Heidebrink JL, Clark CM et al. (2007). FDG-PET improves accuracy in distinguishing frontotemporal dementia and Alzheimer's disease. Brain 130: 2616–2635.
Fox PT, Raichle ME, Mintun MA et al. (1988). Nonoxidative glucose consumption during focal physiologic neural activity. Science 241: 462–464.
Franklin BS, Bossaller L, De Nardo D et al. (2014). The adaptor ASC has extracellular and 'prionoid' activities that propagate inflammation. Nat Immunol 15: 727–737.
Frisch S, Dukart J, Vogt B et al. (2013). Dissociating memory networks in early Alzheimer's disease and frontotemporal lobar degeneration – a combined study of hypometabolism and atrophy. PLoS One 8: e55251.
Galantucci S, Tartaglia MC, Wilson SM et al. (2011). White matter damage in primary progressive aphasias: a diffusion tensor tractography study. Brain 134: 3011–3029.
Galvin JE, Price JL, Yan Z et al. (2011). Resting bold fMRI differentiates dementia with Lewy bodies vs Alzheimer disease. Neurology 76: 1797–1803.
Goker-Alpan O, Masdeu JC, Kohn PD et al. (2012). The neurobiology of glucocerebrosidase-associated parkinsonism: a positron emission tomography study of dopamine synthesis and regional cerebral blood flow. Brain 135: 2440–2448.
Gorno-Tempini ML, Dronkers NF, Rankin KP et al. (2004). Cognition and anatomy in three variants of primary progressive aphasia. Ann Neurol 55: 335–346.
Gorno-Tempini ML, Hillis AE, Weintraub S et al. (2011). Classification of primary progressive aphasia and its variants. Neurology 76: 1006–1014.
Gour N, Ranjeva JP, Ceccaldi M et al. (2011). Basal functional connectivity within the anterior temporal network is associated with performance on declarative memory tasks. Neuroimage 58: 687–697.
Graff-Radford J, Murray ME, Lowe VJ et al. (2014). Dementia with Lewy bodies: basis of cingulate island sign. Neurology 83: 801–809.
Groom GN, Junck L, Foster NL et al. (1995). PET of peripheral benzodiazepine binding sites in the microgliosis of Alzheimer's disease. J Nucl Med 36: 2207–2210.
Guo CC, Gorno-Tempini ML, Gesierich B et al. (2013). Anterior temporal lobe degeneration produces widespread network-driven dysfunction. Brain 136: 2979–2991.
Gurol ME, Viswanathan A Gidicsin C et al. (2013). Cerebral amyloid angiopathy burden associated with leukoaraiosis: a positron emission tomography/magnetic resonance imaging study. Ann Neurol 73: 529–536.
Hahnel S, Stippich C, Weber I et al. (2008). Prevalence of cerebral microhemorrhages in amateur boxers as detected by 3T MR imaging. AJNR Am J Neuroradiol 29: 388–391.
Head D, Bugg JM, Goate AM et al. (2012). Exercise engagement as a moderator of the effects of APOE genotype on amyloid deposition. Arch Neurol 69: 636–643.
Hebb DO (1961). Distinctive features of learning in the higher animal. In: JF Delafresnaye (Ed.), Brain Mechanisms and Learning. Oxford University Press, London.
Hedden T, Van Dijk KR, Becker JA et al. (2009). Disruption of functional connectivity in clinically normal older adults harboring amyloid burden. J Neurosci 29: 12686–12694.
Heister D, Brewer JB, Magda S et al. (2011). Predicting MCI outcome with clinically available MRI and CSF biomarkers. Neurology 77: 1619–1628.
Herholz K (2014). Guidance for reading FDG PET scans in dementia patients. Q J Nucl Med Mol Imaging 58: 332–343.
Hoozemans JJ, Rozemuller AJ, van Haastert ES et al. (2011). Neuroinflammation in Alzheimer's disease wanes with age. J Neuroinflammation 8: 171.
Hua X, Leow AD, Parikshak N et al. (2008). Tensor-based morphometry as a neuroimaging biomarker for Alzheimer's disease: an MRI study of 676 AD, MCI, and normal subjects. Neuroimage 43: 458–469.
Ikeda M, Tashiro Y, Takai E et al. (2014). CSF levels of Abeta1-38/Abeta1-40/Abeta1-42 and (11)C PiB-PET studies in three clinical variants of primary progressive aphasia and Alzheimer's disease. Amyloid 21: 238–245.
Ikonomovic MD, Klunk WE, Abrahamson EE et al. (2008). Post-mortem correlates of in vivo PiB-PET amyloid imaging in a typical case of Alzheimer's disease. Brain 131: 1630–1645.
Jack Jr CR, Lowe VJ, Senjem ML et al. (2008). ^{11}C PiB and structural MRI provide complementary information in imaging of Alzheimer's disease and amnestic mild cognitive impairment. Brain 131: 665–680.
Jack Jr CR, Knopman DS, Jagust WJ et al. (2010a). Hypothetical model of dynamic biomarkers of the Alzheimer's pathological cascade. Lancet Neurol 9: 119–128.
Jack CR, Wiste HJ, Vemuri P et al. (2010b). Brain beta-amyloid measures and magnetic resonance imaging atrophy both predict time-to-progression from mild cognitive impairment to Alzheimer's disease. Brain 133: 3336–3348.
Jack CR, Vemuri P, Wiste HJ et al. (2011). Evidence for ordering of Alzheimer disease biomarkers. Arch Neurol 68: 1526–1535.
Jack Jr CR, Knopman DS, Weigand SD et al. (2012). An operational approach to National Institute on Aging-Alzheimer's Association criteria for preclinical Alzheimer disease. Ann Neurol 71: 765–775.
Jack Jr CR, Knopman DS, Jagust WJ et al. (2013). Tracking pathophysiological processes in Alzheimer's disease: an updated hypothetical model of dynamic biomarkers. Lancet Neurol 12: 207–216.

Jacobs HI, Van Boxtel MP, Heinecke A et al. (2012). Functional integration of parietal lobe activity in early Alzheimer disease. Neurology 78: 352–360.

Jacova C, Hsiung GY, Tawankanjanachot I et al. (2013). Anterior brain glucose hypometabolism predates dementia in progranulin mutation carriers. Neurology 81: 1322–1331.

Jagust W, Thisted R, Devous Sr MD et al. (2001). SPECT perfusion imaging in the diagnosis of Alzheimer's disease: a clinical-pathologic study. Neurology 56: 950–956.

Jagust W, Reed B, Mungas D et al. (2007). What does fluorodeoxyglucose PET imaging add to a clinical diagnosis of dementia? Neurology 69: 871–877.

Jeong Y, Cho SS, Park JM et al. (2005). 18F-FDG PET findings in frontotemporal dementia: an SPM analysis of 29 patients. J Nucl Med 46: 233–239.

Johnson KA, Jones K, Holman BL et al. (1998). Preclinical prediction of Alzheimer's disease using SPECT. Neurology 50: 1563–1571.

Johnson SC, Schmitz TW, Trivedi MA et al. (2006). The influence of Alzheimer disease family history and apolipoprotein E epsilon4 on mesial temporal lobe activation. J Neurosci 26: 6069–6076.

Johnson KA, Gregas M, Becker JA et al. (2007). Imaging of amyloid burden and distribution in cerebral amyloid angiopathy. Ann Neurol 62: 229–234.

Johnson KA, Minoshima S, Bohnen NI et al. (2013a). Appropriate use criteria for amyloid PET: a report of the Amyloid Imaging Task Force, the Society of Nuclear Medicine and Molecular Imaging, and the Alzheimer's Association. J Nucl Med 54: 476–490.

Johnson KA, Sperling RA, Gidicsin CM et al. (2013b). Florbetapir (F18-AV-45) PET to assess amyloid burden in Alzheimer's disease dementia, mild cognitive impairment, and normal aging. Alzheimers Dement 9: S72–S83.

Josephs KA, Whitwell JL, Knopman DS et al. (2009). Two distinct subtypes of right temporal variant frontotemporal dementia. Neurology 73: 1443–1450.

Josephs KA, Hodges JR, Snowden JS et al. (2011). Neuropathological background of phenotypical variability in frontotemporal dementia. Acta Neuropathol 122: 137–153.

Josephs KA, Duffy JR, Strand EA et al. (2014a). Progranulin-associated PiB-negative logopenic primary progressive aphasia. J Neurol 261: 604–614.

Josephs KA, Whitwell JL, Weigand SD et al. (2014b). TDP-43 is a key player in the clinical features associated with Alzheimer's disease. Acta Neuropathol 127: 811–824.

Kadir A, Marutle A, Gonzalez D et al. (2011). Positron emission tomography imaging and clinical progression in relation to molecular pathology in the first Pittsburgh Compound B positron emission tomography patient with Alzheimer's disease. Brain 134: 301–317.

Kanda T, Ishii K, Uemura T et al. (2008). Comparison of grey matter and metabolic reductions in frontotemporal dementia using FDG-PET and voxel-based morphometric MR studies. Eur J Nucl Med Mol Imaging 35: 2227–2234.

Kantarci K, Avula R, Senjem ML et al. (2010). Dementia with Lewy bodies and Alzheimer disease: neurodegenerative patterns characterized by DTI. Neurology 74: 1814–1821.

Kantarci K, Lowe V, Przybelski SA et al. (2012a). APOE modifies the association between Abeta load and cognition in cognitively normal older adults. Neurology 78: 232–240.

Kantarci K, Lowe VJ, Boeve BF et al. (2012b). Multimodality imaging characteristics of dementia with Lewy bodies. Neurobiol Aging 33: 2091–2105.

Kantarci K, Weigand SD, Przybelski SA et al. (2013). MRI and MRS predictors of mild cognitive impairment in a population-based sample. Neurology 81: 126–133.

Kenny ER, Blamire AM, Firbank MJ et al. (2012). Functional connectivity in cortical regions in dementia with Lewy bodies and Alzheimer's disease. Brain 135: 569–581.

Kerklaan BJ, van Berckel BN, Herholz K et al. (2014). The added value of 18-fluorodeoxyglucose-positron emission tomography in the diagnosis of the behavioral variant of frontotemporal dementia. Am J Alzheimers Dis Other Demen 29: 607–613.

Kirkpatrick J, Hayman L (1987). White-matter lesions on MR imaging of clinically healthy brains of elderly subjects: possible pathologic basis. Radiology 162: 509–511.

Kirshner HS (2012). Primary progressive aphasia and Alzheimer's disease: brief history, recent evidence. Curr Neurol Neurosci Rep 12: 709–714.

Kiuchi K, Morikawa M, Taoka T et al. (2009). Abnormalities of the uncinate fasciculus and posterior cingulate fasciculus in mild cognitive impairment and early Alzheimer's disease: a diffusion tensor tractography study. Brain Res 1287: 184–191.

Kloppel S, Stonnington CM, Barnes J et al. (2008). Accuracy of dementia diagnosis: a direct comparison between radiologists and a computerized method. Brain 131: 2969–2974.

Knight WD, Kim LG, Douiri A et al. (2011). Acceleration of cortical thinning in familial Alzheimer's disease. Neurobiol Aging 32: 1765–1773.

Knopman DS, DeKosky ST, Cummings JL et al. (2001). Practice parameter: diagnosis of dementia (an evidence-based review). Report of the Quality Standards Subcommittee of the American Academy of Neurology. Neurology 56: 1143–1153.

Knopman DS, Jack Jr CR, Wiste HJ et al. (2012). Short-term clinical outcomes for stages of NIA-AA preclinical Alzheimer disease. Neurology 78: 1576–1582.

Knopman DS, Jack Jr CR, Wiste HJ et al. (2013a). Brain injury biomarkers are not dependent on beta-amyloid in normal elderly. Ann Neurol 73: 472–480.

Knopman DS, Jack Jr CR, Wiste HJ et al. (2013b). Selective worsening of brain injury biomarker abnormalities in cognitively normal elderly persons with beta-amyloidosis. JAMA Neurol 70: 1030–1038.

Kobylecki C, Langheinrich T, Hinz R et al. (2015). ^{18}F-florbetapir PET in patients with frontotemporal dementia and Alzheimer disease. J Nucl Med 56: 386–391.

Koerte IK, Lin AP, Willems A et al. (2015). A review of neuroimaging findings in repetitive brain trauma. Brain Pathol 25: 318–349.

Koivunen J, Scheinin N, Virta JR et al. (2011). Amyloid PET imaging in patients with mild cognitive impairment. A 2-year follow-up study. Neurology 76: 1085–1090.

Kreisl WC, Fujita M, Fujimura Y et al. (2010). Comparison of [(11)C]-(R)-PK 11195 and [(11)C]PBR28, two radioligands for translocator protein (18 kDa) in human and monkey: implications for positron emission tomographic imaging of this inflammation biomarker. Neuroimage 49: 2924–2932.

Kreisl WC, Jenko KJ, Hines CS et al. (2013a). A genetic polymorphism for translocator protein 18 kDa affects both in vitro and in vivo radioligand binding in human brain to this putative biomarker of neuroinflammation. J Cereb Blood Flow Metab 33: 53–58.

Kreisl WC, Lyoo CH, McGwier M et al. (2013b). In vivo radioligand binding to translocator protein correlates with severity of Alzheimer's disease. Brain 136: 2228–2238.

Kropholler MA, Boellaard R, van Berckel BNM et al. (2007). Evaluation of reference regions for (R)-C-11 PK11195 studies in Alzheimer's disease and mild cognitive impairment. J Cereb Blood Flow Metab 27: 1965–1974.

La Joie R, Perrotin A, Barre L et al. (2012). Region-specific hierarchy between atrophy, hypometabolism, and beta-amyloid (Abeta) load in Alzheimer's disease dementia. J Neurosci 32: 16265–16273.

Lam BY, Halliday GM, Irish M et al. (2014). Longitudinal white matter changes in frontotemporal dementia subtypes. Hum Brain Mapp 35: 3547–3557.

Lambert JC, Ibrahim-Verbaas CA, Harold D et al. (2013). Meta-analysis of 74,046 individuals identifies 11 new susceptibility loci for Alzheimer's disease. Nat Genet 45: 1452–1458.

Landau SM, Marks SM, Mormino EC et al. (2012). Association of lifetime cognitive engagement and low beta-amyloid deposition. Arch Neurol 69: 623–629.

Landau SM, Thomas BA, Thurfjell L et al. (2014). Amyloid PET imaging in Alzheimer's disease: a comparison of three radiotracers. Eur J Nucl Med Mol Imaging 41: 1398–1407.

Lehmann M, Ghosh PM, Madison C et al. (2013a). Diverging patterns of amyloid deposition and hypometabolism in clinical variants of probable Alzheimer's disease. Brain 136: 844–858.

Lehmann M, Madison CM, Ghosh PM et al. (2013b). Intrinsic connectivity networks in healthy subjects explain clinical variability in Alzheimer's disease. Proc Natl Acad Sci U S A 110: 11606–11611.

Leyton CE, Villemagne VL, Savage S et al. (2011). Subtypes of progressive aphasia: application of the International Consensus Criteria and validation using beta-amyloid imaging. Brain 134: 3030–3043.

Lim SM, Katsifis A, Villemagne VL et al. (2009). The ^{18}F-FDG PET cingulate island sign and comparison to 123I-beta-CIT SPECT for diagnosis of dementia with Lewy bodies. J Nucl Med 50: 1638–1645.

Lim YY, Villemagne VL, Laws SM et al. (2013). BDNF Val66Met, Abeta amyloid, and cognitive decline in preclinical Alzheimer's disease. Neurobiol Aging 34: 2457–2464.

Liscic RM, Storandt M, Cairns NJ et al. (2007). Clinical and psychometric distinction of frontotemporal and Alzheimer dementias. Arch Neurol 64: 535–540.

Liu L, Drouet V, Wu JW et al. (2012). Trans-synaptic spread of tau pathology in vivo. PLoS One 7: e31302.

Logothetis NK (2008). What we can do and what we cannot do with fMRI. Nature 453: 869–878.

Luk KC, Kehm V, Carroll J et al. (2012). Pathological alpha-synuclein transmission initiates Parkinson-like neurodegeneration in nontransgenic mice. Science 338: 949–953.

Machulda MM, Jones DT, Vemuri P et al. (2011). Effect of APOE epsilon4 status on intrinsic network connectivity in cognitively normal elderly subjects. Arch Neurol 68: 1131–1136.

Madhavan A, Whitwell JL, Weigand SD et al. (2013). FDG PET and MRI in logopenic primary progressive aphasia versus dementia of the Alzheimer's type. PLoS One 8: e62471.

Maeda J, Zhang MR, Okauchi T et al. (2011). In vivo positron emission tomographic imaging of glial responses to amyloid-beta and tau pathologies in mouse models of Alzheimer's disease and related disorders. J Neurosci 31: 4720–4730.

Mahoney CJ, Ridgway GR, Malone IB et al. (2014). Profiles of white matter tract pathology in frontotemporal dementia. Hum Brain Mapp 35: 4163–4179.

Mahoney CJ, Simpson IJ, Nicholas JM et al. (2015). Longitudinal diffusion tensor imaging in frontotemporal dementia. Ann Neurol 77: 33–46.

Mandelli ML, Caverzasi E, Binney RJ et al. (2014). Frontal white matter tracts sustaining speech production in primary progressive aphasia. J Neurosci 34: 9754–9767.

Marchant NL, Reed BR, Sanossian N et al. (2013). The aging brain and cognition: contribution of vascular injury and abeta to mild cognitive dysfunction. JAMA Neurol 70: 488–495.

Maruyama M, Shimada H, Suhara T et al. (2013). Imaging of tau pathology in a tauopathy mouse model and in Alzheimer patients compared to normal controls. Neuron 79: 1094–1108.

Masdeu J (2008). Neuroimaging of disorders leading to dementia. Continuum (AAN) 14: 144–163.

Masdeu JC, Arbizu J (2008). Brain single photon emission computed tomography technological aspects and clinical applications. Semin Neurol 28: 423–434.

Masdeu JC, Zubieta JL, Arbizu J (2005). Neuroimaging as a marker of the onset and progression of Alzheimer's disease. J Neurol Sci 236: 55–64.

Masdeu JC, Kreisl WC, Berman KF (2012). The neurobiology of Alzheimer disease defined by neuroimaging. Curr Opin Neurol 25: 410–420.

Massey LA, Jager HR, Paviour DC et al. (2013). The midbrain to pons ratio: a simple and specific MRI sign of progressive supranuclear palsy. Neurology 80: 1856–1861.

Mathis CA, Kuller LH, Klunk WE et al. (2013). In vivo assessment of amyloid-beta deposition in nondemented very elderly subjects. Ann Neurol 73: 751–761.

McEvoy LK, Fennema-Notestine C, Roddey JC et al. (2009). Alzheimer disease: quantitative structural neuroimaging for detection and prediction of clinical and structural changes in mild cognitive impairment. Radiology 251: 195–205.

McKee AC, Stein TD, Nowinski CJ et al. (2013). The spectrum of disease in chronic traumatic encephalopathy. Brain 136: 43–64.

McKeith IG, Dickson DW, Lowe J et al. (2005). Diagnosis and management of dementia with Lewy bodies: third report of the DLB Consortium. Neurology 65: 1863–1872.

McKhann GM, Knopman DS, Chertkow H et al. (2011). The diagnosis of dementia due to Alzheimer's disease: recommendations from the National Institute on Aging-Alzheimer's Association workgroups on diagnostic guidelines for Alzheimer's disease. Alzheimers Dement 7: 263–269.

McMillan CT, Brun C, Siddiqui S et al. (2012). White matter imaging contributes to the multimodal diagnosis of frontotemporal lobar degeneration. Neurology 78: 1761–1768.

Mendez MF, Shapira JS, McMurtray A et al. (2007). Accuracy of the clinical evaluation for frontotemporal dementia. Arch Neurol 64: 830–835.

Mesulam MM, Weintraub S, Rogalski EJ et al. (2014). Asymmetry and heterogeneity of Alzheimer's and frontotemporal pathology in primary progressive aphasia. Brain 137: 1176–1192.

Mielke MM, Kozauer NA, Chan KC et al. (2009). Regionally-specific diffusion tensor imaging in mild cognitive impairment and Alzheimer's disease. Neuroimage 46: 47–55.

Miettinen PS, Pihlajamaki M, Jauhiainen AM et al. (2011). Structure and function of medial temporal and posteromedial cortices in early Alzheimer's disease. Eur J Neurosci 34: 320–330.

Miller ZA, Rankin KP, Graff-Radford NR et al. (2013). TDP-43 frontotemporal lobar degeneration and autoimmune disease. J Neurol Neurosurg Psychiatry 84: 956–962.

Mondadori CR, de Quervain DJ, Buchmann A et al. (2007). Better memory and neural efficiency in young apolipoprotein E epsilon4 carriers. Cereb Cortex 17: 1934–1947.

Monsell SE, Mock C, Roe CM et al. (2013). Comparison of symptomatic and asymptomatic persons with Alzheimer disease neuropathology. Neurology 80: 2121–2129.

Montine TJ, Phelps CH, Beach TG et al. (2012). National Institute on Aging-Alzheimer's Association guidelines for the neuropathologic assessment of Alzheimer's disease: a practical approach. Acta Neuropathol 123: 1–11.

Mormino EC, Kluth JT, Madison CM et al. (2009). Episodic memory loss is related to hippocampal-mediated beta-amyloid deposition in elderly subjects. Brain 132: 1310–1323.

Morra JH, Tu Z, Apostolova LG et al. (2009). Automated mapping of hippocampal atrophy in 1-year repeat MRI data from 490 subjects with Alzheimer's disease, mild cognitive impairment, and elderly controls. Neuroimage 45: S3–S15.

Morris JC (2012). Revised criteria for mild cognitive impairment may compromise the diagnosis of Alzheimer disease dementia. Arch Neurol 69: 700–708.

Mosconi L, Brys M, Glodzik-Sobanska L et al. (2007). Early detection of Alzheimer's disease using neuroimaging. Exp Gerontol 42: 129–138.

Mosconi L, Tsui WH, Herholz K et al. (2008). Multicenter standardized 18F-FDG PET diagnosis of mild cognitive impairment, Alzheimer's disease, and other dementias. J Nucl Med 49: 390–398.

Mueller SG, Weiner MW (2009). Selective effect of age, Apo e4, and Alzheimer's disease on hippocampal subfields. Hippocampus 19: 558–564.

Nedelska Z, Ferman TJ, Boeve BF et al. (2015). Pattern of brain atrophy rates in autopsy-confirmed dementia with Lewy bodies. Neurobiol Aging 36: 452–461.

Nelson PT, Head E, Schmitt FA et al. (2011). Alzheimer's disease is not "brain aging": neuropathological, genetic, and epidemiological human studies. Acta Neuropathol 121: 571–587.

Nelson PT, Alafuzoff I, Bigio EH et al. (2012). Correlation of Alzheimer disease neuropathologic changes with cognitive status: a review of the literature. J Neuropathol Exp Neurol 71: 362–381.

Nichols LM, Masdeu JC, Mattay VS et al. (2012). Interactive effect of apolipoprotein e genotype and age on hippocampal activation during memory processing in healthy adults. Arch Gen Psychiatry 69: 804–813.

Nolan KA, Lino MM, Seligmann AW et al. (1998). Absence of vascular dementia in an autopsy series from a dementia clinic. J Am Geriatr Soc 46: 597–604.

O'Brien JL, O'Keefe KM, LaViolette PS et al. (2010). Longitudinal fMRI in elderly reveals loss of hippocampal activation with clinical decline. Neurology 74: 1969–1976.

O'Brien JT, Firbank MJ, Davison C et al. (2014). 18F-FDG PET and perfusion SPECT in the diagnosis of Alzheimer and Lewy body dementias. J Nucl Med 55: 1959–1965.

O'Dwyer L, Lamberton F, Bokde AL et al. (2012). Using support vector machines with multiple indices of diffusion for automated classification of mild cognitive impairment. PLoS One 7: e32441.

Okello A, Edison P, Archer HA et al. (2009a). Microglial activation and amyloid deposition in mild cognitive impairment: a PET study. Neurology 72: 56–62.

Okello A, Koivunen J, Edison P et al. (2009b). Conversion of amyloid positive and negative MCI to AD over 3 years: an ^{11}C-PIB PET study. Neurology 73: 754–760.

Ossenkoppele R, Tolboom N, Foster-Dingley JC et al. (2012). Longitudinal imaging of Alzheimer pathology using [(11) C]PIB, [(18)F]FDDNP and [(18)F]FDG PET. Eur J Nucl Med Mol Imaging 39: 990–1000.

Ossenkoppele R, Schonhaut DR, Baker SL et al. (2015). Tau, amyloid, and hypometabolism in a patient with posterior cortical atrophy. Ann Neurol 77: 338–342.

Ostrowitzki S, Deptula D, Thurfjell L et al. (2012). Mechanism of amyloid removal in patients with Alzheimer disease treated with gantenerumab. Arch Neurol 69: 198–207.

Owen DR, Yeo AJ, Gunn RN et al. (2012). An 18-kDa translocator protein (TSPO) polymorphism explains differences in binding affinity of the PET radioligand PBR28. J Cereb Blood Flow Metab 32: 1–5.

Pascual B, Prieto E, Arbizu J et al. (2010). Brain glucose metabolism in vascular white matter disease with dementia: differentiation from Alzheimer disease. Stroke 41: 2889–2893.

Pascual B, Prieto E, Arbizu J et al. (2012a). Decreased carbon-11-flumazenil binding in early Alzheimer's disease. Brain 135: 2817–2825.

Pascual B, Prieto E, Marti-Climent J et al. (2012b). Decreased 11C-flumazenil binding in early Alzheimer disease. J Neuroimaging 22: 106.

Perez-Nievas BG, Stein TD, Tai HC et al. (2013). Dissecting phenotypic traits linked to human resilience to Alzheimer's pathology. Brain 136: 2510–2526.

Perrotin A, Mormino EC, Madison CM et al. (2012). Subjective cognition and amyloid deposition imaging: a Pittsburgh Compound B positron emission tomography study in normal elderly individuals. Arch Neurol 69: 223–229.

Petersen RC (2004). Dementia. Lippincott Williams & Wilkins, Baltimore, MD.

Petersen RC (2013). Do preclinical Alzheimer's disease criteria work? Lancet Neurol 12: 933–935.

Petersen RC, Aisen P, Boeve BF et al. (2013). Mild cognitive impairment due to Alzheimer disease in the community. Ann Neurol 74: 199–208.

Piolino P, Chetelat G, Matuszewski V et al. (2007). In search of autobiographical memories: a PET study in the frontal variant of frontotemporal dementia. Neuropsychologia 45: 2730–2743.

Power JD, Barnes KA, Snyder AZ et al. (2012). Spurious but systematic correlations in functional connectivity MRI networks arise from subject motion. Neuroimage 59: 2142–2154.

Prusiner SB (2013). Biology and genetics of prions causing neurodegeneration. Annu Rev Genet 47: 601–623.

Putcha D, Brickhouse M, O'Keefe K et al. (2011). Hippocampal hyperactivation associated with cortical thinning in Alzheimer's disease signature regions in non-demented elderly adults. J Neurosci 31: 17680–17688.

Quiroz YT, Budson AE, Celone K et al. (2010). Hippocampal hyperactivation in presymptomatic familial Alzheimer's disease. Ann Neurol 68: 865–875.

Rabinovici GD, Furst AJ, O'Neil JP et al. (2007). ^{11}C-PIB PET imaging in Alzheimer disease and frontotemporal lobar degeneration. Neurology 68: 1205–1212.

Rabinovici GD, Jagust WJ, Furst AJ et al. (2008). Abeta amyloid and glucose metabolism in three variants of primary progressive aphasia. Ann Neurol 64: 388–401.

Rabinovici GD, Rosen HJ, Alkalay A et al. (2011). Amyloid vs FDG-PET in the differential diagnosis of AD and FTLD. Neurology 77: 2034–2042.

Ramlackhansingh AF, Brooks DJ, Greenwood RJ et al. (2011). Inflammation after trauma: microglial activation and traumatic brain injury. Ann Neurol 70: 374–383.

Rascovsky K, Hodges JR, Knopman D et al. (2011). Sensitivity of revised diagnostic criteria for the behavioural variant of frontotemporal dementia. Brain 134: 2456–2477.

Reijmer YD, van Veluw SJ, Greenberg SM (2015). Ischemic brain injury in cerebral amyloid angiopathy. J Cereb Blood Flow Metab. http://dx.doi.org/10.1038/jcbfm.2015.88 (epub ahead of print).

Reiman EM, Caselli RJ, Yun LS et al. (1996). Preclinical evidence of Alzheimer's disease in persons homozygous for the epsilon 4 allele for apolipoprotein E. N Engl J Med 334: 752–758.

Reiman EM, Chen K, Alexander GE et al. (2004). Functional brain abnormalities in young adults at genetic risk for late-onset Alzheimer's dementia. Proc Natl Acad Sci U S A 101: 284–289.

Ringman JM, O'Neill J, Geschwind D et al. (2007). Diffusion tensor imaging in preclinical and presymptomatic carriers of familial Alzheimer's disease mutations. Brain 130: 1767–1776.

Ringman JM, Pope W, Salamon N (2010). Insensitivity of visual assessment of hippocampal atrophy in familial Alzheimer's disease. J Neurol 257: 839–842.

Ringman JM, Medina LD, Braskie M et al. (2011). Effects of risk genes on BOLD activation in presymptomatic carriers of familial Alzheimer's disease mutations during a novelty encoding task. Cereb Cortex 21: 877–883.

Rocher AB, Chapon F, Blaizot X et al. (2003). Resting-state brain glucose utilization as measured by PET is directly related to regional synaptophysin levels: a study in baboons. Neuroimage 20: 1894–1898.

Roman GC, Tatemichi TK, Erkinjuntti T et al. (1993). Vascular dementia: diagnostic criteria for research studies. Report of the NINDS-AIREN International Workshop. Neurology 43: 250–260.

Rosenbloom MH, Alkalay A, Agarwal N et al. (2011). Distinct clinical and metabolic deficits in PCA and AD are not related to amyloid distribution. Neurology 76: 1789–1796.

Rowe CC, Villemagne VL (2011). Brain amyloid imaging. J Nucl Med 52: 1733–1740.

Rowe CC, Ng S, Ackermann U et al. (2007). Imaging beta-amyloid burden in aging and dementia. Neurology 68: 1718–1725.

Rowe CC, Pejoska S, Mulligan RS et al. (2013). Head-to-head comparison of ^{11}C-PiB and ^{18}F-AZD4694 (NAV4694) for beta-amyloid imaging in aging and dementia. J Nucl Med 54: 880–886.

Sabri O, Sabbagh MN, Seibyl J et al. (2015). Florbetaben PET imaging to detect amyloid beta plaques in Alzheimer disease: phase 3 study. Alzheimers Dement 11: 964–974.

Sajjadi SA, Acosta-Cabronero J, Patterson K et al. (2013). Diffusion tensor magnetic resonance imaging for single subject diagnosis in neurodegenerative diseases. Brain 136: 2253–2261.

Salmon E, Garraux G, Delbeuck X et al. (2003). Predominant ventromedial frontopolar metabolic impairment in frontotemporal dementia. Neuroimage 20: 435–440.

Sanchez-Juan P, Ghosh PM, Hagen J et al. (2014). Practical utility of amyloid and FDG-PET in an academic dementia center. Neurology 82: 230–238.

Santillo AF, Martensson J, Lindberg O et al. (2013). Diffusion tensor tractography versus volumetric imaging in the diagnosis of behavioral variant frontotemporal dementia. PLoS One 8: e66932.

Sapolsky D, Bakkour A, Negreira A et al. (2010). Cortical neuroanatomic correlates of symptom severity in primary progressive aphasia. Neurology 75: 358–366.

Savva GM, Wharton SB, Ince PG et al. (2009). Age, neuropathology, and dementia. N Engl J Med 360: 2302–2309.

Scheltens P, Fox N, Barkhof F et al. (2002). Structural magnetic resonance imaging in the practical assessment of dementia: beyond exclusion. Lancet Neurol 1: 13–21.

Schneider JA, Arvanitakis Z, Bang W et al. (2007). Mixed brain pathologies account for most dementia cases in community-dwelling older persons. Neurology 69: 2197–2204.

Schuitemaker A, Kropholler MA, Boellaard R et al. (2013). Microglial activation in Alzheimer's disease: an (R)-[(1)(1)C]PK11195 positron emission tomography study. Neurobiol Aging 34: 128–136.

Seeley WW, Crawford RK, Zhou J et al. (2009). Neurodegenerative diseases target large-scale human brain networks. Neuron 62: 42–52.

Sepulcre J, Masdeu JC (2015). Advanced neuroimaging methods towards characterization of early stages of AD. In: JI Castrillo, SG Oliver (Eds.), Systems Biology of Alzheimer's Disease. Humana Press, London.

Sepulcre J, Sabuncu MR, Johnson KA (2012). Network assemblies in the functional brain. Curr Opin Neurol 25: 384–391.

Serrano-Pozo A, Mielke ML, Gomez-Isla T et al. (2011). Reactive glia not only associates with plaques but also parallels tangles in Alzheimer's disease. Am J Pathol 179: 1373–1384.

Sheline YI, Morris JC, Snyder AZ et al. (2010). APOE4 allele disrupts resting state fMRI connectivity in the absence of amyloid plaques or decreased CSF Abeta42. J Neurosci 30: 17035–17040.

Shin J, Lee SY, Kim SJ et al. (2010). Voxel-based analysis of Alzheimer's disease PET imaging using a triplet of radiotracers: PIB, FDDNP, and FDG. Neuroimage 52: 488–496.

Shin J, Kepe V, Barrio JR et al. (2011). The merits of FDDNP-PET imaging in Alzheimer's disease. J Alzheimers Dis 26: 135–145.

Silverman DH (2004). Brain 18F-FDG PET in the diagnosis of neurodegenerative dementias: comparison with perfusion SPECT and with clinical evaluations lacking nuclear imaging. J Nucl Med 45: 594–607.

Silverman DH, Small GW, Chang CY et al. (2001). Positron emission tomography in evaluation of dementia: regional brain metabolism and long-term outcome. JAMA 286: 2120–2127.

Small GW, Siddarth P, Kepe V et al. (2012). Prediction of cognitive decline by positron emission tomography of brain amyloid and tau. Arch Neurol 69: 215–222.

Smith CD, Chebrolu H, Andersen AH et al. (2010). White matter diffusion alterations in normal women at risk of Alzheimer's disease. Neurobiol Aging 31: 1122–1131.

Sperling RA, Dickerson BC, Pihlajamaki M et al. (2010). Functional alterations in memory networks in early Alzheimer's disease. Neuromolecular Med 12: 27–43.

Sperling RA, Aisen PS, Beckett LA et al. (2011a). Toward defining the preclinical stages of Alzheimer's disease: recommendations from the National Institute on Aging-Alzheimer's Association workgroups on diagnostic guidelines for Alzheimer's disease. Alzheimers Dement 7: 280–292.

Sperling RA, Jack Jr CR, Black SE et al. (2011b). Amyloid-related imaging abnormalities in amyloid-modifying therapeutic trials: recommendations from the Alzheimer's Association Research Roundtable Workgroup. Alzheimers Dement 7: 367–385.

Sperling R, Salloway S, Brooks DJ et al. (2012). Amyloid-related imaging abnormalities in patients with Alzheimer's disease treated with bapineuzumab: a retrospective analysis. Lancet Neurol 11: 241–249.

Sperling RA, Rentz DM, Johnson KA et al. (2014). The A4 study: stopping AD before symptoms begin? Sci Transl Med 6: 228fs213.

Stern RA, Daneshvar DH, Baugh CM et al. (2013). Clinical presentation of chronic traumatic encephalopathy. Neurology 81: 1122–1129.

Stricker NH, Schweinsburg BC, Delano-Wood L et al. (2009). Decreased white matter integrity in late-myelinating fiber pathways in Alzheimer's disease supports retrogenesis. Neuroimage 45: 10–16.

Teune LK, Bartels AL, de Jong BM et al. (2010). Typical cerebral metabolic patterns in neurodegenerative brain diseases. Mov Disord 25: 2395–2404.

Thiele F, Young S, Buchert R et al. (2013). Voxel-based classification of FDG PET in dementia using inter-scanner normalization. Neuroimage 77: 62–69.

Thompson PM, Hayashi KM, de Zubicaray G et al. (2003). Dynamics of gray matter loss in Alzheimer's disease. J Neurosci 23: 994–1005.

Tolboom N, van der Flier WM, Boverhoff J et al. (2010). Molecular imaging in the diagnosis of Alzheimer's disease: visual assessment of (11)C PIB and (18)F FDDNP PET images. J Neurol Neurosurg Psychiatry 81: 882–884.

Trivedi MA, Schmitz TW, Ries ML et al. (2008). fMRI activation during episodic encoding and metacognitive appraisal across the lifespan: risk factors for Alzheimer's disease. Neuropsychologia 46: 1667–1678.

Urs R, Potter E, Barker W et al. (2009). Visual rating system for assessing magnetic resonance images: a tool in the diagnosis of mild cognitive impairment and Alzheimer disease. J Comput Assist Tomogr 33: 73–78.

van der Flier WM, van Straaten EC, Barkhof F et al. (2005). Small vessel disease and general cognitive function in non-disabled elderly: the LADIS study. Stroke 36: 2116–2120.

Vellas B, Carrillo MC, Sampaio C et al. (2013). Designing drug trials for Alzheimer's disease: what we have learned from the release of the phase III antibody trials: a report from the EU/US/CTAD Task Force. Alzheimers Dement 9: 438–444.

Vemuri P, Whitwell JL, Kantarci K et al. (2008). Antemortem MRI based STructural Abnormality iNDex (STAND)-scores correlate with postmortem Braak neurofibrillary tangle stage. Neuroimage 42: 559–567.

Vemuri P, Lesnick TG, Przybelski SA et al. (2012). Effect of lifestyle activities on Alzheimer disease biomarkers and cognition. Ann Neurol 72: 730–738.

Vemuri P, Lesnick TG, Przybelski SA et al. (2015). Vascular and amyloid pathologies are independent predictors of cognitive decline in normal elderly. Brain 138: 761–771.

Villemagne VL, Ong K, Mulligan RS et al. (2011a). Amyloid imaging with (18)F-florbetaben in Alzheimer disease and other dementias. J Nucl Med 52: 1210–1217.

Villemagne VL, Pike KE, Chetelat G et al. (2011b). Longitudinal assessment of Abeta and cognition in aging and Alzheimer disease. Ann Neurol 69: 181–192.

Villemagne VL, Burnham S, Bourgeat P et al. (2013). Amyloid beta deposition, neurodegeneration, and cognitive decline in sporadic Alzheimer's disease: a prospective cohort study. Lancet Neurol 12: 357–367.

Villemagne VL, Fodero-Tavoletti MT, Masters CL et al. (2015). Tau imaging: early progress and future directions. Lancet Neurol 14: 114–124.

Viswanathan A, Gschwendtner A, Guichard JP et al. (2007). Lacunar lesions are independently associated with disability and cognitive impairment in CADASIL. Neurology 69: 172–179.

Vlassenko AG, Mintun MA, Xiong C et al. (2011). Amyloid-beta plaque growth in cognitively normal adults: longitudinal [^{11}C]Pittsburgh compound B data. Ann Neurol 70: 857–861.

Vos SJ, Xiong C, Visser PJ et al. (2013). Preclinical Alzheimer's disease and its outcome: a longitudinal cohort study. Lancet Neurol 12: 957–965.

Wang L, Khan A, Csernansky JG et al. (2009). Fully-automated, multi-stage hippocampus mapping in very mild Alzheimer disease. Hippocampus 19: 541–548.

Wee CY, Yap PT, Zhang D et al. (2012). Identification of MCI individuals using structural and functional connectivity networks. Neuroimage 59: 2045–2056.

Whitwell JL, Josephs KA, Murray ME et al. (2008). MRI correlates of neurofibrillary tangle pathology at autopsy: a voxel-based morphometry study. Neurology 71: 743–749.

Whitwell JL, Przybelski SA, Weigand SD et al. (2009). Distinct anatomical subtypes of the behavioural variant of frontotemporal dementia: a cluster analysis study. Brain 132: 2932–2946.

Whitwell JL, Avula R, Senjem ML et al. (2010). Gray and white matter water diffusion in the syndromic variants of frontotemporal dementia. Neurology 74: 1279–1287.

Whitwell JL, Dickson DW, Murray ME et al. (2012a). Neuroimaging correlates of pathologically defined subtypes of Alzheimer's disease: a case-control study. Lancet Neurol 11: 868–877.

Whitwell JL, Weigand SD, Boeve BF et al. (2012b). Neuroimaging signatures of frontotemporal dementia genetics: C9ORF72, tau, progranulin and sporadics. Brain 135: 794–806.

Whitwell JL, Jack Jr CR, Parisi JE et al. (2013). Midbrain atrophy is not a biomarker of progressive supranuclear palsy pathology. Eur J Neurol 20: 1417–1422.

Whitwell JL, Boeve BF, Weigand SD et al. (2015a). Brain atrophy over time in genetic and sporadic frontotemporal dementia: a study of 198 serial magnetic resonance images. Eur J Neurol 22: 745–752.

Whitwell JL, Duffy JR, Strand EA et al. (2015b). Clinical and neuroimaging biomarkers of amyloid-negative logopenic primary progressive aphasia. Brain Lang 142: 45–53.

Whitwell JL, Jones DT, Duffy JR et al. (2015c). Working memory and language network dysfunctions in logopenic aphasia: a task-free fMRI comparison with Alzheimer's dementia. Neurobiol Aging 36: 1245–1252.

Wolk DA, Price JC, Saxton JA et al. (2009). Amyloid imaging in mild cognitive impairment subtypes. Ann Neurol 65: 557–568.

Wolk DA, Grachev ID, Buckley C et al. (2011). Association between in vivo fluorine 18-labeled flutemetamol amyloid positron emission tomography imaging and in vivo cerebral cortical histopathology. Arch Neurol 68: 1398–1403.

Wolz R, Julkunen V, Koikkalainen J et al. (2011). Multi-method analysis of MRI images in early diagnostics of Alzheimer's disease. PLoS One 6: e25446.

Yasuno F, Kosaka J, Ota M et al. (2012). Increased binding of peripheral benzodiazepine receptor in mild cognitive impairment-dementia converters measured by positron emission tomography with [(1)(1)C]DAA1106. Psychiatry Res 203: 67–74.

Yoder KK, Nho K, Risacher SL et al. (2013). Influence of TSPO genotype on 11C-PBR28 standardized uptake values. J Nucl Med 54: 1320–1322.

Yuan Y, Gu ZX, Wei WS (2009). Fluorodeoxyglucose-positron-emission tomography, single-photon emission tomography, and structural MR imaging for prediction of rapid conversion to Alzheimer disease in patients with mild cognitive impairment: a meta-analysis. AJNR Am J Neuroradiol 30: 404–410.

Zhang Y, Schuff N, Du AT et al. (2009). White matter damage in frontotemporal dementia and Alzheimer's disease measured by diffusion MRI. Brain 132: 2579–2592.

Zhang Y, Tartaglia MC, Schuff N et al. (2013). MRI signatures of brain macrostructural atrophy and microstructural degradation in frontotemporal lobar degeneration subtypes. J Alzheimers Dis 33: 431–444.

Zhou J, Gennatas ED, Kramer JH et al. (2012). Predicting regional neurodegeneration from the healthy brain functional connectome. Neuron 73: 1216–1227.

Handbook of Clinical Neurology, Vol. 135 (3rd series)
Neuroimaging, Part I
J.C. Masdeu and R.G. González, Editors

Chapter 27

Neurocutaneous syndromes

NITASHA KLAR[1], BERNARD COHEN[2], AND DORIS D.M. LIN[1]*

[1]*Division of Neuroradiology, Russell H. Morgan Department of Radiology, Johns Hopkins University School of Medicine, Baltimore, MD, USA*

[2]*Departments of Dermatology and Pediatrics, Johns Hopkins University School of Medicine, Baltimore, MD, USA*

Abstract

Neurocutaneous syndromes (or phakomatoses) are a diverse group of congenital disorders that encompass abnormalities of neuroectodermal and, sometimes, mesodermal development, hence commonly involving the skin, eye, and central nervous system. These are often inherited conditions and typically present in early childhood or adolescence. Some of the abnormalities and clinical symptoms may, however, be progressive, and there is an increased risk of neoplastic formation in many of the syndromes. As a group, neurocutaneous syndromes are characterized by distinctive cutaneous stigmata and neurologic symptomology, the latter often representing the most devastating and debilitating features of these diseases. Many of these syndromes are markedly heterogeneous in nature as they affect many organ systems. Given the incurable nature of these conditions and the broad spectrum of pathologies they comprise, treatments vary on a case-by-case basis and tend to be palliative rather than curative. With the advances in molecular genetics, however, greater understanding of biologic functions of the gene products and the correlative phenotypic expression is being attained, and this knowledge may guide future therapeutic developments. This chapter focuses on the cutaneous and neurologic pathology with emphasis on neuroimaging of selective neurocutaneous syndromes, including tuberous sclerosis, Sturge–Weber syndrome, Klippel–Trenaunay syndrome, ataxia-telangiectasia, and incontinentia pigmenti.

INTRODUCTION

Neurocutaneous syndromes, also known as phakomatoses, represent a diverse group of congenital disorders that encompass abnormalities of neuroectodermal and, at times, mesodermal development, hence preferentially manifesting as malformations in the skin, eye, and central nervous system (CNS). These are often inherited conditions, many have genetic abnormality already identified, although spontaneous mutations are common, and a wide spectrum of phenotypic expression is usually the rule because of variable penetrance. There are also disorders, such as Sturge–Weber syndrome (SWS), that appear to occur sporadically with asymmetric, scattered distributions and variable extent of involvement thought to be characteristic of somatic mutation. Neurocutaneous syndromes are characterized by distinctive cutaneous stigmata and CNS abnormalities, even though many are markedly heterogeneous in nature as they affect multiple organ systems. The abnormalities range from hamartomatous malformations to multiple disseminated neoplasia. Traditionally neurocutaneous syndromes are comprised of neurofibromatosis, tuberous sclerosis (TS), and von-Hippel–Lindau syndrome. We have taken a more liberal and broad definition to include entities with the common involvement of tissues of the neuroectodermal origin. Two of the more frequently encountered entities, neurofibromatosis and von Hippel–Lindau, were discussed in a recent issue of the *Handbook of Clinical Neurology* (Jost and Gutmann, 2012). This chapter will review the cutaneous and CNS

*Correspondence to: Doris D.M. Lin, MD, PhD, Division of Neuroradiology, Russell H. Morgan Department of Radiology, Johns Hopkins University School of Medicine, 600 North Wolfe Street, Phipps B-100, Baltimore MD 21287, USA. Tel: +1-443-287-3079, Fax: +1-410-614-1213, E-mail: ddmlin@jhmi.edu

pathology of these and other phakomatoses, with an emphasis on neuroimaging.

TUBEROUS SCLEROSIS

TS, also known as Bourneville–Pringle disease, is a hereditary neurocutaneous syndrome that involves multiple organ systems, including the brain, kidney, skin, retina, heart, lung, liver, and bone. The disease complex was first described by Bourneville in 1880, while the characteristic triad of seizures, mental retardation, and sebaceous adenoma was later highlighted by Vogt (Rodrigues et al., 2012). The eponym "Pringle disease" is used when there are only dermatologic findings, and "Bonneville disease" when the nervous system is affected (Inoue et al., 1998).

Epidemiology and genetics

TS complex (TSC) has a birth rate of 1/6000 (Osborne et al., 1991) with incidence in children estimated between 1/12 000 and 1/14 000 (Ahlsen et al., 1994; Curatolo et al., 2008). It most often occurs spontaneously as a sporadic mutation (60–75%) (van Slegtenhorst et al., 1997); however, when familial, it is inherited in an autosomal-dominant fashion. Members of the same family often exhibit variable phenotypic penetrance, and there is no racial or sexual predilection.

Up to 85% of the time, the complex results from mutations in two genes and their encoded proteins, TSC1 (hamartin) and TSC2 (tuberin), transmitted on the long arm of chromosome 9 (9q34) (Fryer et al., 1987; van Slegtenhorst et al., 1997) and chromosome 16 (16p13) (Kandt et al., 1992), respectively. The disease is thought to follow Knudson's two-hit model, in which the mutated chromosome must be accompanied by a second somatic mutation in the opposite allele to result in tumor formation (Knudson et al., 1971; Marcotte and Crino, 2006).

The *TSC1* and *TSC2* genes are present in all normal tissues, as well as the affected areas of the brain, kidneys, skin, lung, and liver (Marcotte and Crino, 2006), in effect resulting in hamartomatous growths in numerous organ systems. No significant phenotypic difference has been found between the two gene mutations; however, individuals with *TSC2* mutations are usually affected more severely than those with mutations in *TSC1* (Curatolo et al., 2008). In addition, most sporadic cases are due to somatic mutations of *TSC2*.

The hamartin and tuberin proteins together form a cytoplasmic complex that acts as a tumor suppressor, and also regulates signal transduction critical for multiple downstream cellular development and functions. The most notable of these is the inhibition of the phosphatidylinositol 3-kinase/insulin-activated signaling pathway involving the mammalian target of the rapamycin complex 1 (mTOR1), a kinase that plays a role in promoting cell growth, protein synthesis, and division. Through GTPase activation of Ras homolog enriched in brain (Rheb), the hamartin–tuberin complex mitigates the activation of mTOR. Thus, mutations in either the *TSC1* or *TSC2* genes will affect the regulation of cell growth and proliferation (Marcotte and Crino, 2006).

The mTOR1-induced oncogenic effect can be blocked by rapamycin (an mTOR1 inhibitor) and its derivative everolimus. Both can reduce the size of subependymal giant cell astrocytomas (SEGA) (Franz et al., 2006, 2013; Krueger et al., 2013) and cutaneous administration of rapamycin safely induces regression of the facial angiofibromas (Haemel et al., 2010; DeKlotz et al., 2011).

Diagnosis

Major and minor criteria for TS have been established by the Tuberous Sclerosis Complex Consensus Conference in 1998 for clinical diagnosis (Table 27.1) (Roach et al., 1998). DNA testing aids clinical diagnosis and in some cases can allow for prenatal diagnosis; however, it is

Table 27.1

Diagnostic criteria for tuberous sclerosis

Major features
- Facial angiofibromas or forehead plaque
- Nontraumatic ungula or periungual fibroma
- Hypomelanotic macules (three or more)
- Shagreen patch (connective-tissue nevus)
- Multiple retinal nodular hamartomas
- Cortical tuber
- Subependymal nodule
- Subependymal giant-cell astrocytoma
- Cardiac rhabdomyoma, single or multiple
- Lymphangiomyomatosis
- Renal angiomyolipoma

Minor features
- Multiple, randomly distributed pits in dental enamel
- Hamartomatous rectal polyps
- Bone cysts
- Cerebral white-matter radial migration lines
- Gingival fibromas
- Nonrenal hamartoma
- Retinal achromic patch
- Confetti-like skin lesions
- Multiple renal cysts

Definite tuberous sclerosis complex: either two major features or one major feature with two minor features.
Probable tuberous sclerosis complex: one major plus one minor feature.
Possible tuberous sclerosis complex: either one major feature or two or more minor features.

Adapted from Roach et al. (1998).

fraught with a 15% false-negative rate. The potential for false negatives coupled with the 2% occurrence of germline mosaicism in seemingly unaffected parents creates a challenge for diagnosis in family members (Roach and Sparagana, 2004).

Clinical manifestation

Cutaneous

Up to 96% of patients with TS have dermatologic conditions (Webb et al., 1996) (Fig. 27.1). The most common manifestations include the hypomelanotic macules found in over 90–98% of affected patients, so-called "ash-leaf patches," which may be evident at birth (Roach and Sparagana, 2004). Other common skin lesions include the small stippled hypopigmented 0.2–1-cm pretibial confetti spots, and the facial angiofibromas that are present in up to 75% of cases (Jozwiak et al., 2000). Purple light (Wood's lamp) best depicts the hypomelanotic macules, which often present early in life or infancy but may be difficult to see in light-pigmented individuals.

The facial angiofibromas (for which "adenoma sebaceum" is a misnomer) are hamartomas containing vascular and connective tissue, usually presenting later in childhood with progression through adulthood (O'Callaghan, 2008). Often mistaken for acne papules and comedones, these lesions are comprised of symmetric pink to red papules on the face involving the malar regions and nasolabial folds; however, they can be a deep brown color in dark-pigmented individuals. Laser therapy can be used in the setting of cosmetic disfigurement, or for minimizing the risk of bleeding in older children, where these angiofibromas may become quite large and subject to incidental trauma. Topical sirolimus has also been shown to be safe and effective in reducing symptomatic and disfiguring angiofibromas in recalcitrant cases (Haemel et al., 2010; DeKlotz et al., 2011). Shagreen patches or connective-tissue nevi are well-demarcated pebbly skin-colored, yellowish-red hyperpigmented plaques most commonly found on the trunk, but also can be seen on the thighs. These are often noted at birth and reported in approximately 54% of children older than 5 years old, and are usually evident by puberty (Webb et al., 1996).

The forehead fibrous plaque (also a variant of shagreen plaque) appears as a yellowish or reddish patch on the forehead or scalp. It is sometimes mistaken for a

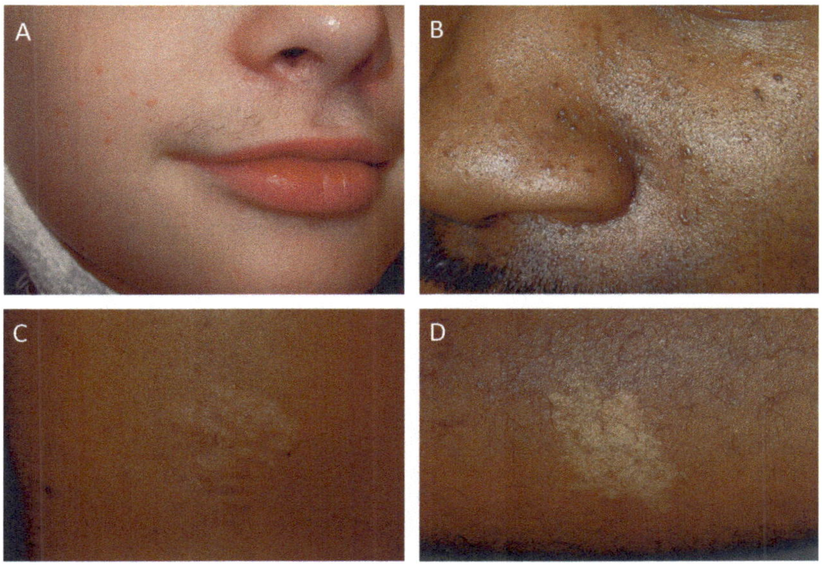

Fig. 27.1. Cutaneous findings in tuberous sclerosis (TS). (**A**) A 13-year-old boy with 1–2-mm smooth dome-shaped red papules on the cheeks, more prominent on the right than left, and around the nose. A skin biopsy revealed an angiofibroma consistent with TS. The family history was negative for similar skin lesions and seizures. (**B**) A 28-year-old man with TS was evaluated for carbon dioxide laser ablation of the angiofibromas on his face, seen as symmetric 2–3-mm hyperpigmented papules. In addition to these angiofibromas, he had several congenital hypopigmented macules on the lower abdomen and thighs, a congenital shagreen patch on the upper chest, and several subungual fibromas that developed during adolescence. (**C**) A 17-year-old boy with a hypopigmented firm superficial plaque comprised of multiple smooth-topped papules on his back characteristic of a shagreen patch. Note also the adjacent scattered 2–3-mm hyperpigmented papules representing angiofibromas. (**D**) An adolescent boy with a congenital ash-leaf macule on his leg, demonstrating a well-demarcated, irregularly shaped hypopigmented macule. He also had multiple hypopigmented macules on his trunk and extremities, collagenomas on his back and chest, subungual fibromas, and a seizure disorder associated with tubers in the brain.

capillary hemangioma or pigmented nevus. Ungual fibromas (seen in 20% of patients) (Roach and Sparagana, 2004) form under the nailbed and tend to leave behind a linear groove on the nail. They may occur posttraumatically. Other dermatologic conditions in TS include skin tags and molluscum fibrosum.

Ocular

Up to 87% of TS patients have retinal lesions, including the classic mulberry lesions adjacent to the optic disc, depigmentation, and plaque-like hamartomas (Roach and Sparagana, 2004). The retinal hamartomas (or retinal astrocytomas) are benign, acquired papillary lesions, which can be multifocal and bilateral. Although these neoplasms are most often clinically silent and nonprogressive, dramatic growth in the setting of TS can occur, resulting in retinal detachment, hemorrhage, and vision loss due to macular obstruction (Shields et al., 2004).

CNS and neuroimaging

Neurologic manifestation includes epilepsy, neurocognitive dysfunction, behavioral problems, and developmental disorders such as autism; however, affected individuals with little or no neurologic impairment are not uncommon. The vast majority of individuals affected by TS exhibit CNS symptoms (Lagos and Gomez, 1967; Curatolo et al., 2008), which are often the most devastating features and are among the most challenging to treat. Seizures are present in up to 80–90% of cases, 70% of which will present within the first year of life, and up to one-third of TS children will experience infantile spasms (Thiele, 2004). The earlier the onset of epilepsy, the more pervasive the autism and developmental problems (Joinson et al., 2003). Some of these symptoms can be correlated with intracranial anatomic findings that manifest as a result of altered proliferation, histogenesis, and migration of neuroglial cells. These include cortical tubers, white-matter migration lines, subependymal nodules (SENs), and SEGAs.

Imaging plays a critical role in the diagnosis, surveillance, and prognostication in TS patients with CNS involvement. It is recommended that affected, asymptomatic children should be monitored by cranial magnetic resonance imaging (MRI) every 1–3 years, and more frequently if they exhibit symptoms. Asymptomatic first-degree relatives should also undergo screening cranial MRI at the time of the affected individual's diagnosis (Hyman and Whittemore, 2000). Detection of anatomic manifestations can be made *in utero*, with early identification of SEN and cardiac rhabdomyomas on fetal ultrasound and MRI. Cortical tubers have been detected as early as 20 weeks of fetal life (Park et al., 1997). Neuroimaging has become an invaluable tool in the diagnosis of the disease, as the CNS abnormalities of TS comprise several of the major criteria required for diagnosis, all easily identifiable by imaging.

Cortical tubers

The tubers in TS are present in 80–95% of cases (Christophe et al., 2000; Marcotte and Crino, 2006) and are strongly associated with epileptogenesis (Thiele, 2004). Symptomatology worsens with increasing number of lesions, potentially leading to more severe autism in adolescents and adults, and intractable epilepsy and cognitive impairment in children. Histopathology of cortical tubers is similar to that of focal cortical dysplasias, consisting of disorganized cortical architecture, dysplastic neurons, enlarged astrocytes, and association with giant cells. The cortex usually demonstrates loss of the normal six-layered arrangement with subpial gliosis, sometimes associated with calcification and cystic change.

The astrocytes within cortical tubers are dysmorphic and greater in both size and number compared to surrounding brain. It follows that the hyperproliferation of the astrocytic cells is likely explained by the disinhibition of cell growth and proliferation mediated by the *TSC1* and *TSC2* mutations (Wong and Crino, 2012).

The pathogenesis behind seizure induction in the presence of tubers remains unclear. The removal of the tubers may improve symptoms, and is usually reserved for intractable seizures; however, whether the tuber itself as a cortical malformation is the epileptogenic source, or whether it induces seizure activity in the perituberal cortex, remains an area of investigation. Epileptogenesis may be related to disinhibition due to altered gamma-aminobutyric acid (GABA) receptors and enhanced excitation by changes in the glutamate receptors occurring selectively in the dysplastic neurons and giant cells found in tubers (White et al., 2001). This notion is supported by the efficacy of vigabatrin, an inhibitor of GABA-transaminase, as an antiepileptic drug in TS.

On MRI, cortical tubers appear as T1 hypointense and T2 hyperintense, expansile lesions in the cortex (and subcortical region) of the brain occurring at the apex of a gyrus, sometimes exhibiting central umbilication (Fig. 27.2). They are often multiple, most often occur in the frontal lobes, and can be associated with cystic change or calcification. The calcification is best seen on computed tomography (CT) as focal hyperdensities (Fig. 27.3), and may be identified on MRI as T2 hypointense areas. Fluid-attenuated inversion recovery (FLAIR) sequence has greater sensitivity in detecting the cortical tubers (Maeda et al., 1995) (Fig. 27.4A, B). As symptomatology worsens with increasing tuber

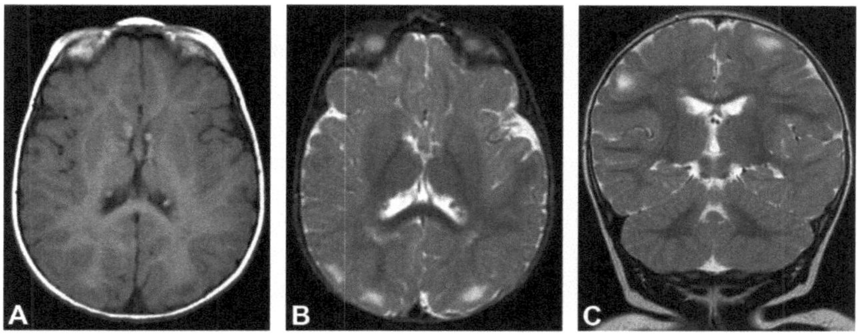

Fig. 27.2. A 1½-year old boy with tuberous sclerosis, epilepsy, autism, and central hypoventilation syndrome. (**A**) Axial T1, (**B**) axial T2, and (**C**) coronal T2-weighted magnetic resonance images show multiple parietal-occipital cortical tubers that appear as expansile regions of T2 hyperintensity, sometimes cyst-like, with umbilication (best seen on coronal images). Each lesion is beneath the broad, shallow cortical gyri and may have a tail of T2 hyperintensity extending towards the ventricles, an appearance characteristic of focal cortical dysplasia. On T1-weighted images these tubers appear hypointense but they are less readily identified. In addition, multiple tiny T1 hyperintense and T2 hypointense nodular lesions cluster along the ventricular margin (often described as "candle guttering" appearance), representing subependymal nodules.

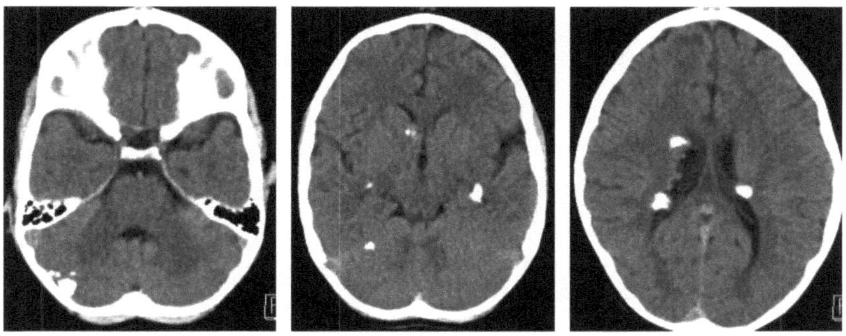

Fig. 27.3. Axial head computed tomography images in the same child as in Figure 27.2, performed at 11 years of age. Multiple hyperattenuated nodules along the ependymal surface represent calcified subependymal nodules. A calcified cortical tuber is also present in the right cerebellar hemisphere.

number, MRI has become a primary tool in the prognostication of CNS disabilities. In older children and adults, cortical tubers with intrinsic T1 shortening may be hidden by the presence of myelination, and advanced imaging sequences such as magnetization transfer can aid traditional spin-echo sequences in better depicting the tubers as well as subtle white-matter abnormalities (Barkovich, 2005). Enhancement of cortical tubers occurs less than 5% of the time (Braffman et al., 1992).

Proton magnetic resonance spectroscopy (MRS) investigation of cortical tubers demonstrates a pattern of decreased ratio of *N*-acetyl aspartate (NAA)/creatine (Cr) due to neuronal loss or dysfunction, and increased myo-inositol/Cr ratio, reflecting gliosis (Yapici et al., 2005). This tool could be particularly helpful in cases where diagnosis is questionable, and the need to distinguish between cortical tubers and neoplasms arises. In addition, correlative analysis between MRS and electroencephalography has identified the tuber as the epileptogenic focus by the presence of a lactate peak (Yapici et al., 2005), serving as a potential guide to surgeons in refractory cases.

The role of diffusion-weighted imaging in TS is still being investigated. Cortical tubers have higher values on apparent diffusion coefficient maps and may be higher still in the epileptogenic tubers (Jansen et al., 2003). Diffusion tensor imaging exploits the microstructure of white-matter tracts to provide information on the integrity of neuronal circuitry and may also be useful in characterization of abnormal white matter (Luat et al., 2007). Cortical tubers are hypometabolic on 2-deoxy-2-[^{18}F] fluoro-D-glucose positron emission tomography (FDG-PET) (Szelies et al., 1983). Alpha-[^{11}C] methyl-L-tryptophan PET shows increased tracer uptake corresponding to areas of epileptogenicity in TS in approximately two-thirds of patients with seizures and is another promising method for noninvasive evaluation (Luat et al., 2007).

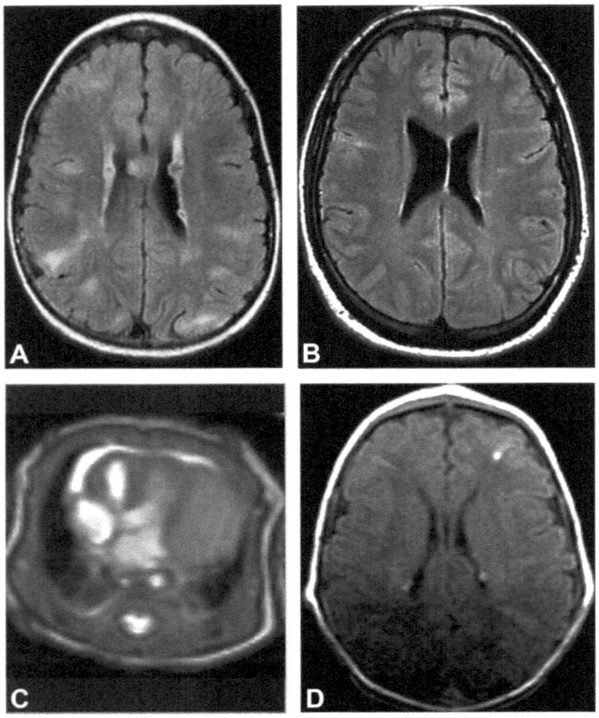

Fig. 27.4. Cortical/subcortical tubers in tuberous sclerosis. (**A**) Fluid-attenuated inversion recovery (FLAIR) is the best sequence demonstrating hyperintense white-matter signal abnormalities in childhood and adults. Note the presence of small subependymal nodules. (**B**) Linear white-matter migration tracks can also be best depicted on FLAIR; these represent the radial migration tracks of the immature neurons that did not reach the cortical destination, and are considered a minor feature in the revised diagnostic criteria. (**C**) A 5-day-old male infant who had multiple cardiac masses detected *in utero* by ultrasound. Axial T1-weighted magnetic resonance image shows a large soft-tissue mass abutting the left cardiac ventricle, consistent with a rhabdomyoma. (**D**) In the same 5-day-old infant, multiple linear radial migration lines and cortical/subcortical tubers are best shown as hyperintensity on T1-weighted images in the neonatal period because of immature myelination. Punctate T1 hyperintense subependymal nodules are also present.

White-matter migration lines

Abnormal white-matter neuronal migration lines are often seen in TS and are believed to represent ectopic neuroglial cells along the path of cortical migration (Griffiths et al., 1998). They are characterized by T2 and FLAIR hyperintense lines, oriented perpendicular to the ventricular axis. Subtle white-matter abnormalities are usually more easily distinguishable in neonates (seen as hyperintensity on T1-weighted images; Fig. 27.4D), as the onset of myelination often obscures these lesions, underlining the utility of imaging at younger ages (Baron and Barkovich, 1999).

Subependymal nodules and subependymal giant cell astrocytoma

SENs are hamartomatous lesions found in 80% of TS cases (Marcotte and Crino, 2006), and are believed to be asymptomatic, with no known relation to epileptogenesis. They are predominantly located along the ependymal surface, but can extend into the periventricular white matter and basal ganglia. They appear in fetal life, normally regressing with age, and are of no known clinical consequence, except for their presumed potential to develop into SEGAs, although the molecular pathogenesis behind this transformation is unknown.

Both SENs and SEGAs are composed of dysmorphic glial cells and giant cells. Lineage studies suggest that cortical tubers and SEN/SEGA may originate from the same progenitor cells derived from the subventricular zone of the lateral ventricles, as evidenced by common expression of cellular markers (Lee et al., 2003; Ess et al., 2005). The major distinguisher between SEGA and SEN is their size. Nodules near the foramen of Monro greater than 5 mm in size have a higher transformation rate to SEGA (Nabbout et al., 1999) compared to smaller nodules in other locations.

SEGAs are of mixed glioneuronal components and are slow growing, usually developing by 20 years of age. They represent the most common brain tumor type in TS patients, occurring in approximately 10–15% of cases (Nabbout et al., 1999; Wong and Crino, 2012). These lesions are nonmalignant tumors with low mitotic index, comprised of spindle cell bundles, gemistocytes, ganglion-like cells, and inflammatory cells, including T lymphocytes and mastocytes (Sharma et al., 2004). They may produce visual impairment, endocrinopathies, and focal neurologic deficits; however, the main concern of these neoplasms ultimately lies within their potential to cause sudden catastrophic obstructive hydrocephalus and intracranial hypertension due to their proximity to the foramen of Monro.

SENs, asymptomatic themselves, do not have much impact clinically; however, their presence aids in the diagnosis of the complex and necessitates monitoring for potential transformation to SEGAs (Fig. 27.5). On imaging, they are associated with calcification 88% of the time. When calcified, they are more easily detected on CT than MRI. In infants, SENs are T1 hyperintense and T2 hypointense, the opposite of what is seen in noncalcified lesions in adults. Enhancement is seen variably in SENs (Altman et al., 1988; Braffman et al., 1992) and therefore is not a reliable indicator for transformation to SEGA, although SEGAs do enhance more commonly (Braffman et al., 1992). SEGAs are distinguished from SEN based on their size and location, as well as their tendency to grow. SENs tend to be less than 1 cm in size (Wong and Crino, 2012)

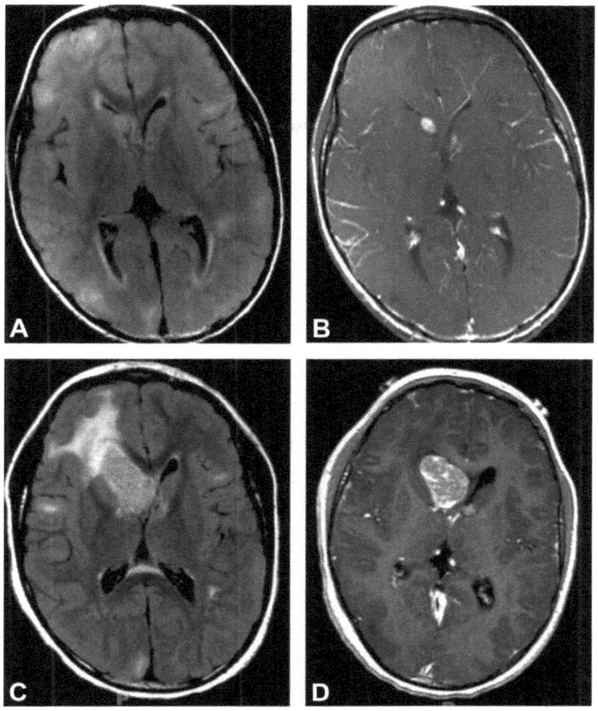

Fig. 27.5. Tuberous sclerosis with subependymal giant cell astrocytomas that grew significantly in a 4-year period in a child. (**A**) Axial fluid-attenuated inversion recovery (FLAIR) and (**B**) postgadolinium T1-weighted magnetic resonance image show a discrete enhancing mass in right frontal horn along the ependymal surface in this child at 7 years of age. Multiple cortical FLAIR hyperintense tubers are also present. (**C, D**) At 11 years of age, the same enhancing mass has grown to fill and expand the right frontal horn, associated with adjacent parenchymal FLAIR hyperintensity, indicating vasogenic edema. Note another small subependymal nodule located at the left foramen of Monro. No obstructive hydrocephalus in this case.

and those located near the foramen of Monro should be monitored for growth over time.

STURGE–WEBER SYNDROME

SWS is also known as encephalotrigeminal angiomatosis, occurring at a frequency ranging between 1 in 20 000 and 50 000 live births (Comi, 2007). It has a sporadic occurrence and was recently found to be caused by a mosaic somatic mutation in *GNAQ* (Shirley et al., 2013), mainly affecting the skin and CNS, occasionally with ophthalmologic manifestations.

Pathogenesis

The etiology and pathogenesis of SWS remain unknown. The presence of skin findings at birth suggests an embryologic insult that manifests itself as a dysplastic vascular malformation in the face, eye, and brain. It is proposed that failure of regression of the embryologic venous plexus in the first trimester constitutes the angiomatous findings in these structures (Comi, 2003). Pathogenesis is likely rooted in the fact that the upper facial neuroectoderm lies in close proximity to the parieto-occipital segment of the neural tube in early stages of embryologic development (Maiuri et al., 1989), explaining the common association between the characteristic stigmata in the homolateral facial skin, eye, and brain. The sporadic nature of the disease belies a genetic explanation; however, familial studies support a somatic gene mutation early in development, with a possible autosomal-dominant mode of inheritance (Comi, 2003) that exhibits an expression pattern characteristic of early somatic mosaicism. This long-held hypothesis of somatic mosaic mutation was recently confirmed by whole-genome sequencing, identifying a unique single-nucleotide mutation in *GNAQ* that was present in affected tissues in SWS and nonsyndromic port-wine stains (Shirley et al., 2013). As *GNAQ* encodes a subunit of G-protein that is involved in signal transduction pathway-regulating cellular activities, including endothelin, it has been postulated that the mutation may provide a mechanism for anomalous vasculogenesis during early embryonic development (Shirley et al., 2013).

Pial angiomatosis with subjacent regional cerebral atrophy represents the hallmark intracranial finding of SWS. The cerebral atrophy is believed to represent involutional changes secondary to a chronic hypoperfused state induced by the pial angioma. The dysplastic vessels within the angiomatous malformation exhibit augmented vascular hyalinization and variable luminal caliber, and induce altered hemodynamics by causing delayed and diminished venous drainage. Slow flow and subsequent thrombotic obstruction in the superficial vessels lead to shunting of blood through aberrant pathways, inducing localized ischemia and intermittent stroke-like episodes. This chronic ischemic state results in regional atrophy, calcification, and gliosis in affected parenchyma (Probst, 1980). Pathology specimens also confirm astrogliosis, neuronal cell loss, and cortical calcification as a result of chronic ischemic injury.

Furthermore, the dysplastic vessels express higher levels of endothelin-1, a vascoconstrictive peptide (Rhoten et al., 1997), and are exposed solely to noradrenergic sympathetic innervation (Cunha e Sa et al., 1997). This unbalanced innervation causes increased constrictor tone and thus impaired cerebral autoregulatory response to blood pressure, which contributes to the chronic ischemia. The ischemia in turn further exacerbates situations of increased oxygen demand, such as with hypotension and seizures (Cunha e Sa et al., 1997).

The altered hemodynamics at the brain surface results in flow diversion to the deeper venous system, which becomes engorged (Probst, 1980), producing the typical venous angiomas. The phenomenon of plethora to the deeper structures is a likely mechanism for the enlarged ipsilateral choroid plexus (glomus) commonly seen in these patients as well.

Clinical manifestation

SWS is subclassified into three types: type 1, the classic form that includes facial and leptomeningeal angiomatosis with or without glaucoma; type 2, facial angioma and possible glaucoma, without intracranial involvement; and type 3, leptomeningeal angioma but no facial angioma or ocular manifestation (Roach, 1992).

Cutaneous

The characteristic skin finding is the port-wine nevus (Fig. 27.6A), a vascular malformation comprised of dilated capillaries, postcapillary venules, and small veins. Skin lesions at birth vary from subtle pink to red blanching patches that demonstrate progressive ectasia, and darken and thicken with age. When present in the setting of SWS, the nevus invariably involves the facial distribution of the ophthalmic division of the trigeminal nerve (V1), sometimes including V2 and V3, and can be bilateral up to 40% of the time (Piram et al., 2012).

While only 6–8% of individuals with port-wine birthmark anywhere on the skin surface are afflicted with SWS (Enjolras et al., 1985; Piram et al., 2012), 25% of people with a V1 malformation demonstrate findings of SWS. Upper-eyelid involvement, large size of the lesion, extension to the contralateral face, or involvement of the V1/V2 distribution increases the diagnostic possibility of SWS in those with the characteristic cutaneous traits (Piram et al., 2012). Notably, 10–15% of individuals with the classic intracranial and ocular stigmata will not display the birthmark (Comi, 2003; Thomas-Sohl et al., 2004). When present, the intracranial and ocular abnormalities are ipsilateral to the skin lesions.

Ocular

The primary ophthalmologic complication is glaucoma (30–70%) (Thomas-Sohl et al., 2004), probably due to a combination of increased venous pressure caused by the vascular malformation of the eye, and alterations in the anterior chamber resulting in impaired drainage (Comi, 2007). This can lead to progressive ocular-globe atrophy and blindness. Other ocular manifestations include hemianopsia (40–45%) (Thomas-Sohl et al., 2004), tortuous and dilated conjunctival or subconjunctival vessels (Fig. 27.6B), and diffuse choroidal hemangiomas (Piram et al., 2012) (Fig. 27.6C).

CNS

Functional morbidity in SWS is related to involvement of the CNS. Neurologic findings include vascular headache (40–60%), developmental delay and mental retardation

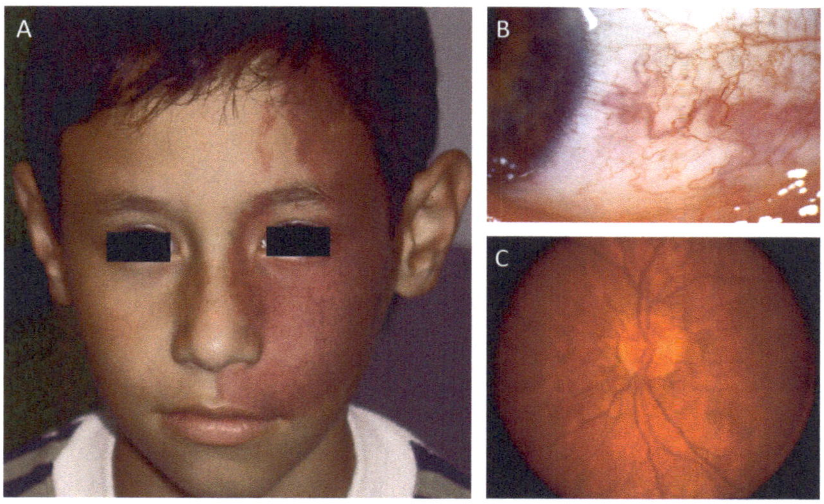

Fig. 27.6. Cutaneous and ocular findings in Sturge–Weber syndrome (SWS). (**A**) An 8-year-old boy with a congenital port-wine stain in the left V1 and V2 distributions, associated with an ipsilateral ocular and pial vascular malformation characteristic of SWS. (Courtesy of Ben Hidalgo-Matlock, MD.) (**B**) A 25-year-old man with SWS had an extensive left facial port-wine stain, elevated intraocular pressure, and seizures. Note the dilated corkscrew conjunctival vessels on the left eye. (**C**) A 6-year-old boy with extensive port-wine stain involving the right face and scalp, and glaucoma in the right eye. The involved right fundus appears bright red due to thickening of the choroidal blood vessels. (**B**, **C** courtesy of Cameron Parsa, MD.)

(50–75%) (Thomas-Sohl et al., 2004), stroke-like symptoms, hemiparesis, and seizures (75%).

Seizures are implicated as a major cause of disability in the affected individuals: 75% occur before the first year of life (Sujansky and Conradi, 1995). It is proposed that epileptogenesis is both due to, and exacerbated by, ischemia caused by the microvascular venous stasis and thrombosis that occur in parenchyma subjacent to the pial angiomatosis. Histopathology sometimes reveals focal cortical dysgenesis, another potential source of seizures (Comi, 2007). The seizures are usually focal in nature, arising from the areas of diseased parenchyma, and incidence increases to 95% when intracranial disease is bilateral (Comi, 2011). Early seizure onset and bilateral disease are both risk factors for developing intractable epilepsy and intellectual impairment (Arzimanoglou and Aicardi, 1992; Roach et al., 1994; Sujansky and Conradi, 1995; Lee et al., 2001). If the seizures are severe and protracted, chances of developmental delay, permanent hemiparesis, and cognitive deficits are increased (Kramer et al., 2000). Epilepsy control is paramount in these patients, as prolonged and even permanent deficits can occur, including hemiparesis, which can affect up to 50–60% of patients (Arzimanoglou and Aicardi, 1992; Kramer et al., 2000).

Patients who obtain seizure control for long periods, either through medical or surgical treatments, may have less intellectual impairment, hemiparesis, and visual field defects (Comi, 2007) than those who do not have successful seizure control. Surgery such as hemispherectomy or lesionectomy should be reserved for severe, medically refractory cases only (Roach et al., 1994; Kramer et al., 2000).

Neuroimaging

In the absence of neurologic symptoms, cerebral imaging is only indicated in cases where the V1 distribution is involved with a port-wine birthmark. It is important to note that imaging may be initially negative in neonates, perhaps because the very early stages of altered venous hemodynamics have not yet reached a threshold for imaging detection, and should be repeated after 6–12 months in at-risk infants with the V1 port-wine birthmark (Boukobza et al., 2000).

The characteristic pial angiomatosis affects the parieto-occipital region most commonly; however, it can sometimes extend to the temporal and frontal lobes. Parallel linear cortical calcifications undulating along the gyral surface yield the characteristic "tram-track" appearance seen both on CT and MR (Smirniotopoulos, 2004). Localized parenchymal atrophy, calcification, and gliosis occur in the gray and white matter subjacent to the angioma. The typical venous angiomas and choroid plexus glomus occur ipsilateral to the pial angioma and cerebral atrophy.

If the hemiatrophy of the brain occurs at an early stage, it can lead to a compensatory hypertrophy of petrous and other structures in the ipsilateral cranium, the so-called Dyke–Davidoff–Maison syndrome. This includes widening of the calvarial diploic space and enlargement of the sinuses and facial musculature. However, whether the diploic space thickening occurs secondarily as part of a compensatory mechanism, or develops on its own due to the anomalous vasculature, is uncertain.

CT is superior to conventional MRI in depicting calcification (Fig. 27.7); however, postcontrast T1-weighted MRI can far better illustrate the leptomeningeal contrast enhancement associated with the pial angiomatosis (Figs 27.8 and 27.9). Contrast-enhanced FLAIR has been promoted as a superior sequence for demonstrating the pial contrast enhancement compared to routine postcontrast T1 sequences, probably due to the suppression of venous signal (Griffiths et al., 2003) (Fig. 27.8). Susceptibility-weighted imaging (SWI) utilizes the inherent T2* effect caused by deoxyhemoglobin within venous structures, which manifests as dark signal

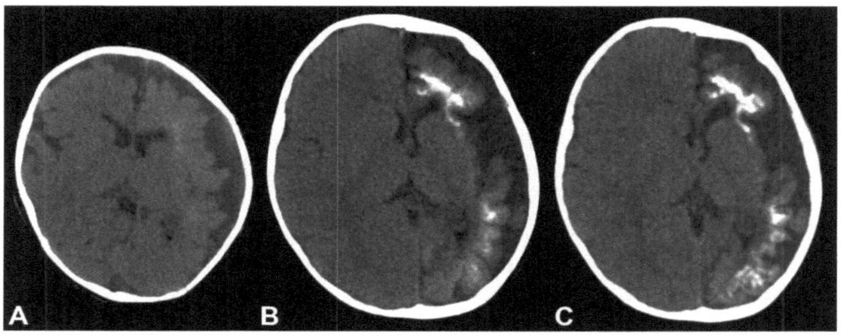

Fig. 27.7. Serial axial head computed tomography examinations in a boy affected by Sturge–Weber syndrome at (**A**) 3 months, (**B**) 1 year, and (**C**) 2½ years of age show progressive cerebral atrophy throughout the left hemisphere, and increasing subcortical and cortical dystrophic calcifications. These changes were subtle during infancy, and dramatically increased within his first year of life.

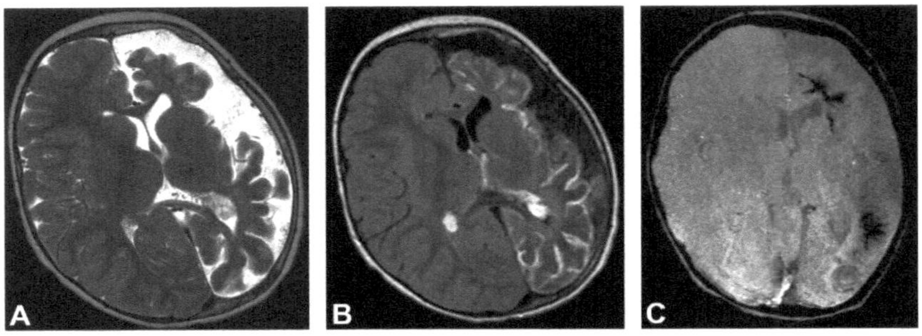

Fig. 27.8. Same boy as Figure 27.7, performed at 2 years of age. (**A**) T2-weighted magnetic resonance image shows marked left cerebral hemisphere volume loss. (**B**) Postgadolinium fluid-attenuated inversion recovery (FLAIR) image demonstrates leptomeningeal enhancement in the affected left cerebral hemisphere, in addition to a prominent enhancing left choroid plexus. (**C**) Susceptibility-weighted imaging reveals patchy areas of dark signal in the left frontal and parietal regions corresponding to calcifications that were more extensively shown on computed tomography.

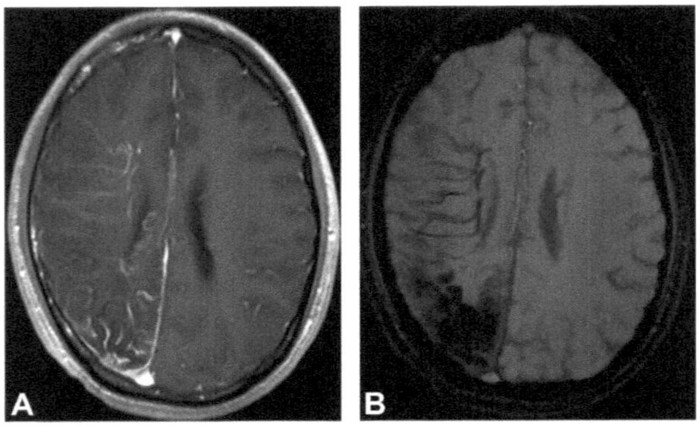

Fig. 27.9. A 15-year-old boy with Sturge–Weber syndrome. (**A**) Postgadolinium T1-weighted image shows leptomeningeal angiomatosis in the right occipital lobe. Prominent enhancing transmedullary veins (venous angiomas) adjacent to the right lateral ventricle serve as a collateral venous drainage pathway. (**B**) Susceptibility-weighted imaging highlights these venous angiomas in the right cerebral hemisphere. In addition, markedly dark signal is present in the right occipital-parietal region, reflecting coarse dystrophic calcification along the site of pial angiomatosis.

(Fig. 27.9). SWI highlights the abnormal parenchymal veins more conspicuously than the postcontrast T1 sequences, and sometimes allows detection of vascular abnormalities that are not seen otherwise (Hu et al., 2008). SWIs provide physiologic, in addition to anatomic, information by characterizing the various degrees of deoxygenation in the brain, potentially illustrating a road map of aberrant venous drainage (Hu et al., 2008), and is also very sensitive for detecting calcifications.

On diffusion-weighted imaging, elevated apparent diffusion coefficient values are seen in the diseased parenchyma, likely due to the increased motion of water molecules after loss of normal cerebral architecture in the setting of gliosis (Cakirer et al., 2005). This is supported by the MRS findings of diminished NAA and elevated choline (Cho), highlighting neuronal cell loss or dysfunction, and breakdown of neuronal tissue (Cunha e Sa et al., 1997; Lin et al., 2006a).

FDG PET reveals disturbances in cerebral glucose uptake, while single-photon emission CT can depict the progressive hypoperfusion of parenchyma underlying the venous angioma, sometimes preceding clinical symptoms and MRI findings (Reid et al., 1997; Lee et al., 2001). Interestingly, Lee and colleagues (2001) demonstrated through PET that regions of brain with relatively mild cerebral hypoperfusion paradoxically correlate more strongly with seizure activity compared to severely hypoperfused brain, exemplifying mildly malfunctioning brain as possessing greater epileptogenic potential than what is likely gliotic brain (Lee et al., 2001).

MR perfusion complements the PET findings as the time–activity curves reveal a normal arterial phase in the majority of the affected brain parenchyma, while venous clearance is delayed, further implicating venous abnormalities as the main culprit in this disease (Lin et al., 2006a). The mean transit time proves the most sensitive parameter on MR perfusion, prolonged in the areas of affected brain (Lin et al., 2006a).

Both functional and anatomic imaging evaluations have a role in prognosis. MRS and MR perfusion may act as functional measures for assessing disease severity, as evidenced by the correlation between diminishing perfusion and metabolite alteration (decreased NAA/Cr and increased Cho/Cr ratios) with worsening neurologic score (Lin et al., 2006a). The presence of disease bilaterality not only portends a worse prognosis, but may also preclude these patients from surgery, especially hemispherectomy, necessitating imaging in treatment stratification. The benefits and timing of surgery remain controversial; however, it is generally believed that early surgery can prevent long-term morbidities associated with SWS (Kramer et al., 2000; Bourgeois et al., 2007).

Thus, functional imaging such as PET may help guide surgical planning early on in cases where morphologic changes have not yet manifested on routine imaging (Lee et al., 2001).

KLIPPEL–TRENAUNAY SYNDROME

Klippel–Trenaunay (KT) syndrome is a sporadic syndrome of mesodermal origin, defined by a characteristic triad of congenital vascular malformation, venous varicosities, and hypertrophy (rarely, hypotrophy) of affected soft tissue and bone. Although not technically a neurocutaneous syndrome due to its lack of predominating CNS pathology, its considerable overlap with SWS in the rare instances when intracranial findings occur deserves mention. Sometimes called Klippel–Trenaunay–Weber syndrome, it has been suggested that this designation should be split into KT and Parkes–Weber (PW) syndromes, representing two distinct entities (Cohen, 2000; Oduber et al., 2008). Both syndromes are characterized by limb enlargement, varicosities, and cutaneous capillary malformations; however, current understanding maintains KT syndrome is a disorder of slow-flow malformations, and should be reserved for those patients with congenital vascular malformations excluding arteriovenous fistulae (AVF), while those with AVFs should be labeled as PW (Cohen, 2000; Oduber et al., 2008). Incidence of KT syndrome is approximately 2–5 per 100 000 (Purkait et al., 2011), although this number should be regarded as an approximation, given the overlap and confusion with other syndromes that contain vascular malformations or tissue hypertrophy, including SWS, PW, Proteus syndrome, and hemihypertrophy (Oduber et al., 2008).

Pathogenesis

The pathogenesis of KT is currently unknown; however, recent discoveries of aberrant *RASA1* expression, involved in mitigating cell proliferation (Renard et al., 2013), and genes involved in angiogenesis, including *AGGF1* (Chen et al., 2013) in affected patients implicate a possible genetic etiology. An alternate hypothesis supports an early embryologic event in fetal development that affects the mesodermal elements as a unifying theory for explaining the various affected cell lines (Star et al., 2010). KT currently has no known heredity and is generally classified as a congenital, noninherited disease. However, cases occurring in multiple family members and in products of consanguinity imply a possible autosomal-recessive inheritance, among other possible inheritance patterns, including somatic mosaicism (Timur et al., 2005; Verhelst and Van Coster, 2005).

Clinical manifestations

Cutaneous and musculoskeletal

Soft-tissue vascular malformations (Fig. 27.10) encountered in KT include capillary malformations (CM, including port-wine stains), venous malformations (VM), lymphatic malformations (LM), and arteriovenous malformations (AVM) (Oduber et al., 2008). The slow-flow types are the most common, and a combination of any of the malformations in the same patient can exist. CMs are seen with greatest frequency, in up to 98% of patients (Jacob et al., 1998). Varicosities or VMs are observed in 72% and LM in 11% (Jacob et al., 1998).

The vascular malformations commonly involve the extremities and trunk, sometimes including visceral organs. Lower-limb involvement occurs in the majority of patients (95%), upper limb less often (5%), and sometimes a combination of the two (15%) (Cohen, 2000). Limb hypertrophy affects 67% of KT syndrome patients (Jacob et al., 1998), usually, but not always, regionally associated with the cutaneous vascular anomaly.

The varicosities typically manifest as the lateral venous anomaly, an embryonic residue found in approximately 72–80% of patients (Jacob et al., 1998; Cohen, 2000). It is distinguished from commonly seen varicose veins by location, size, and age of onset, and can be complicated by thrombophlebitis 19–45% of the time (Jacob et al., 1998). The lateral venous anomaly occurs in infants or children, and is characterized by a plexus of veins beginning on the dorsolateral foot and extending cranially along the lateral leg (Fig. 27.11), sometimes (roughly 33%) involving the entire extremity (Cohen, 2000).

Diagnostic confusion

KT vs PW

The substantial overlap with other syndromes that share many of the same clinical features (such as PW and SWS) creates considerable diagnostic confusion and potential for misdiagnosis. As discussed, the presence of AVF would suggest PW instead of KT. However, there have been rare reports of cerebral (Oyesiku et al., 1988; Dunn and Jaspan, 1993) and spinal AVFs (Dunn and Jaspan, 1993; Rohany et al., 2007) in KT. Many diagnostic criteria have been proposed for KT, some excluding abnormalities of arteriovenous communication (Cohen, 2000), and others allowing for small ones (Oduber et al., 2008). In cases where the presence of AVF or AVM is the predominant feature, PW should be the favored diagnosis. Although digital subtraction angiography is the gold standard, magnetic resonance angiography can noninvasively identify arteriovenous shunting and facilitate categorization of the two conditions (Ziyeh et al., 2004).

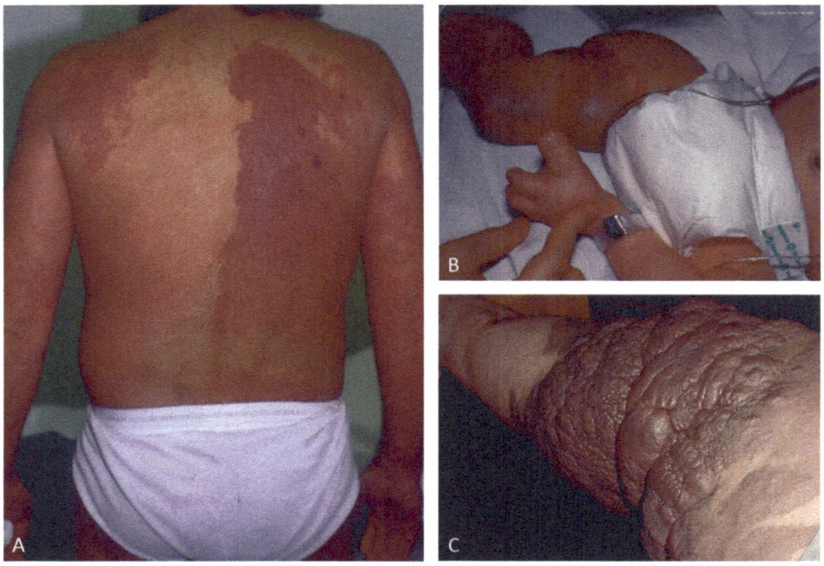

Fig. 27.10. Cutaneous findings in Klippel–Trenaunay–Weber syndrome. (**A**) A 39-year-old man with extensive congenital port-wine stain covering half of his trunk and extending on to both arms and legs. He also had hypertrophy of the soft tissue of the right leg without leg length discrepancy. (Courtesy of Alison Rhein, MD.) (**B**) A 6-month-old baby with hypertrophy of the right leg and left foot associated with malformations of the deep venous system in the right leg. (**C**) A 48-year-old man with congenital right-leg hypertrophy presenting with thick, warty, confluent purple plaques related to a complex congenital venous/lymphatic vascular malformation. He had progressive edema, recurrent infection, and bleeding from the malformation. (Courtesy of Gary Graham, MD.)

Extremity LMs and disorders of the lymphatic system, including lymphatic vesicles and lymphedema, commonly occur in KT and are not seen in PW, a valuable distinguisher (Cohen, 2000). Correctly identifying the appropriate syndrome is important, as patients with PW have a significantly worse prognosis due to the potential for high-output cardiac failure associated with large AVFs.

KT vs SWS

Both KT and SWS are phakomatoses of mesodermal origin with uncertain inheritance, although most cases occur sporadically. In KT, the CM or port-wine nevus is the anomaly seen most frequently, affecting up to 98% of cases (Jacob et al., 1998). They can occur anywhere in the body; however, facial involvement is rarely seen. Understandably, when CMs do involve the face, there is difficulty in distinguishing these patients from SWS, especially in the case of associated ocular and intracranial manifestations, discussed below. Asymmetric limb atrophy in the setting of hemiparesis may occur in SWS, further confounding the issue (Cohen, 2000).

Given the considerable overlap, it is likely that some cases are misdiagnosed as one another, and sometimes patients are diagnosed with both KT and SWS (described as "overlap syndrome": Verhelst and Van Coster, 2005; Rahman et al., 2008; Chhajed et al., 2010; Purkait et al., 2011). While it is uncommon to have CNS involvement in KT, CNS manifestations similar to SWS have been described in more than 40 cases previously (Verhelst and Van Coster, 2005), and a handful reported them as KT-SWS overlap syndromes, with imaging documentation of intracranial involvement (Verhelst and Van Coster, 2005; Rahman et al., 2008; Chhajed et al., 2010; Purkait et al., 2011). However, it is uncertain whether these cases should be regarded as each separate syndrome with unusual presentations, concurrent but distinct etiologic entities, or variant expression of the same syndrome (Vissers et al., 2003; Verhelst and Van Coster, 2005).

Because many of the cerebral stigmata are seen in both disorders, the two should be distinguished by cutaneous findings, with emphasis on the presence of the port-wine stain below the neck attributable to KT and those above the neck designated as SWS, especially when along the V1 distribution. Additionally, the presence of extremity LMs and VMs would support KT over SWS. Clear diagnostic criteria do not exist, and would be necessary in settling the confusion between all these syndromes, which may very well represent a continuum of the same disease (Williams and Elster, 1992).

CNS and neuroimaging

The various CNS findings of KT (Fig. 27.12) include enhancing choroid plexus glomus, cerebral atrophy,

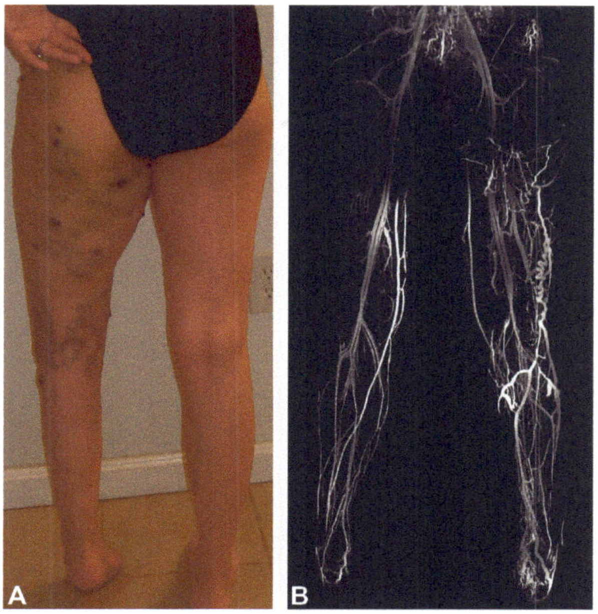

Fig. 27.11. Klippel–Trenaunay–Weber syndrome with venous vascular malformation. (**A**) A 25-year-old woman with a congenital purple patch on her vulvae and new purple linear telangiectasias and nodular lesions gradually appearing in her left hip, genital area, leg, ankle and foot, and left side of her back over years. Her left leg was 3 inches (8 cm) shorter than her right, and her left foot was four shoe sizes smaller than the right. The affected foot swells dramatically episodically. (Courtesy of Laura Essary, MD.) (**B**) A 17-year-old girl with Klippel–Trenaunay. Ablavar (gadofosveset trisodium)-enhanced magnetic resonance angiography shows a tortuous and dilated lateral vein, which is an embryonic residue, coursing along the lateral aspect of the left calf and thigh communicating with the popliteal vein, and with a network of dilated veins in the subcutaneous calf region.

cerebral calcifications, angiomatous leptomeningeal enhancement (Williams and Elster, 1992; Renard et al., 2013), and ischemia (Renard et al., 2012), features that are all demonstrated in SWS. While facial CMs similar to those in SWS may rarely be observed in KT, generally AVM, VM, and LM hardly ever involve the face or brain, although rare cases of cerebral (Huber et al., 1989; Suga et al., 1994) and spinal AVM have been reported (Kojima et al., 1989; Rohany et al., 2007).

Cerebrovascular abnormalities are implicated in the majority of strokes related to KT, including vascular ectasias, dissection, and intracranial aneurysms (Renard et al., 2012). Cerebral aneurysms can have especially catastrophic results in the setting of the known chronic consumptive coagulopathy that sometimes occurs with this condition (Star et al., 2010). It is estimated that noncutaneous vascular abnormalities of the head and neck in KT affect approximately 10% of patients (Star et al., 2010), perhaps warranting consideration of angiographic screening with MR angiography, CT angiography, or conventional angiography in these patients.

The most common CNS finding is alteration in brain size, usually on the same side as the musculoskeletal hypertrophy and skin lesions (Torregrosa et al., 2000). Cerebral (Anlar et al., 1988; Torregrosa et al., 2000) and cerebellar hypertrophy (Anlar et al., 1988) as well as hemimegancephaly have been reported, with the former occurring up to 18% of the time (Torregrosa et al., 2000). The affected brain may be hypometabolic on FDG-PET and display diminished perfusion on perfusion-weighted MRI (Renard et al., 2013). These patients may also be afflicted by seizures, which have been described in the setting of cerebral AVF (Dunn and Jaspan, 1993) and hemimegalencephaly, sometimes with associated cortical gray-matter malformations or cortical heterotopias (Torregrosa et al., 2000; Chhajed et al., 2010).

The calvarium may be diffusely affected by venous vascular malformations, with a picture of hemangiomatosis such as in Figure 27.13. Ophthalmic involvement in KT is uncommon, and may include both retinal and choroidal vascular abnormalities (such as diffuse choroidal angioma), macular telangiectasias, retinal dysplasia, and retinal arteriovenous communications (Brod et al., 1992).

ATAXIA TELANGIECTASIA

Ataxia telangiectasia (A-T) is an autosomal-recessive degenerative neurologic disorder, with incidence estimated between 1 per 40 000 and 300 000 live births (Olsen et al., 2001). Also known as Louis–Bar syndrome, it was first described by Syllaba and Henner in 1926 and 30 years later was defined as its own discrete entity by Boder and Sedgwick (1957).

The disorder is characterized by progressive cerebellar ataxia, oculocutaneous telangiectasia, immunodeficiency resulting in predisposition to recurrent sinopulmonary infections, elevated alpha-fetoprotein levels, endocrine dysfunction, and malignancies. Males and females are equally affected, with estimated life span between 20 and 30 years (Hoche et al., 2012). Patients carry a 30–40% lifetime risk of cancer: hematologic malignancies are the most common (Meyn, 1999). Lymphoma and leukemia typically affect younger patients, whereas solid tumors such as breast, gastric, and basal cell carcinomas are seen in older patients and even heterozygous female carriers have an increased risk for breast cancer (Hoche et al., 2012). Primary CNS tumors have rarely been reported, including pilocytic astrocytoma (Habek et al., 2008), glioblastoma

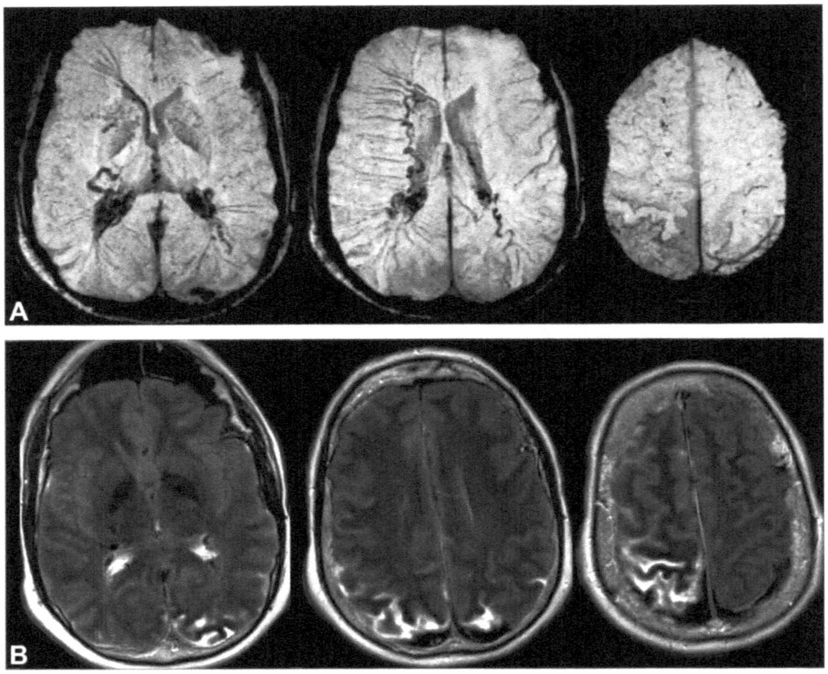

Fig. 27.12. A 28-year-old man with Klippel–Trenaunay syndrome has extensive, complex capillary malformation involving the right chest, abdomen, shoulder, and upper extremities, and some mottled scattered involvement of the left arm and hand, with hypertrophy of the right upper extremity. He also has facial port-wine stain, right-sided glaucoma, seizures, and bilateral intracranial involvement indistinguishable from Sturge–Weber syndrome. (**A**) Susceptibility-weighted imaging shows extensive transmedullary veins draining into enlarged and tortuous deep cerebral veins near the lateral ventricles bilaterally, right more extensive than left. Note also leptomeningeal angiomatosis, most prominent in the high right posterior parietal lobe. (**B**) Gadolinium contrast-enhanced fluid-attenuated inversion recovery (FLAIR) images show enlarged choroid plexus glomus bilaterally, and enhancing pial angiomatosis in the left occipital-parietal region and right parietal lobe.

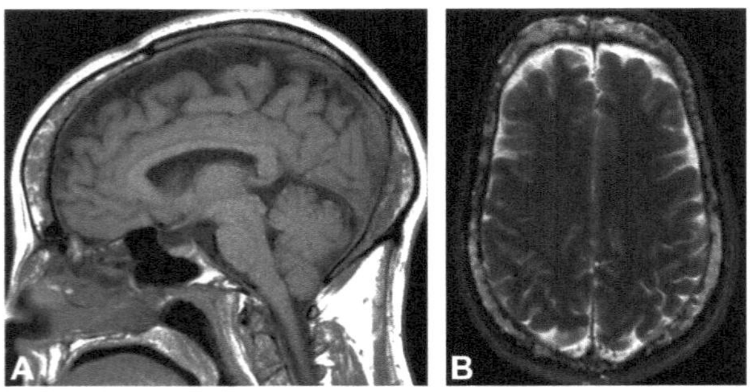

Fig. 27.13. A 43-year-old woman with history of Klippel–Trenaunay complaining of headache and unspecified visual field cut. There was no intracranial involvement. (**A**) Sagittal T1 and (**B**) axial T2-weighted with fat saturation images show diffuse lobular T2 hyperintensity and T1 hypointensity in the calvarial diploic space suggestive of calvarial hemangiomatosis or multiple venous channels. Incidental note was made of mild cerebellar tonsillar ectopia.

(Varan et al., 2004), and medulloblastoma (Hart et al., 1987). The majority (80–90%) of patients with A-T are afflicted by recurrent sinopulmonary infections, which represent a frequent cause of mortality (Sardanelli et al., 1995).

Genetics/pathogenesis

Mutations of the *ATM* gene, mapped to the long arm of chromosome 11, at 11q22–23 are responsible for development of A-T. Over 600 mutations have been identified, located along the length of the gene (Hoche et al., 2012). Most of these mutations are null or missense splice-site mutations, resulting in a dysfunctional or truncated protein (Hoche et al., 2012), leading to either diminished or absent kinase function and thus creating a spectrum from mild (or "variant") to severe ("classic") forms of the disease. The ATM protein has an integral role in signal transduction involved in mediating cellular responses to DNA damage, cell cycle control (Meyn, 1999), and possibly telomeric maintenance (Melcalfe et al., 1996), response to oxidative stress, and mitochondrial homeostasis (Hoche et al., 2012). Individuals with the mutated protein have disabled DNA repair mechanisms, placing them at increased susceptibility to ionizing radiation (IR), and greater propensity to form neoplasms, particularly of lymphoreticular origin.

The ATM gene encodes a serine/threonine kinase, part of the broader family of phosphatidylinositol-3 kinases, which functions as a key signal transducer in the extensive network of downstream DNA repair mechanisms. The ATM kinase is activated by and responds to double-strand breaks in DNA through interactions with the MRN protein complex, the sensor of DNA double-strand breaks. This collaboration results in adenosine diphosphate-dependent phosphorylation of a myriad of proteins involved in DNA repair and replication, cell cycle control, and apoptosis (Lavin, 2008; Tichy et al., 2010). Two such proteins, among numerous others, include the breast cancer susceptibility protein-1 (BRCA1) and p53 binding protein-1 (53BP1), and once recruited, accumulate at the DNA breakage site with a number of other inducible proteins as part of a larger DNA repair machine (Lavin, 2008). p53 and BRCA1 are in and of themselves key players in DNA repair. p53, through activation of a number of target genes, can induce cell-cycle arrest, senescence, or apoptosis (Tichy et al., 2010). The critical interaction of all these proteins is exemplified by this syndrome, as a cardinal feature of A-T includes relative resistance to radiation-induced apoptosis.

Additionally, ATM-dependent phosphorylation events are required for normal cell cycle checkpoint control. The S phase, and thus DNA synthesis, is regulated through ATM-mediated activation of CHK2 (Tichy et al., 2010). Cell cycle arrest can be induced by interactions with p53 and BRCA1, which are factors in modulating the G1/S and G2/M checkpoints, respectively (Tichy et al., 2010). These three proteins are also products of tumor suppressor genes, highlighting the link between ATM signal transduction, cancer, and genetic susceptibility. When defective, this process results in genomic instability, causing subsequent cancer formation and neurodegeneration, the most devastating features of A-T.

Diagnosis

Diagnosis of A-T is relatively simple in patients who present with ataxia and oculocutaneous telangiectasias. However, this disease entity can have highly variable expression, characterized by a tapestry of varying phenotypes and penetrance. Diagnosis can be especially elusive in cases where presentation occurs before the onset of cutaneous telangiectasias, sometimes leading to misdiagnosis with other ataxia syndromes such as Friedreich's ataxia (Sardanelli et al., 1995), ataxia oculomotor apraxias (Taylor and Byrd, 2005), and ataxic cerebral palsy, among others (Cabana et al., 1998). Earlier-presenting, milder cases may have neurologic symptoms that are nonspecific; however they may become more characteristic of the disease over time. Clinical criteria have been established to aid diagnosis in more ambiguous cases (Cabana et al., 1998). Diagnosis can also be confirmed by DNA sequencing, documenting absence or deficiency of the ATM protein through immunoblotting of lymphoblastoid cell lines, or establishing diminished protein activity through kinase assays (Taylor and Byrd, 2005), although these methods are infrequently necessary.

Although no specific therapy exists, early recognition of this disease entity is critical in aiding genetic counseling, guiding symptom management, and identifying heterozygous individuals who may carry an increased risk of developing malignancy (Cabana et al., 1998). Missed diagnosis can also result in inappropriate administration of radiotherapy to cancer patients, resulting in deleterious consequences in these radiosensitive individuals (Hoche et al., 2012).

Clinical manifestation

Oculocutaneous

Cutaneous telangiectasias (Fig. 27.14A) emerge most often on the sun-exposed areas of the face, sclera, and the flexor surface of the extremities by 6–7 years of age (Meyn, 1999), although they can be seen at birth or sometimes never (Tavani et al., 2003). In the majority of cases (approximately 70%) telangiectasias materialize before diagnosis (Cabana et al., 1998). Ocular telangiectasias are seen up to 97% of the time, found on the interpalpebral bulbar conjunctiva (Greenberger et al., 2013). As they do not cause pain or bleed (Cohen et al., 1984), and normal vision is preserved, concern is mostly cosmetic in nature. The pathophysiology behind the development of telangiectasias is not known, although it may include abnormal endothelial and pericyte response to increased expression of vascular endothelial growth factors (Greenberger et al., 2013).

The current understanding maintains that A-T cells are acutely sensitive to IR-induced DNA damage, while ultraviolet (UV)-induced injury repair mechanism remains intact (Sedgwick and Boder, 1991); however, abnormal response of A-T cells to UV radiation has been documented (Oakley et al., 2001). The observation that telangiectasias and pigmented lesions tend to aggregate in sun-exposed areas supports the notion that enhanced UV susceptibility in addition to IR radiosensitivity due to faulty DNA repair are potential underlying mechanisms for cutaneous lesion development.

Other dermatologic manifestations include hypopigmentation (approximately 40%), hyperpigmented macules, known as café-au-lait spots (84%), scaly facial papulosquamous rash (40%), poikiloderma, and seborrheic dermatitis. More rare entities include acanthosis nigricans, hirsutism, and cutaneous granulomas (Greenberger et al., 2013). These granulomas can

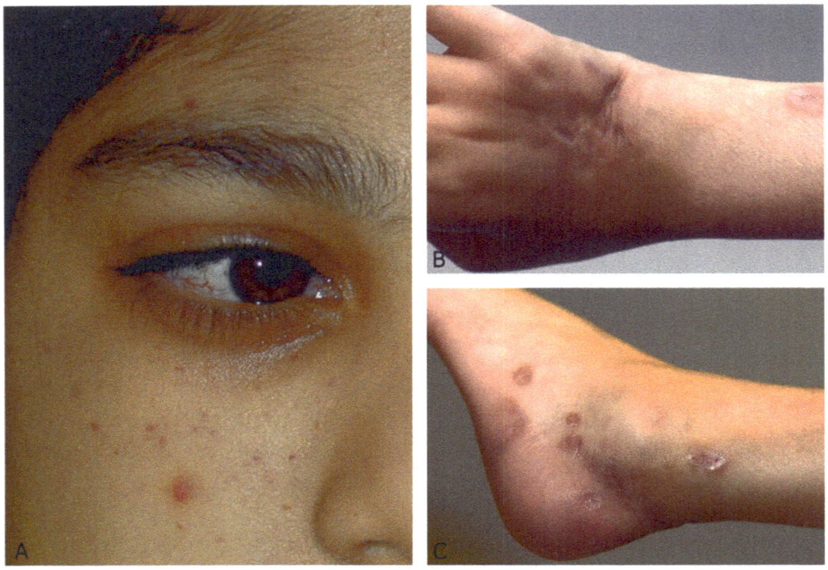

Fig. 27.14. Ataxia-telangiectasia cutaneous findings. (**A**) An 11-year-old girl with conjunctival telangiectasias related to her genodermatosis developed autoimmune thrombocytopenic purpura. Note the scattered facial petechiae related to thrombocytopenia. (**B**) A 12-year-old boy with ataxia-telangiectasia developed progressive violaceous fibrotic atrophic papules and plaques with overlying telangiectasias on his extremities and trunk. These lesions gradually increased in number and size over time. (**C**) Another 12-year-old boy with ataxia-telangiectasia developed painful violaceous plaques on his right hand and wrist since 2 years ago. The lesions slowly progressed and he developed new plaques on his left ankle a year ago (shown here). Multiple biopsies have shown granulomatous changes, but special stains and cultures for bacteria, fungi, and mycobacteria were negative. Despite treatment with antibiotics and topical steroids, the eruption continued to progress.

increase in size, but represent noninfectious chronic granulomatous inflammation (Fig. 27.14B, C), that is also commonly reported in other primary immunodeficiency syndromes (Mitra et al., 2005). Pigmented nevi greater than 5 mm in size occur in up to 40% of patients. Both melanoma and basal cell carcinoma (Cohen et al., 1984) have been reported. However, the risk for skin cancer is yet to be defined, and there are no current consensus guidelines for cancer screening in these individuals.

A progeria-like picture has been described in some cases, characterized by premature graying of the hair, facial lipoatrophy, progeroid facies, senile keratosis, and arcus senilis (Cohen et al., 1984). Although the pathogenesis of the premature aging is unknown at this time, it stands to reason that this process is also due to the underlying defective DNA repair and genomic instability in A-T (Greenberger et al., 2013), and the possible role ATM plays in telomeric maintenance (Melcalfe et al., 1996).

CNS

Out of all the inherited ataxia syndromes, A-T represents the most devastating neurodegenerative process, in which patients are generally normal in infancy and invariably lose cerebellar function over time, most beginning by 2 years of age (Meyn, 1999). Cerebellar dysfunction includes ataxia, ocular apraxia, and dysarthria, sometimes accompanied by extrapyramidal symptoms, including choreoathetoid movements, dystonia, myoclonic jerks, and bradykinesia. The dysfunction initially presents as truncal ataxia and ataxic gait, later spreading to the extremities (Hoche et al., 2012), and patients are eventually wheelchair-dependent by adolescence or early adulthood (Tavani et al., 2003).

Cerebellar and vermian atrophy is the manifest feature, histopathologically characterized by excessive Purkinje and granular cell degeneration in the cerebellum. Supratentorial cerebral volume is relatively preserved. Why the cerebellum and vermis are preferentially involved, and how the neuronal atrophy occurs, remains to be elucidated. Hypotheses of neuronal degeneration include accumulation of unrepaired double-stranded DNA breaks, resulting in buildup of dysfunctional genes and toxic proteins, lack of radiation-induced proapoptotic response, deficiencies in regulating oxidative stress, and dysfunctional mitochondrial respiratory activity (Hoche et al., 2012).

Whether cognitive impairment plays a role in this disease is debated, and current literature in this regard is limited. However, data suggest children with A-T initially maintain normal cognition, as evidenced by infants and toddlers reaching developmental milestones, but later clinically deteriorating over time (Hoche et al., 2012). Peripheral neuropathy and spinal muscular atrophy have also been described (Hoche et al., 2012).

Neuroimaging

MRI serves as the primary and favored modality in neuroimaging, as CT should be avoided in subjects with A-T given their heightened sensitivity to IR. On structural imaging, almost all A-T patients demonstrate cerebellar atrophy (Fig. 27.15) of varying severity (Farina et al., 1994; Sardanelli et al., 1995). Vermian atrophy is observed as the primary feature, while cerebellar hemispheric involvement is more variable (Farina et al., 1994; Sardanelli et al., 1995). Subsequent *ex vacuo* enlargement of the cisterna magna, cerebellar sulci, and the fourth ventricle highlights the posterior fossa volume loss. The degree of atrophy likely parallels clinical disease severity (Farina et al., 1994) and duration (Tavani et al., 2003; Wallis et al., 2007).

The intracranial findings of A-T are usually limited to the cerebellum, without evidence of supratentorial atrophy or signal abnormality (Farina et al., 1994; Lin et al., 2006b; Al-Maawali et al., 2012). When present, supratentorial findings such as microhemorrhages due to telangiectasias (Fig. 27.16) (Ciemens and Horowitz, 2000; Wallis et al., 2007; Habek et al., 2008), foci of coagulation necrosis and, rarely, demyelination are posited to occur predominantly in adult patients (Habek et al., 2008), suggesting an acquired process.

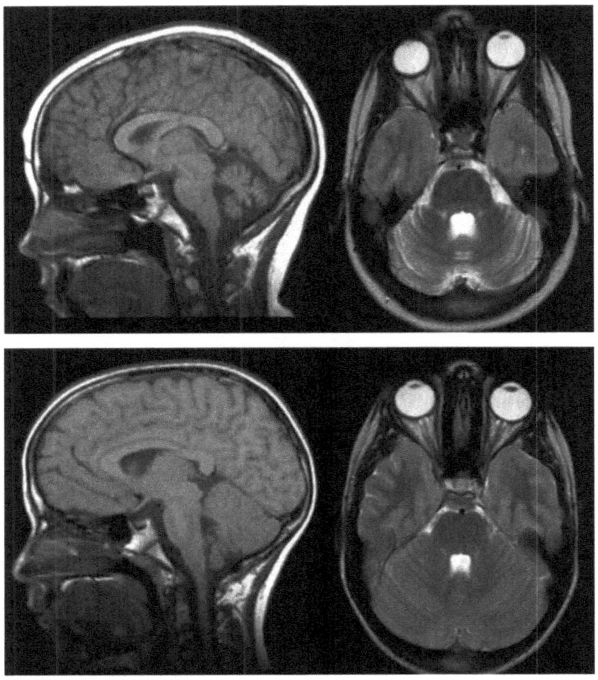

Fig. 27.15. Cerebellar atrophy, particularly paravermian atrophy, can be profound since childhood. Top-sagittal T1 and axial T2-weighted magnetic resonance images of a 9-year-old girl with ataxia-telangiectasia , compared to bottom panel, a 10-year-old normal subject.

In the CNS, telangiectasias affect the brain and conjunctivae (Wallis et al., 2007; Habek et al., 2008). These are best depicted on sequences that exploit the T2-shortening effect of blood products such as T2*, hemosiderin-sensitive gradient recalled echo or SWI, although are also relatively easily detected on postcontrast T1-weighted sequences (Wallis et al., 2007) (Fig. 27.16). Rarely, foci of T2/FLAIR hyperintensity have been reported in the supratentorial white matter (Sardanelli et al., 1995; Habek et al., 2008; Hoche et al., 2012), postulated to represent ischemia, demyelination, or gliosis; however, MRS studies suggest these lesions most likely reflect edema (Lin et al., 2014).

Despite the presence of extrapyramidal symptoms, there is no known abnormality in morphology, signal intensity (Farina et al., 1994), or metabolite composition (as interrogated by MRS) within the basal ganglia (Lin et al., 2006b). Abnormal spectroscopic findings in the cerebellum itself are observed, however, with conflicting results, ranging from universally diminished (Lin et al., 2006b) to normal NAA and elevated Cho (Wallis et al., 2007), potentiating opportunity for future longitudinal studies in order to better elucidate the microcellular metabolic alterations in this disease.

INCONTINENTIA PIGMENTI

Incontinentia pigmenti (IP), also known as Block–Sulzberger disease, is a genodermatosis that affects primarily the systems of ectodermal origin, chiefly the CNS, eyes, hair, teeth, musculoskeletal system, and skin (Carney, 1976). The incidence is reported between 1/10 000 and 1/100 000 and presents almost exclusively in females.

Genetics

IP can occur either as a sporadic mutation or inherited. Up to 55% of affected individuals have a positive family history of IP (Carney, 1976). When familial, IP is inherited as X-linked dominant transmission, affecting the NF-κB essential modulator (NEMO) gene. The NEMO locus has been mapped to chromosome Xq28 (Jin and Jeang, 1999), which is responsible for the majority of IP mutations (Smahi et al., 1994, 2002). The sporadic form has been associated with an Xp11.21 translocation break point (Gorski et al., 1991).

The protein product of the NEMO gene activates the transcription factor, NF-κB, which is involved in

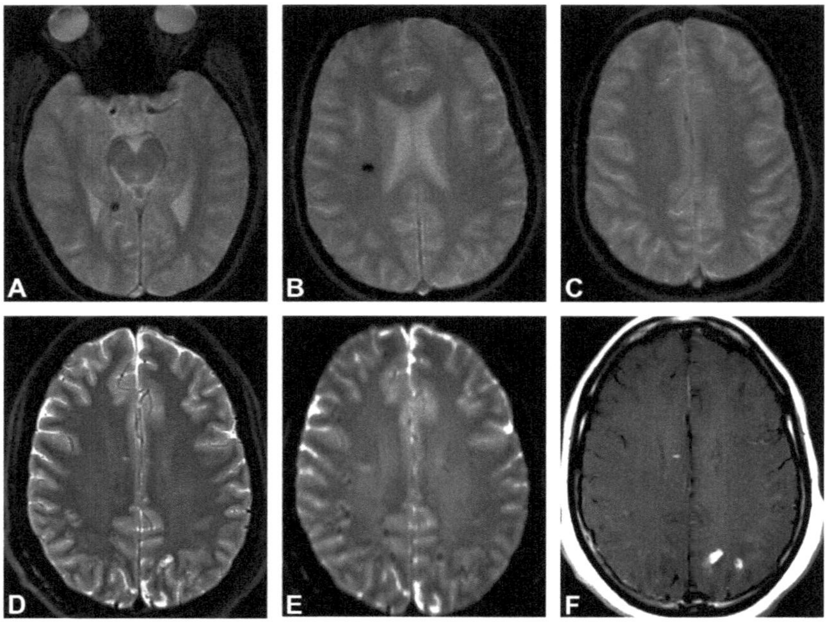

Fig. 27.16. Telangiectasia can be seen in cerebral white matter, best demonstrated on susceptibility-weighted imaging as punctate foci of hemosiderin deposits. These lesions are present in increased number and frequency in older individuals with ataxia-telangiectasia, but apparently are not associated with any clinical symptoms. (**A–C**) Axial hemosiderin-sensitive gradient echo images show several foci of hemosiderin deposits scattered in the right parahippocampal gyral region, right corona radiata, and anterior right centrum semiovale in this 12-year-old female with ataxia-telangiectasia. Ten years later in this same individual, she developed innumerable similar foci that are only vaguely demonstrated on (**D**) axial T2-weighted fast spin-echo, but best shown on (**E**) b_0-echo planar imaging as punctate areas of susceptibility, most concentrated in the posterior frontoparietal white matter and corticomedullary junction bilaterally. Some of these foci show patchy or nodular contrast enhancement on the (**F**) post-gadolinium T1-weighted image.

immune, inflammatory, and apoptotic pathways, and protects against tumor necrosis factor α-induced apoptosis (Yamaoka et al., 1998; Mercurio et al., 1999; Rothwarf and Karin, 1999; Smahi et al., 2000). Cells expressing the mutated gene are eliminated around the time of birth; thus heterozygotes (XX females carrying a single IP mutation) display skewed X-inactivation, favoring cells expressing the wild-type chromosome. This serves as an effective method in counterselection of cells carrying the mutation (Harris et al., 1992; Parrish et al., 1996).

Male hemizygotes (XY) rarely survive *in utero* past the second trimester (Parrish et al., 1996; Smahi et al., 2000). In males who survive to term the mutations are milder, leading to diminished, but not absent, NF-κB activity, and the clinical profile is often accompanied by immunodeficiencies (Smahi et al., 2002). Females with similarly mild mutations may be phenotypically unaffected, due to the function of their coexisting second X-chromosome. IP is also reported in males in unique settings, for instance, due to postzygotic mosaicism or in association with Klinefelter syndrome (XXY) (Fusco et al., 2007).

Clinical manifestation

Cutaneous

IP is characterized by a unique skin rash that progresses through four distinct dermatologic phases, and 90% of cases begin within 2 weeks after birth (Carney, 1976; Hadj-Rabia et al., 2003). Stage I, the vesicular phase, is distinguished by blisters and an inflammatory response alongside epidermal eosinophilic granulocyte infiltration (Fig. 27.17A). The characteristic pattern (a V-shaped rash on the back and S-shaped pattern on anterior trunk) follows the blueprint of embryonic ectodermal cell migration during fetal development, known as the lines of Blaschko. Stage II, the verrucous stage (Fig. 27.17B), is characterized by hyperkeratotic and verrucous lesions which, over time, will evolve into areas of hyperpigmentation due to melanin accumulation marking stage III or hyperpigmented stage (Fig. 27.17C, D). Finally, these will gradually resolve, to be replaced by areas of dermal hypopigmentation and atrophy in stage IV (Cohen, 1987) (Fig. 27.17E). The dermatologic findings are the most common features of the disease, affecting 90% of individuals with IP; however stages

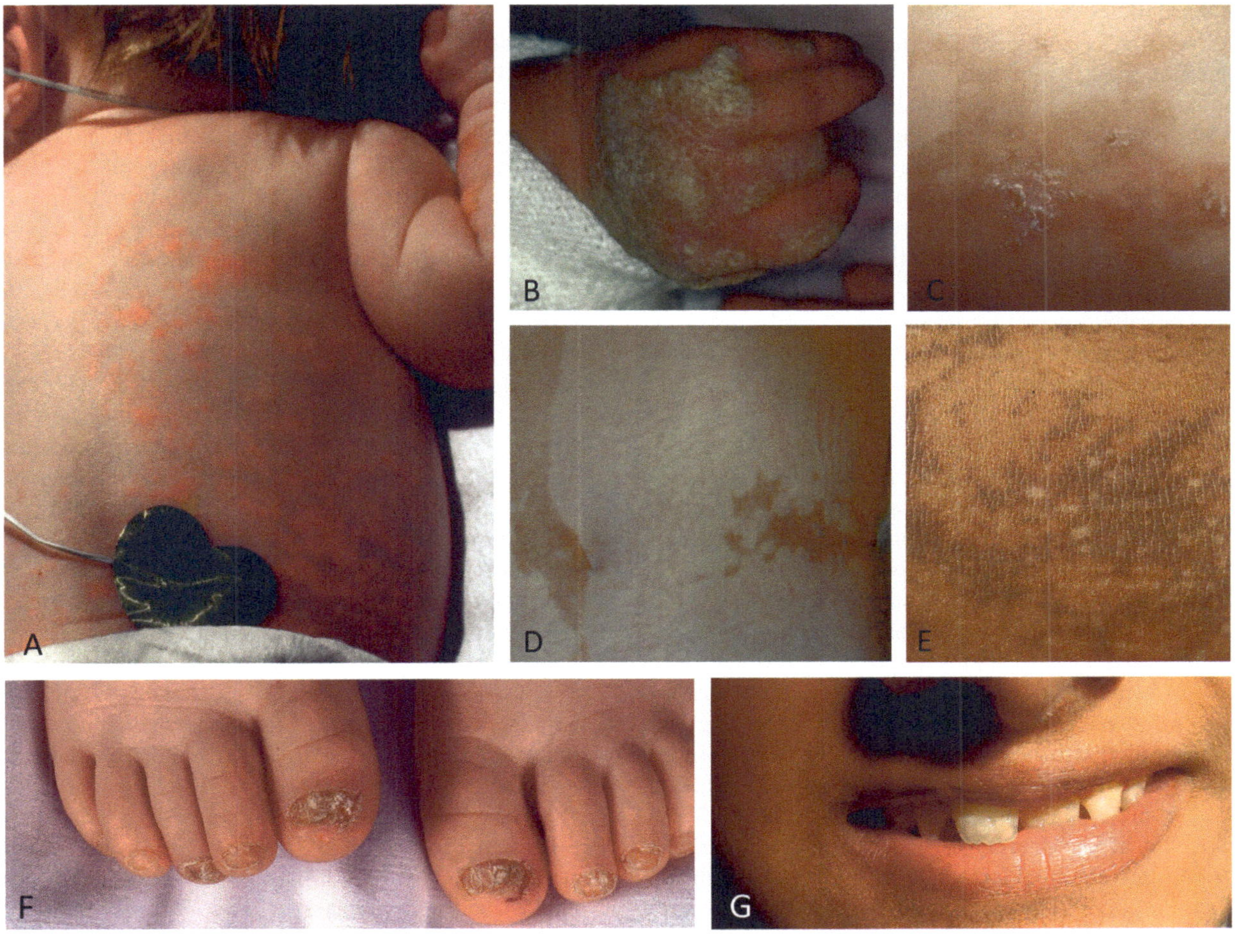

Fig. 27.17. Cutaneous findings in incontinentia pigmenti. (**A**) Erythematous patches along the lines of Blaschko in a 7-day-old female infant. (**B**) Thick linear warty plaques of incontinentia pigmenti in the verrucous stage in a 4-month-old girl. (**C**) Warty crust and swirled hyperpigmentation in an otherwise healthy infant girl. (**D**) Swirled hyperpigmented patches (stage III) in the trunk of a 7-year-old girl. (**E**) Hyperpigmented atrophic swirled patches with scattered round hypopigmented macules in an 8-year-old girl. (**F**) Nail dystrophy: thin, scaly, yellow, split nails in a 5-year-old girl. (**G**) Depressed linear brown plaques and abnormally formed teeth in an 8-year-old girl with incontinentia pigmenti.

may overlap and not all cases will manifest all four stages. The disorder is named for the characteristic hyperpigmented lesions seen in stage III. Nail dystrophy and dental malformation can also be seen (Fig. 27.17F, G).

Ocular

In all, 20–35% of patients have ocular manifestations (Carney, 1976; Hadj-Rabia et al., 2003), and up to 7% suffer from blindness in one or both eyes (Carney, 1976). Among the many ocular findings, including strabismus, nystagmus, cataracts, retinal detachment, and uveitis (Carney, 1976; Goldberg, 1998), the retinal vascular abnormalities are of particular interest. These include peripheral retinal vascular nonperfusion, macular infarction, macular neovascularization, and preretinal neovascularization. The pathogenesis is variable; however, it is often due to retinal arteriolar occlusions and retinal infarction (Lee et al., 1995; Goldberg, 1998). The vascular abnormalities in the eye could result from a similar pathogenetic mechanism that affects the brain as part of a theory that a common vasculopathic and ischemic phenomenon produces both the CNS and ophthalmologic findings in IP (Lee et al., 1995; Hennel et al., 2003).

CNS and neuroimaging

It is the CNS findings in IP that account for the severity of the disease. CNS involvement occurs in approximately 30–50% of cases, with seizures representing the most common symptom (Carney, 1976; Hadj-Rabia et al., 2003), followed by mental retardation, spastic paralysis, and slow motor development (Carney, 1976).

While most patients with CNS abnormalities are affected by seizures, the seizures tend to be either transient or easily treatable. Other known stigmata include motor retardation, microcephaly, cerebral cortical atrophy, hemiparesis, hydrocephalus, cerebellar ataxia, and congenital hearing loss (Carney, 1976). More severe conditions have been described, including infarcts, widespread encephalopathy, and hemorrhagic necrosis (Shuper et al., 1990; Hadj-Rabia et al., 2003; Cartwright et al., 2009).

The pathogenesis of cerebral lesions in IP is unknown. Inflammatory, vascular, destructive, and infectious causes have all been postulated (Hauw et al., 1977; Siemes et al., 1978; Shuper et al., 1990; Lee et al., 1995; Hennel et al., 2003; Lou et al., 2008; Maingay-de Groof et al., 2008). The presence of eosinophilia and leukocytosis in the peripheral blood stream and reports of an overt inflammatory reaction characterized by lymphocytic infiltration in brain parenchyma support the notion of an inflammatory process (Hauw et al., 1977). A second theory implicates vascular abnormalities as the underlying cause, and is supported by the manifestation of hemorrhagic necrosis and infarction. Demonstration of decreased cerebral vascular branching and flow-related enhancement on MRI further reinforces the theory of a vasculopathic and ischemic phenomenon (Lee et al., 1995; Hennel et al., 2003; Hart et al., 2009). MRS in affected areas of the brain reveals reduced NAA and elevated lactate, also supporting ischemia (Lee et al., 1995; Lou et al., 2008). However, the majority of cases fail to demonstrate gross vascular pathology, and it has been postulated that the ischemic findings in those patients could be the sequelae of small-vessel vasculopathy (Lee et al., 1995).

The neuropathologic features of IP include leukodystrophy, microcephaly, polymicrogyria, hypoplasia of the corpus callosum and cerebellum, small cavities in the white matter, focal hemorrhagic necrosis, neuronal loss, hemorrhagic encephalopathy, edema, and ulegyria (Shuper et al., 1990; Hadj-Rabia et al., 2003; Maingay-de Groof et al., 2008; Cartwright et al., 2009). These findings are all identifiable by MRI, and have been reported as early as 3 days of life (Hennel et al., 2003; Wolf et al., 2005). Decreased fractional anisotropy on diffusion tensor imaging in involved brain has been demonstrated (Lou et al., 2008), suggesting impaired or delayed myelination.

CT, ultrasonography, and MRI all have roles in the assessment of neuroanatomic findings in IP. On CT, infarction can be seen as hypodense lesions with mass effect, intermixed with areas of hyperdensity, indicative of associated hemorrhage or cortical laminar necrosis. Nonspecific hyperechogenicity on cranial sonography manifests as a product of both hemorrhage and cytotoxic brain edema (Lee et al., 1995). Hemorrhagic necrosis is best demonstrated on MRI as gyriform T1 hyperintense lesions in the brain, associated with areas of elevated T2 signal and restricted diffusion, reflecting cytotoxic edema (Fig. 27.18). Abnormal congenital developments, such as hypoplasia of the corpus callosum and

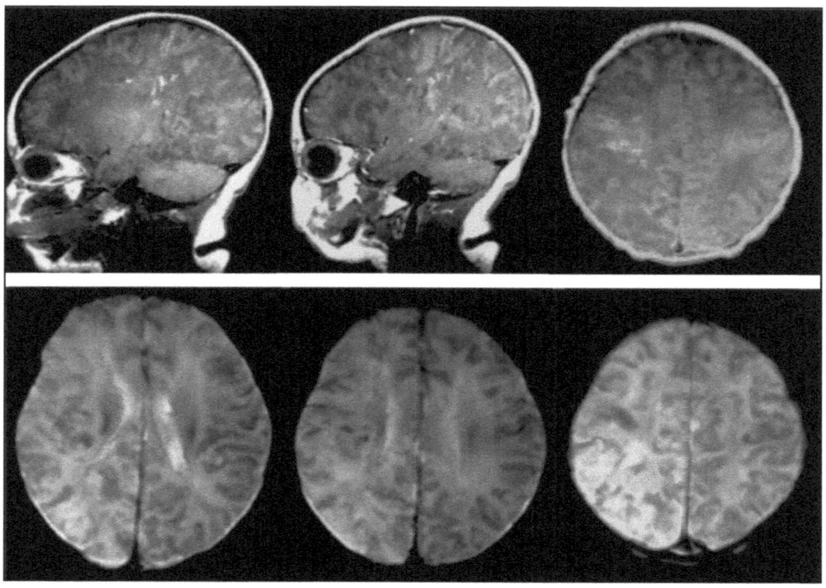

Fig. 27.18. A 3-day-old infant girl with erythematous vesicular skin rash, neonatal encephalopathy, and seizures. Sagittal and axial T1-weighted magnetic resonance images (top panel) show right frontoparietal punctate hyperintensity representing petechial hemorrhage. A larger area of T1 hypointensity, corresponding to T2 hyperintensity (axial T2 images, bottom panel) involving the right parietal occipital lobes with loss of corticomedullary distinction, indicates ischemic infarct.

cerebellum, as well as polymicrogyria, are most easily characterized on MRI. MR angiography may illustrate gross vascular pathology without subjecting the young patients to IR. MRI also has the added advantage of combining spectroscopic and diffusion information.

CONCLUSION

In conclusion, this article has covered symptoms, presentation, and diagnostic criteria of the major neurocutaneous syndromes, with an emphasis on their neuroimaging findings. Neuroimaging plays a very important role in the diagnosis of many of these disorders, and also in determining the degree of cerebral involvement. In the future, it may also play an important role in monitoring the efficacy of new treatments. The considerable variability of these diseases poses a challenge for targeted therapy, and many of these conditions affect multiple organ systems with diverse phenotypic presentations. Due to this complexity, treatment is mainly symptom-specific, tackled in a multidisciplinary approach. Several of these syndromes are genetic, intrinsic to the individual's makeup, which limits curative therapy. Those with unknown pathogenesis, such as SWS and KT, display clinical stigmata at birth, which suggests a possible genetic etiology or an early embryologic insult. The "two-hit" model, conjectured to apply to some of the oncogenic phakomatoses, such as neurofibromatosis, von Hippel–Lindau, and TS, could provide a unifying theory, where an inherent genetic mutation predisposes the individual and a second embryologic insult results in disease manifestation. Familial studies exist in both SWS and KT, and support a somatic inheritance pattern. The lack of obvious heredity in some of these cases may be concealed by somatic mosaicism, as sometimes also seen in TS and IP. Despite the advances in molecular genetic diagnosis and underlying cellular aberrations accounting for several of these syndromes, much remains to be learned. Effective diagnosis, management, and therapy will depend on further discovery into the molecular basis of these conditions. TS is an example where identification of mutated genes and the functionality of their protein products has made great strides towards effective monotherapy for inducing lesion regression across multiple organ systems. It is hoped that future treatment possibilities may be developed as the molecular basis of these diseases is better understood, and that neuroimaging will be able to serve as an objective biomarker of cerebral treatment response.

ACKNOWLEDGMENT

We thank all the contributors for the cutaneous photographs from the Dermatlas.

References

Ahlsen G, Gillberg IC, Lindblom R et al. (1994). Tuberous sclerosis in western Sweden. A population study of cases with early childhood onset. Arch Neurol 51: 76–81.

Al-Maawali A, Blaser S, Yoon G (2012). Diagnostic approach to childhood-onset cerebellar atrophy: a 10-year retrospective study of 300 patients. J Child Neurol 27: 1121–1132.

Altman NR, Purser RK, Post MJ (1988). Tuberous sclerosis: characteristics at CT and MR imaging. Radiology 167: 527–532.

Anlar B, Yalaz K, Erzen C (1988). Klippel–Trenaunay–Weber syndrome: a case with cerebral and cerebellar hemihypertrophy. Neuroradiology 30: 360.

Arzimanoglou A, Aicardi J (1992). The epilepsy of Sturge–Weber syndrome: clinical features and treatment in 23 patients. Acta Neurol Scand Suppl 140: 18–22.

Barkovich AJ (2005). Pediatric Neuroimaging. Lippincott Williams and Wilkins, Philadelphia.

Baron Y, Barkovich AJ (1999). MR imaging of tuberous sclerosis in neonates and young infants. AJNR Am J Neuroradiol 20: 907–916.

Boukobza M, Enjolras O, Cambra M et al. (2000). Sturge–Weber syndrome. The current neuroradiologic data. J Radiol 81: 756–771.

Bourgeois M, Crimmins DW, de Oliveira RS et al. (2007). Surgical treatment of epilepsy in Sturge–Weber syndrome in children. J Neurosurg 106: 20–28.

Braffman BH, Bilaniuk LT, Naidich TP et al. (1992). MR imaging of tuberous sclerosis: pathogenesis of this phakomatosis, use of gadopentetate dimeglumine, and literature review. Radiology 183: 227–238.

Brod RD, Shields JA, Shields CL et al. (1992). Unusual retinal and renal vascular lesions in the Klippel–Trenaunay–Weber syndrome. Retina 12: 355–358.

Cabana MD, Crawford TO, Winkelstein JA et al. (1998). Consequences of the delayed diagnosis of ataxia-telangiectasia. Pediatrics 102: 98–100.

Cakirer S, Yagmurlu B, Savas MR (2005). Sturge–Weber syndrome: diffusion magnetic resonance imaging and proton magnetic resonance spectroscopy findings. Acta Radiol 46: 407–410.

Carney RG (1976). Incontinentia pigmenti: a world statistical analysis. Arch Dermatol 112: 535–542.

Cartwright MS, White DL, Miller ML et al. (2009). Recurrent stroke in a child with incontinentia pigmenti. J Child Neurol 24: 603–605.

Chen D, Li L, Tu X et al. (2013). Functional characterization of Klippel–Trenaunay syndrome gene AGGF1 identifies a novel angiogenic signaling pathway for specification of vein differentiation and angiogenesis during embryogenesis. Hum Mol Genet 22: 963–976.

Chhajed M, Pandit S, Dhawan N et al. (2010). Klippel–Trenaunay and Sturge–Weber overlap syndrome with phakomatosis pigmentovascularis. J Pediatr Neurosci 5: 138–140.

Christophe C, Sékhara T, Rypens F et al. (2000). MRI spectrum of cortical malformations in tuberous sclerosis complex. Brain Dev 22: 487–493.

Ciemens JJ, Horowitz AL (2000). Abnormal white matter signal in ataxia telangiectasia. AJNR Am J Neuroradiol 21: 1483–1485.

Cohen BA (1987). Incontinentia pigmenti. Neurol Clin 5: 361–377.

Cohen Jr MM (2000). Klippel–Trenaunay syndrome. Am J Med Genet 93: 171–175.

Cohen LE, Tanner DJ, Schaefer HG et al. (1984). Common and uncommon cutaneous findings in patients with ataxia-telangiectasia. J Am Acad Dermatol 10: 431–438.

Comi AM (2003). Topical review: pathophysiology of Sturge–Weber syndrome. J Child Neurol 18: 509–516.

Comi AM (2007). Update on Sturge–Weber syndrome: diagnosis, treatment, quantitative measures, and controversies. Lymphat Res Biol 5: 257–264.

Comi AM (2011). Presentation, diagnosis, pathophysiology, and treatment of the neurological features of Sturge–Weber syndrome. Neurologist 17: 179–184.

Cunha E, Sa M, Barrosco CP, Caldas MC et al. (1997). Innervation pattern of malformative cortical vessels in Sturge–Weber disease: a histochemical, immunohistochemical, and ultrastructural study. Neurosurgery 41: 872–876.

Curatolo P, Bombardieri R, Jozwiak S (2008). Tuberous sclerosis. Lancet 372: 657–668.

DeKlotz CM, Ogram AE, Singh S et al. (2011). Successful treatment of angiofibromata of tuberous sclerosis complex with rapamycin. Arch Dermatol 147: 1116–1117.

Dunn WK, Jaspan T (1993). Case report: Cerebral arteriovenous fistula in the Klippel–Trenaunay–Weber syndrome. Clin Radiol 48: 134–136.

Enjolras O, Riche MC, Merland JJ (1985). Facial port-wine stains and Sturge–Weber syndrome. Pediatrics 76: 48–51.

Ess KC, Kamp CA, Tu BP et al. (2005). Developmental origin of subependymal giant cell astrocytoma in tuberous sclerosis complex. Neurology 64: 1446–1449.

Farina L, Uggetti C, Ottolini A et al. (1994). Ataxia-telangiectasia: MR and CT findings. J Comput Assist Tomogr 18: 724–727.

Franz DN, Leonard J, Tudor C et al. (2006). Rapamycin causes regression of astrocytomas in tuberous sclerosis complex. Ann Neurol 59: 490–498.

Franz DN, Belousova E, Sparagana S et al. (2013). Efficacy and safety of everolimus for subependymal giant cell astrocytomas associated with tuberous sclerosis complex (EXIST-1): a multicentre, randomised, placebo-controlled phase 3 trial. Lancet 381: 125–132.

Fryer AE, Chalmers A, Connor JM et al. (1987). Evidence that the gene for tuberous sclerosis is on chromosome 9. Lancet 1: 659–661.

Fusco F, Fimiani G, Tadini G et al. (2007). Clinical diagnosis of incontinentia pigmenti in a cohort of male patients. J Am Acad Dermatol 56: 264–267.

Goldberg MF (1998). Macular vasculopathy and its evolution in incontinentia pigmenti. Ophthalmic Paediatr Genet 19: 141–148.

Gorski JL, Burright EN, Harnden CE et al. (1991). Localization of DNA sequences to a region within Xp11.21 between incontinentia pigmenti (IP1) X-chromosomal translocation breakpoints. Am J Hum Genet 48: 53–64.

Greenberger S, Berkun Y, Ben-Zeev B et al. (2013). Dermatologic manifestations of ataxia-telangiectasia syndrome. J Am Acad Dermatol 68: 932–936.

Griffiths PD, Bolton P, Verity C (1998). White matter abnormalities in tuberous sclerosis complex. Acta Radiol 39: 482–486.

Griffiths PD, Coley SC, Romanowski CA et al. (2003). Contrast-enhanced fluid-attenuated inversion recovery imaging for leptomeningeal disease in children. AJNR Am J Neuroradiol 24: 719–723.

Habek M, Brinar VV, Rados M et al. (2008). Brain MRI abnormalities in ataxia-telangiectasia. Neurologist 14: 192–195.

Hadj-Rabia S, Froidevaux D, Bodak N et al. (2003). Clinical study of 40 cases of incontinentia pigmenti. Arch Dermatol 139: 1163–1170.

Haemel AK, O'Brian AL, Teng JM (2010). Topical rapamycin: a novel approach to facial angiofibromas in tuberous sclerosis. Arch Dermatol 146: 715–718.

Harris A, Collins J, Vetrie D et al. (1992). X inactivation as a mechanism of selection against lethal alleles: further investigation of incontinentia pigmenti and X linked lymphoproliferative disease. J Med Genet 29: 608–614.

Hart RM, Kimler BF, Evans RG et al. (1987). Radiotherapeutic management of medulloblastoma in a pediatric patient with ataxia telangiectasia. Int J Radiat Oncol Biol Phys 13: 1237–1240.

Hart AR, Edwards C, Mahajan J et al. (2009). Destructive encephalopathy in incontinentia pigmenti. Dev Med Child Neurol 51: 159–163.

Hauw JJ, Perie G, Bonnette J et al. (1977). Neuropathological study of incontinentia pigmenti. Anatomical case report (author's transl). Acta Neuropathol 38: 159–162.

Hennel SJ, Ekert PG, Volpe JJ et al. (2003). Insights into the pathogenesis of cerebral lesions in incontinentia pigmenti. Pediatr Neurol 29: 148–150.

Hoche F, Seidel K, Theis M et al. (2012). Neurodegeneration in ataxia telangiectasia: What is new? What is evident? Neuropediatrics 43: 119–129.

Hu J, Yu Y, Juhasz C et al (2008). MR susceptibility weighted imaging (SWI) complements conventional contrast enhanced T1 weighted MRI in characterizing brain abnormalities of Sturge–Weber syndrome. J Magn Reson Imaging 28: 300–307.

Huber M, Longmore DB, Firmin DN et al. (1989). Magnetic resonance tomography flow measurement in cerebral arteriovenous angioma. Digitale Bilddiagn 9: 1–4.

Hyman MH, Whittemore VH (2000). National Institutes of Health consensus conference: Tuberous sclerosis complex. Arch Neurol 57: 662–665.

Inoue Y, Nemoto Y, Murata R et al. (1998). CT and MR imaging of cerebral tuberous sclerosis. Brain Dev 20: 209–221.

Jacob AG, Driscoll DJ, Shaughnessy WJ et al. (1998). Klippel–Trenaunay syndrome: spectrum and management. Mayo Clin Proc 73: 28–36.

Jansen FE, Braun KPJ, Van Nieuwenhuizen O et al. (2003). Diffusion-weighted magnetic resonance imaging and identification of the epileptogenic tuber in patients with tuberous sclerosis. Arch Neurol 60: 1580–1584.

Jin DY, Jeang KT (1999). Isolation of full-length cDNA and chromosomal localization of human NF-kappaB modulator NEMO to Xq28. J Biomed Sci 6: 115–120.

Joinson C, O'Callaghan FJ, Osborne JP et al. (2003). Learning disability and epilepsy in an epidemiological sample of individuals with tuberous sclerosis complex. Psychol Med 33: 335–344.

Jost S, Gutmann DH (2012). Neurofibromatosis and other genetic syndromes. Handb Clin Neurol 105: 569–582.

Jozwiak S, Schwartz RA, Janniger CK et al. (2000). Usefulness of diagnostic criteria of tuberous sclerosis complex in pediatric patients. J Child Neurol 15: 652–659.

Kandt RS, Haines JL, Smith M et al. (1992). Linkage of an important gene locus for tuberous sclerosis to a chromosome 16 marker for polycystic kidney disease. Nat Genet 2: 37–41.

Knudson AG, Di Ferrante N, Curtis JE (1971). Effect of leukocyte transfusion in a child with type II mucopolysaccharidosis. Proc Natl Acad Sci U S A 68: 1738–1741.

Kojima Y, Kuwana N, Sato M et al. (1989). Klippel–Trenaunay–Weber syndrome with spinal arteriovenous malformation. Neurol Med Chir 29: 235–240.

Kramer U, Kahana E, Shorer E et al. (2000). Outcome of infants with unilateral Sturge–Weber syndrome and early onset seizures. Dev Med Child Neurol 42: 756–759.

Krueger D, Care M, Agricola K et al. (2013). Everolimus long-term safety and efficacy in subependymal giant cell astrocytoma. Neurology 80: 574–580.

Lagos JC, Gomez MR (1967). Tuberous sclerosis: Reappraisal of a clinical entity. Mayo Clin Proc 42: 26–49.

Lavin MF (2008). Ataxia-telangiectasia: from a rare disorder to a paradigm for cell signalling and cancer. Nat Rev Mol Cell Biol 9: 759–769.

Lee AG, Goldberg MF, Gillard JH et al. (1995). Intracranial assessment of incontinentia pigmenti using magnetic resonance imaging, angiography, and spectroscopic imaging. Arch Pediatr Adolesc Med 149: 573–580.

Lee JS, Asano E, Muzik O et al. (2001). Sturge–Weber syndrome: correlation between clinical course and FDG PET findings. Neurology 57: 189–195.

Lee A, Maldonado M, Baybis M et al. (2003). Markers of cellular proliferation are expressed in cortical tubers. Ann Neurol 53: 668–673.

Lin DD, Barker PB, Hatfield LA et al. (2006a). Dynamic MR perfusion and proton MR spectroscopic imaging in Sturge–Weber syndrome: correlation with neurological symptoms. J Magn Reson Imaging 24: 274–281.

Lin DD, Crawford TO, Lederman HM et al. (2006b). Proton MR spectroscopic imaging in ataxia-telangiectasia. Neuropediatrics 37: 241–246.

Lin DD, Barker PB, Lederman HM et al. (2014). Cerebral abnormalities in adults with ataxia-telangiectasia. AJNR Am J Neuroradiol 35: 119–123.

Lou H, Zhang L, Xiao W et al. (2008). Nearly completely reversible brain abnormalities in a patient with incontinentia pigmenti. AJNR Am J Neuroradiol 29: 431–433.

Luat AF, Makki M, Chugani HT (2007). Neuroimaging in tuberous sclerosis complex. Curr Opin Neurol 20: 142–150.

Maeda M, Tartaro A, Matsuda T et al. (1995). Cortical and subcortical tubers in tuberous sclerosis and FLAIR sequence. J Comput Assist Tomogr 19: 660–661.

Maingay-de Groof F, Lequin MH, Roofthooft DW et al. (2008). Extensive cerebral infarction in the newborn due to incontinentia pigmenti. Eur J Paediatr Neurol 12: 284–289.

Maiuri F, Gangemi M, Iaconetta G et al. (1989). Sturge–Weber disease without facial nevus. J Neurosurg Sci 33: 215–218.

Marcotte L, Crino PB (2006). The neurobiology of the tuberous sclerosis complex. Neuromolecular Med 8: 531–546.

Melcalfe JA, Parkhill J, Campbell L et al. (1996). Accelerated telomere shortening in ataxia telangiectasia. Nat Genet 13: 350–353.

Mercurio F, Murray BW, Shevchenko A et al. (1999). IkappaB kinase (IKK)-associated protein 1, a common component of the heterogeneous IKK complex. Mol Cell Biol 19: 1526–1538.

Meyn MS (1999). Ataxia-telangiectasia, cancer and the pathobiology of the ATM gene. Clin Genet 55: 289–304.

Mitra A, Pollock B, Gooi J et al. (2005). Cutaneous granulomas associated with primary immunodeficiency disorders. Br J Dermatol 153: 194–199.

Nabbout R, Santos M, Rolland Y et al. (1999). Early diagnosis of subependymal giant cell astrocytoma in children with tuberous sclerosis. J Neurol Neurosurg Psychiatry 66: 370–375.

Oakley GG, Loberg LI, Yao J et al. (2001). UV-induced hyperphosphorylation of replication protein a depends on DNA replication and expression of ATM protein. Mol Biol Cell 12: 1199–1213.

O'Callaghan F (2008). Tuberous sclerosis complex. Paediatr Child Health 18: 30–36.

Oduber CEU, van der Horst CM, Hennekam RC (2008). Klippel–Trenaunay syndrome: diagnostic criteria and hypothesis on etiology. Ann Plast Surg 60: 217–223.

Olsen JH, Hahnemann JM, Borresen-Dale AL et al. (2001). Cancer in patients with ataxia-telangiectasia and in their relatives in the nordic countries. J Natl Cancer Inst 93: 121–127.

Osborne JP, Fryer A, Webb D (1991). Epidemiology of tuberous sclerosis. Ann N Y Acad Sci 615: 125–127.

Oyesiku NM, Gahm NH, Goldman RL (1988). Cerebral arteriovenous fistula in the Klippel–Trenaunay–Weber syndrome. Dev Med Child Neurol 30: 245–248.

Park SH, Pepkowitz SH, Kerfoot C et al. (1997). Tuberous sclerosis in a 20-week gestation fetus: immunohistochemical study. Acta Neuropathol 94: 180–186.

Parrish JE, Scheuerle AE, Lewis RA et al. (1996). Selection against mutant alleles in blood leukocytes is a consistent feature in incontinentia pigmenti type 2. Hum Mol Genet 5: 1777–1783.

Piram M, Lorette G, Sirinelli D et al. (2012). Sturge–Weber syndrome in patients with facial port-wine stain. Pediatr Dermatol 29: 32–37.

Probst FP (1980). Vascular morphology and angiographic flow patterns in Sturge–Weber angiomatosis: facts, thoughts and suggestions. Neuroradiology 20: 73–78.

Purkait R, Samanta T, Sinhamahapatra T et al. (2011). Overlap of Sturge–Weber syndrome and Klippel–Trenaunay syndrome. Indian J Dermatol 56: 755–757.

Rahman M, Rahman S, Rahman M et al. (2008). Overlapping of Sturge Weber syndrome and Klippel Trenaunay Weber syndrome. Mymensingh Med J 17: 78–81.

Reid DE, Maria BL, Drane WE et al. (1997). Central nervous system perfusion and metabolism abnormalities in Sturge–Weber syndrome. J Child Neurol 12: 218–222.

Renard D, Larue A, Taieb G et al. (2012). Recurrent cerebral infarction in Klippel–Trenaunay–Weber syndrome. Clin Neurol Neurosurg 114: 1019–1020.

Renard D, Campello C, Taieb G et al. (2013). Neurologic and vascular abnormalities in Klippel–Trenaunay–Weber syndrome. JAMA Neurol 70: 127–128.

Rhoten RL, Comair YG, Shedid D et al. (1997). Specific repression of the preproendothelin-1 gene in intracranial arteriovenous malformations. J Neurosurg 86: 101–108.

Roach ES (1992). Neurocutaneous syndromes. Pediatr Clin North Am 39: 591–620.

Roach E, Sparagana S (2004). Diagnosis of tuberous sclerosis complex. J Child Neurol 19: 643–649.

Roach ES, Riela AR, Chugani HT et al. (1994). Sturge–Weber syndrome: recommendations for surgery. J Child Neurol 9: 190–192.

Roach E, Gomez MR, Northrup H (1998). Tuberous sclerosis complex consensus conference: revised clinical diagnostic criteria. J Child Neurol 13: 624–628.

Rodrigues DA, Gomes CM, Costa IM (2012). Tuberous sclerosis complex. An Bras Dermatol 87: 184–196.

Rohany M, Shaibani A, Arafat O et al. (2007). Spinal arteriovenous malformations associated with Klippel–Trenaunay–Weber syndrome: a literature search and report of two cases. AJNR Am J Neuroradiol 28: 584–589.

Rothwarf DM, Karin M (1999). The NF-kappa B activation pathway: a paradigm in information transfer from membrane to nucleus. Sci STKE 5: R1.

Sardanelli F, Parodi RC, Ottonello C et al. (1995). Cranial MRI in ataxia-telangiectasia. Neuroradiology 37: 77–82.

Sedgwick R, Boder E (1991). Ataxia-telangiectasia. In: PJ Vinken, G Bruyn, H Klawans (Eds.), Handbook of Clinical Neurology. Elsevier, New York, USA.

Sharma MC, Ralte AM, Gaekwad S et al. (2004). Subependymal giant cell astrocytoma – a clinicopathological study of 23 cases with special emphasis on histogenesis. Pathol Oncol Res 10: 219–224.

Shields JA, Demirci H, Marr BP et al. (2004). Sebaceous carcinoma of the eyelids: Personal experience with 60 cases. Ophthalmology 111: 2151–2157.

Shirley MD, Tang H, Gallione CJ et al. (2013). Sturge–Weber syndrome and port-wine stains caused by somatic mutation in GNAQ. N Engl J Med 368: 1971–1979.

Shuper A, Bryan N, Singer H (1990). Destructive encephalopathy in incontinentia pigmenti: a primary disorder? Pediatr Neurol 6: 137–140.

Siemes H, Schneider H, Dening D et al. (1978). Encephalitis in two members of a family with incontinentia pigmenti (Bloch–Sulzberger syndrome). The possible role of inflammation in the pathogenesis of CNS involvement. Eur J Pediatr 129: 103–115.

Smahi A, Hyden-Granskog C, Peterlin B et al. (1994). The gene for the familial form of incontinentia pigmenti (IP2) maps to the distal part of Xq28. Hum Mol Genet 3: 273–278.

Smahi A, Courtois G, Vabres P et al. (2000). Genomic rearrangement in NEMO impairs NF-kappaB activation and is a cause of incontinentia pigmenti. The international incontinentia pigmenti (IP) consortium. Nature 405: 466–472.

Smahi A, Courtois G, Hadj Rabi S et al. (2002). The NF-kappaB signalling pathway in human diseases: from incontinentia pigmenti to ectodermal dysplasias and immune-deficiency syndromes. Hum Mol Genet 11: 2371–2375.

Smirniotopoulos JG (2004). Neuroimaging of phakomatoses: Sturge–Weber syndrome, tuberous sclerosis, von Hippel–Lindau syndrome. Neuroimaging Clin N Am 14 (171–183): vii.

Star A, Fuller CE, Landas SK (2010). Intracranial aneurysms in Klippel–Trenaunay/Weber syndromes: case report. Neurosurgery 66: 1027–1028.

Suga T, Yasuda J, Okudaira Y et al. (1994). A case of Klippel–Trenaunay–Weber syndrome associated with intracranial multiple angiomas. No To Shinkei 46: 889–894.

Sujansky E, Conradi S (1995). Sturge–Weber syndrome: age of onset of seizures and glaucoma and the prognosis for affected children. J Child Neurol 10: 49–58.

Szelies B, Herholz K, Heiss WD et al. (1983). Hypometabolic cortical lesions in tuberous sclerosis with epilepsy: demonstration by positron emission tomography. J Comput Assist Tomogr 7: 946–953.

Tavani F, Zimmerman RA, Berry GT et al. (2003). Ataxia-telangiectasia: the pattern of cerebellar atrophy on MRI. Neuroradiology 45: 315–319.

Taylor AM, Byrd PJ (2005). Molecular pathology of ataxia telangiectasia. J Clin Pathol 58: 1009–1015.

Thiele EA (2004). Managing epilepsy in tuberous sclerosis complex. J Child Neurol 19: 680–686.

Thomas-Sohl KA, Vaslow DF, Maria BL (2004). Sturge–Weber syndrome: a review. Pediatr Neurol 30: 303–310.

Tichy A, Vavrova J, Pejchal J et al. (2010). Ataxia-telangiectasia mutated kinase (ATM) as a central regulator of radiation-induced DNA damage response. Acta Medica 53: 13–17.

Timur AA, Driscoll DJ, Wang Q (2005). Biomedicine and diseases: The Klippel-Trenaunay syndrome, vascular anomalies and vascular morphogenesis. Cell Mol Life Sci 62: 1434–1447.

Torregrosa A, Marti-Bonmati L, Higueras V et al. (2000). Klippel–Trenaunay syndrome: frequency of cerebral and cerebellar hemihypertrophy on MRI. Neuroradiology 42: 420–423.

van Slegtenhorst M, de Hoogt R, Hermans C et al. (1997). Identification of the tuberous sclerosis gene TSC1 on chromosome 9q34. Science 277: 805–808.

Varan A, Buyukpamukcu M, Ersoy F et al. (2004). Malignant solid tumors associated with congenital immunodeficiency disorders. Pediatr Hematol Oncol 21: 441–451.

Verhelst H, Van Coster R (2005). Neuroradiologic findings in a young patient with characteristics of Sturge–Weber syndrome and Klippel–Trenaunay syndrome. J Child Neurol 20: 911–913.

Vissers W, Van Steensel M, Steijlen P et al. (2003). Klippel–Trenaunay syndrome and Sturge–Weber syndrome: variations on a theme? Eur J Dermatol 13: 238–241.

Wallis LI, Griffiths PD, Ritchie SJ et al. (2007). Proton spectroscopy and imaging at 3 T in ataxia-telangiectasia. AJNR Am J Neuroradiol 28: 79–83.

Webb DW, Clarke A, Fryer A et al. (1996). The cutaneous features of tuberous sclerosis: a population study. Br J Dermatol 135: 1–5.

White R, Hua Y, Scheithauer B et al. (2001). Selective alterations in glutamate and GABA receptor subunit mRNA expression in dysplastic neurons and giant cells of cortical tubers. Ann Neurol 49: 67–78.

Williams 3rd DW, Elster AD (1992). Cranial CT and MR in the Klippel–Trenaunay–Weber syndrome. AJNR Am J Neuroradiol 13: 291–294.

Wolf NI, Kramer N, Harting I et al. (2005). Diffuse cortical necrosis in a neonate with incontinentia pigmenti and an encephalitis-like presentation. AJNR Am J Neuroradiol 26: 1580–1582.

Wong M, Crino PB (2012). Tuberous sclerosis and epilepsy: role of astrocytes. Glia 60: 1244–1250.

Yamaoka S, Courtois G, Bessia C et al. (1998). Complementation cloning of NEMO, a component of the IkappaB kinase complex essential for NF-kappaB activation. Cell 93: 1231–1240.

Yapici Z, Dincer A, Eraksoy M (2005). Proton spectroscopic findings in children with epilepsy owing to tuberous sclerosis complex. J Child Neurol 20: 517–522.

Ziyeh S, Spreer J, Rossler J et al. (2004). Parkes Weber or Klippel–Trenaunay syndrome? Non-invasive diagnosis with MR projection angiography. Eur Radiol 14: 2025–2029.

Handbook of Clinical Neurology, Vol. 135 (3rd series)
Neuroimaging, Part I
J.C. Masdeu and R.G. González, Editors

Chapter 28

Cerebrospinal fluid flow in adults

WILLIAM G. BRADLEY[1]*, VICTOR HAUGHTON[2], AND KENT-ANDRE MARDAL[3]

[1]*Department of Radiology, University of California San Diego Health System, San Diego, CA, USA*

[2]*Section of Neuroradiology, Department of Radiology, University of Wisconsin, Madison, WI, USA*

[3]*Department of Mathematics, University of Oslo, Oslo, Norway*

Abstract

This chapter uses magnetic resonance imaging phase-contrast cerebrospinal fluid (CSF) flow measurements to predict which clinical normal-pressure hydrocephalus (NPH) patients will respond to shunting as well as which patients with Chiari I are likely to develop symptoms of syringomyelia.

Symptomatic NPH patients with CSF flow (measured as the aqueductal CSF stroke volume) which is shown to be hyperdynamic (defined as twice normal) are quite likely to respond to ventriculoperitoneal shunting. The hyperdynamic CSF flow results from normal systolic brain expansion compressing the enlarged ventricles. When atrophy occurs, there is less brain expansion, decreased aqueductal CSF flow, and less likelihood of responding to shunting.

It appears that NPH is a "two-hit" disease, starting as benign external hydrocephalus in infancy, followed by deep white-matter ischemia in late adulthood, which causes increased resistance to CSF outflow through the extracellular space of the brain.

Using computational flow dynamics (CFD), CSF flow can be modeled at the foramen magnum and in the upper cervical spine. As in the case of NPH, hyperdynamic CSF flow appears to cause the signs and symptoms in Chiari I and can provide an additional indication for surgical decompression. CFD can also predict CSF pressures over the cardiac cycle. It has been hypothesized that elevated pressure pulses may be a significant etiologic factor in some cases of syringomyelia.

CSF FLOW IN THE BRAIN

Cerebrospinal fluid (CSF) is formed primarily in the choroid plexus within the ventricles at a rate of 500 cc/day. It usually flows out of the ventricular system via the foramina of Lushka and Magendie into the subarachnoid space (SAS). Once in the SAS, the CSF either flows down around the spinal cord or flows up over the cerebral convexities, eventually to be primarily absorbed by the arachnoid granulations (macroscopic) and arachnoidal villi (microscopic) on either side of the superior sagittal sinus. Obstruction from the point of CSF production to the point of uptake leads to ventricular enlargement and hydrocephalus (Fig. 28.1). Obstruction proximal to the outlet foramina of the fourth ventricle is termed "obstructive" hydrocephalus and obstruction distal to the fourth ventricle is called "communicating."

Superimposed on the slow egress from the ventricles to the SAS is a more prominent pulsatile motion due to the beating of the heart. During systole blood flows into the brain, causing it to expand inwards, compressing the ventricles, and outwards, compressing the cortical veins and SAS. The inward expansion leads to pulsatile outflow of CSF through the aqueduct and the rest of the ventricular system. This results in a normal CSF flow void in the aqueduct on magnetic resonance imaging (MRI). The systolic expansion forces CSF and venous blood

*Correspondence to: William G. Bradley, Jr, MD, PhD, FACR, Professor and Chair, Department of Radiology, University of California San Diego Health System, 402 Dickinson St #454, San Diego, CA 92103-8224, USA. Tel: +1-619-543-2890, Fax: +1-619-543-2889, E-mail: wgbradley@ucsd.edu

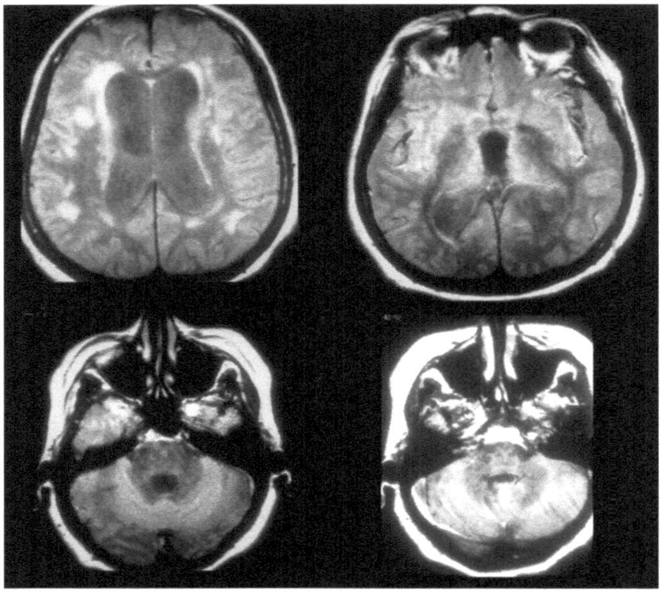

Fig. 28.1. Normal-pressure hydrocephalus on older proton density-weighted conventional spin echo shows ventriculomegaly, deep white-matter ischemia, and a cerebrospinal fluid flow void that extends from the third ventricle to the obex of the fourth ventricle.

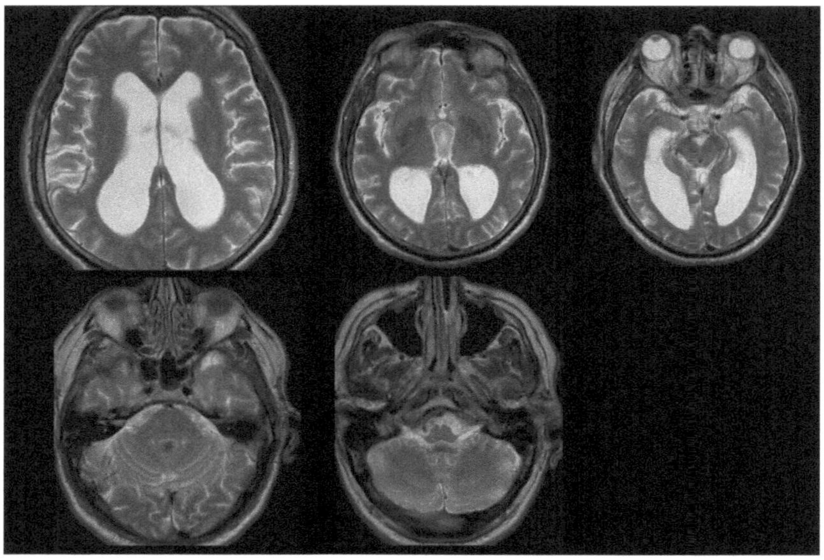

Fig. 28.2. Normal-pressure hydrocephalus on a current T2-weighted fast spin-echo image shows less conspicuous cerebrospinal fluid flow void extending from foramen of Munro to obex. Although less conspicuous than in the past, this finding is now more specific for hyperdynamic flow, albeit less sensitive.

out of the fixed volume of the skull by the Monro–Kellie hypothesis. This results in the systolic outflow of CSF at the foramen magnum and from there down the SAS of the spinal canal. During diastole, the volume of the brain decreases and CSF flows in a reverse direction through the aqueduct and the foramen magnum.

In communicating hydrocephalus, the lateral and third ventricles are enlarged, with the brain eventually expanding out to the inner of the calvarium. During systole, the brain can only expand inwards against the larger drum head of the lateral and third ventricles, leading to much more CSF outflow through the aqueduct, producing a much darker CSF flow void (Figs 28.1 and 28.2). This was an early sign of hyperdynamic CSF flow, indicating that, although communicating hydrocephalus was present, there was minimal atrophy (Bradley et al., 1991b). Most causes of communicating hydrocephalus are due to subarachnoid hemorrhage or meningitis, the former obstructing the arachnoidal villi and the latter often obstructing more proximally at the level of basal cisterns, particularly with viscous fungal, tubercular, or other granulomatous meningidites. A subset of communicating hydrocephalus seen in the elderly is termed "normal-pressure hydrocephalus (NPH)" and is defined by enlarged ventricles and the clinical triad of gait disturbance, dementia, and incontinence.

A subset of communicating hydrocephalus seen in infants aged 6–12 months is termed "benign external hydrocephalus" due to decreased uptake of CSF by the arachnoidal granulations (Fig. 28.3). Since their sutures are still open, such children present with a head circumference increasing at a faster percentile rate than body weight or length and are referred for imaging to exclude a brain tumor. CSF accumulates over the frontal convexities as the head enlarges, leading to a characteristic imaging appearance (Fig. 28.3). Since this condition has been attributed to immature arachnoidal granulations which will eventually catch up to the production of CSF, these children do not need to be shunted – although recent findings suggest that this condition may not be as benign as previously thought (see below) and that their CSF uptake may never be normal.

NORMAL-PRESSURE HYDROCEPHALUS

NPH was first described by Hakim and Adams in 1965 (Adams et al., 1965). At that time, the cause was not known, i.e., the disease was considered "idiopathic." Since that time, patients with known causes of chronic communicating hydrocephalus have also been included as part of NPH. These known cases tend to be younger and respond better to shunting than the idiopathic variety, possibly because of poor historic selection criteria for the latter.

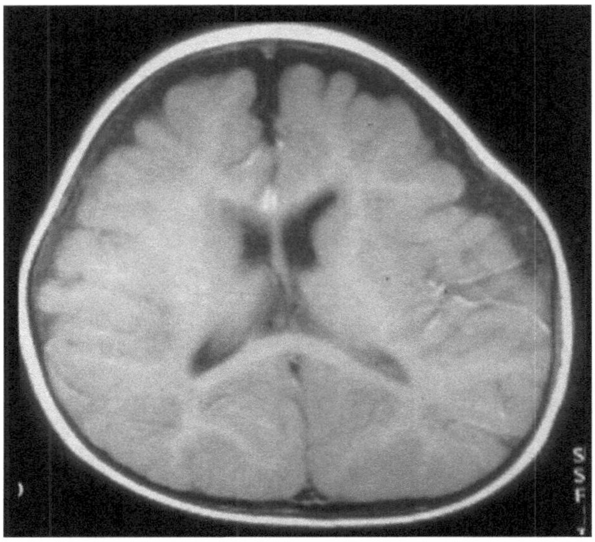

Fig. 28.3. Benign external hydrocephalus in a 7-month-old with mild ventriculomegaly and increased cerebrospinal fluid in the frontal subarachnoid space.

When an elderly patient presents with a gait disturbance and dementia suggestive of NPH, the first diagnostic test is usually an MRI looking for ventricular dilatation out of proportion to any sulcal enlargement, i.e., the pattern of communicating hydrocephalus rather than atrophy (Fig. 28.1). The amount of interstitial edema surrounding the lateral ventricles should be minimal to absent (which goes along with the normal mean intraventricular pressure). There is frequently associated evidence of deep white-matter ischemia (DWMI), a.k.a. small-vessel ischemia (Fig. 28.1), a.k.a. leukoaraiosis (Bradley et al., 1991a). The third ventricle is often bowed out and may have a prominent CSF flow void which extends down through the aqueduct to the obex of the fourth ventricle (Figs 28.1 and 28.2).

The CSF flow void is indicative of hyperdynamic CSF flow similar to the flow voids seen in arteries on MRI. The extent of the CSF flow void on conventional proton density-weighted spin-echo images in the past (Fig. 28.1) was found to correlate with successful response to ventriculoperitoneal shunting for NPH (Bradley et al., 1991b). Unfortunately, the more modern MRI techniques such as fast/turbo spin echo are much more intrinsically flow-compensated, thus the flow void is less conspicuous now than in the early days of MRI; however, when present it means the flow is extremely hyperdynamic (Fig. 28.2). This led to the development of more sophisticated phase-contrast (PC) MRI techniques to evaluate CSF flow for the selection of appropriately symptomatic patients for possible ventriculoperitoneal shunting for NPH (Nitz et al., 1992).

PHASE-CONTRAST CSF VELOCITY IMAGING

With PC-MRI, the slice is positioned in an angled axial plane so it is perpendicular to the aqueduct (Fig. 28.4). The higher the resolution the better, since the aqueduct is such a small structure. We use a 512 × 512 matrix over a 16-cm field of view, achieving spatial resolution of 312 microns (0.312 mm) (Fig. 28.5), although some use lower spatial resolution to save time. Like PC MR angiography, the encoding velocity (V_{enc}) needs to be specified prior to the study being performed. Since most of these studies are performed by the MR technologists without physician supervision, we use V_{enc} of 10, 20, and 30 cm/s to balance velocity aliasing with sensitivity. We also use retrospective cardiac gating with either chest (electrocardiogram) leads or finger plethysmography. Most MRI systems today have automated software which converts the PC-MRI data into the volume of CSF flowing

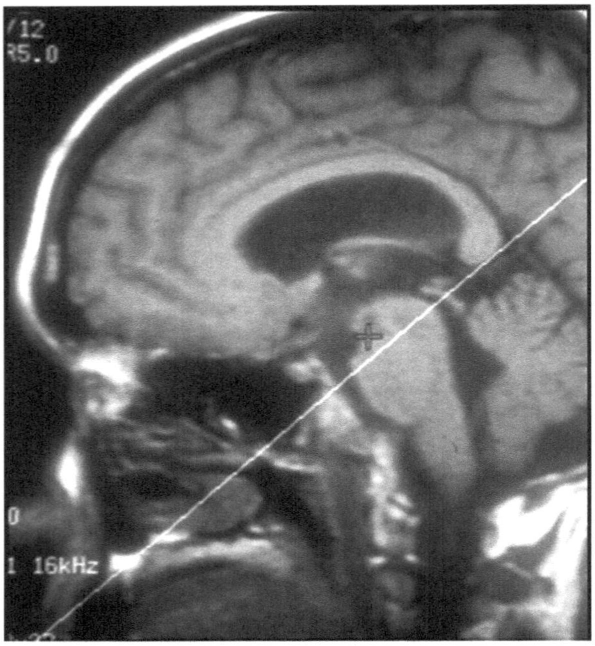

Fig. 28.4. Slice positioning perpendicular to the midaqueduct for phase-contrast cerebrospinal fluid flow study.

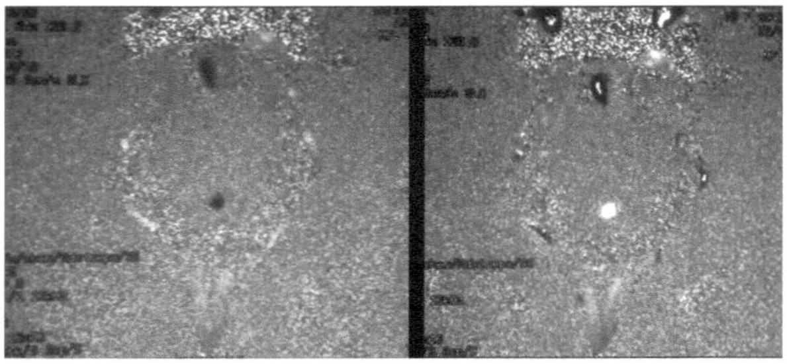

Fig. 28.5. Phase-contrast images showing aqueductal flow up during diastole (black) and flow down during systole (white). CSF, cerebrospinal fluid.

craniocaudad during systole and caudocraniad during diastole (Fig. 28.6). Since the flow down and the flow up are within 5% of each other (with a small net forward motion), we take the average and call it the aqueductal CSF stroke volume (ACSV). Elevated ACSV has been associated with a favorable response to shunting for NPH (Bradley et al., 1996).

Different investigators have used different values for the minimum ACSV appropriate for shunting, since it is highly machine- and technique-dependent. Therefore, it is recommended that anyone wishing to use PC-MRI to diagnose shunt-responsive NPH first perform CSF flow studies on a number of normal elderly patients without dilated ventricles to determine what is normal on your scanner. Then when a "r/o NPH" patient is evaluated, an ACSV twice that value should be sought prior to recommending shunting.

It is important to evaluate the quality of the PC-CSF flow technique. Lower V_{encs} tend to be more accurate but are more susceptible to velocity aliasing, while higher V_{encs} are less sensitive to aliasing but are noisier. The sinusoidal volumetric CSF flow curve (Fig. 28.6) should be evaluated for both aliasing and to be certain that the area under the curve above the zero-flow line (diastole) approximately equals the area below the line (systole). If systolic flow is much greater than diastolic flow, it is possible that the retrospective cardiac gating is not adequately sampling diastole.

If the ACSV is not twice normal in a patient with symptomatic NPH, it is likely that the patient has already gone on to develop atrophy and will be less likely (but not impossible!) to improve with a shunt. On the other hand, symptomatic patients very early in their disease may not have developed hyperdynamic CSF flow yet and may benefit from a repeat study in 6 months (Scollato et al., 2008).

When we perform MRI to rule out NPH we perform a routine MRI of the brain, a PC-MRI CSF flow study and a bright CSF thin-slice sagittal image to evaluate for possible aqueductal stenosis. Depending on the MR vendor, this could be FIESTA (GE), TrueFISP (Siemens), or bFFE (Philips), but it is important to get a slice thickness less than a millimeter (Fig. 28.7). Since aqueductal stenosis presents with the same clinical triad as NPH – plus chronic headaches – these patients are

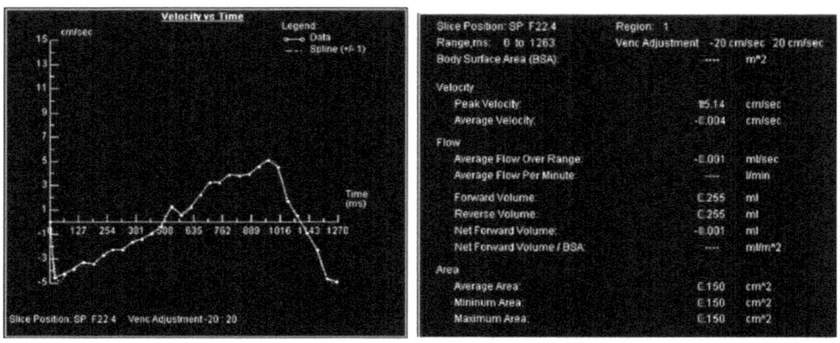

Fig. 28.6. Volumetric, almost sinusoidal, cerebrospinal fluid (CSF) flow through the aqueduct over one cardiac cycle. Integrating the areas under and over the horizontal zero flow line yields the volumes of CSF going caudad in systole and cephalad in diastole, respectively, as shown in the chart. These should be within 5% and their average is the aqueductal CSF stroke volume (ACSV).

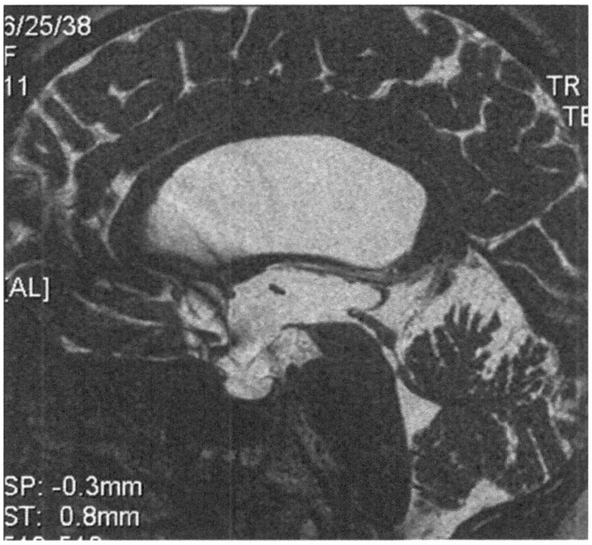

Fig. 28.7. Midsagittal fast imaging employing steady-state acquisition (FIESTA) image showing web in distal aqueduct, i.e., aqueductal stenosis.

often referred for imaging to exclude NPH. As part of the routine MRI, we also perform a coronal sequence (either T1- or T2-weighted) looking for the disproportionately enlarged SAS hydrocephalus (DESH) pattern (Hashimoto et al., 2010), which is large Sylvian cisterns and a tight superior convexity SAS (Fig. 28.8).

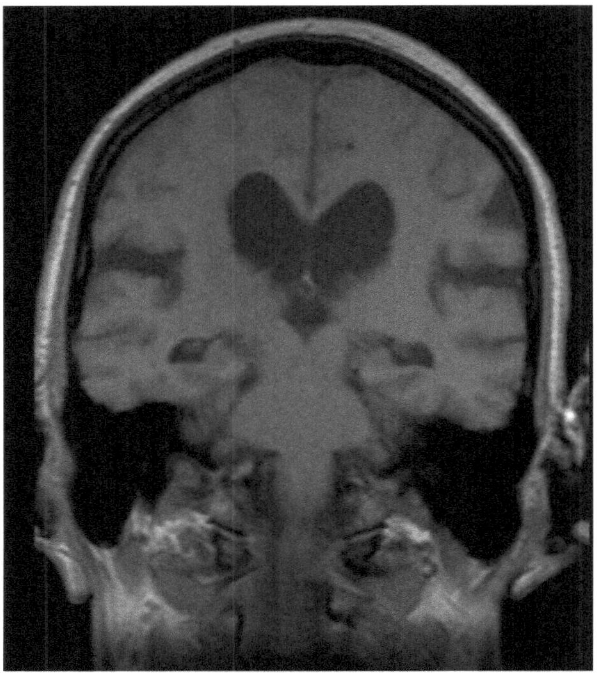

Fig. 28.8. Disproportionately enlarged subarachnoid space hydrocephalus (DESH) pattern of normal-pressure hydrocephalus with ventriculomegaly, prominent Sylvian cisterns, and tight superior convexities.

POSSIBLE ETIOLOGY OF IDIOPATHIC NPH

Having used MRI to study NPH for over 30 years now, it is tempting to speculate on the etiology of the "idiopathic" form. We know that patients with shunt-responsive NPH have both hyperdynamic CSF flow and DWMI (Fig. 28.1). We also know that NPH patients have larger intracranial volumes than age- and sex-matched controls (Bradley et al., 2004) and have had dilated ventricles for years prior to becoming symptomatic (Fig. 28.9). The enlarged intracranial volume raises the possibility that perhaps these patients had benign external hydrocephalus as infants (Bradley et al., 2006).

With decreased CSF outflow via the fourth ventricle, such patients might have developed a parallel pathway for CSF resorption, similar to a parall electrical circuit with a fixed voltage drop that is now able to conduct twice as much current (Bradley et al., 2006). A potential parallel pathway for CSF resorption would be the extracellular space of the brain. Thus CSF would cross the ependyma and be resorbed by the brain parenchyma per se, be transported out the Virchow–Robin spaces via aquaporin 4 receptors, or punch through the pia to get into the SAS. The patients would continue with this dual pattern of CSF resorption, with the extracellular CSF gliding over the myelin lipid, until their elderly years when they develop DWMI.

The histopathologic hallmark of DWMI is myelin pallor (Marshall et al., 1988). With less lipid, there is more water and, therefore, high signal on T2-weighted and fluid-attenuated inversion recovery (FLAIR) images. The outward-flowing CSF in the extracellular space of the brain is now attracted to the denuded myelin protein. This attraction between the polar water molecules of the CSF and the charged side groups of the myelin protein increases the resistance to CSF outflow via the extracellular space of the brain. The outflowing CSF is slowed by the DWMI and backs up, leading to NPH (Bradley et al., 2006).

In support of the above hypothesis is the finding that there is more water in the extracellular space of the brain in patients with NPH than in age-matched controls. This finding comes from the fact that the apparent diffusion coefficient from diffusion-weighted imaging is elevated compared to normal (Bradley et al., 2006). While DWMI has a higher water content than normal brain, as noted above, the apparent diffusion coefficient is statistically higher for a given degree of DWMI in NPH patients than in normal elderly patients (Fig. 28.10). It is also highest in the periventricular region, supporting the concept that the DWMI is damming up the CSF (Fig. 28.11).

Note that the right-hand columns in Figure 28.10 are labeled "pre-NPH." These are patients who were

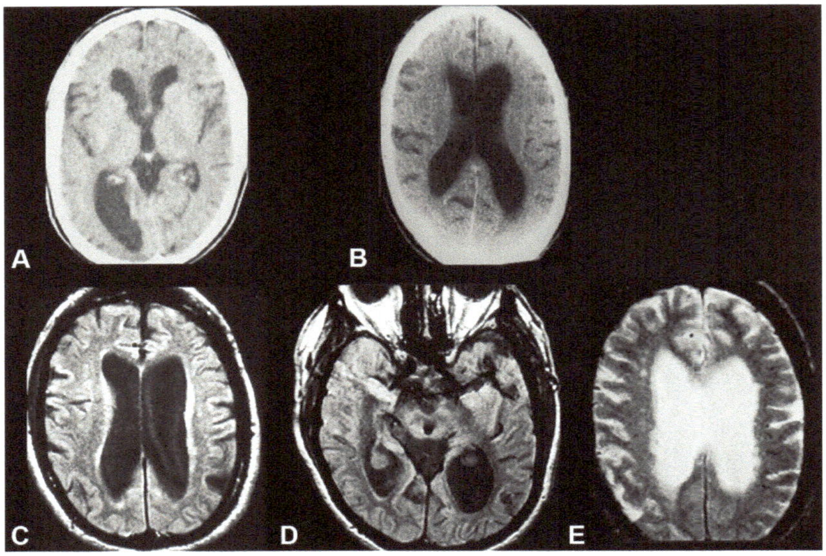

Fig. 28.9. Future normal-pressure hydrocephalus (NPH) patient with 19 years of earlier imaging showing ventriculomegaly before symptoms of NPH. (Reproduced from Bradley et al., 2006, with permission from *Journal of Magnetic Resonance Imaging*.)

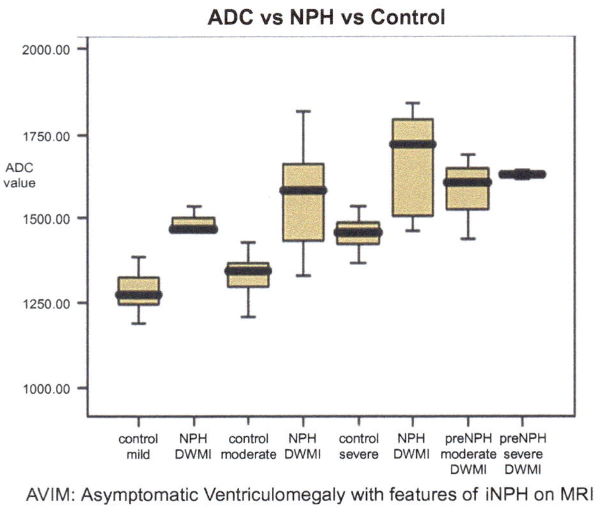

Fig. 28.10. Apparent diffusion coefficient (ADC) vs degree of deep white-matter ischemia (DWMI) in normal-pressure hydrocephalus (NPH) and age-matched controls, showing significantly higher ADC (indicating higher water content) in NPH vs controls for a given degree of DWMI. (Reproduced from Bradley et al., 2006, with permission from *Journal of Magnetic Resonance Imaging*.)

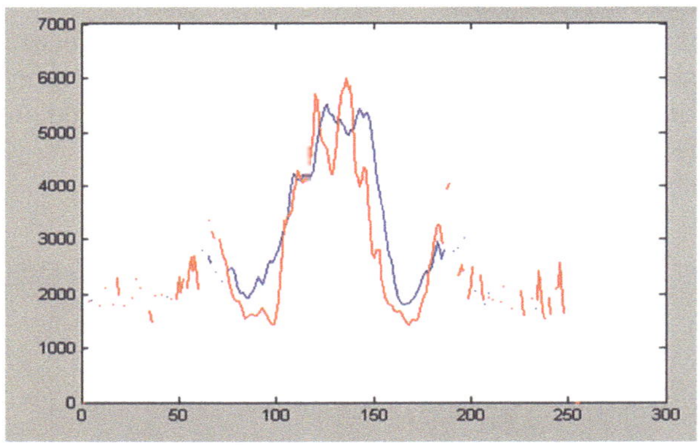

Fig. 28.11. Apparent diffusion coefficient (ADC) profile in midcoronal plane in normal subjects (red) and normal-pressure hydrocephalus (NPH) patients (blue). The central double peak is the lateral ventricles. Note the higher water content in the extracellular space next to the ventricles, possibly due to impaired centrifugal flow from deep white-matter ischemia. (Reproduced from Bradley et al., 2006, with permission from *Journal of Magnetic Resonance Imaging*.)

considered normal elderly controls without symptoms of NPH. They may fall into the same category as the patient illustrated in Figure 28.9, who had enlarged ventricles 19 years before he developed symptoms of NPH. This has been called AVIM: asymptomatic ventriculomegaly with features of idiopathic NPH on MRI. It is important to observe these patients for the potential development of a future gait disturbance.

CSF FLOW IN THE SPINE

CSF in the spinal canal oscillates, due to the expansion of the brain in systole (Monro-Kellie hypothesis). The use of oily intrathecal contrast media provided radiologists with the first opportunity to observe the oscillatory movement of CSF. The movement of the oily contrast medium pantopaque in the cervical SAS suggested a very simple pattern of plug flow because the contrast medium which was immiscible with CSF concealed the complexity of CSF movement. The movement of water-soluble contrast media and radioisotopes in the

SAS also failed to display the complex cyclic movement of CSF with the cardiac cycle. Oscillatory movement of CSF has become an important topic because of its theoretic role in the pathogenesis of syringomyelia. MRI and computational fluid dynamics have demonstrated complex patterns of CSF flow and suggested mechanisms by which syringomyelia develops.

CSF OSCILLATORY FLOW RELATED TO THE CARDIAC CYCLE

CSF in the spinal canal has an oscillatory flow pattern, moving caudally when the arterial systolic pulse wave reaches the brain and moving cephalad during diastole. Caudal flow (systole) has shorter duration and greater velocities than cephalad flow (Fig. 28.12) (Armonda et al., 1994). The CSF cycles at the same rate as the heart beats, i.e., on average about 50–70 bpm. Movement of CSF into the spine displaces venous blood from the epidural venous plexus. CSF flux therefore decreases along the cervical and thoracic spinal canal. CSF flow correlates with CSF pressure fluctuations. Due to inertial effects in the CSF, peak CSF flow appears about 90 degrees out of phase with the pressure oscillations.

The oscillatory motion of CSF explains the familiar slow convection pattern of radionuclides observed in the SAS. The elastic properties of the SAS enable pressure waves, which may also contribute to the development of syringomyelia and to neurologic signs and symptoms in Chiari I patients (Loth et al., 2001). To date the pressure waves are not adequately characterized since direct measurements are invasive. Simulations in patient-specific models when available will improve this characterization.

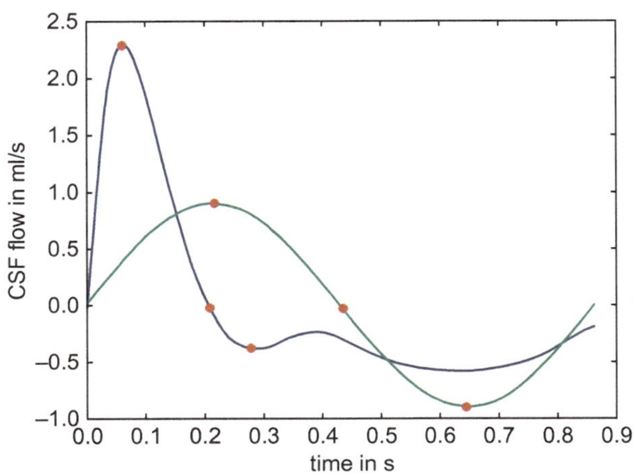

Fig. 28.12. Plot of cerebrospinal fluid (CSF) velocity versus time in the cycle. The idealized physiologic flow is shown in blue and, for comparison, a sinusoidal wave is shown in red. The positive (systolic flow) has a shorter duration and a greater peak magnitude than the negative flow (diastole).

NORMAL PATTERN OF CSF FLOW IN THE SPINE

Inertial and viscous effects determine CSF flow patterns. CSF flow in the spinal canal usually conforms to a laminar pattern, meaning that the fluid flows more rapidly in the center of a channel and less rapidly near a boundary, due to the frictional effects in a viscous fluid. The complex anatomy of the SAS produces a complex flow pattern in the CSF. One feature of CSF flow, evident in PC-MR, is the inhomogeneity of velocities throughout the SAS and the cardiac cycle. The peak CSF flow velocities in any axial section of the spine are located anterolateral to the spinal cord. The anterior midline and posterior SASs have slower velocities (Fig. 28.13). Another feature is an increase in peak velocities in the cervical spine from C1 to C4 (Shah et al., 2010), as the cross-sectional area of the SAS velocity decreases. Fluid flows along the long axis of the spinal canal and radial to it. PC-MR techniques demonstrate multidirectional flow, large vortices, and countercurrents (Fig. 28.14). Simultaneous flow in both a caudad and a cephalad direction occurs during some phases of the cycle, typically near the time when fluid flow reverses. Synchronous bidirectional flow occurs with sufficient volume in symptomatic Chiari I patients that it is detected in PC-MR, but not in normal human subjects.

PHYSIOLOGIC FACTORS AFFECTING CSF FLOW

How physiologic changes in the body and especially exercise affect CSF flow has interest because some patients with the Chiari malformation experience exertional headaches. The oscillatory CSF flow is affected by the pulse rate. As the pulse rate increases, the length of the diastolic phase of CSF flow decreases to a greater extent than does systole phase. One study shows that increasing the heart rate from 80 to 120 bpm in Chiari I patients or controls approximately doubles the average pressure gradients, while peak values remain unchanged. In addition, the volume of synchronous bidirectional flow velocities increased (Linge et al., 2011). Tonsillar herniation elevates both peak and average pressure gradients during rest and exertion.

SPINAL PATHOLOGY EFFECTS ON SPINAL FLUID FLOW

The descent of the cerebellar tonsils into the cervical spinal canal (Chiari I malformation) affects CSF flow. In Chiari patients CSF flow has greater velocities, complexity, and periods of synchronous bidirectional flow than it does in normal subjects. Caudad flow velocities at the foramen magnum reach 12 cm/s in Chiari I patients compared to 5 cm/s in healthy adults (Heiss et al., 1999).

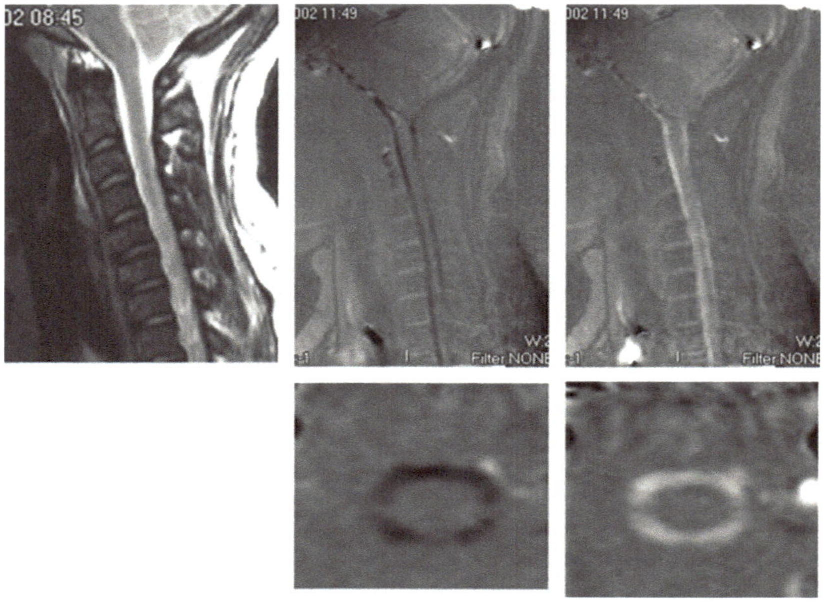

Fig. 28.13. Axial magnetic resonance (MR) image at C2 acquired with phase-contrast (PC) MR shows inhomogeneous flow in the subarachnoid space. The sagittal MR (top left) image shows less than 5 mm of tonsillar herniation. A sagittal PC MR image (top middle) shows caudal cerebrospinal fluid flow (black, negative sign) anterior and posterior to the cord. A sagittal image later in the cycle (top right) shows cephalad flow anterior and posterior to the cord. Axial images (bottom row) show caudad flow (left) and cephalad flow (right) at the same times in the cycle. The axial images show inhomogeneous flow with greater velocities anterolateral to the spinal cord. (Reproduced from Shah et al., 2010, with permission of *American Journal of Neuroradiology*.)

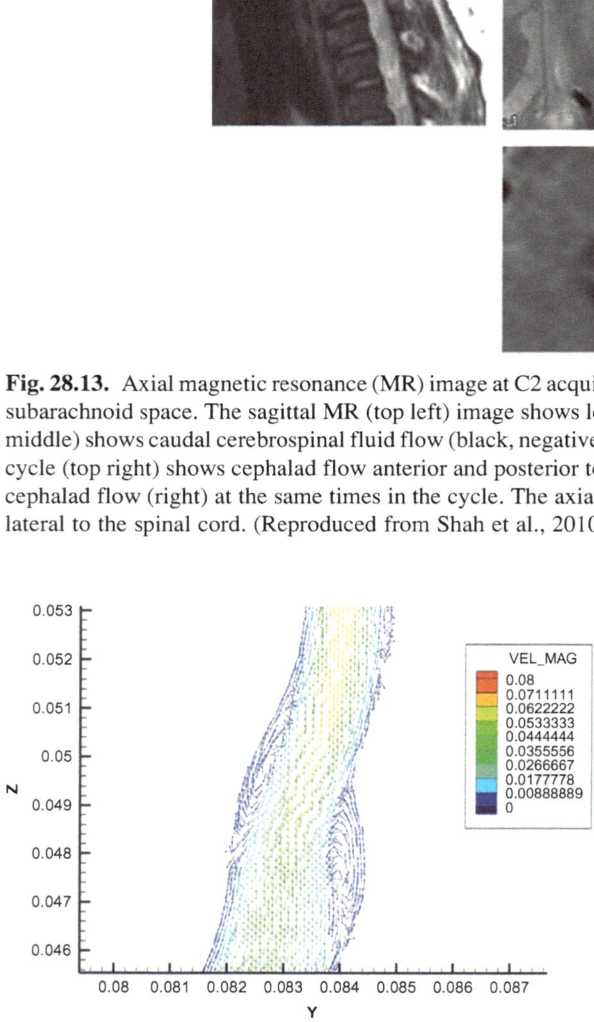

Fig. 28.14. Coronal image cerebrospinal fluid flow patterns demonstrated by means of "streamlines" which indicate the direction and magnitude of flow in the subarachnoid space. The image shows multidirectional flow with vortices and countercurrents.

Cephalad (diastolic) velocities are also elevated in Chiari I, although to a lesser extent. The Chiari I malformation may produce syringomyelia and neurologic signs and symptoms, although the degree of tonsillar descent does not predict the type or presence of symptoms (Meadows et al., 2000). Some patients with tonsils extending less than 5 mm into the foramen magnum are symptomatic, while others with descent greater than 5 mm are not. MRI with cardiac gated PC-MR, developed to image blood and CSF flow, provides physiologic information that complements the anatomic information obtained with MR. PC-MR in Chiari I patients shows that CSF flow posterior to the cord is partially obstructed and anterior to the cord is accelerated by the position of the tonsils (Armonda et al., 1994; Hofmann et al., 2000; Quigley et al., 2004). PC-MR demonstrates greater complexity of flow with larger jets and increased inhomogeneity of flow (Quigley et al., 2004) (Fig. 28.15). In some regions, such as the anterolateral SAS, CSF velocities are greatly elevated, while in other regions, such as the posterior SAS and the midline region of the anterior SAS, CSF flow is reduced. Large jets of flow in the posterior-lateral SAS present in both a craniad and a caudad direction at the same time are observed in some regions within the SAS (Quigley et al., 2004). How fine structure in the SAS such as denticulate ligament and nerve roots affect flow requires additional study. These observations, and the improvement in syringomyelia and symptoms after craniocervical decompression, support the theory that hyperkinetic CSF flow causes neurologic signs and symptoms in the Chiari I malformation.

Flow imaging has limitations. If images are obtained in the sagittal plane, flow is imaged over much of the cervical spine, but only in the midline, where the most extreme velocities are not found. If the axial plane is

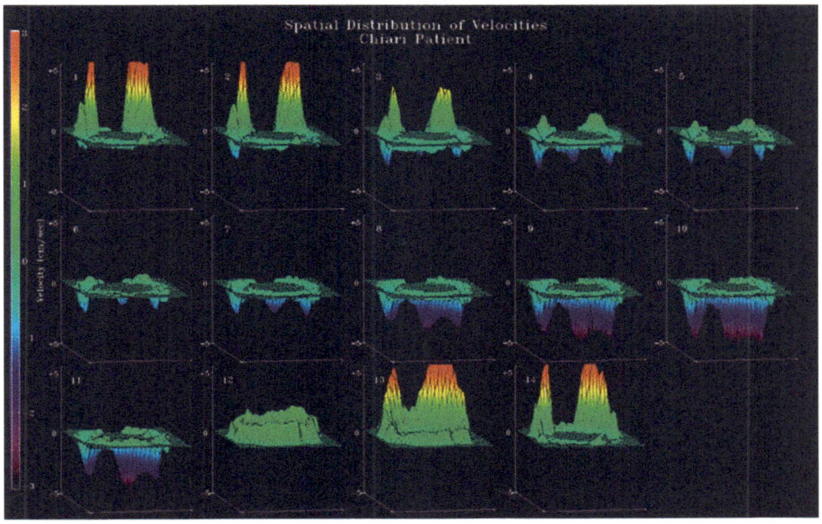

Fig. 28.15. A contour plot of cerebrospinal fluid (CSF) velocities at an axial slice through C1 through the cardiac cycles in a Chiari I patient demonstrating complexity of CSF flow. The plot shows the velocity of flow at each picture element in the subarachnoid space at this level at each of 14 phases of the cardiac cycle. Anterior to the cord are large jets, larger than in healthy subjects. (Reproduced from Quigley et al., 2004, with permission of *Radiology*.)

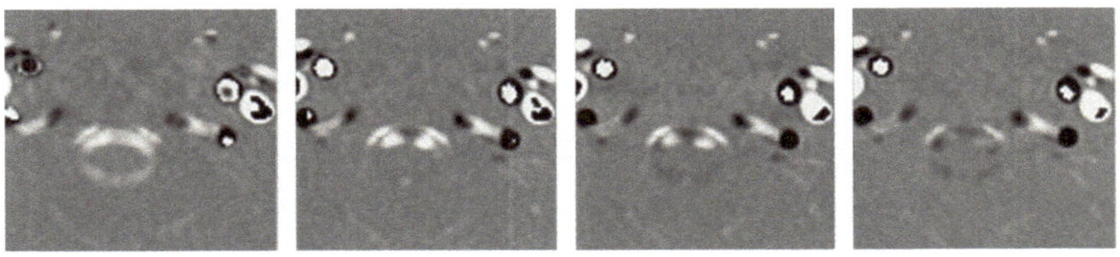

Fig. 28.16. Four sequential axial phase-contrast (PC) magnetic resonance images at the upper end of the cervical spinal canal illustrating synchronous bidirectional flow. The first image shows flow in the caudad direction (white). The next image shows continued flow in the caudad direction with cephalad flow in the craniad direction in the midline anterior to the cord. The fourth image shows flow in both cephalad and caudad directions. The four images encompass about 28% of the cardiac cycle. (Reproduced from Hofkes et al., 2007, with permission of *American Journal of Neuroradiology*.)

selected, flow is measured only at the foramen magnum or one segment of the spinal canal, and the most extreme velocities lateral to the midline are detected. Compared with normal volunteers, Chiari I patients have abnormal CSF flow profiles (Ellenbogen et al., 2000).

The goal of imaging in the Chiari I malformation is to select patients who will benefit from craniocervical decompression. The measurement of tonsillar ectopia does not predict improvement from surgical decompression. PC-MRI may provide additional evidence that a Chiari malformation requires surgical treatment. Used to distinguish patients who are symptomatic from the malformation from those who are asymptomatic, PC-MRI has an accuracy of about 60–70% (Hofkes et al., 2007). The flow pattern that is found exclusively in the symptomatic patients is synchronous bidirectional flow, that is the simultaneous presence of a jet (high velocity in one region) and a counter jet in an adjacent location in the SAS, in other words, the simultaneous presence of flow in caudad and cephalad directions (Fig. 28.16).

Processes that modify the tissue within or around the SAS may affect CSF flow. A simulation shows that arachnoiditis, which presumably stiffens or roughens the external boundaries of the SAS, increases flow resistance and pressure pulses in the CSF (Bilston et al., 2006). Investigators hypothesize that the elevated CSF pressure may be a significant factor in the pathogenesis of some types of syringomyelia.

BIOMECHANICS OF CSF FLOW

With mathematical equations such as Navier-Stokes, the pressure and velocity of a moving fluid can be calculated, with greater spatial and temporal resolution than achieved with PC-MR. Very sophisticated programs have been developed based on fluid mechanics, termed computational flow dynamics or CFD. These have been

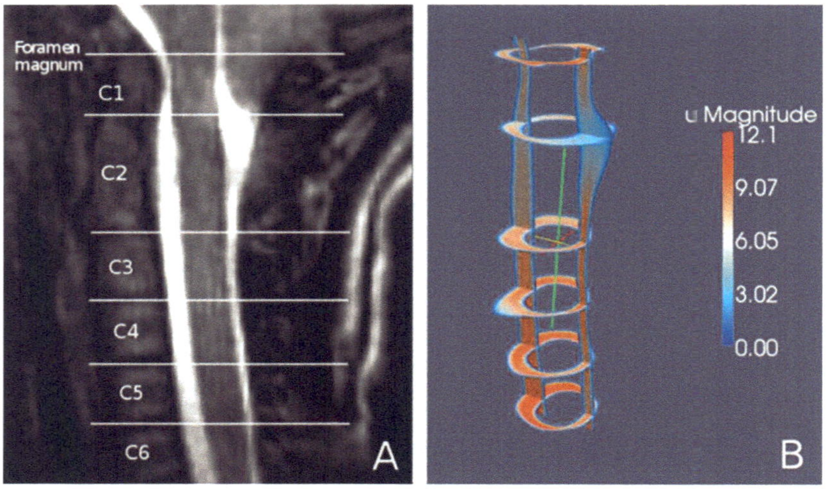

Fig. 28.17. Cerebrospinal fluid flow demonstrated by simulation visualized in 3D by means of a sagittal and selected axial images. Flow has greater velocities at C5 than at C1 and has greatest velocities anterolateral in the subarachnoid space. (Reproduced from Rutkowska et al., 2012, by permission of *American Journal of Neuroradiology*.)

applied to the flow of CSF in the spinal canal in healthy adults and in patients with the Chiari I malformation. In one study, exact mathematic models were created of the SAS in a normal adult and a Chiari I patient, in which pressures and velocities were calculated for each point within the SAS throughout the cardiac cycle (Fig. 28.17). The calculations showed that fluid flowing in the foramen magnum of the patient with Chiari I malformation has jets anterior to the spinal cord, in the location where they are shown with PC-MR (Fig. 28.5). The authors also showed that CSF pressures increased with distance along the upper spinal canal, in correspondence with velocities (Roldan et al., 2009). Computational scientists have been able to model CSF flow throughout the cardiac cycle in an idealized model of the SAS (Alperin et al., 2001). In the idealized model, the introduction of the tonsils into the upper cervical spinal canal flow caused different flow patterns. This study confirmed that CSF velocities increase between the foramen magnum and C4 (Shah et al., 2010). CFD promises to improve our understanding of CSF flow, because it has extremely good spatial and temporal resolution, because it provides both flow and pressure measurements, and because it demonstrates the internal structure of flow.

EFFECT OF SPINAL SURGERY ON CSF FLOW

Craniovertebral decompression, an effective treatment for syrinx in Chiari patients, reduces peak CSF velocities (Dolar et al., 2004) and reduces CSF pressure gradients. At the foramen magnum, pressures and velocities diminish toward normal; lower in the cervical spine the surgery normalizes pressures and velocities (Linge et al., 2013); it also lowers the pressures to which the spinal cord is subjected. Laminectomy to treat cervical spinal stenosis may also reduce CSF pressures and velocities.

CONCLUSIONS

The flow of CSF is not simple "plug flow" in and out of the cranial vault but complex flow due to the complex anatomy and to viscous and inertial effects in fluid streams (Hentschel et al., 2010). Furthermore, the spinal canal is not a rigid structure but an elastic one, so that moving fluids produce pressure waves. These pressure waves may also contribute to the development of syringomyelia and to neurologic signs and symptoms in Chiari I patients (Loth et al., 2001). Additional CFD studies will enhance understanding of CSF flow and will guide efforts to design simple and accurate clinical and imaging tests to determine which symptoms result from the malformation and which patients will benefit from surgical decompression. CFD creates the possibility of performing a "virtual decompression" on a patient to determine the size and dimension of the surgical intervention in order to restore normal CSF flow to the spinal canal.

Spinal CSF has a complex oscillatory flow pattern resulting from the displacement of cranial CSF. MR flow imaging shows cyclic changes in spinal fluid flow related to the cardiac cycle, spinal fluid flow jets related to the complex spinal anatomy, i.e., flow vortices. It shows hyperdynamic CSF flow in the presence of tonsillar ectopia. CFD simulations show these complex flow patterns and provide measurements of the CSF pressure gradients through the cardiac cycle. Engineering calculations suggest that the inertial and viscous forces in CSF have similar proportions to blood flowing in the aorta. Ongoing studies suggest how CSF flow may have a role in the development of syringomyelia and how surgical management may be optimized.

References

Adams RD, Fisher CM, Hakim S et al. (1965). Symptomatic occult hydrocephalus with normal cerebrospinal-fluid pressure. N Engl J Med 273: 117–126.

Alperin N, Kulkarni K, Roitberg B et al. (2001). Analysis of magnetic resonance imaging-based blood and cerebrospinal fluid flow measurements in patients with Chiari I malformation: a system approach. Neurosurg Focus 11: 1–10.

Armonda RA, Citrin CM, Foley KT et al. (1994). Quantitative cine-mode magnetic resonance imaging of Chiari I malformations: an analysis of cerebrospinal fluid dynamics. Neurosurgery 35: 214–224.

Bilston L, Fletcher D, Stoodley M (2006). Focal spinal arachnoiditis increases subarachnoid space pressure: a computational study. Clin Biomech 21: 579–584.

Bradley W, Whittemore A, Watanabe A et al. (1991a). Association of deep white matter infarction with chronic communicating hydrocephalus: implications regarding the possible origin of normal-pressure hydrocephalus. AJNR Am J Neuroradiol 12: 31–39.

Bradley WG, Whittemore AR, Kortman KE et al. (1991b). Marked cerebrospinal fluid void: indicator of successful shunt in patients with suspected normal-pressure hydrocephalus. Radiology 178: 459–466.

Bradley WG, Scalzo D, Queralt J et al. (1996). Normal-pressure hydrocephalus: evaluation with cerebrospinal fluid flow measurements at MR imaging. Radiology 198: 523–529.

Bradley WG, Safar FG, Hurtado C et al. (2004). Increased intracranial volume: a clue to the etiology of idiopathic normal-pressure hydrocephalus? AJNR Am J Neuroradiol 25: 1479–1484.

Bradley WG, Bahl G, Alksne JF (2006). Idiopathic normal pressure hydrocephalus may be a "two hit" disease: benign external hydrocephalus in infancy followed by deep white matter ischemia in late adulthood. J Magn Reson Imaging 24: 747–755.

Dolar MT, Haughton VM, Iskandar BJ et al. (2004). Effect of craniocervical decompression on peak CSF velocities in symptomatic patients with Chiari I malformation. AJNR Am J Neuroradiol 25: 142–145.

Ellenbogen RG, Armonda RA, Shaw DW et al. (2000). Toward a rational treatment of Chiari I malformation and syringomyelia. Neurosurg Focus 8: 1–10.

Hashimoto M, Ishikawa M, Mori E et al. (2010). Diagnosis of idiopathic normal pressure hydrocephalus is supported by MRI-based scheme: a prospective cohort study. Cerebrospinal fluid res 7: 1–10.

Heiss JD, Patronas N, Devroom HL et al. (1999). Elucidating the pathophysiology of syringomyelia. J Neurosurg 91: 553–562.

Hentschel S, Mardal K-A, Løvgren AE et al. (2010). Characterization of cyclic CSF flow in the foramen magnum and upper cervical spinal canal with MR flow imaging and computational fluid dynamics. AJNR Am J Neuroradiol 31: 997–1002.

Hofkes SK, Iskandar BJ, Turski PA et al. (2007). Differentiation between symptomatic Chiari I malformation and asymptomatic tonsillar ectopia by using cerebrospinal fluid flow imaging: initial estimate of imaging accuracy 1. Radiology 245: 532–540.

Hofmann E, Warmuth-Metz M, Bendszus M et al. (2000). Phase-contrast MR imaging of the cervical CSF and spinal cord: volumetric motion analysis in patients with Chiari I malformation. AJNR Am J Neuroradiol 21: 151–158.

Linge SO, Haughton V, Løvgren AE et al. (2011). Effect of tonsillar herniation on cyclic CSF flow studied with computational flow analysis. AJNR Am J Neuroradiol 32: 1474–1481.

Linge S, Mardal K-A, Haughton V et al. (2013). Simulating CSF flow dynamics in the normal and the Chiari I subarachnoid space during rest and exertion. AJNR Am J Neuroradiol 34: 41–45.

Loth F, Yardimci MA, Alperin N (2001). Hydrodynamic modeling of cerebrospinal fluid motion within the spinal cavity. J Biomech Eng 123: 71–79.

Marshall V, Bradley JR W, Marshall C et al. (1988). Deep white matter infarction: correlation of MR imaging and histopathologic findings. Radiology 167: 517–522.

Meadows J, Kraut M, Guarnieri M et al. (2000). Asymptomatic Chiari type I malformations identified on magnetic resonance imaging. J Neurosurg 92: 920–926.

Nitz WR, Bradley WG, Watanabe AS et al. (1992). Flow dynamics of cerebrospinal fluid: assessment with phase-contrast velocity MR imaging performed with retrospective cardiac gating. Radiology 183: 395–405.

Quigley MF, Iskandar B, Quigley MA et al. (2004). Cerebrospinal fluid flow in foramen magnum: temporal and spatial patterns at MR imaging in volunteers and in patients with Chiari I malformation. Radiology 232: 229–236.

Roldan A, Wieben O, Haughton V et al. (2009). Characterization of CSF hydrodynamics in the presence and absence of tonsillar ectopia by means of computational flow analysis. AJNR Am J Neuroradiol 30: 941–946.

Rutkowska G, Haughton V, Linge S et al. (2012). Patient-specific 3D simulation of cyclic CSF flow at the craniocervical region. AJNR Am J Neuroradiol 33 (9): 1756–1762.

Scollato A, Tenenbaum R, Bahl G et al. (2008). Changes in aqueductal CSF stroke volume and progression of symptoms in patients with unshunted idiopathic normal pressure hydrocephalus. AJNR Am J Neuroradiol 29: 192–197.

Shah S, Haughton V, Del Rão AMO (2010). Flow through the upper cervical spinal canal in Chiari I malformation. AJNR Am J Neuroradiol 32: 1149–1153.

Handbook of Clinical Neurology, Vol. 135 (3rd series)
Neuroimaging, Part I
J.C. Masdeu and R.G. González, Editors

Chapter 29

Inherited or acquired metabolic disorders

FLORIAN EICHLER[1]*, EVA RATAI[2], JASON J. CARROLL[2], AND JOSEPH C. MASDEU[3]

[1]*Department of Neurology, Massachusetts General Hospital, Boston, MA, USA*

[2]*Department of Radiology, Massachusetts General Hospital, Boston, MA, USA*

[3]*Department of Neurology, Houston Methodist Hospital, Houston, TX, USA*

Abstract

This chapter starts with a description of imaging of inherited metabolic disorders, followed by a discussion on imaging of acquired toxic-metabolic disorders of the adult brain. Neuroimaging is crucial for the diagnosis and management of a number of inherited metabolic disorders. Among these, inherited white-matter disorders commonly affect both the nervous system and endocrine organs. Magnetic resonance imaging (MRI) has enabled new classifications of these disorders that have greatly enhanced both our diagnostic ability and our understanding of these complex disorders. Beyond the classic leukodystrophies, we are increasingly recognizing new hereditary leukoencephalopathies such as the hypomyelinating disorders. Conventional imaging can be unrevealing in some metabolic disorders, but proton magnetic resonance spectroscopy (MRS) may be able to directly visualize the metabolic abnormality in certain disorders. Hence, neuroimaging can enhance our understanding of pathogenesis, even in the absence of a pathologic specimen. This review aims to present pathognomonic brain MRI lesion patterns, the diagnostic capacity of proton MRS, and information from clinical and laboratory testing that can aid diagnosis. We demonstrate that applying an advanced neuroimaging approach enhances current diagnostics and management. Additional information on inherited and metabolic disorders of the brain can be found in Chapter 63 in the second volume of this series.

INHERITED METABOLIC DISORDERS

Most inherited metabolic disorders of the brain are monogenetic disorders in which the mutant gene encodes an aberrant enzyme involved in lipid or protein metabolism. The inability to degrade or synthesize substrate leads to an upstream excess or downstream lack of vital lipids. This can cause a wide range of pathology, ranging from inflammatory demyelination to axonal degeneration and microglial activation. Hence, the often-cited prominent demyelination is only one manifestation in leukodystrophies, and myelin-forming oligodendrocytes are not the only cells affected in these disorders.

Leukodystrophies are hereditary disorders of white matter that impair a brain that is initially normally formed and without obvious structural defect (Costello et al., 2009; Kohlschutter et al., 2010). They can affect brain myelin throughout life and are commonly progressive in nature. First manifestations are often cognitive deterioration, followed by motor and balance as well as visual abnormalities. Classic leukodystrophies typically lead to a vegetative state or death within months to years. In general, the earlier the onset of symptoms, the more progressive the disease course.

Yet, there are some common characteristics that distinguish the pathology in leukodystrophies from that of other disorders. This is where magnetic resonance imaging (MRI) has played a seminal role in visualization of the lesion pattern (van Der Knaap, 2005). The demyelinating lesions are usually confluent and symmetric. Many of the classic disorders, such as X-linked

*Correspondence to: Dr. Florian Eichler, Massachusetts General Hospital, 55 Fruit Street, ACC 708, Boston MA 02114, USA. Tel: +1-617-724-7121, Fax: +1-617-726-9422, E-mail: feichler@partners.org

adrenoleukodystrophy (X-ALD), metachromatic leukodystrophy (MLD), and Krabbe disease, show relative sparing of subcortical fibers. Yet other disorders have early involvement of the U-fibers and other unique characteristics, such as cystic rarefaction and degeneration.

In addition, an increasing number of hereditary leukoencephalopathies are being recognized. While these disorders also affect myelin, they generally follow a more static course. These include hereditary disorders that do not show demyelination, but rather hypomyelination (Steenweg et al., 2010). Common neurologic features in hypomyelinating disorders are developmental delay, nystagmus, cerebellar ataxia, and spasticity. One of the better-characterized hypomyelinating disorders is Pelizaeus–Merzbacher disease. Beyond this classic disorder, a multitude of other hypomyelinating disorders exist. Only about half of patients with evidence of hypomyelination on MRI are definitively diagnosed with a specific disorder. Yet, specific clinical and MRI features can be pathognomonic and lead to diagnosis.

There are, however, several metabolic brain disorders not associated with obvious white-matter abnormalities on brain MRI. Some of these disorders, such as defects in creatine metabolism, can be detected by proton magnetic resonance spectroscopy (MRS). Cerebral creatine deficiency syndromes (CCDSs) are a group of inborn errors of creatine metabolism comprising two autosomal-recessive disorders that affect the biosynthesis of creatine – arginine:glycine amidinotransferase deficiency and guanidinoacetate methyltransferase deficiency – and an X-linked defect that affects the creatine transporter, SLC6A8 deficiency. The common clinical presentation in CCDS includes mental retardation, expressive speech and language delay, autistic-like behavior, and epilepsy. Importantly, treatment of creatine biosynthesis defects can result in clinical improvement, emphasizing the importance of early diagnosis.

This chapter aims to present the diagnostic MRI lesion patterns of inherited metabolic disorders of the brain, as well as the utility of advanced MR techniques. Some of the techniques described have already been established in clinical practice, while others are experimental in nature and subject to ongoing research.

Conventional brain MRI: metabolic disorders causing demyelination

Most metabolic disorders cause selective damage to the nervous system that can be detected by MRI. These imaging patterns are in many cases pathognomonic. Both demyelinating and hypomyelinating disorders carry distinct features, listed in Table 29.1. While the patterns of maturation of white matter are similar on T1- and T2-weighted images, the time at which white matter appears to mature is delayed on T2-weighted images. Therefore, T1-weighted imaging may be more sensitive to immature myelin than T2-weighted imaging.

X-ALD is a lethal neurodegenerative disorder with manifestations ranging from inflammatory demyelination to a chronic axonopathy of the spinal cord. In X-ALD, a defect in peroxisomal beta-oxidation causes accumulation of very-long-chain fatty acids in tissue and plasma, in particular the central nervous system and adrenal glands. At least four clinical phenotypes have been delineated: childhood cerebral, adult cerebral, adrenomyeloneuropathy (AMN), and female heterozygotes for X-ALD.

The posterior regions of the brain are involved in 80–90% of childhood cerebral ALD and the frontal regions in 5–10% (Melhem et al., 1999; Moser et al., 2000). The lesion evolves in a symmetric confluent fashion, starting in the splenium or genu of the corpus callosum and spreading into the periventricular white matter (Fig. 29.1). The arcuate fibers are initially spared. In the acute phase, a garland of contrast enhancement is present. This pattern is markedly different from that seen in the adult form of the disease, AMN, a noninflammatory chronic axonopathy. However, all phenotypes display a systematic progression that that can be quantified using a 34-point scoring system (Loes et al., 1994, 2003).

Parieto-occipital white-matter lesions are also present in Krabbe disease (globoid cell leukodystrophy), but there is no garland of contrast enhancement (Loes et al., 1999; Wenger et al., 2001). MLD shows more diffuse involvement of both frontal and posterior regions of the brain (Eichler et al., 2009). Involvement of the corpus callosum is seen early in MLD, although not as striking as that seen in ALD or globoid cell leukodystrophy. A tigroid pattern is often apparent in the centrum semiovale. In contrast to ALD, the outer subarachnoid spaces are not enlarged in MLD, even in the most advanced stages of disease.

Other disorders have characteristic early involvement of the U-subcortical fibers. Children with Canavan disease present with an enlarged brain (megalencephaly) (Surendran et al., 2003; Kumar et al., 2006). Their MRI shows diffuse white-matter involvement, including the subcortical U-fibers (Janson et al., 2006). There is also involvement of the basal ganglia and other deep gray nuclei. Alexander disease is another leukodystrophy that often manifests with megalencephaly (van der Knaap et al., 2001). Imaging studies typically show cerebral white-matter abnormalities affecting the frontal regions, although unusual variants are increasingly recognized (van der Knaap et al., 2005, 2006).

Table 29.1

Examples of Characteristic Neuroimaging in Inherited Metabolic and Endocrine Disorders

Disease	Mutated genes	Characteristics on Brain MRI
Aicardi- Goutières Syndrome (AGS)	*ADAR1, RNASEH2A, RNASEH2B, RNASEH2C, SAMHD1, TREX1*	Temporal lobe swelling followed by atrophy with temporal horn dilatation, early global cerebral atrophy and visible calcifications
Canavan Disease	*ASPA*	Macrocephaly, subcortical U-fibers and basal ganglia involved
Cerebrotendineous Xanthomatosi	*CYP27A1*	Cerebellar lesions, calcifications visible on CT or susceptibility weighted MRI
Creatine Deficiency of the Brai	*GAMT, AGAT*	Absent Creatine peak on MRS
FA2H related disorders		Pontocerebellar atrophy, mild cerebral atrophy, and thinning of the corpus callosum, on T2-weighted images hypointensities of the globus pallidus and hyperintensities of subcortical/periventricular white matter
Fabry Disease	*GALA*	Multiple small infarcts, high signal in the pulvinar
Fucosidosis	*FUCA1*	T2 hypointensity globus pallidus
Globoid Leukodystrophy (Krabbe Disease)	*GALC*	Posterior predominance, no contrast enhancement
Glutaric Aciduria	*GCDH*	Subdural hygromas, delayed myelination
GM2 gangliosidoses	*GM2 gangliosides*	Hypomyelination.; in infants decreased or cholineand in late onset patients decreased N-acetylaspartate on MRS
Hypomyelination with congenital cataracts	*FAM126A*	Hypomyelination, T1 hypointensity in central white matter and T1 hyperintensity in subcortical white matter
Hypomyelination, Hypodontia, Hypogonadotropic Hypogonadism	*POLR3A, B*	Early cerebellar atrophy with absence of putamen
Kearns Sayre Syndrome	Mitochondrial DNA deletions	On CT calcium deposits in globus pallidum and caudate, MRI: subcortial white matter abnormalities on T2 weighted images
Leukoencephalopathy with Brain Stem and Spinal Cord Involvement and Elevated Lactate	*DARS2*	Characteristic brainstem pattern: pyramidal tracts, cerebellar connections and intraparenchymal trajectories of trigeminal nerve. Decreased N-acetylaspartate and increased myo-inositol, choline and lactate on MRS
Leukoencephalopathy associated with a disturbance in the metabolism of polyols	*RPIA*	Elevated levels of arabinitol and ribitol (coupled resonances between 3.5 and 4ppm) on MRS
Metachromatic leukodystrophy	*ARSA*	Diffuse with initial; subcortical sparing, "tigroid pattern" in centrum semiovale
Peroxisomal Biogenesis disorders	*PEX* genes	Migrational abnormalities (e.g. perisylvian polymicrogyria)
Sialic acid storage disorders	*SLC17A5*	Thin corpus callosum and cerebelllar atrophy, myelin deficiency
Sjogren Larsson Syndrome	*FALDH or ALDH3A2*	In complete myelination. T2 hyperintensities in periventricular and deep white matter
Vanishing White Matter Disease	*EIF2B1-5*	Confluent cystic degeneration, white matter signal appears CSF-like
Wilsons Disease	*ATP7B*	Lesions in thalamus, putamen and caudate, also in globus pallidum, claustrum and subthalamic nucleus
X-Linked Adrenoleukodystrophy	*ABCD1*	CCALD: posterior predominance with contrast enhancement in acute phase, elevated Cho at lesion edge on MRS AMN: corticospinal tracts and dorsal columns, no contrast enhancement, decreased N-acetylaspartate on MRS

MRI, magnetic resonance imaging; CSF, cerebrospinal fluid; CT, computed tomography; MRS, magnetic resonance spectroscopy; CCALD, childhood cerebral adrenoleukodystrophy; AMN, adrenomyeloneuropathy.

MRI of vanishing white-matter disease demonstrates progressive rarefaction of white matter over time on proton density and fluid-attenuated inversion recovery (FLAIR) images (van der Knaap et al., 1997, 2002; Leegwater et al., 2001). Autopsy findings have confirmed the white-matter rarefaction and cystic degeneration suggested by MRI. Regions of relative sparing include the subcortical U-fibers, corpus callosum, internal capsule, and the anterior commissure. The cerebellar white matter and brainstem show variable degrees of involvement, but do not undergo cystic degeneration.

Cerebrotendinous xanthomatosis (CTX) is a rare, but treatable, disorder characterized by a defect in the

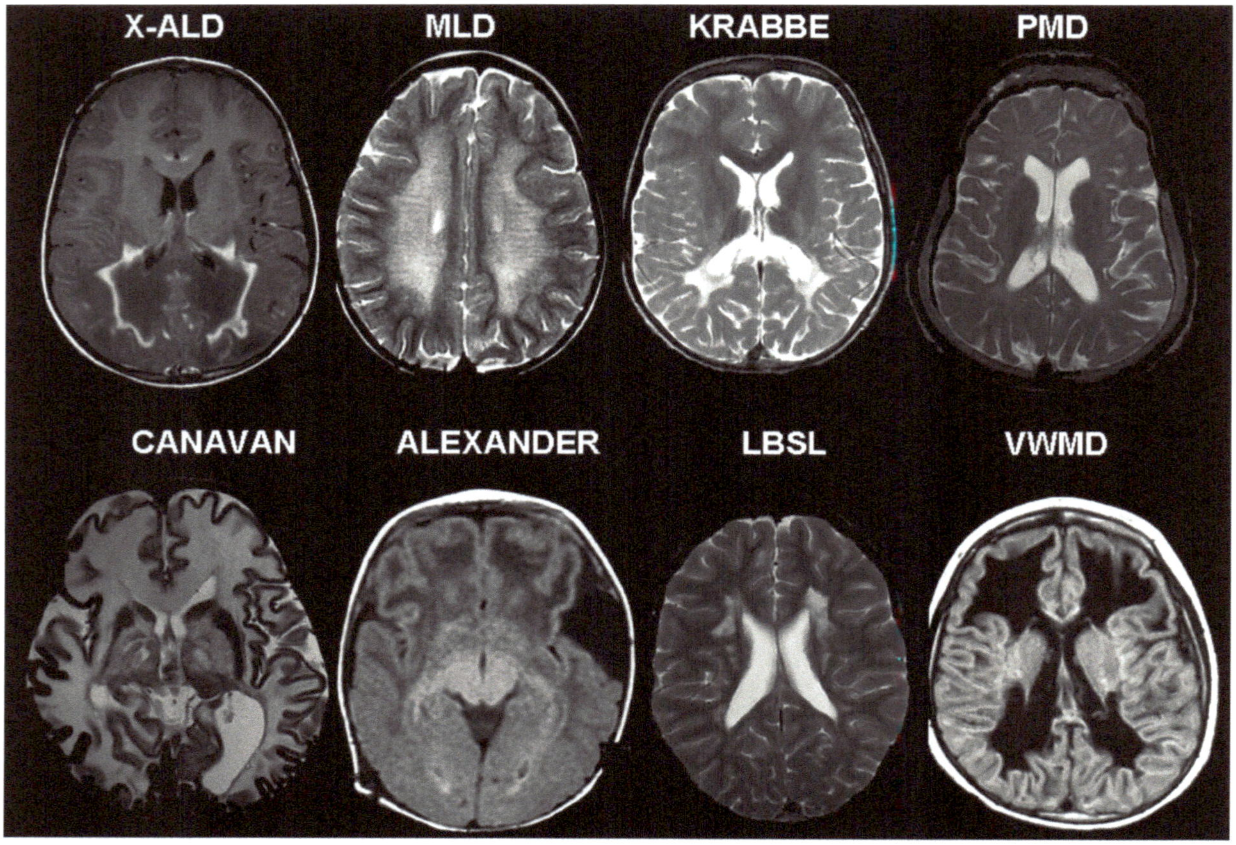

Fig. 29.1. Lesion patterns on conventional magnetic resonance imaging in leukodystrophies and hypomyelinating disorders, including: X-linked adrenoleukodystrophy (X-ALD); metachromatic leukodystrophy (MLD); Krabbe's disease; Pelizaeus–Merzbacher disease (PMD); Canavan's disease; Alexander's disease; leukoencephalopathy with brainstem and spinal cord involvement and elevated white-matter lactate (LBSL); and vanishing white-matter disease (VWMD). (Reproduced from Ratai et al., 2012.)

metabolic pathway of cholesterol (Salen et al., 1987). Symptoms in infancy include diarrhea, cataracts, and psychomotor retardation. In adulthood, the spectrum of neurologic dysfunction includes mental retardation leading to dementia, psychiatric symptoms, premature retinal aging, and epileptic seizures. The most distinctive MRI abnormalities are symmetric bilateral T2 hyperintensity in the dentate nuclei and adjacent cerebellar white matter (De Stefano et al., 2001).

Brainstem lesion patterns can often provide critical clues to an accurate diagnosis. Leukoencephalopathy with brainstem and spinal cord involvement and elevated white-matter lactate (LBSL) has recently been described and shows distinct involvement of the pyramidal tracts, medial lemniscus, mesencephalic trigeminal tracts, intraparenchymal trigeminal nerves, and superior cerebellar peduncles (Scheper et al., 2007; van Berge et al., 2014; van der Knaap et al., 2003). This distinct lesion pattern led to the identification of the responsible gene, DARS2, which encodes mitochondrial aspartyl-tRNA synthetase.

Conventional brain MRI: metabolic disorders causing hypomyelination

In hypomyelinating disorders, the boundaries between gray and white matter often appear "blurred" (Steenweg et al., 2010). The T2 hypointensity of the white matter is milder in hypomyelination than in demyelination and other white-matter pathology. Overall, the brain MRI in hypomyelination looks like that of a young child, with less well-distinguished gray and white matter. As opposed to "delayed myelination," the pattern on brain MRI is unchanged, i.e., myelination is "stuck" on two MRIs 6–12 months apart in a child older than 1 year of age. While at first glance hypomyelinating disorders may all have a similar MRI appearance, there are a group of disorders in which the MRI can provide important clues to the diagnosis (Table 29.2). In these individual disorders, attention to the deep gray-matter structures will often reveal a characteristic "signature" (Steenweg et al., 2010).

Table 29.2

Brain metabolite abnormalities on proton magnetic resonance spectroscopy (MRS)

Leukodystrophy or hypomyelinating disorder	Systemic metabolites	Brain metabolites abnormalities on proton MRS
Canavan disease	Urine *N*-acetylaspartate	Highly elevated *N*-acetylaspartate
Cerebrotendineous xanthomatosis	Plasma cholestanol	Lipid peaks seen in cerebellum
Creatine deficiency of the brain		Absent creatine peak
Globoid leukodystrophy (Krabbe disease)	Plasma glucocerebrosides, psychosine	Choline and myo-inositol elevations, decreased *N*-acetylaspartate
GM2 gangliosidoses	GM2 gangliosides	Infantile: variable choline, myoinositol, and *N*-acetylaspartate. Late onset: decreased *N*-acetylaspartate
Hypomyelination with atrophy of the basal ganglia and cerebellum	Unknown	Increased myo-inositol and creatine
Megalencephalic leukodystrophy with cysts	Unknown	Decreased ratio of *N*-acetylaspartate to creatine
Pelizaeus–Merzbacher disease	Unknown	Variable reports on changes in *N*-acetylaspartate and choline
Vanishing white-matter disease	Decreased ratio of asialotransferrin to transferrin in CSF	Within cystic white matter, complete absence of all metabolites
X-linked adrenoleukodystrophy	Plasma very-long-chain fatty acids	CCALD: choline elevations within normal-appearing white matter, elevations of lactate within the lesion AMN: decreased *N*-acetylaspartate in adrenomyeloneuropathy

CSF, cerebrospinal fluid; CCALD, childhood cerebral adrenoleukodystrophy; AMN, adrenomyeloneuropathy.

Advanced MRI techniques, such as proton MRS and diffusion tensor imaging (DTI), permit the investigation of changes in metabolite levels and water diffusion parameters in leukodystrophy patients. Both metabolite levels and water diffusion parameters offer an opportunity to assess the degree of axonal loss and demyelination in the leukodystrophies.

Proton MRS in demyelinating metabolic disorders

MRS offers the unique ability to measure metabolite levels *in vivo* in a noninvasive manner (Barker and Horska, 2004; Barker et al., 2010) (Fig. 29.2). These metabolite quantifications can be used to identify disease, measure the severity of an injury, or monitor a patient's response to treatment. Table 29.2 shows the most well-characterized metabolite abnormalities detected by MRS in leukodystrophies.

The resonances seen in the brain by MRS are typically low-weight molecules. In the normal brain, the most prominent peak arises from *N*-acetylaspartate (NAA) at 2.0 ppm. Therefore, decreased NAA peaks are sensitive for neuronal damage, although extremely nonspecific. The other major peaks include creatine and phosphocreatine, as well as choline-containing compounds, and are observed at 3.0 and 3.3 ppm, respectively. ^{1}H MR spectra acquired with short echo times are characterized by additional resonances from myo-inositol at 3.5 ppm, and glutamate and glutamine, which overlap with each other, so that they are often referred to as Glx, at ~2.5 ppm. Under normal conditions, the lactate concentration is very low in the adult brain. This resonance (observed as a doublet) occurs at 1.32 ppm.

NAA within the adult brain is found exclusively in neurons, serving as a marker of neuronal density and viability and reported to be decreased in a number of neurologic disorders. NAA is the source of acetyl in myelin membrane biosynthesis (Chakraborty et al., 2001) and is coupled to lipid metabolism and energy generation (Moffett et al., 2007). Creatine serves as a marker for energy-dependent systems in cells, and it tends to be low in processes that have low metabolism, such as necrosis and infarction. However, creatine and phosphocreatine are in equilibrium, and thus the creatine peak remains stable in size despite bioenergetic abnormalities that occur with multiple pathologies. Consequently, the creatine resonance is often used as an internal standard.

The choline resonance arises from signals of several soluble components that resonate at 3.2 ppm. This resonance contains contributions primarily from

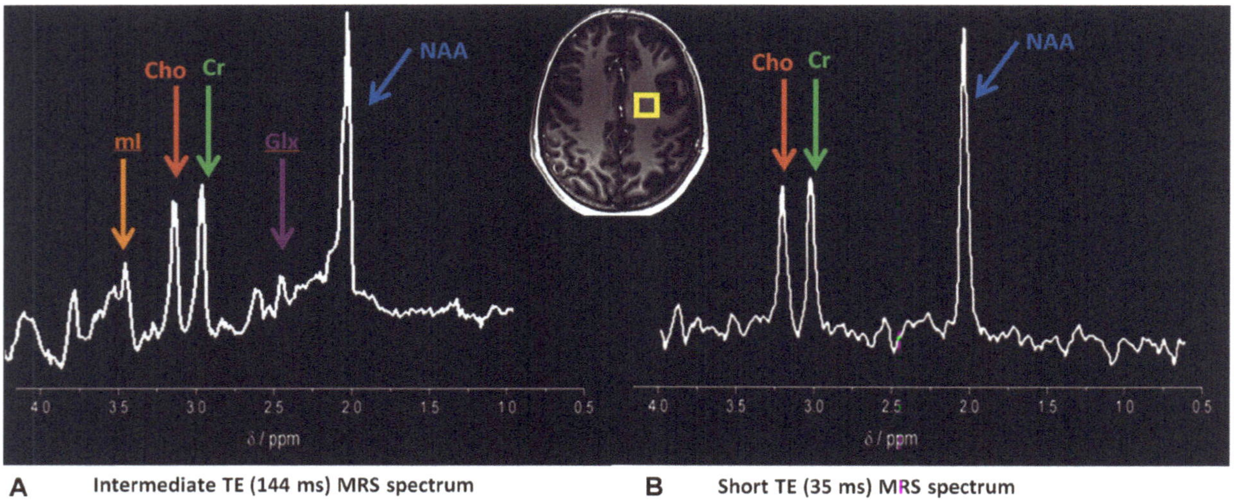

Fig. 29.2. Magnetic resonance spectroscopy (MRS) of white matter in a normal brain. (**A**) Obtained from an 8-cm^3 voxel using PRESS localization (TE/TR = 35/1500 ms, 128 averages). Detectable metabolites include *N*-acetylaspartate (NAA), glutamine and glutamate (Glx), creatine (Cr), choline-containing compounds (Cho), and myo-inositol (mI). (**B**) Obtained from the same voxel using an intermediate echo time of 144 ms. Intermediate TE spectra have less baseline distortion and are easy to process and analyze, but show fewer metabolites than short TE spectra. Lactate (1.3 ppm) (doublet) are inverted, which makes it easier to differentiate them from lipids/macromolecules. Note that short TE demonstrates peaks attributable to more metabolites, including lipids and macromolecules, glutamine and glutamate, and myo-inositol.

glycerophosphocholine, phosphocholine, and choline. Changes in this resonance are commonly seen with diseases that have alterations in membrane turnover as well as inflammatory and gliotic processes (Tzika et al., 1993; Pouwels et al., 1998).

The function of myo-inositol is not fully understood, although it is believed to be an essential requirement for cell growth, an osmolyte, and a storage form for glucose (Ross, 1991). Myo-inositol is primarily located in glia, and an increase in myo-inositol is commonly thought to be a marker of gliosis (Brand et al., 1993). Lactate is produced by anaerobic metabolism, and increased lactate has been found during hypoxia (Kreis et al., 1996), mitochondrial diseases (Mathews et al., 1993; Castillo et al., 1995), seizures (Breiter et al., 1994), and in the first hours after birth (Barkovich et al., 2001, 2006). Of note, lactate peaks are inverted at 1.3 ppm with intermediate echo times (typically TE 135–144 ms). Lipids are associated with the breakdown of tissue and as such are typically seen in myelin destruction or necrosis. Due to their short T2 relaxation time, their presence is most obvious at short TE (30–35 ms). Lipids may obscure the presence of lactate or alanine; consequently, intermediate-TE (135–144 ms) or long-TE (270–288 ms) studies are often preferred to detect lactate or alanine more reliably.

In X-ALD, proton MRS depicts more extensive brain abnormalities than does conventional MRI (Kruse et al., 1994). The white-matter lesion in children with X-ALD shows reduced NAA/creatine and increased choline/creatine, myo-inositol/creatine, and Glx/creatine (Tzika et al., 1993). Spectroscopic changes in normal-appearing white matter that precede disease progression in patients with X-ALD have been described (Eichler et al., 2002). The changes are an increase in choline and a decrease in NAA. They occur in areas where subsequent lesion progression is observed, but not in the remainder of the brain. These areas may represent a zone of impending or beginning demyelination (Fig. 29.3).

AMN is the adult variant of X-ALD. The disease pathology is usually limited to the spinal cord and peripheral nerves ("pure AMN"), but usually shows cerebral involvement on histopathology. MRS studies showed reduced global NAA/choline and NAA/creatine in adults with AMN compared with controls. These changes are most prominent in the internal capsule and parieto-occipital white matter. Decreased ratios of NAA in the absence of choline/creatine elevation suggest prominent axonal involvement (Dubey et al., 2005). Furthermore, Expanded Disability Status Scale scores may inversely correlate with global NAA/creatine, suggesting a potential role of axonal injury in clinical disability in pure AMN (Dubey et al., 2005). Brain involvement demonstrable by MRI is rare in female subjects heterozygous for X-ALD, including those who have clinical evidence of spinal cord involvement. Nevertheless, NAA levels are reduced in the corticospinal projection fibers in female subjects with normal results on conventional MRI sequences, suggesting axonal dysfunction (Fatemi et al., 2003).

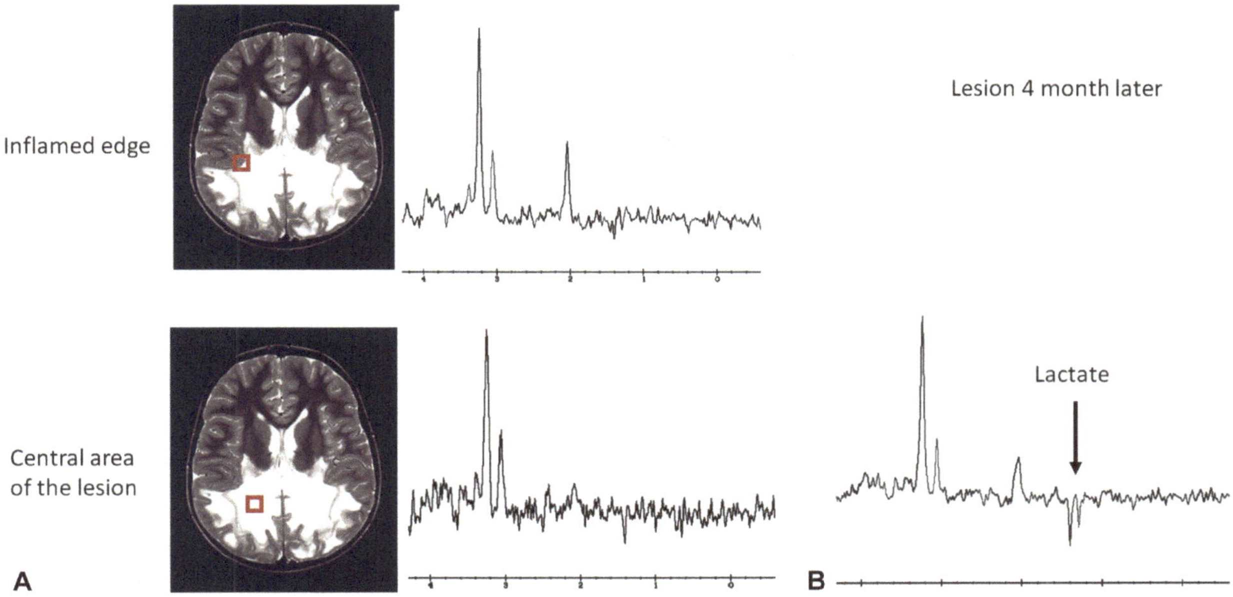

Fig. 29.3. Magnetic resonance spectroscopy (MRS) of a boy with X-linked adrenoleukodystrophy. A 6-year-old boy presented with behavioral abnormalities, followed by gait and speech difficulties and hearing loss. Posterior periventricular lesions are seen on T2-weighted images. (**A**) MRS spectra show increased choline/*N*-acetylaspartate ratios form in peripheral, inflamed edge and central area of the lesion. (**B**) Follow-up MRS 4 month later shows increased levels of lactate. (Adapted from Ratai and Gonzalez, 2009.)

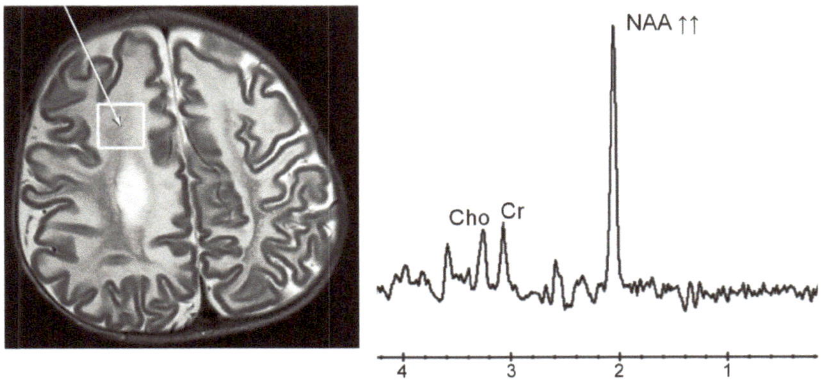

Fig. 29.4. Magnetic resonance imaging (MRI) and magnetic resonance spectroscopy (MRS) of a patient with Canavan disease. T2-weighted MR image (left) and single-voxel MRS of the frontal white matter of a 21-month-old boy with Canavan disease. Patient was born without complications after an uncomplicated pregnancy, but failed to achieve expected developmental milestones, and developed nystagmus and poor muscular head control. Physical examination showed generalized hypotonia and macrocephaly. MRS shows prominent *N*-acetylaspartate (NAA) peak due to a mutation in the enzyme aspartoacylase, which results in the inability to catabolize NAA. Cho, choline; Cr, creatine. (Adapted from Ratai et al., 2012.)

Canavan disease is caused by a deficiency in aspartoacylase, an enzyme involved in the process of degrading NAA to aspartate and acetate. Deficiency leads to the accumulation of toxic levels of NAA, which impairs normal myelination and results in spongiform degeneration of the brain (Grodd et al., 1991; Tsai and Coyle, 1995). The elevations in NAA can be detected by MRS *in vivo* (Fig. 29.4), a diagnostic clue that can then be confirmed by urine measurement of NAA. The distinctly higher NAA peak can even be detected in the newborn, although a radiologist only familiar with MR spectra in adults may not recognize the elevation in the newborn as pathologic.

LBSL is an autosomal-recessive disorder clinically characterized by slowly progressive signs of pyramidal, cerebellar, and dorsal column dysfunction due to mutations in the DARS2 gene. LBSL shows a very distinct MRI pattern, with selective involvement of cerebral and cerebellar white matter as well as brainstem and spinal tracts, while the subcortical U-fibers are spared (Fig. 29.1). In LBSL, MRS characteristically reveals decreased NAA and increased lactate, choline and myo-inositol peaks in the white matter, suggesting axonal damage and gliosis (Uluc et al., 2008).

CTX is a rare disorder due to an inherited defect in the metabolic pathway of cholesterol. Early diagnosis of the disease is particularly important, as patients benefit from therapy with chenodeoxycholic acid. Although the disease is clinically characterized by the concomitant presence of tendon xanthomas, juvenile cataracts, progressive neurologic impairment, and chronic diarrhea, clinical features may vary greatly (Federico et al., 2013). Characteristic biochemical abnormalities include high plasma and tissue cholestanol concentration, normal-to-low plasma cholesterol concentration, decreased chenodeoxycholic acid, increased concentration of bile alcohols and their glyconjugates, and increased concentrations of cholestanol and apolipoprotein B in cerebrospinal fluid. *CYP27A1* is the only gene in which mutations are known to cause CTX (Federico et al., 2013). MRS in CTX shows a reduction in NAA levels and the presence of a lactate peak and/or lipids (Fig. 29.5). NAA decreases are attributed to neuroaxonal damage due to neurotoxic deposition of cholesterol (Pilo de la Fuente et al., 2008). A recent case report described the presence of abnormal lipid peaks at 0.9 and 1.3 ppm in the cerebellar hemisphere (Embirucu et al., 2010). These peaks can either be attributed to membrane breakdown or they may serve as surrogate markers of major lipid storage, and they may have a potential role in monitoring therapeutic response. In addition, one patient had an increase in MI concentration, pointing to gliosis and astrocytic proliferation (Embirucu et al., 2010).

Alexander disease is an autosomal-dominant disorder characterized clinically by megalencephaly in infancy accompanied by progressive spasticity and cognitive and behavioral regression. Younger patients typically present with seizures, megalencephaly, developmental delay, and spasticity. In older patients, bulbar or pseudobulbar symptoms predominate, frequently accompanied by spasticity. The disease in childhood is progressive, with most infant patients dying within a decade of onset. Later-onset cases may have a longer clinical course. Imaging studies of the brain typically show cerebral white-matter abnormalities, predominantly involving the frontal regions (Fig. 29.1). Advanced cases typically show extensive cerebral white-matter changes with frontal predominance, a periventricular rim with high signal on T1-weighted images (which may enhance with contrast) and low signal on T2-weighted images, abnormalities of basal ganglia and thalami, as well as brainstem abnormalities (van der Knaap et al., 2001). On T2-weighted images, the cerebellar vermis and all portions of the cerebellar hemispheres may appear abnormally hyperintense. MRS of the cerebellum reveals markedly decreased NAA levels (Fig. 29.6). Alexander disease is caused by a mutation in the gene for glial fibrillary acid protein, which encodes an intermediate filament protein for astrocytes.

The lack of hexosaminidase A in Tay–Sachs disease impairs degradation of the ganglioside GM2, leading to excessive storage in neurons. In infancy, normal myelin development is also impaired. This leads to progressive weakness and loss of motor skills in the first year of life. Only one-half of all patients learn to sit independently, and one-half of those patients lose the ability within a year. Infrequently, patients with

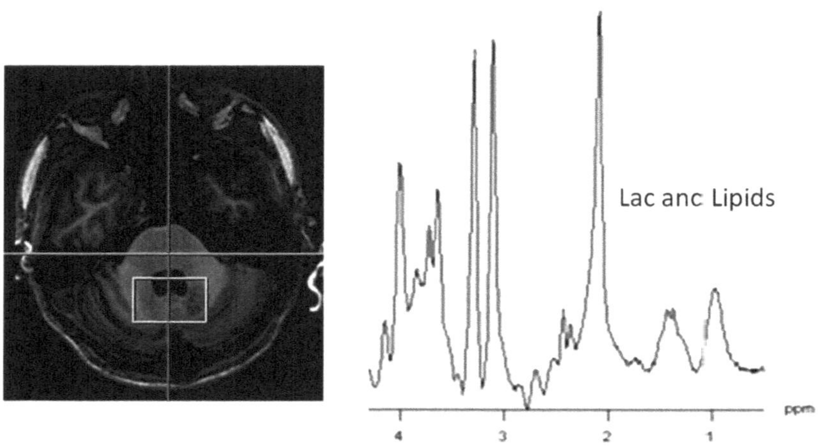

Fig. 29.5. A magnetic resonance spectroscopy study in cerebrotendinous xanthomatosis (CTX) showed a reduction in *N*-acetylaspartate levels and the presence of lactate (Lac) and lipid peaks. (Adapted from Ratai et al., 2012.)

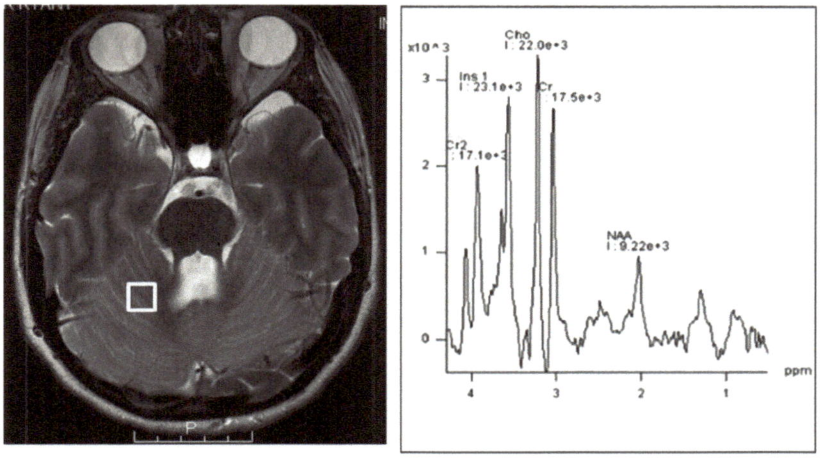

Fig. 29.6. Alexander's disease. Magnetic resonance spectroscopy imaging (MRSI) and magnetic resonance imaging (MRI) of a 29-year-old male patient recently diagnosed with Alexander disease. On T2-weighted MR images, the cerebellar vermis and all portions of the cerebellar hemispheres appear abnormally hyperintense. MRSI of the cerebellum reveals markedly decreased *N*-acetylaspartate levels.

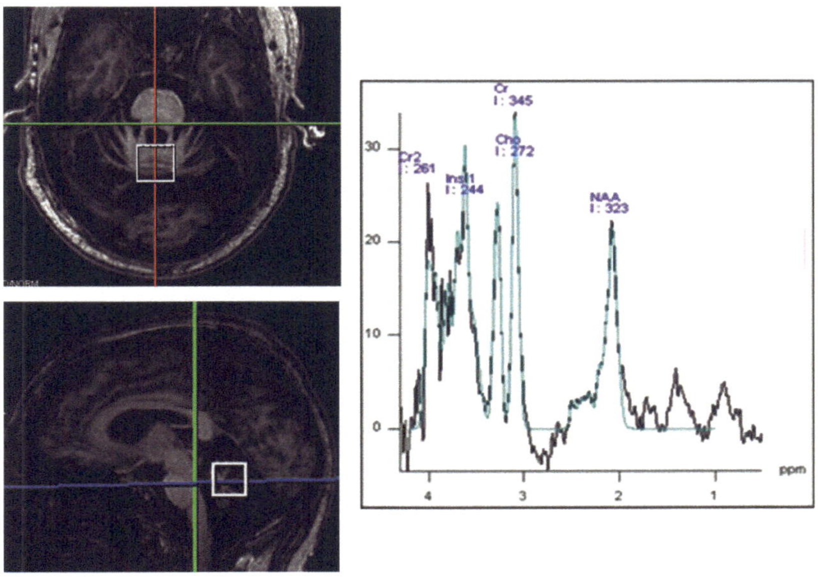

Fig. 29.7. Tay–Sachs disease. Single-voxel spectroscopy acquisition of a 30-year-old male late-onset Tay–Sachs patient, showing decrease in *N*-acetylaspartate/creatine (NAA/Cr) and increase in myo-inisitol (mI)/Cr ratio.

mutations in the *G269S* gene can present in adulthood, manifesting motor dysfunction, cerebellar dysfunction, or psychosis, with gait abnormalities also occurring frequently (Neudorfer et al., 2005). MRI findings in patients with gangliosidoses include T2 hypointense and T1 hyperintense changes in the ventral thalami, T2 hyperintensity in the basal ganglia, and white-matter hypomyelination (Figs 29.1 and 29.7). The infantile forms of GM1 and GM2 gangliosidoses are very difficult to differentiate on the basis of MRI findings.

Proton MRS in hypomyelinating metabolic disorders

In the developing brain, choline and myo-inositol are the dominant peaks in the MR spectrum. Their levels are high compared to creatine. In contrast, NAA levels are low in newborns and increase with age, while choline and myo-inositol decrease with age. During the first 6 months of life, these metabolic changes are most rapid, leveling off at about 30 months of age (Holshouser et al., 1997). These changes are crucial,

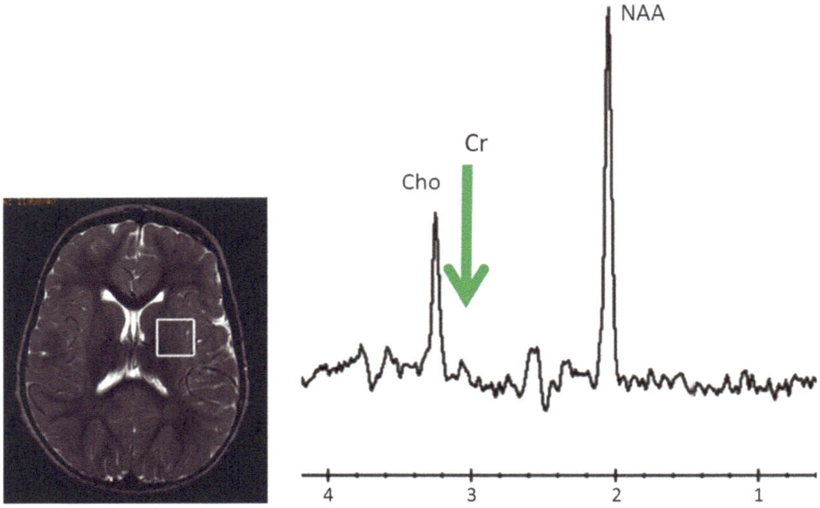

Fig. 29.8. Magnetic resonance imaging (MRI) and magnetic resonance spectroscopy (MRS) of a child with creatine deficiency. MRI and MRS of a 2.5-year-old child with mental retardation, seizures, and speech delay. Conventional MRI showed two 3-mm nonspecific hyperintensities deep to the facial colliculi (not shown here) and was otherwise normal. ^{1}H MRS in the outlined voxel, at 1.5 T and TE 144, showed absence of the normal creatine resonance at 3.0 ppm (arrow). Serologic testing showed low levels of creatine (Cr) and guanidinoacetate consistent with arginine:glycine amidinotransferase (AGAT) deficiency. Cho, choline; NAA, *N*-acetylaspartate.

as both hypomyelination and delayed myelination produce abnormalities in these metabolites.

The MR spectra of patients with 4H-syndrome, a rare form of hypomyelinating leukodystrophy, reveal low choline/creatine and NAA/creatine, and a prominent myo-inositol peak can be observed (Wolf et al., 2005; Outteryck et al., 2010). Low choline levels are indicative of hypomyelination due to decreased membrane synthesis and turnover.

In the syndrome characterized by hypomyelination with atrophy of the basal ganglia and cerebellum, myo-inositol and creatine levels are found to be elevated in the cerebral white matter, while NAA and choline levels are normal (van der Knaap et al., 2007). These findings suggest that neither axonal loss nor active demyelination occurs in the setting of gliosis.

In Pelizaeus–Merzbacher disease, another hypomyelinating disorder, there have been discrepant reports on metabolite abnormalities detected by MRS. In part these findings may be explained by the concurrent pathophysiologic processes of hypomyelination, gliosis, and neuronal loss over time (Cecil, 2006).

Proton MRS in metabolic disorders with normal imaging

The biochemical hallmarks of CCDS include cerebral creatine deficiency, as detected *in vivo* by ^{1}H MRS of the brain, and specific disturbances in metabolites of creatine metabolism in body fluids. In urine and plasma, abnormal guanidinoacetic acid (GAA) levels are found in AGAT deficiency (reduced GAA) and GAMT deficiency (increased GAA). In urine of males with SLC6A8 deficiency, an increased creatine/creatinine ratio is detected. CCDSs may be responsible for a considerable fraction of children and adults affected with mental retardation of unknown etiology. Thus, screening for this group of disorders should be considered in this population (Fig. 29.8).

ADVANCED MR TECHNOLOGY IN INHERITED METABOLIC DISORDERS

High-field-strength imaging has been a major technical advance in the imaging of the leukodystrophies and hypomyelinating disorders compared with 1.5 T. MRI at 4 and 7 T allows for better visualization of lesion architecture, white-matter tracts, and gray–white-matter differentiation. The field of proton MRS has also benefited from higher field strength (Oz et al., 2005; Ratai et al., 2008). Better spectral resolution results from improved signal-to-noise ratio and chemical shift dispersion, and this in turn leads to more reliable detection of metabolites such as myo-inositol and glutamine.

Using 7 T MRS, decreased NAA in the cortex of X-ALD patients can be detected, and this appears greater in male hemizygotes than in female heterozygotes and most pronounced with the occurrence of white-matter lesions in males (Ratai et al., 2008). Although the cytoarchitecture of the cerebral cortex generally appears normal in X-ALD, scattered neuronal loss can be seen in gray matter during a pathologic examination. Both ratios of myo-inositol and choline to creatine were found to be higher in normal-appearing white matter of adult ALD patients with brain lesions compared to those without lesions. Yet the interpretation of 7 T MRS data also poses challenges. The quantification of spectral data in the presence of substantial radiofrequency excitation field (B1) variations is difficult. Therefore focus has shifted on using adiabatic pulses to compensate for radiofrequency inhomogeneity and reduce the chemical shift displacement error (Tannus and Garwood, 1997; Andronesi et al., 2010).

Overcoming some of the shortcomings of DTI, novel methods now exist to map complex fiber architectures of white matter and other brain tissue. Diffusion spectrum imaging (DSI) allows resolution of regions of three-way fiber crossings (Schmahmann et al., 2007; Wedeen et al., 2008; Hagmann et al., 2010). On DTI this was not possible, as fiber crossing led to decreases in fractional anisotropy (FA), making it difficult to distinguish pathologic changes from normal fiber crossings. The years ahead will likely bring more studies employing DSI in leukodystrophy patients.

Other advances in MR technology have brought great practical benefits. Sedation and anesthesia represent risks in advanced brain disease of leukodystrophy patients. Using new techniques such as propeller MRI, it has become possible to oversample k space and thereby compensate for motion to allow follow-up MRI without sedation (Forbes et al., 2003; Tamhane and Arfanakis, 2009). As an alternative to these retrospective motion-correction techniques, it is also possible to prospectively correct motion in structural imaging and single-voxel spectroscopy using image-based navigators (White et al., 2010; Hess et al., 2011; Tisdall et al., 2012).

In patients with more advanced leukodystrophies, these advances may allow for imaging without sedation and thereby give insight into the more advanced stages of disease.

To avoid long sedation periods, fast imaging is of paramount importance. Fast chemical shift imaging (CSI) concepts have evolved from concepts related to spatial encoding using gradient switching during acquisition (Mansfield, 1984; Guilfoyle et al., 1989). The proton echo planar spectroscopic imaging (PEPSI) sequence uses standard-phase encoding in the x direction, while phase encoding in the y direction is replaced by bipolar gradients, switching during data acquisition (Posse et al., 1995). Spiral trajectories in k space allow even faster encoding of spatial information due to faster gradient duty cycle (Adalsteinsson et al., 1998; Adalsteinsson and Spielman, 1999). In spiral imaging k space is filled by spiral readouts that are produced by sinusoidally varying gradients in both the x and y axes. Recently, Andronesi et al. (2012) implemented a three-dimensional volumetric *in vivo* MRS sequence using spiral trajectories at a spatial resolution of 1 cm^3 with a total scan time of < 2.5 minutes. These improvements in image quality and imaging time allow more routine acquisition of spectroscopic data in the clinical setting.

Overall, no single advanced imaging technology is expected to bring about a breakthrough in the leukodystrophies. Rather, longitudinal repeat imaging with a multimodal approach and coregistration of high-resolution imaging with advanced spectroscopic and diffusion imaging will lead to new pathophysiologic insights in the years to come. Different diseases and varying phenotypes and stages within the disease will require varying imaging modalities.

ACQUIRED TOXIC-METABOLIC DISORDERS OF THE ADULT BRAIN[1]

Although genetic predisposition plays a key role in the susceptibility of the brain to toxic and metabolic insults, the diseases that follow are different from the ones discussed above, where a single mutation can be responsible for the disorder. In contrast, the disorders that follow are caused by mechanisms ranging from severe brain hypoxia caused by carbon monoxide poisoning to autoimmune or viral disease damaging the liver or other organs and, secondarily, the brain. Here, the imaging changes are also relatively symmetric, affecting similar structures on both sides of the brain, and can adopt several predominant patterns: (1) lasting changes in the gray matter, including cortex and basal ganglia; (2) lasting changes predominantly in the basal ganglia; (3) transient changes in cortex and basal ganglia; (4) lasting changes in white matter; and (5) transient changes in white matter. These groupings only indicate the regions predominantly affected and the most common evolution: lasting refers to imaging changes that typically do not resolve in a few days or weeks. Also the type of imaging changes may depend on the severity of the insult produced by the same mechanism. For instance, a mild osmotic disorder may cause transient changes, while a more severe one may cause lasting changes. Finally, several toxic substances, such as amphetamines, by damaging endothelial cells and raising blood pressure can induce intracerebral hemorrhages, discussed in Chapter 18. Other drug abuse has been linked to an increased incidence of ischemic stroke (Kelly et al., 1992), discussed in Chapters 16 and 17. However, substance abuse may only be a factor and other underlying causes of stroke, such as preexisting arteriovenous malformations, should be considered in the management of these patients (McEvoy et al., 2000).

[1]The previous sections were written by Drs. F. Eichler and E. Ratai; this section is written by Drs. J.J. Caroll and J.C. Masdeu.

LASTING GRAY-MATTER CHANGES

This group is well exemplified by anoxic encephalopathy. Anoxic encephalopathy causes cytotoxic edema, which can be appreciated on computed tomography (CT) and MRI. Cytotoxic edema implies a failure of the sodium-potassium pump in the cell membrane and is most often associated with cell necrosis, causing lasting changes. In addition, the metabolically most active regions of the brain, namely the cortex and deep gray nuclei, are most often affected because these regions suffer most from the impairment in aerobic metabolism.

Anoxic encephalopathy

A severe reduction in the availability of oxygen to the entire brain, as in the case of cardiac arrest or carbon monoxide poisoning, causes necrosis with a preference for the depth of the cortical sulci, globus pallidus, and superior portion of the cerebellar cortex (Figs 29.9 and 29.10). On MRI, the earliest changes can be appreciated on diffusion-weighted imaging, depicting restricted diffusion in the gray matter, both deep and cortical (Arbelaez et al., 1999) (Fig. 29.9). As the days go by and the lesions become more organized, necrotic areas become hyperintense on T2 and may show enhancement after gadolinium infusion, reflecting a breakdown of the blood–brain barrier in the organizing infarcted tissue (Fig. 29.10). This disseminated injury pattern is most frequent in younger patients with intact brain vasculature; anoxic events in older people with arterial stenosis may manifest with the MRI characteristics of acute strokes, with focal ischemic changes in the stenotic arterial territory (see Chapters 16 and 17).

Hypoglycemic brain injury

Just as the lack of oxygen can damage the brain, the lack of the only energy source the brain uses, namely glucose, can result in brain damage. Not surprisingly, the pattern

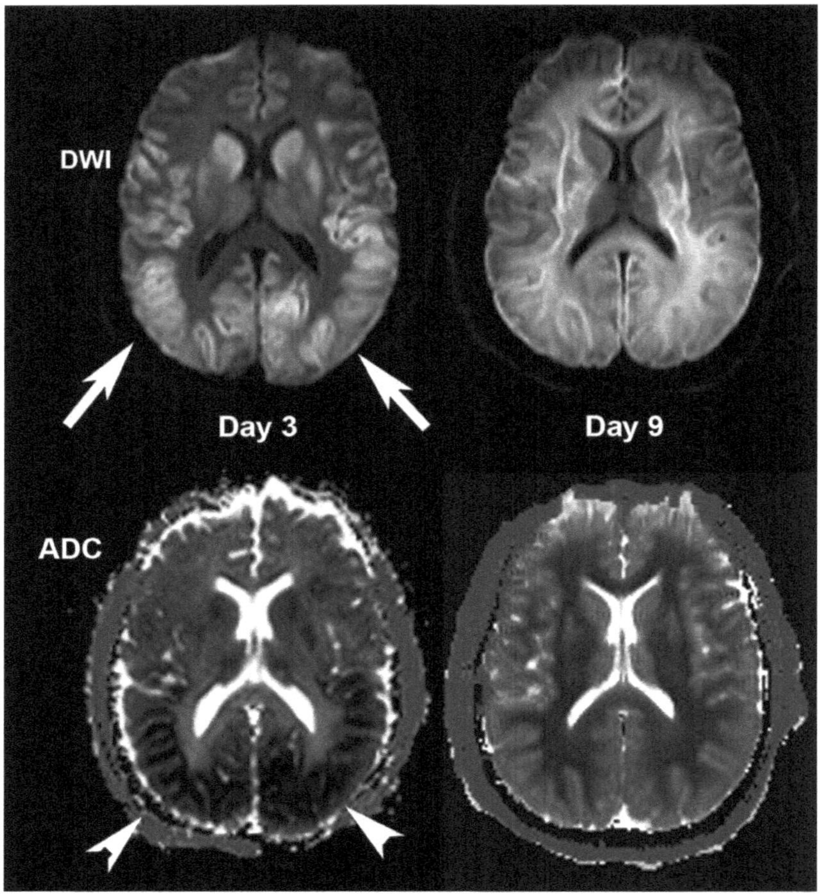

Fig. 29.9. Anoxic brain damage. Diffusion-weighted imaging (DWI) and apparent diffusion coefficient (ADC) map from an unconscious 35-year-old man, obtained 3 and 9 days after a severe anoxic event. Diffusion restriction is noticeable in caudate nuclei, right putamen, and multiple areas of the cortical ribbon bilaterally, with a posterior predominance. In the same areas the ADC map shows abnormally low values, indicating cytotoxic edema and necrosis. This finding has disappeared by day 9.

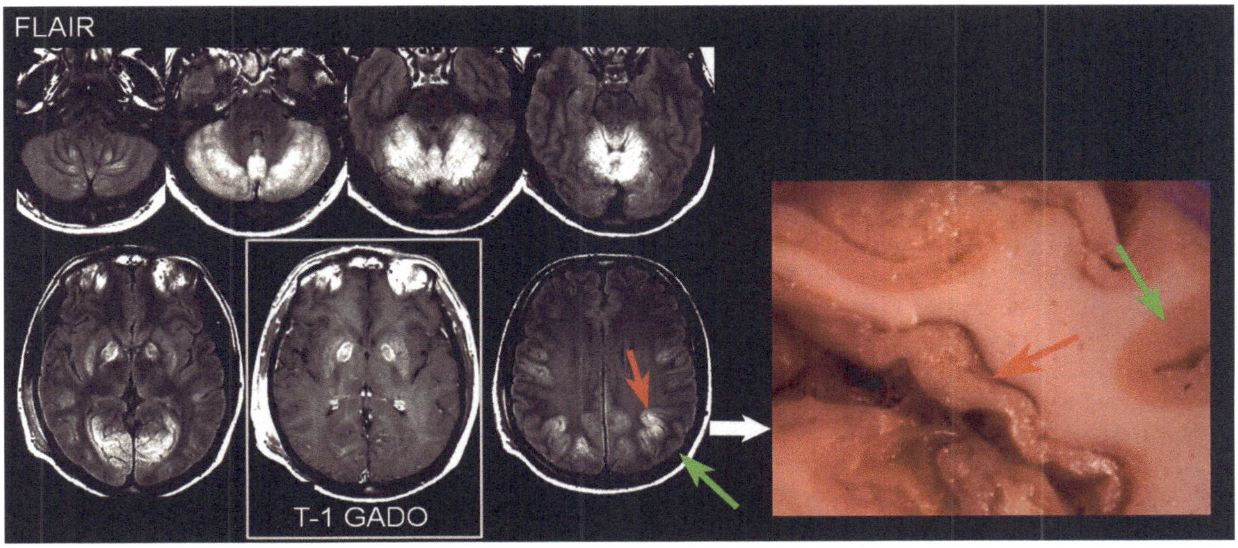

Fig. 29.10. Anoxic brain damage. Magnetic resonance imaging (MRI) from a 39-year-old man obtained 7 days after a severe anoxic event. Fluid-attenuated inversion recovery (FLAIR) images show areas of hyperintensity most marked in the superior portion of the cerebellum, globus pallidus, and depth of the cortical sulci. The pattern is bilateral. The globus pallidus enhances after gadolinium administration (T-1 GADO). Note that cortical involvement is spotty, with areas markedly affected (red arrows) and others that appear spared (green arrows). Even areas that appear spared on MRI may have sustained some degree of neuronal damage, particularly in layers III and V (laminar necrosis).

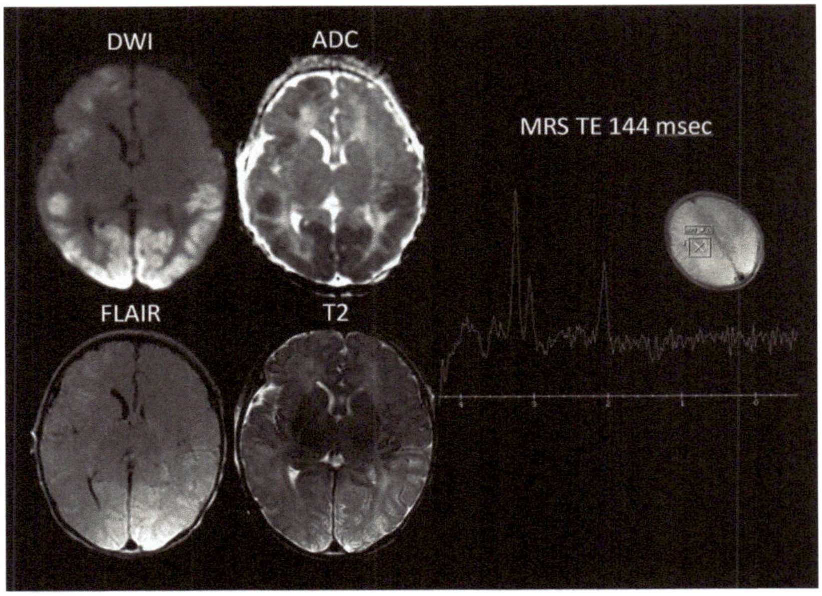

Fig. 29.11. Hypoglycemic brain injury. Magnetic resonance imaging (MRI) and magnetic resonance spectroscopy (MRS) from a 6-day-old male born full-term with generalized tonic-clonic seizure due to profound hypoglycemia (blood glucose 21) in the setting of adrenal insufficiency. Brain MRI demonstrates cortical and subcortical restricted diffusion and T2 hyperintensity involving posteriorly both cerebral hemispheres. MRS at TE 144 ms demonstrates depressed *N*-acetylaspartate peaks consistent with neuronal injury. DWI, diffusion-weighted imaging; ADC, apparent diffusion coefficient; FLAIR, fluid-attenuated inversion recovery.

of involvement on MRI or CT resembles the pattern found in anoxic encephalopathy: both are acute disturbances of energy availability (Bakshi et al., 2000; Yong et al., 2012) (Fig. 29.11).

Mitochondrial encephalopathies

These disorders also interfere with energy metabolism, but they have a much stronger genetic component than the disorders just mentioned. They include mitochondrial myopathy, encephalopathy, lactic acidosis and stroke-like episodes (MELAS), discussed in Chapter 17, and the Leigh's syndrome complex, discussed in Chapter 63 of the second neuroimaging volume.

Vitamin availability disorders

Two disorders of vitamin availability present with characteristic imaging findings: vitamin B_1 or thiamine deficiency causes Wernicke's encephalopathy and B_{12} deficiency causes subacute combined degeneration of the spinal cord, discussed in Chapter 38 of the second neuroimaging volume.

Wernicke's encephalopathy typically presents with a subacute gait disorder, memory impairment, and ophthalmoparesis in patients at risk for thiamine deficiency, classically those with chronic alcohol abuse or malnutrition (Sechi and Serra, 2007). Cases have also been described after bariatric surgery for obesity (Samanta, 2015), cancer chemotherapy (Macri et al., 2015), or hyperemesis gravidarum (Yahia et al., 2015). Areas of the brain most affected by the disorder are the mammillary bodies and periventricular gray matter of the third and fourth ventricles as well as the cerebral aqueduct (Fig. 29.12). Less frequently affected are the caudate nuclei, posterior putaminal nuclei, and perirolandic cortex (Santos Andrade et al., 2010) (Fig. 29.12). In these regions, Wernicke's encephalopathy primarily affects the capillary endothelium, which appears swollen (Torvik, 1985). Loss of blood–brain barrier is evidenced by contrast enhancement after gadolinium administration (Fig. 29.13). Frequent on neuropathologic observation (Torvik, 1985), but less frequent on imaging, are perivascular hemorrhagic changes, which can result in frank intracranial hemorrhage (Fig. 29.14). It could be argued that this entity should be listed among the transient gray-matter disorders, because it recedes with the appropriate treatment (Sechi and Serra, 2007). However, when the lesions are present on imaging, some degree of permanent damage is not infrequent; the Wernicke's encephalopathy picture may yield to a more chronic amnesic syndrome, Korsakoff's syndrome (Isenberg-Grzeda et al., 2012).

Toxic encephalopathies

Many of the cerebral manifestations of inhaled or ingested toxic substances reflect the metabolic damage caused by the dysfunction of heart, lungs, or liver produced by the toxin or by the interference with energy metabolism that results in imaging patterns similar to

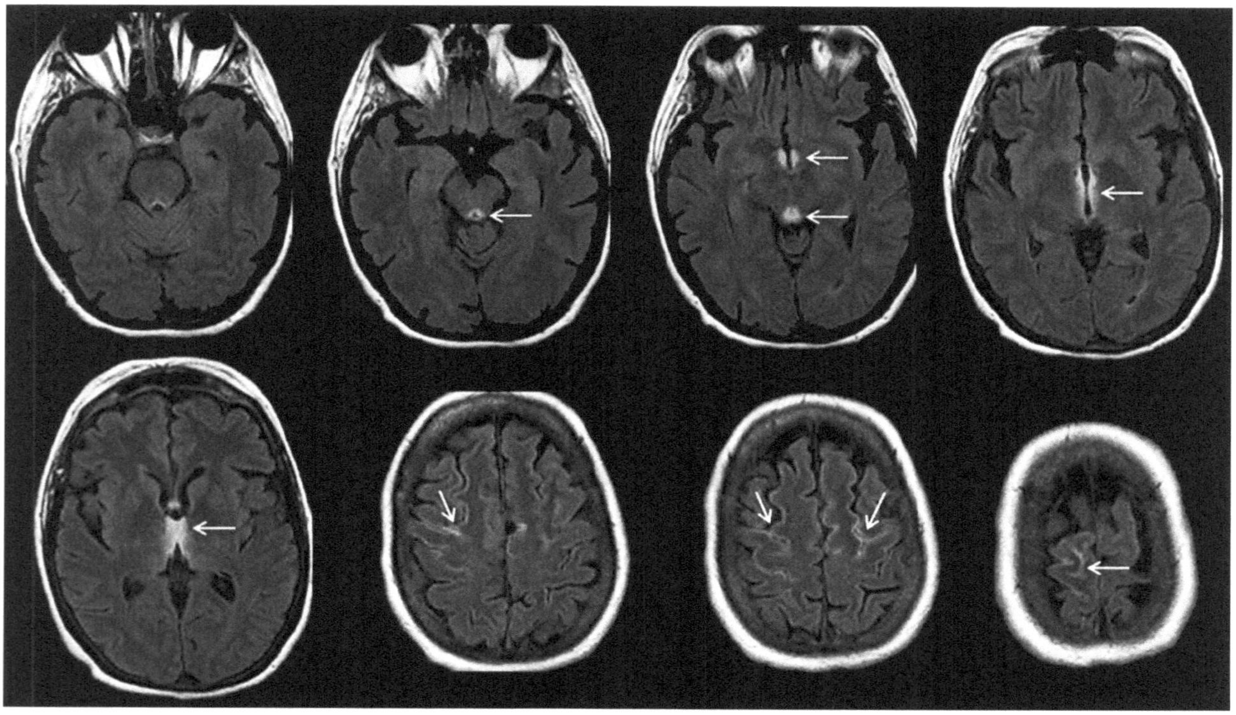

Fig. 29.12. Wernicke's encephalopathy: topography. Fluid-attenuated inversion recovery images show characteristic hyperintense lesions (arrows) around the Sylvian aqueduct, in the mammillary bodies and walls of the third ventricle, and in the perirolandic cortex.

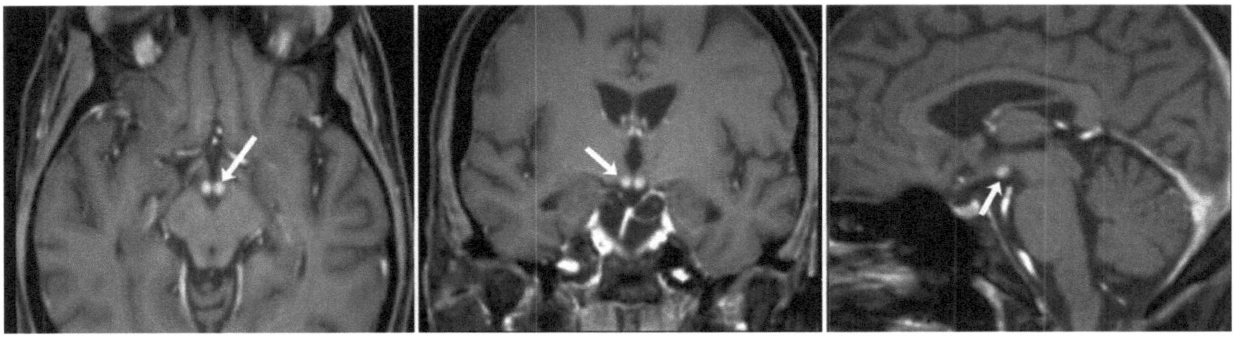

Fig. 29.13. Wernicke's encephalopathy: enhancement. T1 postgadolinium images show contrast enhancement in the mammillary bodies (arrows).

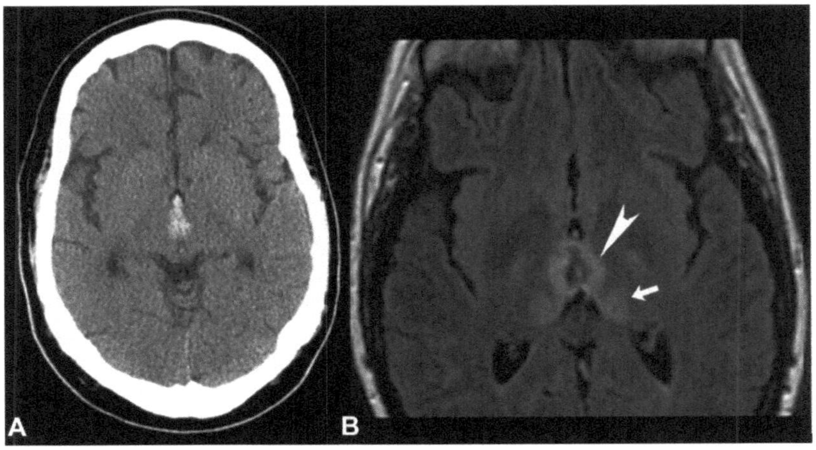

Fig. 29.14. Wernicke's encephalopathy: hemorrhage. (**A**) Computed tomography (CT) scan discloses a hemorrhage as a hyperdense area in the inferior portion of the third ventricle. (**B**) Fluid-attenuated inversion recovery magnetic resonance imaging at the level of the lesion shows a rounded area (arrowhead) in the same region of the CT hemorrhage; its core is bright, likely corresponding to remaining extracellular methemoglobin, surrounded by dark hemosiderin, and more peripherally there is a bright, donut-like halo, likely corresponding to edema in the surrounding thalamic tissue. In addition and more posteriorly located, there are bilateral hyperintense areas in the pulvinar nucleus of the thalamus (arrow).

ischemia or hypoxia. For instance, a typical anoxic pattern (Fig. 29.10) results from carbon monoxide poisoning or from cyanide poisoning.

LASTING BASAL GANGLIA CHANGES

Toxic encephalopathies

Some toxins characteristically damage the basal ganglia.

Manganese poisoning

Manganese poisoning affects most often welders and smelter workers poorly protected from manganese-containing fumes (Sriram et al., 2015), causing a parkinsonian syndrome, similar to Parkinson's disease but with a greater incidence of psychiatric manifestations and gait impairment (Racette, 2014). On MRI, there is bilaterally increased T1 signal in the globus pallidus (Fig. 29.15) and, to a lesser extent, the putamen, thalamus, midbrain, and other areas of the brain, such as the hippocampus (Long et al., 2014; Racette, 2014). A similar MRI pattern is present in chronic liver failure, also likely reflecting increased manganese levels in the brain. T1 hyperintensity on MRI is so characteristic that it has been used as an index or biomarker of manganese brain content (Criswell et al., 2012b; Li et al., 2014). In addition to the striking MRI findings, MRS in manganese toxicity has revealed decreased levels of myo-inositol in the thalamus and globus pallidus (Long et al., 2014).

Methanol or ethylene glycol poisoning: severe metabolic acidosis

Intoxication with either of these compounds causes a metabolic acidosis. In addition, their metabolism yields

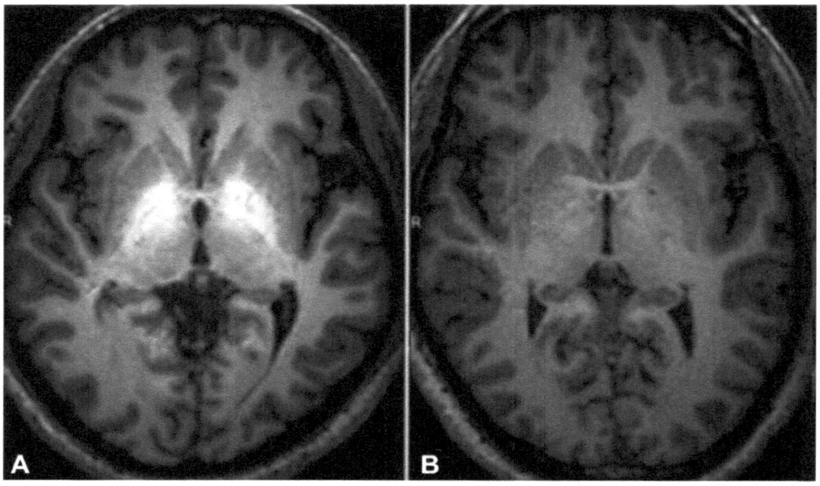

Fig. 29.15. Manganese toxicity, magnetic resonance imaging (MRI). (**A**) T1 MRI from a welder showing hyperintense signal in the globus pallidus bilaterally. Compare with a control (**B**). (Modified from Long et al., 2014.)

substances that are cytotoxic: formate from methanol metabolism and glycolate, glyoxylate and calcium oxalate, the last a potent nephrotoxic, from ethylene glycol metabolism (Kruse, 2012). Formate exerts its cytotoxic effects, at least in part, by inhibiting cytochrome aa3 and cytochrome c oxidase and thereby interfering with intramitochondrial electron transport. Critical degrees of interference with these cytochromes result in cellular injury and death. Retinal ganglion cells and the putamen seem to be particularly susceptible to this kind of injury, which results in impaired vision or even blindness. Imaging changes occur only in the more severe cases (Blanco et al., 2006; Takao et al., 2006; Arora et al., 2007), with characteristic involvement of the putamen, the center of which may become necrotic and hemorrhagic (Fig. 29.16). Some days after the injury, the margins of the lesion may enhance with contrast, offering a peculiar appearance that has been termed the "lentiform fork sign" (Grasso et al., 2014). The subcortical white matter can also be affected (Fig. 29.17).

Organophosphate poisoning

There are few imaging cases reported and they show widely divergent findings, suggesting that the imaging characteristics are not specific. Imaging patterns described have included lenticular nucleus lesions (Fig. 29.18) (Panda et al., 2014), including the "eye of the tiger" sign (Srinivasan et al., 2010a) (see Chapter 25, Figs 25.5 and 25.6), but also brainstem and cerebellar lesions (Teke et al., 2004), posterior reversible encephalopathy (Phatake et al., 2014), a reversible lesion in the splenium of the corpus callosum (Wang et al., 2015), and chronic atrophy in the insula and inferomedial temporal regions of individuals exposed to sarin (Yamasue et al., 2007).

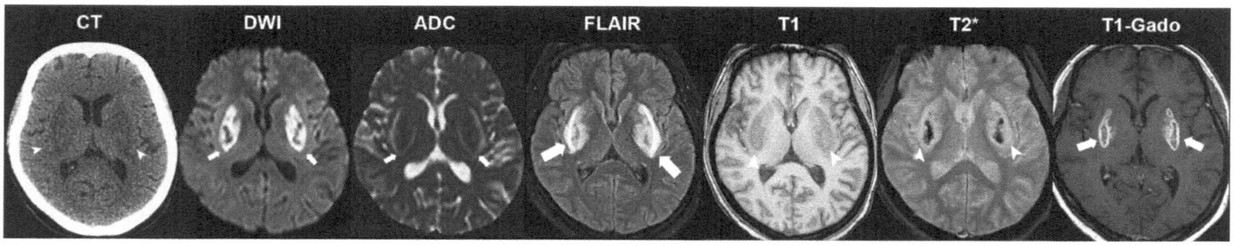

Fig. 29.16. Methanol intoxication. Acute metabolic acidosis. Computed tomography (CT) and magnetic resonance imaging (MRI) findings in a case of severe metabolic acidosis, as caused by methanol intoxication. The findings are bilateral and quite symmetric. On CT, there is decreased attenuation of the putamen (arrowheads), which may become less obvious when the hemorrhagic component of the lesion increases after the acute event. On MRI, the striking changes in the putamen are noticeable first on diffusion-weighted imaging (DWI). Both on this sequence and on fluid-attenuated inversion recovery (FLAIR) images, the outer portion of the putamen appears brightest (arrows); this has been termed the "lentiform fork sign." These peripheral areas of the lesion may enhance after gadolinium infusion (T1-Gado, arrows). The core of the lesion has a mixed signal on FLAIR and many contain blood products, most obvious on T2* imaging. (Modified from Grasso et al., 2014.)

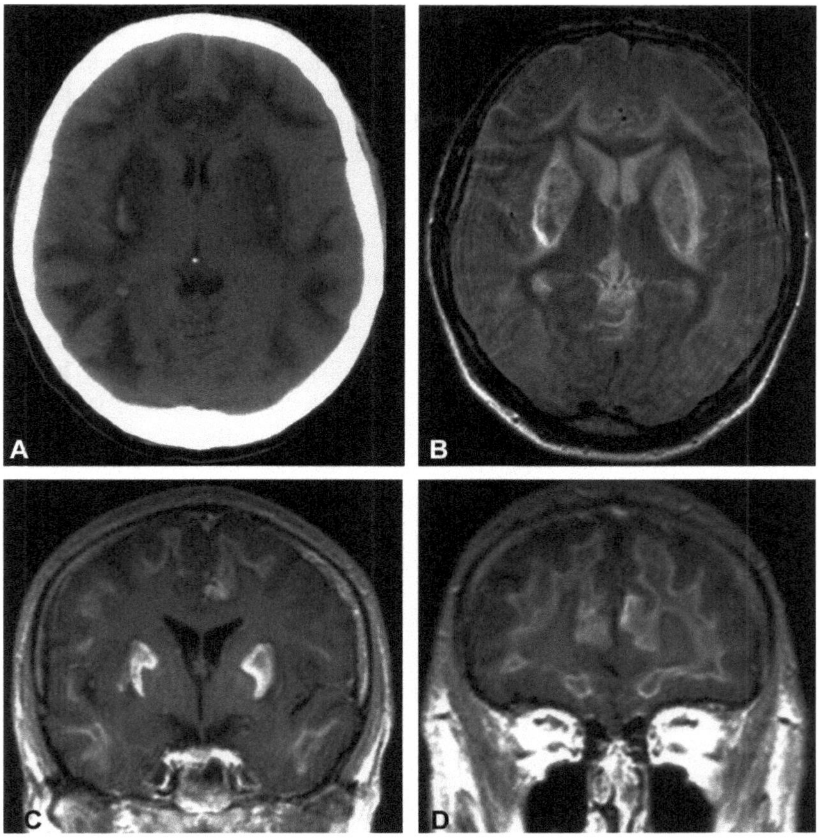

Fig. 29.17. Methanol intoxication. Subcortical white-matter lesions. (**A**) Computed tomography (CT) from a 35-year-old man 5 days after methanol intoxication, showing hypodense areas in the putamen and subcortical white matter bilaterally. In the posterior portion of the putamen there are hyperdense areas, suggesting a hemorrhagic component. (**B**) On this T2-weighted magnetic resonance imaging, obtained on day 7, the areas that appeared hypodense on CT appear hyperintense; areas of low intensity within putamen suggest a hemorrhagic component. (**C, D**) Gadolinium-enhanced images showing enhancement of the subcortical white matter and putamen. (Adapted from Blanco et al., 2006.)

Hepatic disease

Patients with advanced liver disease are at risk for manganese neurotoxicity secondary to impaired biliary clearance (Criswell et al., 2012a), and for this reason their T1 MRI may show bilateral high signal in the globus pallidus (Fig. 29.19), as found with manganese intoxication (Fig. 29.15). The differential diagnosis of this finding includes not only all diseases causing liver failure, such as Wilson's disease, but in addition basal ganglia mineralization, idiopathic as a consequence of a prior hypoxic-ischemic event, hyperalimentation (Aschner et al., 2015), and retained gadolinium contrast. Patients may develop a parkinsonian syndrome. Interestingly, unlike in Parkinson's disease, where the loss of presynaptic dopamine storage affects mostly the tail of the putamen, in chronic liver disease dopamine loss has been described (Criswell et al., 2012a) to be most marked in the anterior portion of the putamen and in the caudate nucleus (Fig. 29.20).

Wilson's disease

The findings in Wilson's disease, an autosomal-recessive disorder of copper metabolism, are discussed in Chapter 25 (Fig. 25.2) and in Chapter 63 in the second volume (Fig. 63.15). Most patients have signal abnormalities in the putamen, caudate, thalamus, and midbrain. Patients with predominant liver disease may have increased deposition of manganese in the brain, with resultant high T1 signal in the globus pallidus. About one-third of all patients have globus pallidus hypointensity on T2-weighted MRI. The midbrain "face of the giant panda" sign on T2-weighted MRI (Fig. 25.2B) is present in about 15% of patients and is considered pathognomonic for Wilson's disease.

Pantothenic kinase-associated neurodegeneration

Mutations in the *PANK2* gene, on chromosome 20p13, are associated with progressive gait and postural problems. On T2-weighted MRI images, there is bilateral

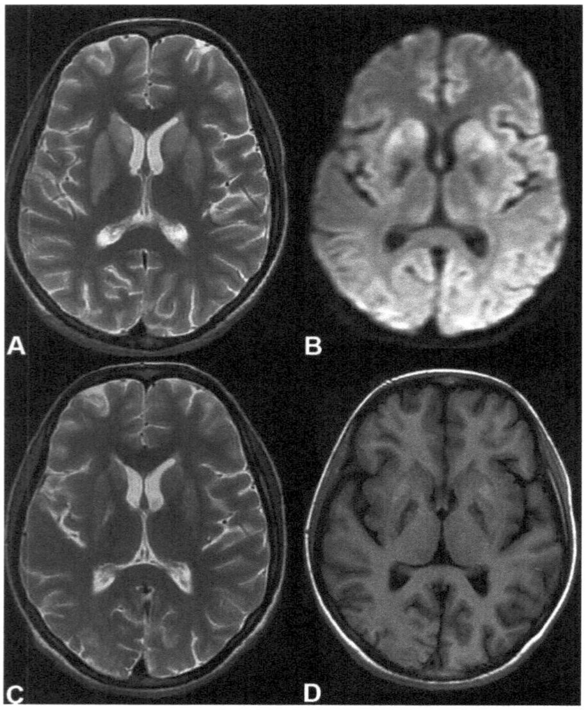

Fig. 29.18. Organophosphate poisoning by pesticide ingestion in a 14-year-old girl. Putamen and caudate are hyperintense on first T2 exam (**A**) and show diffusion restriction (**B**). A month later they are less hyperintense (**C**). The globus pallidus is markedly hypointense on T1 (**D**). From (Panda et al., 2014).

hypointensity in the globus pallidus, with a central area of hyperintensity, giving the appearance of an eye of a tiger. This entity is discussed in Chapters 25 (Figs 25.5 and 25.6) and 63 in the second volume (Fig. 63.16).

Basal ganglia calcification and iron deposition

On CT, some degree of calcification in the globus pallidus is present in about 15% of individuals who are 40–60 years of age and in 30% of those older than 60 years (Nicolas et al., 2013). This finding has no clinical correlates and is due to the deposition of calcium in the media of perforating arterioles. However, calcification in the disorders that follow, while typically affecting earlier and more extensively the basal ganglia, most often affects other structures as well, including the dentate nucleus of the cerebellum, thalamus, and cerebellar and cerebral white matter. In addition to calcium, iron deposits in the same areas. Increased iron deposition in the basal ganglia has been described with hemochromatosis (Berg et al., 2000), which may also be associated with the brain MRI changes characteristic of liver disease (Fig. 29.19), and with many neurodegenerative disorders, including Alzheimer disease (Chapter 26) and parkinsonian syndromes (Chapters 24 and 25).

Fahr's disease

This disorder has also been known as idiopathic striopallidodentate calcinosis, nonarteriosclerotic cerebral calcification, or idiopathic basal ganglia calcification (Cavalcanti-Mendes et al., 2009). In Fahr's disease, associated with mutations in the *SLC20A2* and *PDGFRB* genes (Nicolas et al., 2013), the calcifications are not restricted to the globus pallidus, but more widespread, involving the cerebellum, basal ganglia, thalamus, and hemispheric white matter (Figs 29.21 and 29.22). In addition to calcium, there is iron deposition in the media of small arteries (Kimura et al., 2015) (Fig. 29.23). Regarding the clinical findings, in one series (Nicolas et al., 2013), 71% of the patients with idiopathic basal ganglia calcification were symptomatic (mean age of clinical onset: 39 ± 20 years), most often with cognitive impairment (58.8%), psychiatric symptoms (56.9%), and movement disorders (54.9%).

Parathyroid disorders

The morphology and distribution of cerebral calcification that may be present in any parathyroid disorder, but most often in hypoparathyroidism, are similar to those in Fahr's disease (Goswami et al., 2012). In addition to genetic risk factors (Kurozumi et al., 2013; Choi et al., 2015), this syndrome has been associated with thalassemia (Koutsis et al., 2015) and postsurgical hypoparathyroidism (Tsai et al., 2013).

Postradiation changes

Possibly related to radiation-induced changes in perforating arterioles, cerebral calcification has been described in the radiation fields of patients with a longer survival, mostly radiated during childhood and particularly in association with methotrexate chemotherapy (Pearson et al., 1983; Lewis and Lee, 1986; Legido et al., 1988; Fernandez-Bouzas et al., 1992; Srinivasan et al., 2010b). The basal ganglia are most often affected, but the cerebral white matter may also be involved. The pattern of brain involvement resembles more the two disorders described above than the nodular, asymmetric calcifications seldom described with germ cell or other tumors (Almubarak et al., 2009).

TRANSIENT GRAY-MATTER CHANGES

Posterior reversible encephalopathy syndrome (PRES)

On imaging, this syndrome most often presents with striking white-matter changes (Hinchey et al., 1996; Lee et al., 2008) and for this reason it is discussed more fully below, among the disorders causing transient

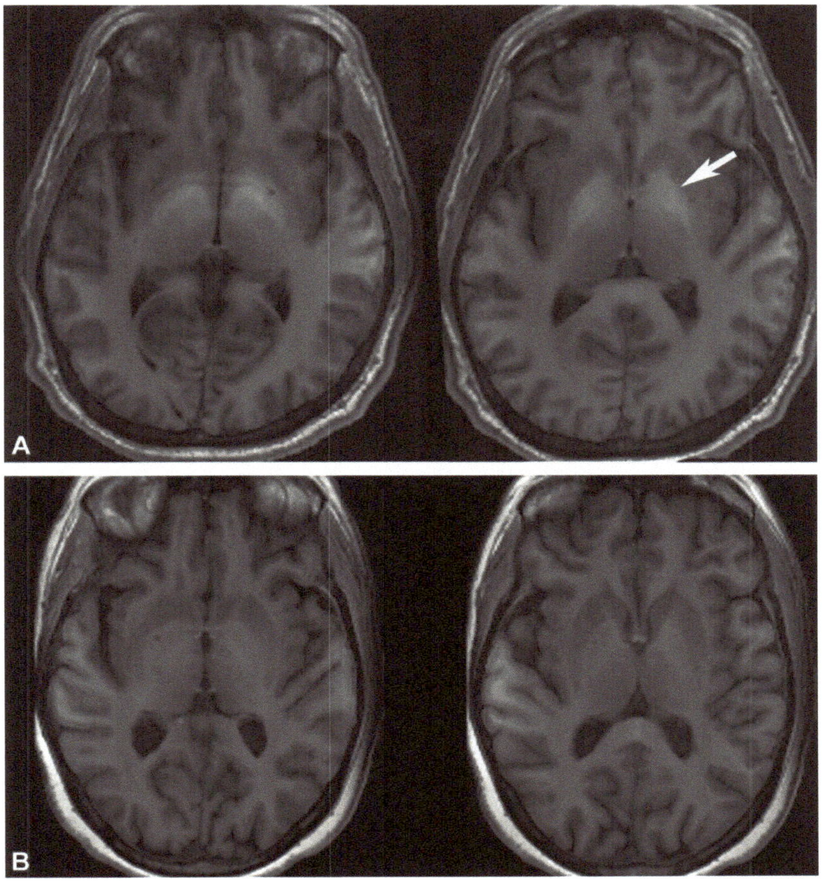

Fig. 29.19. Chronic liver disease. (**A**) T1-weighted magnetic resonance imaging (MRI) from a 51-year-old man with a 10-year history of liver disease and a transjugular intrahepatic portosystemic shunt performed 5 years prior to MRI shows a hyperintense signal in the globus pallidus bilaterally. (**B**) For comparison, MRI obtained with the same technique in a patient without liver disease.

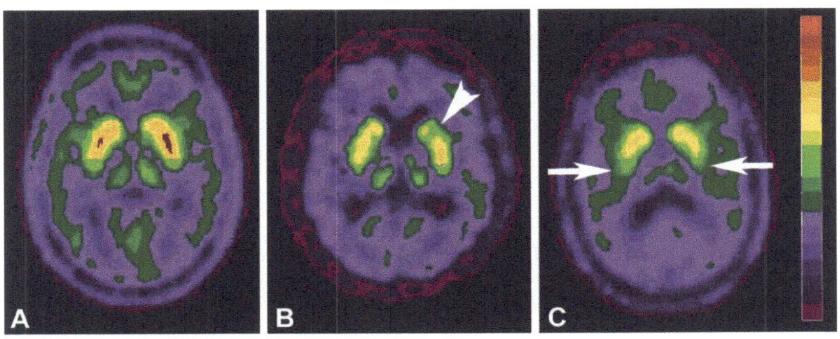

Fig. 29.20. Chronic liver failure with manganese toxicity, [18 F]fluoroDOPA (FDOPA) positron emission tomography (PET). FDOPA PET in (**A**) a healthy control; (**B**) a patient with chronic liver failure causing manganese toxicity and reduced FDOPA uptake in the anterior portion of the striatum (arrowhead); and (**C**) a patient with Parkinson's disease, with the characteristically decreased FDOPA uptake in the posterior portion of the putamen (arrows). (Modified from Criswell et al., 2012a.)

white-matter changes. However, even on imaging, some patients may have predominant involvement of gray-matter structures, such as the caudate nuclei or the thalamus (Kumai et al., 2002), and most patients present with seizures, a manifestation of cortical dysfunction. This is a disorder of gray matter as much as it is of white matter. But, unlike in cases of anoxia, attended by cytotoxic edema and necrosis, PRES is characterized by

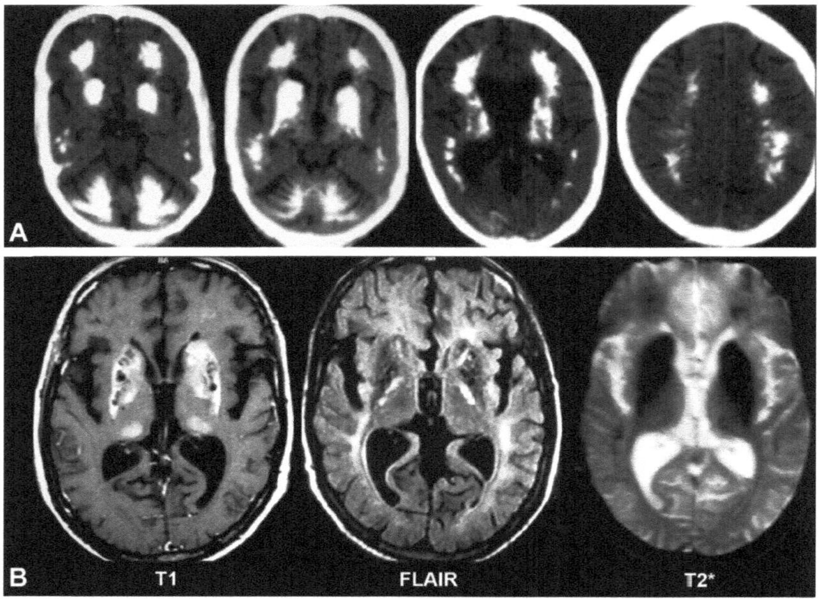

Fig. 29.21. Severe Fahr's disease. (**A**) Computed tomography (CT) and (**B**) magnetic resonance imaging from a 57-year-old man with Fahr's disease. Note the extensive calcifications on CT, involving cerebellar deep nuclei and white matter, basal ganglia, thalamus, and the hemispheric white matter. On the T1 image after gadolinium, the appearance of the basal ganglia and thalami was identical to the precontrast scan, showing abnormally increased intensity. The darker areas in the basal ganglia correspond to heavier calcification or to perivascular spaces, noticeable also in the fluid-attenuated inversion recovery (FLAIR) image. On FLAIR, the whiter matter is hyperintense, particularly in the internal capsule. A T2*, gradient echo image shows markedly reduced signal in the basal ganglia, suggestive of iron deposition. (Reproduced from Cavalcanti-Mendes et al., 2009.)

vasogenic edema due to increased capillary permeability. More than in the cortex or subcortical U-fibers, edema tends to accumulate in the white matter deeper to the subcortical U-fibers (Feigin and Budzilovich, 1980) and for this reason the changes on MRI are more apparent in the white matter than the gray matter. The gray matter, however, is involved as well, and, when the injury is severe enough, involved gray matter may show restricted diffusion, which is evidence of a transition from reversible vasogenic edema to the cytotoxic edema that characterizes necrosis (Schaefer et al., 2001; Covarrubias et al., 2002).

Nonketotic hyperglycemic hemichorea

A few patients with nonketotic hyperglycemia have been reported to present with a hyperintense lesion on T1-weighted MRI (Fig. 29.24) in the putamen contralateral to the side of the body with chorea (Wintermark et al., 2004; Felicio et al., 2008). Typically, the lesion recedes with treatment. Hyperintensity on T1-weighted images may be caused by hemorrhagic lesions, including hemorrhagic infarction, and these should be excluded. However, several of these cases with follow-up studies have ruled out hemorrhagic or ischemic pathology (Wintermark et al., 2004; Felicio et al., 2008).

LASTING WHITE-MATTER CHANGES

Anoxic and toxic leukoencephalopathies

A delayed leukoencephalopathy is an uncommon complication of hypoxic-anoxic events (Zamora et al., 2015), including carbon monoxide intoxication (Choi, 1983; Geraldo et al., 2014). Typically the episode of hypoxia has been mild and the patient may have had a brief loss of consciousness, but few or no acute imaging findings. A few days or weeks later there is clinical worsening and the appearance of white-matter lesions (Fig. 29.25).

Toluene poisoning

Toluene poisoning, occurring most often as the result of chronic occupational or purposeful inhalation, causes diffuse pallor of the white matter, particularly noticeable on T2-weighted sequences, with loss of gray–white-matter demarcation (Fig. 29.26), and atrophy of the corpus callosum and cerebellum (Rosenberg et al., 1988; Kamran and Bakshi, 1998). Toluene poisoning may cause abnormal T2 hyperintense signal in the thalamus (Fig. 29.26), basal ganglia, and cortex (particularly paracentral and visual cortex), which may appear hyperintense (Suzuki et al., 2009) or hypointense (Rosenberg et al., 1988; Kamran and Bakshi, 1998), in the second instance probably related to iron deposition in more severe or longer-standing cases.

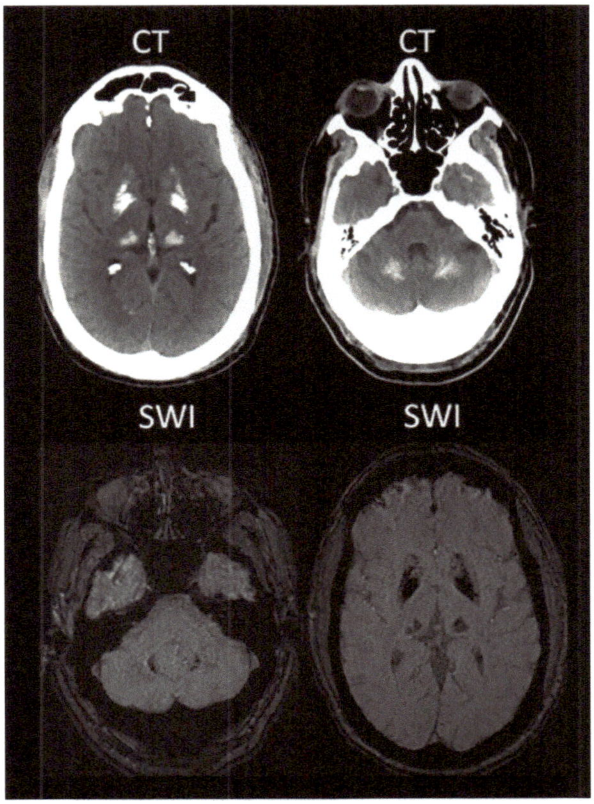

Fig. 29.22. Fahr's disease. Computed tomography (CT) and susceptibility-weighted imaging (SWI) from a 49-year-old male with progressive cognitive impairment and parkinsonian features. Head CT demonstrates symmetric calcification of both basal ganglia, thalami, and dentate nuclei. Brain magnetic resonance imaging with high-resolution SWI demonstrates abnormal susceptibility artifact in a similar distribution to the head CT.

Late delayed radiation injury or radiation necrosis

While transient white-matter changes, in the form of FLAIR hyperintensity, can be seen from days to weeks (acute radiation injury) or 1–6 months (early delayed radiation injury) after radiation, later-appearing changes (early delayed radiation injury) have worse prognosis because they correspond to white-matter necrosis from arteriolar injury. The gross pathology consists of areas of white-matter necrosis that spares the cortex (Fig. 29.27A). The margin of the lesion typically has a dotted appearance secondary to small petechial hemorrhages. On histology (Fig. 29.27B), white-matter arterioles display fibrinoid wall necrosis, with vessel occlusion and perivascular hemorrhages. While vascular damage is the most prominent finding on histology, and could explain the necrosis of the white matter on an ischemic basis, whether the vascular damage is caused directly by radiation, or by other mechanisms, including autoimmunity, is still unclear (Na et al., 2014).

Involved areas have high signal on T2 and low signal on T1-weighted images (Fig. 29.28). The T1 contrast enhancement patterns in radiation necrosis probably depend on the stage of the lesion and degree of necrosis. Two patterns have been described (Reddy et al., 2013): (1) hazy mesh-like diffuse enhancement; and (2) rim enhancement with feathery indistinct margins (Fig. 29.28), likely at the margin between the necrotic and healthy tissue. By contrast, recurrent tumor enhancement typically presents as focal solid nodules and solid uniform enhancement with distinct margins (Reddy et al., 2013). Radiation necrosis is an ischemic lesion and therefore perfusion is decreased (Fig. 29.28), while the nonnecrotic areas of recurrent high-grade tumors have increased vascularity and increased perfusion. Thus, perfusion techniques like dynamic susceptibility contrast material-enhanced

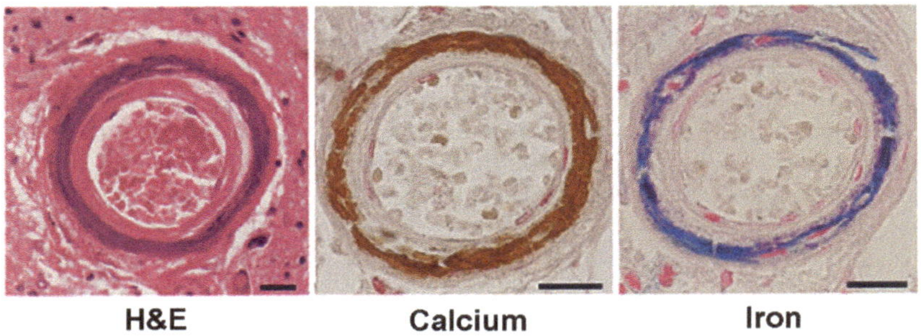

Fig. 29.23. Fahr's disease histology. Sections of a small artery from the basal ganglia of a 62-year-old man with a SLC20A2 mutation and extensive calcifications in the brain. On hematoxylin and eosin (H&E) staining, the media of the vessel appears strongly basophilic and glassy. Calcium and iron stains reveal a deposition of both in the media of the vessel. (Reproduced from Kimura et al., 2015.)

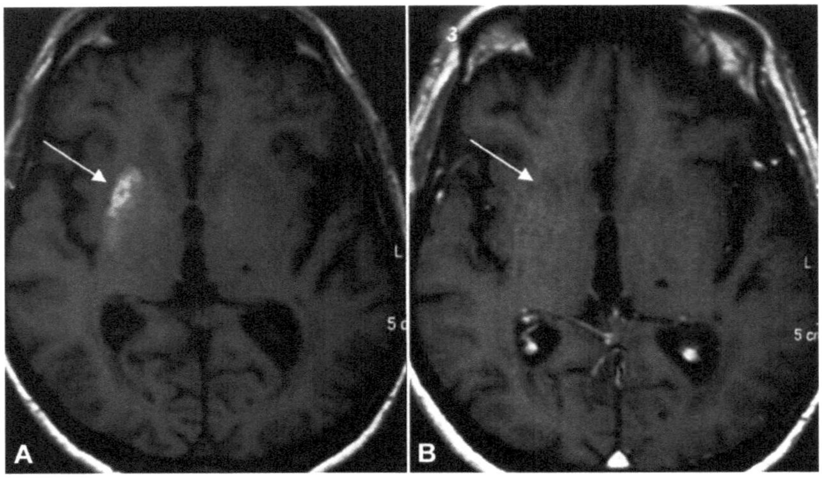

Fig. 29.24. Nonketotic hyperglycemia with unilateral chorea. (**A**) Noncontrast T1-weighted magnetic resonance imaging (MRI) from a 70-year-old man with hyperglycemia (560 mg/dL) and unilateral chorea in the left side of the body, opposite to the hyperintense signal observed in the right putamen (arrow). (**B**) Gadolinium-enhanced T1-weighted MRI, 9 months after the prior MRI, once the hyperglycemia had been corrected, was unremarkable. (Reproduced from Felicio et al., 2008.)

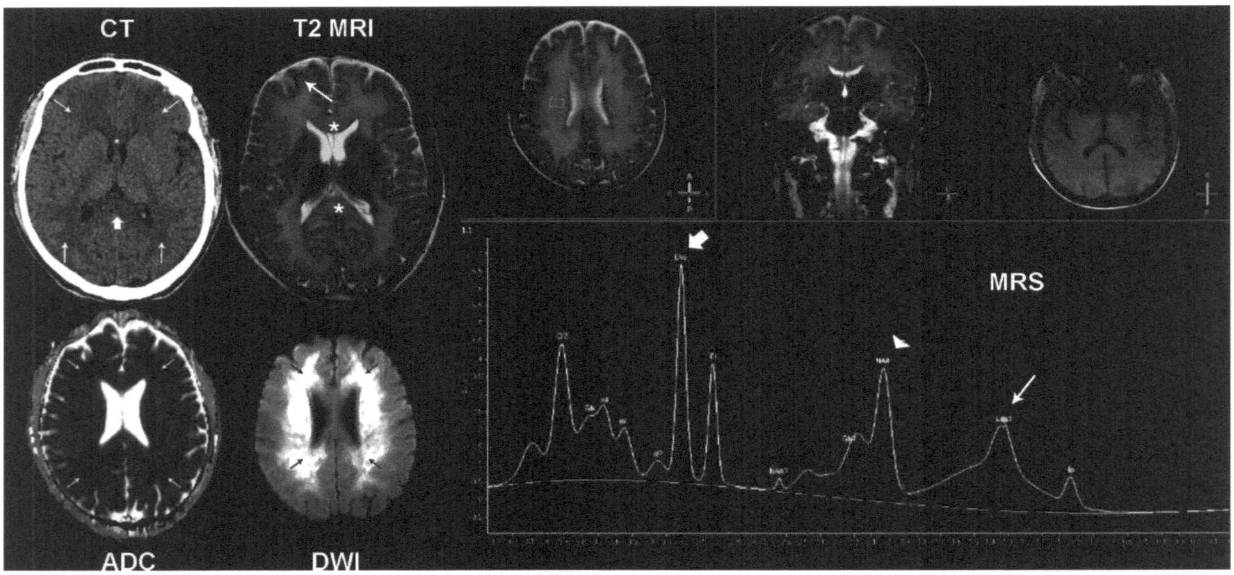

Fig. 29.25. Delayed leukoencephalopathy after carbon monoxide poisoning. A 40-year-old male with diffuse posthypoxic demyelination (1 month after the initial event and before treatment). Axial noncontrast computed tomography (CT) scan shows diffuse hypodensity in the periventricular white matter (small arrows), the splenium (large arrow), and the genu (asterisks) of the corpus callosum. Axial T2 and coronal T2 (above magnetic resonance spectroscopy: MRS) show a diffuse, confluent hyperintensity of the white matter, including the corpus callosum (white asterisks), and the internal (black arrow) and the external (black asterisks) capsules. Axial diffusion-weighted imaging (DWI) shows diffuse hyperintensity in the white matter with corresponding hypointensity on the axial apparent diffusion coefficient (ADC) map (2d), reflecting restricted diffusion. MRI, magnetic resonance imaging. (Reproduced from Geraldo et al., 2014.)

(CE) T2*-weighted perfusion MRI and dynamic CE T1-weighted perfusion MRI may be helpful in distinguishing these lesions (Kim et al., 2014). As discussed in Chapter 13, MRS may also be helpful in differentiating radiation necrosis from tumor recurrence. On PET imaging, the uptake of [^{18}F]fluorodioxyglucose, [^{18}F]FDOPA (Karunanithi et al., 2013), and [^{11}C] methionine (Minamimoto et al., 2015) is reduced in radiation necrosis (Fig. 29.29), but increased in tumor recurrence.

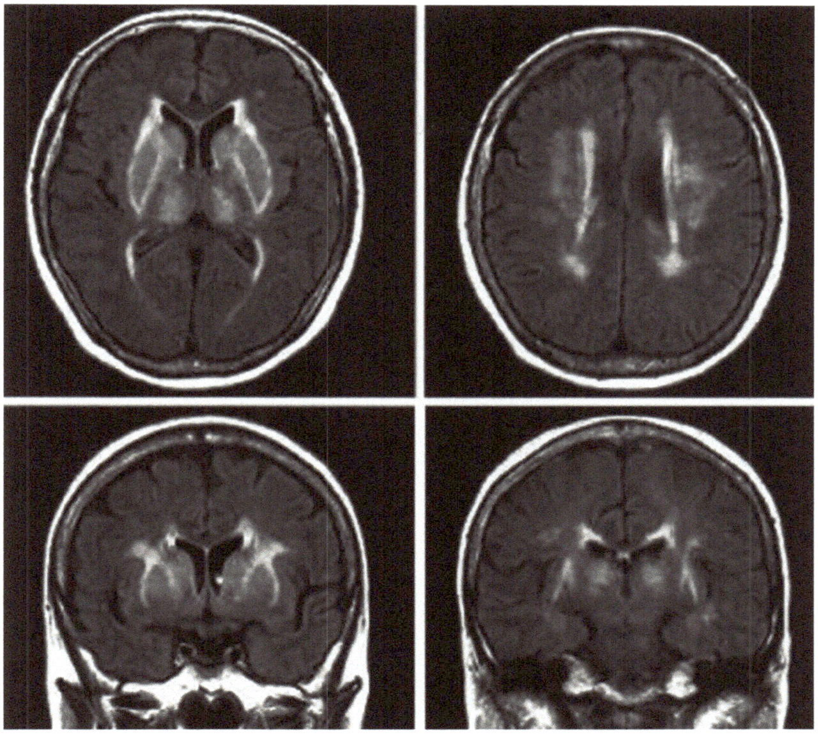

Fig. 29.26. Toluene poisoning. Fluid-attenuated inversion recovery images from a 63-year-old woman with a history of chronic inhalation of organic solvents. Notice the loss of gray–white demarcation, suggesting loss of the normal white-matter signal, and frankly increased white-matter signal in periventricular white matter, as well as internal and external capsules. Increased signal is also present in the thalami and, to a lesser extent, in the striatum. (Adapted from Suzuki et al., 2009.)

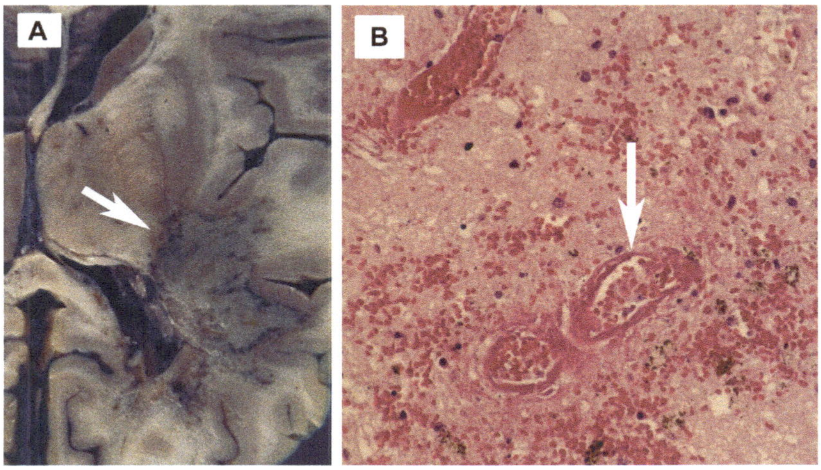

Fig. 29.27. Radiation necrosis. Pathology. (**A**) Gross pathology from a 23-year-old man with radiation necrosis following irradiation of a middle-fossa meningioma. The core of the lesion (arrow) is discolored with a greenish hue and corresponds to white-matter necrosis. The margins of the lesion, from where the histology to the right was obtained, show petechial hemorrhages. Notice how the lesion abuts the cortex but spares it. (**B**) Histology shows fibrinoid necrosis of arteriolar walls (arrow), with vessel occlusion and perivascular hemorrhages, evidenced by extravasated erythrocytes and brownish deposits of hemosiderin.

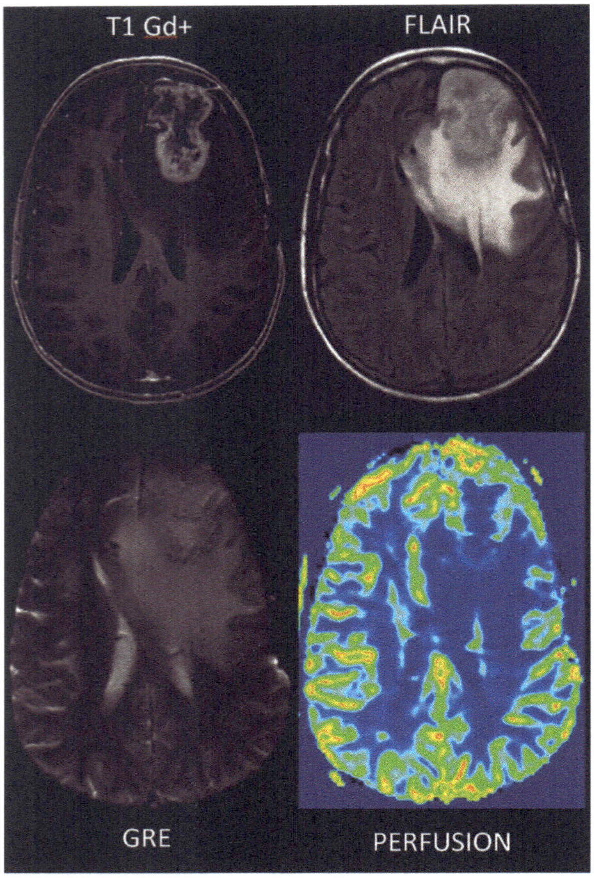

Fig. 29.28. Radiation necrosis: magnetic resonance imaging (MRI). Postgadolinium T1 (T1 Gd+), fluid-attenuated inversion recovery (FLAIR), gradient echo (GRE), and perfusion MRI images from a 47-year-old woman with a left frontal glioblastoma treated with subtotal resection followed by concurrent radiation and temazolomide. MRI 3 months after radiation completion demonstrates a large region of lace-like enhancement in the anterior left frontal lobe adjacent to the resection cavity with a thick peripheral rim of enhancement, central petechial hemorrhage, extensive surrounding vasogenic edema and mass effect, as well as decreased cerebral blood flow on perfusion MRI.

Osmotic demyelination syndrome

Subacute demyelination in the basis pontis or central pontine myelinolysis (Fig. 29.30) may be related to severe hyperosmolality (McKee et al., 1988) or, more often, the rapid correction of severe hyponatremia (Alleman, 2014). In the setting of hyponatremia, cells swell and lose organic osmolytes (myo-inositol, taurine, glutamine, glutamate, creatine, phosphocreatine, and glycerophosphorylchlorine). With sodium supplementation, these organic osmolytes (with the exception of glycerophosphorylchlorine) reaccumulate in the cell slowly (5 days to a week). Rapid serum sodium correction is associated with a relative overshoot of brain sodium and chloride levels in the presence of low organic osmolyte concentration, resulting in central pontine myelinolysis in experimental animals (Alleman, 2014). Neuropathologically, there is loss of oligodendrocytes and myelin, with a variable amount of axonal loss (McKee et al., 1988; Alleman, 2014).

Osmotic demyelination can also involve extrapontine sites, most often the cerebellum and lateral geniculate body, but also the external and extreme capsules, basal ganglia, thalamus, gray–white junction of the cerebral cortex, and hippocampi. On CT the lesion may pass unnoticed. On MRI, the pontine area of demyelination appears hypointense on T1- and hyperintense on T2-weighted images (Fig. 29.30), and often demonstrates restricted diffusion on DWI (Fig. 29.31). Milder lesions do not enhance with contrast, but may show decreased signal on susceptibility-weighted imaging (Fig. 29.30), which may represent iron deposition (Alleman, 2014). As this abnormality may reverse after the acute stage (Fig. 29.30), an alternative explanation would be increased perfusion through the area. More severe lesions may display contrast enhancement (Alleman, 2014). Reported MRS features include low choline levels, increased choline-creatine ratio, low NAA levels, and low lipid levels (Alleman, 2014). Although pontine involvement may be present both in this entity and Wernicke's encephalopathy, central pontine myelinolysis tends to involve the basis pontis, while Wernicke's encephalopathy tends to involve the pontine tegmentum.

Marchiafava–Bignami disease

Originally described neuropathologically in red-wine drinkers as a necrotic lesion of the corpus callosum (Marchiafava and Bignami, 1903), similar lesions have been reported repeatedly on CT and MRI studies (Hillbom et al., 2014). Rather than a disease it is a syndrome, caused by a multiplicity of etiologies (Hillbom et al., 2014). Thiamine deficiency, possibly coupled with toxicity from alcohol or substances associated with it, is probably the main cause (Hillbom et al., 2014). However, the Marchiafava–Bignami appellative has been applied to similar callosal lesions probably caused by acute disseminated encephalomyelitis (Dujmovic et al., 2015), extrapontine osmotic demyelination (Duray et al., 2014), and all the etiologies associated with the reversible splenial lesion syndrome (RESLES), described in the next section (Kakkar et al., 2014; Nakamura et al., 2015). On CT the callosal lesion appears hypodense or the corpus callosum may simply appear thinner than normal (Hillbom et al., 2014). On MRI, the affected areas of the corpus callosum appear hypointense on T1- and hyperintensense on T2-weighted images, with restricted diffusion on DWI often seen in the acute stage (Fig. 29.31).

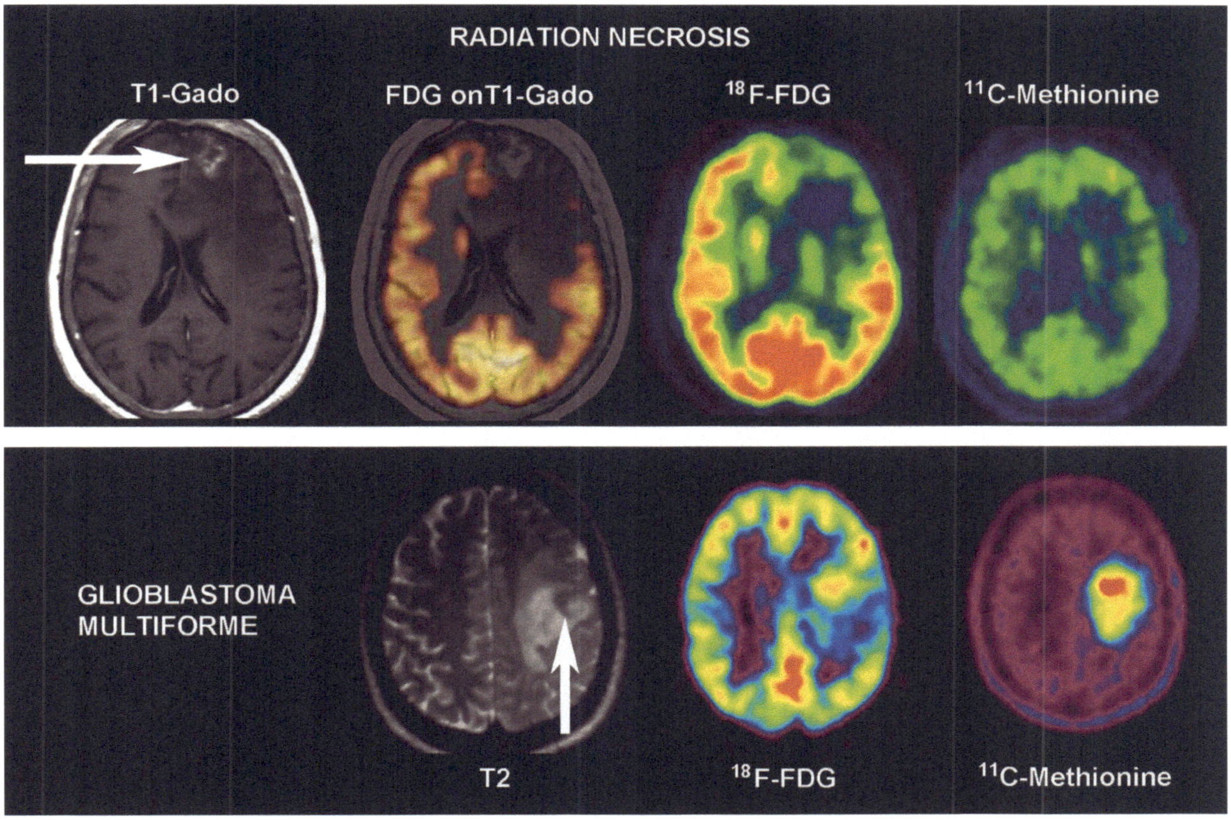

Fig. 29.29. Radiation necrosis: positron emission tomography (PET). Findings in a case of radiation necrosis (top row, arrow) are contrasted with those from a tumor, a glioblastoma multiforme (bottom row, arrow). On postgadolinium T1 (T1-Gado) magnetic resonance imaging (MRI) there is an enhancement pattern similar to the one found in Figure 29.28 MRI. ^{18}F-fluorodeoxyglucose (FDG) PET showed decreased metabolism in the area of radiation necrosis (see the metabolism image superimposed on the MRI – FDG on T1-Gado), but there is increased metabolism in the area of the tumor. Similarly, on ^{11}C-methionine PET, there is little uptake in radiation necrosis, but very marked uptake in the tumor.

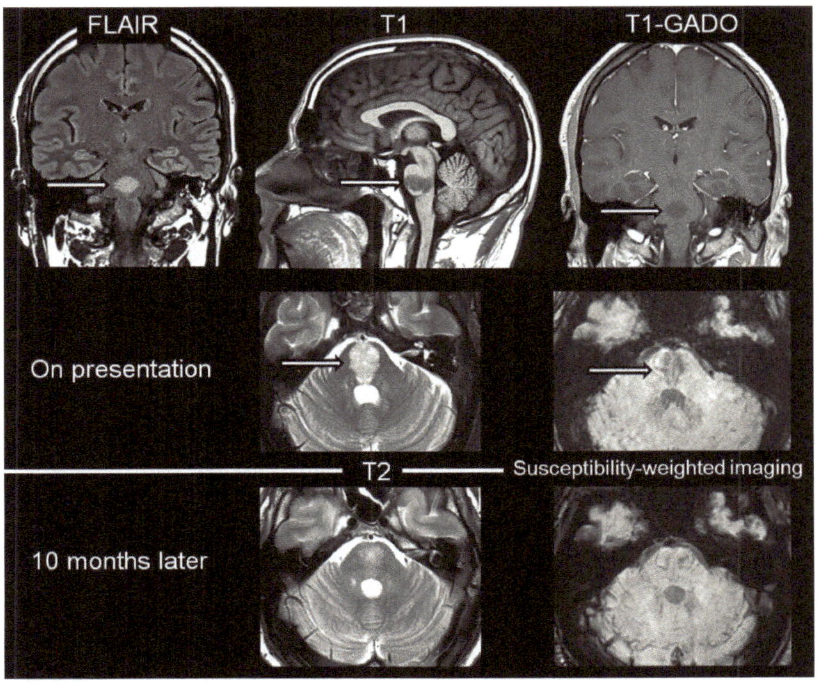

Fig. 29.30. Osmotic demyelination. Central pontine myelinolysis. Magnetic resonance imaging from a 36-year-old man who the previous week had ingested 10 cans daily of high-energy drinks; he had ataxia, dysarthria, vertigo, and upper-extremity paresthesias. FLAIR, fluid-attenuated inversion recovery; T1-GADO, postgadolinium T1. (Courtesy of Darin T. Okuda, M.D., F.A.A.N., and Braeden D. Newton, B.S., UT Southwestern Medical Center at Dallas, Dallas, TX, USA.)

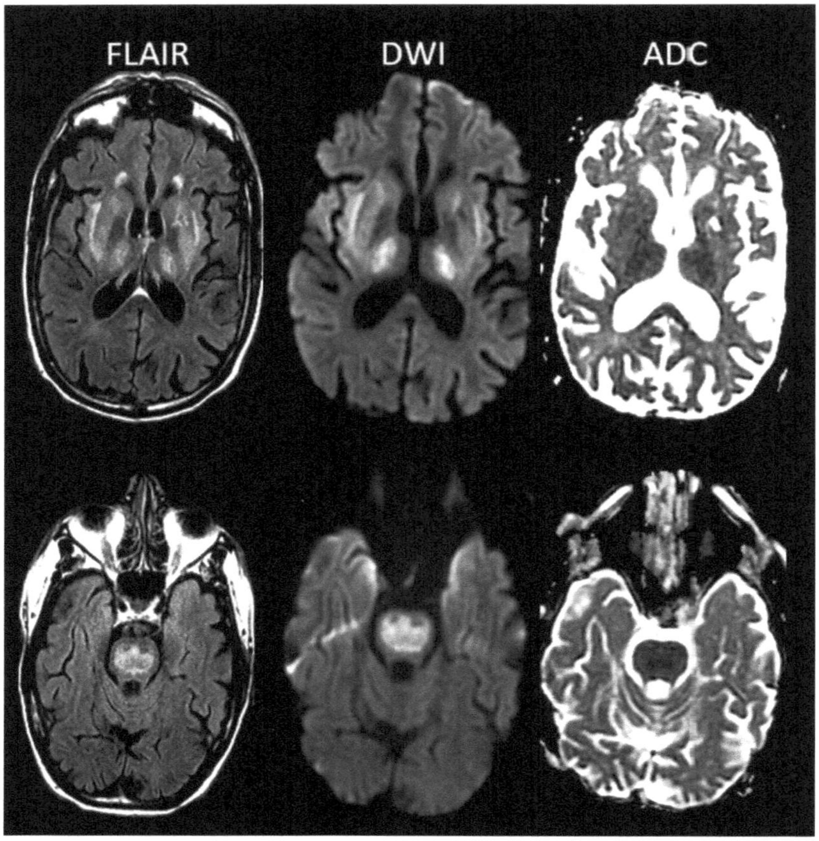

Fig. 29.31. Osmotic demyelination. Pontine and extrapontine myelinolysis. Magnetic resonance imaging (MRI) from a 49-year-old male with a history of polysubstance abuse found next to a crack pipe and alcohol bottle. The serum sodium was 108 mEq/L on admission, and was rapidly corrected to 130 mEq/L over 48 hours. Brain MRI demonstrates symmetric abnormal T2 (see fluid-attenuated inversion recovery (FLAIR) image) hyperintense signal in basal ganglia and thalami as well as the central pons, with associated restricted diffusion in the central pons and both thalami. DWI, diffusion-weighted image; ADC, apparent diffusion coefficient map.

FLAIR images may show a hyperintense rim around a cavitary lesion in the core of the corpus callosum (Fig. 29.32). The lesions usually do not enhance after gadolinium, but this may depend on when in the process the study is obtained. With prompt thiamine therapy, the lesion may improve and MRI can be used to document the favorable evolution and study the metabolic changes occurring in the tissue (Gass et al., 1998; Gambini et al., 2003). In severe cases, diffusion tractography has been used to document elegantly the loss of crossing fibers in the corpus callosum (Fig. 29.33).

TRANSIENT WHITE-MATTER CHANGES

Posterior reversible encephalopathy syndrome

This syndrome is also discussed in Chapter 16 (Fig. 16.24). Well known from previous literature discussing MRI and CT changes with acute hypertension, particularly in association with eclampsia (Raroque et al., 1990), this syndrome was popularized by a frequently cited study (Hinchey et al., 1996) that described "a reversible posterior leukoencephalopathy syndrome." The evolution in the literature from leukoencephalopathy to simply encephalopathy resulted from ample evidence of involvement of the cortical or deep gray matter, not only on imaging – 40% of cases in a large series (Lee et al., 2008) – but also from the clinical symptomatology, characterized by seizures in more than 80% of cases (Datar et al., 2015). However, we have placed this entity among the reversible white-matter disorders because on MRI subcortical white-matter involvement tends to be most obvious.

In the Mayo Clinic experience (Lee et al., 2008), the most common causes were hypertension (53%), renal disease (45%), dialysis dependency (21%), malignancy (32%), and transplantation (24%). Of course the causes listed are not exclusive of each other. For instance, many patients with kidney disease have hypertension; transplanted patients are often on cyclosporine or tacrolimus,

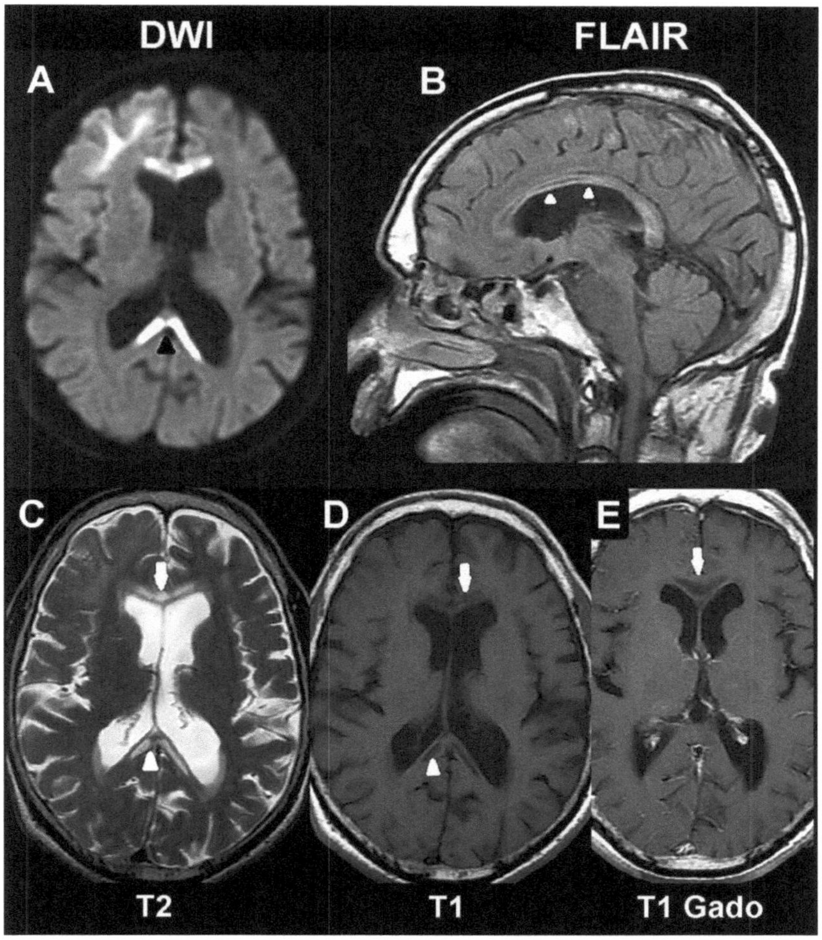

Fig. 29.32. Marchiafava–Bignami syndrome. Magnetic resonance imaging from a 50-year-old man with chronic alcoholism, seizures, and a gait disorder. On diffusion-weighted imaging (DWI), restricted diffusion is present in the rostrum and posterior portion of the body of the corpus callosum (**A**, arrowhead). On fluid-attenuated inversion recovery (FLAIR), there is cavitation in the anterior portion of the corpus callosum (**B**, arrowheads), with a normal appearance of the splenium. The callosal lesion appears hyperintense on T2 (**C**, arrows) and hypointense on T1 (**D**, arrows), but does not enhance after gadolinium infusion (**E**, arrow). (Reproduced from Paidipati Gopalkishna Murthy, 2014.)

which have been linked to this syndrome (Agarwal et al., 2015; Giussani et al., 2016). Other causes include eclampsia, systemic lupus erythematosus, allergic purpura, and acute intermittent porphyria (Maramattom et al., 2005; Ni et al., 2011). In the Mayo Clinic series (Lee et al., 2008), presenting symptoms included clinical seizures (87%), encephalopathy (92%), visual symptoms (39%), and headache (53%). Mean peak systolic blood pressure at presentation was 187 mmHg. Clinical symptoms resolved after a mean of 5.3 days.

The most common imaging finding is increased subcortical white-matter signal on FLAIR images (Fig. 29.34). Abnormal white-matter signal corresponds to vasogenic edema, as evidenced by the lack of restricted diffusion, rather, facilitated diffusion on apparent diffusion coefficient (Fig. 16.24) (Schaefer et al., 2001; Covarrubias et al., 2002). The apparently greatest involvement of the white matter may simply reflect the underlying pathology, vasogenic edema, which is more pronounced in the white matter than in the cortex, even when the primary pathology affects both or is mostly cortical (Feigin and Budzilovich, 1980; Milhorat, 1992). Because of the arrangement of their vascular network, ground substances, including mucopolysaccharides, and elastic fiber structure, the cortex and subcortical U-fibers, are less likely to accumulate as large an amount of vasogenic edema fluid as is the white matter deeper to the U-fibers (Feigin and Budzilovich, 1980).

Contrast enhancement happens rarely, affects only some areas, and typically occurs concomitantly with restricted diffusion (the precontrast apparent diffusion

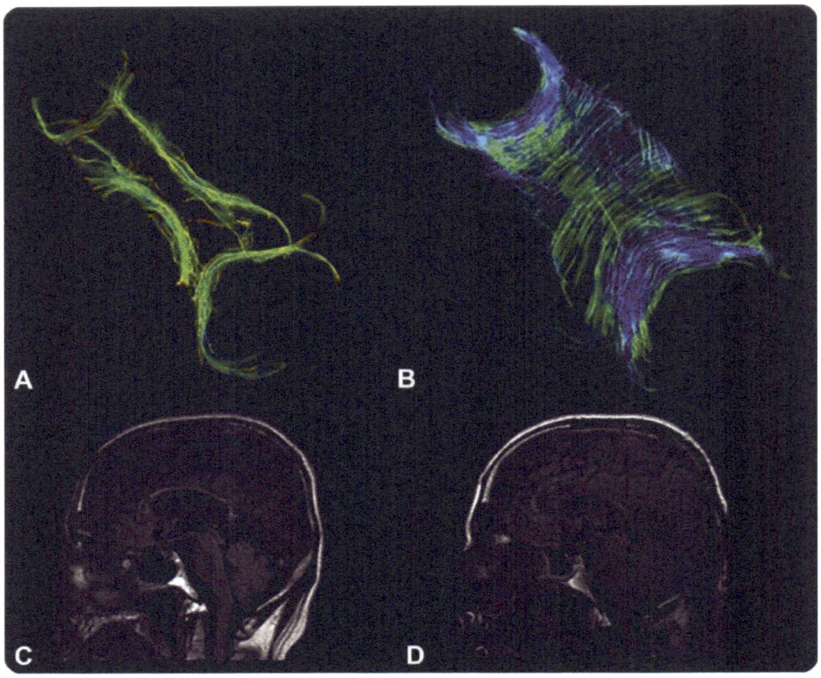

Fig. 29.33. Marchiafava–Bignami syndrome diffusion tensor imaging. Magnetic resonance imaging (MRI) corpus callosum tractography and sagittal T1 MRI from a 57-year-old man, a chronic alcoholic, with Marchiafava–Bignami disease (**A** and **C**) and a healthy control (**B** and **D**). Note the cavitation in the corpus callosum on (**C**) and the loss of crossing callosal fibers on tractography (**A**). (Reproduced from Lakatos et al., 2014.)

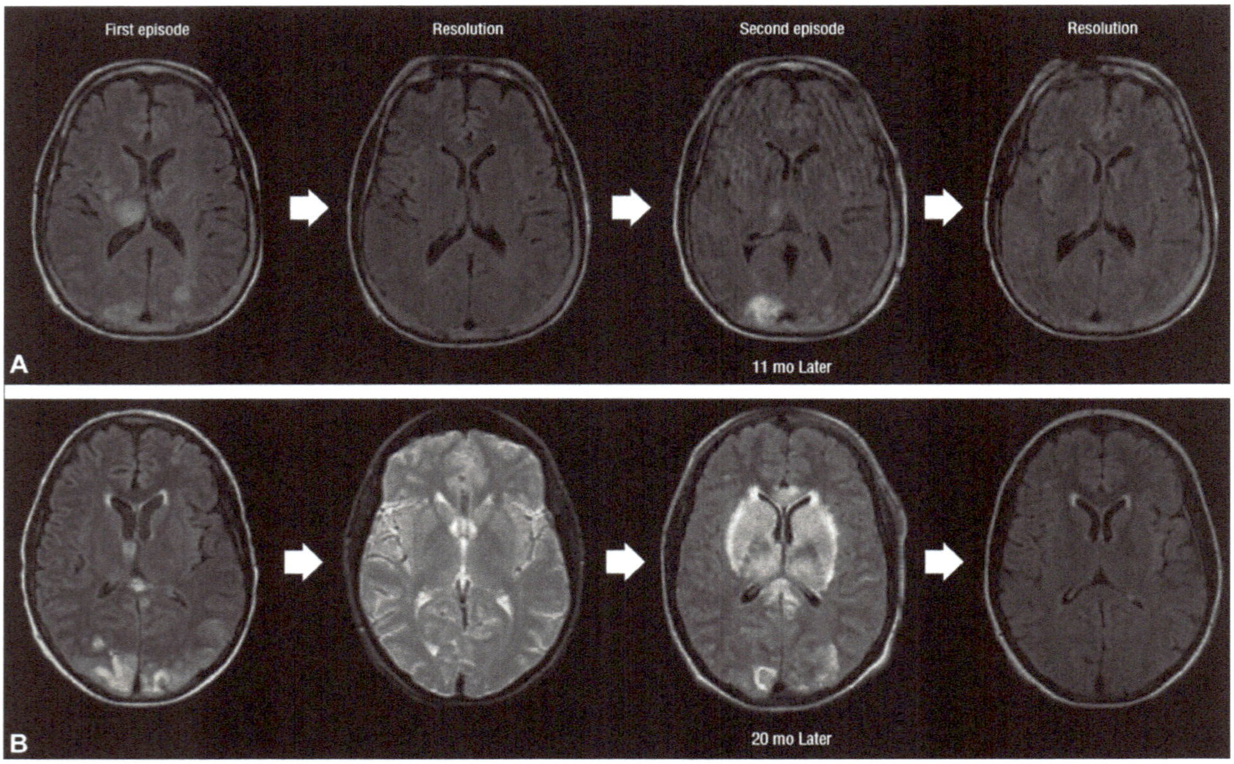

Fig. 29.34. Posterior reversible encephalopathy syndrome (PRES). T2-weighted images from 2 patients: (**A**), a 15-year-old man with non-Hodgkin's lymphoma, end-stage kidney disease, and hypertension; and (**B**), a 37-year-old quadriplegic man with hypertensive episodes. Note the resolution of the changes with treatment but the recurrence in these cases. The thalami are involved in both patients. The splenium of the corpus callosum is involved in (**B**). (Reproduced from Lee et al., 2008.)

coefficient map may show hyperintensity) (Schaefer et al., 2001; Covarrubias et al., 2002; Lee et al., 2008) and may reflect severe endothelial damage with necrosis. As to the topography of the imaging changes, they most often involve the occipital, parietal, and posterior temporal regions (Fig. 29.34). Increased signal in the cerebellum, brainstem, and thalami is also frequent (Fig. 29.34). Although the posterior regions of the brain are most often affected, involvement of the anterior portion of the brain was observed in 50–90% of cases (Covarrubias et al., 2002; Lee et al., 2008). With the appropriate treatment, the imaging changes typically recede in a few days to weeks (Hinchey et al., 1996; Lee et al., 2008), but in some cases gray-matter areas may undergo necrosis and have permanent changes, or the syndrome may recur (Lee et al., 2008) (Fig. 29.34).

Reversible splenial lesion syndrome

Transient lesions in the splenium of the corpus callosum have been described with antiepileptic drug withdrawal, infection, high-altitude cerebral edema, or metabolic disorders, including hypoglycemia and hypernatremia (Garcia-Monco et al., 2011). Complete resolution after a variable lapse is the rule. Clinical presentation is nonspecific, without evidence of callosal disconnection syndromes. Neuroimaging shows a nonenhancing, round-shaped lesion centered in the splenium of the corpus callosum that disappears after a variable lapse (Fig. 29.35). The lesion often demonstrates restricted diffusion, suggestive of cytotoxic edema (Fig. 29.35). In a few patients, mostly those with high-altitude cerebral edema, the lesion had high apparent diffusion coefficient values, consistent with vasogenic edema (Garcia-Monco et al., 2011). These findings suggest that, as the name implies, the pathogenesis of this MRI finding is varied, ranging from pure edema to transient damage of oligodendrocytes. It is conceivable that some of these cases represent osmotic demyelination.

A similar splenial lesion has been reported after organophosphate poisoning (Wang et al., 2015) and with metronidazole encephalopathy, but in this entity there is often additional involvement of the periaqueductal gray and dentate nucleus (Kim et al., 2007); as the reported patients had complex systemic disorders, the possibility of other metabolic causes for the reported lesions is not completely ruled out.

CONCLUSIONS

MRI has allowed for much progress in the field of inherited metabolic disorders. Before the advent of MRI, metabolically vulnerable brain was not well understood. Today MRI has helped define disorders through the recognition of specific lesion patterns and their evolution over time. This has also led to identification of novel leukodystrophies and the genes underlying these disorders. Even in previously well-characterized disorders, MRI patterns have shed light on disease mechanisms.

The understanding of the pathology and molecular basis of metabolic disorders has in turn allowed for new insight into the significance of MRI changes and elucidated the capabilities of MR techniques. Brain MRI today is a valuable tool in monitoring disease progression and the success of therapeutic interventions in leukodystrophies and other metabolic brain disorders. A multimodal approach employs a variety of sequences sensitive to different brain tissue characteristics. Together these techniques will be able to provide clues to the important early presymptomatic stages of the inherited diseases, beyond what pathology revealed in the past.

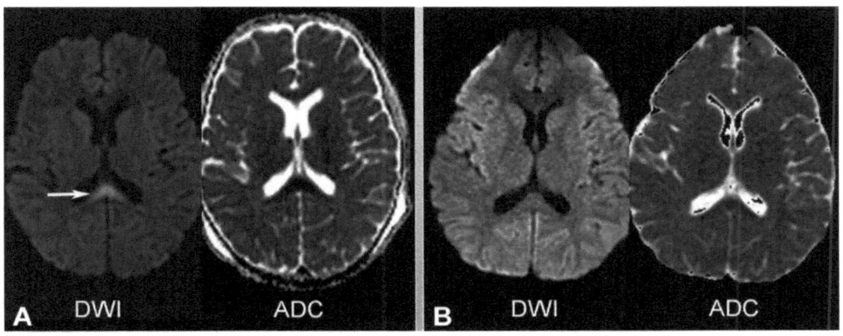

Fig. 29.35. Isolated and reversible splenial lesion syndrome (RESLES). Diffusion-weighted imaging (DWI) and apparent diffusion coefficient (ADC) map before (**A**) and 1 month later (**B**), after treatment with intravenous immunoglobulin. Diffusion restriction present in the first study (A, arrow) is not present in the follow-up study. The patient was a 7-year-old boy presenting with fever, conjunctivitis, mucosal erythema, and a rash, consistent with Kawasaki's disease. Initial serum sodium was 120 mEq/L. (Courtesy of Dr. Venu Parachuri, Medical College of Wisconsin Affiliated Hospitals, Milwaukee, WI, USA.)

References

Adalsteinsson E, Spielman DM (1999). Spatially resolved two-dimensional spectroscopy. Magn Reson Med 41: 8–12.

Adalsteinsson E, Irarrazabal P, Topp S et al. (1998). Volumetric spectroscopic imaging with spiral-based k-space trajectories. Magn Reson Med 39: 889–898.

Agarwal A, Kapur G, Altinok D (2015). Childhood posterior reversible encephalopathy syndrome: magnetic resonance imaging findings with emphasis on increased leptomeningeal FLAIR signal. Neuroradiol J 28: 638–643.

Alleman AM (2014). Osmotic demyelination syndrome: central pontine myelinolysis and extrapontine myelinolysis. Semin Ultrasound CT MR 35: 153–159.

Almubarak S, Gan YC, Steinbok P et al. (2009). Occurrence of basal ganglia germ cell tumors without a mass. Arch Neurol 66: 789–792.

Andronesi OC, Ramadan S, Ratai EM et al. (2010). Spectroscopic imaging with improved gradient modulated constant adiabaticity pulses on high-field clinical scanners. J Magn Reson 203: 283–293.

Andronesi OC, Gagoski BA, Adalsteinsson E et al. (2012). Correlation chemical shift imaging with low-power adiabatic pulses and constant-density spiral trajectories. NMR Biomed 25: 195–209.

Arbelaez A, Castillo M, Mukherji SK (1999). Diffusion-weighted MR imaging of global cerebral anoxia. AJNR Am J Neuroradiol 20: 999–1007.

Arora V, Nijjar IB, Multani AS et al. (2007). MRI findings in methanol intoxication: a report of two cases. Br J Radiol 80: e243–e246.

Aschner JL, Anderson A, Slaughter JC et al. (2015). Neuroimaging identifies increased manganese deposition in infants receiving parenteral nutrition. Am J Clin Nutr 102: 1482–1489.

Bakshi R, Morcos MF, Gabryel TF et al. (2000). Is fluid-attenuated inversion recovery MRI more sensitive than conventional MRI for hypoglycemic brain injury? Neurology 55: 1064–1065.

Barker PB, Horska A (2004). Neuroimaging in leukodystrophies. J Child Neurol 19: 559–570.

Barker PB, Bizzi A, De Stefano N et al. (2010). Clinical MR Spectroscopy: Techniques and Applications. Cambridge University Press, Cambridge.

Barkovich AJ, Westmark KD, Bedi HS et al. (2001). Proton spectroscopy and diffusion imaging on the first day of life after perinatal asphyxia: preliminary report. AJNR Am J Neuroradiol 22: 1786–1794.

Barkovich AJ, Miller SP, Bartha A et al. (2006). MR imaging, MR spectroscopy, and diffusion tensor imaging of sequential studies in neonates with encephalopathy. AJNR Am J Neuroradiol 27: 533–547.

Berg D, Hoggenmuller U, Hofmann E et al. (2000). The basal ganglia in haemochromatosis. Neuroradiology 42: 9–13.

Blanco M, Casado R, Vazquez F et al. (2006). CT and MR imaging findings in methanol intoxication. AJNR Am J Neuroradiol 27: 452–454.

Brand A, Richter-Landsberg C, Leibfritz D (1993). Multinuclear NMR studies on the energy metabolism of glial and neuronal cells. Dev Neurosci 15: 289–298.

Breiter SN, Arroyo S, Mathews VP et al. (1994). Proton MR spectroscopy in patients with seizure disorders. AJNR Am J Neuroradiol 15: 373–384.

Castillo M, Kwock L, Green C (1995). MELAS syndrome: imaging and proton MR spectroscopic findings. AJNR Am J Neuroradiol 16: 233–239.

Cavalcanti-Mendes Gde A, Carvalho GT, Christo PP et al. (2009). An unusual case of Fahr's disease. Arq Neuropsiquiatr 67: 516–518.

Cecil KM (2006). MR spectroscopy of metabolic disorders. Neuroimaging Clin N Am 16: 87–116. viii.

Chakraborty G, Mekala P, Yahya D et al. (2001). Intraneuronal N-acetylaspartate supplies acetyl groups for myelin lipid synthesis: evidence for myelin-associated aspartoacylase. J Neurochem 78: 736–745.

Choi IS (1983). Delayed neurologic sequelae in carbon monoxide intoxication. Arch Neurol 40: 433–435.

Choi KH, Shin CH, Yang SW et al. (2015). Autosomal dominant hypocalcemia with Bartter syndrome due to a novel activating mutation of calcium sensing receptor, Y829C. Korean J Pediatr 58: 148–153.

Costello DJ, Eichler AF, Eichler FS (2009). Leukodystrophies: classification, diagnosis and treatment. Neurologist 15: 319–328.

Covarrubias DJ, Luetmer PH, Campeau NG (2002). Posterior reversible encephalopathy syndrome: prognostic utility of quantitative diffusion-weighted MR images. AJNR Am J Neuroradiol 23: 1038–1048.

Criswell SR, Perlmutter JS, Crippin JS et al. (2012a). Reduced uptake of FDOPA PET in end-stage liver disease with elevated manganese levels. Arch Neurol 69: 394–397.

Criswell SR, Perlmutter JS, Huang JL et al. (2012b). Basal ganglia intensity indices and diffusion weighted imaging in manganese-exposed welders. Occup Environ Med 69: 437–443.

Datar S, Singh T, Rabinstein AA et al. (2015). Long-term risk of seizures and epilepsy in patients with posterior reversible encephalopathy syndrome. Epilepsia 56: 564–568.

De Stefano N, Dotti MT, Mortilla M et al. (2001). Magnetic resonance imaging and spectroscopic changes in brains of patients with cerebrotendinous xanthomatosis. Brain 124: 121–131.

Dubey P, Fatemi A, Barker PB et al. (2005). Spectroscopic evidence of cerebral axonopathy in patien with "pure" adrenomyeloneuropathy. Neurology 64: 304–310.

Dujmovic I, Nikolic I, Gavric-Kezic M et al. (2015). Teaching NeuroImages: Reversible widespread brain MRI lesions in Marchiafava-Bignami disease. Neurology 84: e81–e82.

Duray MC, De Maeseneire C, Rutgers MP et al. (2014). Acute reversible Marchiafava-Bignami disease with hypernatremia: a "callosal myelinolysis"? Rev Neurol (Paris) 170: 232–234.

Eichler FS, Barker PB, Cox C et al. (2002). Proton MR spectroscopic imaging predicts lesion progression on MRI in X-linked adrenoleukodystrophy. Neurology 58: 901–907.

Eichler F, Grodd W, Grant E et al. (2009). Metachromatic leukodystrophy: a scoring system for brain MR imaging observations. AJNR Am J Neuroradiol 30: 1893–1897.

Embirucu EK, Otaduy MC, Taneja AK et al. (2010). MR spectroscopy detects lipid peaks in cerebrotendinous xanthomatosis. AJNR Am J Neuroradiol 31: 1347–1349.

Fatemi A, Barker PB, Ulug AM et al. (2003). MRI and proton MRSI in women heterozygous for X-linked adrenoleukodystrophy. Neurology 60: 1301–1307.

Federico A, Dotti M, Gallus G (2013). Cerebrotendinous xanthomatosis. In: R Pagon, M Adam, H Ardinger (Eds.), GeneReviews® [Internet]. University of Washington, Seattle, WA.

Feigin I, Budzilovich GN (1980). The influence of the ground substance on the extracellular water of normal and edematous human brain: focal edema and the demyelinating diseases, including multiple sclerosis. J Neuropathol Exp Neurol 39: 13–29.

Felicio AC, Chang CV, Godeiro-Junior C et al. (2008). Hemichorea-hemiballism as the first presentation of type 2 diabetes mellitus. Arq Neuropsiquiatr 66: 249–250.

Fernandez-Bouzas A, Ramirez Jimenez H, Vazquez Zamudio J et al. (1992). Brain calcifications and dementia in children treated with radiotherapy and intrathecal methotrexate. J Neurosurg Sci 36: 211–214.

Forbes KP, Pipe JG, Karis JP et al. (2003). Brain imaging in the unsedated pediatric patient: comparison of periodically rotated overlapping parallel lines with enhanced reconstruction and single-shot fast spin-echo sequences. AJNR Am J Neuroradiol 24: 794–798.

Gambini A, Falini A, Moiola L et al. (2003). Marchiafava-Bignami disease: longitudinal MR imaging and MR spectroscopy study. AJNR Am J Neuroradiol 24: 249–253.

Garcia-Monco JC, Cortina IE, Ferreira E et al. (2011). Reversible splenial lesion syndrome (RESLES): what's in a name? J Neuroimaging 21: e1–e14.

Gass A, Birtsch G, Olster M et al. (1998). Marchiafava-Bignami disease: reversibility of neuroimaging abnormality. J Comput Assist Tomogr 22: 503–504.

Geraldo AF, Silva C, Neutel D et al. (2014). Delayed leukoencephalopathy after acute carbon monoxide intoxication. J Radiol Case Rep 8: 1–8.

Giussani A, Ardissino G, Belingheri M et al. (2016). Posterior reversible encephalopathy syndrome after kidney transplantation in pediatric recipients: two cases. Pediatr Transplant 20: 68–71.

Goswami R, Sharma R, Sreenivas V et al. (2012). Prevalence and progression of basal ganglia calcification and its pathogenic mechanism in patients with idiopathic hypoparathyroidism. Clin Endocrinol (Oxf) 77: 200–206.

Grasso D, Borreggine C, Perfetto F et al. (2014). Lentiform fork sign: a magnetic resonance finding in a case of acute metabolic acidosis. Neuroradiol J 27: 288–292.

Grodd W, Krageloh-Mann I, Klose U et al. (1991). Metabolic and destructive brain disorders in children: findings with localized proton MR spectroscopy. Radiology 181: 173–181.

Guilfoyle DN, Blamire A, Chapman B et al. (1989). PEEP – a rapid chemical-shift imaging method. Magn Reson Med 10: 282–287.

Hagmann P, Sporns O, Madan N et al. (2010). White matter maturation reshapes structural connectivity in the late developing human brain. Proc Natl Acad Sci U S A 107: 19067–19072.

Hess AT, Tisdall MD, Andronesi OC et al. (2011). Real-time motion and B0 corrected single voxel spectroscopy using volumetric navigators. Magn Reson Med 66: 314–323.

Hillbom M, Saloheimo P, Fujioka S et al. (2014). Diagnosis and management of Marchiafava-Bignami disease: a review of CT/MRI confirmed cases. J Neurol Neurosurg Psychiatry 85: 168–173.

Hinchey J, Chaves C, Appignani B et al. (1996). A reversible posterior leukoencephalopathy syndrome. N Engl J Med 334: 494–500.

Holshouser BA, Ashwal S, Luh GY et al. (1997). Proton MR spectroscopy after acute central nervous system injury: outcome prediction in neonates, infants, and children. Radiology 202: 487–496.

Isenberg-Grzeda E, Kutner HE, Nicolson SE (2012). Wernicke-Korsakoff-syndrome: under-recognized and under-treated. Psychosomatics 53: 507–516.

Janson CG, McPhee SW, Francis J et al. (2006). Natural history of Canavan disease revealed by proton magnetic resonance spectroscopy (1H-MRS) and diffusion-weighted MRI. Neuropediatrics 37: 209–221.

Kakkar C, Prakashini K, Polnaya A (2014). Acute Marchiafava-Bignami disease: clinical and serial MRI correlation. BMJ Case Rep. pii: bcr2013203442.

Kamran S, Bakshi R (1998). MRI in chronic toluene abuse: low signal in the cerebral cortex on T2-weighted images. Neuroradiology 40: 519–521.

Karunanithi S, Sharma P, Kumar A et al. (2013). 18 F-FDOPA PET/CT for detection of recurrence in patients with glioma: prospective comparison with 18 F-FDG PET/CT. Eur J Nucl Med Mol Imaging 40: 1025–1035.

Kelly MA, Gorelick PB, Mirza D (1992). The role of drugs in the etiology of stroke. Clin Neuropharmacol 15: 249–275.

Kim E, Na DG, Kim EY et al. (2007). MR imaging of metronidazole-induced encephalopathy: lesion distribution and diffusion-weighted imaging findings. AJNR Am J Neuroradiol 28: 1652–1658.

Kim HS, Goh MJ, Kim N et al. (2014). Which combination of MR imaging modalities is best for predicting recurrent glioblastoma? Study of diagnostic accuracy and reproducibility. Radiology 273: 831–843.

Kimura T, Miura T, Aoki K et al. (2015). Familial idiopathic basal ganglia calcification: Histopathologic features of an autopsied patient with an SLC20A2 mutation. Neuropathology. http://dx.doi.org/10.1111/neup.12280.

Kohlschutter A, Bley A, Brockmann K et al. (2010). Leukodystrophies and other genetic metabolic leukoencephalopathies in children and adults. Brain Dev 32: 82–89.

Koutsis G, Karadima G, Panas M (2015). Symptomatic striopallidodentate calcinosis (Fahr's syndrome) in a thalassemic patient with hypoparathyroidism. Ann Hematol 94: 897–899.

Kreis R, Arcinue E, Ernst T et al. (1996). Hypoxic encephalopathy after near-drowning studied by quantitative 1H-magnetic resonance spectroscopy. J Clin Invest 97: 1142–1154.

Kruse JA (2012). Methanol and ethylene glycol intoxication. Crit Care Clin 28: 661–711.

Kruse B, Barker PB, van Zijl PC et al. (1994). Multislice proton magnetic resonance spectroscopic imaging in X-linked adrenoleukodystrophy. Ann Neurol 36: 595–608.

Kumai Y, Toyoda K, Fujii K et al. (2002). Hypertensive encephalopathy extending into the whole brainstem and deep structures. Hypertens Res 25: 797–800.

Kumar S, Mattan NS, de Vellis J (2006). Canavan disease: a white matter disorder. Ment Retard Dev Disabil Res Rev 12: 157–165.

Kurozumi A, Okada Y, Arao T et al. (2013). Extrapyramidal symptoms and advanced calcification of the basal ganglia in a patient with autosomal dominant hypocalcemia. Intern Med 52: 2077–2081.

Lakatos A, Kosta P, Konitsiotis S et al. (2014). Marchiafava-Bignami disease: An acquired callosotomy. Neurology 83: 1219.

Lee VH, Wijdicks EF, Manno EM et al. (2008). Clinical spectrum of reversible posterior leukoencephalopathy syndrome. Arch Neurol 65: 205–210.

Leegwater PA, Vermeulen G, Konst AA et al. (2001). Subunits of the translation initiation factor eIF2B are mutant in leukoencephalopathy with vanishing white matter. Nat Genet 29: 383–388.

Legido A, Zimmerman RA, Packer RJ et al. (1988). Significance of basal ganglia calcification on computed tomography in children. Pediatr Neurosci 14: 64–70.

Lewis E, Lee YY (1986). Computed tomography findings of severe mineralizing microangiopathy in the brain. J Comput Tomogr 10: 357–364.

Li SJ, Jiang L, Fu X et al. (2014). Pallidal index as biomarker of manganese brain accumulation and associated with manganese levels in blood: a meta-analysis. PLoS One 9e93900.

Loes DJ, Hite S, Moser H et al. (1994). Adrenoleukodystrophy: a scoring method for brain MR observations. AJNR Am J Neuroradiol 15: 1761–1766.

Loes DJ, Peters C, Krivit W (1999). Globoid cell leukodystrophy: distinguishing early-onset from late-onset disease using a brain MR imaging scoring method. AJNR Am J Neuroradiol 20: 316–323.

Loes DJ, Fatemi A, Melhem ER et al. (2003). Analysis of MRI patterns aids prediction of progression in X-linked adrenoleukodystrophy. Neurology 61: 369–374.

Long Z, Jiang YM, Li XR et al. (2014). Vulnerability of welders to manganese exposure – a neuroimaging study. Neurotoxicology 45: 285–292.

Macri A, Fleres F, Ieni A et al. (2015). Wernicke encephalopathy as rare complication of cytoreductive surgery and hyperthermic intraperitoneal chemotherapy. Int J Surg Case Rep 16: 29–32.

Mansfield P (1984). Spatial mapping of the chemical shift in NMR. Magn Reson Med 1: 370–386.

Maramattom BV, Zaldivar RA, Glynn SM et al. (2005). Acute intermittent porphyria presenting as a diffuse encephalopathy. Ann Neurol 57: 581–584.

Marchiafava E, Bignami A (1903). Sopra un'alterazione del corpo calloso osservata in soggetti alcoolisti. Riv Patol Nerv Ment 8: 544–549.

Mathews PM, Andermann F, Silver K et al. (1993). Proton MR spectroscopic characterization of differences in regional brain metabolic abnormalities in mitochondrial encephalomyopathies. Neurology 43: 2484–2490.

McEvoy AW, Kitchen ND, Thomas DG (2000). Intracerebral haemorrhage and drug abuse in young adults. Br J Neurosurg 14: 449–454.

McKee AC, Winkelman MD, Banker BQ (1988). Central pontine myelinolysis in severely burned patients: relationship to serum hyperosmolality. Neurology 38: 1211–1217.

Melhem ER, Barker PB, Raymond GV et al. (1999). X-linked adrenoleukodystrophy in children: review of genetic, clinical, and MR imaging characteristics. AJR Am J Roentgenol 173: 1575–1581.

Milhorat TH (1992). Classification of the cerebral edemas with reference to hydrocephalus and pseudotumor cerebri. Childs Nerv Syst 8: 301–306.

Minamimoto R, Saginoya T, Kondo C et al. (2015). Differentiation of brain tumor recurrence from post-radiotherapy necrosis with 11C-methionine PET: visual assessment versus quantitative assessment. PLoS One 10: e0132515.

Moffett JR, Ross B, Arun P et al. (2007). N-Acetylaspartate in the CNS: from neurodiagnostics to neurobiology. Prog Neurobiol 81: 89–131.

Moser HSK, Watkins P, Powers J, Moser A (2000). X-linked adrenoleukodystrophy. McGraw Hill, New York.

Na A, Haghigi N, Drummond KJ (2014). Cerebral radiation necrosis. Asia Pac J Clin Oncol 10: 11–21.

Nakamura Y, Matsuya M, Ikeda K, et al. (2015). A case of Marchiafava-Bignami disease suggesting vasogenic edema. Rinsho Shinkeigaku (in press).

Neudorfer O, Pastores GM, Zeng BJ et al. (2005). Late-onset Tay-Sachs disease: phenotypic characterization and genotypic correlations in 21 affected patients. Genet Med 7: 119–123.

Ni J, Zhou LX, Hao HL et al. (2011). The clinical and radiological spectrum of posterior reversible encephalopathy syndrome: a retrospective series of 24 patients. J Neuroimaging 21: 219–224.

Nicolas G, Pottier C, Charbonnier C et al. (2013). Phenotypic spectrum of probable and genetically-confirmed idiopathic basal ganglia calcification. Brain 136: 3395–3407.

Outteryck O, Devos D, Jissendi P et al. (2010). 4H syndrome: a rare cause of leukodystrophy. J Neurol 257: 1759–1761.

Oz G, Tkac I, Charnas LR et al. (2005). Assessment of adrenoleukodystrophy lesions by high field MRS in non-sedated pediatric patients. Neurology 64: 434–441.

Paidipati Gopalkishna Murthy K (2014). Magnetic resonance imaging in marchiafava-bignami syndrome: a cornerstone in diagnosis and prognosis. Case Rep Radiol 2014: 609708.

Panda AK, Bala K, Bhirud L (2014). Extrapyramidal syndrome. BMJ Case Rep 2014.

Pearson AD, Campbell AN, McAllister VL et al. (1983). Intracranial calcification in survivors of childhood medulloblastoma. Arch Dis Child 58: 133–136.

Phatake R, Desai S, Lodaya M et al. (2014). Posterior reversible encephalopathy syndrome in a patient of organophosphate poisoning. Indian J Crit Care Med 18: 250–252.

Pilo de la Fuente B, Ruiz I, Lopez de Munain A et al. (2008). Cerebrotendinous xanthomatosis: neuropathological findings. J Neurol 255: 839–842.

Posse S, Tedeschi G, Risinger R et al. (1995). High speed 1H spectroscopic imaging in human brain by echo planar spatial-spectral encoding. Magn Reson Med 33: 34–40.

Pouwels PJ, Kruse B, Korenke GC et al. (1998). Quantitative proton magnetic resonance spectroscopy of childhood adrenoleukodystrophy. Neuropediatrics 29: 254–264.

Racette BA (2014). Manganism in the 21st century: the Hanninen lecture. Neurotoxicology 45: 201–207.

Raroque Jr HG, Orrison WW, Rosenberg GA (1990). Neurologic involvement in toxemia of pregnancy: reversible MRI lesions. Neurology 40: 167–169.

Ratai EM, Gonzalez RG (2009). Magnetic resonance spectroscopy and the biochemical basis of neurological disease. In: SW Atlas (Ed.), Magnetic resonance imaging of the brain and spine. Lippincott Williams and Wilkins, Philadelphia, PA.

Ratai E, Kok T, Wiggins C et al. (2008). Seven-Tesla proton magnetic resonance spectroscopic imaging in adult X-linked adrenoleukodystrophy. Arch Neurol 65: 1488–1494.

Ratai E, Caruso P, Eichler F (2012). Advances in MR imaging of leukodystrophies. In: P Bright (Ed.), Neuroimaging – clinical applications. Available online at: http://www.intechopen.com/books/neuroimaging-clinical-applications/advances-in-mr-imaging-of-leukodystrophies.

Reddy K, Westerly D, Chen C (2013). MRI patterns of T1 enhancing radiation necrosis versus tumour recurrence in high-grade gliomas. J Med Imaging Radiat Oncol 57: 349–355.

Rosenberg NL, Kleinschmidt-DeMasters BK, Davis KA et al. (1988). Toluene abuse causes diffuse central nervous system white matter changes. Ann Neurol 23: 611–614.

Ross BD (1991). Biochemical considerations in 1H spectroscopy. Glutamate and glutamine; myo-inositol and related metabolites. NMR Biomed 4: 59–63.

Salen G, Berginer V, Shore V et al. (1987). Increased concentrations of cholestanol and apolipoprotein B in the cerebrospinal fluid of patients with cerebrotendinous xanthomatosis. Effect of chenodeoxycholic acid. N Engl J Med 316: 1233–1238.

Samanta D (2015). Dry beriberi preceded Wernicke's encephalopathy: Thiamine deficiency after laparoscopic sleeve gastrectomy. J Pediatr Neurosci 10: 297–299.

Santos Andrade C, Tavares Lucato L, da Graca Morais Martin M et al. (2010). Non-alcoholic Wernicke's encephalopathy: broadening the clinicoradiological spectrum. Br J Radiol 83: 437–446.

Schaefer PW, Gonzalez RG, Hunter G et al. (2001). Diagnostic value of apparent diffusion coefficient hyperintensity in selected patients with acute neurologic deficits. J Neuroimaging 11: 369–380.

Scheper GC, van der Klok T, van Andel RJ et al. (2007). Mitochondrial aspartyl-tRNA synthetase deficiency causes leukoencephalopathy with brain stem and spinal cord involvement and lactate elevation. Nat Genet 39: 534–539.

Schmahmann JD, Pandya DN, Wang R et al. (2007). Association fibre pathways of the brain: parallel observations from diffusion spectrum imaging and autoradiography. Brain 130: 630–653.

Sechi G, Serra A (2007). Wernicke's encephalopathy: new clinical settings and recent advances in diagnosis and management. Lancet Neurol 6: 442–455.

Srinivasan KG, Praveen Kumar M, Ushanandhini KP et al. (2010a). MRI eye-of-the-tiger sign in organophosphate poisoning. A case report. Neuroradiol J 23: 407–411.

Srinivasan KG, Ramprabananth S, Ushanandhini KP et al. (2010b). Radiation-induced mineralizing microangiopathy in a case of recurrent craniopharyngioma. A case report. Neuroradiol J 23: 412–415.

Sriram K, Lin GX, Jefferson AM et al. (2015). Modifying welding process parameters can reduce the neurotoxic potential of manganese-containing welding fumes. Toxicology 328: 168–178.

Steenweg ME, Vanderver A, Blaser S et al. (2010). Magnetic resonance imaging pattern recognition in hypomyelinating disorders. Brain 133: 2971–2982.

Surendran S, Matalon KM, Tyring SK et al. (2003). Molecular basis of Canavan's disease: from human to mouse. J Child Neurol 18: 604–610.

Suzuki S, Suzuki K, Hirata K (2009). Pictures in clinical medicine. Brain magnetic resonance imaging in chronic trichloroethylene and toluene exposure. Intern Med 48: 861–862.

Takao H, Doi I, Watanabe T (2006). Serial diffusion-weighted magnetic resonance imaging in methanol intoxication. J Comput Assist Tomogr 30: 742–744.

Tamhane AA, Arfanakis K (2009). Motion correction in periodically-rotated overlapping parallel lines with enhanced reconstruction (PROPELLER) and turboprop MRI. Magn Reson Med 62: 174–182.

Tannus A, Garwood M (1997). Adiabatic pulses. NMR Biomed 10: 423–434.

Teke E, Sungurtekin H, Sahiner T et al. (2004). Organophosphate poisoning case with atypical clinical survey and magnetic resonance imaging findings. J Neurol Neurosurg Psychiatry 75: 936–937.

Tisdall MD, Hess AT, Reuter M et al. (2012). Volumetric navigators for prospective motion correction and selective reacquisition in neuroanatomical MRI. Magn Reson Med 68: 389–399.

Torvik A (1985). Two types of brain lesions in Wernicke's encephalopathy. Neuropathol Appl Neurobiol 11: 179–190.

Tsai G, Coyle JT (1995). N-acetylaspartate in neuropsychiatric disorders. Prog Neurobiol 46: 531–540.

Tsai DR, Huang SH, Lin SH (2013). Bilateral striopallidodentate calcinosis secondary to postsurgical hypoparathyroidism. BMJ Case Rep. http://dx.doi.org/10.1136/bcr-2013-200591.

Tzika AA, Ball Jr WS, Vigneron DB et al. (1993). Childhood adrenoleukodystrophy: assessment with proton MR spectroscopy. Radiology 189: 467–480.

Uluc K, Baskan O, Yildirim KA et al. (2008). Leukoencephalopathy with brain stem and spinal cord involvement and high lactate: a genetically proven case with distinct MRI findings. J Neurol Sci 273: 118–122.

van Berge L, Hamilton EM, Linnankivi T et al. (2014). Leukoencephalopathy with brainstem and spinal cord involvement and lactate elevation: clinical and genetic characterization and target for therapy. Brain 137: 1019–1029.

van Der Knaap MS (2005). Magnetic resonance of myelination and myelin disorders, 3rd edition. Springer, New York.

van der Knaap MS, Barth PG, Gabreels FJ et al. (1997). A new leukoencephalopathy with vanishing white matter. Neurology 48: 845–855.

van der Knaap MS, Naidu S, Breiter SN et al. (2001). Alexander disease: diagnosis with MR imaging. AJNR Am J Neuroradiol 22: 541–552.

van der Knaap MS, Leegwater PA, Konst AA et al. (2002). Mutations in each of the five subunits of translation initiation factor eIF2B can cause leukoencephalopathy with vanishing white matter. Ann Neurol 51: 264–270.

van der Knaap MS, van der Voorn P, Barkhof F et al. (2003). A new leukoencephalopathy with brainstem and spinal cord involvement and high lactate. Ann Neurol 53: 252–258.

van der Knaap MS, Salomons GS, Li R et al. (2005). Unusual variants of Alexander's disease. Ann Neurol 57: 327–338.

van der Knaap MS, Ramesh V, Schiffmann R et al. (2006). Alexander disease: ventricular garlands and abnormalities of the medulla and spinal cord. Neurology 66: 494–498.

van der Knaap MS, Linnankivi T, Paetau A et al. (2007). Hypomyelination with atrophy of the basal ganglia and cerebellum: follow-up and pathology. Neurology 69: 166–171.

Wang J, Shao Y, Shi K et al. (2015). Restricted diffusion in the splenium of the corpus callosum in organophosphate induced delayed neuropathy: case report and review of literatures. Int J Clin Exp Med 8: 14246–14250.

Wedeen VJ, Wang RP, Schmahmann JD et al. (2008). Diffusion spectrum magnetic resonance imaging (DSI) tractography of crossing fibers. Neuroimage 41: 1267–1277.

Wenger DA, Suzuki K, Suzuki Y et al. (2001). Galactosylceramide lipidosis: globoid cell leukodystrophy (Krabbe disease). In: CR Schriver, AL Beaudet, WS Sly, D Valle (Eds.), Metabolic and Molecular Bases of Inherited Disease. McGraw-Hill, New York, pp. 3669–3694.

White N, Roddey C, Shankaranarayanan A et al. (2010). PROMO: real-time prospective motion correction in MRI using image-based tracking. Magn Reson Med 63: 91–105.

Wintermark M, Fischbein NJ, Mukherjee P et al. (2004). Unilateral putaminal CT, MR, and diffusion abnormalities secondary to nonketotic hyperglycemia in the setting of acute neurologic symptoms mimicking stroke. AJNR Am J Neuroradiol 25: 975–976.

Wolf NI, Harting I, Boltshauser E et al. (2005). Leukoencephalopathy with ataxia, hypodontia, and hypomyelination. Neurology 64: 1461–1464.

Yahia M, Najeh H, Zied H et al. (2015). Wernicke's encephalopathy: a rare complication of hyperemesis gravidarum. Anaesth Crit Care Pain Med 34: 173–177.

Yamasue H, Abe O, Kasai K et al. (2007). Human brain structural change related to acute single exposure to sarin. Ann Neurol 61: 37–46.

Yong AW, Morris Z, Shuler K et al. (2012). Acute symptomatic hypoglycaemia mimicking ischaemic stroke on imaging: a systemic review. BMC Neurol 12: 139.

Zamora CA, Nauen D, Hynecek R et al. (2015). Delayed posthypoxic leukoencephalopathy: a case series and review of the literature. Brain Behav 5: e00364.

Handbook of Clinical Neurology, Vol. 135 (3rd series)
Neuroimaging, Part I
J.C. Masdeu and R.G. González, Editors

Chapter 30

Imaging of skull base lesions

HILLARY R. KELLY[1]* AND HUGH D. CURTIN[2]

[1]*Department of Radiology, Harvard Medical School and Massachusetts Eye and Ear Infirmary; and Division of Neuroradiology, Massachusetts General Hospital, Boston, MA, USA*

[2]*Department of Radiology, Harvard Medical School and Massachusetts Eye and Ear Infirmary, Boston, MA, USA*

Abstract

Skull base imaging requires a thorough knowledge of the complex anatomy of this region, including the numerous fissures and foramina and the major neurovascular structures that traverse them. Computed tomography (CT) and magnetic resonance imaging (MRI) play complementary roles in imaging of the skull base. MR is the preferred modality for evaluation of the soft tissues, the cranial nerves, and the medullary spaces of bone, while CT is preferred for demonstrating thin cortical bone structure. The anatomic location and origin of a lesion as well as the specific CT and MR findings can often narrow the differential diagnosis to a short list of possibilities. However, the primary role of the imaging specialist in evaluating the skull base is usually to define the extent of the lesion and determine its relationship to vital neurovascular structures. Technologic advances in imaging and radiation therapy, as well as surgical technique, have allowed for more aggressive approaches and improved outcomes, further emphasizing the importance of precise preoperative mapping of skull base lesions via imaging. Tumors arising from and affecting the cranial nerves at the skull base are considered here.

INTRODUCTION

A thorough knowledge of the normal anatomy is essential to radiologic evaluation of the skull base. In certain locations, small lesions can have profound neurologic implications, while in others, lesions can grow to a very large size before coming to clinical attention. Although location and imaging characteristics can often narrow the differential diagnosis down to a few possibilities, the role of the imaging specialist is usually to define the exact margins of the lesion and its relationship to vital neurovascular structures in the skull base. This chapter will focus on the foramina of the skull base, the neurovascular structures that traverse them, and a few major entities that affect these structures. More detailed discussions of differential diagnosis and primary tumors of the clivus, sella, and orbits can be found in other chapters in this volume.

ANATOMY

The skull base is the inferior surface of the cranial vault, made up of five bones, the frontal, ethmoid, sphenoid and occipital bones and the paired temporal bones (Fig. 30.1). The skull base can be divided into three regions: the anterior skull base, central skull base, and posterior skull base. The definitions presented here are based on anatomic references (Lang 1987 a, b, c; Rhoton, 2000 a, b, c, 2002), although these anatomic divisions are not absolute and may vary by institution and in the literature. When used uniformly by a multidisciplinary team in the evaluation of skull base lesions, such divisions can be useful for narrowing the differential diagnosis, as well as planning a surgical approach or radiation therapy.

*Correspondence to: Hillary R. Kelly, MD, Massachusetts General Hospital, Division of Neuroradiology, 55 Fruit St, GRB-273A, Boston MA 02114, USA. Tel: +1-617-726-8320, Fax: +1-617-724-3338, E-mail: hillary.kelly@mgh.harvard.edu

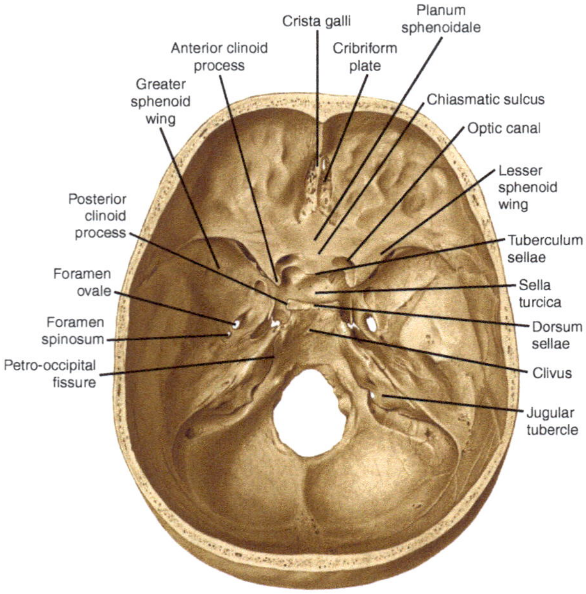

Fig. 30.1. Endocranial view of the skull base.

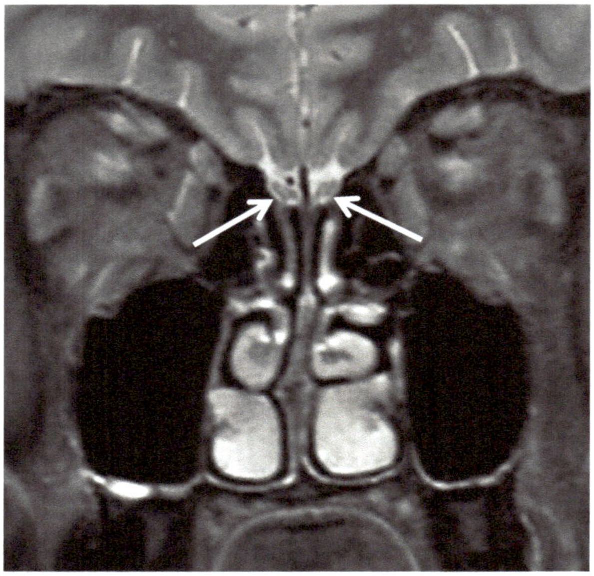

Fig. 30.2. Cranial nerve I. Coronal short tau inversion recovery (STIR) image demonstrating the position of the olfactory nerves (white arrows) along the superior aspect of the cribriform plate.

Anterior skull base

The anterior skull base forms the floor of the anterior cranial fossa and the roof for the nasal cavity, ethmoid sinuses, and orbits. Anteriorly, the anterior skull base is bounded by the frontal bone and posterior walls of the frontal sinuses. Posteriorly, the lesser wings and chiasmatic groove/tuberculum sellae of the sphenoid bone form the boundary between the anterior skull base and the central skull base.

The olfactory bulbs and tracts of cranial nerve I lie along the planum sphenoidale and the cribriform plate of the ethmoid bone, which form the medial part of the anterior cranial fossa (Fig. 30.2). Multiple small perforations in the cribriform plate transmit the fibers of the olfactory nerves from the nasal mucosa to the olfactory bulbs. The foramen cecum is a small pit just anterior to the crista galli that is often closed, but when patent transmits an emissary vein from the nasal cavity to the superior sagittal sinus.

Central skull base

The sphenoid bone forms most of the central skull base. As stated above, the central skull base is divided from the anterior skull base by the lesser wings of the sphenoid laterally and the tuberculum sellae medially. The posterior boundary of the central skull base is formed by the petrous ridges of the temporal bone laterally and the dorsum sellae of the sphenoid medially. The central skull base forms the floor of the middle cranial fossa and the roof of the sphenoid sinus and nasopharynx. There are numerous foramina and fissures in the central skull base and a detailed understanding of their relationships as well as the important adjacent intracranial and extracranial soft-tissue structures is crucial for skull base imaging (Figs 30.1 and 30.3).

The optic canal is formed by the lesser wing of the sphenoid and transmits cranial nerve II (the optic nerve) and the ophthalmic artery. The optic canal is superior to the superior orbital fissure (SOF), formed by a cleft between the lesser and greater wings of the sphenoid. The SOF transmits cranial nerves III, IV, V_1, and VI (oculomotor, trochlear, ophthalmic, and abducens nerves), as well as the superior and inferior ophthalmic veins.

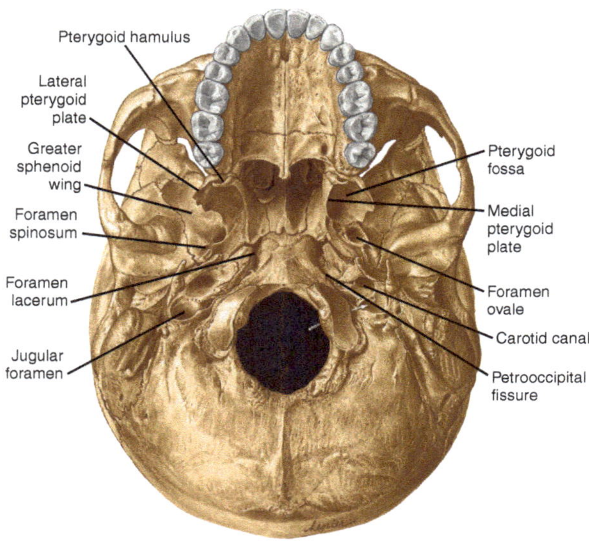

Fig. 30.3. Exocranial view of the skull base.

Together the optic canal and SOF form an important pathway between the intracranial and extracranial compartments at the orbital apex.

The foramen rotundum is found immediately inferior to the SOF and transmits the second division of the trigeminal nerve (V_2), connecting the gasserian ganglion at the inferolateral margin of Meckel's cave to the pterygopalatine fossa (PPF), at the level of the inferior orbital fissure (IOF). The IOF is formed by a cleft between the greater wing of the sphenoid and the body of the maxilla at the orbital floor and transmits the infraorbital artery, vein, and nerve (from V_2). The vidian canal is inferomedial to the foramen rotundum and transmits the vidian artery and nerve, connecting the foramen lacerum posteriorly to the PPF anteriorly. The foramen lacerum is not a true foramen but forms the cartilaginous junction between the sphenoid bone and the petrous apex of the temporal bone. The foramen lacerum forms the medial aspect of the floor of the horizontal petrous internal carotid canal and is also continuous with the petro-occipital fissure (petroclival synchondrosis) posteriorly.

The foramen ovale and foramen spinosum are located within the greater wing of the sphenoid and are oriented almost perpendicular to the foramen rotundum and vidian canal. The foramen ovale transmits the third division of the mandibular nerve (V_3), connecting the Meckel's cave in the middle cranial fossa to the masticator space. The foramen spinosum is located posterolateral to the foramen ovale and transmits the middle meningeal artery and vein.

Posterior skull base

The posterior skull base and posterior cranial fossa are comprised of the temporal bones posterior to the petrous ridges, the body of the sphenoid posteroinferior to the dorsum sellae, and the occipital bone. The temporal bones are often considered separately from the posterior skull base, sometimes referred to as the posterolateral skull base. A detailed discussion of the temporal bone is beyond the scope of this chapter but will be briefly covered here with the remainder of the posterior skull base.

The internal auditory canal (IAC) is located within the petrous temporal bone and transmits cranial nerves VII and VIII, the nervus intermedius and the labyrinthine artery (internal auditory artery), and at times a loop of the anterior inferior cerebellar artery. The stylomastoid foramen is found on the external surface of the posterolateral skull base, between the mastoid tip and the styloid process, and transmits cranial nerve VII from the temporal bone into the parotid gland (Figs 30.3 and 30.4).

The jugular foramen is inferior to the IAC, located at the posterior aspect of the petro-occipital fissure, between the temporal and occipital bones. The jugular foramen is most often described as having two compartments: an anteromedial pars nervosa and a posterolateral pars vascularis, partially separated by bony prominences on opposite surfaces of the temporal and occipital bones, the intrajugular processes. Cranial nerve IX and its tympanic branch (Jacobson nerve) as well as the inferior petrosal sinus typically travel in the medial aspect of the jugular foramen, while cranial nerve X, its auricular branch (Arnold nerve), cranial nerve XI, and the internal jugular vein travel in the lateral aspect. However, the anatomy can be variable and, in some cases, both cranial nerves IX and X travel in the medial aspect. In simplified terms, the nerves and the inferior petrosal sinus travel medially while the internal jugular vein always travels laterally, although the relationship of the nerves to the intrajugular processes can vary. Given this variability, we prefer not to use the terms pars nervosa and pars vascularis. At its exit from the skull

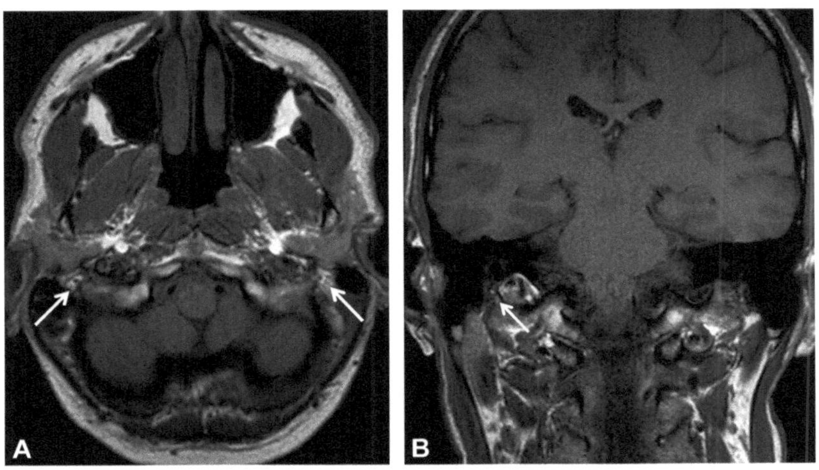

Fig. 30.4. Stylomastoid foramen. Axial (**A**) and coronal (**B**) noncontrast T1-weighted image of the skull base demonstrates normal fat signal in the stylomastoid foramen (arrows).

base, the jugular foramen communicates with the post-styloid parapharyngeal (carotid) space.

The hypoglossal canal is inferomedial to the jugular foramen, located between the jugular tubercle and the condyle of the occipital bone. The hypoglossal canal transmits cranial nerve XII. The occipital bone also forms the foramen magnum centrally, which transmits the medulla oblongata, the ascending portion of cranial nerve XI, and the vertebral arteries.

Extracranial soft tissues

The fat in the soft tissues bordering the extracranial openings of the foramina and fissures of the skull base is especially important in central skull base imaging as this fat provides excellent contrast between normal tissue and lesions. Obliteration of these extracranial fat planes at the skull base is often the earliest sign of involvement by malignant, inflammatory, or infectious processes (Curtin, 1998; Curtin and Hagiwara, 2011; Morani et al., 2011; Moonis et al., 2012).

In the central skull base, there are three major locations that should be evaluated. At the orbital apex, there is sufficient fat between the optic nerve and extraocular muscles to allow for detection of most lesions. A small amount of orbital fat also protrudes through the SOF (cranial nerves (CN) III, IV, V_1, and VI) at the level of the anterior cavernous sinus (Fig. 30.5). The PPF (V_2), mentioned above, is a narrow cleft located posterior to the posterior wall of the maxillary sinus and is also almost entirely filled by fat. This fat-filled space is an extremely important area to evaluate in skull base imaging as it connects with five spaces, creating a potential route of spread of disease processes in the deep face (Fig. 30.6). The PPF connects with the orbit via the IOF, with the infratemporal fossa via the pterygomaxillary fissure, the central skull base and middle cranial fossa via vidian canal and foramen rotundum, the nasal cavity via the sphenopalatine foramen, and the oral cavity via lesser palatine foramina and the pterygopalatine canal leading to the greater palatine foramina. Lastly, there is a layer of fat along the medial margin of the lateral pterygoid muscle that is contiguous with foramen ovale as it exits the skull base (Fig. 30.7). This "trigeminal fat pad" contains V_3 as it enters the masticator space and can be obliterated by disease spread along the mandibular nerve (Curtin and Hagiwara, 2011).

In the posterolateral skull base, the fat at the stylomastoid foramen is an important marker for spread of tumor along cranial nerve VII (Fig. 30.4). Fat also surrounds cranial nerves IX, X, XI, and XII just below the skull base at the jugular foramen and hypoglossal canal.

Intracranial soft tissues

In the central skull base, the majority of the foramina communicate with the cavernous sinus or Meckel's cave. The gasserian ganglion (the convergence of the divisions of cranial nerve V) lies along the inferior lateral aspect of Meckel's cave, with the remainder of this space filled with cerebrospinal fluid. Obliteration of the normal cerebrospinal fluid signal in Meckel's cave is an important marker for disease involving the trigeminal nerve, especially V_2 and V_3.

IMAGING PROTOCOLS AND CONSIDERATIONS

Imaging modalities and protocols

Computed tomography (CT) and magnetic resonance (MR) play complementary roles in imaging evaluation of lesions of the skull base (Chong et al., 2004; Glenn, 2005; Borges, 2008a; Parmar et al., 2009) and are often both required for defining the full extent of disease. CT provides excellent bony anatomic detail and is useful for evaluating the bony margins of the skull base foramina, as well as in diagnosis of primary bony lesions of the

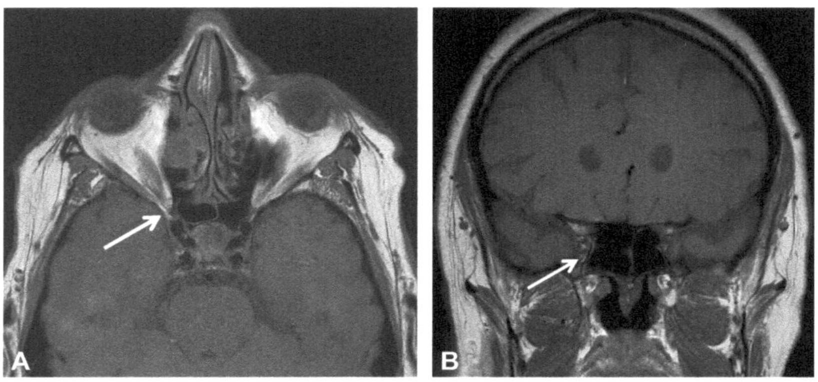

Fig. 30.5. Superior orbital fissure. Axial (**A**) and coronal (**B**) noncontrast T1-weighted images demonstrate normal hyperintense fat signal protruding through the superior orbital fissure towards the anterior cavernous sinus (arrows).

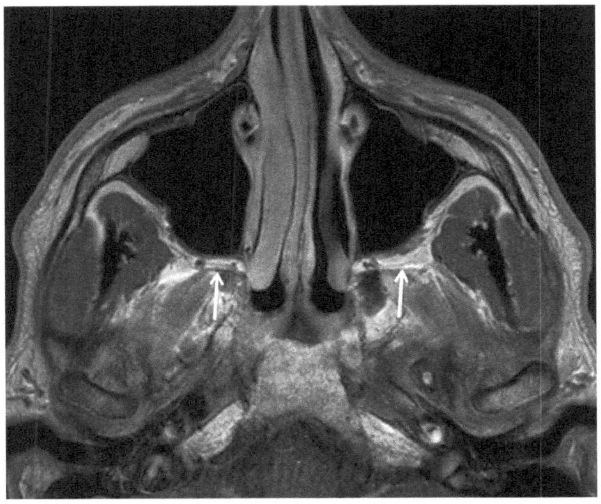

Fig. 30.6. Pterygopalatine fossa. Axial postcontrast T1-weighted image demonstrates normal hyperintense fat signal within the pterygopalatine fossae (arrows).

skull base. CT can also provide information regarding the rate of growth of a lesion and may help categorize disease as aggressive or benign by pattern of growth (Curtin and Chavali, 1998; Borges, 2008a). CT is also superb for evaluating subtle changes in the important fat planes at the extracranial openings of the various foramina. However, MR is usually considered to be the optimum imaging modality for evaluation of the soft tissues, including the cranial nerves, and is important to exclude or evaluate the extent of intracranial pathology. Bone marrow invasion can be seen on MR prior to the erosive changes evident on CT (Tomura et al., 1998; Parmar et al., 2009). MR imaging (MRI) is also key in discriminating between tumor and either benign mucosal thickening or retained sinus secretions when paranasal sinus involvement is suspected (Borges, 2008a; Parmar et al., 2009).

Since the development and widespread use of multidetector CT, a single-volume acquisition in the axial plane is typically obtained (slice thickness of 0.625–1.25 mm), with subsequent creation of multiplanar reformats in soft tissue and bone algorithm as needed (Borges, 2008a; Parmar et al., 2009; Curtin and Hagiwara, 2011). Contrast is typically used when evaluating a mass lesion or the cavernous sinus; however, if the patient is undergoing concurrent MRI, a noncontrast CT may be considered to be sufficient.

MRI can be performed in any plane; however, the axial and coronal planes are most frequently used in skull base imaging. Most protocols include conventional or fast spin-echo T1-weighted images in axial and coronal planes, axial and/or coronal T2-weighted images, and postcontrast T1-weighted images in multiple planes, with or without fat saturation (Borges, 2008a; Curtin and Hagiwara, 2011; Morani et al., 2011). Although many imaging specialists advocate for the use of fat saturation techniques in skull base imaging, caution should be used as susceptibility effect resulting in artifact at the interface between the air in the sphenoid sinus and its bony wall and contiguous soft tissues can obscure the adjacent structures, including the cavernous sinus and foramen rotundum (Fig. 30.8) (Borges, 2008a; Curtin and Cunnane, 2009). An alternative method is to compare nonfat-saturated pre- and postcontrast images with a high-matrix, small field-of-view technique to maximize resolution. The relatively higher T1 signal of fat compared to tumor can usually be differentiated on such high-resolution T1-weighted images with the use of wide windows (Borges, 2008a; Curtin and Cunnane, 2009; Curtin and Hagiwara, 2011). In either case, the imaging

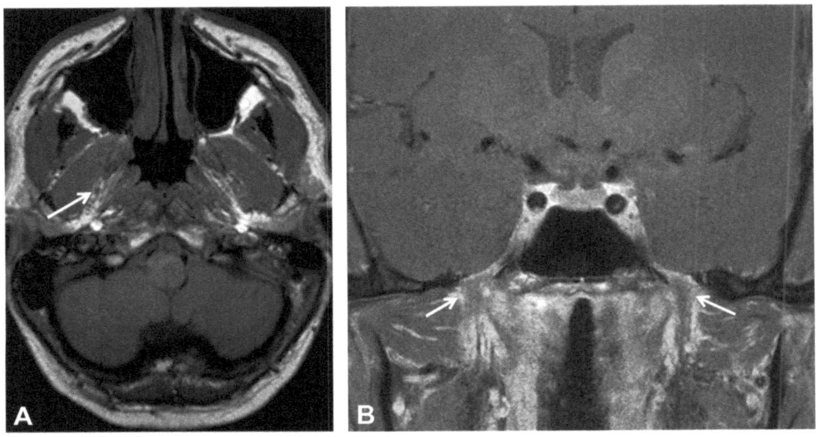

Fig. 30.7. Pterygoid fat pad. Axial (**A**) noncontrast T1-weighted image demonstrates normal hyperintense fat signal surrounding the mandibular nerve (V3) in the pterygoid fat pad (arrow). Coronal (**B**) postcontrast T1-weighted image demonstrates V3 exiting through foramen ovale into the pterygoid fat pad in the masticator space (arrows).

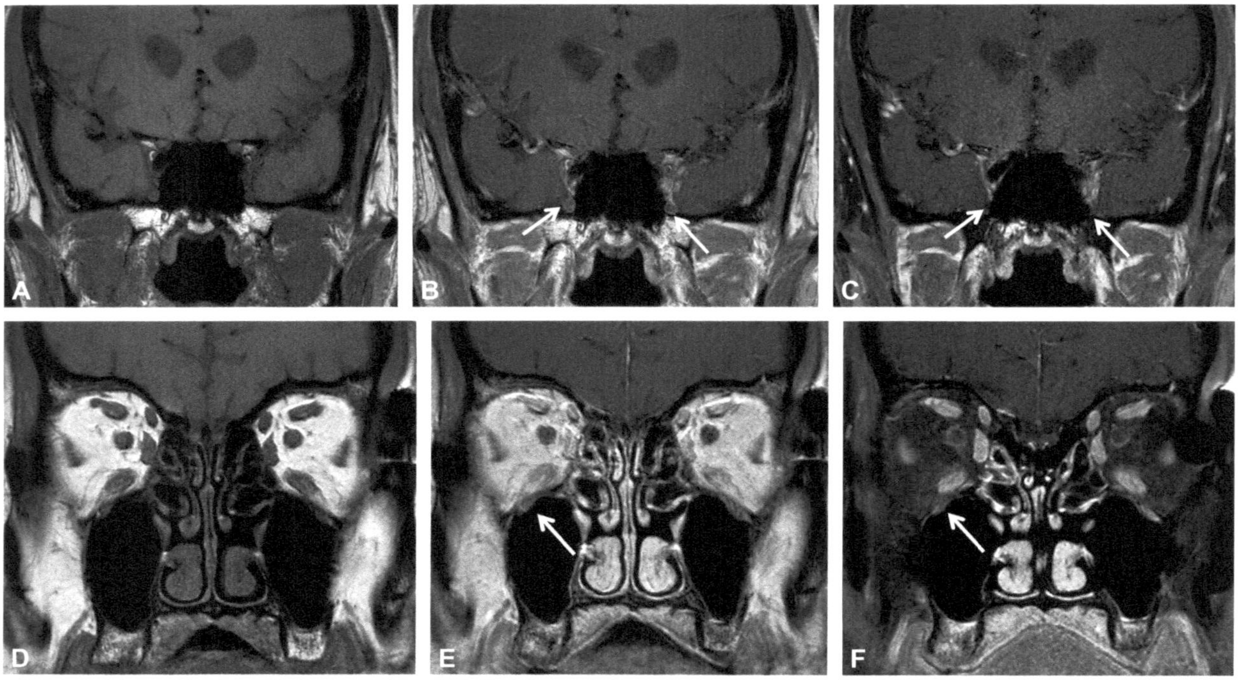

Fig. 30.8. Coronal T1-weighted precontrast (**A** and **D**), T1-weighted postcontrast without fat saturation (**B** and **E**), and T1-weighted postcontrast with fat saturation (**C** and **F**) images through foramen rotundum (**A**, **B**, and **C**) and the infraorbital foramen (**D**, **E**, and **F**). Susceptibility artifact due to the interface between the air in the sphenoid sinus and the adjacent soft tissues obscures V_2 within foramen rotundum bilaterally (arrows: **C**) and V_1 on the right within the infraorbital foramen (arrow: **F**) on the fat-saturated images. The nerves are well seen on the postcontrast T1-weighted images without fat saturation (arrows in **B** and **E**).

specialist must be careful to document that the foramina are well seen.

Fat suppression can be helpful for evaluation of subtle bony involvement of disease at the skull base. Tumor extending into bone can usually be visualized on precontrast T1-weighted imaging, although on the postcontrast T1-weighted images the enhancing tumor may be difficult to differentiate from normal marrow. In this case fat suppression may be helpful in accentuating subtle changes in the marrow. Fat suppression is frequently used with the T2-weighted sequences for the same reason.

Critical imaging questions

Imaging plays a critical role in diagnosis and treatment planning for lesions of the skull base. Advances in imaging techniques and surgical tools over the past few decades have allowed for more aggressive approaches to skull base lesions, with surgeons accessing disease previously thought to be unresectable (Curtin and Chavali, 1998; Glenn, 2005). Adoption of collaborative multidisciplinary team approaches to therapy has also resulted in improved outcomes and prognosis in patients with skull base neoplasms (Durden and Williams, 2001; Borges, 2008a). MR in particular is crucial for precise mapping of tumor extent, both for preoperative purposes and in planning focused high-energy radiation approaches.

The imaging specialist plays a critical role in answering the following questions when evaluating lesions of the skull base: What is the most likely diagnosis? Is the lesion resectable? What are the safe routes to biopsy? Which structures would need to be sacrificed to achieve complete resection? What is the best surgical approach? If radiation therapy is necessary, what are the exact margins of the lesion and what is the relationship to vital neurovascular structures?

TUMORS INVOLVING THE SKULL BASE FORAMINA

As mentioned in the introduction, this chapter is primarily focused on the foramina of the skull base, the major neurovascular structures that traverse them, as well as a few important pathologic entities affecting these structures. We have divided these pathologic entities into tumors arising from nerves, tumor following nerves (perineural tumor spread), and tumors arising outside of nerves and affecting them secondarily.

Neurogenic tumors

SCHWANNOMAS

Schwannomas are benign tumors arising from the nerve sheath composed of differentiated neoplastic Schwann cells (Scheithauer et al., 1999). Schwannomas are the most common primary tumors of the cranial nerves (Zabel et al., 2001) and can arise as sporadic isolated lesions or associated with neurofibromatosis type II. Although they can arise from any nerve, over 90–95% are vestibular schwannomas involving cranial nerve VIII (Zabel et al., 2001). These lesions are discussed in greater detail in another chapter in this volume.

The trigeminal nerve is the second most commonly affected cranial nerve after the vestibular nerve and the most commonly affected nerve in the central skull base (Fishbein and Kaplan, 1999; Borges and Casselman, 2007). Trigeminal schwannomas can arise anywhere along the nerve, from its cisternal segment to the main extracranial branches (Samii et al., 1995; Borges, 2008b; Zhang et al., 2009). Tumors involving both the middle cranial fossa and posterior fossa often have a dumbbell appearance (Fig. 30.9), with an anterior component enlarging the cavernous sinus and the posterior component protruding beneath the tentorium into the posterior fossa (Borges, 2008b; Razek and Castillo, 2009).

Schwannomas arising from cranial nerves IX, X, and XI typically involve the medial aspect of the jugular foramen at the posterior skull base. Hypoglossal schwannomas are also uncommon, but can involve the basiocciput, extending intra- and extracranially. Schwannomas of cranial nerves III, IV, and VI are rare in the absence of neurofibromatosis type II, but can involve the cisternal segments of these nerves, the cavernous sinus, and/or the orbit (Figs 30.10–30.12).

On MRI, schwannomas are typically low to intermediate in signal intensity on T1-weighted imaging, high signal intensity on T2-weighted images, and enhance heterogeneously. When large, these tumors often contain cystic or necrotic components (Fig. 30.9). When extending through neural foramina, they tend to cause smooth bony enlargement rather than erosion, best appreciated by CT. Extracranial extension of trigeminal schwannomas can involve and enlarge the foramen ovale, the foramen rotundum, or the SOF. Enlargement of the facial nerve canal and/or stylomastoid foramen in the temporal bone can be seen with cranial nerve VII schwannomas

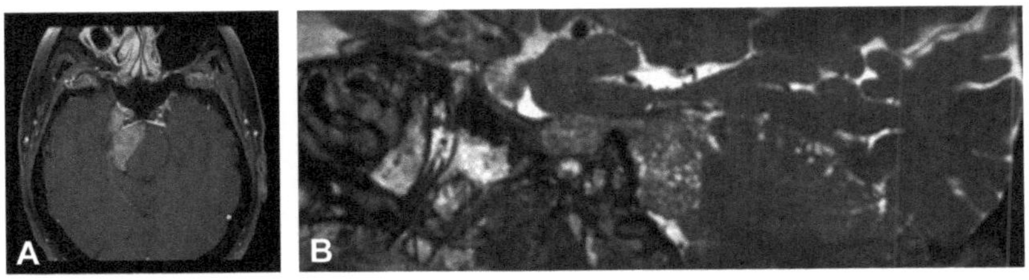

Fig. 30.9. Trigeminal schwannoma. Axial postcontrast T1-weighted fat-saturated image (**A**) demonstrates an enhancing lesion in the right prepontine cistern and extending into Meckel's cave on the right, with mild bulging of the lateral margin of the right cavernous sinus into the right middle cranial fossa. The tumor has a bilobed appearance, also seen on the sagittal high-resolution T2-weighted image (**B**).

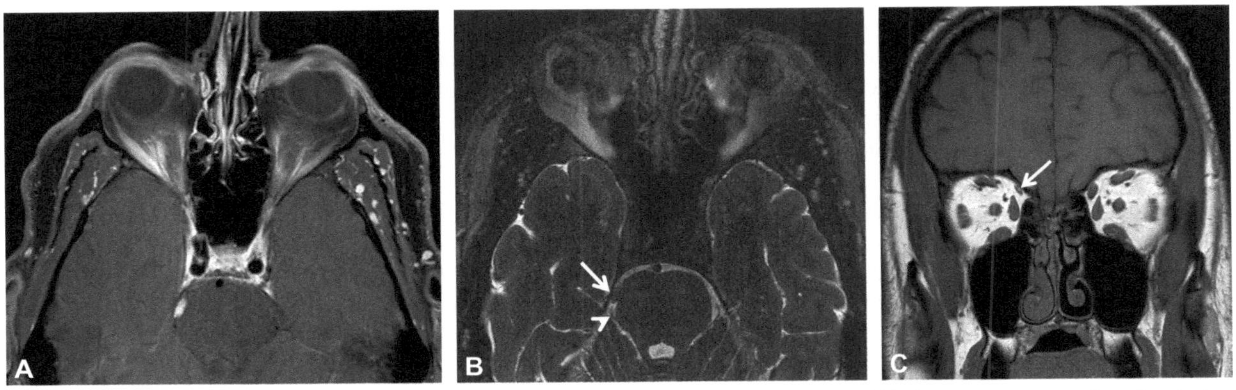

Fig. 30.10. Trochlear schwannoma. Axial postcontrast T1-weighted fat-saturated image (**A**) demonstrates an enhancing lesion along the lateral aspect of the pons. On the axial high-resolution T2-weighted image (**B**), the lesion (arrow) is seen along the course of the cisternal segment of the right trochlear nerve (arrowhead). Atrophy of the right superior oblique muscle (arrow) can be seen on the coronal T1-weighted image (**C**) through the orbits.

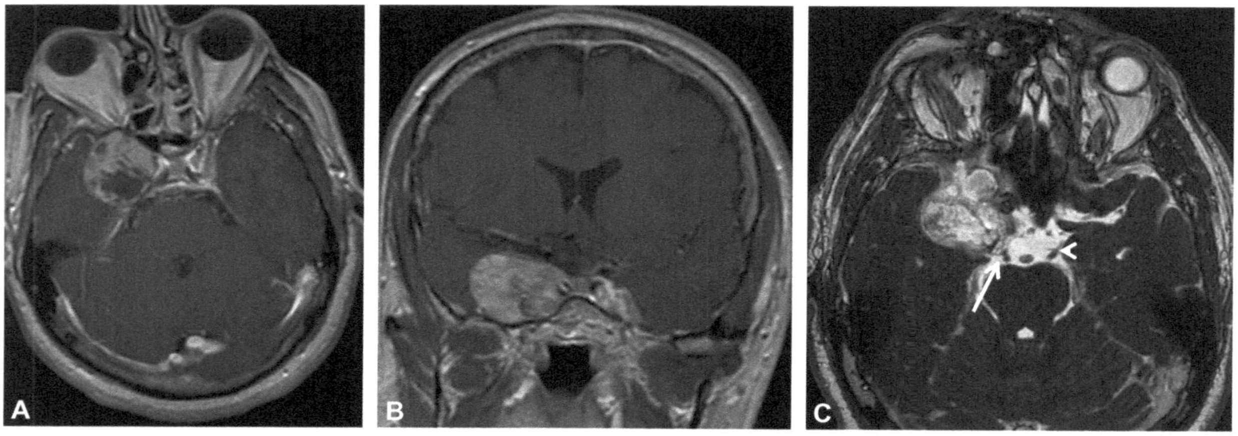

Fig. 30.11. Oculomotor schwannoma. Axial (**A**) and coronal (**B**) postcontrast T1-weighted images demonstrate a heterogeneous enhancing lesion with central nonenhancing cystic components expanding the right cavernous sinus and involving the right middle cranial fossa. Axial high-resolution T2-weighted image (**C**) demonstrates that the lesion involves the right oculomotor nerve, extending to its cisternal segment (arrow). The normal left oculomotor nerve is seen in the prepontine cistern (arrowhead).

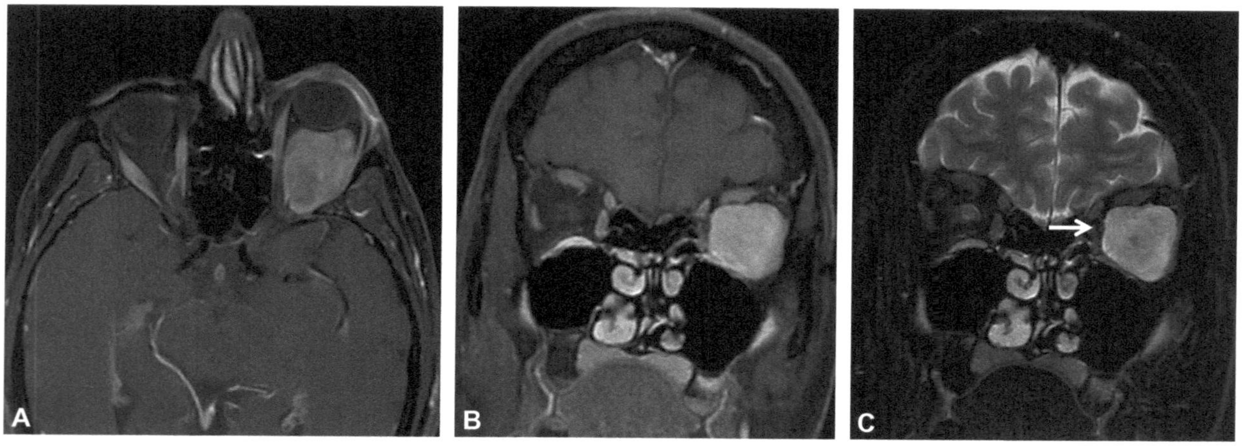

Fig. 30.12. Orbital schwannoma. Axial (**A**) and coronal (**B**) T1-weighted fat-saturated postcontrast images and coronal T2-weighted fat-saturated image (**C**) demonstrating a lobulated enhancing lesion in the left orbit that was separate from and displaced the left optic nerve medially (white arrow). At surgery a schwannoma was found.

(Fig. 30.13). Jugular foramen schwannomas may result in changes of the superolateral jugular tubercle, while slow growth of a hypoglossal schwannoma will typically expand the hypoglossal foramen and undermine the jugular tubercle from below (Fig. 30.14). Extracranial extension through the foramina can efface the important fat pads bordering the skull base foramina. A schwannoma arising from cranial nerves III, IV, or VI may obliterate the fat signal at the SOF. A trigeminal schwannoma can extend through foramen rotundum and efface the fat in the PPF, or, if extending along V_3 through foramen ovale, will efface the fat in the trigeminal fat pad along the lateral pterygoid muscle. Lack of fat signal at the stylomastoid foramen is an important indicator of a tumor involving the extracranial segment of cranial nerve VII (Fig. 30.13B). Lesions of cranial nerves IX, X, XI, or XII may efface the fat surrounding these nerves just inferior to the skull base at the jugular foramen and/or hypoglossal canal.

Denervation fatty muscle atrophy can be seen when imaging schwannomas of the cranial nerves. Unilateral fatty atrophy of the muscles of mastication may be an initial clue to an underlying schwannoma of V_3 (Fig. 30.15). Ipsilateral fatty denervation changes in the tongue can also be seen with hypoglossal schwannomas (Fig. 30.14). Rarely, volume loss can be seen in the extraocular muscles with lesions of cranial nerves III, IV, or VI (Fig. 30.10).

NEUROFIBROMAS

Although schwannomas account for approximately 85% of primary tumors of the cranial nerves (Borges and Casselman, 2007), neurofibromas are the second most

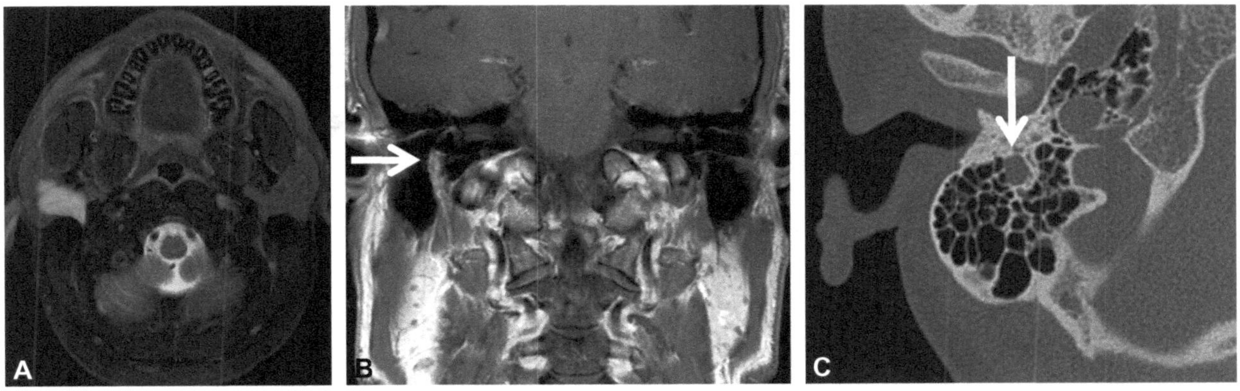

Fig. 30.13. Facial schwannoma. Axial T2-weighted fat-saturated image (**A**) demonstrating a lobulated T2 hyperintense lesion in the right parotid gland extending through the widened right stylomastoid foramen. Enlargement of the facial nerve canal in the mastoid is seen on the coronal postcontrast T1-weighted image (**B**) and the axial CT image (**C**) through the right temporal bone (arrows).

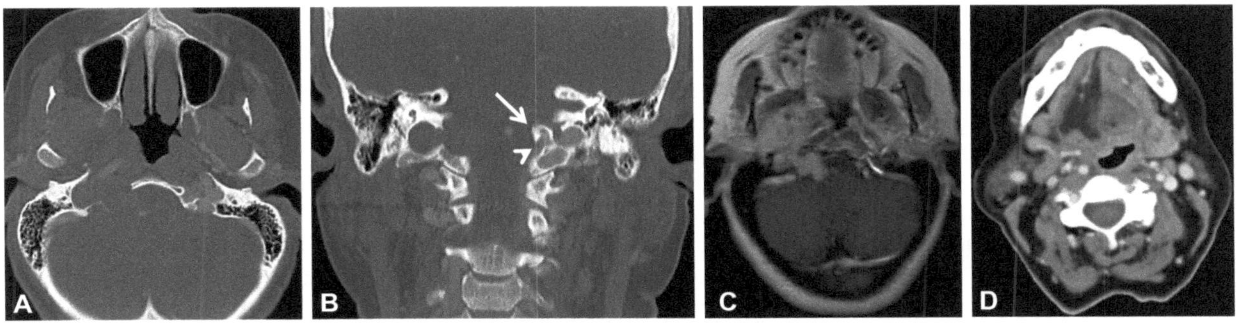

Fig. 30.14. Hypoglossal schwannoma. Axial computed tomography (CT) image (**A**) demonstrates smooth expansion of the right hypoglossal canal. On the coronal CT image (**B**), the right jugular tubercle has been eroded from below; the normal appearance of the hypoglossal canal (arrowhead) and jugular tubercle (arrow) can be seen on the contralateral side. Axial postcontrast T1-weighted image (**C**) demonstrates the enhancing lesion expanding the right hypoglossal canal with large intracranial and extracranial components. Axial CT image (**D**) demonstrates fatty atrophy of the muscles of the right tongue due to hypoglossal paresis.

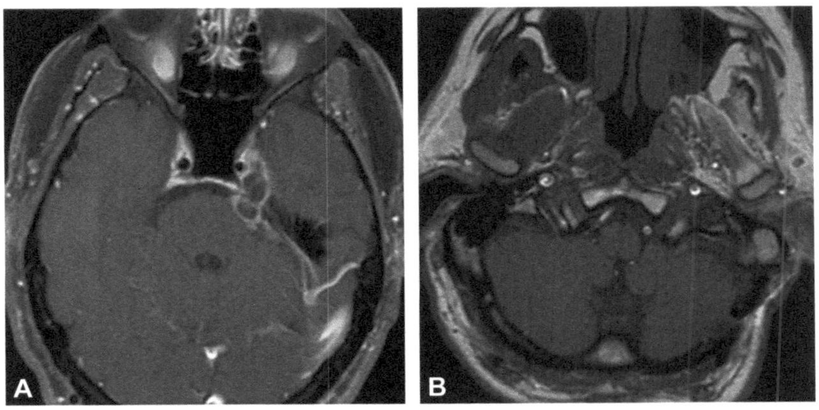

Fig. 30.15. Trigeminal schwannoma. Axial postcontrast T1-weighted fat-saturated image (**A**) demonstrating a heterogeneously enhancing lesion in the left prepontine cistern and left Meckel's cave. Axial noncontrast T1-weighted image (**B**) demonstrates fatty atrophy of the left-sided muscles of mastication.

common tumor of the cranial nerves (Majoie et al., 1999). These lesions are derived from several layers of the nerve sheath including Schwann cells, fibroblasts, and perineural-like cells (Scheithauer et al., 1999). Neurofibromas can affect the cranial nerves sporadically, but are typically seen in the setting of neurofibromatosis type I. Neurofibromas enlarge the nerve and may incorporate axons. At the skull base, neurofibromas

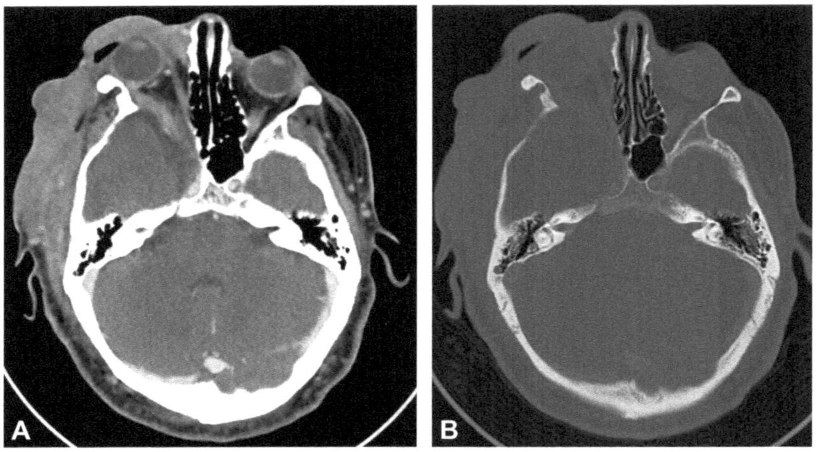

Fig. 30.16. Plexiform neurofibroma. Axial contrast-enhanced computed tomography in soft-tissue (**A**) and bone (**B**) windows demonstrating a large enhancing lesion involving the right face and orbit. Hypoplasia of the right sphenoid wing is also demonstrated, with a large meningocele involving the anterior margin of the right middle cranial fossa.

are typically plexiform and occur almost exclusively in neurofibromatosis type I (Scheithauer et al., 1999). These lesions are infiltrative and unencapsulated, most often involving V_1 and V_2 when occurring in the skull base (Majoie et al., 1999; Razek and Castillo, 2009). Such plexiform neurofibromas can involve the orbit, with enlargement of the SOF and underdevelopment of the greater wing of the sphenoid, which are also characteristic bony findings of neurofibromatosis type I (Fig. 30.16) (Curtin et al., 2011).

Malignant peripheral nerve sheath tumors

Malignant schwannomas of the skull base have been reported in the literature but are extremely rare (Majoie et al., 1999). Plexiform neurofibromas can undergo malignant degeneration, with a 10% lifetime risk of malignant peripheral nerve sheath tumors in patients with neurofibromatosis type I (Bredella et al., 2007).

Perineural tumor spread

Tumors of the head and neck can spread via the cranial nerves into and through the skull base. The term "perineural tumor spread" (PNS) must be distinguished from the term "perineural invasion," which is a histologic finding at the primary tumor site. PNS follows the nerve itself into the skull base, allowing for distant spread of tumor, with an impact on prognosis and treatment approach (Curtin, 1998; Moonis et al., 2012). Salivary malignancies, especially adenoid cystic carcinoma, are the most common primary tumors; however, this pattern of spread has also been described with squamous cell carcinoma, nasopharyngeal carcinoma, desmoplastic melanoma, myeloma, leukemia, and lymphoma (Curtin and Cunnane, 2009; Moonis et al., 2012).

PNS typically involves the second and third divisions of the trigeminal nerve and the descending mastoid segment of the facial nerve, though other nerves may be involved (Ginsberg, 1999; Moonis et al., 2012). Cutaneous malignancies of the nose or cheek can involve V_2 via the infraorbital nerve. Primary tumors of the maxillary sinuses may spread to the PPF and V_2 via the retromaxillary fat pad. Spread to the PPF and V_2 can occur from primary palate lesions that travel along the greater and lesser palatine nerves. Tumors of the retromolar trigone, oral cavity, or mandible can gain access to V_3 via the inferior alveolar nerve or the lingual nerve. Parotid malignancies can also spread to V_3 via the auriculotemporal nerve, which travels within this salivary gland just posterior to the mandibular ramus. Nasopharyngeal carcinoma can invade directly into the PPF with subsequent involvement of V_2 or can invade the masticator space and involve V_3. (In our experience, involvement of the cranial nerves by nasopharyngeal carcinoma is often due to direct extension rather than PNS.) PNS along the facial nerve is typically due to tumors arising in the parotid gland (Ginsberg, 1999; Moonis et al., 2012).

Connections exist between cranial nerves V and VII that facilitate spread from one cranial nerve to another (Moonis et al., 2012). The greater superficial petrosal nerve is a branch of the facial nerve that exits the temporal bone and passes near Meckel's cave before joining the deep petrosal nerve to form the vidian nerve and continuing into the PPF. PNS spread along trigeminal branches reaching either the PPF or Meckel's cave can spread in a retrograde fashion to the facial nerve via this pathway. The auriculotemporal nerve arises from V_3 just inferior to foramen ovale at the skull base. This nerve travels along the posterior margin of the mandible and communicates via its rami with branches of the facial nerve in the parotid gland. PNS can occur from V to VII or vice versa within the parotid gland (Moonis et al., 2012).

MR is more sensitive for detection of PNS, although findings at CT can include obliteration of the fat planes adjacent to the skull base foramina, specifically the PPF, the pterygoid or trigeminal fat pad, and the stylomastoid foramen (Fig. 30.17). Effacement of these fat planes and foraminal enlargement can also be seen by MR (Fig. 30.18); however, more subtle findings include nerve enlargement and enhancement (Moonis et al., 2012). Additional MR findings include effacement of the fluid signal in Meckel's cave, bulging of the walls of the cavernous sinus, and/or enhancement of the nerves running through these structures (Fig. 30.18). Once tumor reaches the PPF, cavernous sinus, or Meckel's cave, it can spread in an antegrade fashion along the other branches of the trigeminal nerve or facial nerve, or may extend retrograde towards the pons (Fig. 30.19). The nerves should be evaluated in their entirety, as skip lesions can occur.

Tumors with secondary involvement of the cranial nerves

Many tumors can arise at the skull base and involve the nerves secondarily. Although space does not permit an extensive review of these lesions, the major entities are discussed here.

Meningiomas

Meningiomas are the most common nonglial brain tumors and are covered in detail in another chapter in this volume. This section will focus on meningiomas of the skull base that affect the cranial nerves.

Meningiomas arise from meningothelial arachnoid cells (arachnoid "cap" cells) and are most common along the cerebral convexities or parasagittally (Buetow et al., 1991; Curtin et al., 2011). However, approximately 20% of meningiomas involve the skull base and tend to be symptomatic due to proximity and compression of the adjacent cranial nerves or vascular structures (McGregor and Sarkar, 2009). Meningiomas of the skull base can either arise intracranially and extend through neural foramina or can arise directly from the arachnoid cells that accompany the cranial nerves along their nerve sheaths (Sanna et al., 2007). Rarely, meningiomas can arise extradurally, presumably also due to arachnoid cells along cranial nerve sheaths or due to ectopic cells left behind during development. Extradural meningiomas have been reported to arise in the outer table of the skull and overlying skin, the intradiploic space, inside the paranasal sinuses, the parotid gland, and the parapharyngeal space (Buetow et al., 1991).

In the anterior cranial fossa, meningiomas arising along the planum sphenoidale may cause olfactory symptoms (Fig. 30.20). More posteriorly, lesions that arise along the tuberculum sellae or chiasmatic sulcus can cause visual symptoms or pituitary dysfunction. Meningiomas in the medial middle cranial fossa are also prone to result in visual symptoms, involving the optic nerve directly or due to involvement of the cavernous sinus and the cranial nerves that traverse it (Fig. 30.21). Tumors of the sphenoid bone can also involve Meckel's cave and affect the trigeminal nerve (Fig. 30.22). In the posterior skull base, meningiomas can arise at the jugular foramen or foramen magnum, with associated cranial neuropathies of cranial nerves IX, X, XI, and/or XII.

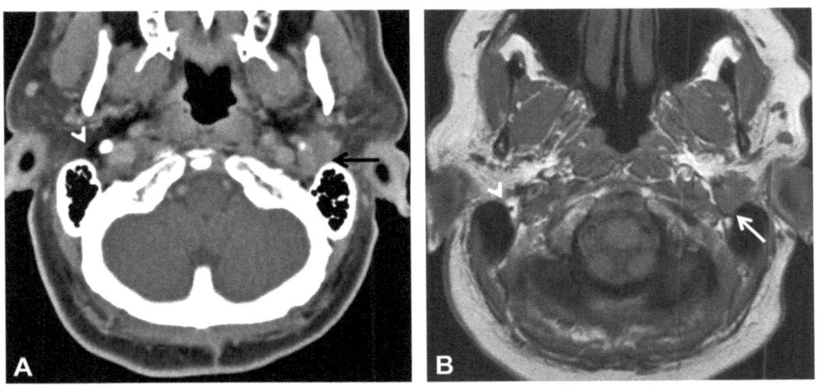

Fig. 30.17. Perineural spread of tumor along cranial nerve VII. Axial contrast-enhanced computed tomography of the skull base (**A**) and axial precontrast T1-weighted (**B**) images demonstrate a nodular lesion in the left parotid gland extending into the stylomastoid foramen (arrows). Normal fat density/intensity is seen in the right stylomastoid foramen (arrowheads). The primary tumor was an adenoid cystic carcinoma arising in the left parotid gland with perineural spread of tumor into the mastoid segment of the left facial nerve.

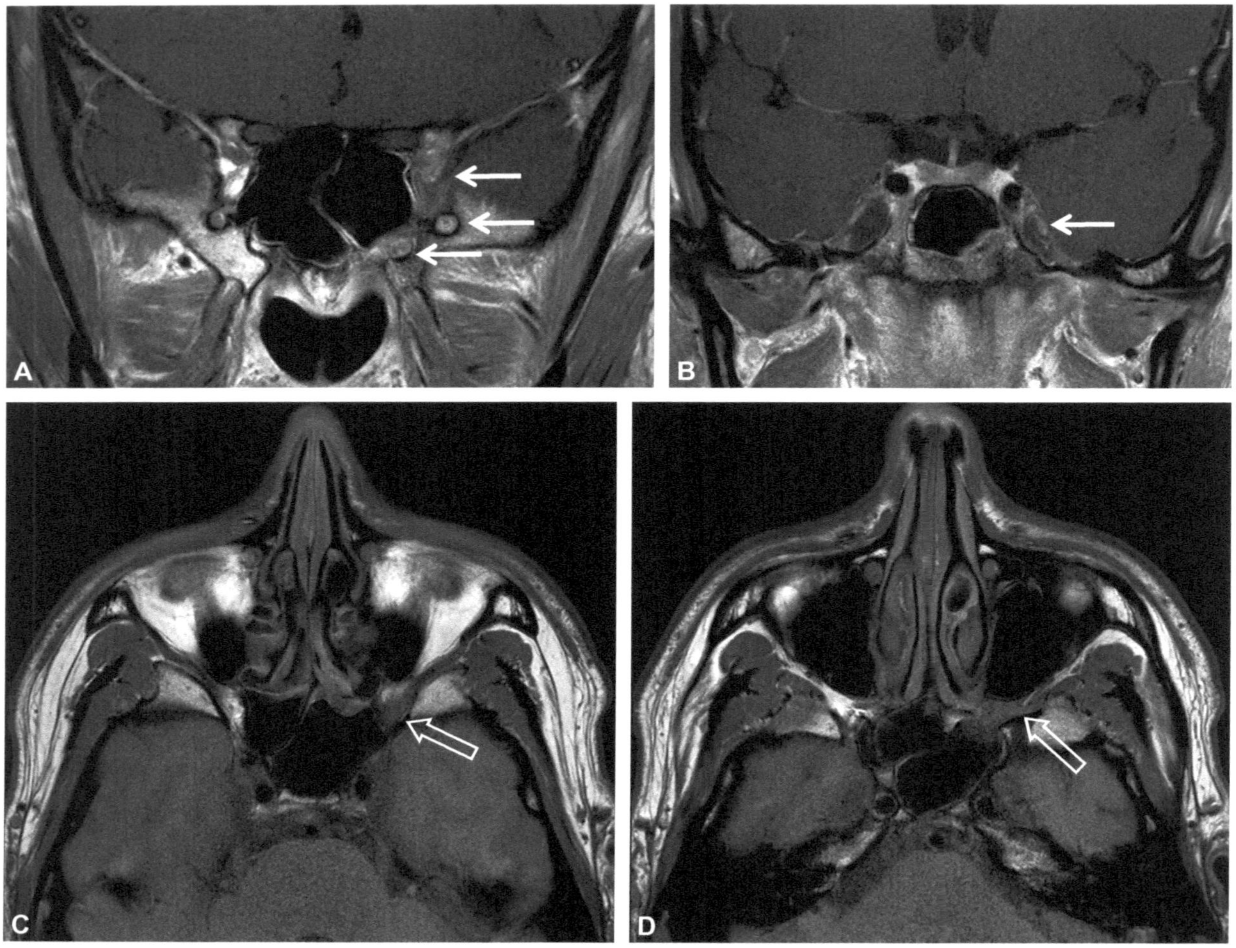

Fig. 30.18. Perineural spread of adenoid cystic carcinoma arising in the palate. Coronal postcontrast T1-weighted images demonstrate enlargement and enhancement within superior orbital fissure, foramen rotundum, and vidian canal on the left (arrows: **A**), with extension along V2 into Meckel's cave on the left (arrow: **B**). Axial precontrast T1-weighted images in the same patient demonstrate effacement of the normal fat at the superior orbital fissure (open arrow: **C**) and pterygopalatine fossa (open arrow: **D**) on the left.

On noncontrast CT, meningiomas are hyperdense and may demonstrate calcifications. The soft-tissue components of the tumor will enhance after contrast administration. Hyperostosis of the adjacent bone is more commonly seen than other patterns of bony change and is highly suggestive of a meningioma. Tumors involving the neural foramina can mimic nerve sheath tumors due to enlargement of the foramina; however, a permeative sclerotic pattern of bony foraminal involvement is more suggestive of a meningioma. Upward "blistering" of the planum sphenoidale and/or pneumosinus dilatans of the sphenoid sinus (enlargement of the sinus adjacent to the tumor) can occur with planum sphenoidale tumors (Fig. 30.23) (Curtin et al., 2011).

On MR, meningiomas are typically hypo- or isointense to the brain parenchyma on T1- and T2-weighted images and typically enhance avidly after contrast administration. An enhancing "dural tail" can be seen along the margins of the tumor. When involving the cavernous sinus, a meningioma will typically enhance less avidly than the uninvolved venous sinus (Curtin et al., 2011).

MR or CT angiography may be performed to assess the effect of the tumor on the internal carotid artery, as meningiomas of the central skull base may encase and narrow this vessel (Fig. 30.24). As mentioned above, extradural meningiomas have been reported to arise within the parapharyngeal space, although primary extracranial meningiomas in this location are very rare. Extradural meningiomas arising at the vagus nerve can be predominantly extracranial, with mass effect on the internal carotid artery and internal jugular vein in the poststyloid parapharyngeal space inferior to the skull base (Fig. 30.25).

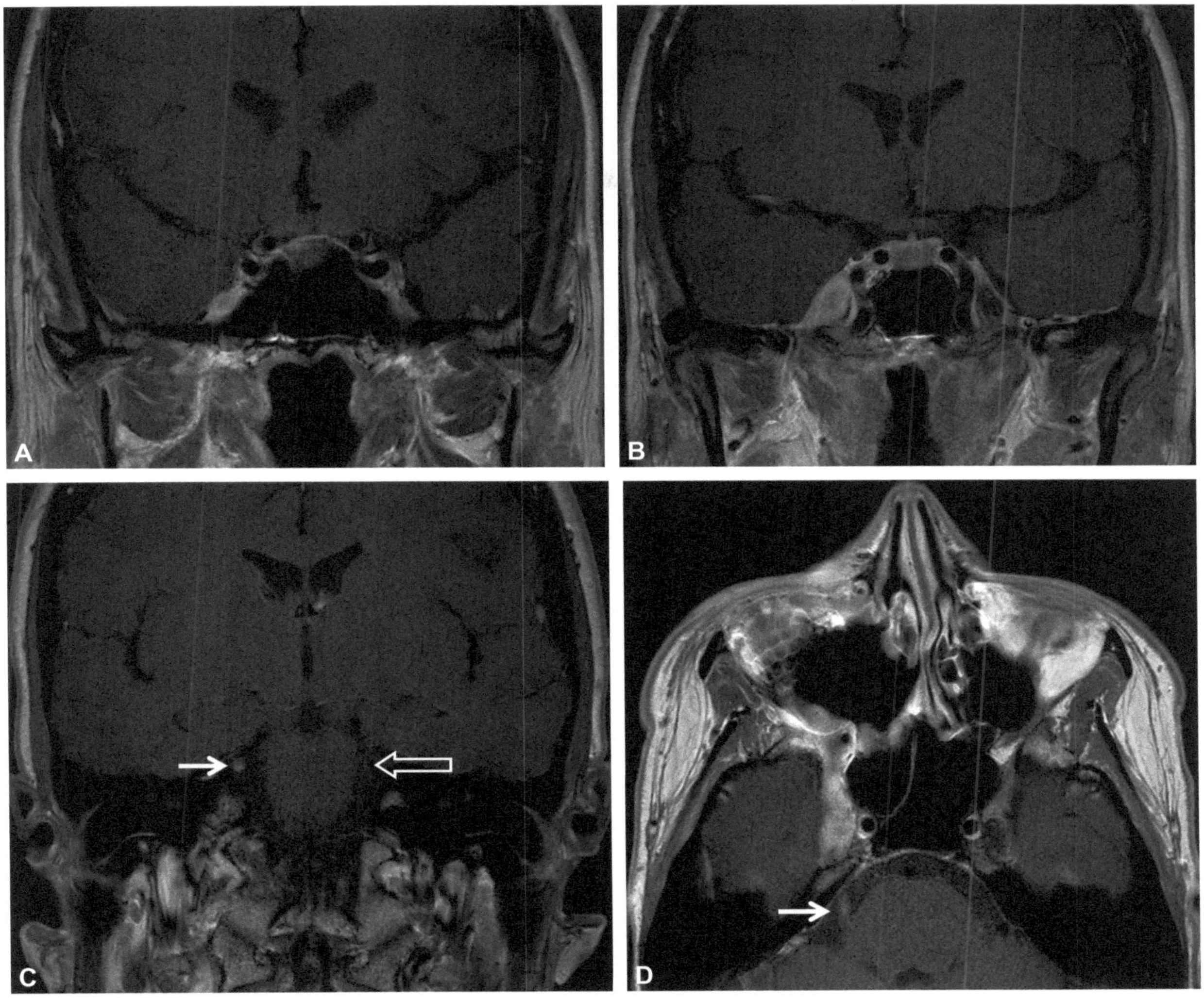

Fig. 30.19. Coronal (**A**, **B**, and **C**) and axial (**D**) T1-weighted postcontrast images in a patient with a low-grade sarcoma of the floor of the orbit demonstrate expansion and enhancement within foramen rotundum (**A**, **D**) and Meckel's cave (**B**, **D**) consistent with perineural spread of tumor. Retrograde spread of tumor continued along the cisternal segment of cranial nerve V (arrows: **C** and **D**). The normal nonenhancing cisternal segment of cranial nerve V on the left is faintly seen in **C** (open arrow).

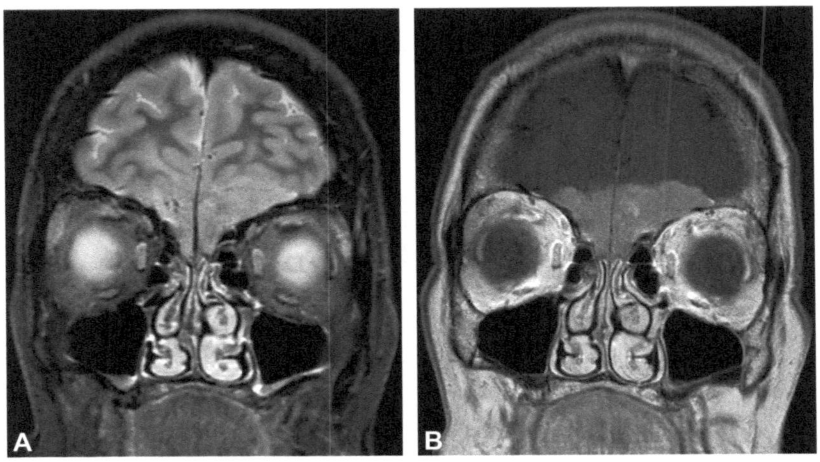

Fig. 30.20. Planum sphenoidale meningioma. Coronal T2-weighted fat-saturated (**A**) and T1-weighted postcontrast (**B**) images demonstrate an extra-axial enhancing lesion abutting the cribriform plate, with mass effect on the adjacent inferior frontal lobes. The olfactory nerves are not seen and are likely compressed by this meningioma.

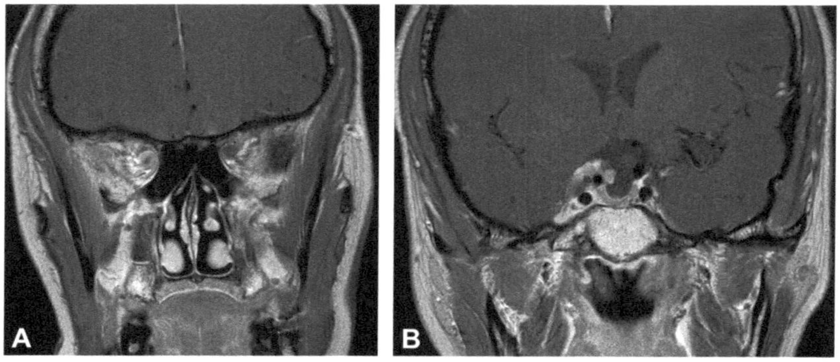

Fig. 30.21. (**A**, **B**) Meningioma of the optic nerve sheath, cavernous sinus, and Meckel's cave. Coronal T1-weighted postcontrast images demonstrate an enhancing lesion circumferentially surrounding the right optic nerve in the orbit. The right optic nerve is much smaller in caliber than the left due to compression. This meningioma also involved the right cavernous sinus and Meckel's cave.

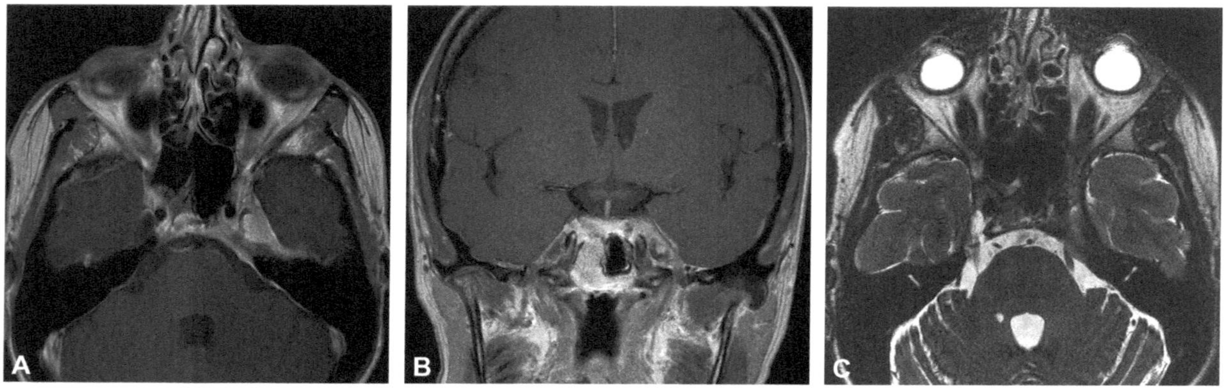

Fig. 30.22. Meningioma. Axial (**A**) and coronal (**B**) postcontrast T1-weighted images demonstrate an enhancing lesion involving Meckel's cave on the left, with enhancing dural tails extending along the tentorium and left middle cranial fossa. The lesion extended up to, but not through, foramen ovale on the left. Axial high-resolution T2-weighted image (**C**) demonstrates loss of the normal fluid signal in Meckel's cave on the left due to the meningioma.

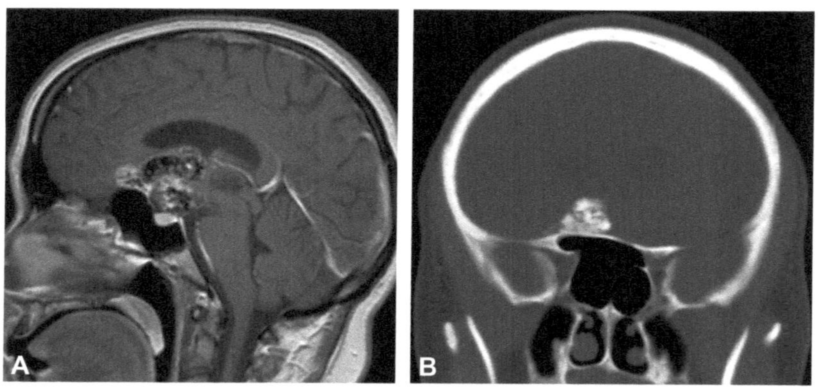

Fig. 30.23. (**A**, **B**) Pneumosinus dilatans. Sagittal postcontrast T1-weighted image demonstrates a heterogeneously enhancing extra-axial lesion (meningioma) centered along the dorsum sellae, with upward bulging ("blistering") of the roof of the sphenoid sinus. Coronal computed tomography demonstrates that the lesion is heavily calcified and the sphenoid sinus extends superiorly over the right superior orbital fissure.

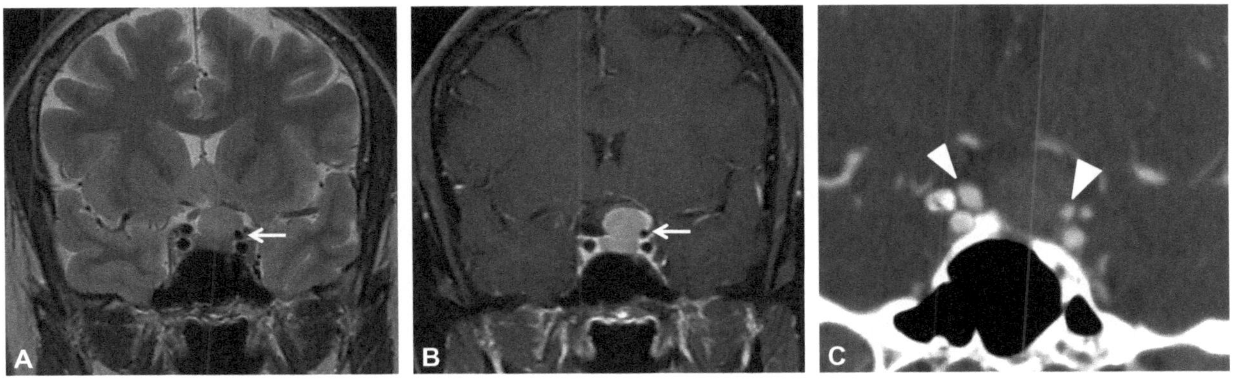

Fig. 30.24. Suprasellar meningioma. Coronal T2-weighted (**A**) and T1-weighted fat-saturated postcontrast (**B**) images demonstrate a homogeneously enhancing lesion in the sella and suprasellar cistern partially encasing and narrowing the left cavernous carotid artery flow void (arrows). Coronal reformatted image from a computed tomography angiogram (**C**) demonstrates the marked asymmetry in caliber of the cavernous internal carotid arteries (arrowheads).

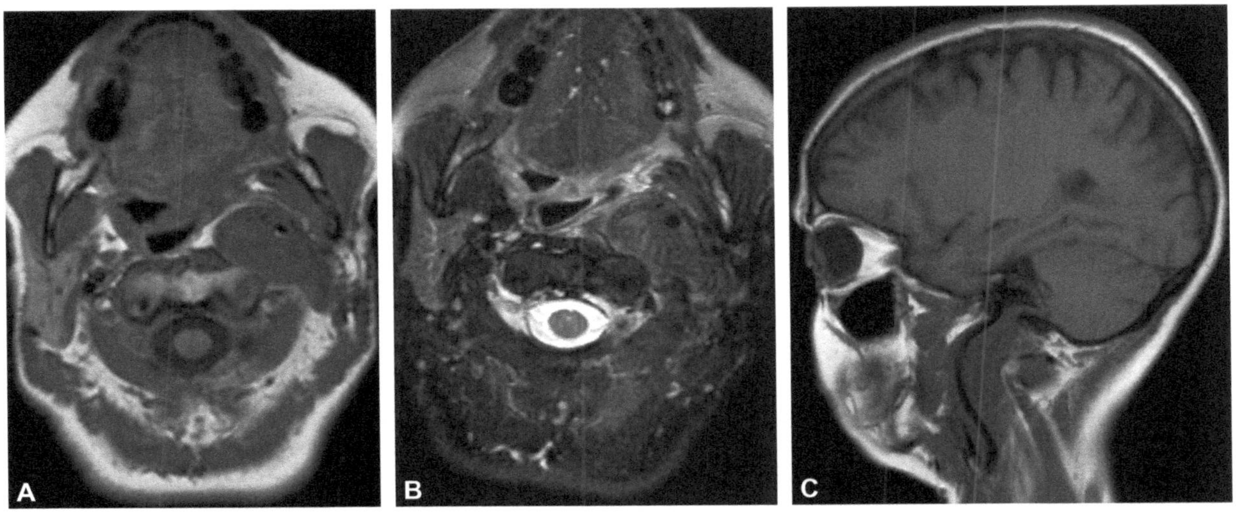

Fig. 30.25. Jugular foramen meningioma with a large extracranial component. Axial precontrast T1-weighted (**A**) and postcontrast T1-weighted fat-saturated (**B**) images demonstrate a heterogeneously enhancing lesion in the left poststyloid parapharyngeal space that encases the left internal carotid artery and displaces it anterolaterally. The sagittal precontrast T1-weighted image (**C**) demonstrates that the lesion is contiguous with the jugular foramen but is predominantly extracranial.

Paragangliomas

Paragangliomas (also called "glomus tumors") are highly vascular tumors arising from paraganglionic cells of neural crest origin, many of which are distributed along the cranial nerves and their branches (Rao et al., 1999; Borges and Casselman, 2007). At the skull base the most common sites of involvement are the jugular foramen, the middle ear, and along the vagus nerve (Rao et al., 1999; Boedeker et al., 2005). With the exception of paragangliomas of cranial nerve X, these lesions are extrinsic to the cranial nerves and deficits tend to occur late in the disease course (Rao et al., 1999; Borges and Casselman, 2007). Glomus vagale paragangliomas are associated with a higher rate of cranial neuropathies than paragangliomas arising elsewhere in the head and neck (Rao et al., 1999; Zanoletti and Mazzoni, 2006; Lozano et al., 2008).

The characteristic imaging features of this tumor are largely due to hypervascularity, with intense homogeneous enhancement on both CT and MR. Vascular flow voids can also be seen as hypointense structures within the lesion on T2-weighted images. In contrast to schwannomas and meningiomas, paragangliomas involving the jugular foramen and adjacent skull base tend to demonstrate a more aggressive or infiltrative pattern of bony erosion, often described as a "moth-eaten"

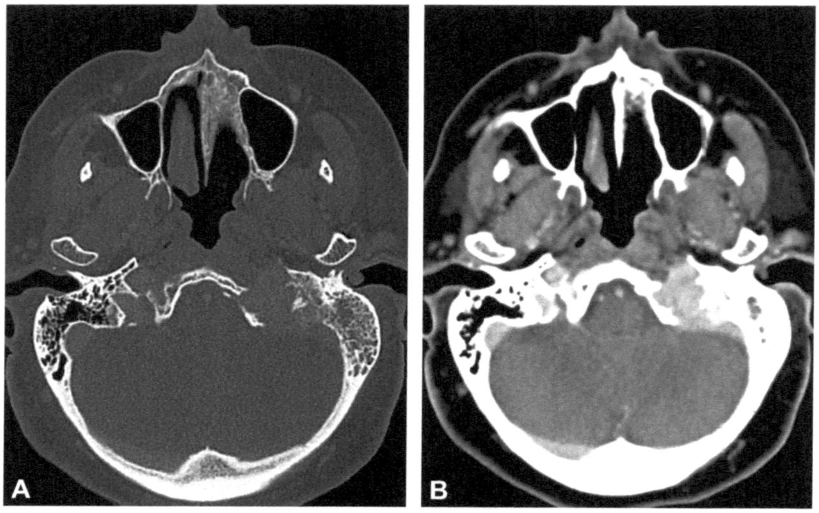

Fig. 30.26. (**A**, **B**) Glomus jugulare. Axial computed tomography images demonstrate an enhancing lesion centered in the left jugular foramen. The bony margins are irregular with an eroded permeative pattern typical of paragangliomas.

appearance (Fig. 30.26) (Rao et al., 1999; Borges and Casselman, 2007).

Paragangliomas of the vagus nerve (glomus vagale) are reported to occur at two sites: at the inferior (nodose) ganglion, typically appearing as a spindle-shaped mass within the poststyloid parapharyngeal space, compressing the internal jugular vein, displacing the internal carotid artery anteromedially and the lateral pharyngeal wall medially, with minimal skull base destruction; while lesions at the superior (jugular) ganglion have been described as "dumbbell-shaped," extending superiorly into the posterior fossa and inferiorly into the poststyloid parapharyngeal space, with a "waist" at the enlarged jugular foramen (Rao et al., 1999; Borges and Casselman, 2007), although in our experience this appearance is rare.

In the middle ear and jugular foramen paragangliomas are thought to arise from three discrete bodies that are anatomically related to the tympanic branch of the glossopharyngeal nerve (Jacobson nerve), the auriculotemporal branch of the vagus nerve (Arnold nerve), or the jugular bulb (Rao et al., 1999; Borges and Casselman, 2007). Glomus tympanicum tumors are confined to the middle ear (Fig. 30.27), while glomus jugulare tumors involve the jugular foramen. Almost all glomus jugulare tumors involve both the middle ear and jugular foramen and so the term glomus jugulotympanicum is often preferred (Fig. 30.28). The key finding is erosion or demineralization of the lateral plate of the jugular foramen. With a glomus tympanicum, the jugular plate is intact. The most common location is in the

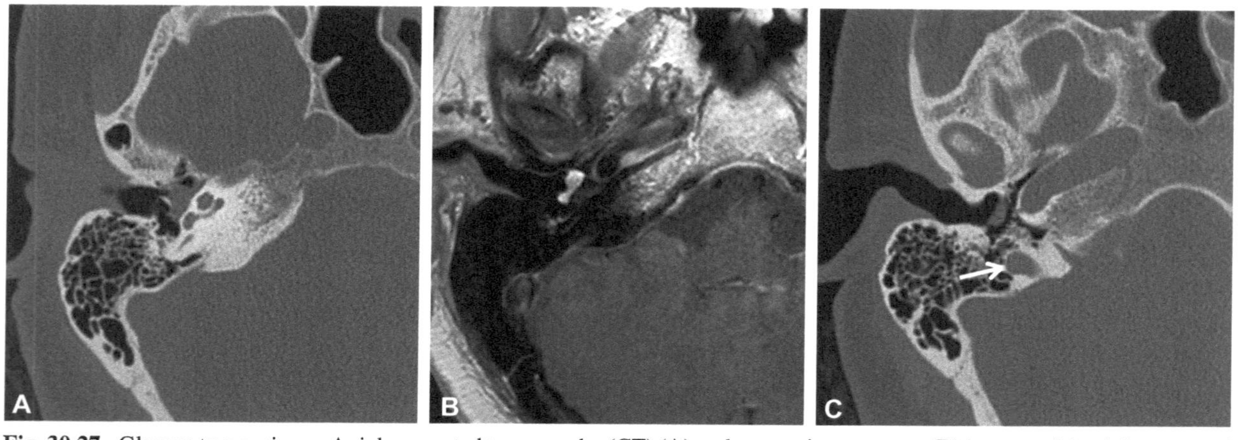

Fig. 30.27. Glomus tympanicum. Axial computed tomography (CT) (**A**) and magnetic resonance (**B**) images of the right temporal bone demonstrate a lobulated lesion centered on the cochlear promontory that avidly enhances. Axial CT image (**C**) at a slightly more inferior level confirms that the lesion is confined to the middle ear and the lateral jugular plate is intact (arrow).

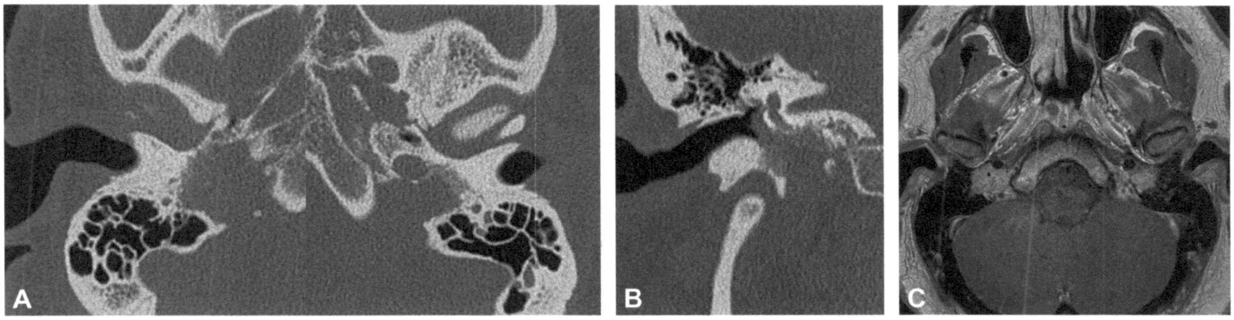

Fig. 30.28. Glomus jugulotympanicum. Axial computed tomography (CT) images of the right and left temporal bones (**A**) demonstrate erosive permeative changes at the jugular foramina bilaterally. Coronal CT of the right temporal bone (**B**) demonstrates that the right lesion involves the right middle-ear cavity with loss of the lateral jugular plate. Axial postcontrast T1-weighted image (**C**) demonstrates enhancing lesions involving the jugular foramina bilaterally in this patient with bilateral glomus jugulotympanicum tumors.

middle ear along the cochlear promontory (Fig. 30.27). Regardless of the terms used, the extent of tumor must be well delineated as the surgical approaches to these lesions vary greatly (Borges and Casselman, 2007).

Involvement of cranial nerve VII is most often due to invasion by large paragangliomas arising from the middle ear or jugular foramen. Rarely, primary paragangliomas can arise from the facial nerve itself (glomus faciale), typically within the descending facial nerve canal in the mastoid (Kania et al., 1999; Wippold et al., 2004), although there are also reports of lesions involving the labyrinthine and geniculate segments (Mafee et al., 2000).

Lesions that appear to arise in bone

Lesions arising in bone at the skull base can secondarily involve the cranial nerves. As all regions of the skull base contain bone, many osseous lesions may involve any of the anatomic compartments discussed previously. These include fibrous dysplasia, Paget disease, metastases, plasmacytomas, non-Hodgkin's lymphoma, giant cell lesions, Langherhans cell histiocytosis, and aneurysmal bone cysts.

Fibrous dysplasia is a disorder of bone involving abnormal development and formation of fibroblasts resulting in abnormal mineralization and expansion (Hullar and Lustig, 2003). These expansile lesions may involve and narrow the neural foramen and can compromise cranial nerve function. On MR fibrous dysplasia is often hypointense to isointense on T2-weighted images, hypointense on precontrast T1-weighted images, and can enhance avidly, mimicking an aggressive tumor (Fig. 30.29). However, the diagnosis is usually relatively straightforward by CT, with intact cortex and medullary expansion with an internal "ground-glass" matrix (Curtin and Chavali, 1998; Hullar and Lustig, 2003; Curtin and Cunnane, 2009).

Paget disease is a primary metabolic disorder of bone of unknown etiology comprised of abnormal activity of

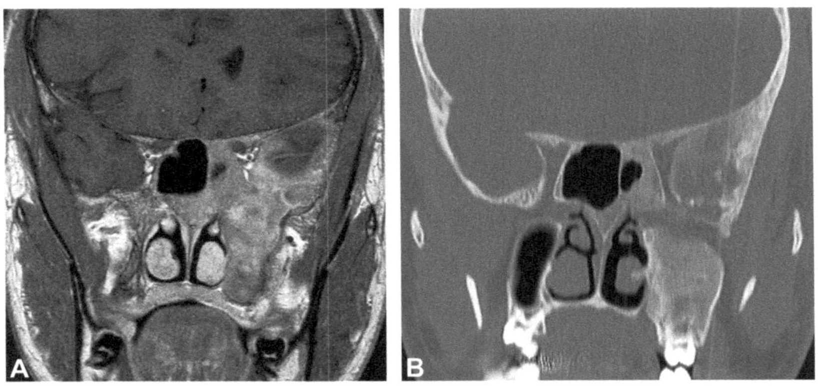

Fig. 30.29. Fibrous dysplasia. Coronal T1-weighted postcontrast image (**A**) demonstrates an apparent expansile enhancing lesion involving the left skull base, filling the left maxillary and sphenoid sinuses and involving the walls of the left orbit, with narrowing of the left optic canal. There is also mild mass effect on the left optic nerve. However, the appearance on the coronal computed tomography (**B**) confirms that this is fibrous dysplasia, with the characteristic expansile ground-glass matrix in the involved bone.

osteoblasts and osteoclasts resulting in excessive bone remodeling (Smith et al., 2002; Hullar and Lustig, 2003). The excessive osteoblastic reaction to abnormal osteoclastic resorption of bone results in course, thick bone that is more vascular and softer than normal bone. Complications in the skull base include cranial neuropathies, hearing loss, and basilar invagination. Secondary sarcomas can also arise within this abnormal bone.

Metastases and plasmacytomas can occur anywhere but tend to affect bones with medullary space more frequently, including the body and greater wing of the sphenoid. Langherhans cell histiocytosis typically occurs in pediatric patients, classically appearing as a "punched-out" lesion with nonsclerotic margins (Fig. 30.30). In the skull base, the temporal bone is the most common site of involvement (D'Ambrosio et al., 2008).

In the central skull base, there are tumors that are relatively specific for certain anatomic locations. Pituitary adenomas and craniopharyngiomas are discussed in detail in other chapters, but are mentioned here given their close relationship to the skull base. Invasive pituitary adenomas can involve the clivus and/or cavernous sinuses. Though uncommon, pituitary adenomas can expand through the sellar floor inferiorly rather than expanding superiorly into the sella and suprasellar cistern. In these cases the lesion may appear to reside predominantly within the sphenoid body (Nishio et al., 2001) (Fig. 30.31). Similarly, craniopharyngiomas are most commonly found in the sella or suprasellar cistern, but can grow into or rarely occur completely within the sphenoid bone (Arndt et al., 2007).

Chordomas are malignant primary bone tumors found at the midline as they arise from the remnants

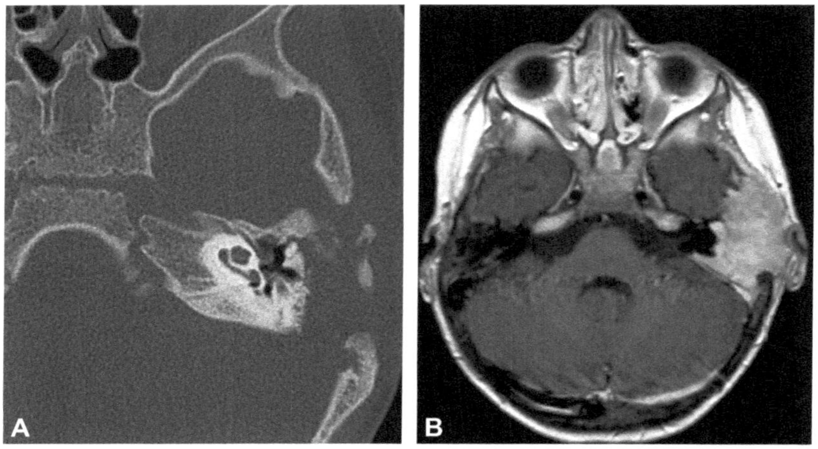

Fig. 30.30. Langerhans cell histiocytosis. Axial computed tomography image through the left temporal bone of a pediatric patient (A) demonstrates a lytic lesion in the left mastoid and middle-ear cavity extending to the squamosal portion of the temporal bone with "punched-out" sharp margins. Axial T1-weighted postcontrast image (B) of a magnetic resonance scan in the same patient demonstrates an avidly enhancing lesion involving the majority of the left temporal bone.

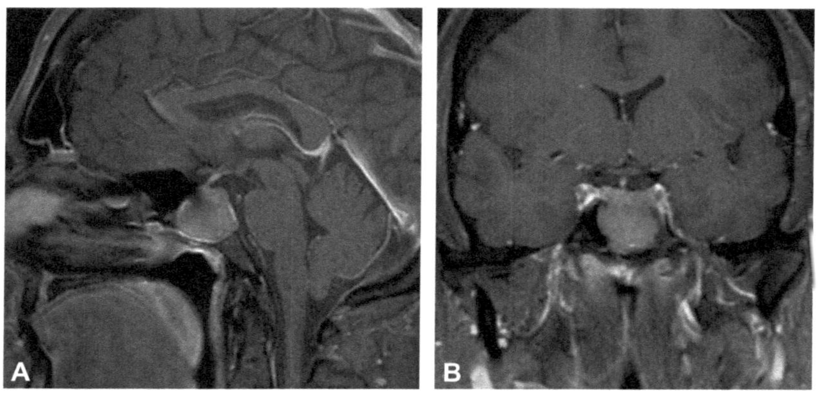

Fig. 30.31. Invasive pituitary macroadenoma. Sagittal and coronal postcontrast T1-weighted fat-saturated images demonstrate a lesion that has eroded through the sellar floor and is predominantly involving the basisphenoid of the clivus. There is no suprasellar extension or mass effect on the optic nerve or chiasm.

of the notochord. Approximately one-third of cases involve the skull base, arising almost exclusively from the clivus (Chugh et al., 2007). On CT, these lesions are expansile with erosive sharp bony margins and islands of residual cortical bone. The MR appearance is variable and can be homogeneous; however, there are typically areas of T1 hyperintense signal representing cyst-like areas with internal hemorrhage or proteinaceous fluid. Chordomas are typically markedly T2 hyperintense (Fig. 30.32) (Curtin and Chavali, 1998; Borges, 2008b).

In contrast to chordomas, chondrosarcomas of the skull base tend to occur just lateral to midline, typically centered at the petro-occipital fissure (Fig. 30.33), although they can also arise at the midline in the posterior nasal septum or at the spheno-occipital synchondrosis. There has been significant controversy in the literature in differentiating chordomas and chondrosarcomas of the central skull base given overlap in their histologic patterns, radiologic appearance, and clinical presentation. Precise diagnosis is important as prognosis and outcome are markedly different, and advances in immunohistochemical staining have clarified the issue (Rosenberg et al., 1999). For the purposes of imaging diagnosis, lesions arising parasagittally at the petro-occipital synchondrosis are almost always cartilaginous, while chordoma is much more likely at the midline than chondrosarcoma (Curtin and Cunnane, 2009; Curtin et al., 2011).

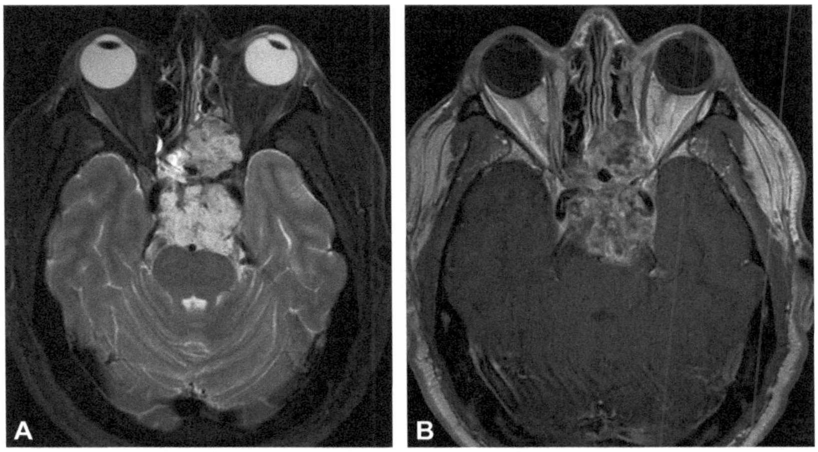

Fig. 30.32. Chordoma. Axial T2-weighted fat-saturated image (**A**) demonstrates a markedly T2 hyperintense midline lesion replacing the clivus and sphenoid body and extending into the ethmoid and prepontine cistern. Axial postcontrast T1-weighted image (**B**) at the same level demonstrates a heterogeneously enhancing lesion.

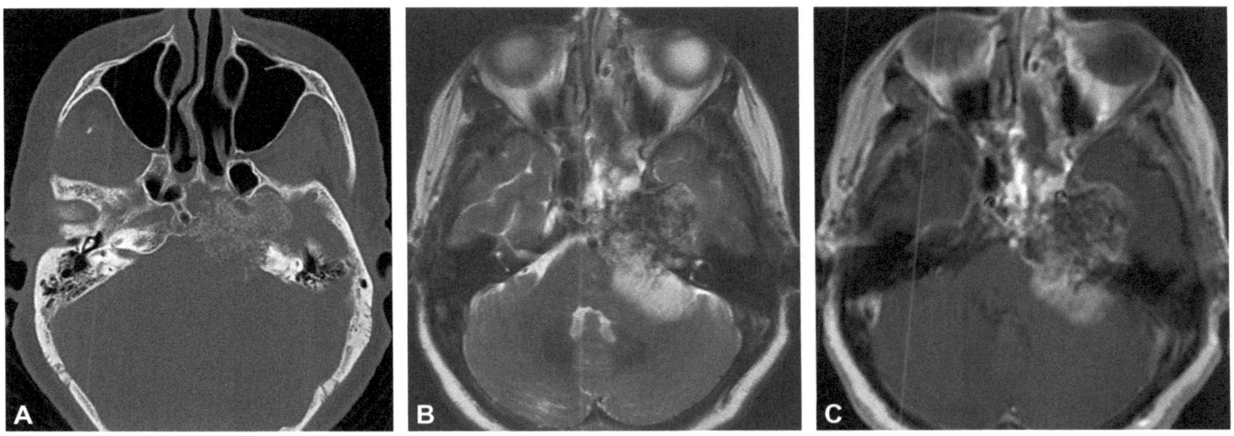

Fig. 30.33. Chondrosarcoma. Axial computed tomography (CT) image (**A**) demonstrating an expansile lesion centered at the left petro-occipital fissure with a chondroid matrix. Axial T2-weighted (**B**) and postcontrast T1-weighted (**C**) images demonstrate avid enhancement and areas of T2 hyperintensity. The hypointense areas on magnetic resonance imaging correspond to the chondroid matrix on the CT.

CONCLUSIONS AND FUTURE DEVELOPMENTS

The anatomy of the skull base is complex and a thorough knowledge of its fissures and foramina, the cranial nerves and vascular structures that traverse them, as well as the adjacent extracranial soft tissues is critical when imaging and evaluating lesions of this region. Although MR is often the preferred imaging modality, CT plays a complementary role as patterns of bony involvement can further narrow the differential diagnosis. Advances in both imaging and surgical technology, as well as the advent of focused radiation techniques in the past few decades, have resulted in better treatment options and prognoses for skull base lesions, with surgeons operating in spaces previously thought to be inaccessible. Tumors involving the skull base foramina typically arise from the cranial nerves themselves or from cells or tissues that follow the course of these nerves. PNS is an important pathway for metastatic tumor spread into the central nervous system via the skull base.

Further advancements in imaging technology are on the horizon, including molecular imaging of tumors based on cell biology and viability, as well as targeted contrast agents, and will likely lead to greater diagnostic specificity. MR/positron emission tomography scanning and higher field-strength MRI may allow early identification of recurrent or metastatic disease. Image-guided therapies may also allow for less invasive treatment and presumably improved outcomes.

References

Arndt S, Wiech T, Mader I et al. (2007). Entire infrasellar craniopharyngioma simulating clival chordoma. Otolaryngol Head Neck Surg 137: 981–983.

Boedeker CC, Ridder GJ, Schipper J (2005). Paragangliomas of the head and neck: diagnosis and treatment. Fam Cancer 4: 55–59.

Borges A (2008a). Skull base tumours part I: imaging technique, anatomy and anterior skull base tumours. Eur J Radiol 66: 338–347.

Borges A (2008b). Skull base tumours part II: Central skull base tumours and intrinsic tumours of the bony skull base. Eur J Radiol 66: 348–362.

Borges A, Casselman J (2007). Imaging the cranial nerves: part II: primary and secondary neoplastic conditions and neurovascular conflicts. Eur Radiol 17: 2332–2344.

Bredella MA, Torriani M, Hornicek F et al. (2007). Value of PET in assessment of patients with neurofibromatosis type I. Am J Roentgenol 189: 928–935.

Buetow MP, Buetow PC, Smirniotopoulos JG (1991). Typical, atypical, and misleading features of meningioma. Radiographics 11: 1087–1106.

Chong VF, Khoo JB, Yoke-Fun F (2004). Imaging of the nasopharynx and skull base. Neuroimaging Clin N Am 14: 695–719.

Chugh R, Tawbi H, Lucas DR et al. (2007). Chordoma: the nonsarcoma primary bone tumor. Oncologist 12: 1344–1350.

Curtin HD (1998). Detection of perineural spread: fat is a friend. AJNR Am J Neuroradiol 19: 1385–1386.

Curtin HD, Chavali R (1998). Imaging of the skull base. Radiol Clin North Am 36: 801–817.

Curtin HD, Cunnane MB (2009). The skull base. In: SW Atlas (Ed.), Magnetic Resonance Imaging of the Brain and Spine, 4th Edn. Lippincott Williams and Wilkins, Philadelphia, pp. 1088–1119.

Curtin HD, Hagiwara M (2011). Embryology, anatomy, and imaging of the central skull base. In: PM Som, HD Curtin (Eds.), Head and Neck Imaging, 5th Edn. Elsevier, St. Louis, pp. 927–946.

Curtin HD, Hagiwara M, Som PM (2011). Pathology of the central skull base. In: PM Som, HD Curtin (Eds.), Head and Neck Imaging, 5th Edn., Elsevier, St. Louis, pp. 947–1016.

D'Ambrosio N, Soohoo S, Warshall C et al. (2008). Craniofacial and intracranial manifestations of Langerhans cell histiocytosis: report of findings in 100 patients. AJR Am J Roentgenol 191: 589–597.

Durden DD, Williams DW (2001). Radiology of skull base neoplasms. Otolaryngol Clin North Am 34: 1043–1064.

Fishbein NJ, Kaplan MJ (1999). Magnetic resonance imaging of the central skull base. Top Magn Reson Imaging 10: 325–346.

Ginsberg LE (1999). Imaging of perineural tumor spread in head and neck cancer. Semin Ultrasound CT MR 20: 175–186.

Glenn LW (2005). Innovations in neuroimaging of skull base pathology. Otolaryngol Clin North Am 38: 613–629.

Hullar TE, Lustig LR (2003). Paget's disease and fibrous dysplasia. Otolaryngol Clin North Am 36: 707–732.

Kania RE, Bouccara D, Colombani JM et al. (1999). Primary facial canal paraganglioma. Am J Otolaryngol 20: 318–322.

Lang J (1987a). Anterior cranial base anatomy. In: LN Sekhar, VL Schramm (Eds.), Tumor of the Cranial Base: Diagnosis and Treatment, Futura Publishing Company, Mount Kisco, NY, pp. 247–264.

Lang J (1987b). Middle cranial base anatomy. In: LN Sekhar, VL Schramm (Eds.), Tumor of the Cranial Base: Diagnosis and Treatment, Futura Publishing Company, Mount Kisco, NY, pp. 313–334.

Lang J (1987c). Posterior cranial base anatomy. In: LN Sekhar, VL Schramm (Eds.), Tumor of the Cranial Base: Diagnosis and Treatment, Futura Publishing Company, Mount Kisco, NY, pp. 441–460.

Lozano FS, Gomez JL, Mondillo MC et al. (2008). Surgery of vagal paragangliomas: six patients and review of the literature. Surg Oncol 17: 281–287.

Mafee MF, Raofi B, Kumar A et al. (2000). Glomus faciale, glomus jugulare, glomus tympanicum, glomus vagale, carotid body tumors, and simulating lesions. Role of MR imaging. Radiol Clin North Am 38: 1059–1076.

Majoie CB, Hulsmans FJ, Castelijns JA et al. (1999). Primary nerve-sheath tumours of the trigeminal nerve: clinical and MRI findings. Neuroradiology 41: 100–108.

McGregor JM, Sarkar A (2009). Stereotactic radiosurgery and stereotactic radiotherapy in the treatment of skull base meningiomas. Otolaryngol Clin North Am 42: 677–688.

Moonis G, Cunnane MB, Emerick K et al. (2012). Patterns of perineural tumor spread in head and neck cancer. Magn Reson Imaging Clin N Am 20: 435–446.

Morani AC, Ramani NS, Wesolowski JR (2011). Skull base, orbits, temporal bone, and cranial nerves: Anatomy on MR imaging. Magn Reson Imaging Clin N Am 19: 439–456.

Nishio S, Morioka T, Fujiwara S et al. (2001). Prolactinoma with preferential infrasellar extension: a report of two cases. J Clin Neurosci 8: 287–289.

Parmar H, Gujar S, Shah G et al. (2009). Imaging of the anterior skull base. Neuroimaging Clin N Am 19: 427–439.

Rao AB, Koeller KK, Adair CF (1999). From the archives of the AFIP. Paragangliomas of the head and neck: radiologic-pathologic correlation. Radiographics 19: 1605–1632.

Razek AA, Castillo M (2009). Imaging lesions of the cavernous sinus. AJNR Am J Neuroradiol 30: 444–452.

Rhoton Jr AL (2000a). The foramen magnum. Neurosurgery 47 (3 Suppl): S155–S193.

Rhoton Jr AL (2000b). Jugular foramen. Neurosurgery 47 (3 Suppl): S267–S285.

Rhoton Jr AL (2000c). The posterior fossa cisterns. Neurosurgery 47 (3 Suppl): S287–S297.

Rhoton Jr AL (2002). The anterior and middle cranial base. Neurosurgery 51 (4 Suppl): S273–S302.

Rosenberg AE, Nielsen GP, Keel SB et al. (1999). Chondrosarcoma of the base of the skull: a clinicopathologic study of 200 cases with emphasis on its distinction from chordoma. Am J Surg Pathol 23: 1370–1378.

Samii M, Migliori MM, Tatagiba M et al. (1995). Surgical treatment of trigeminal schwannomas. J Neurosurg 82: 711–718.

Sanna M, Bacciu A, Falcioni M et al. (2007). Surgical management of jugular foramen meningiomas: a series of 13 cases and review of the literature. Laryngoscope 117: 1710–1719.

Scheithauer BW, Woodruff JM, Erlandson RA (1999). Tumors of the peripheral nervous system. In: Atlas of Tumor Pathology, Third Series., Armed Forces Institute of Pathology, Washington, DC.

Smith SE, Murphey MD, Motamedi K et al. (2002). From the archives of the AFIP. Radiologic spectrum of Paget disease of bone and its complications with pathologic correlation. Radiographics 22: 1191–1216.

Tomura N, Hirano H, Sashi R et al. (1998). Comparison of MR imaging and CT in discriminating tumor infiltration of bone and bone marrow in the skull base. Comput Med Imaging Graph 22: 41–51.

Wippold FJ, Neely JG, Haughey BH (2004). Primary paraganglioma of the facial nerve canal. Otol Neurotol 25: 79–80.

Zabel A, Debus J, Thilmann C et al. (2001). Management of benign cranial nonacoustic schwannomas by fractionated stereotactic radiotherapy. Int J Cancer 96: 356–362.

Zanoletti E, Mazzoni A (2006). Vagal paraganglioma. Skull Base 16: 161–167.

Zhang L, Yang Y, Xu S et al. (2009). Trigeminal schwannomas: A report of 42 cases and reviews of the relevant surgical approaches. Clin Neurol Neurosurg 111: 261–269.

Handbook of Clinical Neurology, Vol. 135 (3rd series)
Neuroimaging, Part I
J.C. Masdeu and R.G. González, Editors

Chapter 31

Imaging of orbital disorders

MARY BETH CUNNANE[1,2]* AND HUGH DAVID CURTIN[1]

[1]*Department of Radiology, Harvard Medical School and Massachusetts Eye and Ear Infirmary, Boston, MA, USA*

[2]*Division of Neuroradiology, Massachusetts General Hospital, Boston, MA, USA*

Abstract

Diseases of the orbit can be categorized in many ways, but in this chapter we shall group them according to etiology.

Inflammatory diseases of the orbits may be infectious or noninfectious. Of the infections, orbital cellulitis is the most common and typically arises as a complication of acute sinusitis. Of the noninfectious, inflammatory conditions, thyroid orbitopathy is the most common and results in enlargement of the extraocular muscles and proliferation of the orbital fat. Idiopathic orbital inflammatory syndrome is another cause of inflammation in the orbit, which may mimic thyroid orbitopathy or even neoplasm, but typically presents with pain.

Masses in the orbit may be benign or malignant and the differential diagnosis primarily depends on the location of the mass lesion, and on the age of the patient. Lacrimal gland tumors may be lymphomas or epithelial lesions of salivary origin. Extraocular muscle tumors may represent lymphoma or metastases. Tumors of the intraconal fat are often benign, typically hemangiomas or schwannomas. Finally, globe tumors may be retinoblastomas (in children), or choroidal melanomas or metastases in adults.

INTRODUCTION

There are a large variety of diseases which involve the orbit and the discussion of these disorders can be organized according to etiology (e.g., infection, inflammation, neoplasm) or by anatomic location. In this chapter we will consider disease entities predominantly by etiology. However, in deference to the fact that the anatomic location of an abnormality may be the most straightforward thing to determine during the initial evaluation, the section on tumors will be subcategorized by anatomic site.

INFECTION

Preseptal cellulitis

Preseptal disorders are abnormalities of the eyelids. The orbital septum, together with the tarsal plates, makes up the fibrous layer that supports the structure of the eyelids. Superiorly, the orbital septum attaches to the orbital rim, and extends from there to the aponeurosis of the levator palpebrae muscle. Inferiorly, the orbital septum extends from the bony orbit to the tarsal plate (Bron et al., 1997). In general the orbital septum provides a strong barrier to the spread of infection from the lids into the orbits.

Preseptal cellulitis may arise from sinus disease, or from trauma, such as abrasions or insect bites. Many of these patients do not present for imaging, as they are easily diagnosed via physical exam. Imaging is reserved for those patients in whom orbital cellulitis is suspected either because the patient has failed to improve after 24 hours of antibiotics or when there are clinical features which raise concern for orbital involvement, such as proptosis or restricted motility (Howe and Jones, 2004). Imaging features include skin thickening and subcutaneous soft-tissue stranding (Fig. 31.1). Occasionally abscesses may develop in the preseptal soft

*Correspondence to: Mary Beth Cunnane, M.D., Staff Radiologist, Massachusetts Eye and Ear Infirmary, Instructor in Radiology, Harvard Medical School, 243 Charles St., Boston MA 02114, USA. Tel: +1-617-573-3842, Fax: +1-617-573-3490, E-mail: MaryBeth_Cunnane@MEEI.HARVARD.EDU

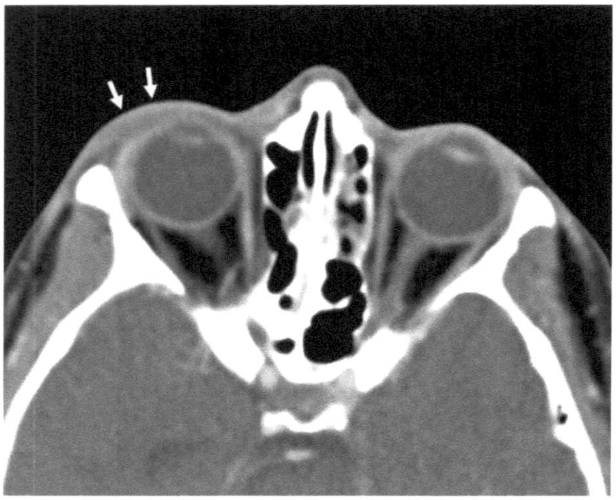

Fig. 31.1. Preseptal cellulitis. Soft-tissue swelling and skin thickening (arrows) are identified in this patient with preseptal cellulitis. There is no evidence of extension through the septum into the orbital fat.

tissues; these are recognized as rim-enhancing fluid collections on contrast-enhanced computed tomography (CT) or magnetic resonance imaging (MRI) (Fig. 31.2).

Orbital cellulitis

Orbital cellulitis occurs when there is spread of infection into the orbit, most frequently from the ethmoid sinuses. Though orbital cellulitis can be seen on either MRI or CT, contrast-enhanced CT is most practical in the initial evaluation as it accurately depicts both the orbits and the paranasal sinuses, and can be used for image-guided sinus surgery for patients who fail to respond to antibiotics. MRI is an appropriate adjunct to CT in patients in whom intracranial involvement is suspected, as it allows the most sensitive evaluation for epidural, subdural, leptomeningeal, and cortical infection/inflammation.

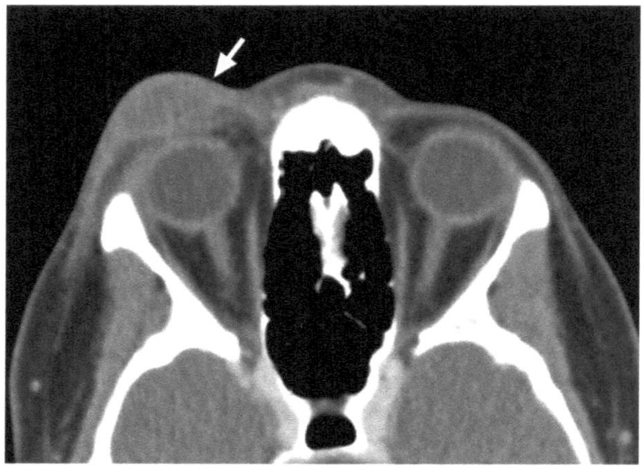

Fig. 31.2. Preseptal abscess. A lenticular soft-tissue density is seen (arrow) in the preseptal soft tissues on this noncontrast computed tomography image. This was incised and purulent fluid was evacuated.

The orbital complications of sinusitis range in severity (Chandler et al., 1970). In the least severe cases, CT will demonstrate soft-tissue stranding, indicative of edema. Subperiosteal abscesses are recognized as lenticular, rim-enhancing fluid collections bordering an opacified sinus. Frequently these lie against the lamina papyracea but they may also lie along the orbital roof, if infection has spread to the orbit from a supraorbital ethmoid air cell. More severe complications of orbital cellulitis include intraconal abscess, and cavernous sinus thrombosis (Chandler et al., 1970) (Fig. 31.3).

Invasive fungal sinusitis

Patients who are immunocompromised secondary to diabetes, chemotherapy, or immunosuppression for transplants are susceptible to invasive fungal infection extending from the paranasal sinuses into the orbits. This diagnosis requires a high degree of clinical suspicion

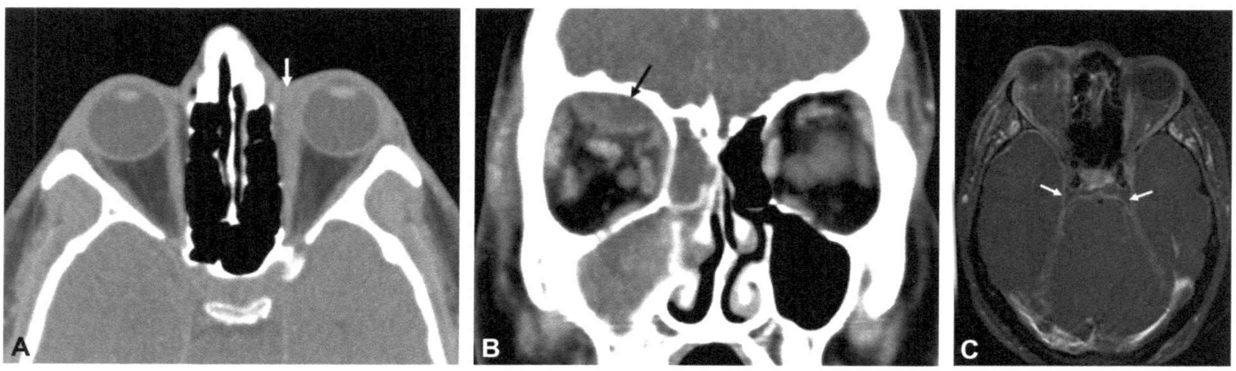

Fig. 31.3. Spectrum of orbital cellulitis. (**A**) Soft tissue is identified medial to the left medial rectus muscle (arrow). No focal fluid collection is identified. (**B**) Lenticular collection of fluid (arrow) representing a subperiosteal abscess. (**C**) In this case, facial and orbital infection has led to cavernous sinus thrombosis. Only the anterior portion of the left cavernous sinus fills with blood. There is no enhancement in the right cavernous sinus (arrow) or the posterior aspect of the left cavernous sinus (arrow), due to thrombus.

as the findings on imaging may be very subtle, especially in comparison to the clinical presentation (Chandrasekharan et al., 2012). Whereas there is frequently complete opacification of adjacent sinuses in bacterial orbital cellulitis, in invasive fungal disease, the sinus opacification may be mild, and frank abscesses are rare. Both CT and MRI may demonstrate soft tissue external to the maxillary sinus as the fungi pass through intact bone (Silverman and Mancuso, 1998; Mossa-Basha et al., 2013) (Figs 31.4 and 31.5). Osseous erosion may also be seen (Fig. 31.5). Wide surgical debridement is performed for treatment, but cavernous sinus involvement precludes complete resection and therefore is the most important finding to detect in patients considered for surgery. This can be evaluated with either contrast-enhanced CT or MRI, depending on the severity of the patient's illness and whether the underlying medical condition allows the administration of gadolinium (Fig. 31.6).

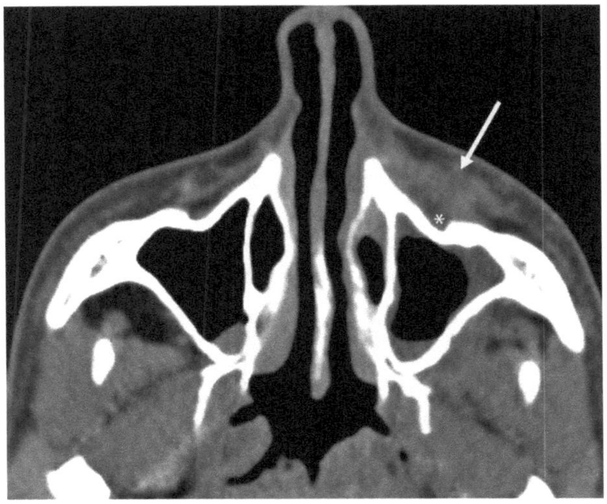

Fig. 31.4. Invasive fungal sinusitis. The left maxillary sinus is only partially opacified. However, there is soft tissue external to the sinus (arrow) which extends to the infraorbital nerve canal (asterisk). This finding of extra-sinus soft tissue is suggestive of invasive fungal disease rather than bacterial infection. This patient had a biopsy confirming mucormycosis.

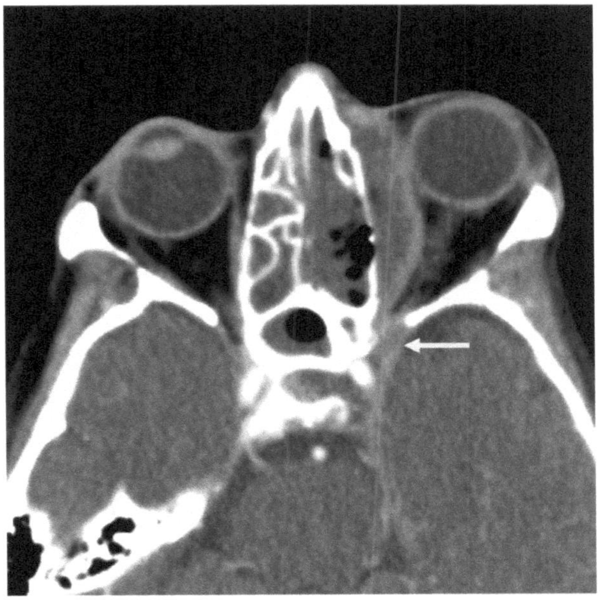

Fig. 31.6. Invasive fungal sinusitis. Contrast-enhanced computed tomography demonstrates an abscess in the medial left orbit. In addition, there is expansion of the anterior portion of the left cavernous sinus by tissue which demonstrates less enhancement than the normal cavernous sinus (arrow), indicating cavernous sinus invasion. This finding indicates that the infection is unresectable.

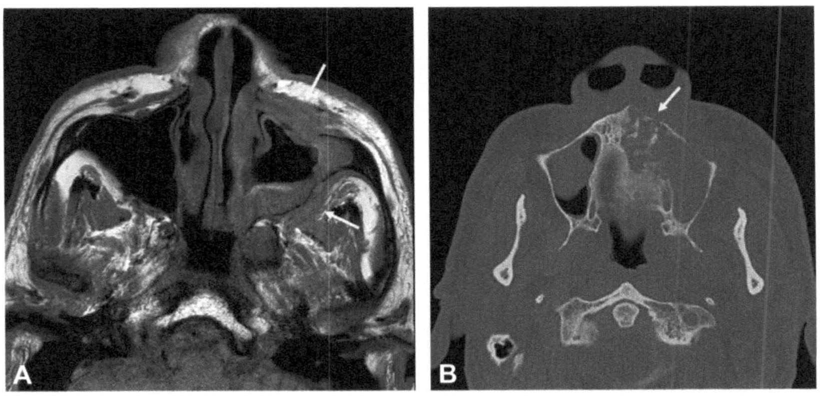

Fig. 31.5. Invasive fungal sinusitis. (**A**) On this T1-weighted magnetic resonance imaging, there is abnormal soft tissue surrounding the left maxillary sinus (arrows). (**B**) Computed tomography in the same patient demonstrates mottled bony destruction of the maxilla (arrow).

NONINFECTIOUS INFLAMMATION OF THE ORBITS

Thyroid orbitopathy

Thyroid orbitopathy is an autoimmune disease in which there is production of autoantibodies leading to inflammatory changes in the orbit. The autoantibodies presumably target a protein which is shared by both the orbit and thyroid. Although most patients with thyroid orbitopathy are known to have thyroid disease, most commonly Graves disease, a minority are euthyroid at presentation (Bartalena and Tanda, 2009).

Patients with thyroid orbitopathy have enlargement of the extraocular muscles which occurs in a characteristic progression – first inferior rectus, then medial rectus, then superior muscle complex (superior rectus and levator palpebrae), followed by the lateral rectus and the obliques (Lacey et al., 1999). When examining the images of a patient with thyroid orbitopathy, attention should be directed to the orbital apex, where enlarged muscle tissue may crowd the optic nerve, resulting in compressive optic neuropathy (Fig. 31.7).

A minority of patients with thyroid orbitopathy have increased orbital fat, without much in the way of extraocular muscle enlargement. These patients demonstrate proptosis as well, with straightening of the optic nerve. These cases are examples of what is termed the lipogenic form of thyroid orbitopathy (Nunery, 1991; Rubin et al., 1998) (Fig. 31.8).

Thyroid orbitopathy is the most common cause of extraocular muscle enlargement; however, when encountering a patient with enlarged extraocular muscles, other diagnoses, such as cavernous-carotid fistula, the myositis form of orbital pseudotumor, and metastases should also be considered (Rothfus and Curtin, 1984). Table 31.1 lists the differential diagnosis of extraocular muscle enlargement.

Idiopathic orbital inflammatory syndrome/orbital pseudotumor

Another common cause of orbital inflammation is idiopathic orbital inflammatory syndrome or orbital psuedotumor. Orbital pseudotumor occurs due to an infiltration of the orbital structures with lymphocytes and fibroblasts. Frequently patients present with acute pain and

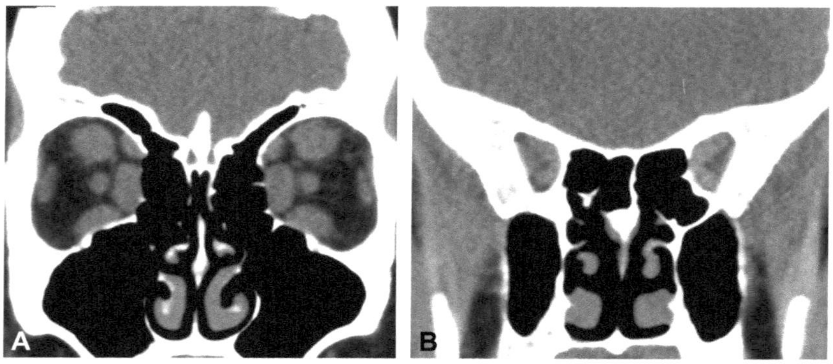

Fig. 31.7. Thyroid orbitopathy. (**A**) Coronal computed tomography through the orbits demonstrates marked enlargement of the inferior rectus muscles, the medial rectus muscles, and the superior muscle complex bilaterally in a symmetric fashion. (**B**) There is crowding of the optic nerve at the orbital apex, a phenomenon which may result in compressive optic neuropathy.

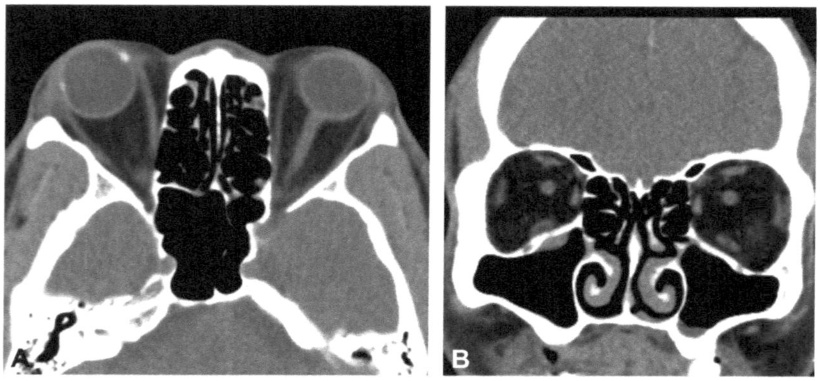

Fig. 31.8. Lipoid variant of thyroid orbitopathy. In this less common form of thyroid orbitopathy, the orbital fat has proliferated. This proliferation of fat results in proptosis (**A**), despite the normal size of the extraocular muscles (**B**).

Table 31.1

Causes of extraocular muscle enlargement

Thyroid orbitopathy
Myositis form of idiopathic orbital inflammatory syndrome (orbital pseudotumor)
Metastatic disease (breast, lung cancer)
Lymphoma
Schistosomiasis
Carotid-cavernous fistula
Acromegaly

Table 31.2

Causes of lacrimal gland enlargement

Dacryoadenitis due to orbital pseudotumor
Infectious dacryoadenitis
Sarcoidosis
Lymphoma
Pleomorphic adenoma
Adenoid cystic
Mucoepidermoid carcinoma

inflammatory signs such as erythema and swelling. Patients with orbital pseudotumor may have a variety of clinical presentations, and generally the presentation mirrors the location on which inflammation is centered. Accordingly, the varieties of pseudotumor are often organized according to the center of inflammation into anterior, dacroadenitis, myositis, posterior/perineuritis, and diffuse, patterns of involvement which may be recognized at imaging (Yuen and Rubin, 2003).

In anterior pseudotumor, inflammation lies along the globe and is particularly noticeable at the junction of the globe and the optic nerve (a finding called episcleritis). In dacryoadenitis there is diffuse enlargement of the lacrimal gland as well as soft-tissue stranding surrounding the gland (See Table 31.2 for other causes of lacrimal gland enlargement to consider in the differential diagnosis.) In posterior pseudotumor, abnormal soft tissue surrounds the optic nerve and may extend into the cavernous sinus. In diffuse pseudotumor, soft tissue diffusely infiltrates the orbital fat. Finally in myositis there is enlargement of extraocular muscles with soft-tissue stranding in the surrounding fat (Fig. 31.9).

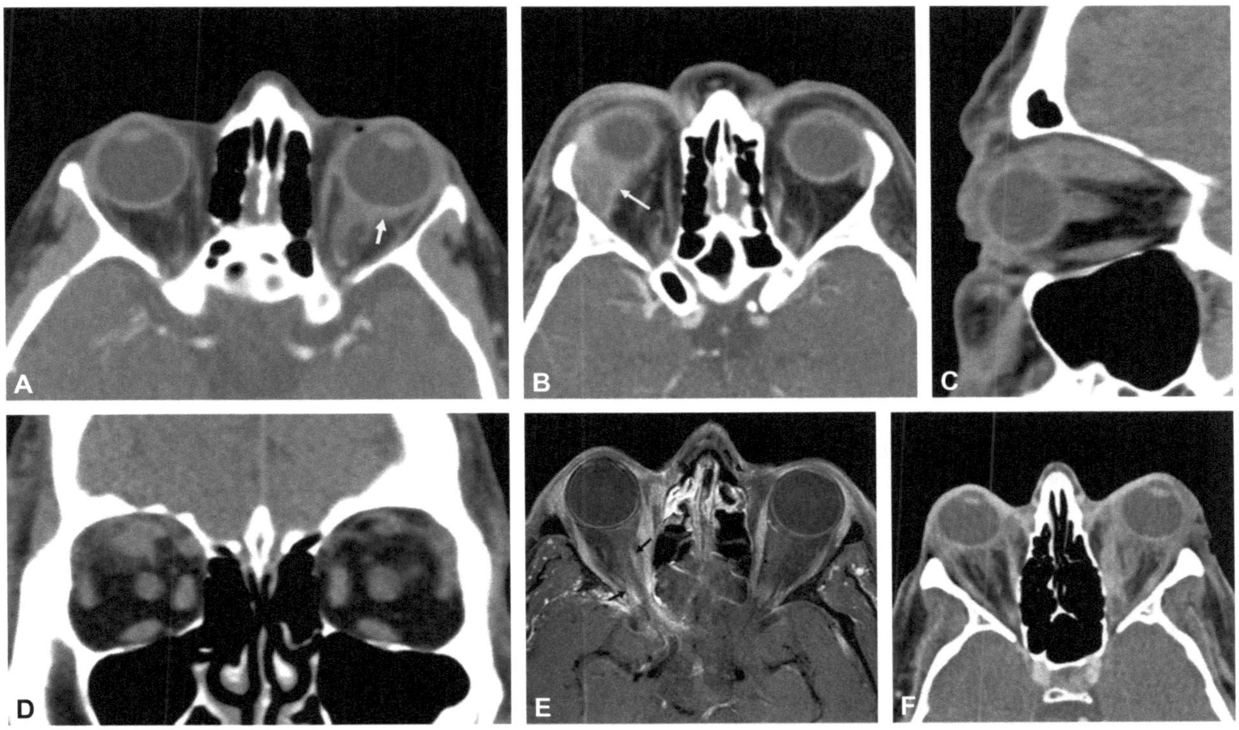

Fig. 31.9. Orbital pseudotumor. (**A**) Anterior form: note the soft-tissue stranding along the posterior aspect of the left globe (arrow). There is also a mild degree of preseptal soft-tissue swelling laterally. (**B**) Dacryoadenitis. The right lacrimal gland is enlarged (arrow) and demonstrates an ill-defined border due to inflammatory soft-tissue stranding which surrounds it. Note also the soft-tissue stranding in the preseptal fat on the right. (**C**) Myositis. There is significant enlargement of the superior muscle complex, involving both the muscle belly and the tendinous insertion on the globe. Note the soft-tissue stranding surrounding the superior muscle complex on the coronal images (**D**), indicating inflammation. (**E**) Posterior. There is abnormal linear enhancement surrounding the right optic nerve (arrows) at the orbital apex. (**F**) Diffuse. Soft-tissue stranding extends diffusely throughout the intraconal fat bilaterally, leading to proptosis. There is also enlargement of the left medial rectus muscle.

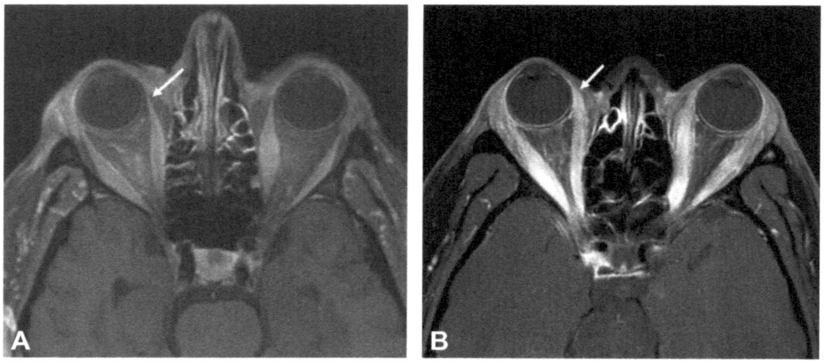

Fig. 31.10. Comparison of the appearance of the myotendinous junction (arrow), which is typically thin in thyroid orbitopathy (**A**), and thickened in orbital pseudotumor (**B**).

A typical feature of pseudotumor is the soft-tissue stranding that it causes in the orbital fat, and this finding can help suggest this diagnosis. Depending on the location of inflammation, pseudotumor is in the differential diagnosis with a wide variety of entities. A typical question that arises is whether an extraocular muscle is enlarged due to pseudotumor or due to thyroid orbitopathy. When considering these cases it is useful to remember that thyroid orbitopathy tends to be bilateral, symmetric, involve the medial and inferior rectus muscles before any additional muscles, and causes spindle-shaped enlargement of the muscle, with sparing of the myotendinous junction. The myositis form of pseudutumor, however, is often unilateral, and may involve muscles in any order. In addition there is typically involvement of the myotendinous junction (Fig. 31.10) (Rothfus and Curtin, 1984).

Other less common inflammatory diseases that can involve the orbits include sarcoidosis, Sjögren's disease, and Wegener's granulomatosis. Sarcoidosis is characterized histologically by the presence of noncaseating granulomas. It may affect the eye and ocular adnexa in 10–50% of patients. Ocular manifestations such as anterior uveitis are the most common manifestations (Smith and Foster, 1996); however, in a minority of patients orbital and adnexal involvement may occur as well. In patients with orbital and adnexal involvement, lacrimal involvement is the most common abnormality (Prabhakaran et al., 2007; Demirci and Christianson, 2011) (Fig. 31.11). These patients may have involvement of the salivary glands as well, which can be a radiographic clue to the diagnosis.

Granulomatosis with polyangiitis (Wegener's) is another inflammatory disease which can affect the orbit. Up to half of patients with Wegener's disease will have involvement of the eye or orbit (Fauci et al., 1983). Ocular involvement includes conjunctivitis, scleritis, uveitis, and optic nerve vasculitis (Fauci et al., 1983). Orbital involvement may occur secondary to extension from the adjacent paranasal sinuses, and may lead to nasolacrimal duct obstruction or proptosis (Santiago and Fay, 2011) (Fig. 31.12).

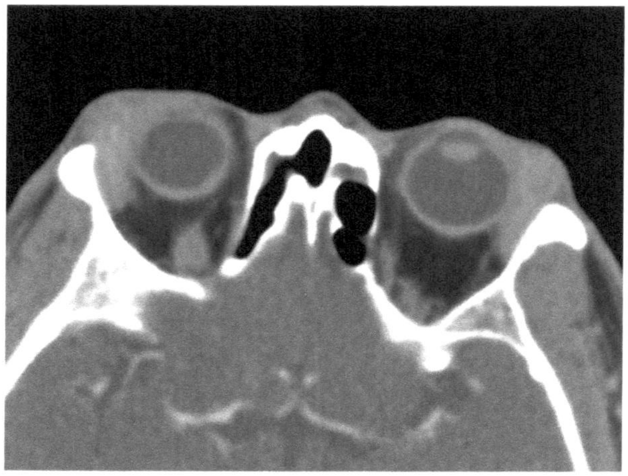

Fig. 31.11. Sarcoidosis. Bilateral enlargement of the lacrimal glands is seen. The patient also had mediastinal lymphadenopathy consistent with sarcoidosis.

SPACE-OCCUPYING LESIONS

Vascular lesions

The space-occupying lesions of the orbit can generally be divided into two categories: vascular lesions and nonvascular neoplasms. In Shields' large series of over 1000 patients presenting with orbital tumors or conditions simulating orbital tumors, vasculogenic lesions accounted for 17% of the total number of cases (Shields et al., 2004b). Vascular malformations may involve any part of the orbit.

Infantile hemangiomas develop within the first 3 months after birth and then proliferate over the first year, after which time they regress. They demonstrate lobulated margins, avidly enhance, and have significant

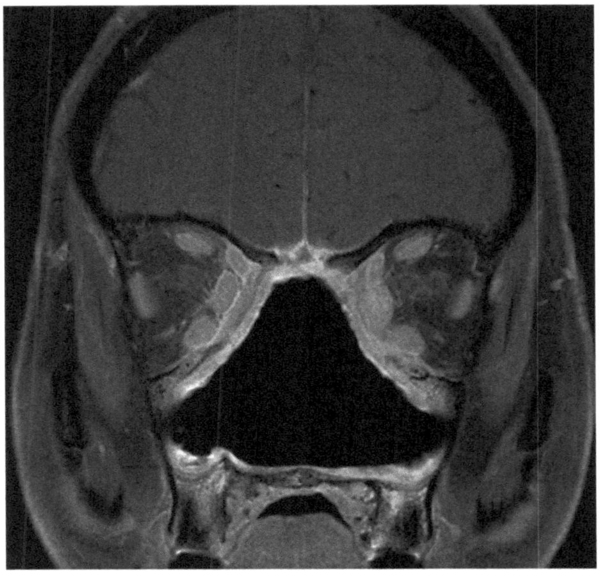

Fig. 31.12. Wegener's disease extending into the orbits. Coronal postcontrast magnetic resonance imaging demonstrates extensive destruction of the paranasal sinuses and nasal cavity (the patient had no history of prior surgery). Enhancing soft tissue is seen infiltrating into the medial orbits bilaterally, as well as across the floor of the anterior cranial fossa.

blood flow, which may be reflected on MRI by the presence of flow voids (Rootman, 2003; Smoker et al., 2008) (Fig. 31.13).

Older children and adults may have low-flow vascular malformations (venolymphatic). These do not demonstrate flow voids, and have variable enhancement. They may expand during upper respiratory illnesses and may also hemorrhage, which can be seen as fluid–fluid levels on MRI (Smoker et al., 2008) (Fig. 31.14).

Dilations of the orbital veins, termed varices, may cause intermittent proptosis, triggered by Valsalva. Frequently these are collapsed at the time of imaging, but asking the patient to Valsalva will reproduce the symptoms, and imaging following Valsalva will show a newly dilated enhancing structure, when compared with earlier sequences (Rootman, 2003).

Cavernous hemangiomas are one of the most common lesions occurring in the orbital fat in adults. They are round tumors with sharp margins. They are T2 hyperintense and lobulated with patchy enhancement that becomes more uniform with the passage of time (Fig. 31.15) (Rootman, 2003; Smoker et al., 2008).

Solid tumors of the orbit

The differential diagnosis of neoplasms involving the orbits depends on the age of the patient and the location of the tumor. However, rhabdomyosarcoma can occur anywhere in the pediatric orbit and lymphoma anywhere in the adult orbit.

Preseptal soft tissues

Tumors of the preseptal soft tissues tend to be skin cancers (squamous cell carcinoma, basal cell carcinoma, melanoma) and tumors of the conjunctiva (most frequently, lymphoma). High-resolution imaging demonstrates orbital involvement and provides a map for surgical treatment and radiation therapy of these tumors (Fig. 31.16). When evaluating patients with preseptal tumors it is important to examine the submental, submandibular, and intraparotid lymph nodes for metastatic disease (Fig. 31.16). The infraorbital nerve (a branch of V2) and the supraorbital nerve (a branch of V1) should also be examined for thickening and enhancement, signs of perineural tumor spread.

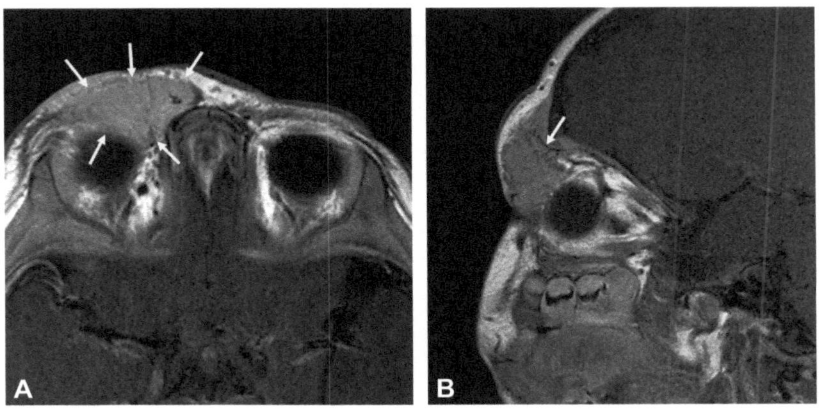

Fig. 31.13. Infantile hemangioma. (**A**) Axial postcontrast T1-weighted magnetic resonance imagingdemonstrates an avidly enhancing lobulated mass in the preseptal soft tissues of the right orbit (arrows). (**B**) On this sagittal image one can appreciate the serpiginous flow voids extending through the lesion (arrow).

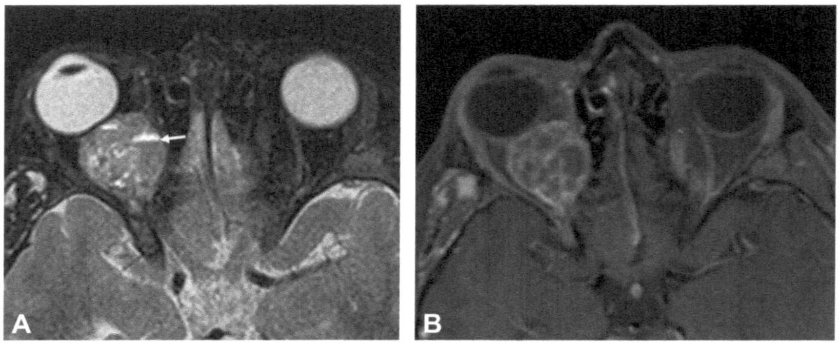

Fig. 31.14. Venolymphatic malformation. Magnetic resonance imaging with contrast was performed in this child with sudden proptosis. (**A**) T2-weighted image demonstrates fluid–fluid levels (arrow) due to recent hemorrhage. (**B**) Postcontrast image demonstrates mostly fluid-filled lesion with multiple enhancing septations.

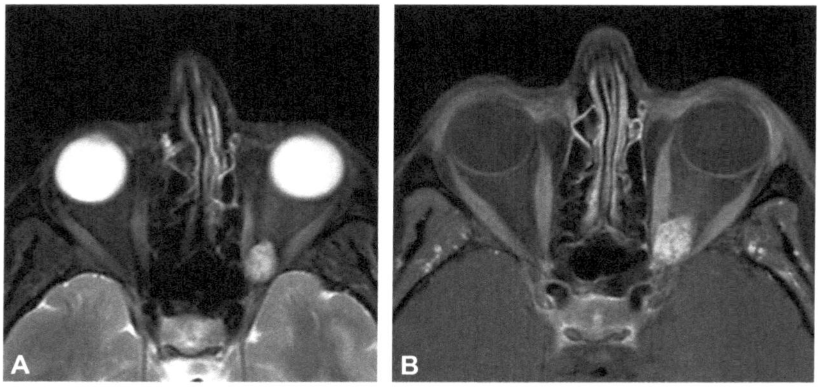

Fig. 31.15. (**A, B**) Cavernous hemangioma. Well-demarcated mass in the posterior left orbit with mildly lobulated margins. This is T2 hyperintense (**A**) and demonstrates enhancement which is mildly heterogeneous (**B**). In larger lesions, enhancement may progress from initial to delayed images as the lesion fills in with contrast.

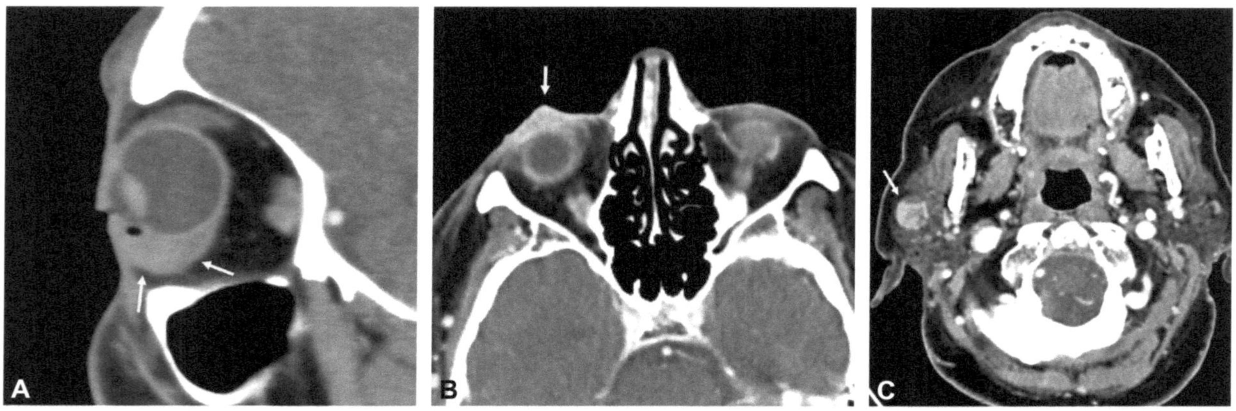

Fig. 31.16. Preseptal tumors. (**A**) Sagittal image of this patient with conjunctival lymphoma shows postseptal extension into the orbit abutting the inferior globe (arrows). (**B**) Nodular soft tissue along the right lid (arrow) represents a squamous cell carcinoma. (**C**) Additional images in the same patient show a metastatic intraparotid lymph node (arrow).

Lacrimal gland

Lacrimal gland tumors account for approximately 10% of all orbital tumors. Twenty percent are epithelial in origin, whereas 80% are lymphoproliferative. Of the epithelial tumors, 55% are benign (most commonly pleomorphic adenoma). Of the 45% which are malignant, adenoid cystic carcinoma is the most common pathology (Shields et al., 2004a). Tumors arising from the lacrimal gland will present in the superotemporal orbit. Examination of the interface between the tumor and the globe will assist in differential diagnosis. Epithelial lesions of the lacrimal gland tend to be round tumors which push on the globe, like a marble or a ball (Fig. 31.17). Lymphoproliferative lesions, including lymphoma, are softer and will mold to the globe (Figs 31.18 and 31.19). In addition, epithelial lesions tend to arise from the orbital portion of the lacrimal gland, whereas lymphoproliferative lesions involve both the orbital and palpebral portions of the lacrimal gland (Gao et al., 2013). Finally, lymphomas of the lacrimal gland may be bilateral, whereas epithelial lesions of the lacrimal gland are unilateral.

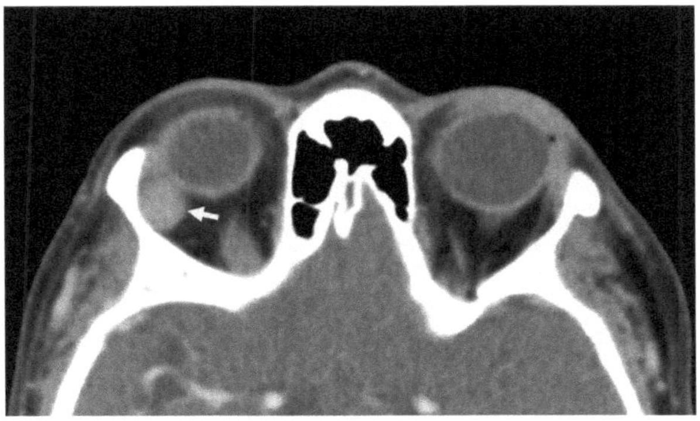

Fig. 31.17. Mucoepidermoid cancer of the lacrimal gland. Computed tomography demonstrates a right lacrimal gland tumor which is confined to the orbital lobe and looks like a marble pushing on the globe (arrow), a characteristic of epithelial tumors.

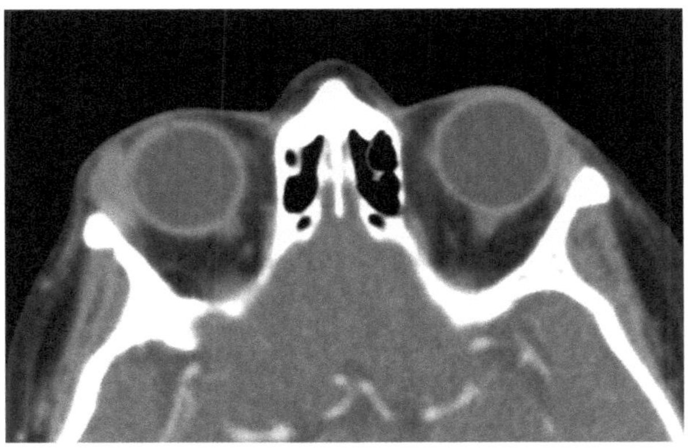

Fig. 31.18. Lacrimal gland lymphoma. Both the orbital and palpebral portions of the right lacrimal gland are enlarged by soft tissue which molds to the globe rather than pushing on the globe in this patient with lacrimal gland lymphoma.

Extraocular muscles

Neoplasia is an unusual cause of extraocular muscle enlargement which nevertheless must be considered in older patients and in patients whose pattern of muscle enlargement is atypical for thyroid disease. Metastases to the extraocular muscles are rare (Weiss et al., 1984). These are most commonly seen in the setting of cutaneous melanoma and breast cancer (Fig. 31.20) (Lacey et al., 1999). In the case of breast cancer, patients will often present with enophthalmos, rather than proptosis, due to this schirrous nature of breast cancer metastases in the orbit. The extraocular muscles may also be involved by leukemia and lymphoma (Lacey et al., 1999).

Intraconal lesions

Some orbital masses appear to lie simply within the orbital fat rather than localized to any orbital structure such as the optic nerve, globe, muscles, or lacrimal gland. These include neurogenic lesions, such as schwannomas. Schwannomas comprise 1–2% of all orbital tumors. They are more common superiorly within the orbit and may be seen in the intraconal fat as well-demarcated ovoid or cone-shaped lesions. They most commonly demonstrate peripheral or uniform enhancement (rather than patchy progressive enhancement, as a cavernous hemangioma would) (Wang and Xiao, 2008) (Fig. 31.21). They arise from branches of the cranial nerves or the autonomic nerves extending through the orbit, rather than the optic nerve itself, which instead gives rise to meningiomas.

Optic nerve

The optic nerve may be infiltrated by or compressed by tumor. Optic gliomas are tumors of the optic nerve itself. They are most commonly grade I pilocytic astrocytomas with a benign clinical course. They may be associated with neurofibromatosis type 1. Patients with optic gliomas have enlargement and signal abnormality of the optic nerve (Fig. 31.22), which may also involve the chiasm and optic tracts. There may be patchy enhancement of the nerve as well. The enlargement of the optic nerve distinguishes optic nerve glioma from inflammatory optic neuritis.

Optic nerve meningiomas arise from the dural covering of the optic nerve or represent extensions of intracranial meningiomas (Eddleman and Liu, 2007). They most

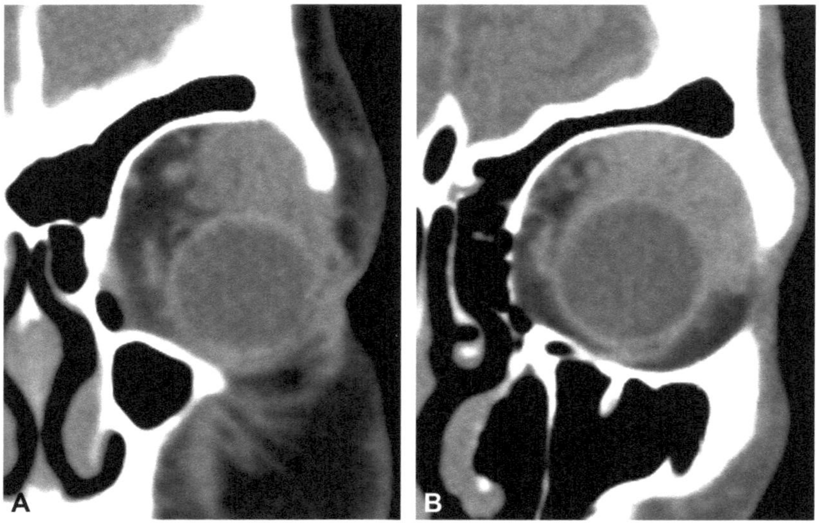

Fig. 31.19. Comparison of interface between lacrimal tumor and globe. (**A**) This pleomorphic adenoma, like other epithelial lesions, pushes on the globe. (**B**) This lacrimal gland lymphoma molds to the globe.

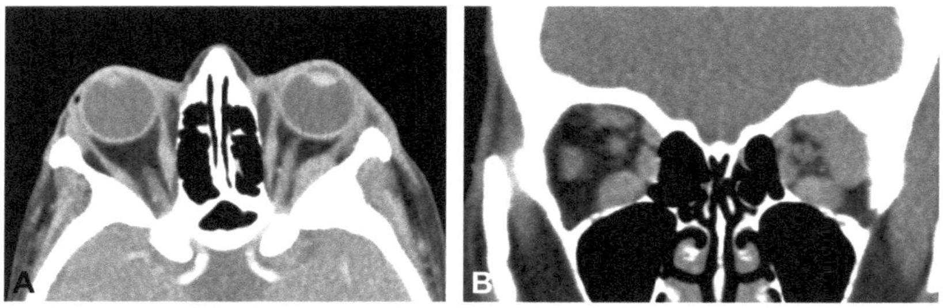

Fig. 31.20. Metastases to extraocular muscles. Axial (**A**) and coronal (**B**) computed tomography images through the orbit demonstrate enlargement of the extraocular muscles in an asymmetric pattern. On the left there is greater involvement of the lateral rectus than the medial rectus, a finding which would be atypical for thyroid orbitopathy. These muscles are enlarged by breast cancer metastases.

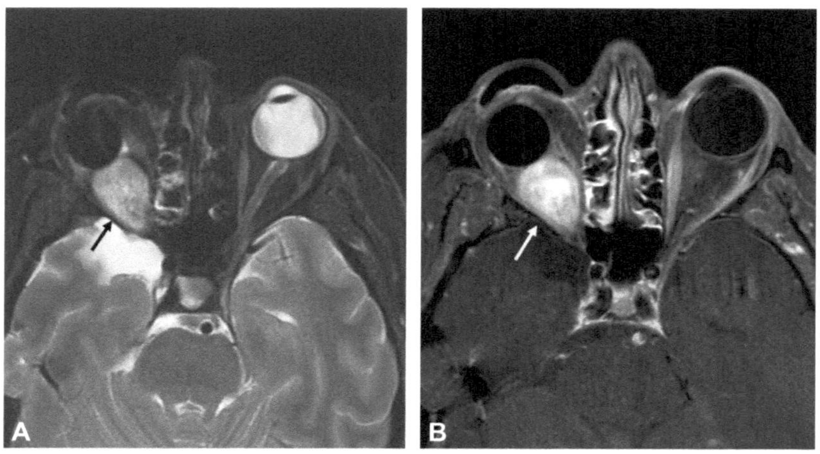

Fig. 31.21. Schwannoma of the right orbit. Recurrent schwannoma of the right orbit in a patient with resection. (**A**) T2-weighted images demonstrate an intermediate signal ovoid mass in the posterior right orbit (arrow). A spacer and scleral shell are also present anteriorly in this patient who is status postenucleation. (**B**) There is uniform enhancement of this mass. The borders are very smooth, unlike the cavernous hemangiomas, which tend to have a somewhat more lobulated appearance.

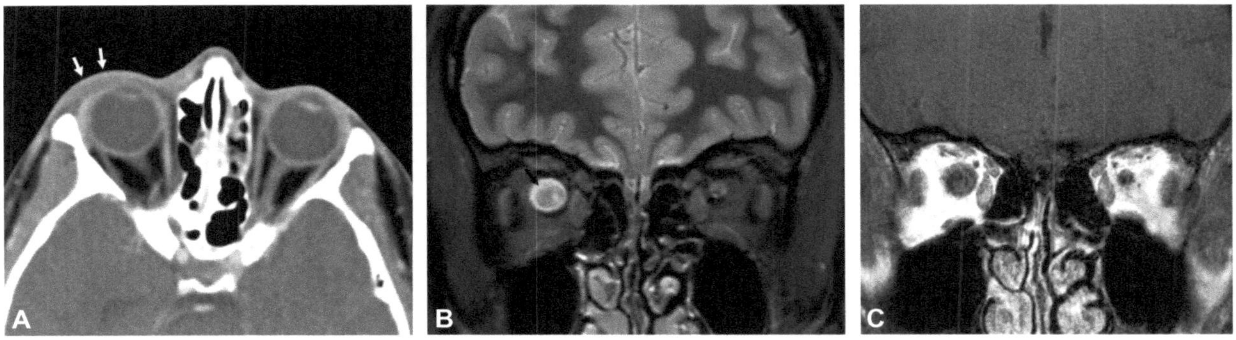

Fig. 31.22. Right optic nerve glioma. Axial T2 (**A**) and coronal short tau inversion recovery (STIR) (**B**) images through the orbits demonstrate expansion and signal abnormality of the optic nerve (arrows). On gadolinium-enhanced images (**C**) there is minimal enhancement, consistent with the low-grade nature of these tumors.

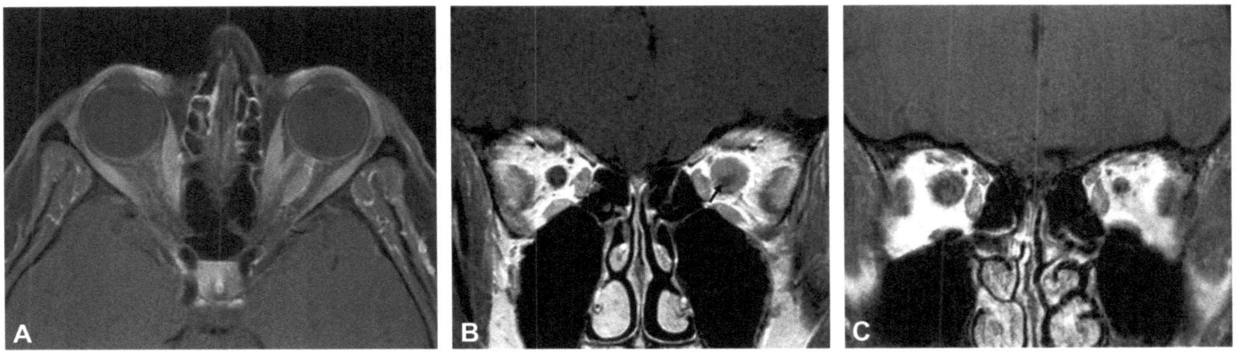

Fig. 31.23. Left optic nerve meningioma. Axial (**A**) gadolinium-enhanced images demonstrates tram-track enhancement surrounding the left optic nerve. On coronal images (**B** and **C**), the nerve can be identified (arrow) surrounded by enhancing tumor arising from the dura.

commonly extend along the nerve in a tubular pattern with tram-track enhancement (Fig. 31.23). They may also demonstrate a more globular configuration, with tumor extending eccentrically from the nerve (Dutton, 1992; Saeed et al., 2003). Like other intracranial meningiomas, they can calcify, which may indicate a more indolent course (Saeed et al., 2003). Most frequently these are unilateral; however 5% of cases are bilateral (Dutton, 1992). Because the meningioma typically lies between the optic nerve and its blood supply, resection leads to ischemia of the optic nerve, typically causing blindness. These tumors are therefore diagnosed radiographically, and managed conservatively, with radiotherapy if vision declines, in order to halt progression (Eddleman and Liu, 2007).

Globe

Most disorders of the globe are adequately investigated via history and physical exam and are only seen by radiologists as incidental findings. However, patients with ocular cancers may undergo imaging in order to evaluate for extension beyond the globe.

In the child, the most common intraocular tumor is retinoblastoma. This may occur sporadically or in the setting of a congenital abnormality of the tumor suppressor RB1 gene (Balmer et al., 2006). Patients with abnormalities of the RB1 gene will have multiple bilateral tumors and are also at risk of intracranial tumors occurring in the pineal or suprasellar regions (so-called trilateral retinoblastoma) (Kivelä, 1999).

Retinoblastomas appear hyperintense to vitreous on T1-weighted images, hypointense to vitreous on T2-weighted images, and enhance after the administration of contrast. Tumors will display susceptibility artifact on gradient echo images due to calcification (Fig. 31.24). MRI is particularly useful in determining involvement of the optic nerve, which can occur as tumor spread across the lamina cribrosa into the substance of the nerve, or as spread along the dura of the optic nerve sheath (Fig. 31.25). Optic nerve spread significantly increases the risk of metastases in this tumor (Balmer et al., 2006).

Retinoblastomas, like other primitive neuroectodermal tumors, demonstrate restricted diffusion, with

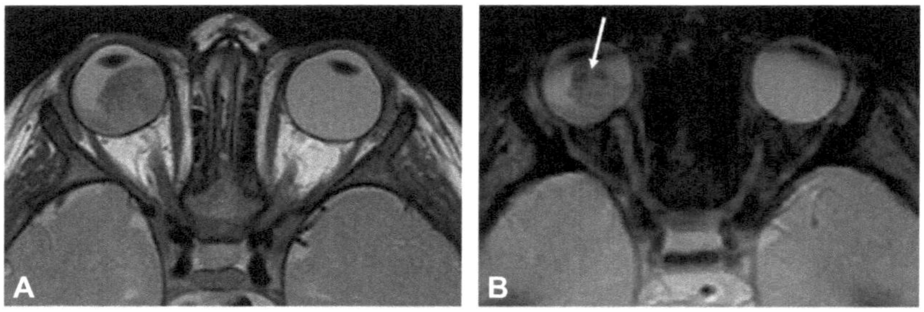

Fig. 31.24. Retinoblastoma. (**A**) Axial T2-weighted image demonstrates a hypointense mass in the right globe. (**B**) This demonstrates increased susceptibility artifact on susceptibility-weighted images, due to the presence of calcification (arrow).

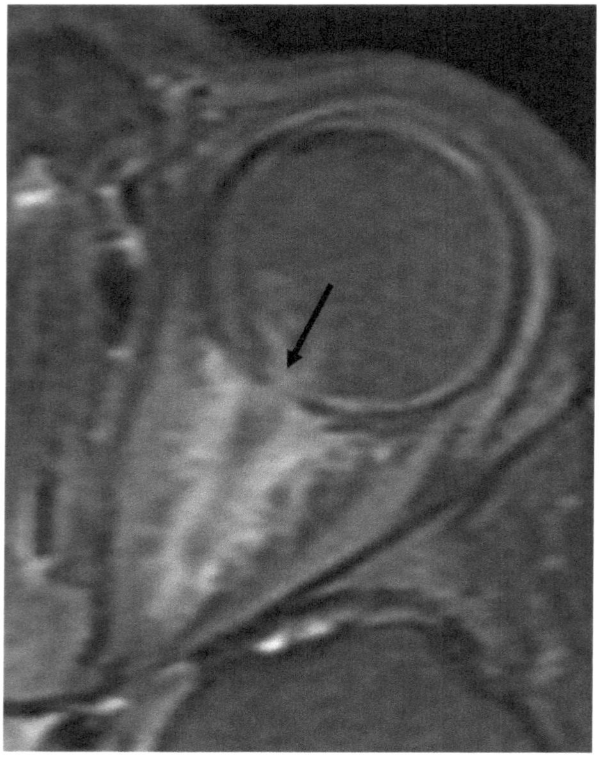

Fig. 31.25. Retinoblastoma with extension along the optic nerve. In this magnified view of a postcontrast T1-weighted magnetic resonance imaging, the arrow points to enhancing tumor which extends through the lamina cribrosa into the optic nerve itself. In addition, enhancing tumor extends along the dura of the optic nerve sheath.

lower apparent diffusion coefficient values compared to vitreous. The lowest apparent diffusion coefficient values correspond to viable tumor, whereas more intermediate values correspond to necrotic portions within the tumor (de Graaf et al., 2012).

Retinoblastomas are the most common cause of leukocoria, or loss of the red reflex, on physical exam. However, an important confounder in the evaluation of the patient with leukocoria is the diagnosis of persistent hyperplastic primary vitreous (PHPV) (Fig. 31.26). PHPV results from failure of the embryonic blood vessels to regress, and typically causes microphthalmia. Fibrovascular tissue lies posterior to the lens, and there may be intraocular hemorrhage or proteinaceous fluid. PHPV does not cause calcification, a feature which may distinguish it from retinoblastoma.

Choroidal melanomas are the most common intraocular tumor in adults, though metastases (typically from lung and breast cancer) and lymphoma may also present with intraocular tumors. Choroidal melanomas may be intrinsically T1 hyperintense due to the presence of melanin (amelanotic melanomas may not demonstrate this feature). These tumors are often hypointense on T2-weighted images and enhance avidly. Melanomas may extend through the sclera into the orbit.

Rhabdomyosarcoma

Rhabdomyosarcoma generally occurs in children and often lies in the superior orbit. Although the tumor contains muscle cells, it does not arise from the extraocular muscles. Most patients present with proptosis, and the mass may demonstrate rapid growth (Shields and Shields, 2003). On CT the masses often appear extraconal, are ovoid, and are typically well circumscribed. There may be associated bone reaction or frank destruction, particularly with larger tumors (Sohaib et al., 1998; Shields and Shields, 2003). On MRI tumors demonstrate avid enhancement (Shields and Shields, 2003; Conneely and Mafee, 2005) and may show restricted diffusion, as do many small round blue-cell tumors (Fig. 31.27).

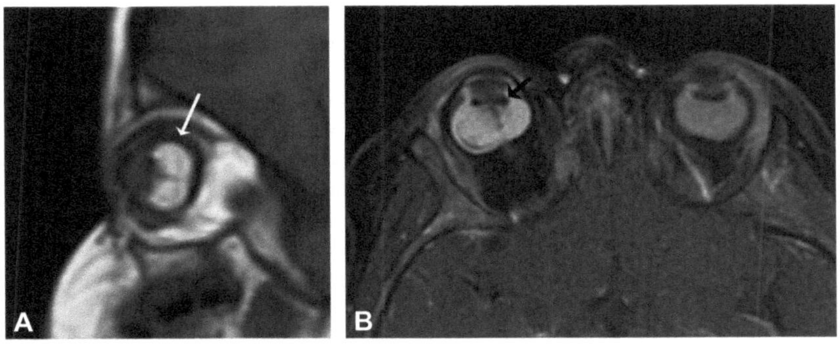

Fig. 31.26. Persistent hyperplastic primary vitreous (PHPV). This patient, who was ultimately determined to have Norrie's disease (a genetic syndrome which features PHPV), was initially evaluated for retinoblastoma due to bilateral leukocoria. Sagittal (**A**) precontrast T1-weighted images demonstrate a small eye with T1 hyperintense material in the posterior chamber, likely reflecting hemorrhage or proteinaceous fluid (arrow). Postcontrast axial (**B**) images demonstrate no additional enhancement to suggest tumor. Hypointense tissue posterior to the lens (arrow) is the fibrovascular tissue, which fails to regress in these patients. A linear channel extending from this tissue posteriorly is presumed to represent Cloquet's canal, through which the fetal vessels traveled through the posterior chamber to reach the lens.

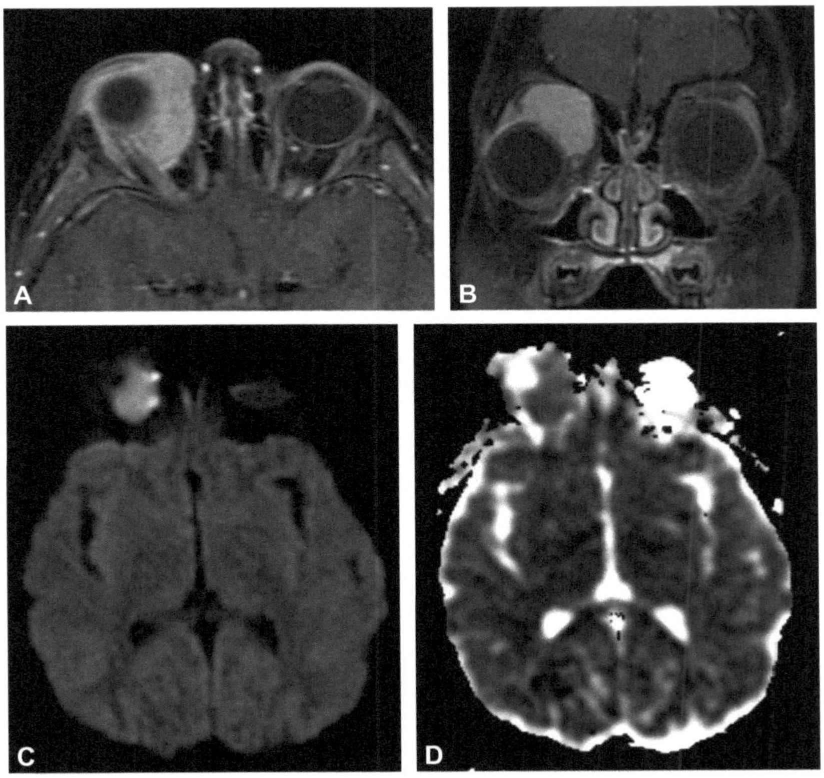

Fig. 31.27. Orbital rhabdomyosarcoma. Axial (**A**) and coronal (**B**)-enhanced magnetic resonance images demonstrate an avidly enhancing tumor involving the superomedial orbit. Diffusion-weighted imaging (**C**) and apparent diffusion coefficient (**D**) images show the mass to have restricted diffusion of water, a finding often seen in small round blue-cell tumors such as rhabdomyosarcomas.

References

Balmer A, Zografos L, Munier F (2006). Diagnosis and current management of retinoblastoma. Oncogene 25: 5341–5349.

Bartalena L, Tanda M (2009). Clinical practice. Graves' ophthalmopathy. N Engl J Med 360: 994–1001.

Bron A, Wolff E, Tripathi R et al. (1997). Wolff's anatomy of the eye and orbit. Chapman & Hall, London.

Chandler J, Langenbrunner D, Stevens E (1970). The pathogenesis of orbital complications in acute sinusitis. Laryngoscope 80: 1414–1428.

Chandrasekharan R, Thomas M, Rupa V (2012). Comparative study of orbital involvement in invasive and non-invasive fungal sinusitis. J Laryngol Otol 126: 152–158.

Conneely MF, Mafee MF (2005). Orbital rhabdomyosarcoma and simulating lesions. Neuroimaging Clin N Am 15: 121–136.

De Graaf P, Pouwels P, Rodjan F et al. (2012). Single-shot turbo spin-echo diffusion-weighted imaging for retinoblastoma: initial experience. AJNR Am J Neuroradiol 33: 110–118.

Demirci H, Christianson M (2011). Orbital and adnexal involvement in sarcoidosis: analysis of clinical features and systemic disease in 30 cases. Am J Ophthalmol 151: 1074–1080.

Dutton J (1992). Optic nerve sheath meningiomas. Surv Ophthalmol 37: 167–183.

Eddleman C, Liu J (2007). Optic nerve sheath meningioma: current diagnosis and treatment. Neurosurg Focus 23.

Fauci AS, Haynes BF, Katz P et al. (1983). Wegener's granulomatosis: prospective clinical and therapeutic experience with 85 patients for 21 years. Ann Intern Med 98: 76–85.

Gao Y, Moonis G, Cunnane M et al. (2013). Lacrimal gland masses. AJR Am J Roentgenol 201: 81.

Howe L, Jones N (2004). Guidelines for the management of periorbital cellulitis/abscess. Clin Otolaryngol Allied Sci 29: 725–728.

Kivelä T (1999). Trilateral retinoblastoma: a meta-analysis of hereditary retinoblastoma associated with primary ectopic intracranial retinoblastoma. J Clin Oncol 17: 1829–1837.

Lacey B, Chang W, Rootman J (1999). Nonthyroid causes of extraocular muscle disease. Surv Ophthalmol 44: 187–213.

Mossa-Basha M, Ilica A, Maluf F et al. (2013). The many faces of fungal disease of the paranasal sinuses: CT and MRI findings. Diagn Interv Radiol 19: 195–200.

Nunery W (1991). Ophthalmic Graves' disease: a dual theory of pathogenesis. Ophthalmol Clin North Am 4.

Prabhakaran V, Saeed P, Esmaeli B et al. (2007). Orbital and adnexal sarcoidosis. Arch Ophthalmol 125: 1657–1662.

Rootman J (2003). Vascular malformations of the orbit: hemodynamic concepts. Orbit 22: 103–120.

Rothfus WE, Curtin HD (1984). Extraocular muscle enlargement: a CT review. Radiology 151: 677–681.

Rubin P, Watkins L, Rumelt S et al. (1998). Orbital computed tomographic characteristics of globe subluxation in thyroid orbitopathy. Ophthalmology 105: 2061–2064.

Saeed P, Rootman J, Nugent R et al. (2003). Optic nerve sheath meningiomas. Ophthalmology 110: 2019–2030.

Santiago Y, Fay A (2011). Wegener's granulomatosis of the orbit: a review of clinical features and updates in diagnosis and treatment. Semin Ophthalmol 26: 349–355.

Shields J, Shields C (2003). Rhabdomyosarcoma: review for the ophthalmologist. Surv Ophthalmol 48: 39–57.

Shields J, Shields C, Epstein J et al. (2004a). Review: primary epithelial malignancies of the lacrimal gland: the 2003 Ramon L. Font lecture. Ophthal Plast Reconstr Surg 20: 10–21.

Shields J, Shields C, Scartozzi R (2004b). Survey of 1264 patients with orbital tumors and simulating lesions: the 2002 Montgomery Lecture, part 1. Ophthalmology 111: 997–1008.

Silverman C, Mancuso A (1998). Periantral soft-tissue infiltration and its relevance to the early detection of invasive fungal sinusitis: CT and MR findings. AJNR Am J Neuroradiol 19: 321–325.

Smith J, Foster C (1996). Sarcoidosis and its ocular manifestations. Int Ophthalmol Clin 36: 109–125.

Smoker W, Gentry L, Yee N et al. (2008). Vascular lesions of the orbit: more than meets the eye. Radiographics 28: 185.

Sohaib S, Moseley I, Wright J (1998). Orbital rhabdomyosarcoma – the radiological characteristics. Clin Radiol 53: 357–362.

Wang Y, Xiao L (2008). Orbital schwannomas: findings from magnetic resonance imaging in 62 cases. Eye 22: 1034–1039.

Weiss R, Grisold W, Jellinger K et al. (1984). Metastasis of solid tumors in extraocular muscles. Acta Neuropathol 65.

Yuen S, Rubin P (2003). Idiopathic orbital inflammation: distribution, clinical features, and treatment outcome. Arch Ophthalmol 121: 491–499.

Index

NB: Page numbers in *italics* refer to figures and tables.

B

F

H

I

J

K

L

M

N

O

Q

T

U

V

W

X

Z

FSC
www.fsc.org
MIX
Papier | Fördert
gute Waldnutzung
FSC® C083411

Kolibri 360 GmbH
Ferdinand-Jühlke-Straße 7
99095 Erfurt, Deutschland
produktsicherheit@kolibri360.de